Nursing Assessment
and Diagnosis

The Jones and Bartlett Series in Nursing

Adult Emergency Nursing Procedures, Proehl

Basic Steps in Planning Nursing Research, Third Edition, Brink/Wood

Bone Marrow Transplantation, Whedon

Cancer Chemotherapy: A Nursing Process Approach, Barton Burke et al.

Cancer Nursing: Principles and Practice, Second Edition, Groenwald et al.

Chemotherapy Care Plans, Barton Burke

A Clinical Manual for Nursing Assistants, McClelland/Kaspar

Children's Nutrition, Lifshitz/Finch/Lifshitz

Chronic Illness: Impact and Intervention, Second Edition, Lubkin

Clinical Nursing Procedures, Belland/Wells

A Comprehensive Curriculum for Trauma Nursing, Bayley/Turcke

Comprehensive Maternity Nursing, Second Edition, Auvenshine/Enriquez

Concepts in Oxygenation, Ahrens/Rutherford

Critical Care Review, Wright/Shelton

Emergency Care of Children, Thompson

Essential Medical Terminology, Stanfield

Family Life: Process and Practice, Janosik/Green

Fundamentals of Nursing with Clinical Procedures, Second Edition, Sundberg

1991-1992 Handbook of Intravenous Medications, Nentwich

Handbook of Oncology Nursing, Johnson/Gross

Health Assessment in Nursing Practice, Third Edition, Grimes/Burns

Health and Wellness, Fourth Edition, Edlin/Golanty

Healthy People 2000, U.S. Department of Health & Human Services

Human Development: A Life-Span Approach, Fourth Edition, Freiberg

Instruments for Clinical Nursing Research, Oncology Nursing Society

Intravenous Therapy, Nentwich

Introduction to the Health Professions, Stanfield

Introduction to Human Disease, Third Edition, Crowley

Journal of Perinatal Education, ASPO

Management and Leadership for Nurse Managers, Swansburg

Management of Spinal Cord Injury, Second Edition, Zejdlik

Math for Health Professionals, Third Edition, Whisler

Medical Terminology, Stanfield

Memory Bank for Chemotherapy, Preston

Memory Bank for IVs, Second Edition, Weinstein

Memory Bank for Medications, Second Edition, Kostin/Evans

Mental Health and Psychiatric Nursing: A Caring Approach, Davies/Janosik

The Nation's Health, Third Edition, Lee/Estes

Nursing and the Disabled: Across the Lifespan, Fraley

Nursing Assessment and Diagnosis, Second Edition, Bellack/Edlund

Nursing Diagnosis Care Plans for Diagnosis-Related Groups, Neal/Paquette/Mirch

Nursing Management of Children, Servonsky/Opas

Nursing Pharmacology, Second Edition, Wallace

Nursing Research: A Quantitative and Qualitative Approach, Roberts/Burke

Nutrition and Diet Therapy: Self-Instructional Modules, Second Edition, Stanfield

Pediatric Emergency Nursing Procedures, Bernardo/Bove

Perioperative Nursing Care, Fairchild

Perioperative Patient Care, Second Edition, Kneedler/Dodge

A Practical Guide to Breastfeeding, Riordan

Psychiatric Mental Health Nursing, Second Edition, Janosik/Davies

Ready Reference of Common Emergency and Prehospital Drugs, Cummings

Ready Reference for Critical Care, Strawn

The Research Process in Nursing, Third Edition, Dempsey/Dempsey

Understanding/Responding, Second Edition, Long/Prophit

Writing a Succesful Grant Application, Second Edition, Reif-Lehrer

Second Edition

Nursing Assessment and Diagnosis

JANIS P. BELLACK

BARBARA J. EDLUND

Medical University of South Carolina

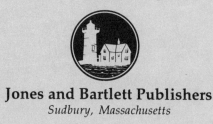

Jones and Bartlett Publishers
Sudbury, Massachusetts

Boston   London   Singapore

Editorial, Sales, and Customer Service Offices
Jones and Bartlett Publishers
40 Tall Pine Drive
Sudbury, MA 01776
(978) 443-5000
(800) 832-0034
info@jbpub.com
http://www.jbpub.com

Jones and Bartlett Publishers International
Barb House, Barb Mews
London W6 7PA
UK

Library of Congress Cataloging-in-Publication Data

Bellack, Janis P.
  Nursing assessment and diagnosis
Janis P. Bellack and Barbara J. Edlund. — 2nd ed.
    p.   cm.
  Rev. ed. of: Nursing assessment [edited by] Janis P. Bellack.
Penny A. Bamford. c1987.
  Includes bibliographical references and index.
  ISBN 0-86720-436-2
  1. Nursing assessment.   2. Nursing diagnosis.   I. Edlund,
Barbara.   II. Nursing assessment.   III. Title.
  [DNLM. 1. Nursing Assessment.   WY 100 B435n]
RT48.N875   1992
610.73—dc20
DNLM/DLC
for Library of Congress   91-35361
                                                  CIP

ISBN 0-86720-436-2

Production Services: WordCrafters Editorial Services, Inc.
Interior Design: Laura Cleveland
Cover Designer: Melinda Grosser
Cover Illustration: Margaret Petterson, Mt. Pleasant, SC

Printed in the United States of America

02 01 00 99 98   10 9 8 7 6 5 4 3

To my parents, Elaine and Loren Peacock,
whose ideals, integrity, and commitment to excellence
provided valuable lessons that continue to inspire me.
Love, Jan

To my family—
my husband Bill and son Bret,
the wonderful women I call Mom,
and the special men I call Dad.
With love, Barb

Contents

Foreword

This second edition of *Nursing Assessment and Diagnosis* is a timely book that reflects the dynamic changes taking place in our society. Multiple external influences have given impetus and direction to the evolution and expansion of nursing practice. Issues of cost containment, quality improvement, and accountability confront today's health care practitioners and place special demands on the professional nurse.

Not only must nurses be able to deliver quality nursing care, they must also do so with an understanding of the social context in which nursing takes place. This context is both contemporary and futuristic, and it emphasizes the nurse's accountability for the scope, quality, and cost effectiveness of nursing care services. Thus, the ever-expanding knowledge base required for professional nursing practice has enhanced the importance and value of nursing assessment and diagnosis in the delivery of comprehensive health care.

The authors portray nursing assessment and diagnosis with a clear understanding of the larger social and health care contexts in which nurses practice. At the same time, the practical aspects of assessment and diagnosis provide the central focus for the book.

Theory-based knowledge, research, and examples from clinical practice are incorporated throughout. There is a wealth of valuable information in this text, including the essential knowledge nurses need—as well as specific approaches and techniques nurses can use—to conduct a comprehensive assessment.

Perhaps the most important feature of the book is its multidimensional approach to assessing and diagnosing people's responses to health problems and life situations. People are viewed as dynamic, integrated beings with physiological, psychosocial, and developmental dimensions, who function within their respective family, cultural, and environmental contexts.

The changes in this edition and what is covered are included in the authors' preface. Certain features, however, deserve special mention. The universal needs of clients are addressed fully in the chapters dealing with physiological and psychosocial assessment. Family, cultural, and environmental influences on health are explored, with recognition that these influences are continually evolving and changing, eliciting a range of human responses—sometimes favorable, sometimes not.

A particular strength of the book is the new chapters that focus on assessment of special clients. As someone whose particular interest is maternal-child health, I was especially pleased to see chapters dealing with the childbearing woman, the newborn, the infant and child, and the adolescent. The added chapter on the older client is also welcome, considering the growing number of elderly in our society.

The numerous illustrations, tables, and guides enhance understanding of the text. References are excellent, and the authors do a creditable job of supporting their points of view. Other learning features, such as chapter objectives, practice activities, and chapter highlights add to the value of the book.

The authors present a comprehensive approach that not only helps the nurse develop and refine the ability to assess diverse clients in a variety of health care settings, but also addresses the profession's commitment to providing effective and responsive nursing care within an ever-changing social context.

This important and timely book will help students of nursing—both undergraduate and graduate—and practicing nurses gain the knowledge and skills they need to become proficient in nursing assessment and diagnosis. As such, it has the potential for enhancing the quality of care delivered to culturally diverse clients of all ages and in a variety of health care settings, ultimately improving health outcomes.

Juanita W. Fleming, Ph.D., R.N., F.A.A.N.
University of Kentucky, Lexington

Preface

Nursing Diagnosis and Assessment presents a comprehensive approach to assessment and diagnosis from a nursing perspective. Many changes in nursing practice and health care delivery have taken place since the first edition of the book was published. The increased acuity of hospitalized clients, early discharge, home care, the aging of the population with a concommitant rise in chronic illnesses, complex technologies, and changing standards of health care are placing special demands on professional nursing practice.

Today's nurses are assuming greater responsibility and accountability for client assessment, decision making, and health outcomes in all types of settings—hospitals, ambulatory care centers, outreach clinics, long-term care facilities, schools, industry, and homes. More than ever before, nurses must be prepared to perform comprehensive assessments of clients as a basis for making accurate nursing diagnoses, designing and implementing cost-effective interventions, and improving health outcomes.

This second edition is both a revision and an expansion of the first edition, with greater emphasis placed on nursing diagnosis. Together, assessment and diagnosis are the cornerstones of the nursing process. A careful and adequate assessment and the formulation of nursing diagnoses are crucial to client welfare. Without a comprehensive data base and valid and appropriate nursing diagnoses, nursing care is at risk of becoming routinized and insensitive to the uniqueness of the individual client. Because nursing assessment and diagnosis are so essential to the delivery of safe, competent, and knowledgeable care, we have chosen to devote this book to an in-depth look at these first critical phases of the nursing process.

The first edition, Nursing Assessment: A Multidimensional Approach (1984), pioneered a nursing model for assessment, in contrast to the body systems models presented in most texts. As nurses became eager to learn physical examination techniques, the techniques themselves were often disproportionately emphasized and valued. In the process, the nursing perspective was lost and practitioners were left to figure out on their own how to place physical examination in a context relevant for nursing. This new edition continues to emphasize the importance of using a nursing model to systematically structure the assessment to derive appropriate nursing diagnoses as a basis for delivering optimal care.

We contend that when assessment is equated with physical examination (i.e., body systems, head-to-toe approach), a view of human beings emerges that is more suited to the practice of medicine than the practice of nursing. While physical assessment data are important, they should be collected as part of a comprehensive nursing assessment and for the purpose of formulating nursing diagnoses.

Nursing assessment should be structured in a way that is conceptually consistent with nursing's view of human beings. Such a view is multidimensional and incoporates the diverse yet interrelated aspects of human behavior and functioning—family, cultural, environmental, developmental, psychosocial, and physiological. This book provides such an approach.

FEATURES OF THE SECOND EDITION

This edition has been retitled to reflect its expanded scope. It has also been completely revised. The latest nursing knowledge, including theory and research related to the various parameters of nursing assessment and diagnosis, is incorporated throughout. The applicability of content to people with consideration of their ages, cultural diversity, and health has been preserved.

The organizational framework has been revised to achieve greater consistency among chapters. A chapter outline appears at the beginning of each chapter. For Chapters 7 through 24, this outline serves as a checklist of assessment parameters related to the particular dimension. In addition, each chapter includes a content outline, objectives, practice activities, and recommended readings to supplement and enhance chapter material, as well as numerous tables, figures, and photographs to enhance understanding of text material. Chapter Highlights have replaced chapter summaries; they are designed to emphasize key points.

Chapters 10 through 24 are organized consistently around four themes: the knowledge needed to assess the particular dimension, the nursing history, clinical appraisal and screening, and related nursing diagnoses. Tables are included that outline the nursing history and clinical appraisal for each dimension of the nursing assessment.

Other noteworthy features of the second edition include:

■ Expansion of the introductory chapter to provide a framework for nursing assessment and diagnosis, including beliefs about nursing, the nursing process, standards of nursing practice, and the knowledge, skills, and values needed to conduct a comprehensive assessment and formulate nursing diagnoses.

■ In-depth treatment of nursing diagnosis as both process and outcome, with an emphasis on data analysis and synthesis and the formulation of nursing diagnostic statements.

■ Placement of the chapters on family, cultural, and environmental assessment earlier in the book to emphasize the social and contextual factors that influence human health.

■ Modification of the chapters on psychosocial and physiological assessment to focus primarily on the adult client.

■ Addition of an entirely new section on nursing assessment and diagnosis of clients across the lifespan, including chapters on the pregnant woman, the neonate, the infant and child, the adolescent, and the older adult.

■ Inclusion of a color-edged reference section of nursing diagnoses included in the North American Nursing Diagnosis Association's *Taxonomy I Revised—1990*, complete with defining characteristics and related factors. (An alphabetized index is provided inside the front cover for easy reference.)

■ Incorporation of approaches and techniques for physical examination within the appropriate chapters (for example, physical assessment of the heart and lungs is included in the chapter on oxygenation assessment).

■ A concluding chapter that provides a case example of an adult client to illustrate integration of nursing assessment and diagnosis. The chapter is written as a self-guided learning module to help readers synthesize and apply their knowledge to a specific case situation.

ORGANIZATION OF THE SECOND EDITION

Part I provides an overview of the knowledge that underpins nursing assessment and diagnosis. An organizing framework, including the knowledge, skills, and values needed for nursing assessment and diagnosis, is considered in the first chapter. A complete overview of the nursing process is also provided. Chapters 2 and 3 focus on the collection of assessment data, beginning with interviewing and the nursing history, followed by clinical appraisal and screening. Documentation is thoroughly examined in Chapter 4, with emphasis on effective reporting and recording of assessment information and nursing diagnoses.

Chapters 5 and 6 are devoted to nursing diagnosis. Chapter 5 focuses on the analysis and synthesis of assessment data, with special consideration of clinical reasoning. Nursing diagnosis as the outcome of a comprehensive nursing assessment is examined in Chapter 6, including a review of the history, advantages, and limitations of using nursing diagnoses to categorize the domain of nursing practice.

Part II focuses on assessment of the client's family, culture, and environment as social and contextual forces that influence health. Family assessment is considered in Chapter 7, with an emphasis on family theory and selected approaches and tools for assessing families. Chapter 8 addresses cultural assessment, with a special focus on the relationship of culture to health values, beliefs, and practices. Environmental assessment is examined in Chapter 9. Assessment of home, work, or school and health care environments is emphasized. Health risk appraisal has been added to this chapter because of current concerns with environmental and lifestyle influences on health.

Developmental assessment is considered in Part III. Chapter 10 focuses on assessing the development of children, including developmental history, clinical appraisal of developmental capabilities, and screening for possible delays. Sections on assessing child-parent interaction and children's health knowledge and behaviors have been added. Theories of adult development, the aging process, life review, appraisal of developmental changes, and adults' health knowledge and practices are examined in Chapter 11.

Part IV focuses on dimensions of psychosocial assessment. Chapter 12 emphasizes the assessment of intrapersonal functioning (including self-concept, motivation, cognition, affect and mood, and temperament) and interpersonal functioning (including social roles and relationships, stressors and stress responses, and coping strategies). Sexuality assessment is explored in Chapter 13, including approaches to assessing sexuality and the relationship of age, culture, and health to sexual development and functioning. Physical assessment of the breasts and external genitalia is included in this chapter because of its close relationship to human sexuality.

Physiological assessment is considered in Part V. This section preserves the dimensions from the first edition, although the sequence of the chapters has been reorganized. Chapters 14 through 19 include, respectively, assessment of physical integrity (general appraisal, physical growth, vital signs, skin integrity, and the immune system), sensory-perceptual-neurologic functioning (including pain assessment), activity-sleep (mobility, fitness, rest, and sleep), oxygenation (breathing and circulation), nutrition, and fluid–electrolyte balance and elimination.

Part VI is an entirely new section devoted to nursing assessment and diagnosis of special clients, with a primary emphasis on physiological dimensions of their health. Chapters are included on the pregnant woman, the neonate, the infant and child, the adolescent, and the older adult. Each chapter is organized according to the same framework used in Part V. Behavioral responses are also incorporated where appropriate. Part VI concludes with a chapter that illustrates the integration of nursing assessment and diagnosis, using an adult client as a case example.

We do not expect that as thorough and complete an assessment as is presented in this book can be conducted on all clients for whom the nurse cares. Clearly, this would be impossible—and not very cost effective! Instead our intent is to present a solid framework in the theory and practice of a comprehensive, multidimensional nursing assessment of clients across the lifespan. With experience, you will become proficient in focusing on those aspects of assessment and diagnosis that are essential for each client. You will also become more

adept at recognizing those dimensions which require special or more detailed attention in a given client within a particular clinical context.

This book is designed to build on your knowledge of human physiology, psychology, sociology, and human growth and development throughout the lifespan. The content and scope of the book will be useful to undergraduate students who are learning nursing assessment and diagnosis for the first time, as well as to graduate students and practicing nurses, who will find the book a valuable learning guide and resource.

Use of a multidimensional, *nursing* approach to assessment and diagnosis fosters an appreciation of each client as a unique person and emphasizes the dynamic interaction among the many dimensions that influence health and well-being. While each dimension is considered separately in this book for learning purposes, it is critical to remember that all dimensions interact with and influence each other in many ways. *It is the whole person who counts.* The whole person, therefore, must be assessed if an appropriate plan of nursing care is to be developed.

ACKNOWLEDGMENTS

Our writing would not be complete without acknowledging the many wonderful people whose efforts and support have been instrumental in helping us prepare this second edition.

We are grateful to our colleagues and students at the Medical University of South Carolina for the enthusiastic support and encouragement they gave us throughout this project. We owe special thanks to Mary Inman, our research assistant; Marcia Higaki, Gloria Reid, and George Campbell, our superb and dedicated typists; and Pam Poe, who provided expert assistance with processing copyright permissions.

We are particularly indebted to Jim Keating, vice-president and publisher at Jones and Bartlett, whose wisdom, faith, and support kept moving us steadily toward our goal.

Margaret Petterson, a local artist whose work we have long admired, deserves special recognition for her beautiful rendering of an original painting for the book's cover that symbolizes our view of nursing assessment and diagnosis—a journey along a winding path, seeking the unknown.

We also want to thank the following people:

■ The contributors to the first edition, including Jane Balint, Karen Bickel, Kathy Blomquist, Sandy Campbell, Lynne Goodykoontz, Carolyn

Fore, Phyllis Healy, Patti Hunsicker, Ann Jessop, Beverly Kopala, Esther Matassarin-Jacobs, JoAnn Wever, Julia Morris, Patti Moschel, Carol Macnee, Kay Robinson, Julie Sebastian, Marsha Starr, Barbara Teague, Fran Thurber, Sherry Warden, and Pat Woodard, whose original works provided a solid foundation for our revisions.

■ Dan Bellack and Tracy Harler for many of the additional photographs in this edition.

■ And the editorial and production staff of Jones and Bartlett and WordCrafters, especially Ann Mohan, for their assistance and responsiveness throughout the editing and production process.

A special thanks is owed Jorge Grimes, Elizabeth Burns, Martha Auvenshine, Martha Enriquez, Jane Servonsky, and Susan Opas for permission to use original material from their books, and the North American Nursing Diagnosis Association for granting use of its complete *Taxonomy I Revised—1990*.

Most especially, we are deeply appreciative of our husbands and sons, for their patience, tolerance, humor, and love, which sustained us through many, many months of writing and editing.

Contributors

Janis P. Bellack, PhD, RN
Associate Professor of Nursing and Assistant
  Dean for Undergraduate Programs
Medical University of South Carolina
College of Nursing
Charleston, SC

Barbara J. Edlund, PhD candidate, RN, MNP
Associate Professor of Nursing
Medical University of South Carolina
College of Nursing
Charleston, SC

Daniel R. Bellack, PhD
Visiting Assistant Professor of Psychology
College of Charleston
Charleston, SC

M. Suzanne Doscher, MS, RN
Associate Professor of Nursing
Medical University of South Carolina
College of Nursing
Charleston, SC

Barbara Kavanagh Haight, DrPH, RN, C, FAAN
Professor of Nursing
Medical University of South Carolina
College of Nursing
Charleston, SC

Ellen H. Janosik, MS, RN
Associate Professor Emeritus
Department of Nursing
Alfred University
Alfred, NY

Carolyn H. Jenkins, MS, MSN, CDE, RD, RN, C
Assistant Professor of Nursing
Medical University of South Carolina
College of Nursing
Charleston, SC

Toni Tripp-Reimer, PhD, RN, FAAN
Professor of Nursing
University of Iowa
College of Nursing
Iowa City, IA

Marybeth Young, PhD, RN, C
Assistant Professor of Nursing
Niehoff School of Nursing
Loyola University
Chicago, IL

PART I

Introduction to Nursing Assessment and Diagnosis

1

A Framework for Nursing Assessment and Diagnosis

OBJECTIVES

Upon completion of this chapter, you should be able to:

■ Describe the changing role of the nurse in health care.

■ Explain nursing beliefs about *person, environment, health,* and *nursing.*

■ Articulate the knowledge, skills, values, professional behaviors, and attitudes that enable a nurse to perform a multidimensional nursing assessment.

■ Examine legal and ethical issues related to nursing assessment and diagnosis.

In its early days, nursing was characterized by two aims: care of the sick and the promotion of health. Both were accomplished with little or no direction from physicians. In caring for the sick, nurses concentrated on providing comfort and modifying the environment so that health could be resorted. In promoting health, nurses were concerned primarily with teaching women how to create environments conducive to healthy living for their families, thereby reducing the risk of illness (Ellis, 1982).

THE NURSE'S CHANGING ROLE IN HEALTH CARE

As the practice of modern medicine began to take shape, the disease-oriented model of health care emerged. This "medical model," with its emphasis on illness and cure, provided the framework for nursing care as well. Physicians gained control of hospitals and, thereby, nursing in hospital settings. Nursing centered on carrying out medical orders prescribed by a physician to cure disease. Independent nursing, such as modifying the environment and giving emotional support, remained part of nursing practice, but became secondary.

In the last 25 years, however, nursing has become an independent, creative force in health care. Many external influences have given impetus and direction to the evolution of contemporary nursing.

Since World War II, tremendous scientific and technological advances have brought radical changes in society and, consequently, in the delivery of health-care services. Physiology, molecular biology, pharmacology, epidemiology, and the social sciences have advanced. Increasing specialization and mushrooming technology have changed the face and direction of health care—and continue to do so.

Societal changes also have exerted a major influence on health care and consequently on nursing practice. Increasing population, shifts in demographics (more elderly, fewer young, more ethnic diversity), urbanization, changing roles of women, concern for human rights and welfare, and economic constraints are some of the forces shaping modern health-care practices. The doctor–nurse–client triad has evolved into a multifaceted, complex, and expensive health-care system.

One particularly noteworthy trend in the last decade has been the increasing emphasis that health-care providers, consumers, and insurance companies have placed on the promotion of health and the prevention of illness. Today's *clients* know more about their bodies and their mental and physical health than the *patients* of an earlier era. They are assuming active, decision-making roles in seeking and accepting health-care services. As individuals and in groups, people are saying that they want—and have a right—to be treaed as whole human beings, not as diseases.

Although the health-care system remains disease-oriented with its predominant focus on treatment and cure, greater emphasis now is given to keeping people healthy. Health maintenance organizations (HMOs), family practice centers, primary care centers, rural health-care clinics, fitness centers in business and industrial settings, and other similar services geared to promoting and maintaining health are multiplying. Nursing curricula almost universally incorporate content related to primary health care of the well person while continuing to emphasize the multidimensional needs of those who are ill or hospitalized. In fact, as Ellis (1982) notes,

> As nursing has moved from doing *for* [clients] to working with [clients], helping people to care for themselves and involving them in their care and decisions about their health, the modes of nursing are increasingly those of educating, guiding, or motivating not only the identified . . . [client] but his [or her] family and/or community. (p. 407)

Nursing always has concerned itself with each client's comprehensive needs. As knowledge proliferated and the population increased, however, it become evident that no single discipline could be all or do all for the client. Consequently, numerous other health-care disciplines—physical therapy, pharmacy, social work—have emerged, each with its own clearly defined role. In one sense, this multidisciplinary approach to health care is desirable because, ideally, it ensures that the various and many needs of the client are met. However, as more and more disciplines become involved with each client's treatment, health care becomes fragmented, services are duplicated, and clients often feel divided into bits and pieces.

Fortunately, as the health-care system grows in size and complexity, nursing continues to maintain its perspective of the client as a complex human being with interrelated, multidimensional needs: developmental, psychological, social, cultural, and physiological. Thus, the unique contribution of nursing remains its concern with the whole person within a sometimes overwhelming health-care system.

PHILOSOPHY AND BELIEFS ABOUT NURSING

Historically, nursing has embraced certain beliefs about its service and the value of that service to society. All health disciplines, including nursing, espouse the common goals of preserving and restoring health. Some disciplines are concerned primarily with a certain aspect of health: dentists and dental hygienists with oral health, or respiratory therapists with respiratory functioning. Others, such as nursing and certain medical specialties (e.g., family medicine, internal medicine, pediatrics), are concerned with multiple facets of health. What differentiates nursing from those medical specialties, however, is its unique view of the person. Medicine is concerned with a peron's body, or body sysems, whereas nursing views a person from a holistic and multidimensional perspective: the context of a person's physical and sociocultural environment as it influences health.

Nursing is guided by a philosophical and conceptual framework that gives structure and meaning to nursing practice, as well as to nursing education and research. This framework includes certain beliefs about the phenomena of concern to nursing, and there is a general agreement that they are fourfold: *person, environment, health,* and *nursing* (see Figure 1-1). These concepts comprise what has been called the "metaparadigm of nursing" (Fawcett, 1984).

More definitively, the four concepts of central concern to nursing include:

the *person* who is the recipient of nursing care,

the *environment* within which the person develops, lives, and interacts with others,

health, a state that reflects the person's general well-being and daily functioning, and

nursing, those actions and interactions aimed at promoting, maintaining, or restoring the person's optimal health.

These concepts provide a framework within which nursing practice, including assessment and diagnosis, takes place.

There are numerous conceptual models within the discipline of nursing that offer varying perspectives for viewing nursing's framework. Examples of commonly used conceptual models include Roy's adaptation model, Orem's self-care model, Neuman's health-care systems model, Johnson's behavioral systems model, Roger's life process model, Travelbee's interaction model, and Parse's man-living-health model, among others. Each interprets the four concepts in a different way. Table 1-1 illustrates the different perspectives of each.

Certain beliefs about each of the four concepts form the basis of the framework for nursing assessment and diagnosis presented in this book. The perspective presented here is intended to serve as a guide for acquiring the knowledge and skills to perform a comprehensive, multidimensional nursing assessment.

Person

Throughout this book, person is viewed as having interrelated developmental, cognitive, emotional, social, cultural, and physiologic characteristics and abilities and as functioning as an integrated, active whole from conception to death. A person also continuously interacts (exchanges energy) with the environment. A change in one dimension will have an impact, to a greater or less degree, on all other dimensions. For example, when a person experiences an emotionally traumatic event, the ability to think logically and to enjoy social relationships often is disrupted, as are such bodily functions as digestion and sleep.

Further, although people are characterized by many dimensions that can be studied individually, the dimensions cannot be understood separately.

Each person develops behaviors in response to such drives or needs as hunger, elimination, rest, affiliation, and safety. The responses develop as a person grows older and become regular and predictable. These patterned responses help us cope with the daily demands of living.

Environment

Environment refers to all the conditions, circumstances, and forces that influence human functioning, behavior, and development. The concept

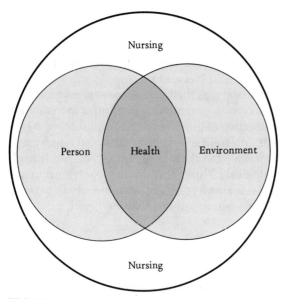

FIGURE 1-1. Nursing's Major Concepts.

TABLE 1-1
Views of Nursing's Metaparadigm—Conceptual Models

Model	Person	Environment	Health	Nursing (Goal)
Sr. Callista Roy's adaptation model	A biopsychosocial adaptive system that functions holistically in four modes: physiologic needs, self-concept, role function, and interdependence.	All internal and external stimuli (focal, contextual, residual) that influence a person.	A state of adaptation viewed on a continuum.	To promote and support adaptation in the four modes and decrease ineffective responses.
Dorothea Orem's self-care model	A self-care agent with universal, developmental, and health deviation self-care requisites, capabilities, and deficits.	Physical and psychosocial conditions and surroundings; external to the person.	Self-care ability; state of structural and functional integrity and wholeness; a wellness–illness dichotomy.	To assist client to achieve, maintain, or restore self-care capabilities in order to meet self-care requisites.
Betty Neuman's health-care systems model	An open system of physiologic, psychological, sociocultural, and developmental variables.	Internal and external forces or stressors surrounding a person at any point in time.	A condition of harmony and balance viewed on a wellness–illness continuum.	To help the client attain and maintain stability and "total wellness" by reducing stressors and adverse conditions.
Dorothy Johnson's behavioral systems model	A behavioral system with seven integrated, interdependent subsystems: achievement, affiliative, aggressive, dependence, eliminative, ingestive, and sexual; functional whole striving to maintain a steady state (behavioral system balance).	Internal and external forces that impinge on a person; no clear definition of environment.	Efficient and effective system functioning; behavioral system balance and stability.	To attain, maintain, or restore behavioral balance and stability at the highest possible level.
Martha Roger's life process model	A unitary human being; an open system; a patterned energy field that changes continuously. Change is unidirectional (forward) and negentropic, toward increasing complexity and diversity. A person interacts continuously, mutually, and simultaneously with the environment.	An energy field consisting of all that is external to any given human field.	An expression of the life process that emerges from the mutual, simultaneous interaction of human and environmental fields; health and illness are part of the same continuum.	To facilitate "symphonic inter-interaction" between person and environment through directing and redirecting patterning of the human and environmental fields.
Joyce Travelbee's interpersonal model	A unique, biopsychosocial, irreplaceable being who can	The arena in which a person experiences the full range	A person's subjective interpretation of his or her physical,	An interpersonal process to assist a person to find hope

(continued)

TABLE 1-1 (Continued)

Model	Person	Environment	Health	Nursing (Goal)
	be perceived only through his or her own eyes; always in the process of evolving and becoming; capable of free choice.	of the human condition.	mental, and social state.	and meaning in illness and suffering.

incorporates a peron's internal systems and characteristics (such as physical health, intellectual capability, and temperament) and external context (including contagious diseases, where and how the person lives, and his or her sociocultural background). The interactions of people and their environments are major determinants of health.

Florence Nightingale recognized the importance of the environment to health as reflected in her belief (1859) that the role of the nurse is to "put the [person] in the best condition for *nature* to act upon him." Her concern with creating a conducive environment, through proper nutrition, sanitation, air, and hygiene, emphasized the importance of the natural environment to health.

Health

In its social policy statement, the American Nurses Association (ANA) identifies health as "the center of nursing attention, not as an end in itself, but as a means to life that is meaningful and manageable" (ANA, 1980, p. 6). Health is a dynamic state that reflects a person's developmental and behavioral capabilities (as well as limitations) and is a manifestation of that person's interaction with the environment. Health is a continually evolving and changing pattern; it is not static.

There are no universal, culture-free norms of health (Phillips, 1990). Individuals define and perceive health (and illness) in many ways. Health consists both of objective indicators, which can be observed or measured, and subjective meaning, which must be reported by the person (Pender, 1990). Objective indicators of health include behaviors or responses that indicate an alteration in one or more dimensions of physical or mental functioning. Health also encompasses how a person interprets or perceives his or her objective state. The meaning and importance that people attribute to health depend on many factors and vary across cultures and situations.

Pender (1990) proposes a five-dimension sys-

tem for classifying human expressions of health: *affect, attitudes, activity, aspirations,* and *accomplishments*—some of which can be measured and some of which rely on what the person says. The five dimensions are described in Table 1-2.

Tripp-Reimer (1985) recommends a health grid using the dimensions of *disease–nondisease* and *wellness–illness* as axes (see Figure 1-2) for plotting a person's health. The disease–nondisease axis represents the observable, measurable state of health; the wellness–illness axis represents a person's subjective interpretation of his or her disease–nondisease state.

Tripp-Reimer (1985) suggests that conceptualizing health in this way allows the nurse to understand when there is a mismatch of a diagnosed health state (disease–nondisease) and the client's perception of it (wellness–illness). Quadrants I and III represent agreement between objective state and subjective perception. However, quadrants II and IV represent disagreement. In quadrant II, the client perceives illness in the absence of objective indidators of disease, as in those who persist in believing they have dreased diseases (cancer, AIDS) that cannot be confirmed empirically. In quadrant IV, people with diagnosed diseases perceive themselves as well (healthy), as do those individuals with physical disabilities or chronic diseases (diabetes, arthritis) who participate fully and capably in daily life. However, people with diagnosed disease who deny their diagnoses, such as a person with Type I diabetes who refuses to administer daily insulin injections, also fall within this quadrant.

Nursing

Nursing's primary concern is the health of people within the context of their internal and external environments (Donaldson & Crowley, 1978). This concern is reflected in Florence Nightingale's 1859 definition of nursing as having "charge of the personal health of somebody." Virginia Henderson's

TABLE 1-2
Classification System for Expressions of Health

Affect			
Serenity	Harmony	Vitality	Sensitivity
Calm	Close to God	Energetic	Aware
Relaxed	Contemplative	Vigorous	Connected
Peaceful	At one with the universe	Zestful	Intimate
Content		Alert	Loving
Comfortable		Fit	
Glowing		Buoyant	
Happy		Exhilarated	
Joyous		Powerful	
Pleasant		Courageous	
Satisfied			

Attitudes		
Optimism	Relevancy	Competency
Hopeful	Useful	Purposive
Enthusiastic	Contributing	Initiating
Open	Valued	Self-motivating
Reverent	Caring	Self-affirming
Trustful	Committed	Innovative
	Involved	Masterful
		Challenged

Activity		
Positive life patterns	Meaningful work	Invigorating play
Eating a healthy diet	Setting realistic goals	Having meaningful hobbies
Exercising regularly	Varying activities	Engaging in satisfying leisure activities
Managing stress	Undertaking challenging tasks	Planning energizing diversions
Obtaining adequate rest	Assuming responsibility for self	
Avoiding harmful substances	Collaborating with coworkers	
Building positive relationships	Receiving intrinsic or extrinsic rewards	
Seeking and using health information		
Monitoring health		
Coping constructively		
Maintaining a health-strengthening environment		

Aspirations	
Self-actualization	Social contribution
Growth or emergence	Enhancement of global harmony and interdependence
Personal effectiveness	Preservation of the environment
Organismic efficiency	

Accomplishments		
Enjoyment	Creativity	Transcendence
Pleasure from daily living	Maximum use of capacities	Freedom
Sense of achievement	Innovative contribution	Expansion of consciousness
		Optimized harmony between man and environment

Note. From "Expressing Health Through Lifestyle Patterns" by N.J. Pender, 1990, *Nursing Science Quarterly, 3*(3), p. 118. Copyright 1990, Chestnut House Publications, Inc. Reproduced with permission.

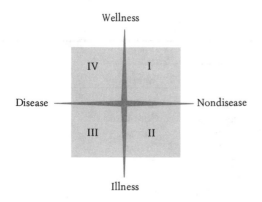

FIGURE 1-2. Health Grid. (*Note.* From "Expanding Four Essential Concepts in Nursing Theory" by T. Tripp-Reimer, in J. C. McCloskey & H. K. Grace [Eds.], *Current Issues in Nursing* [2nd ed.], St. Louis: The C. V. Mosby Co. Reprinted by permission.)

1964 definition of nursing, widely adopted and still evident, suggests that nursing's role is "to assist the individual, sick or well, in the performance of those activities contributing to health or its recovery (or to a peaceful death) that he [or she] would perform unaided if he [or she] had the necessary strength, will or knowledge. And to do this in such a way as to help him [or her] gain independence as rapidly as possible" (p. 42).

Reflecting the influence of nursing's attempts to define its domain, the ANA's document, *Nursing: A Social Policy Statement* (1980), offers the following contemporary definition of nursing:

> Nursing is the diagnosis and treatment of human responses to actual or potential health problems.

This document also suggests that the human responses with which nursing is concerned are wide-ranging and tend to be "multiple, episodic or continuous, fluid and varying, and . . . less discrete or circumscribed than medical diagnostic categories" (ANA, 1980, p. 10). The ANA *Social Policy Statement* identifies the defining characteristics of nursing practice as *nursing phenomena, theory application, nursing actions,* and *effects* (outcomes).

Nursing phenomena are the person's responses to actual or potential health problems. These responses may be health-restoring responses to actual health problems or health-supporting responses to potential health problems. It is important to note that nursing focuses on a person's responses to a health problem, not the health problem itself. Some examples of human responses with which nursing is concerned include self-care limitations, impaired functioning, pain and discomfort, self-image changes, and problems with relationships (ANA, 1980).

Theory application encompasses a nurse's use of concepts, principles, and processes to explain or interpret a person's responses to actual or potential health problems. Theory also provides the basis for implementing nursing actins and evaluating client outcomes. Nurses draw upon many theories from nursing and other disciplines in order to assure that the multidimensional needs and concerns of people are not overlooked.

Nursing actions promote health, prevent illness, and restore health and require a range of intellectual, interpersonal, and technical competencies to succeed. Nurses must be able to describe and explain their actions.

Effects, or outcomes, result from nursing actions and, ideally, are beneficial to the client, Effects should indicate that progress is being made toward or has been achieved in resolving harmful responses or promoting positive responses to an actual or potential health problem.

These four characteristics of nursing practice—phenomena, theory application, nursing actions, and effects—are reflected in *the nursing process,* nursing's systematic framework for nursing practice.

THE NURSING PROCESS

Nurses are prepared through education and experience to care for people in need of nursing care. Contemporary nursing practice is guided by a broad theoretical framework that draws from the humanities, the biological and social sciences, and an ever-expanding body of nursing knowledge. Nursing applies this knowledge to the care of clients by means of a systematic framework called *the nursing process.* The nursing process is logcal and deliberate, yet fluid and dynamic. The nursing process occurs within the context of nurse–client interaction and is, therefore, a human-to-human experience, not a scientifically controlled event.

The nursing process provides the nurse with a framework for approaching clients and addressing their responses to actual or potential health problems in a conscious, careful, deliberate manner. Such an approach avoids nursing care based on imitation ("That's how everyone does it"), hunches ("This seems like a good way to do it"), or tradition ("We've always done it this way.").

Generally, the nursing process involves five sequential, interrelated steps or phases: (1) *assessment* (data collection), (2) *diagnosis,* (3) *planning,* (4) *implementation* (treatment), and (5) *evaluation.* Although the phases of the nursing process occur sequentially, they are not necessarily linear. Rather, each phase influences and is influenced by the others. Each phase builds on previous phases and influences subsequent phases. For example, a nurse cannot develop a plan of care and select interventions from that plan until valid nursing diagnoses have been formulated from an adequate assessment. A nurse cannot evaluate outcomes of care unless the expected or desired outcomes have been specified in the care plan. Thus, while the phases are artificially separated for purposes of study, in actual practice a nurse moves fluidly among them. For instance, while a nurse is carrying out a planned nursing intervention such as relieving pain (implementation), additional information may be collected (assessment) to further validate a nursing diagnosis of pain (diagnosis), alternative measures to relieve the client's pain may be identified (planning), and the client's responses to the nursing measures may be noted (evaluation). In collecting additional data, the nurse may determine that sufficient evidence exists to warrant a new nursing diagnosis, such as sleep pattern disturbance related to pain. Thus, during every nurse–client interaction, a nurse continuously gathers information that may suggest additional nursing diagnoses or be used to plan, implement, evaluate, or revise nursing care.

The five phases of the nursing process and their components are depicted in Figure 1-3. The model illustrates the dynamic, cyclical, interdependent, and often overlapping nature of the five nursing process phases.

The nursing process is flexible and can be used with any client in any context—hospital, home, school, or clinic, and regardless of the client's age, health status, or cultural background. The nursing process also may be applied to families and communities as well as individual clients. The five phases of the nursing process are described more fully below.

Assessment

Assessment is the act of appraising or reviewing. In the context of the nursing process, assessment involves collecting information from and about a client and identifying relevant cues along the way. Data collection is a continuous process throughout the duration of the nurse–client relationship.

A nurse begins assessing the moment he or she meets a client. Assessment involves obtaining information, within a specified conceptual or theoretical framework, about a client's functioning, patterns, strengths and limitations, and concerns. The information is obtained through observation, interview—both structured and sponatenous—and through examination or clinical appraisal of the cli-

ent. Additional information may be obtained by reviewing the client's health records, laboratory tests, and in consultation with others, such as family members or other health professionals. Chapters 2 and 3 provide an overview of the approaches and methods a nurse uses to assess a client's health status and responses.

Diagnosis

Diagnosis involves the analysis and synthesis of available data to formulate impressions about a client's responses. These impressions are called *nursing diagnoses*. Therefore, diagnosis is first a process of analyzing and interpreting data and second the development of nursing diagnostic statements that specify a client's particular response and its contributing, or etiological, factors. Nursing diagnoses are a client's responses to actual or potential health problems, not the health problems themselves. Although nurses engage in collaborative interventions related to medical diagnoses, such as administering medication and intravenous fluids, nursng diagnoses are concerned only with clients' health responses, which nurses are legally, educationally, and experientially qualified to treat.

As a nurse collects data about a given client, the information is interpreted continually to determine if there are certain patterns. The data are sorted, clustered, and analyzed by the nurse. Tentative diagnostic hypotheses (inferences) are developed, which then are validated to assure accuracy. Once confirmed, diagnostic hypotheses are formulated as nursing diagnostic statements. When possible, nursing diagnoses should be selected from the most recent nursing diagnosis taxonomy approved by the North American Nursing Diagnosis Association (NANDA). This taxonomy specifes not only nursing diagnoses, but their defining characteristics and possible related factors. The defining characteristics are useful in validating a particular nursing diagnosis.

The process of analyzing and synthesizing information is reviewed in depth in Chapter 5. Chapter 6 focuses on the development of the nursing diagnostic statement and includes the 1990 NANDA-approved taxonomy (classification) of nursing diagnoses with defining characteristics and related factors.

Planning

Once nursing diagnoses have been formulated, the planning phase begins. A nurse can seldom try to resolve all a client's nursing diagnoses simultaneously, so they must be assigned priorities. Several factors should be considered when establishing the

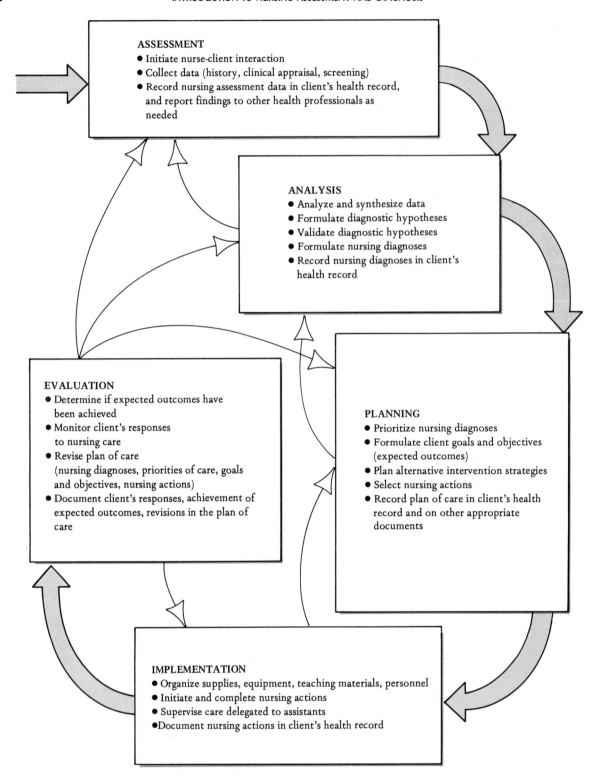

ASSESSMENT
- Initiate nurse-client interaction
- Collect data (history, clinical appraisal, screening)
- Record nursing assessment data in client's health record, and report findings to other health professionals as needed

ANALYSIS
- Analyze and synthesize data
- Formulate diagnostic hypotheses
- Validate diagnostic hypotheses
- Formulate nursing diagnoses
- Record nursing diagnoses in client's health record

EVALUATION
- Determine if expected outcomes have been achieved
- Monitor client's responses to nursing care
- Revise plan of care (nursing diagnoses, priorities of care, goals and objectives, nursing actions)
- Document client's responses, achievement of expected outcomes, revisions in the plan of care

PLANNING
- Prioritize nursing diagnoses
- Formulate client goals and objectives (expected outcomes)
- Plan alternative intervention strategies
- Select nursing actions
- Record plan of care in client's health record and on other appropriate documents

IMPLEMENTATION
- Organize supplies, equipment, teaching materials, personnel
- Initiate and complete nursing actions
- Supervise care delegated to assistants
- Document nursing actions in client's health record

FIGURE 1-3. Phases of the Nursing Process.

priority of nursing diagnoses, including the client's need for biological survival and functioning, the urgency of the need, the client's perceptions and values, and the nature of the nurse–client relationship.

Certain basic human needs, such as oxygena-

tion, fluid and electrolyte balance, temperature regulation, avoiding pain, nutrition, elimination, and protection from injury take precedence over such needs as activity, sexuality, emotional security, attachment, and self-esteem. For example, a burned client's need for an open airway, prevention of hypovolemic shock, and pain control must be attended to immediately. Concerns about the client's alteration in body image and the interfences with sexuality and self-esteem that may develop must wait until the client's physiological functioning has been stabilized.

The urgency of the nursing diagnosis also must be considered. The potential threat to the safety of an infant whose crib rail has been left down or of an elderly and disoriented client who tries to leave a nursing home unattended takes precedence (at least temporarily) over the infant's nutritional needs or the elderly client's pain from arthritis.

The client's perceptions and values are also important determinants in setting priorities for nursing care. Unfortunately, they often are overlooked in favor of the diagnosis or diagnoses that the nurse believes should take priority. When the client's perceptions of priority are ignored, however, the desired outcomes of care are not likely to be achieved. For instance, a young mother brings her 2-year-old to a clinic for a checkup. A nurse observes the child drinking cola from a baby bottle, and the mother acknowledges that the child consumes about three 8-ounce bottles of the cola a day. This is a pressing problem. But the mother's chief concern is not being able to control the child's aggressive, manipulative behavior. Unless the nurse focuses first on the mother's priority, success in changing the child's nutritional habits is likely to be thwarted.

The nature of the nurse–client relationship also will determine the order in which the nurse attempts to deal with the client's diagnoses. Suppose the client's problems are interpersonal or sexual. Effective interventions will depend on a close and trusting relationship between the nurse and the client. Such relationships take time to develop. Consequently, these nursing diagnoses may be given a lower priority until mutual rapport, trust, and respect have developed.

After nursing diagnoses have been ranked, goals and objectives are developed with the client to clearly delinate the expected outcomes of care. A *goal* is a broadly stated outcome, such as "Client will breathe comfortably and without distress," or "Client will cope effectively with altered body image." Specific objectives then are written for each goal, specifying changes in client behaviors that should result from nursing interventions. Objectives should include measurable criteria that provide parameters for determining whether objectives have been achieved. For example, a hospitalized client's nursing diagnosis is "sleep pattern disturbance related to environmental noise and interruptions for nursing care." The goal may state, "Client will rest and sleep comfortably," whereas an objective will specify, "Client will sleep for at least two uninterrupted periods of 3 hours each during the night."

It is important to formulate client objectives that are both measurable *and* realistic. An objective that specifies a hospitalized client will sleep for eight uninterrupted hours is probably unrealistic. Realistic objectives take into account the client's usual patterns and motivation; the health-care setting; resources available to client and nurse; and the client's age, cultural background, and health status. Goals and objectives that are inconsistent with the client's usual patterns or that contradict the client's cultural practices probably will not be achieved.

Objectives may be short-term or long-term. Short-term objectives make it easier to evaluate a client's progress toward long-term objectives. For example, a long-term objective for an obese woman might state, "Client will lose 50 pounds in 1 year." A short-term statement then might be, "Client will lose approximately 1 pound per week."

Goals and objectives are most likely to be useful and effective when they are:

- mutually established and acceptable to both client and nurse,
- measurable,
- realistic in terms of human and material resources,
- congruent with the client's developmental level, health status, cultural background, and behavioral patterns.

Once goals and objectives have been stated, the next step in planning is to formulate alternatives for achieving the stated goals and objectives. Alternative strategies are those nursing actions that are likely to facilitate desired outcomes. For example, alternatives for a postoperative client experiencing pain may include distraction and relaxation techniques, positioning for comfort, or administration of a prescribed analgesic.

After identifying alternatives, the nurse selects a course of action. In a sense, selection of nursing actions parallels the process of prioritizing nursing diagnoses. The actions the nurse selects, and the order in which they are implemented, depend on the following factors:

Known effectiveness of the action (based on theoretical and clinical knowledge and the nurse's experience)

Time and resources available

Possible side effects

Client preferences

In the case of pain relief, the nurse might decide to help the client learn relaxation techniques. This action requires time, however, and if the client is having acute, intense pain and is requesting "a pain shot," the nurse probably will choose to administer the prescribed analgesic first and to teach the client relaxation techniques once the pain has subsided. This will help the client cope with recurrence of the pain. If the pain begins to recur, the nurse then may select relaxation as the first alternative nursing action.

Implementation

Implementation is the "doing" or intervening phase of the nursing process. It involves organizating and actually delivering nursing care, the aim of which is to accomplish stated goals and objectives.

Nursing interventions should be purposeful and supported with rationale. Sound rationale is derived from the nurse's knowledge, prior experience, and the individualized assessment of the client. Confidence, proficiency, and efficiency are especially important attributes for the nurse to possess and to convey during the implementation phase. These attributes are gained through education, practice, and self-appraisal.

Nurses are professionally and legally accountable to their clients for the nursing care rendered. The actual nursing care delivered and the outcomes of that care are often the means used to judge nursing competence. Safe and effective nursing interventions depend on a sound nursing assessment and care plan.

The implementation phase of the nursing process involves a variety of nursing actions, including:

- performing or assisting a client to perform activities of daily living and to meet basic physiological needs,

- fostering a client's self-care and independence,

- teaching and counseling a client about the health promotion and health restoration,

- promoting a safe, comfortable environment,

- assisting a client to carry out the health-care plans, such as medications and therapeutic treatments, of other health-care providers,

- initiating interventions in selected client emergencies,

- promoting a client's psychosocial and spiritual well-being,

- stimulating and supporting client growth and development,

- ensuring a client's legal rights are protected and ethical concerns are addressed,

- referring a client to appropriate health and social resources in the community.

Nursing actions also may be concerned with meeting the needs, such as information, health teaching, and emotional support, of a client's family members and significant others. Nursing interventions should be responsive to a client's ethnic/cultural context and take into consideration a client's developmental level, cognitive ability, financial resources, and expressed wishes related to the plan of care.

Nurses may delegate portions of a client's care to such assistants as licensed practical or vocational nurses (LPN/LVN), nurse's aides, or other patient-care assistants. However, the professional nurse retains responsibility and accountability for a client's nursing care and thus should ensure adequate supervision of assistants.

Evaluation

Evaluation focuses on the client's behavioral changes and compares them with the outcome criteria stated in the objectives. Evaluations are made throughout the nursing process. As a nurse works with a client, the client's responses to nursing interventions are monitored and appraised to determine if the desired outcomes (objectives) have been accomplished, For example, if the objective states the client "will walk with assistance for 15 minutes four times a day," it is measured (evaluated) easily by monitoring the client's activity, reviewing the nurses' notes for the day, or confirming with the client that the objective has been met. Such feedback helps determine a client's progress toward long-term goals and resolution of the nursing diagnosis. If progress toward desired outcomes is not evident, the nurse should try to determine (1) if the nursing diagnosis is correct, (2) if stated goals and objectives are reasonable and realistic, (3) if nursing interventions are appropriate, and (4) if any revisions or modifications in the plan are indicated.

It may be that insufficient information was obtained during the nursng assessment and, therefore, a faulty nursing diagnosis was formulated. For example, a nursing diagnosis of "noncompliance with taking prescribed oral contraceptives related to forgetfulness" may actually reflect "fear related to misinformation about oral contraceptives." Goals and objectives determined to be unacceptable to the client or unrealistic in terms of the client's usual patterns and lifestyles, available resources, or other factors should be revised accordingly.

Nursing interventions should be evaluated in terms of their effectiveness, efficiency, and cost. if a selected nursing action does not achieve the intended outcome, another should be tried. If the prescribed nursing action is inefficient (requires too much time or too many resources, given human and material constraints) or too costly, alternatives should be developed.

Finally, the nursing care plan should be revised on the basis of information obtained from the evaluation. Revisions may be indicated for any of the reasons already discussed, or they may reflect changes in the client's health status. A short-term objective for a client's first postoperative day may state, "Will walk with assistance for 15 minutes two times today." On the third postoperative day, the objective may be revised to state, "Will walk unassisted at least four times today."

Evaluation and modification of the nursing care plan often occur in response to a client's increased or decreased ability to provide self-care.

Planned nursing interventions that may be appropriate for a 72-year-old woman who is critically ill following a cerebral vascular accident should be revised to reflect her ability to care for herself as she recovers.

Evaluation is a crucial phase of the nursing process because it provides the basis for improving nursing care. It indicates those nursing diagnoses that have been resolved, but may also lead to further assessment and the development of new nursing diagnoses.

STANDARDS OF NURSING PRACTICE

The *ANA Standards of Nursing Practice*, first published in 1973, provide an excellent framework for evaluating the quality of nursing care. These standards emphasize the nursing process as the framework for professional nursing practice, regardless of the practice setting. The standards were developed to establish or define parameters that indicate an acceptable level of nursing in order to determine the quality of care a client receives.

There are eight general standards of nursing practice. There is a format for the standards; each is accompanied by a statement of rationale, and a list of assessment factors for determining whether

---

American Nurses Association Standards of Nursing Practice

STANDARD I

The collection of data about the health status of the client/patient is systematic and continuous. The data are accessible, communicated, and recorded.

Rationale: Comprehensive care requires complete and ongoing collection of data about the client/patient to determine the nursing care needs of the client/patient. All health status data about the client/patient must be available for all members of the health care team.

Assessment Factors:

1. Health status data include:
   - Growth and development
   - Biophysical status
   - Emotional status
   - Cultural, religious, socioeconomic background
   - Performance of activities of daily living
   - Patterns of coping
   - Interaction patterns
   - Client's/patient's perception of and satisfaction with his [or her] health status
   - Client/patient health goals

   - Environment (physical, social, emotional, ecological)
   - Available and accessible human and material resources
2. Data are collected from:
   - Client/patient, family, significant others
   - Health care personnel
   - Individuals within the immediate environment and/or community
3. Data are obtained by:
   - Interview
   - Examination
   - Observation
   - Reading records, reports, etc.
4. There is a format for the collection of data which:
   - Provides for a systematic collection of data
   - Facilitates the completeness of data collection
5. Continuous collection of data is evident by:
   - Frequent updating
   - Recording of changes in health status
6. The data are:
   - Accessible on the client/patient records

(continued)

- Retrievable from record-keeping systems
- Confidential when appropriate

STANDARD II

Nursing diagnoses are derived from health status data.

Rationale: The health status of the client/patient is the basis for determining the nursing care needs. The data are analyzed and compared to norms when possible.

Assessment Factors:

1. The client's/patient's health status is compared to the norm in order to determine if there is a deviation from the norm and the degree and direction of deviation.

2. The client's/patient's capabilities and limitations are identified.

3. The nursing diagnoses are related to and congruent with the diagnoses of all other professionals caring for the client/patient.

STANDARD III

The plan of nursing care includes goals derived from the nursing diagnoses.

Rationale: The determination of the results to be achieved is an essential part of planning care.

Assessment Factors:

1. Goals are mutually set with the client/patient and pertinent others:
   - They are congruent with other planned therapies.
   - They are stated in realistic and measurable terms.
   - They are assigned a time period for achievement.

2. Goals are established to maximize functional capabilities and are congruent with:
   - Growth and development
   - Biophysical status
   - Behavioral patterns
   - Human and material resources

STANDARD IV

The plan of nursing care includes priorities and the prescribed nursing approaches or measures to achieve the goals derived from the nursing diagnoses.

Rationale: Nursing actions are planned to promote, maintain and restore the client's/patient's well-being.

Assessment Factors:

1. Physiological measures are planned to manage (prevent or control) specific patient problems and are related to the nursing diagnoses and goals of care, e.g. ADL, use of self-help devices, etc.

2. Psychosocial measures are specific to the client's/patient's nursing care problem and to the nursing care goals, e.g., techniques to control aggression, motivation.

3. Teaching-learning principles are incorporated into the plan of care and objectives for learning stated in behavioral terms, e.g. specification of content for learner's level, reinforcement, readiness, etc.

4. Approaches are planned to provide for a therapeutic environment:
   - Physical environmental factors are used to influence the therapeutic environment, e.g. control of noise, control of temperature, etc.
   - Psychosocial measures are used to structure the environment for therapeutic ends, e.g. paternal participation in all phases of the maternity experience.
   - Group behaviors are used to structure interaction and influence the therapeutic environment, e.g. conformity, ethos, territorial rights, locomotion, etc.

5. Approaches are specified for orientation of the client/patient to:
   - New roles and relationships
   - Relevant health (human and material) resources
   - Modifications in plan of nursing care
   - Relationship of modifications in nursing care plan to the total care plan

6. The plan of nursing care includes the utilization of available and appropriate resources:
   - Human resources—other health personnel
   - Material resources
   - Community

7. The plan includes an ordered sequence of nursing actions.

8. Nursing approaches are planned on the basis of current scientific knowledge.

STANDARD V

Nursing actions provide for client/patient participation in health promotion, maintenance and restoration.

Rationale: The client/patient and family are continually involved in nursing care.

Assessment Factors:

1. The client/patient and family are kept informed about:
   - Current health status
   - Changes in health status
   - Total health care plan
   - Nursing care plan
   - Roles of health care personnel
   - Health care resources

2. The client/patient and family are provided with the information needed to make decisions and choices about:
   - Promoting, maintaining and restoring health
   - Seeking and utilizing appropriate health care personnel
   - Maintaining and using health care resources

STANDARD VI

Nursing actions assist the client/patient to maximize his [or her] health capabilities.

Rationale: Nursing actions are designed to promote, maintain and restore health.

Assessment Factors:

1. Nursing actions:
   - Are consistent with the plan of care.
   - Are based on scientific principles.
   - Are individualized to the specific situation.
   - Are used to provide a safe and therapeutic environment.
   - Employ teaching-learning opportunities for the client/patient.
   - Include utilization of appropriate resources.

2. Nursing actions are directed by the client's/patient's physical, physiological, psychological and social behavior associated with:
   - Ingestion of food, fluid, and nutrients
   - Elimination of body wastes and excesses in fluid
   - Locomotion and exercise
   - Regulatory mechanisms—body heat, metabolism
   - Relating to others
   - Self-actualization

STANDARD VII

The client/patient's progress or lack of progress toward goal achievement is determined by the client/patient and the nurse.

Rationale: The quality of nursing care depends upon comprehensive and intelligent determination of nursing's impact upon the health status of the client/patient. The client/patient is an essential part of this determination.

Assessment Factors:

1. Current data about the client/patient are used to measure his [or her] progress toward goal achievement.

2. Nursing actions are analyzed for their effectiveness in the goal achievement of the client/patient.

3. The client/patient evaluates nursing actions and goal achievement.

4. Provision is made for nursing follow-up of a particular client/patient to determine the long-term effects of nursing care.

STANDARD VIII

The client/patient's progress or lack of progress toward goal achievement directs reassessment, reordering of priorities, new goal setting and revision of the plan of nursing care.

Rationale: The nursing process remains the same, but the input of new information may dictate new or revised approaches.

Assessment Factors:

1. Reassessment is directed by goal achievement or lack of goal achievement.

2. New priorities and goals are determined and additional nursing approaches are prescribed appropriately.

3. New nursing actions are accurately and appropriately initiated.

Note. From *Standards of Nursing Practice*, American Nurses' Association, 1973. Reprinted with permission, American Nurses' Association, Kansas City, MO.

---

the standard has been achieved, thus indicating the quality of nursing care rendered the client.

All eight standards appear in the box. Of particular importance to this book are standards I and II, which emphasize the collection of information and the development of nursing diagnoses.

The general *Standards of Nursing Practice* are applicable to all specialties of clinical nursing practice. However, the various ANA divisions have formulated standards specific to each clinical specialty. Each division's standards parallel the general standards but are written to specify the scope and nature of nursing practice in a particular clinical specialty, such as maternal-child health nursing practice, gerontologic nursing practice, community health nursing practice, and so on. All, however, include standards related to nursing assessment and nursing diagnosis as essential components of professional nursing practice.

Figure 1-4 illustrates the relationship of the ANA's definition of nursing practice, the *Standards of Nursing Practice*, and the phases of the nursing process.

KNOWLEDGE NEEDED FOR NURSING ASSESSMENT AND DIAGNOSIS

Certain knowledge and abilities are necessary for a nurse to perform a comprehensive, multidimensional nursing assessment. The essential knowledge for professional nursing practice is obtained through education as well as experience.

Nursing is a caring process that relies on knowledge from the liberal arts, the sciences, and

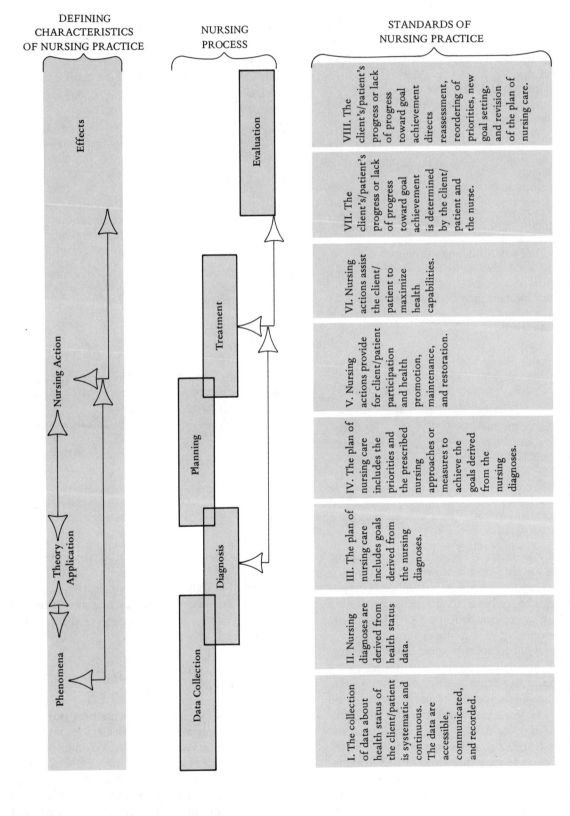

FIGURE 1-4. Defining Characteristics of Nursing Practice: Relationship to the Nursing Process and the Standards of Nursing Practice. (*Note.* From *Nursing: A Social Policy Statement* by American Nurses Association, 1980, Kansas City, MO: ANA, pp. 14–15. Reprinted by permission.)

the discipline of nursing. All three are essential for professional nursing practice and, more specifically, for conducting a comprehensive, multidimensional nursing assessment.

Liberal Arts Knowledge

Knowledge of the liberal arts is civilizing knowledge—it helps a nurse become a fully participating human being. The liberal arts include philosophy, ethics, religious studies, language, literature, history, and the fine and performing arts. Such knowledge prepares a nurse to understand, appreciate, and participate as a free and contributing member of society. Studying the liberal arts facilitates the development of a variety of intellectual, affective, and sometimes physical abilities that can be applied to solving problems associated with the human condition. Such broad learning is especially important for nursing because of its concern for people and their responses to human situations and experiences.

The American Association of Colleges of Nursing (AACN) (1986) describes the abilities that enable a liberally educated person to "responsibly challenge the status quo and anticipate and adapt to change "(p. 4). Such qualities are necessary for

TABLE 1-3
Knowledge and Abilities from the Liberal Arts

Write, read, and speak English clearly and effectively in order to acquire knowledge, convey and discuss ideas, evaluate information, and think critically.

Think analytically and reason logically using verifiable information and past experience in order to select or create solutions to problems.

Understand a second language, at least at an elementary level, in order to widen access to the diversity of world cultures.

Comprehend life and time from historical and contemporary perspectives and draw from past experiences to influence the present and future.

Comprehend the meaning of human spirituality in order to recognize the relationship of beliefs to culture, behavior, health, and healing.

Appreciate the role of the fine and performing arts in stimulating individual creativity, expressing personal feelings and emotions, and building a sense of the commonality of human experience.

Understand the nature of human values and develop a personal philosophy in order to make ethical judgments in both personal and professional life.

Note. From Essentials of College and University Education for Professional Nursing by American Association of Colleges of Nursing, 1986, Washington, DC: AACN, pp. 4–5. Reprinted by permission.

personal well-being and growth and for contributing to the well-being of others. The kinds of abilities acquired through a liberal education are described in Table 1-3.

Scientific Knowledge

Knowledge of the biological and social sciences, such as biology, chemistry, physics, environmental science, mathematics, statistics, psychology, sociology, anthropology, political science, and economics, is essential for understanding human physiological and psychosocial responses. It also is essential for comprehending and negotiating the complexities of the health-care system on behalf of the people for whom a nurse cares. Historically, nurses have relied heavily on knowledge from the sciences as a basis for providing nursing care.

The AACN (1986) delineates the abilities based on scientific knowledge that professional nurses should possess (see Table 1-4). These abilities enable a nurse to understand the basis of much of human behavior.

Nursing Knowledge

Nursing has been categorized as both art and science. Carper (1978) identifies four fundamental types of knowledge that she terms nursing's "patterns of knowing." These patterns include (1) empirics, the science of nursing, (2) esthetics, the art of nursing, (3) personal knowledge, and (4) ethical knowledge. Carper notes that "the body of knowl-

TABLE 1-4
Knowledge and Abilities from the Sciences

Understand other cultural traditions in order to gain a perspective on personal values and the similarities and differences among individuals and groups.

Use mathematical concepts, interpret quantitative data, and use computers and other information technology in order to analyze problems and develop positions that depend on numbers and statistics.

Use concepts from the behavioral and biological sciences in order to understand oneself and one's relationships with other people and to comprehend the nature and function of communities.

Understand the physical world and its relationship with human activity in order to make decisions that are based on scientific evidence and responsive to the values and interests of the individual and society.

Gain a perspective on social, political, and economic issues for resolving societal and professional problems.

Note. From Essentials of College and University Education for Professional Nursing by American Association of Colleges of Nursing, 1986, Washington, DC: AACN, pp. 4–5. Reprinted by permission.

edge that serves as the rationale for nursing practice has patterns, forms, and structure that . . . exemplify characteristic ways of thinking about [nursing] phenomena "(p. 13).

Benner (1983) distinguishes between *theoretical nursing knowledge*, which is developed through research, and *clinical nursing knowledge*, which is acquired through the practice of nursing. She points out that the difference between the two types of nursing knowledge is "knowing *that*" versus "knowing *how*."

Nursing knowledge thus can be summarized as incorporating three types of knowledge: theoretical and scientific, esthetic, and clinical.

Theoretical and Scientific Knowledge

A body of nursing theory and science has been emerging over the last 25 years. Theoretical and scientific knowledge within the discipline of nursing involves the development and testing of empirical knowledge to describe, explain, and predict human responses. This body of knowledge is "factual, descriptive, and ultimately aimed at developing abstract and theoretical explanations" of these responses (Carper, 1978).

As early as 1859, Nightingale emphasized the importance of research in building nursing's body of knowledge. She was instrumental in laying the groundwork for the systematic study of conditions affecting the sick, with particular attention to nursing actions that were effective in restoring health. She was a meticulous data keeper and believed fervently in a systematic approach to nursing care.

In the last quarter century, nurses have focused on building a body of scientific knowledge for validating and improving nursing practice. Currently, the development of scientific knowledge in nursing is focused on three major areas: health promotion and disease prevention, human responses to acute and chronic illness, and systems for delivering nursing care. The National Center for Nursing Research has selected several priorities for nursing science research, including low birth weight (mothers and infants); human immunodeficiency virus (HIV)-positive patients, partners, and families; long-term care; symptom (e.g., pain, fatigue, nausea) management; information systems, including standardized data sets and a taxonomy for classifying nursing's concerns; health promotion; and dependence on technology for preserving and prolonging life (Hinshaw, Heinrich, & Block, 1988).

Thus, the theoretical and scientific knowledge needed for nursing assessment and diagnosis includes knowledge from the traditional scientific disciplines as well as nursing's own unique body of knowledge. Scientific knowledge continues to proliferate at a pace that boggles the human mind. Therefore, it is essential that nurses are acquainted with the broad concepts of scientific knowledge in order to connect new advances with previous learning.

Esthetic Knowledge

Esthetic knowledge often has been referred to as the art of nursing. Esthetic knowledge encompasses that which is concerned with the self (personal awareness), interpersonal relationships ("therapeutic use of self"), communication, caring, empathy, and advocacy, among others. Esthetic knowledge is expressive and allows the nurse to enter into genuine, meaningful relationships with people who need nursing services. In contrast to the abstract, theoretical knowledge of nursing science, esthetic knowledge helps the nurse understand and respond to each client as a unique human being within a particular context or situation.

From an esthetic perspective, nursing involves an encounter with another person. The goal of nurse–client interaction is to enhance the health and well-being of the client, help the client cope with health and illness situations, and facilitate the client's ability to find meaning in and grow from life experiences. Esthetic knowledge enables a nurse to consider each encounter with a client as a unique, mutual, and subjective experience.

Clinical Knowledge

Clinical knowledge is developed when a nurse applies theoretical knowledge within the context of a nurse–client interaction or relationship. What emerges as the nurse gains experience is an ability to respond to clients holistically, rather than relying on theoretical propositions or scientific maxims.

Benner (1982) proposes that clinical knowledge is developed as a nurse acquires practical experience with clients and offers a five-level model for developing clinical knowledge (see box). Benner notes that the levels reflect differences in two ways: movement from dependence on abstract, theoretical knowledge to the use of previous experience (clinical knowledge), and transformation of a nurse's perception of a clinical situation from bits and pieces to a perception of the whole. Thus, clinical knowledge is embedded in and derived from actual clinical encounters.

Levels of Clinical Knowledge

Novice: Uses context-free rules and norms to guide actions. Unable to use discretionary judgment. Appraises clinical situations in terms of objective attributes.

Advanced Beginner: Able to identify recurrent aspects of clinical situations. Ability to recognize relevant aspects depends on past experiences. All aspects and attributes are treated as equally important. Needs help in sorting out most important aspects and in setting priorities.

Competent: Able to judge relative importance of different aspects or attributes of the clinical situation. Plans care with consideration of long-term goals. Thinks ana-

lytically and contemplatively about clinical problems. Able to cope with and manage many contingencies. Efficient and organized.

Proficient: Perceives clinical situations as wholes. Performance is guided by clinical maxims derived from prior experience. Able to "hone in "on key aspects of situation. Responsive to contextual variables and uniqueness of each situation.

Expert: Intuitively grasps the situation. Focuses quickly and accurately on the problem without having to plod through a host of alternative possibilities. Uses rich descriptive phrases to describe own practice and decision-making.

Note. Adapted from "Novice to expert," by P. Benner, 1982, *American Journal of Nursing, 82,* pp. 402–407. Adapted by permission.

SKILLS NEEDED FOR NURSING ASSESSMENT AND DIAGNOSIS

Quality nursing practice requires many skills. A nurse must acquire competencies in three domains: *cognitive* (intellectual), *interpersonal*, and *technical*.

Cognitive Skills

Intellectual, or cognitive, competencies include a nurse's basic knowledge, derived from life experiences and formal education; the ability to solve problems; and the ability to think critically and to examine clinical phenomena. A nurse also must possess analytical skills, decision-making abilities, judgment, and insight. In order to assess a client or a clinical situation, a nurse must know what to look for and how to look for it. A nurse must be able to ask the right questions, make sense of the information received, be perceptually aware of client and environmental cues, and attend to the relevant ones. A nurse also must be able to use a systematic approach for identifying a client's problems or needs, and to sort out, organize, and cluster pieces of information in order to make clinical nursing judgments.

Nursing assessment demands that a nurse think critically and analytically about clinical phenomena. Critical thinking is a cognitive process that "involves weighing the accuracy and logic of the evidence—an understanding of the nature of valid inferences, abstractions, and generalizations" (Miller & Malcolm, 1990, p. 67). Critical thinking is

goal-directed and purposeful and requires a degree of skepticism and persistence in seeking solutions to problems. Critical thinking, as applied to nursing assessment and diagnosis, involves exploring and gathering information about nursing concerns, examining the data collected, analyzing the relationships among the data, and drawing conclusions about the client's needs and problems. A nurse's conclusions take into account all available information and can be justified by the evidence.

Nursing assessment and diagnosis also require a nurse to maintain a sense of curiosity—a willingness to pursue and investigate available avenues of information about the various dimensions of human functioning. Curiosity is related closely to inquisitiveness, a process of seeking answers to questions to satisfy one's curiosity (Sneed, 1990). Inquisitiveness about clinical phenomena, such as a client's failure to adhere to prescribed treatments or a mother's perceptions of her newborn infant, is an important dimension of curiosity and an essential requisite for comprehensive, valid nursing assessments and diagnoses.

Two other important cognitive competencies are creativity and adaptability. Creativity refers to a nurse's ability to use imagination—to develop and test new and original approaches to nursing care when more traditional approaches do not produce the desired outcomes or changes in clients' behaviors. Adaptability, or flexibility, is a nurse's ability to adapt or adjust to a variety of clinical situations. Adaptability implies that a nurse is willing to consider alternative approaches or strategies in all phases of the nursing process. For example, during an interview a client expresses a particular concern about one of the nurse's questions about health status. The nurse should be sufficiently flexible to modify or adapt the nursing history interview to explore this concern with the client, while not losing sight of the original focus or goal.

An important process that enhances a nurse's cognitive competencies is reflection. Saylor (1990) defines reflection as a "process of reviewing one's repertoire of clinical experience and knowledge to invent novel approaches to complex clinical problems "(p. 8). Nurses need time in their practices to reflect on what they encounter in order to develop effective and innovative approaches to care. Reflection also provides an opportunity for evaluating one's own competencies as a stimulus for continued growth, as a person and a professional. Reflection is an essential process for nursing assessment and diagnosis. As nurses collect data during the assessment phase, they reflect on the data—what they mean, what nursing diagnoses they suggest, what solutions may help resolve those diagnoses—and in so doing, begin to generate creative responses to what they have observed clinically. As Saylor (1990) quotes Richert (1988):

> Practice in any profession requires the processing of technical and scientific knowledge for use in a context that is rapidly changing and uncertain. The ability to think about what one does and why—assessing past actions, current situations, and intended outcomes—is vital to intelligent practice that is reflective rather than routine or reflexive. Reflection influences how one grows as a professional by influencing how successfully one is able to learn from one's experiences. (p. 11)

Interpersonal Skills

Interpersonal skills refer to a nurse's ability to develop a relationship and rapport with a client and family and to interact with the client in a meaningful, goal-directed manner. To be effective, a nurse must employ appropriate verbal and nonverbal communication skills, including empathetic listening. A nurse must also be able to transmit a sense of concern, caring, and commitment to a client, thus helping to foster an atmosphere of mutual trust and respect.

In order to develop effective interpersonal skills and be able to respond constructively, a nurse must develop a certain degree of self-awareness. Understanding and accepting one's self enables a nurse to acknowledge and value a client's

uniqueness. Becoming self-aware is a self-initiated process—a willingness to get in touch with one's own thoughts, feelings, and perceptions, and with how they influence one's interactions with others. Self-awareness involves continual self-development and an openness to new opportunities.

Authenticity is another interpersonal skill essential to effective nurse–client relationships. Authenticity involves being truthful, open, and willing to share one's self with another in a human-to-human relationship. Authenticity is a hallmark of a genuine, caring relationship between nurse and client and facilitates a client's openness and willingness to disclose important information to a nurse.

Thus, a nurse's attitudes, disposition, and manner influence the quality of the nurse–client relationship and affect how the nurse approaches the client, seeks information, and responds to the client's disclosures. Interpersonal skills can therefore foster or inhibit a nurse's ability to perform a comprehensive nursing assessment.

Technical Skills

Technical competencies needed for nursing assessment and diagnosis include those techniques, procedures, or tools that involve the use or manipulation of special equipment or instruments or sometimes simply the nurse's own motor skills or abilities. Examples of technical skills that a nurse may employ when conducting a nursing assessment include measurement of vital signs, examination of the ears using an otoscope, testing of neurological reflexes, administering developmental screening tests, and testing a urine specimen with a dipstick. A nurse always should keep in mind, however, that technical competencies should be grounded in nursing knowledge and thus are used in conjunction with a nurse's intellectual skills. Interpersonal competencies also are used with technical competencies. For example, when auscultating breath sounds, the nurse should explain to the client the reason for the procedure, what it will feel like ("This may feel cold"), and what the client is expected to do to help ("Breathe deeply when I tell you"). A nurse also should be sensitive to how the client responds to a technical procedure, such as anxiety about the unknown, fear of anticipated pain, or embarrassment when asked to expose certain areas of the body.

Careful and deliberate use of cognitive, interpersonal, and technical skills enables a nurse to conduct a more comprehensive, sensitive, valid, and efficient nursing assessment.

VALUES NEEDED FOR NURSING ASSESSMENT AND DIAGNOSIS

Nurses should ascribe to the values of professional nursing and reflect these values in their attitudes, behaviors, and personal qualities (American Association of Colleges of Nursing, 1986). Values are those ideals to which a person is committed, and that serve as a guide for behavior (American Association of Colleges of Nursing, 1986).

In an age of rapid change, increasing diversity of the population, greater technological dependence, and the emergence of heretofore unknown and unimagined ethical dilemmas, awareness of one's own values is essential. In health-care situations, the values of the nurse, the client, the profession of nursing, and of society interface and sometimes conflict. Nurses work with clients who often are very different from themselves—different in color, socioeconomic status, religious and spiritual beliefs, lifestyle, cultural values, education, and language. The values of a client who engages repeatedly in high-risk behaviors, despite health education, may conflict with those of a nurse who values health and risk-reduction. A nurse who supports a person's right to refuse life-prolonging treatment may have difficulty working with a physician who initiates artificial ventilation despite the client's wishes. In order to work effectively with clients within the context of a particular health-care system and the larger society, nurses should strive to clarify the values they hold about people, health, health care, and the values the nursing profession has embraced.

Professional values often are expressed in a formal code of ethics. Curtin and Flaherty (1982) identify acceptance of a code of ethics as one hallmark of professional nurses. The American Nurses Association, Canadian Nurses Association, and International Council of Nurses each have adopted a code of ethics that reflects the values embraced by members of the profession (see boxed inserts).

The American Association of Colleges of Nursing (1986) identifies seven essential values for the professional nurse: (1) altruism, (2) equality, (3) esthetics, (4) freedom, (5) human dignity, (6) justice, and (7) truth. Each is defined, and examples of attitudes, personal qualities, and professional behaviors are provided in Table 1-5.

ISSUES IN NURSING ASSESSMENT AND DIAGNOSIS

A profession exists for the purpose of providing service to the public. Inherent in this definition is the concept of accountability. A profession and, therefore, professionals are accountable to the public for their services. Recipients of a profession's services have a right to knowledgeable, competent,

---

American Nurses Association Code of Ethics

- The nurse provides services with respect for human dignity and the uniqueness of the client unrestricted by considerations of social or economic status, personal attributes, or the nature of health problems.

- The nurse safeguards the client's right to privacy by judiciously protecting information of a confidential nature.

- The nurse acts to safeguard the client and the public when health care and safety are affected by the incompetent, unethical, or illegal practice of any person.

- The nurse assumes responsibility and accountability for individual nursing judgments and actions.

- The nurse maintains competence in nursing.

- The nurse exercises informed judgment and uses individual competence and qualifications as criteria in seeking consultation, accepting responsibilities, and delegating nursing activities to others.

- The nurse participates in activities that contribute to the ongoing development of the profession's body of knowledge.

- The nurse participates in the profession's efforts to implement and improve standards of nursing.

- The nurse participates in the profession's efforts to establish and maintain conditions of employment conducive to high quality nursing care.

- The nurse participates in the profession's effort to protect the public from misinformation and misrepresentation and to maintain the integrity of nursing.

- The nurse collaborates with members of the health professions and other citizens in promoting community and national efforts to meet the health needs of the public.

Note. From *Code for Nurses with Interpretive Statements* by American Nurses Association, Kansas City, MO, 1985. Reprinted by permission.

Canadian Nurses Association Code of Ethics

The body of the code is divided into the following sources of nursing obligations:

CLIENTS

- A nurse is obliged to treat clients with respect for their individual needs and values.

- Based on respect for clients and regard for their rights to control their own care, nursing care should reflect respect for clients' right of choice.

- The nurse is obliged to hold confidential all information about a client learned in the health care setting.

- The nurse has an obligation to be guided by consideration for the dignity of clients.

- The nurse is obligated to provide competent care to clients.

- The nurse is obliged to represent the ethics of nursing before colleagues and others.

- The nurse is obligated to advocate clients' interests.

- In all professional settings, including education, research, and administration, the nurse retains a commitment to the welfare of clients. The nurse has an obligation to act in a fashion that will maintain trust in nurses and nursing.

HEALTH TEAM

- Client care should represent a cooperative effort, drawing on the expertise of nursing and other health professions. By acknowledging personal or professional limitations, the nurse recognizes the perspective and expertise of colleagues from other disciplines.

- The nurse, as a member of the health care team, is obliged to take steps to ensure that the client receives competent and ethical care.

SOCIAL CONTEXT OF NURSING

- Conditions of employment should contribute to client care and to the professional satisfaction of nurses. Nurses are obliged to work toward securing and maintaining conditions of employment that satisfy these goals.

RESPONSIBILITIES OF THE PROFESSION

- Professional nurses' organizations recognize a responsibility to clarify, secure, and sustain ethical nursing conduct. The fulfillment of these tasks requires professional organizations to remain responsive to the rights, needs, and interests of clients and nurses.

Note. From *Code of Ethics for Nursing.* Reprinted with permission from Canadian Nurses Association, February 1985.

---

safe care and a right to participate actively in that care. According to Gordon (1989), the consumer has "the right to receive the best possible quality of care, care grounded in a firm knowledge base and performed by those who can make use of that knowledge base through the application of sound judgment and a clear and appropriate value system" (p. 253).

Today's health-care consumers know their rights within the health-care system, including what services professionals are able to provide, and thus are able to articulate their needs and wishes. It is within this context that nursing is practiced today. Therefore, it is extremely important for a nurse to recognize that clients have a right to know about their nursing care and that the nurse has a responsibility to provide that information and respond to the client's questions and concerns.

Inherent in the concept of a client's right to know is the issue of informed consent. Informed consent means that clients are informed about a particular procedure to be performed, such as data

collection, a medical treatment, or a surgical procedure, and consent to the procedure based on the information provided. In nonemergency situations, informed consent must be obtained prior to any procedure, and it is the responsibility of the person performing the procedure to obtain the consent. Therefore, before initiating the nursing assessment, the client has a right to know what the purpose and scope of the questions will be and a right to choose to participate. Clients also may refuse to respond to the nurse's assessment questions, although they also have a right to know how that refusal might affect the nurse's ability to provide comprehensive nursing care.

The nurse should keep in mind that informed consent means that the client (1) voluntarily consents, (2) is competent and capable of giving consent, and (3) that adequate information for making a decision has been given to the client. Certain clients may require others to provide consent on their behalf: minors and those who are mentally or physically incapacitated to such a degree that they are unable to understand what is expected of them.

International Council of Nurses Code for Nurses

The fundamental responsibility of the nurse is four-fold: to promote health, to prevent illness, to restore health, and to alleviate suffering.

The need for nursing is universal. Inherent in nursing is respect for life, dignity, and rights of man. It is unrestricted by considerations of nationality, race, creed, color, age, sex, politics, or social status.

Nurses render health services to the individual, the family, and the community and coordinate their services with those of related groups.

NURSES AND PEOPLE

The nurse's primary responsibility is to those people who require nursing care.

The nurse, in providing care, promotes an environment in which the values, customs and spiritual beliefs of the individual are respected.

The nurse holds in confidence personal information and uses judgment in sharing this information.

NURSES AND PRACTICE

The nurse carries personal responsibility for nursing practice and for maintaining competence by continual learning. The nurse maintains the highest standards of nursing care possible within the reality of a specific situation.

The nurse uses judgment in relation to individual competence when accepting and delegating responsibilities.

The nurse when acting in a professional capacity should at all times maintain standards of personal conduct which reflect credit upon the profession.

NURSES AND SOCIETY

The nurse shares with other citizens the responsibility for initiating and supporting action to meet the health and social needs of the public.

NURSES AND CO-WORKERS

The nurse sustains a cooperative relationship with co-workers in nursing and other fields. The nurse takes appropriate action to safeguard the individual when his care is endangered by a co-worker or any other person.

NURSES AND THE PROFESSION

The nurse plays the major role in determining and implementing desirable standards of nursing practice and nursing education.

The nurse is active in developing a core of professional knowledge.

The nurse, acting through the professional organization, participates in establishing and maintaining equitable social and economic working conditions in nursing.

Note. From *ICN Ethical Code for Nurses: Ethical Concepts Applied to Nursing* by International Council of Nurses, Geneva, 1973, Imprimeries Populaires. Reprinted by permission.

Another critical issue related to conducting the nursing assessment is the client's right to privacy. Many times the issue of privacy is forgotten when a person enters the health-care system. Too often the client becomes a number or a diagnostic label. Discussions are held and decisions made about and for the client instead of *with* the client. While it is often necessary to obtain a large amount of information from a client to ensure a comprehensive nursing assessment and valid diagnoses, the process does intrude on the client's privacy. The amount of information sought, coupled with the examinations, tests, and procedures performed often contribute to the client's feeling "exposed "to unfamiliar persons in an unfamiliar setting. Amid all the data collection, health-care professionals can easily lose sight of the person who has sought their help.

Nurses are not immune to this type of thinking nor the type of care that results when one operates with this mind-set. Such thinking, however, is not in keeping with the essence of what it means to be a professional nurse. For the nurse to function in a truly professional manner, the values of competence in practice, trust, shared respect, and client participation in decision-making must be assured. Great care must be taken to preserve a client's dignity and sense of privacy. When data are collected in a competent, sensitive, caring, and efficient manner, the client's dignity and humanity are protected, and the nurse's respect and concern for the client are evident.

As a member of the health-care team, the nurse collaborates with other professionals in caring for clients, including collecting assessment information related to the client's health care. Collaboration ensures that the total picture is considered and that those with the needed expertise are involved in the client's care. Collaboration minimizes unnecessary duplication, an important con-

TABLE 1-5
Essential Values for the Professional Nurse

Essential Values*	Examples of Attitudes and Personal Qualities	Examples of Professional Behaviors
1. ALTRUISM Concern for the welfare of others.	Caring Commitment Compassion Generosity Perseverance	Gives full attention to the patient/client when giving care. Assists other personnel in providing care when they are unable to do so. Expresses concern about social trends and issues that have implications for health care.
2. EQUALITY Having the same rights, privileges, or status.	Acceptance Assertiveness Fairness Self-esteem Tolerance	Provides nursing care based on the individual's needs irrespective of personal characteristics.** Interacts with other providers in a non-discriminatory manner. Expresses ideas about the improvement of access to nursing and health care.
3. ESTHETICS Qualities of objects, events, and persons that provide satisfaction.	Appreciation Creativity Imagination Sensitivity	Adapts the environment so it is pleasing to the patient/client. Creates a pleasant work environment for self and others. Presents self in a manner that promotes a positive image of nursing.
4. FREEDOM Capacity to exercise choice.	Confidence Hope Independence Openness Self-direction Self-discipline	Honors individual's right to refuse treatment. Supports the rights of other providers to suggest alternatives to the plan of care. Encourages open discussion of controversial issues in the profession.
5. HUMAN DIGNITY Inherent worth and uniqueness of an individual.	Consideration Empathy Humaneness Kindness Respectfulness Trust	Safeguards the individual's right to privacy. Addresses individuals as they prefer to be addressed. Maintains confidentiality of patients/clients and staff. Treats others with respect regardless of background.
6. JUSTICE Upholding moral and legal principles.	Courage Integrity Morality Objectivity	Acts as a health-care advocate. Allocates resources fairly. Reports incompetent, unethical, and illegal practice objectively and factually.**
7. TRUTH Faithfulness to fact or reality.	Accountability Authenticity Honesty Inquisitiveness Rationality Reflectiveness	Documents nursing care accurately and honestly. Obtains sufficient data to make sound judgments before reporting infractions of organizational policies. Participates in professional efforts to protect the public from misinformation about nursing.

*The values are listed in alphabetic rather than priority order.
**From *Code for Nurses*, American Nurses' Association, 1976.
Note. From *Essentials of College and University Education for Professional Nursing* by American Association of Colleges of Nursing, 1986, Washington, DC: AACN, pp. 6–7. Reprinted by permission.

sideration when so many professionals may be involved in responding to the client's needs. As a vital member of the health-care team, the nurse offers a broad, holistic perspective that considers the impact of health and illness, as well as the effects of treatment, on the client's quality of life. It is a perspective that considers the client's family as an integral part of the health-care process, that values all members of the health-care team, and sees the client at the center of this effort. Finally, it is a perspective that recognizes the importance of shared communication and creative problem-solving on the client's behalf.

Nurses play a key role in helping people achieve their optimum health potentials and to live lives to their fullest, regardless of the presence of disease or disability. Within this framework, the nurse is in a prime position to coordinate and monitor the care of clients so the very best comprehensive and humane care is provided.

Chapter Highlights

- In the last 25 years, nursing has become an independent and creative force in health care.

- The concepts of interest to the discipline and profession of nursing are fourfold: *person, environment, health,* and *nursing,* which together comprise nursing's "metaparadigm."

- Philosophical beliefs and theoretical perspectives about each of the concepts provide a framework for nursing practice, including nursing assessment and diagnosis.

- Nurses apply knowledge to the care of clients by means of a systematic framework called the nursing process. This process involves five sequential and interrelated phases: assessment, diagnosis, planning, implementation, and evaluation.

- The *Standards of Nursing Practice* (ANA, 1973) define parameters for determining the quality of nursing care.

- Nursing assessment and diagnosis are guided by three kinds of knowledge: liberal arts, scientific knowledge, and nursing knowledge. Nursing knowledge incorporates three types of knowledge: theoretical and scientific knowledge, esthetic knowledge, and clinical knowledge.

- To perform a comprehensive nursing assessment, a nurse must integrate and use skills from three domains: cognitive, interpersonal, and technical.

- Nurses should ascribe to the values of professional nursing and reflect these values in their attitudes, behaviors, and personal qualities as they interact with others, both personally and professionally.

- Important issues that should be considered when conducting a comprehensive nursing assessment include the nurse's accountability to the client and the client's right to informed consent, privacy, knowledgeable and competent care, and active participation in the assessment and diagnostic process.

- The professional nurse plays a primary role in coordinating and monitoring the care of clients in collaboration with other health professionals, thus ensuring a comprehensive nursing assessment and the formulation of nursing diagnoses unique to the client and to the domain of nursing practice.

Recommended Readings

Benner, P. (1982). From novice to expert. *American Journal of Nursing, 82,* 402–407.

Benner, P. (1983). Uncovering the knowledge embedded in clinical practice. *Image: The Journal of Nursing Scholarship, XV*(2), 36–41.

Corcoran, S.A. (1986). Planning by expert and novice nurses in cases of varying complexity. *Research in Nursing and Health, 9,* 155–162.

Diers, D. (1986). To profess—To be a professional. *Journal of Nursing Administration, 16*(3), 25–30.

Meleis, A.I. (1990). Being and becoming healthy: The core of nursing knowledge. *Nursing Science Quarterly, 3*(3), 107–114.

Saylor, C.R. (1990). Reflection and professional education: Art, science, and competency. *Nurse Educator, 15*(2), 8–11.

Sneed, N.V. (1990). Curiosity and the yen to discover. *Nursing Outlook, 38,* 36–39.

Tripp-Reimer, T. (1984). Reconceptualizing the construct of health. *Research in Nursing and Health, 7,* 101–109.

References

American Association of Colleges of Nursing. (1986). *Essentials of college and university education for professional nursing.* Washington, DC: Author.

American Nurses Association. (1973). *Standards: Nursing practice.* Kansas City: Author.

American Nurses Association. (1980). *Nursing: A social policy statement.* Kansas City: Author.

Benner, P. (1982). From novice to expert. *American Journal of Nursing, 82,* 402–407.

Benner, P. (1983). Uncovering the knowledge embedded in clinical practice. *Image: The Journal of Nursing Scholarship, XV*(2), 36–41.

Carper, B.A. (1978). Fundamental patterns of knowing in nursing. *Advances in Nursing Science, 1*(1), 13–23.

Curtin, L., & Flaherty, M.J. (1982). *Nursing ethics: Theories and pragmatics*. Bowie, MD: Brady.

Donaldson, S.K., & Crowley, D.M. (1978). The discipline of nursing. *Nursing Outlook, 26*, 113–120.

Ellis, R. (1982). Conceptual issues in nursing. *Nursing Outlook, 30*, 406–410.

Fawcett, J. (1984). *Analysis and evaluation of conceptual models of nursing*. Philadelphia: F.A. Davis.

Gordon, S.E. (1989). Accountability to the public, the profession, the employer, and the self. In S. Leddy & J.M. Pepper (Eds.), *Conceptual bases of professional nursing* (2nd ed., pp. 249–264). Philadelphia: J.B. Lippincott.

Henderson, V. (1964). *The nature of nursing*. New York: Macmillan.

Hinshaw, A.S., Heinrich, J., & Block, D. (1988). Evolving clinical nursing research priorities: A national endeavor. *Journal of Professional Nursing, 4*, 458–459.

Miller, M.A., & Malcolm, N.S. (1990). Critical thinking in the nursing curriculum. *Nursing Outlook, 38*, 67–73.

Nightingale, F. (1859). *Notes on nursing: What it is and what it is not*. London: Harrison.

Pender, N.J. (1990). Expressing health through lifestyle patterns. *Nursing Science Quarterly, 3*(3), 115–122.

Phillips, J.R. (1990). The different views of health. *Nursing Science Quarterly, 3*(3), 103.

Richert, A. (1988). *Teaching teachers to reflect: A consideration of program structure*. Unpublished doctoral dissertation, Stanford University, Palo Alto, CA.

Saylor, C.R. (1990). Reflection and professional education: Art, science, and competency. *Nurse Educator, 15*(2), 8–11.

Sneed, N.V. (1990). Curiosity and the yen to discover. *Nursing Outlook, 38*, 36–39.

Tripp-Reimer, T. (1985). Expanding four essential concepts in nursing theory: The contribution of anthropology. In J.C. McCloskey & H.K. Grace (Eds.), *Current issues in nursing* (2nd ed., pp. 91–103), Boston: Blackwell.

Collecting Assessment Data: Interviewing and the Nursing History

OBJECTIVES

Upon completion of this chapter, you should be able to:

- Describe the characteristics of the three phases (introduction, working, termination) of an interview.
- Describe the influence of nonverbal behaviors on the interview.
- Differentiate between successful and inhibiting interviewing techniques, giving examples of each.
- Explain variables that influence the interview process, including the environment and the client's age, language, literacy, and health.
- Explain the purposes of the nursing history interview.
- Differentiate between a nursing history and a medical history.
- Describe the components of a comprehensive nursing history.
- Obtain a complete nursing history, using the format provided in this book.

Nursing involves interaction between people. Therefore, a nurse needs skill in communication to complete the steps of the nursing process, i.e., assessment, analysis, planning, implementation, and evaluation. The interview is a principal tool for obtaining and validating the assessment. Although a nurse can collect basic physical data by inspection, palpation, percussion, and auscultation, a client's own description is needed to complete these findings. Furthermore, a nurse obtains psychological, social, cultural, and spiritual data almost entirely by interviewing or observing behavior. An organized framework for gathering this significant information is the nursing history.

Efficiency in obtaining a thorough and useful nursing history is acquired through practice and by using interviewing skills that foster a relationship in which thoughts, feelings, and experiences can be shared. The nurse's communication skills are central to creating such an environment.

This chapter discusses the definition, types, and purposes of the interview and differentiates the assessment interview from a therapeutic interview. The process and several communication techniques are described, as are variables that influence the interview. Also included are types of nursing histories as well as guidelines for structuring the history-taking interview.

THE ASSESSMENT INTERVIEW

In our society, the word *interview* frequently connotes two people communicating, with the primary connecting force being the agenda of the interviewer. Telephone interviews and sidewalk opinion polls are examples of such interviews. The focus is on the interviewer as the owner and director of the interview and on successfully gathering responses to questions. The interviewee's role is primarily passive, simply answering questions. The focus of such interviews is the factual aspect of messages exchanged by the two individuals. The latent, implicit messages and how the interview unfolds is of little, if any, significance.

Within the context of the nurse–client relationship, the word *interview* has a broader, more complex, and perhaps more significant meaning. Any nurse–client interview is a goal-oriented, purposeful interaction between nurse and client in which the client is always the focus. There is shared participation and mutual ownership, regardless of the specific goal or purpose of the interview. The nurse actively participates and observes. The key to the nurse's participation is knowledge and skillful, helpful communication. The nurse's role as observer requires developing and using a keen sense of focus on the client's latent messages and on the process: the client's and nurse's reactions to what is occurring between them. The latter assists significantly in making valid interpretations of assessment data and in building a trusting, open, nurse–client relationship.

Interviews may be formal or informal. Formal interviews generally are structured—a predetermined guide or interview schedule delineates the kinds of information to be gathered or given. For example, the initial interview is formal because the nursing history format serves as a guide or tool. A particular challenge for the nurse during this interview is to not lose sight of the interpersonal aspect. A monotonous, investigative approach to interviewing may end with words written in all the blanks of the nursing history form, with the nurse missing a critical opportunity to initiate a meaningful relationship that will benefit the client.

Another example of a formal interview is one conducted for the purpose of gathering data for research. The structure for this interview may be very rigid; however, the data collector always must be responsive to the client as a person and not as an object to be used simply for achieving the purposes of the study.

Informal interviews are not prestructured but they are goal-oriented. Most of the interactions between nurse and client are informal interviews: The contact is not structured but emerges spontaneously and centers on the client's needs.

Whether the interview is formal or informal, nurse–client interviews can be further classified according to their primary purpose—assessment or treatment.

Assessment interviews help the nurse learn what care the client needs and how best to deliver it. During assessment interviews significant attention is given to appraising the client's responses to actual or potential health problems. Assessment interviews are the foundation for diagnosing and planning nursing care that addresses the client's unique responses to the human experience.

Treatment-centered, or therapeutic, interviews relate primarily to the implementation phase of the nursing process. The therapeutic interview occurs when the nurse actively assists, supports, or guides the client in coping with an actual or potential health problem. Thus, nurses teach or counsel during treatment interviews.

Principles that underpin nurse–client interviews are the same for all interviews. Aside from knowing and using these principles as guides, the nurse also must be very clear about the purpose of the interview. The nurse's clarity of purpose should in turn help make the purpose of the interview clear to the client.

In general, an interview has one of the following purposes: (1) *to gain information,* (2) *to give information,* or (3) *to motivate.* Gaining information is the most common reason for the assessment interview, whether in the initial assessment or during ongoing care. Giving information is associated primarily with treatment interviews. For example, teaching (e.g., about medication or discharge instructions) focuses on providing information to the client or sometimes to significant others for achieving established goals. Interviews in which motivation is the central purpose focus on changing behavior and thus are therapeutic in nature. Assisting a client to adhere to a treatment regimen or introducing a special diet or an exercise program are examples of motivating interviews.

THE INTERVIEW PROCESS

An interview can be divided into three phases: introduction, working, and termination. Although each is described separately here, it is important to remember that they constitute a process, with each phase contributing to and dependent upon the others. All three phases occur in virtually every interview, though the length of each may vary, and each phase may not be a discrete entity. An interview is a dynamic process; hence, intertwining of phases is characteristic.

Introduction Phase

The introduction phase is one of negotiation and data collection. During an initial interview, nurse and client are getting to know each other, introducing themselves and establishing rapport. The nurse obtains identifying data such as name, age, and address, and client and nurse try to find out about each other. The interaction may seem like aimless social chit-chat, but this period is important both in an initial interview and later. Frequently, the chit-chat serves as an ice-breaker and can provide the astute nurse with an entree to more meaningful communication with the client. It provides a basis for the rapport necessary to achieve goals.

The nurse's self-introduction is important because it legitimizes the interview. The nurse's name, role, and reason for being there all should be stated clearly. It is not reasonable to expect clients to share information, particularly of a personal nature, with someone whose name or role is un-

clear and whose purpose is unknown. Describing and discussing the purpose of an informal interview may be particularly challenging for the novice. However, open discussion of purpose is critical to establishing the interview as a professional one rather than a social one.

The introductory phase also establishes the interview contract, an implicit agreement between nurse and client that establishes rules and norms for the relationship. The contract should include the length of this and subsequent interviews, the time and place of subsequent interviews, confidentiality, purpose, role expectations, and cost to the client, if appropriate. The contract may be negotiated for one interview or for a series of interviews. The contract negotiated with a client in a walk-in clinic may be for one interview, whereas the contract established with a client in a hospital probably will be for the duration of the client's stay.

Contracts must be negotiated carefully. If the rules and purposes are unclear to the client, the nurse, or both, the interview or relationship is unlikely to progress as anticipated.

Working Phase

During the working phase, nurse and client move toward fulfilling the stated purpose of the interview. For example, in an initial interview, the portion concerned with obtaining information related to history and assessment constitutes the work. If rapport and trust were established during the introduction, the work will go well.

Lack of rapport or feelings of discomfort will diminish both quality and quantity of information obtained. A client who does not clearly understand the purposes of the interview, or who feels uncomfortable, may be less willing to disclose and listen. The information obtained may be sparse or even inaccurate.

During the working phase, the nurse is responsible for maintaining rapport and trust and for keeping the interview goal-oriented. Listening to the client, responding to manifest and latent messages, giving the client undivided and uninterrupted attention, and treating the client with respect help maintain rapport. Respect involves recognizing that the client is an individual with inherent needs and rights. Using a title and the client's surname, unless another preference is indicated, and recognizing the client's need for privacy are but two ways that respect can be communicated.

Progress toward the goal of the interview is maintained by a number of techniques, such as refocusing the client with phrases like "you mentioned earlier" when the interview has drifted from the topic at hand. Another technique is to move at the client's pace. Begin where the client is by first discussing topics the client explicitly or implicitly introduces. It is not helpful to push the client to discuss topics that the nurse considers pertinent before the client gives cues of readiness.

Beginning the working phase of the history-taking interview with an open question—"What brings you into the hospital today?"—will elicit information that the client, at least theoretically, will be willing to discuss. This information then may be used to move toward the stated goal.

Termination Phase

The termination phase is the closure of the interview. Termination should be planned and discussed when the contract is established. Some interviews may last an hour or more, whereas others last only a few minutes. Whatever duration was decided on, the client should be reminded when the end of the interview is approaching. Statements such as "Our time will be up in five more minutes," "I will be leaving in a few minutes," or "I think that what you've told me gives me a fairly good picture of how you're feeling" signal termination.

During termination it is frequently useful to summarize what has occurred. Summarizing helps the client to reflect and share the salient features of the interview from his or her perspective and allows the nurse to do the same. This activity can be very useful for adjusting the client's plan of care. The termination phase also should include specific plans for future interviews or information about where the client can obtain assistance if no further visits are planned.

APPROACHES TO INTERVIEWING

The two major approaches to interviewing are direct and indirect. The direct interview is structured, employing specific questions posed by the interviewer. The interview has a predetermined goal and purpose. This type of structure requires that the interviewer be creative and imaginative to accomplish the agenda while not ignoring the client's right to help set the pace. Direct interviews are useful both for giving and gathering information.

The indirect interview has less structure. The client and nurse share a mutually agreed upon purpose, which is client-centered. The pace is set by the client. Interviews intended to motivate (e.g., counseling or problem-solving) frequently use the indirect approach.

Sometimes a highly structured interview schedule has to be strictly maintained, as when gathering data for research. But using the direct approach exclusively produces a disjointed question–answer session that may or may not elicit the information needed. Conversely, using only the indirect approach may consume great quantities of time without eliciting the desired information.

When the indirect approach is used, the nurse should distinguish between "indirect" and "nonresponsive." It is easy to confuse the two, because the indirect approach requires less verbalization by the interviewer, who says "Yes," "Um," "Go on," "You feel angry?" or nods instead of asking formal questions. But in being indirect the nurse is helping clients share what concerns them most. This requires considerable effort and responsiveness.

Usually, combining direct and indirect approaches during the interview leads to optimal results. The indirect approach might be used to elicit the client's perception of problems, whereas the direct approach is used to obtain facts and to keep the interview focused on the desired goal. For example, in the history-taking interview, an open question like "Can you tell me what brings you into the clinic today?" elicits the client's point of view. It encourages the client to express the problem at his or her level of readiness. Once the problems are voiced, they may be explored by direct questions, e.g., "Do you only become nauseated after you eat?" "Has this ever been a problem for you before?"

NONVERBAL CONSIDERATIONS IN THE INTERVIEW PROCESS

Communication involves complex verbal and nonverbal cues that influence each other. Discussing the two separately therefore is artificial in terms of what really happens, but it is useful for purposes of discussion.

Communication involves much more than the spoken word. Tone of voice, body movements, facial expression, and use of personal space all influence meaning. When a wife assures her husband through tightly pursed lips that "everything is just fine," or when a nurse tells the client "everything is just fine" but avoids eye contact, both are delivering messages in which the nonverbal message contradicts the words being spoken. When such a contrast occurs, the person receiving the communication tends to respond to the nonverbal message. Thus, nonverbal communication can strongly influence the outcome of an interview.

Defining interviewing as a goal-oriented interaction between nurse and client implies awareness of what is being communicated. Yet nonverbal communication may be at least partially beyond the range of awareness, and this lack of awareness can result in misunderstanding and misinterpretation. The nurse who is aware of his or her nonverbal behaviors is taking the first step toward consistent verbal and nonverbal communication.

Besides the issue of consistent messages, other aspects of nonverbal communication are especially pertinent to interviewing. Birdwhistle (1979) estimates that only 35 percent of the meaning of social interchanges is conveyed verbally. If a client who is experiencing severe chest pain demonstrates body, facial, and vocal expressions that are different than what is expected for the pain described, others may minimize or dismiss the pain. The client's words mean less to the observer than grimacing, clutching the chest or arm, bending over, or groaning.

The context of behavior determines its social meaning. Nonverbal behavior should be interpreted in terms of the culture in which it was learned. A nurse who is accustomed to dealing with the nuclear family may be very unnerved when a client from a different culture constantly is surrounded by many generations of distant family members. Similarly, a nurse raised in the Anglo-Saxon tradition of the "stiff upper lip" may be startled if news of a patient's death is received by the family with wailing, shrieking, keening, or tearing of hair. Yet to omit such overt expressions in some cultures connotes lack of respect for the dead.

Nonverbal messages are generally clear and truthful; they convey feelings and emotions more accurately than do words. The nonverbal message may be clearly apparent despite conscious effort to control it. For example, when a client who had recently noticed a lump in her breast was admitted to the hospital for a biopsy, she smiled frequently and kept repeating, "I'm not worried. They're almost positive it's a cyst." She talked rapidly, tapped her foot, and kept twisting a ring on her finger. The nurse who took the history noted that the client's actions belied her words.

Nonverbal behaviors frequently communicate more efficiently than verbal statements. Movements and gestures are shortcuts. The face of a parent whose child has just died expresses in a few seconds what might not be said in an hour's conversation.

Specific components of nonverbal behavior include body motion, vocal cues, touch, body appearance, and use of silence.

Body Motion

Body motion, or kinesic behavior, is culturally determined and includes gestures, eye behavior, facial expressions, body movement, and posture. Maintaining eye contact helps communicate attentiveness and trustworthiness. The client who looks away when a specific topic is mentioned may be communicating discomfort in discussing that subject. Eye contact also may communicate anger or aggression. The expression "if looks could kill" conjures up the image of one person staring angrily at another. Whether staring communicates anger or not, it makes interview participants uncomfortable and should be avoided. Eye contact should be relaxed. Smiling—if it is genuine—is a reinforcing response. Forced smiling is usually obvious and conveys a message of its own. Congruence between the client's facial expressions and words should be noted, keeping in mind that the cultural meanings attached to smiling and eye contact are not universal. For example, in some cultural groups the smile may denote anger, while in others direct eye contact may connote lack of respect. Among some Asian groups, prolonged eye contact is considered impolite. Thus, what appears "shifty-eyed" to an American may be intended by the Asian client as a courtesy.

A relaxed posture provides information about the client's comfort level. A rigid posture in the interview usually indicates anxiety. The shaking of a crossed leg also can indicate anxiety, as can frequent hand motions. Shifts in body position or posture should be observed throughout. In general, relaxed, natural movement toward the interviewer indicates feelings of warmth and trust, whereas movement away from the interviewer communicates discomfort or a desire to escape the interaction. It is also important to note at what point in the interview such behaviors occur. A client who suddenly turns partially away when plans for discharge are mentioned may be communicating a lack of readiness.

Vocal Cues

Vocal characteristics add meaning to the spoken word. A flat voice with little or no inflection may suggest depression or some other affective disturbance. A rise in volume frequently indicates anger or aggressiveness; forced or grunting speech indicates pain. Familiar examples are anxious persons whose speech is slow and filled with pauses or who talk very rapidly. In either case the rate of speech may make understanding difficult.

Appearance

Appearance also communicates. At first meeting, people notice such factors as apparent age, sex, general body structure, eye and hair color, race, and manner of dress, all of which influence the impressions one person forms about another. Although nurses are taught to observe and describe clients in objective terms, cultural bias may be so ingrained that a nurse is not even aware that judgments about a client are being made. Yet the nurse's approach, demeanor, and manners are based on this unconscious judgment. A poorly dressed client may encounter quite a different attitude than a client who is dressed in well-tailored and obviously expensive clothes. Keep in mind that clients, too, have cultural biases and are applying them to the nurse.

Silence

Silence can be a useful interview tool. As with any human behavior, silence has many meanings. Silence may communicate thoughtfulness, comfort, embarrassment, anger, sadness, or anxiety. Silence that occurs because the interviewer is unsure how to proceed can produce considerable anxiety. In such cases it may be helpful to remain silent for a few moments and then summarize what has occurred up to that point. This strategy gives the interviewer time to reflect upon what has happened and to see the situation more clearly. Summarizing also affords the client an opportunity to validate or clarify the interviewer's perceptions.

Sometimes silence or the threat of silence makes an interviewer talk more, shooting numerous, rapid-fire, direct questions. Dealing with silence in this manner creates tremendous obstacles. Additionally, the client may feel bombarded and may find that there is not enough time to think about what has been asked and to formulate responses.

Listening to another person requires being silent. If the interviewer does most of the talking, establishing or maintaining a nurse–client relationship based upon the client's needs is not likely to occur.

Touch

Touch is the first form of communication we experience and remains one of the most powerful. When words fail, touch often communicates. An arm around the shoulder of someone who is grieving communicates deeper and more personal feelings than saying "I'm sorry."

As health-care professionals, nurses have permission to touch, even though touching among strangers generally is unacceptable in our culture. In the nursing situation, touch is considered legitimate.

Touch that occurs while the nurse provides direct personal care is often called "procedural touch" to distinguish it from more spontaneous touching not related to direct physical care. Bathing, giving an injection, massaging the back, palpating the abdomen, or checking reflexes provide opportunities for assessment but also convey the nurse's feelings toward the client. One client said, "I don't like to have Ms. X give me a bath. She is so rough." Ms. X's touch told the client that she was uncaring and hurried.

Nonprocedural touch provides additional opportunities for communicating acceptance, caring, and hope. A hand on the arm of a client who is anxious can offer support (Figure 2-1). The nurse must be sensitive to the client's readiness and willingness to be touched. Clients who are uncomfortable with touching and being touched may resent it, or in some cases fall apart. Additionally, the nurse must be clear on the intended purpose of touch. For example, using touch prematurely may block the client's further expression of feelings. Premature use of touch often occurs out of the nurse's own sense of anxiety and helplessness.

People vary widely in their use and acceptance of touch. Because use of touch is culturally regulated, the effects of early learning may be difficult

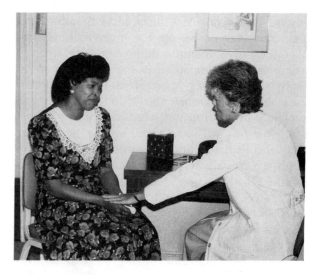

FIGURE 2-1. The appropriate use of touch can be a powerful and effective way to communicate with a client during an interview.

to change. However, the nurse who knows the potentially positive outcomes of touching may be motivated to use it often. Used with caring and discrimination, touch can greatly enhance the interview process.

Specific use of touch in the interview will vary according to context. What is acceptable for one client may not be acceptable for another. The handshake, however, is generally appropriate in the initial interview. This initiates human contact with the client and also provides assessment data related to skin temperature, anxiety, and muscle strength.

SUCCESSFUL INTERVIEWING TECHNIQUES

Successful interviewing depends, in part, upon the expertise of the interviewer in using several specific techniques. Principles, rules, and descriptions of techniques can be learned by reading, but integrating the techniques and applying them in real interview situations takes supervised experience. What follows is an overview of interview techniques that are especially applicable to assessment.

Encouraging Verbalization

During the interview, the nurse helps the client discuss concerns in a manner that provides a basis for planning and implementing optimum care. Both verbal and nonverbal techniques help accomplish this goal.

Questioning

Questioning is a valuable tool that is frequently misused or overused. Of course, questions are important, but using too many questions—particularly direct ones—can defeat the purpose of most interviews. In one study, interviewers perceived as being the least empathetic asked the most questions (Statler, 1977). Nurses who are not empathetic frequently perceived by clients as asking irrelevant or poorly conceived questions.

Questions are useful for obtaining information ("How long have you been bothered by indigestion?"), clarifying ("Are you saying that the indigestion has become almost constant?"), and identifying the client's perceptions and feelings ("Can you describe how the constant indigestion has affected you?"). Questions may be classified as open or closed.

Open questions elicit perceptions and feelings and encourage clients to express what they see as important and are comfortable in discussing. Examples of open questions are: "What have you

tried for your indigestion?" or "How does the pain you're having now differ from the pain you described earlier?"

Open questions help establish rapport by indicating interest and a willingness to listen, but responses to open questions may be too long and not relevant to the topic under discussion. If time is very limited, extensive use of open questions may severely reduce the amount of information collected.

Closed questions are used to elicit facts. Closed questions are structured to elicit one- or two-word responses, frequently "yes" or "no." Examples of closed questions are: "How old are you?" and "Have you ever been hospitalized before?"

Inexperienced or anxious interviewers tend to use closed questions to keep the interview sequence predictable and thus increase their own comfort. Information obtained this way may be limited; many topics are covered but the data are superficial. This is not to suggest that the nurse avoid the use of closed questions. A combination of open and closed questions is likely to yield the best information.

When obtaining assessment data, it is frequently useful to begin with broad, open questions and to use closed or direct questions to narrow the line of inquiry. For example:

NURSE: What happens when you begin to have pain?

CLIENT: I begin to hurt real bad. The pain just gets worse and worse. Then I start to sweat and pretty soon I feel nauseated.

NURSE: Can you describe where the pain starts and how it progresses?

CLIENT: It starts here [points] right under my ribs on the right side, then it feels like it shoots through to my back and up between my shoulder blades.

NURSE: Does it always progress in that order?

In this instance, the nurse began the interaction with two open questions. A closed question then was used to obtain specific information about the progression of the client's pain.

Encouraging the Client to Continue

There are several verbal and nonverbal behaviors that may encourage a client to continue talking. Nodding the head, sounds such as "Um-hm," short statements such as "Go on" or "And then?" and repeating several of the client's own words, such as "You're feeling depressed," indicate that the client should continue. Like questions, they are extremely useful but can easily be overused. If used too frequently, these behaviors may actually indicate inattention.

Reflection

By using reflection (stating one's perception of the client's message in different words), the nurse provides feedback that allows the client to assess the nurse's view. Perceptions then can be validated or corrected, often leading to greater clarification.

Reflection can be stated in terms of content or feelings. Reflection of content involves restating the cognitive portion of the message to clarify what the client has said, or to assist the client in approaching the problem from a different viewpoint. For example:

CLIENT: Sometimes the pain starts in my back and sometimes in my stomach. It may move from one place to another. It just depends.

NURSE: There's no consistent pattern to the pain.

Feeling is reflected by stating the feelings implied by the client. Reflection of feeling relies heavily on such nonverbal aspects of communication as facial expression, eye contact, body movement and position, tone of voice, and rate of speech. For example:

CLIENT: Jill isn't walking yet. At 13 months all of my other children had been walking for at least a month. [Looks at hands.]

NURSE: You're afraid that there might be something wrong with her.

Sometimes either content or feeling can be reflected, and a choice must be made:

CLIENT: I fed Jimmy an egg yesterday. Then about an hour later he began having all of this vomiting and diarrhea. And it hasn't stopped. He wasn't supposed to have eggs until next week.

NURSE: (Content) You think maybe there's a connection between your giving him the egg and the diarrhea.

(Feeling) You feel concerned about giving Jimmy eggs before he was supposed to have them.

Jessop (1979) suggests several factors to consider when deciding whether to reflect feelings or content.

Phase of the nurse–client relationship. Most people consider discussing feelings to be more intimate and revealing than discussing content. If reflection of feeling is used too early in the relationship, the client may become uncomfortable and may exaggerate normal defenses to the point where communication is inhibited.

Client level of readiness. Because of our cultural attitudes toward feelings, clients need extra time to establish a relationship with the nurse before discussing feelings than before discussing content.

Goals of the interview. Goals related to specific tasks, such as teaching a client self-care skills, usually require more emphasis on paraphrasing (reflection of content). When discussing implications of and adjustments to chronic illness, the nurse probably will need to use more reflection of feeling.

Appropriateness of the techniques. Remember that communication with a client should be goal-oriented and techniques should be chosen to move the interview along. Overusing reflection or paraphrasing or using one technique to the exclusion of others is likely to be detrimental.

Active Listening

Too often listening is thought of as a passive activity. Lewis (1973) differentiates between listening and hearing:

> "To hear" means specifically to become aware of sounds. It is essentially a passive thing, occurring automatically when sound waves stimulate the auditory nerves. "To listen" requires one to make an active, conscious effort to attend closely to the auditory stimuli. The distinction between the two words lies in the "conscious effort" required for listening, which makes it more active than just hearing a sound. (p. 37)

Active listening, then, is not automatic; it requires paying close attention. Active listening conveys respect and caring; it involves attention to meaning, not simply to words. When clients say, "You're not listening" or "If someone would only listen," they are probably referring to the meaning.

Too often, interviewers emphasize talking instead of listening. Most interviewers could improve their results by listening more and talking less. Listening allows the nurse to understand what is happening, to make sense of the information being presented by the client—to concentrate on the *meaning* of the interaction. Active listening is not easy. It requires patience, concentration, and an ability to view the interaction objectively.

Besides listening for content and feelings, the nurse should listen for set or pattern. Whereas listening for content or feelings involves the here and now, listening for a set involves being alert for a predisposition to respond in a certain way over time. Such phrases as "I've always felt that way," "I never seem to win," "Nobody can keep me down" are cues to the presence of a "set." Such cues may indicate how the client will respond to a particular situation, such as illness or hospitalization.

Responses that convey active listening help to develop the rapport and empathy necessary for meaningful interaction. These essential ingredients in the interview process tend to be somewhat elusive. Empathy has been described as being able to enter into another person's life and accurately perceive feelings and their meanings. Empathy also may be described as a process that involves both perceiving feelings and their meanings and communicating what is being experienced to the other individual. Hence, an empathic person can experience a situation from another's frame of reference and also can communicate that perception to the other individual.

Rapport relates to feelings of cooperation and harmony between nurse and client. Since empathy promotes feelings of cooperation and harmony, rapport can be said to develop as a result of empathy.

Strategies for developing empathy involve both verbal and nonverbal behaviors, although specific behaviors are difficult to identify. Active listening seems to be an important component of empathically perceiving meaning. By using reflection of content and reflection of feelings, the interviewer conveys his or her perception of the interaction to the client and affords the client the opportunity to validate or correct the perception. Statements such as "You're very angry about having to be readmitted to the hospital," "It sounds as if things are pretty overwhelming right now," "The decision about whether to have surgery has been a difficult one" enhance communication, whereas telling the client, "I understand," frequently shuts off communication. Understanding occurs within each individual and can truly be felt only by that individual.

INHIBITING INTERVIEWING TECHNIQUES

Just as there are techniques that promote communication there are also techniques that inhibit the interview process. Some have been described previously; others are described below.

Leading or Biased Questions

Leading questions suggest that one answer is more desirable than another. Asking, "You don't have any heart disease in your family, do you?" in-

creases the probability of a "no" because the question indicates that "no" is the response expected. Clients may be intimidated by leading questions, or they may respond as they believe they "should" in an effort to please the interviewer. In either case, the information obtained may be inaccurate.

The nurse should avoid asking more than one question at a time. For example, "Are you married or not?" is confusing because it is difficult to know for which question an answer is expected.

Giving Advice or Opinions

The questions "What would you do?" and "What do you think?" are familiar to most nurses. Clients who ask these questions may be seeking more information on which to base their own decisions. But they also may be asking the nurse to make the decision for them. The nurse who tries to help by providing the information directly in the form of advice or an opinion may produce negative consequences. "I would have the surgery" may be translated by the client into "You should have the surgery." The client who does not follow the advice may feel inadequate or guilty. Moreover, telling the client what you would do or what should be done relieves the client of both responsibility and accountability for the decision. The client may perceive the nurse as making the decision and then blame the nurse for negative outcomes.

A more useful technique in helping the client reach a decision is to reflect what has been heard, then redirect the discussion to the client's frame of reference. This technique not only provides the opportunity to clarify and validate what has been heard but also offers insight into areas in which the client may lack information.

CLIENT (6 months pregnant): I've heard a lot about breast-feeding recently but my mother bottle-fed all her children, and we all did well. What would you do?

NURSE: You're unsure about whether to breast-feed or bottle-feed your baby. Let's look at the pros and cons of both methods.

The nurse reflected the client's perceived feelings back to her and then redirected the interaction to the client's frame of reference by suggesting that the nurse and client together examine the pros and cons of breast- and bottle-feeding. During the ensuing discussion, the nurse can determine the client's level of knowledge and provide accurate information as needed. The actual decision, however, is both the right and responsibility of the client.

Defense-Producing Techniques

Defense-producing techniques make the client feel put down or angry. Perhaps the most familiar example is the use of why: "Why did you do that?" "Why do you feel that way?" Questions phrased this way seem to ask for the client's underlying motivation for a particular behavior or feeling, and they are difficult to answer. The client may not know the underlying motives or may not wish to discuss them. Indeed, underlying motivation often is not what the nurse really wants to know. In any event, asking why tends to make the client feel threatened and defensive. Once this occurs, the client's energy probably will become focused on justifying or defending the behavior or feelings in question. The information the nurse seeks will not be obtained.

Questions that begin with "How . . . ?" "Can you describe . . . ?" or "What . . . ?" generally encourage an answer. For example, instead of asking, "Why did you stop taking your medication?", try asking, "What happened that made you decide to stop taking your medicine?" "What kept you from coming to the clinic sooner?" is less threatening than "Why didn't you come to the clinic sooner?" "Can you describe how you feel useless?" is more likely to yield a useful response than "Why do you feel that way?"

Statements such as "I understand what you're going through" or "I know just how you feel" also may make the client feel put down or angry. As previously discussed, telling a person "I know just how you feel" is, in fact, not true. Clients often react negatively to such statements, although they may not say so. Responses such as "You can't possibly understand" or "You couldn't possibly know how I feel" should not be unexpected. The client who feels put down becomes defensive, and further communication is inhibited. It is better to employ skillful use of reflection to communicate what you perceive to be the client's thoughts and feelings without introducing your own personal experience or cultural bias.

Providing Unrealistic Reassurance

Providing reassurance is frequently misinterpreted to mean, "You have nothing to worry about, everything is going to be all right." There are situations, however, in which everything is *not* going to be all right. Using unrealistic statements to soothe a troubled client is likely to inhibit the development of a therapeutic relationship.

Realistic reassurance involves letting the client know the nurse has heard what has been said, then intervening with appropriate words and actions. For example, the nurse observes that a client is fearful of getting out of bed for the first time after surgery. An appropriate reassuring response might be:

Nurse: You're afraid that you might get lightheaded and fall when you get out of bed. Ms. J. and I will be here to help you as you get up. We'll help you back into bed right away if you feel dizzy.

The nurse acknowledges the client's fear and provides the client with the assistance necessary to feel more secure in getting out of bed.

VARIABLES THAT INFLUENCE THE INTERVIEW PROCESS

In addition to the fact that the nurse's communication skills are a significant variable in the conduct of any interview, other variables also influence the nurse–client interview. Six major variables influence the interview's content, process, and structure—environment, culture, use of personal space, age, language and literacy, and the client's health.

Environment

The setting for the interview can have a profound impact on both the process and the content of any interview. Nurse–client interviews are conducted in many different settings (e.g., a semi-private hospital room, a crowded and busy out-patient clinic, or a client's home). Each setting brings with it a unique set of challenges for the nurse and client during the interview.

Creating a perfect interview environment rarely is possible. However, it is an important part of the nurse's responsibility to see that the environment is as conducive and comfortable as possible. Many times this requires that the nurse engage in some preparatory work prior to the actual interview. For example, a crowded clinic may not have space designated for nurse–client interviews and the nurse may have to search for space to even meet with the client. The search should occur prior to inviting the client to join the nurse for an interview. If the nurse does not plan, clients are likely to immediately perceive the nurse as disorganized, hurried, and not truly interested in their welfare.

Indeed, privacy is a critical factor for the conduct of any nurse–client interview. However, circumstances may not allow for the nurse and client to be alone in a quiet room. In such cases, every effort should be made to assure as much privacy as possible so that confidential information is not overheard and so the client feels comfortable disclosing information. Drawing the curtains around the client's bed or placing a sign on the door that states "Interview in process: Please do not disturb" can provide a significant sense of privacy and security and minimize distractions and noise.

The physical distance between the nurse and client and the seating arrangement are critical environmental variables. The concept of distance and its relationship to the interview was explored earlier in this chapter. If the nurse and client are seated in chairs during the interview, the chairs should be placed at right angles. This arrangement facilitates eye contact and physical comfort for each person. Conducting the interview if the client is in bed presents an additional consideration for the nurse. It is advisable for the nurse to be at eye level with the client. Hence, sitting in a chair at a 45-degree angle to the bed is useful. If the nurse stands during the interview, it is apt to communicate that the nurse has a superior position and is in charge of the interview and that the client is expected to function in a submissive role.

Other significant environmental factors relate primarily to esthetics (American Association of Colleges of Nursing [AACN], 1986). For example, proper lighting and a comfortable temperature are two factors over which the nurse generally has some control. Additionally, it is crucial for the nurse's manner to communicate genuine interest and caring. Transmission of caring and interest can have a tremendous impact on helping the client to become psychologically comfortable with sharing.

Indeed, the environment in which the interview takes place can foster or detract significantly from its meaning and value. Addressing the environment as a critical variable requires that the nurse possess creativity, imagination, sensitivity, and appreciation (AACN, 1986).

Culture

The rules about interacting with others that people learn are culturally determined. How an American shares thoughts and feelings, maintains closeness and separateness, or responds to illness differs from the customs of a person from, for example, an Arab nation or China. Although the idea of cultural differences seems obvious and rational when read from the printed page, the same differences are apt to be approached much less rationally in real life. Culture permeates the entire being. Human beings are immersed in it and tend to judge all others' behavior in terms of their own beliefs and values. This ethnocentric approach is not conducive to establishing the rapport necessary for accurate assessment. Changing response patterns may not be an easy task, however.

None of this is meant to imply that nurses should not try to become aware of their own cultural biases as well as those of others. The point is that the nurse's cultural heritage is as deeply ingrained as is the cultural heritage of each client with whom the nurse interacts. Becoming aware of personal values, the values of other cultural groups, and the differences between the two is an important step in providing sensitive, multidimensional nursing care (see chap. 8).

Cultural differences form the basis of many of the barriers to effective nurse–client discussions, especially the interview process. In fact, the crux of miscommunication within the nurse–client relationship oftentimes is related to culturally disparate beliefs and values. Clinton (1986) asserts that nurses must broaden their awareness of the impact of disparate cultures on the interview process, otherwise "professional manipulation" is apt to occur. In such an event, the nurse may attempt to convince clients that their views are wrong or are not acceptable. As people, nurses cannot help but view the client through the cultural lenses of their own heritages; however, as professionals, they must broaden their perspectives and strive diligently to understand the client's cultural perspective.

Several factors that have a high cultural component were discussed in the section related to nonverbal communication. Additionally, the cultural use of space and culturally determined responses to illness are specifically related to the interview process.

Use of Personal Space

The rules that relate to how we use space and distance to maintain closeness and separateness vary from culture to culture. Hall (1966) uses the term *proxemics* to describe this use and enumerates four distances employed by middle-class Americans: intimate, personal, social, and public. Intimate and personal distances are frequently used in the health-care situation.

Intimate Distance

Intimate distance involves the areas closest to the body and extends about one-and-one-half feet. All close physical activity, including sexual activity, is carried out in this zone. The senses of touch, sight, hearing, and smell are highly involved. Body sounds such as breathing can be heard, and there is an intense awareness of body odors. Squinting and distortion may occur as the individual tries to focus on an object within the visual field.

Many nursing activities, like bathing, back rubs, and physical assessments, are carried out at this distance. Americans tend to feel uncomfortable if anyone other than an intimate intrudes into this space. Although exceptions are granted to health-care providers, feelings of discomfort and uneasiness may persist. Explaining procedures and the reasons for their use and establishing rapport with the client are an important prelude to entering the intimate body space. Brief yes-or-no questions are appropriate during the assessment examination or while carrying out other close-range activities. For lengthy discussion, distance should be increased to allow eye contact and to avoid the visual distortion that occurs at close range.

Personal Distance

The limits of personal distance are one-and-one half to four feet. At one-and-one half feet, touching is easy. Reassuring gestures, such as putting a hand on the shoulder, can be accomplished from this distance. The ability to touch decreases as one approaches the periphery. Vocalization varies from speaking quietly at the close range to soft, normal tones as one approaches four feet.

Most nursing interviews take place within the zone of personal distance (Figure 2-2). The client is close enough so that nonverbal behaviors can be observed closely. Voice tones can be kept low enough to maintain some semblance of privacy,

even in a multibed unit. Trust and closeness can be established at this distance.

Social Distance

Social distance encompasses the area from four to twelve feet. The interactions between people are less personal, becoming more formal as the distance increases. Taking a nursing history while separated from the client by a large desk may shift the interaction from personal to social distance, thus creating a barrier to the development of trust and rapport (Figure 2-3). Nonverbal messages of caring and involvement are conveyed less easily.

To be heard, vocal tones need to be in the normal range, making confidentiality difficult if others are in the room. Such details as pupil responses are difficult to see, but the entire body can be observed easily. This is not possible at intimate or personal distance.

Public Distance

Public distance includes distances beyond twelve feet. Close interaction with another person does not occur at public distance; rather, interaction becomes much more formal, as in a public-speaking situation.

The foregoing discussion relates primarily to the way middle-class people in the United States use space and distance. The distances described and the way space is used may be different for other cultures. For example, many U.S. cultural groups require more distance for comfort than Latin Americans do. Thus, during an interview a

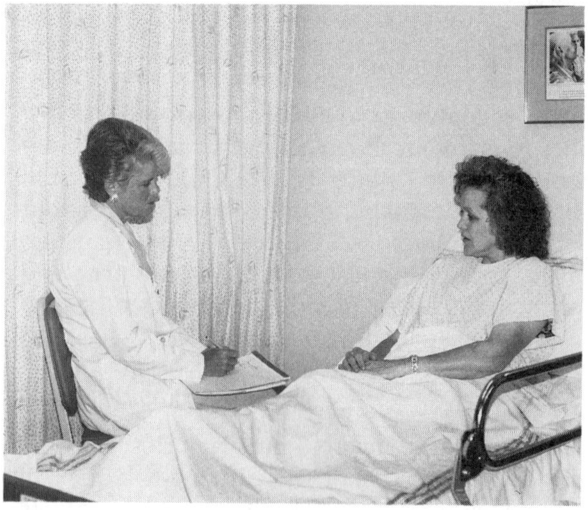

FIGURE 2-2. Most nurse–client interviews take place within the zone of personal distance (1½ to 4 feet between nurse and client).

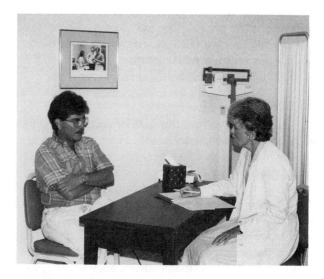

FIGURE 2-3. Taking a nursing history while separated from the client can shift personal distance to social distance and create a barrier to trust and rapport.

Latin American client may inadvertently invade the intimate space of a nurse from the United States. The nurse, feeling uncomfortable, is likely to move away. Similarly, the client is likely to withdraw if the nurse exceeds the client's culturally defined inner limit of conversational distance. In either instance, the effort to maintain a culturally appropriate distance is apt to be perceived as rejecting and decreases the effectiveness of the interview.

Activities carried out in intimate and personal space that involve physical closeness or touch vary among cultures. A nurse raised in a culture in which spontaneous touch is the norm may find that unless the client was raised in a similar environment, use of nonprocedural touch, such as putting an arm around the client's shoulder or sitting in close proximity, produces anxiety in the client and outcomes other than those planned.

The point to keep in mind is that the cultural orientation of *both* nurse and client affects and in some instances interferes with development of rapport or a positive interview environment.

Age

Age, or developmental level, is a variable that influences both the process and the structure of the interview. Although the principles remain constant, they differ in several aspects for children and older people.

Interviewing the Child and Parent

Though the amount of the child's verbal participation in the interview varies tremendously with age, even the youngest child should be included. Infants and young children require someone, usually the parent, to provide factual information and to receive health-care teaching in their behalf. However, children themselves can provide a good deal of verbal and nonverbal information.

Because of limited verbal activities, children below the age of seven use nonverbal communication extensively. In addition, regardless of the child's age, it is the nonverbal communication that conveys the most salient messages. The feelings and needs of the child are likely to be expressed behaviorally. Fear of treatments or of being in the hospital may be communicated by such behaviors as acting out or withdrawing. The nurse is encouraged to determine, by observation, or interview with a parent, specific behavioral cues.

Play is one of the major forms of communication for children. Informal observation of a child's play or use of planned games can provide a wealth of assessment data. Simple games such as peek-a-

boo, pat-a-cake, or "this little piggy" are particularly useful in assessing young children. When carried out in a nonthreatening manner, they promote rapport and trust that will allow the nurse to conduct a complete assessment.

Puppets can help older children express feelings and provide information (Figure 2-4). Events such as "going to the hospital" or "being sick" can be described and talked about from the relatively safe vantage point of another person, the puppet. Telling stories about pictures or drawing pictures can be used in the same manner. The nurse often can obtain more valid information about a child's perceptions and responses by observing a child's reenactment of hospital procedures, such as admission or diagnostic testing, than by questioning the child directly.

The child's sensitivity to the nurse's nonverbal behaviors also has implications for the interview. Feelings of anxiety or anger may be readily picked up by the child and responded to as the child has responded to similar feelings in the past. Children are highly sensitive to their environments and may make incorrect interpretations about words, gestures, and voice tone. Their interpretations are influenced by their developmental level and their previous experiences. The nurse should be careful to use words that do not instill fear in the child. For example, explaining to the child that the nurse is going to "check your temperature" instead of "take your temperature" avoids the possibility that the child may interpret that something will be taken

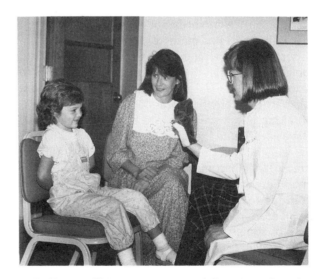

FIGURE 2-4. Using a puppet or doll to interview the child can be a more effective means of getting the youngster to express thoughts and feelings than direct questioning. Direct questions may threaten or confuse young children.

away. It is best to approach the child in a calm, unhurried manner, allowing the child to make the first overture. Broad smiles and other facial gestures should be avoided.

Seating in the interview should be arranged so that face-to-face interaction is possible. To children, an adult, especially one who is towering over them, is a giant. Whenever possible, the nurse should be at the child's eye level.

Verbal interactions with children follow the same principles as interactions with adults. Language should be clear and concise. Vocabulary should be at the child's level of comprehension. Medical terminology should be avoided. An honest explanation of treatments and events is imperative. For small children, the explanation should not be provided too far in advance, as the child may forget or may become increasingly anxious. Explanations that are less than honest will jeopardize any trust that has been built in the relationship. Similarly, if the child is given a choice, the nurse must be prepared to accept the child's decision. If there is no choice, do not ask the child, "Do you want to . . . ?" This is extremely important when trying to enlist the child's cooperation, as in the assessment examination. A positive approach such as, "I'll help you take off your shirt," is more likely to gain the child's cooperation than, "Will you take off your shirt?"

Communication with a child varies according to the child's stage of growth and development. Thinking processes of young children tend to be egocentric and concrete. They view everything from their own frame of reference; the idea of an alternative viewpoint is not even considered. Verbalization contains many references to "me." Consider how frightening the hospital or clinic would be if everything in the environment were related to you personally. The nurse should be careful about abstract or idiomatic expressions; a child's concrete thinking may translate expressions like "the walls have ears" quite literally.

As children grow and as their verbal skills increase, they become more able to participate in the interview themselves. Older children need opportunities to present their views of the situation, apart from the parental figure. This is particularly true of adolescents, who may be unwilling to provide sensitive information or to discuss feelings with a parent present (Figure 2-5). The adolescent needs support and privacy. Listening without interjecting your own values is also important. Avoiding such phrases as "You should . . ." and "You have to . . ." promotes trust in the relationship.

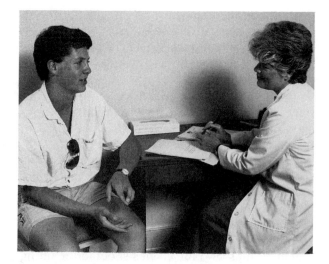

FIGURE 2-5. Adolescents should be given an opportunity to meet privately with the nurse during the history interview.

The communication skills used in any interview with an adult are appropriate for parents. The difference is the parents are present on behalf of the child, not themselves. During the course of the interview, interaction between the child and the parents should be observed. Take notice of who does the talking; is it shared or does the parent always speak for both? Is the child listened to? Are touching behaviors observed? How is unruly behavior handled?

Parents may experience strong feelings of guilt about their child being sick. Repeated questioning by the parents about the cause of the child's illness or statements like "If only I had . . ." or "Maybe I should have . . ." indicate the presence of these feelings. Using biased or leading questions to obtain information will reinforce them. The nurse should use every opportunity to commend parents for appropriate care.

Parental expectations also influence the interview. Satisfaction and compliance are related to how well expectations are met. Attentiveness may decrease dramatically if the parent does not perceive that concerns and expectations are being heard. Manifestations of attention loss include decrease in eye contact, increased body movement, silence, or an increase in such verbalizations as "Yes" and "Uh-hm." It is important that parents and children perceive that the nurse is listening to them and values what they have to say.

Interviewing the Older Client

The physiological and psychological effects of aging may require the nurse to modify the interview.

Hearing loss and a slowing of the ability to process information can be countered by an increase in speech volume (not pitch) and a slight decrease in speech rate (Figure 2-6). The nurse should never shout at the elderly client. In addition to being demeaning, shouting usually results in an increase in pitch, which accentuates the tones most likely to have been lost. Face-to-face interaction makes lip reading possible and may help offset a hearing deficit. For female nurses, bright lipstick may make lip movement more apparent.

The client with a severe hearing deficit is apt to have trouble understanding the nurse's words and may react with irritation and frustration. Enunciating clearly and using simple language works best. It may be necessary to speak loudly near the client's ear. In addition, when interviewing the elderly client with a hearing deficit, ask only those questions necessary to obtain required information.

It also helps to sit close to clients who have visual problems. The proximity allows the partially sighted client to see the nurse as clearly as possible.

Touch is an important avenue of communication with the elderly client. Sensation tends to decrease with age, but touch communicates the caring and support so important in establishing a relationship. Remember, though, to use touch in ways appropriate to the client's cultural background. People who always have maintained distance will not enjoy touching simply because they have become elderly.

The elderly client may move more slowly and may speak more slowly than a younger client. An unhurried interview, affording the client enough time to answer questions, is imperative. Hurrying the client will decrease the quality and quantity of information and interfere with establishing rapport.

The life review engaged in by an elderly person can be used to advantage in the interview. The client who likes to reminisce will provide much useful data. The nurse should be particularly attuned to information related to family, cultural background, and lifestyle. Observations about such factors as confusion, memory, orientation, or self-esteem also can be made at this time. The nurse, however, must be able to verify the facts before making judgments about normal or abnormal findings.

Language and Literacy

The nurse–client interview is greatly influenced by their similarities and differences in language and level of literacy. When the nurse and client do not speak the same language, there is limited common ground for communication. Nurses who are not bilingual but who practice in locales where there is more than one predominant language should learn at least the basics of the second language and learn the nuances of communications in that language (Longo & Williams, 1978). Otherwise, it is necessary to use interpreters. Since many nurse–client interviews are informal, not sharing a common language can be a tremendous barrier to the relationship.

But a common language is no insurance that a meaningful interview will occur. Nurses constantly must remind themselves that the jargon of health-care professionals often is equivalent to a foreign language for clients. This is true for well-educated clients as well as for those with limited educations. Using jargon or using words out of context may be perceived as disinterest and unwillingness by the nurse to communicate and may alienate the client (Doak, Doak & Root, 1985). Questions such as, "When did you first start having symptoms of gastritis?" or "Do you only get diaphoretic if you skip lunch?" should be phrased as "When did your stomach start bothering you?" and "Do you only start sweating if you don't eat lunch?" The use of plain words and a level of vocabulary in keeping with the client's understanding is essential to successful interviewing.

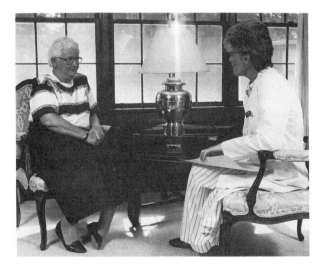

FIGURE 2-6. When interviewing the elderly client, the nurse should face the client and speak directly. It may be necessary to use a louder-than-normal tone of voice if the client has a hearing deficit, but the nurse should never shout at the client.

Health

The client's health is another important factor that influences the conduct of an interview. A client who is seriously ill, in pain, anxious, or unable to concentrate may find it impossible to participate in the give-and-take of the interview as it has been described. Alteration in length and structure of the interview may be necessary (Figure 2-7).

As the level of illness increases, the client's ability to participate tends to decrease. The seriously ill client who has numerous tubes and machines attached will be unable to provide a long, detailed history. Short conversations that require less talking can be used to obtain data from a seriously ill client, and additional data can be obtained from family members or other sources.

Obtaining information from the family is necessary, too, when the client is in no condition to participate. Serious illness or a decreased level of consciousness, however, does not negate the necessity of maintaining contact with the client. The client may not be able to talk, or may talk very little, but nonverbal communication still will be possible. The nurse can help by interpreting the client's behaviors or apparent feelings. Therefore, it is important to develop skill at recognizing and interpreting behavioral cues.

People in extreme pain or with high levels of anxiety will be unable to participate fully in a long interview. The nurse should assess the sources of discomfort and try to relieve the pain before beginning the interview. Short, direct conversations help the client provide information without further increasing pain or anxiety. A direct approach pro-

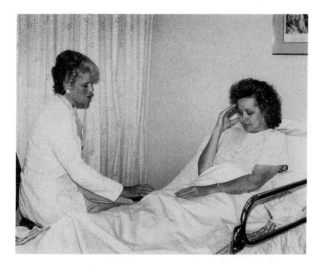

FIGURE 2-7. The nurse should be attentive and responsive to cues that indicate the client is unable to continue the interview.

vides structure that helps the client whose concentration span is limited.

THE NURSING HISTORY

The previous section on interviewing considers the process for collecting assessment data, the "how-to's" of gathering clinical information. This section focuses on the content of the nursing assessment, specifically the nursing history. The nursing history is a structured format for obtaining the relevant clinical information in the assessment interview.

The nursing history is a critical component of a comprehensive nursing assessment, contributing 80 to 90 percent of the clinical data obtained from a client. The history provides a systematic framework for gathering subjective data about a client's health patterns and status. The data are considered subjective because they are the client's stated perceptions about his or her own health. This information helps the nurse develop accurate nursing diagnoses and plan, implement, and evaluate appropriate nursing care. Specifically, the nursing history allows the nurse to plan and modify nursing actions in accordance with a client's wishes.

The nursing history is a deliberate plan for collecting and organizing clinical information. It is an important tool of the nursing assessment. It is, however, a means to a goal, not an end in itself. The goal of the nursing history is to gain as comprehensive and accurate a picture as possible of a client's health in order to make judgments. Judgments are formed on the basis of the client's descriptions and responses to purposeful questioning, as well as the nurse's observations of the client during the interview.

Skill and efficiency in obtaining a nursing history and making systematic observations of a client during the interview are acquired with practice. As the nurse gains knowledge and experience, he or she becomes increasingly able to anticipate and respond appropriately to cues that help focus the nursing history interview. Thus, the nurse's efficiency is enhanced and valuable time is saved. This is not to suggest that the nursing history interview ought to be a hurried process. Rather, the nurse who is proficient at collecting information is able to focus questioning to elicit data pertinent to an individual client's case. The expert nurse is less likely to spend time gathering unnecessary or extraneous information. The novice must rely on structured tools for history-taking and often has difficulty knowing which questions are important and which are not. Thus, all questions are pursued with a client, and the nursing history typically commands a great deal of the inexperienced nurse's time. Expert nurses, on the other hand, rely on experience and clinical cues to gather data and are able to collect more relevant and valid information in less time (Benner, 1984). The beginner should not become discouraged, but realize that proficiency will be gained with experience.

The nursing history provides an excellent way to establish initial rapport with a client. The history is a relatively nonthreatening way to get to know a client and gain the client's trust and confidence, since clients in health-care settings expect to be asked questions about their health. As trust is established, the client becomes more willing to disclose intimate information.

Types of Histories

The type of nursing history obtained from a client is determined by several factors: the nature of the client's contact with the health-care setting, the client's current health, and the particular setting or context. Generally speaking, there are three types of nursing histories: initial or comprehensive, problem-oriented, and update.

An initial, or comprehensive, nursing history typically is obtained upon a client's entry into a particular health system, such as a hospital, ambulatory facility, or home health setting. The initial nursing history is a comprehensive review of a client's health. It allows the nurse to gain an appreciation of the client as a person and to assess the client's general health. The initial, complete history also serves as a basis for future comparison. A comprehensive nursing history results in the identification of a client's strengths as well as actual or potential nursing diagnoses that may require intervention. A nurse also may identify actual or potential health problems that lie outside the scope of nursing and require referral to another health professional. Examples of clients from whom a nurse should collect a comprehensive nursing history are a pregnant woman during her first prenatal visit, a client admitted to the hospital for medical treatment or surgery, or a client newly referred to a home health agency for nursing care.

A second type of nursing history is the problem-oriented history, which is obtained when a client has a particular, usually acute, health problem. A problem-oriented history should be obtained, for example, on a child brought to a pediatric clinic with vomiting and fever, or from a client admitted to the emergency room with chest pains and shortness of breath. The problem-oriented history should focus on the immediate problem, events that led to the problem, home or emergency treatment, the client's responses to treatment, effects of the problem on the client, and so forth. Depending on the outcome, it may be necessary to obtain a complete nursing history at some later point. It would be inappropriate, and in some instances unsafe, to take time to obtain a complete nursing history from a client who is experiencing an acute problem requiring immediate attention and intervention.

A third type of nursing history is an update history, which is concerned with documenting changes that have occurred in the client's health since the client's last contact with the nurse or the particular health system. Information obtained in an update builds on the initial comprehensive nursing history. For example, an update obtained from a preschool child may include achievement of developmental milestones, changes in daily patterns, readiness for school, and family changes since the child's previous visit.

The Nursing History Versus the Medical History

The nursing history differs from the medical history, although some of the information obtained in each may overlap. The focus of the medical history is the collection of information that assists in detecting potential or actual pathological conditions. The outcome of the medical history is the formulation of medical diagnoses and a plan for medical or surgical intervention. The medical history has a relatively standard format and includes a history of the client's present and past health problems, their treatment, a family medical history, and a review of body systems.

The nursing history, on the other hand, focuses on physiological, psychosocial, cultural, and developmental patterns and characteristics that affect or are affected by a client's health. It is concerned with a client's responses to alterations in health that may require nursing intervention. Information obtained in the nursing history is used as a basis for formulating nursing diagnoses and for planning nursing care.

An example will help clarify the differences between the medical and nursing histories. The physician may make a medical diagnosis of myocardial infarction in a 56-year-old man, admit him to the coronary care unit, and prescribe appropriate medical treatment. In this instance, the physician's history focuses on:

The client's signs and symptoms
The chronology of events that led to the client's admission

Alleviating or aggravating factors

Family medical history

Contributing habits, such as smoking, and

A general review of systems.

The *nursing* history for this client focuses on:

The client's perception of what is happening to him

The client's understanding of his treatment

How the client is coping with his symptoms, diagnosis, hospitalization, and treatment

Any interferences with the client's work and financial situation

Alterations in the client's self-concept, self-esteem, and activity

Impact of the client's illness on his family

Available support systems and resources, and so forth.

Because the nursing history differs from a medical history, the client may express surprise at the nurse's interest in the client's responses to health problems. Clients expect to be asked about specific signs and symptoms they are experiencing, effectiveness of particular treatments, and other medical concerns. They are less familiar with being questioned about what they are feeling, how they are coping, what effect the particular problem is having on their daily lives, and how they are managing the problem. Some clients may be suspicious of the nurse's inquiries, either because they may interpret the nurse's questions to mean that something is seriously wrong or because their cultural pattern is one of self-protection and unwillingness to share with outsiders. Therefore, the nurse should describe the purpose of the nursing history and how it differs from a medical history, and explain to the client how the information will be used to individualize care.

The Nursing History Format

The nursing history can be obtained through interview, a written questionnaire, or a combination of the two. The advantages of gathering clinical information via interview are that it provides a context for face-to-face nurse–client interaction and allows the nurse to respond to the client's cues as they occur. For instance, if a client says she has no particular concerns about her health, but nonverbal cues indicate otherwise, the nurse can acknowledge the nonverbal expressions and explore further the client's feelings and perceptions. In addition, during a history interview, the nurse can clarify the client's

responses or ask questions to gather further information. Gordon (1987) suggests that a successful nursing history interview is characterized by the nurse guiding the interview 20 percent of the time, with the client talking the remaining 80 percent. The nurse's role is to initiate the interview, help focus the client's narrative, and terminate the session.

Written questionnaires completed by the client prior to coming to the health system allow the client to respond at his or her own pace and save valuable professional time. However, they have the disadvantages of not providing an opportunity for nurse–client interaction and for clarification of the client's responses.

A written questionnaire combined with a follow-up interview to clarify and amplify the client's responses saves time while providing an opportunity for the nurse to have personal contact with the client. The questionnaire and combination questionnaire–interview approaches are most likely to be used for initial, comprehensive health visits, elective hospital admissions, or same-day surgery settings.

Structure of the Nursing History

The structure of the nursing history will depend on the philosophical and conceptual views of nurses in a particular health-care setting. For instance, if people are seen as a set of body systems (medical model), then the nursing history probably will be structured similarly to, or may even be the same as, the medical history. If clients are viewed as multidimensional beings, then the nursing history will include categories that encompass the physiological, psychosocial, cultural, and developmental patterns that characterize a human being.

If nursing is to make a unique contribution to client care, then a *nursing* format should be used. Historically, nursing assessments have paralleled those of the medical profession. The inherent danger is that nurses who assess clients with a medical model are more likely to view them as diseases than as people. For example, a 52-year-old man with a medical diagnosis of diabetes mellitus may be seen as "the diabetic" rather than "Mr. Jones, a person who has diabetes." Nurses who learn to assess clients from a nursing perspective value people and prefer to use a nursing history that addresses all dimensions of human functioning.

Whatever particular conceptual framework is used in a given setting—adaptation model, self-care model, general systems model, life process model, need hierarchy, or developmental model—the structure of the nursing history should provide categories for collecting clinical information. Such categories enable the nurse to organize data in any health-care setting, irrespective of clients' medical diagnoses or health. All nursing frameworks have the purpose of identifying client strengths and de-

riving nursing, not medical, diagnoses. Table 2-1 illustrates a comprehensive nursing history structured according to the assessment categories used in this book. Table 2-2 presents Gordon's (1987) functional health patterns format.

TABLE 2-1
Nursing History Guide

Client profile:
Name
Residence
Birthdate; current age
Sex
Race; ethnic/cultural group
Marital status; number of children
Religious preference
Education/occupation
Usual health care provider
Reason for health contact
Source of history information; reliability

Sociocultural history:
Family
Family members, significant others (Who are most significant persons to client; on whom does client depend?)
Family roles, interaction patterns, power relationships (Who makes family decisions?)
Achievement of family developmental tasks
Family strengths
Family stressors/crisis; effect of illness on family roles and functioning
Coping strategies

Cultural
Ethnic/cultural group affiliation
Value orientation (present/future)
Health/illness beliefs: How does client explain illness occurrences?
Health-related customs: Dietary practices/restrictions, communication patterns, etc.; illness behaviors (home or folk remedies, responses to pain)
Religious membership and practices; sources of spiritual hope and strength

Environmental
Biological: exposure to organisms, allergens; allergies—food, medication, other
Physical: pollution hazards (air, water, noise); climate; sensory stimuli (overload or deprivation) in home, work/school, or health-care environment; personal health habits—immunizations, childhood or recent illnesses/injuries, health checkups, use of coffee, tea, alcohol, tobacco, marijuana; medications—type, dosage, frequency
Socioeconomic: employment/occupational status; economic status (sources of income, ability to meet living expenses and pay for health care); social support (friends, participation as a neighborhood and community member); home environment—living facilities,

space, satisfaction with living environment, actual or potential safety hazards; work/school environment—physical facilities, organizational network, exposure to hazards, satisfaction with work or school; perceived stressors; health-care environment—physical environment, space, comfort, exposure to stressors or hazards

Developmental history:
Family health history (hereditary factors)—parents, grandparents, siblings, children

Child
Prenatal, perinatal, and postnatal history
Achievement of developmental milestones (motor, language-cognition, personal-social)
Parents' perceptions of child's developmental progress; concerns

Adult
Achievement of developmental tasks (physical, sensory-cognition, psychosocial)
Satisfaction with life stage; problems or concerns

Psychosocial history:
Intrapersonal
Body image development and concerns; changes in body image
Self-esteem (perception of self-worth)
Cognition: Educational level; thought processes (coherence, continuity), abstract reasoning (if child, level of cognitive development, school achievement), judgment and insight, reality orientation, literacy (ability to read)
Affect/mood: General feeling tone; occurrences of anxiety, anger, depression (In response to what? How managed?)
Temperament: emotional behavioral style, impulsivity, sociability, activity level

Interpersonal
Communication patterns (verbal, nonverbal); ability to convey ideas and feelings effectively
Roles (ascribed, achieved); interpersonal relationships (friends, work/school associates)—ability to get along with others; social activities
Stressors (life changes, illness, etc.)
Coping strategies (How does client cope with stressors?)

Sexuality
Gender identity; if older child or adolescent, onset of primary and secondary sex characteristics (puberty)
Sexual knowledge/education: sources of information, questions or concerns

(continued)

TABLE 2-1 (Continued)

Sexual activity: use of contraception; concerns or problems

Reproductive history: gravida, para, aborta; infertility; menopause

Breast or testicular self-exam: knowledge, frequency of practice

History of sexually transmitted disease (how treated; questions or concerns)

Health problems that interfere with sexuality

Physiological history:

Physical Integrity:

Hygiene practices (bath, shower—frequency and time of day, hair and nail care, use of deodorant, lotion, oils; shaving, use of makeup); availability of bath facilities, soap and water

Growth patterns—recent weight loss or gain; growth spurts (i.e., puberty)

Skin—color changes, rashes, lesions, excessive dryness or oiliness, pruritus, excessive perspiration or odor

Hair—condition of hair and scalp, hair loss, pigment changes

Sensory/Perceptual/Neurologic Functioning:

Senses—any disturbances of vision, hearing, smell, taste, or touch; use of corrective aids (eyeglasses, contact lenses, hearing aids)

Neurological status—level of consciousness, coordination, balance, muscle tone; reflexes; any interferences (convulsions, weakness, tremors, etc.)

Pain—occurrence of pain (type, location, duration, intensity, precipitating and alleviating factors); how managed

Activity/Sleep:

Ability to carry out activities of daily living, exercise patterns (type, frequency), leisure activities; special abilities (creative, athletic)

Daily sleep patterns (number of hours slept daily, bed-time and arising time, naps); sleep environment (number of pillows, blankets; security object[s], light, noise, etc.); use of sleeping aids or bedtime rituals

Any interferences with sleep or recent changes in sleep patterns

Muscle strength and endurance; problems with gait, posture, range of motion, movement; assistance or equipment needed for mobility (walker, prosthesis, wheelchair, crutches, transport)

Oxygenation:

Usual respiratory and pulse rates; usual blood pressure (if known)

Any known problems with breathing, heart, blood pressure, or blood circulation (palpitations, epigastric distress, cyanosis, dizziness, headache, varicosities, bleeding tendencies, chronic cough); medications (type, dosage, frequency) or other aids used for relief

Nutrition:

Dietary intake (24-hour recall or 3- or 7-day food record)—food types and amounts; use of vitamin and mineral supplements; food preferences

Self-feeding and food preparation abilities (Who purchases food?); ability to meet food expenses

Number of teeth, eruption of teeth, teething discomfort, dental hygiene and dental care practices (brushing, flossing, denture care, dental visits, cavities); use of fluoride supplements

Special dietary needs—restrictions, practices, food intolerances

Fluid/Electrolytes and Elimination:

Usual daily fluid intake and output; voiding and bowel patterns, maintenance of patterns (laxatives, diet), changes in patterns; achievement of bowel and bladder control

Interferences (edema, constipation, diarrhea, nausea, vomiting, enuresis, incontinence, urgency, ostomy)—how managed

---

Regardless of which nursing format is used, the nurse should individualize the timing and sequence of the interview according to the particular needs of each client. Although it is important to conduct the nursing history interview systematically, rigid adherence to a form may inhibit a client's disclosure of significant information. The client should feel that the nurse is inquiring out of a sense of genuine concern for the client's welfare, not because of a need to get through the interview as quickly as possible. Questions should not be read from a list. Rather, the nurse should attempt to reframe suggested questions and topics. Instead of asking, "Do you have any dietary restrictions?",

the nurse might say, "You mentioned earlier that you are an Orthodox Jew. What particular foods should we avoid serving you during your hospital stay?" The latter tells the client that the nurse acknowledges him or her as a person and recognizes that the client has unique needs, which will be taken into account when planning care.

In order to ensure accuracy, the nurse should take brief notes during the history interview to avoid omitting important information when the history is fully recorded for the client's health record. A consistent format makes it easier to take notes, recall important information, and accurately document the history. The nurse should explain

TABLE 2-2
Gordon's Functional Health Patterns Assessment

1. *Health Perception–Health Management Pattern*
   a. How has general health been?
   b. Any colds in past year?
   c. Most important things to do to keep healthy? Think these things make a difference to health? (Include family folk remedies, if appropriate). Use of cigarettes, alcohol, drugs? Breast self-exam?
   d. In past, been easy to find ways to follow things doctors or nurses suggest?
   e. If appropriate: What do you think caused this illness? Actions taken when symptoms perceived? Results of action?
   f. If appropriate: Things important to you while you're here? How can we be most helpful?

2. *Nutritional–Metabolic Pattern*
   a. Typical daily food intake? (Describe.) Supplements?
   b. Typical daily fluid intake? (Describe.)
   c. Weight loss/gain? (Amount)
   d. Appetite?
   e. Food or eating: Discomfort? Diet restrictions?
   f. Heal well or poorly?
   g. Skin problems: Lesions, dryness?
   h. Dental problems?

3. *Elimination Pattern*
   a. Bowel elimination pattern (Describe.) Frequency? Character? Discomfort? Control?
   b. Urinary elimination pattern. (Describe.) Frequency? Problem in control?
   c. Excess perspiration? Odor problems?

4. *Activity–Exercise Pattern*
   a. Sufficient energy for desired/required activities?
   b. Exercise pattern? Type? Regularity?
   c. Spare time (leisure) activities? Child: Play activities?
   d. Perceived ability for: (code for level)
      Feeding ____   Grooming ____
      Bathing ____   General mobility ____
      Toileting ____   Cooking ____
      Bed mobility ____   Home maintenance ____
      Dressing ____   Shopping ____
      Functional Levels Code
      Level 0:   Full self-care
      Level I: Requires use of equipment or device
      Level II: Requires assistance or supervision from another person
      Level III: Requires assistance or supervision from another person and equipment or device
      Level IV: Is dependent and does not participate

5. *Sleep–Rest Pattern*
   a. Generally rested and ready for daily activities after sleep?
   b. Sleep onset problems? Aids? Dreams (nightmares)? Early awakening?

6. *Cognitive–Perceptual Pattern*
   a. Hearing difficulty? Aid?
   b. Vision? Wear glasses? Last checked?
   c. Any change in memory lately?
   d. Easiest way for you to learn things? Any difficulty learning?
   e. Any discomfort? Pain? How do you manage it?

7. *Self-Perception–Self-Concept Pattern*
   a. How would you describe yourself? Most of the time, feel good (not so good) about yourself?
   b. Changes in your body or the things you can do? Problem to you?
   c. Changes in way you feel about yourself or your body (since illness started)?
   d. Find things frequently make you angry? Annoyed? Fearful? Anxious? Depressed? What helps?

8. *Role–Relationship Pattern*
   a. Live alone? Family? Family structure (diagram)?
   b. Any family problems you have difficulty handling? (nuclear/extended)
   c. How does family usually handle problems?
   d. Family depend on you for things? How managing?
   e. If appropriate: How family/others feel about your illness/hospitalization?
   f. If appropriate: Problems with children? Difficulty handling?
   g. Belong to social groups? Close friends? Feel lonely (frequency)?
   h. Things generally go well for you at work? (School)? If appropriate: Income sufficient for needs?
   i. Feel part of (or isolated in) neighborhood where living?

9. *Sexuality–Reproductive Pattern*
   a. If appropriate: Any changes or problems in sexual relations?
   b. If appropriate: Use of contraceptives? Problems?
   c. Female: When menstruation started? Last menstrual period? Menstrual problems? Para? Gravida?

10. *Coping–Stress Tolerance Pattern*
    a. Tense a lot of the time? What helps? Use any medicines, drugs, alcohol?
    b. Who's most helpful in talking things over? Available to you now?
    c. Any big changes in your life in the last year or two?
    d. When (if) have big problems (any problems) in your life, how do you handle them?

(continued)

TABLE 2-2 (Continued)

e. Most of the time, is this (are these) way(s) successful?

11. *Value–Belief Pattern*
   a. Generally get things you want out of life?
   b. Religion important in your life? If appropriate: Does this help when difficulties arise?

c. If appropriate: Will being here interfere with any religious practices?

12. *Other*
   a. Any other things that we haven't talked about that you'd like to mention?
   b. Questions?

Note. Reproduced by permission from Gordon, Marjory: Nursing diagnosis: Process and application, ed. 2, New York, 1987, McGraw-Hill Book Co.; copyrighted by Mosby-Year Book, Inc., St. Louis.

the purpose of note-taking. It is essential, however, that the nurse maintain regular eye contact with the client, to convey interest and concern as well as to observe the client's nonverbal responses.

When concluding the nursing history interview, the client should be given an opportunity to add information or express further concerns (Gordon, 1987). The nurse should summarize the assessment data and note particular areas of strength or concern. Clients should be asked to identify which areas are of greatest concern to them and be reassured that their perceptions are important. Clients have a right to know that the information gathered will be used to help them in some way. The nurse then should terminate the interview according to the guidelines provided earlier in this chapter.

Chapter Highlights

■ Nurse–client interviews may be formal or informal and assess or respond to the client's needs.

■ The purposes of the interview include gaining information from the client, giving information to the client, and motivating the client to make a behavioral change.

■ The phases of the interview process include the introduction, working, and termination phases.

■ The two major approaches to interviewing are direct and indirect.

■ Interviewing requires a nurse to be aware of her or his own verbal and nonverbal communications and those of the client.

■ Successful interviewing techniques include encouraging verbalization, questioning, reflection, and active listening.

■ Techniques that impede the interview process including leading or biased questions, giving advice, defense-producing questions, and providing unrealistic reassurance.

■ Many variables influence the content and process of the interview, including the cultures of the nurse and client, the setting in which the interview occurs, the age of the client, the language and literacy level of the nurse and client, and the client's health.

■ The nursing history provides a structured format for the conduct of the assessment interview.

■ Factors that influence the type of nursing history obtained from the client include the nature of a client's contact with the health-care setting, the client's health, and the particular setting or context.

■ The nursing history focuses on physiological, psychosocial, cultural, environmental, and developmental characteristics that relate to a client's health.

■ The conceptual framework for nursing in a particular health-care setting influences the format used for the nursing history.

Practice Activities

1. Obtain at least three nursing history forms currently in use in local health agencies. Analyze the forms in terms of content and structure, types of categories, comprehensiveness, applicability to clients of all ages or in other settings, and use of a nursing versus medical framework. Discuss advantages and disadvantages of each form.

2. Role-play a history-taking interview, with the "client" in the role of:
   a. A 6-year-old who is having a school checkup
   b. A 16-year-old who is requesting birth control pills
   c. A 22-year-old pregnant woman during her first prenatal visit
   d. An elderly person who has had a stroke
   e. A person who speaks little English
   f. A person who is deaf
   g. A person in acute pain

Discuss the feelings and responses of the nurse and the client in each of these situations.

3. Obtain a nursing history from at least two of the following clients using one of the frameworks from this chapter:
   a. A healthy child
   b. A healthy adult
   c. An elderly client in a nursing home or senior citizens center
   d. A hospitalized child or adult
   e. A client with a chronic illness (e.g., diabetes, heart disease, rheumatoid arthritis, cerebral palsy)
   f. A pregnant woman

Recommended Readings

Braverman, B.G. (1990). Eliciting assessment data from the patient who is difficult to interview. *Nursing Clinics of North America, 25*(4), 743–750.

Brown, M.A. (1988). A comparison of health responses of expectant mothers and fathers. *Western Journal of Nursing Research, 10,* 527–542.

Hanna, D.V., & Wyman, N.B. (1987). Assessment + diagnosis = care planning: A tool for coordination. *Nursing Management, 18,* 106–109.

Hughes, C., Blackburn, S., & Wargo, M. (1986). On masking among clients. *Topics in Clinical Nursing, 8*(1), 83–89.

McConnell, E.A. (1988). Seeing your patient as a mosiac. *Nursing, 18*(12), 50–51.

Morrison, E.G. (1989). Nursing assessment: What do nurses want to know? *Western Journal of Nursing Research, 11,* 469–476.

Norris, L. (1986). Coaching the question. *Nursing, 16*(5), 100.

Price, B. (1987). First impressions: Paradigms for patient assessment. *Journal of Advanced Nursing, 12,* 699–705.

Rosenthal, T.T. (1982). The construction of a relationship. *Health Values, 6,* 28–30.

References

American Association of Colleges of Nursing. (1986). *Essentials of college and university education for professional nursing.* Washington, DC: Author.

Benner, P. (1984). *From novice to expert: Excellence and power in clinical practice.* Menlo Park, CA: Addison-Wesley.

Birdwhistle, R.L. (1979). *Kinesics & context: Essays on body motion communication.* Philadelphia: University of Pennsylvania Press.

Clinton, J. (1986). Sociocultural issues relevant to health care. In C. Edelman & C. Mandle (Eds.). *Health promotion throughout the lifespan* (pp. 570–583). St. Louis: C.V. Mosby.

Doak, C., Doak, L. & Root, J. (1985). *Teaching patients with low level literacy skills.* Philadelphia: Lippincott.

Gordon, M. (1987). *Nursing diagnosis: Process and application* (2nd ed.). New York: McGraw-Hill.

Jessop, A.L. (1979). *Nurse–patient communication: A skills approach.* North Amherst, MA: Microtraining Associates.

Lewis, G.K. (1973). *Nurse–patient communication.* Dubuque, IA: William C. Brown.

Longo, D. & Williams, R. (1978). *Clinical practice in psychosocial nursing: Assessment & intervention.* New York: Appleton-Century-Crofts.

Statler, C.B. (1977). Relationship of perceived empathy to nurses' communication. *Nursing Research, 26,* 437–440.

3

Collecting Assessment Data: Clinical Appraisal and Screening

CHAPTER OUTLINE

- Sources of Information
- Types of Information
  Subjective and Objective   Current and Historical
- Methods of Collecting Information
  Nursing History   Observation   Inspection
  Palpation   Percussion   Auscultation
  Consultation
- Using Data Collection Methods
- Screening
  Purposes of Screening   Criteria for
  Screening   Types of Screening   The Screening
  Process   Selected Examples of Screening

OBJECTIVES

Upon completion of this chapter, you should be able to:

- Recognize the importance of information as the foundation of the nursing process.
- Identify guidelines for collecting information.
- Differentiate among the following types of data: subjective, objective, current, and historical.
- Describe each of the following methods of collecting information and identify the type (objective or subjective) generated:
  1. nursing history
  2. observation
  3. inspection
  4. palpation
  5. percussion
  6. auscultation
  7. consultation
- Describe the correct techniques for inspection, palpation, percussion, and auscultation.
- Obtain objective and subjective data (as appropriate) using each of the methods of collecting information.
- Recognize the importance of screening as a component of the nursing assessment of any client.
- Explain the purposes, criteria, and types of screening.
- Identify selected health risks and the available methods for early detection.
- Incorporate appropriate screening methods in the nursing assessment of a client.

Gathering information is the foundation of the nursing process. It is the base on which nursing care is built. The critical role of this phase of the nursing process has been outlined clearly in the *Standards of Nursing Practice* developed by the American Nurses Association (ANA). The first standard specifies the need for the systematic collection of data about the health of the client (ANA, 1973). "The fact that this standard is the first of the eight standards is significant in reinforcing its importance as key to the remaining steps of the nursing process," write Iyer, Taptich, and Bernocchi-Losey (1986, p. 19).

Data, in the context of nursing assessment, refers to the pertinent and necessary information gathered from a variety of sources about the client's present or projected health needs and problems. The nature and quantity of the data may vary, but the system used to collect it is basically the same in all situations.

SOURCES OF INFORMATION

The nurse uses two kinds of sources when collecting clinical information: primary sources and secondary sources.

The *primary source* of data is the client. Most information the client supplies is not readily available from any other source. Clients are the experts about their needs, their feelings about health problems, their expectations about care, treatment, and recovery. The nurse recognizes that the information supplied by the client will be influenced by a variety of factors, such as the client's culture and social background, physical and emotional well-being, past experiences, level of knowledge, sources of motivation, and environment.

While collecting health information from the client, the nurse continually "analyzes, sorts, and labels the information received" (Hughes, Blackburn & Wargo, 1986, p. 83). The nurse also decides when to probe, when to accept information as accurate, and when to question the accuracy of the data. It is important for nurses to recognize when clients may be "masking" (Hughes et al., 1986) or providing incomplete information. Henry (1973) notes that individuals may exhibit masking behavior when they feel vulnerable and threatened. Masking behavior is therefore, self-protective. Families may also use masking as "a kind of collective covering up" (Hughes et al., 1986, p. 85).

Masking or withholding information is an aspect of being human. Therefore, the nurse should be alert to certain cues that may indicate masking. The cues include incongruity between objective and subjective data and physical assessment findings not supported by the client's history (Hughes et al., 1986). Additionally, if the nurse and client differ in age, ethnic background or education, the client may feel a need to limit or modify the information disclosed. The nurse should make every effort to minimize the need for masking on the part of the client. Of utmost importance is establishing a therapeutic relationship with the client. It is through this relationship that the nurse can reduce the barriers to the sharing of information. By demonstrating empathy and a positive regard, a nurse encourages open, honest self-disclosure from the client.

If a nurse senses that a client is masking, various techniques can be used to point out discrepancies and incongruities (see chap. 2). However, a nurse must exercise sound clinical judgment, including attending to the contextual nature of the relationship, when deciding whether to confront masking behavior or note the behavior as a coping style. A nurse carefully collects data in an objective and accepting manner, respecting the separateness and uniqueness of the other person.

The factors that influence the information supplied by the client are the same ones that influence the nurse's ability to effectively and objectively gather data. Great care should be taken to avoid assigning personal meanings or interpretations to the data. A nurse whose previous experience indicates that all colostomy clients initially are reluctant to look at their stomas may approach every colostomy client with this preconception. This belief will interfere with unbiased information gathering regarding a particular client's feelings about the stoma. "The nurse can develop the ability to differentiate actual data from personal interpretation through an adequate knowledge base, self-awareness, and conscious attention to potential misinterpretations," writes Christensen (1986, p. 61).

The nurse may use *secondary sources* to supplement data gathered from the client. Secondary sources include family and significant others, health-care professionals, the client's health records, and the nurse's own knowledge.

The client's family and other close persons such as friends and co-workers can contribute meaningful information about how the client functions in his or her usual home or work environment. In addition, family or friends often have information regarding a client's past responses to illness. For example, six hours after undergoing a hemorrhoidectomy, a 35-year-old man denies pain and refuses medication. The nurse observes that his fists are clenched and his face is taut. His pulse rate is elevated in comparison to his preoperative rate. The nurse suspects that the client is in pain. When questioned, his wife tells the nurse that at home her husband won't even take an aspirin for a headache because he believes a man should "grin and bear it." The wife, in this instance, provides data about her husband's usual response to pain that the client did not share with the nurse. This information will assist the nurse in planning care to meet this client's need for pain relief. Family and significant others often are a willing and valuable source of information and usually are eager to be involved in the care of their loved ones.

Other health-care professionals also may be consulted for additional information. The nurse may contact a client's physician to find out what medications have been prescribed or a physical therapist to determine a client's physical and emotional response to weight-bearing exercises. Each health-care professional, as an expert in a particular field, can provide valuable insights and information that the nurse may not have.

The client's current and previous health records contain a wealth of useful information. The health record may include social information (religion, occupation, insurance coverage), a complete medical history and physical examination findings, laboratory and x-ray results, and notations by other health-care professionals who have been in contact with the client. Health-care records, therefore, warrant the nurse's careful study because they add another dimension.

The nurse's knowledge also is a source of important information that constantly is drawn upon in assessment. Knowledge of the normal, or deviations from the normal, be it anatomy and physiology, growth and development, or psychodynamics, helps the nurse ask the right questions and look for the right things. This knowledge not only allows the nurse to make an initial assessment of the client's health, but provides the basis for recognizing a change in status on subsequent assessments (Iyer et al., 1986). The nurse's ability to solve problems and make decisions about the relevance and significance of the information also is essential for effective data collection. Alfaro (1986) stresses that data collection is only one component of the assessment phase. She notes that as data is collected the nurse must be concerned with validating it. This involves making sure which information is fact and which is questionable. Verifying information with secondary sources is helpful in assuring that accurate data has been obtained.

Once the information has been validated, the nurse organizes it, clustering it into groups to as-

sist in identifying patterns of health or illness. For example, a nurse identifies a pattern of lack of adherence to diet and medication in the initial assessment of a client with hypertension. The nurse recognizes that additional information must be obtained to better determine what the pattern means (Alfaro, 1986). Is the lack of adherence due to a lack of knowledge, lack of skill in food preparation, or a lack of motivation? Gathering more information will provide the answer.

Secondary sources should be used liberally in nursing assessment, but "the nurse must carefully consider the client's rights to privacy and confidentiality when obtaining information from secondary sources" (Iyer et al., 1986, p. 27). Data from secondary sources always should be viewed as supplementing data from the client. Information obtained from secondary sources is useful for clarifying, amplifying, or substantiating the data the nurse obtains from the client.

TYPES OF INFORMATION

Gathering data during an assessment can be classified according to a number of characteristics. Two of the commonly used classification systems will be examined here. Data may be categorized as subjective or objective and as current or historical.

Subjective and Objective

Subjective data can be experienced or perceived only by the client and not by the observer. This information is gathered through conversation and cannot be observed directly or examined by the nurse. *Subjective data are what the client says, perceives, or feels.* Pain, nausea, weakness, blurring of vision, feelings of depression, and a description of one's home life are examples. None of these can be observed directly by the nurse. Subjective data are unique to the client and have diagnostic value because they assist the nurse in understanding the client's perspective. Subjective information is valued "because the nurse's primary emphasis is on people and their total situation, including, but not limited to disease" (Gordon, 1987, p. 194). One of the primary sources of subjective data is the nursing history, the structured interview that focuses on all the pertinent and necessary information that influence an individual's health. Since the client is the informant, the information collected while taking a nursing history is subjective. The nursing history as a data collection tool is covered in Chapter 2.

Objective data consist of behaviors, activities,

and events that can be observed or measured by another person by means of the five senses. *Objective data are factual: They can be seen, heard, touched, smelled, and in rare instances tasted.* Examples of objective data are a rash, the respiratory rate, halitosis, a flushed face, edema, and a slouched posture. Each can be observed directly by the nurse. The results of laboratory or clinical tests also are objective since they can be verified by the senses of the person performing the test. For example, in doing a complete blood count (CBC), the laboratory personnel use their sight to count and describe blood cells. The results of a CBC are, therefore, objective. The nurse uses observation as the major source of objective information.

Objective data often may be found to support subjective data and subjective data to support objective data. Some examples may clarify this point. A client complains of leg pain (subjective). The nurse notes that the client's pulse rate is 100 beats per minute and that the client is clutching her leg (objective). The nurse realizes that a pulse of 100 is rapid and that a rapid pulse often accompanies pain; thus, the objective data substantiate the client's subjective complaint of pain. On the other hand, the nurse may feel a client's abdomen and note that the bladder is full (objective). The client may validate this finding by expressing the need to urinate (subjective). By analyzing the information and categorizing it as objective or subjective, a nurse is able to substantiate the data collected initially.

By separating data into subjective and objective categories, a nurse often can identify discrepancies. For instance, a client states, "I'm not the least bit worried about my operation tomorrow" (subjective). The nurse observes that the client is biting his nails, perspiring, and has smoked six cigarettes in 30 minutes (objective). In this case, there appears to be a discrepancy between the subjective and objective. Further assessment is indicated to resolve this discrepancy.

Subjective and objective information are equally important in a comprehensive nursing assessment. Gordon (1987) notes that it is important to realize that there are two value systems associated with subjective and objective data. Objective data are valued for diagnostic significance. When a nurse provides a physician with data on a client's health, the focus is frequently on objective data. "The physician considers subjective reports to be tentative until verification can be obtained by objective measures," Gordon writes (1987, p. 194).

Subjective and objective data are equally important to the nurse in the conduct of a compre-

hensive nursing assessment. When assessing a client, a nurse should try to elicit objective data that correspond with subjective data and subjective data that correspond with objective data. By categorizing data as subjective or objective, the nurse is better able to validate data and to identify and resolve discrepancies.

Current and Historical

Another way of viewing information is in terms of time: whether it is current or historical. Current data pertain to what is happening now. Historical data relate to what has happened in the past. Historical information may relate to what happened yesterday, last year, or many years ago. An example may clarify: A client is admitted for surgery. On return from the recovery room, the client's blood pressure is 98/72 (current data). Concerned that this reading might be indicative of hypotension, the nurse refers to the client's health record to determine the preoperative blood pressure. The nurse determines that three days ago, on admission, the client's blood pressure was 100/76 (historical data). By comparing current and historical data, the nurse can conclude that the client's blood pressure is not a cause for alarm. Using current data in conjunction with historical data provides more comprehensive information about a client's health and is particularly useful in determining and understanding patterns of behavior.

The various types of information collected during assessment (subjective and objective, current and historical), when combined and interpreted, provide a complete base on which to plan and implement nursing care. Because nurses are concerned with collecting all relevant data about a client, they should gather all four types whenever possible.

METHODS OF COLLECTING INFORMATION

The nursing history, observation, inspection, palpation, percussion, auscultation, and consultation are the seven basic methods of collecting information during a nursing assessment. Each method requires special skill; as with any skill, effective and efficient use is achieved through regular practice.

Nursing History

The nursing history is one of the primary means of collecting information (Chapter 2). It is important to remember that the nursing history serves simply as a guide that directs the nurse to areas that should be covered. The questions do not ensure a meaningful interview all by themselves. The usefulness of the guide and its ability to elicit worthwhile information are determined by the nurse's interviewing skills and the nurse's ability to create an interpersonal climate and environment conducive to client participation. The nursing history is supplemented by several other methods of collecting information.

Observation

The second important method of gathering data about a client is observation. Observation is a general term referring to the process of gathering information that can be perceived by one or more of the senses. The senses are used in a number of ways to observe the client's general appearance and physical function, content and process of interactions, and environment (Christensen, 1986). Observation, therefore, yields objective rather than subjective information. The sense most frequently associated with observation is sight. The nurse can often see meaningful behaviors or signs. For example, a nurse may see a client lying motionless in bed or a dressing saturated with blood. These visual observations will lead the nurse to investigate further. In another situation, the nurse may observe behaviors or signs that substantiate subjective data. A nurse may observe a respiratory rate of 28 per minute and use it to substantiate a client's subjective report of shortness of breath. When observation is used to collect information, the other senses often come into play, too. The nurse may hear a wheeze or hear a client crying. Touch may be used to determine texture, moisture, temperature, and density. The nurse may feel an enlarged lymph node or palpate a mass. Smell may be used to detect such odors as a wound infection or acetone breath. Observation, then, refers to the use of all the senses in data collection.

Skillful observation is guided by knowledge and requires purposeful use of the senses. A nurse must consciously use sight, hearing, smell, and touch in the pursuit of relevant data. People may sit in a classroom day after day and yet not know the color of the walls. They have not observed their surroundings purposefully, even though they have seen them daily. Although observation requires no special maneuvers or instruments, its importance in gathering information should not be underestimated. Nurses learn observation skills through practice; they need not rely on intuition (Hogstel, 1987). To assist in developing observational skills, Hogstel (1987) offers a number of suggestions:

■ Initially, look globally. Scan the immediate environment, observing the client, the equipment in the room, furniture, windows, floors, and bathroom. This can be done within a few seconds.

■ Observe from the general to the specific. After observing a patient's leg in a cast, look closely at the color of the toes to be sure circulation is adequate in the extremities.

■ Note the details of what you are observing by silently describing what you are seeing.

■ Use all senses to observe. Listen, look, feel, smell and in rare instances taste. Each of the senses can provide additional and corroborative information.

■ Jot down the specific observations as you make them. This will guard against forgetting pertinent information when you later record your findings. It also will provide a basis for comparison.

■ Be specific and objective in making observations. Avoid personal interpretation of behavior; document the behavior that is observed.

■ Validate observations with another registered nurse. (p. 90)

Perfecting observational skills takes practice. A nurse should take every opportunity to gain experience in this very important method of gathering data. All assessment builds on observation.

Inspection

Inspection is a specific type of observation. While observation involves the use of all the senses in gathering data, inspection primarily refers to a more systematic and thorough visual examination of the client. Inspection is "active looking" without any motor activity. It is used by the nurse to collect information about significant behaviors or physical features. Inspection specifies such characteristics as shape, position, size, symmetry, color, anatomical location, and movement. Inspection may, for example, reveal a deformity of the chest contour such as a "barrel chest," abdominal distention, an umbilical hernia, clubbing of the nails, or discoloration of the sclera. More than any other method of examination, inspection depends upon the knowledge of the observer. We have a tendency to see only those things that have meaning to us. A nurse also is likely to perceive more of what is looked for than what is looked at. A nurse will obtain approximately 90% of all the information a physical examination will yield through inspection. Palpation, percussion, or auscultation rarely will uncover an abnormality that doesn't exhibit some sign on careful inspection (King, 1983).

Therefore, inspection should be used purposefully as a data collection method and should be completed prior to palpation, percussion, or auscultation of body parts or systems. Adequate lighting and full exposure of the part are essential.

General usage of the term *inspection* restricts it to looking with the unaided eye. However, inspection in a broader sense includes use of such instruments as an otoscope or ophthalmoscope to visualize otherwise inaccessible body parts. These instruments enhance inspection, thus ensuring greater accuracy. The otoscope facilitates inspection of the ear, whereas the ophthalmoscope is used to inspect the eye. Inspection combined with the use of instruments permits the nurse to determine more thorough information.

Inspection by Ophthalmoscope

The *ophthalmoscope* (Figure 3-1) provides a means of illuminating and viewing the internal structure of the eye: the fundus or that portion of the eye posterior to the lens. When an ophthalmoscopic examination is performed, the room should be darkened. The ophthalmoscope should be set on 0 diopters (a lens that neither converges nor diverges light rays) by rotating the lens selector with the index finger. Use the right hand and right eye to examine the client's right eye and the left hand and left eye to examine the client's left eye. The ophthalmoscope is held firmly against the examiner's face with the eye directly behind the sight hole. The thumb of the examiner's free hand holds the client's upper eyelid open (Figure 3-2), and the examination proceeds:

- Ask the client to look straight ahead and gaze fixedly at some distant point that is at eye level.

- Keep your index finger on the lens selector dial, ready to change lenses as necessary to bring the structures being examined into focus.

- From a position approximately 12 to 15 inches from the client and 15 degrees lateral to the client's line of vision, shine the light beam on the pupil and note the orange glow in the pupil—the red retinal reflex.

- Move toward the client along the 15-degree line until your forehead is almost touching your thumb, which you had previously placed on the client's eyebrow.

- At this point, you should be able to visualize the retina in the vicinity of the optic disc (a yellowish round or oval body).

- If you cannot locate the disc, follow a blood vessel toward the center of the eye until the disc is found.

- Rotate the lens selector dial with your index finger to find optimal magnification for a distinct view of the retina.

- If the client is nearsighted, rotate the lens counterclockwise to the red numbers indicating minus diopters.

- If the client is farsighted, rotate the lens to the plus diopters, indicated by the black numbers.

- After you achieve sharp focus, inspect the optic disc and retinal blood vessels carefully. The appearance of these structures is discussed in Chapter 15.

Inspection by Otoscope

The *otoscope* (Figure 3-3) provides a source of light and means of magnification for inspecting the external auditory canal and tympanic membrane (Figure 3-4). To perform the examination:

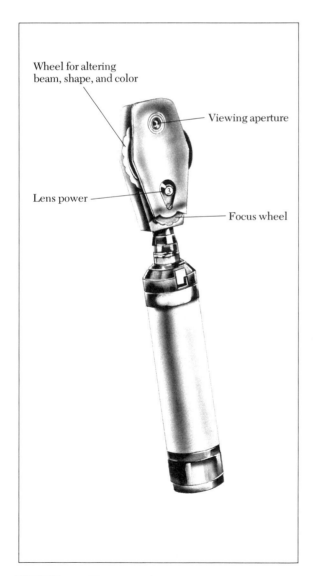

Wheel for altering beam, shape, and color

Viewing aperture

Lens power

Focus wheel

FIGURE 3-1. The Parts of an Ophthalmoscope.

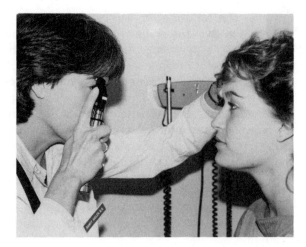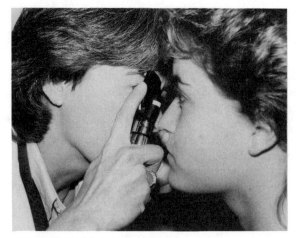

FIGURE 3-2. The Correct Technique for Examining the Internal Eye Structures.

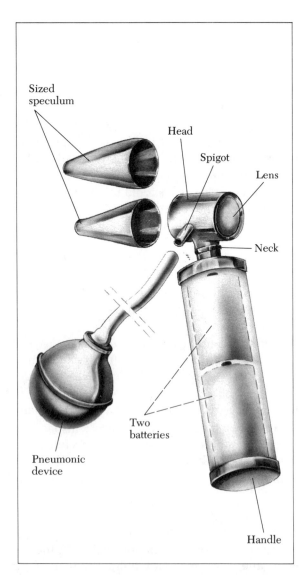

FIGURE 3-3. The Parts of an Otoscope.

- Select the largest speculum that will comfortably fit the external meatus of the client's ear.
- Hold the otoscope in your dominant hand.
- Instruct the client to tilt the head to the side opposite the ear being inspected. (Thus, if you are examining the right ear, the client tilts the head to the left.)

For adults, grasp the auricle firmly between your thumb and index finger, and pull it upward, back, and slightly out from the body before you insert the speculum. For infants and young children, pull the auricle downward and slightly out from the body. These maneuvers straighten the external auditory canal and thus enhance inspection.

- Check for patency of the external meatus before inserting the speculum of the otoscope.
- Gently insert the speculum of the otoscope slightly down and forward.
- Inspect the ear canal for redness, swelling, presence of cerumen (ear wax), and discharge or foreign bodies.
- Visualize the eardrum, identify landmarks, and note the color and sheen of the membrane. The appearance of these ear structures and landmarks will be discussed in Chapter 15.

The pneumatic device of the otoscope (Figure 3-3) is used to evaluate the mobility of the tympanic membrane. To use this type of otoscope effectively, the nurse should be sure that the speculum inserted into the external canal seals the canal from outside air. Positive and negative pressure then is gently applied by squeezing and releasing the bulb of the device. This technique will enable the nurse to observe the membrane moving

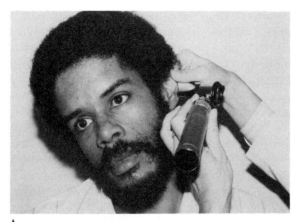

A

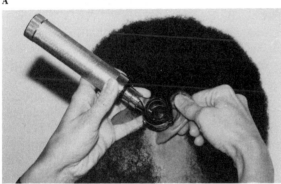

B

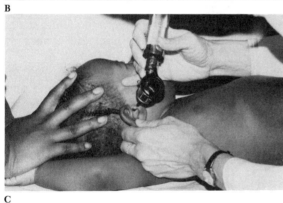

C

FIGURE 3-4. The Otoscopic Examination. A. Client is asked to tilt head to one side. B. Auricle is pulled upward, back, and slightly outward, and the speculum of the otoscope is inserted gently. C. Otoscopic examination of a child.

in and out as evidenced by a change in the appearance of the cone of light.

Palpation

Palpation is the fourth method used to gather information and involves the use of touch. Palpation follows a thorough inspection and is used, for instance, to determine the texture of the hair, the temperature of the skin, and the extent of tenderness in any accessible body tissue. The position, size, shape, consistency, and mobility of organs

and other masses may be palpated. A distended bladder, enlarged liver, and the presence of pedal pulses may be detected by palpation.

Generally, the fingertips are used for palpation (Figure 3-5). The concentration of nerve endings in the fingertips makes them most sensitive to fine tactile discrimination. Temperature changes are detected more accurately with the dorsum (back) of the hand, whereas the palm, specifically the palmar surface of the metacarpophalangeal joints, is most sensitive to vibration. The nurse therefore uses the fingertips to palpate an enlarged lymph node, the dorsum of the hand to determine if a reddened area on the skin is warmer than the surrounding skin, and the palm to detect vibration, such as a thrill from a heart murmur.

Light palpation generally is preferred for examination of most body parts and always should precede deep palpation. Heavy pressure on the fingertips or continued pressure over a period of time will dull the examiner's sense of touch. When using light palpation, the nurse's dominant hand is held parallel to the body's surface with fingers ex-

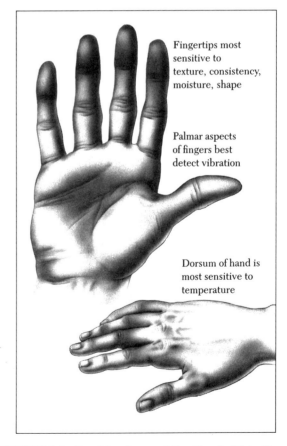

Fingertips most sensitive to texture, consistency, moisture, shape

Palmar aspects of fingers best detect vibration

Dorsum of hand is most sensitive to temperature

FIGURE 3-5. Sensitive Areas of the Hand. (*Note.* From Grimes/Burns: *Health Assessment in Nursing Practice,* Second Edition, © 1987. Jones and Bartlett, Publishers, p. 135.)

tended, and pressure is gently exerted downward as the hand is moved in a circular motion (Figure 3-6). When it is necessary to increase pressure to distinguish, for example, the size and shape of a mass, better discrimination is achieved by pushing down several times rather than holding the fingertips down for a long time.

When deep palpation is indicated, as in examination of the abdomen to locate organs and masses, the nurse should place the fingers of the

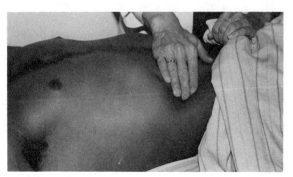

FIGURE 3-6. Light Palpation. The nurse's hand is held parallel to the body's surface with fingers extended. Pressure is exerted gently downward as hand is moved in a circular motion.

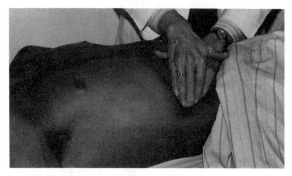

FIGURE 3-7. Bimanual Deep Palpation.

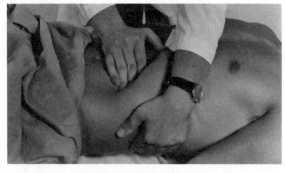

FIGURE 3-8. Deep Palpation of the Spleen. (*Note.* From Grimes/Burns: *Health Assessment in Nursing Practice*, Second Edition, © 1987. Boston: Jones and Bartlett Publishers.)

dominant hand over the area to be palpated. The fingers of the nondominant hand then should be placed on the distal phalangeal joints of the examining hand (Figure 3-7). When using bimanual deep palpation, pressure is applied primarily with the top hand while the more passive bottom hand is relaxed and is therefore better able to perceive the tactile sensations. Deep palpation may be performed using only the examiner's dominant hand (Figure 3-8). However, when deep palpation is difficult due to obesity or muscular resistance, for example, the bimanual technique should be used.

The best sequence for palpation is symmetrical; corresponding areas on each side of the body are compared sequentially. Deviations from the normal are detected more readily this way, and the normality of a finding can be validated, since it is unlikely that corresponding parts would have identical abnormalities.

The effectiveness of palpation, especially deep palpation of internal organs, depends to some extent on the client's state of relaxation. Muscular tension interferes with palpation, often limiting the amount of information the nurse can glean or distorting the findings. To help clients relax, they should be positioned comfortably and properly gowned. In the case of a client who is particularly tense, placing a pillow under the knees will slightly flex the lower extremities and reduce the tension on the abdominal wall. Initially palpating the client's abdomen with the client's hand under the examiner's hand may further reduce tension. As the examination proceeds, the examiner can slip one hand beneath the client's hand to directly palpate the abdomen. This technique also is useful with a client who is very ticklish. The nurse's hands should be warmed by briskly rubbing them together or running warm water over them before initiating palpation. Painful or tender areas should be palpated last. The nurse should monitor the client's facial expressions to determine whether palpation elicits pain or tenderness.

Percussion

Percussion is the method of gathering information in which the surface of the body is struck to produce sounds that can be heard and vibrations that can be felt. These sounds and vibrations vary according to the density of the underlying tissue. Percussion is used to determine whether the underlying tissue is air-filled, fluid-filled, or solid. It also is used to determine the size and shape of internal organs by assisting in location of the borders. For example, a nurse may percuss a client's bladder to determine if it is full or percuss the liver to determine if it is enlarged. Percussion is effective only in gathering information about structures lying near the body's surface. It has been estimated that the vibrations produced by percussion will not be detected if structures are deeper than 5 to 7 cm below the skin. It is important for the nurse to know that percussion is not as helpful with the obese client because organs or masses beyond a depth of 5 to 7 cm usually are not detected.

The most frequently used percussion method is *mediate*, or *indirect*, percussion. It is commonly used to assess a client's thorax and abdomen. Mediate percussion is done by striking a stationary finger placed on the client's body:

- Place your nondominant hand on the client directly over the part to be percussed.

- Only the distal phalanx of the middle finger of this hand should be in contact with the body. The remaining fingers and palm of the hand are raised off the area.

- This finger, called the *pleximeter*, should be placed flat and held firmly against the area to be percussed.

- Use the tip of the flexed middle finger of your dominant hand, called the *plexor*, to strike the pleximeter between the fingernail and the distal interphalangeal joint of the middle finger.

- Your fingernail must be short to avoid using the pad of the finger, which produces a sound of poorer quality.

- Keep your forearm stationary, with the motion coming from your wrist.

- Maintain a 90-degree angle between the plexor and pleximeter during percussion.

- To elicit clear, unmuffled sounds, the blows should be firm, short, and rapid with immediate removal of the plexor (Figure 3-9).

- Proper percussion technique is dependent upon correct positioning of the hands and wrist action, not the power used to elicit the sound.

This percussion technique is best learned by demonstration and supervised practice.

Another percussion method less commonly used is *immediate*, or *direct*, percussion. To perform this type of percussion, the nurse strikes or taps the body with one or more fingers of one hand. Immediate percussion will elicit tenderness if an underlying organ is inflamed. For example, immediate percussion over an infected sinus will induce pain.

Five distinct notes can be distinguished by skillful percussion (Table 3-1). Flatness is the note elicited when muscle or bone is percussed. Very dense tissue, such as the liver or spleen, produces a thudding dull sound.

Percussion of the normal, air-filled lungs produces a hollow, resonant note. An air-filled stomach or puffed-out cheek produces a tympanic, or drumlike, sound. Hyperresonance is a note not normally percussed in the body. It is a sound between resonance and tympany and occurs when percussing an emphysematous lung, for example.

In general, the less dense the tissue (the more air it contains), the louder and longer the sound will be. The more compact the tissue (the less air it contains), the fainter and shorter the sound will be. Percussion of the least dense tissue produces tympany, and percussion of the most dense tissue produces flatness. The five percussion notes can be viewed as a continuum, with flatness representing one end and tympany the opposite end (Figure 3-10). The other notes, dullness, resonance, and

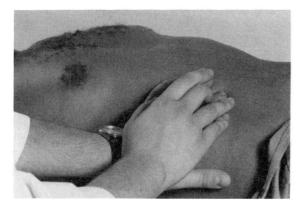
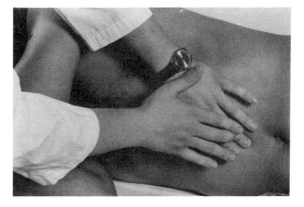

FIGURE 3-9. Indirect (Mediate) Percussion. The flexed middle finger of the dominant hand, the plexor, strikes and bounces off the pleximeter, the middle finger of the opposite hand. (*Note.* From Grimes/Burns: *Health Assessment in Nursing Practice,* Second Edition, © 1987. Boston: Jones and Bartlett Publishers.)

TABLE 3-1
Notes Produced by Percussion

	Intensity	Pitch	Duration	Area or Organ Where Percussion Sound May Occur
Flat	Soft	High	Short	Muscle, bone, thigh
Dull	Medium	Medium	Medium	Liver, spleen
Resonant	Loud	Low	Long	Lung
Hyperresonant	Very loud	Very low	Very long	Emphysematous lung
Tympanic	Loud	High	Medium	Gastric air bubble

hyperresonance, fall in between; their exact position on the continuum is determined by their relationship to the density of the tissue being percussed.

Auscultation

Auscultation is listening to sounds produced by the body. Auscultation may be direct (immediate) or indirect (mediate). With direct auscultation, the nurse uses the unaided ear near or on the body surface to listen to a sound. For example, an expiratory wheeze or nasal congestion may be detected by direct auscultation. Generally, though, auscultation is mediate; the nurse listens with a stethoscope, which amplifies the internal body sounds and transmits them to the nurse's ear. The nurse uses a stethoscope primarily to auscultate sounds from the heart, blood vessels, lungs, and stomach. The heart can be auscultated for its various heart sounds, the lungs for breath sounds, and the abdomen for bowel sounds.

The auscultated sounds are described in terms of their pitch, intensity, duration, and quality. The pitch is the frequency of vibration of the sound waves; high-pitched sounds have a greater number of vibrations per second than low-pitched sounds. Intensity refers to the loudness of the sound. Body sounds may be loud, as in tracheal breath sounds, or soft, as in most heart sounds. The duration of the sound (long or short) should be noted when appropriate. Finally, the quality of the sound

should be determined. Quality refers to a subjective description of the sound: rumbling, blowing, or musical.

Stethoscopes used in auscultation should have both a bell and a diaphragm. The funnel-shaped, open bell is used to detect low-pitched sounds, such as diastolic heart murmurs. The bell has the advantage of conducting sound with no distortion of pitch. However, the diameter of the bell does restrict the volume of sound that can be transmitted. The bell should be applied lightly to the body surface, with just enough pressure to seal the edges. If the bell is applied too firmly, it will act as a diaphragm. The diaphragm is used to detect high-pitched sounds such as normal or abnormal lung sounds. The diaphragm filters out low frequencies, so that sounds heard through the diaphragm are higher pitched than sounds heard through the bell. Because of its greater size, the diaphragm is more sensitive to faint sound. For example, breath sounds, friction rubs, heart sounds, and crepitus are best heard with the diaphragm, while venous hums, bruits, and heart murmurs are best heard with the bell. The stethoscope's earpieces must fit snugly enough to occlude the ear canals and prevent any interference of environmental noise.

Effective auscultation requires a systematic approach, with the nurse proceeding from one area of the body to another and comparing areas symmetrically. For instance, in auscultating the lungs, the nurse should listen posteriorly from the apex (top) to the base of the lungs, then proceed to the

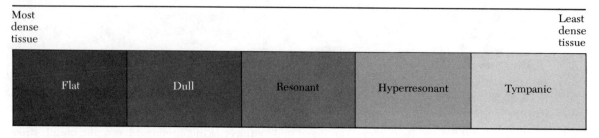

FIGURE 3-10. The Continuum of Percussion Notes.

anterior chest, always comparing sounds heard at corresponding areas of the chest wall. The nurse should concentrate on one sound at a time in each location. While examining, it is generally best to concentrate on normal sounds first, as this will make detection of abnormal sounds easier.

Auscultation should be performed in a quiet environment. The nurse should attempt to remove all interfering sounds by closing the door, turning off the radio or television, and asking the client not to talk. Auscultation should not be done over hair or clothing, as the rubbing of the chestpiece will distort the findings. False sounds also may be produced by inadvertently sliding the chestpiece over the skin or by rubbing or jarring the tubing or chestpiece.

Consultation

These six methods of collecting information all involve interaction with the client. One additional method, consultation, takes place away from the client. Consultation involves the exchange of information such as asking the advice or opinion of another person who is considered an expert in a particular area. A nurse frequently consults other health-care professionals. For example, a psychiatric nurse might be consulted when planning care for a postoperative client who is hostile and withdrawn. A physician might be asked to explain the rationale for insulin dosage for an uncontrolled diabetic client who is being taught home management. Consultation also may be used to gather information from the client's family, friends, teachers, or coworkers, who see the client in everyday life. To obtain an accurate diet history, the nurse caring for a cardiac client on a restricted sodium diet may consult the client's spouse. The teacher of a child with learning disabilities may be consulted for his or her impression of the child's capabilities. Health records also may be consulted. An outpatient health record can provide the history of a hypertensive client's blood pressure prior to hospital admission. Finally, the nurse may refer to textbooks, journals, or research reports to gather information helpful in planning a client's nursing care.

Consultation as a means of gathering information must be employed with strict attention to protecting confidentiality. A consultation conference should be planned so that it takes place in a setting that ensures privacy. Only information that is pertinent should be shared with the consultant. In some instances, it may be appropriate to ask the client for permission to consult a family member, coworker, or teacher. The purpose of consultation

is to gather information that will aid the nurse in planning care, not simply to obtain or share confidential information concerning the client.

USING DATA COLLECTION METHODS

By employing any combination of the seven methods described here, a nurse can collect a great deal of objective and subjective information. Which methods yield subjective data and which provide objective data? The nursing history is the primary means of gathering subjective information, whereas observation is the primary source of objective information. Inspection, palpation, percussion, and auscultation provide objective data, since each technique employs one or more of the nurse's senses to elicit information. Consultation generally provides subjective information since it is given by another individual either orally or in writing, as on a health record, and is influenced by that person's perception of the situation. Some forms of consultation, such as laboratory test results on a health record, do yield objective data.

The seven methods seldom are used separately or sequentially. The nurse can gather objective information during the nursing history and subjective data during inspection: A client may talk about pain when the nurse palpates a tender area. A comprehensive nursing assessment will include all seven methods in varying proportions, depending on the clinical setting and situation. During an assessment, one method may validate findings gathered by another method. Inspection may reveal evidence of an enlarged lymph node that the nurse can confirm by palpation. The nurse may sense a dull area in the abdomen that normally would be tympanic when percussed. By palpating the same area, the nurse notes an enlarged liver.

Whatever method is used, the nurse's own knowledge will influence its effectiveness. The broader the nurse's knowledge, the more meaningful information becomes. Knowing what questions to ask and how to ask them and what to look for, listen to, and feel for undoubtedly influence the quality and quantity of the information gathered. For example, by knowing the usual symptoms of diabetic ketoacidosis (polyuria, excessive thirst, nausea and vomiting, abdominal pain), the nurse can ask the right questions to obtain meaningful information from the client.

When gathering information, the nurse must strive to be objective and to note and record only what is said or observed. The nurse recognizes that the information must be validated and organized, which will enable the nurse to identify patterns, gather additional information if necessary, and then determine what it all means. This process is essential if accurate and appropriate nursing diagnoses are to be formulated.

SCREENING

Screening is an important component of the total nursing assessment of any client. This process can be described as assessing for potential or probable health problems to promote early detection and intervention. Screening methods, including laboratory tests, contribute to the information the health professional collects as part of the total assessment.

Screening is defined as the *process of identifying unrecognized or preclinical disease in asymptomatic, apparently healthy individuals.* Tests, examinations, or other procedures are used to distinguish apparently healthy persons who do not have a disease from those who probably do have disease (Mausner & Kramer, 1985; Valanis, 1986). It is important to note that screening is not diagnostic. Rather, screening is used to identify persons who probably have health problems and therefore warrant further, specific diagnostic evaluation. In addition, the focus of screening is on unrecognized health problems—those problems that are not causing noticeable signs and symptoms. In general, screening tests are less expensive, less accurate, simpler, more acceptable, and less risky to a presumably healthy population than are diagnostic tests (Table 3-2).

Purposes of Screening

Screening serves several purposes in addition to the primary one of identifying early (i.e., prior to symptoms) those individuals who are at risk for a particular health problem (Table 3-3). Secondary purposes of screening are to provide the nurse with an opportunity to educate a client about health risk factors and the importance of periodic future screening, assuming the results are negative (i.e., no indication of a potential health problem at present). Further, screening affords a chance to provide guidance about behaviors or practices that can lower the client's risk of developing a particular disease; counseling about the importance of diet, exercise, and not smoking to lessen the risk of cardiovascular disease.

Criteria for Screening

There are certain criteria for deciding if screening is appropriate, accurate, and efficient. When evaluating the need for any screening, the following criteria (Anderson & McFarlane, 1988; Wilson & Jungner, 1968) should be used where feasible for a given individual or population group:

- The disease to be screened for must have an asymptomatic period during which detection and treatment significantly reduce morbidity and mortality.

- The disorder must be common and/or have a significant impact on the quality or quantity of life.

TABLE 3-2
Comparison of Screening and Diagnostic Procedures

Factors	Screening Tests	Diagnostic Procedures
Purpose	To identify the possibility of a condition or disease.	To firmly rule in/out a condition or disease.
Complexity	Simple; time-efficient.	Simple to very complex; usually more time-consuming.
Expense	Minimal to moderate cost.	Moderate to high cost.
Accuracy	Low-moderate degree of accuracy.	High degree of accuracy.
Safety	Highly safe.	High-low degree of safety.
Acceptability	Highly acceptable.	Moderate-low acceptability.

TABLE 3-3
Purposes of Screening

Purpose	Example
Health education	Education about risk factors, use of the health-care system, and the importance of periodic screening.
Anticipatory guidance	Guidance about behaviors of practices that can help prevent future health problems.
Enhancement of the information	Whether results are positive or negative, results of screening add information to the nursing assessment.
Identification of the incidence of disease	Identifying the incidence of a disease in a population facilitates health program planning for care of those with the problem and prevention of the health problem in the remainder of the population.

■ Tests must be available that are acceptable to the client and screener. Factors to consider include cost, time involved, convenience, discomfort, and risk associated with the screening tests.

■ There should be an agreement/policy about which test values will result in referral of individuals for diagnosis and subsequent treatment.

■ Diagnostic tests must be available that can differentiate disease from nondisease.

■ Treatment modalities for the disease must be available and acceptable to the client and health professional.

■ The long-term benefits of therapeutic treatment of the disease must outweigh the long-term detriments of the condition and the costs of screening and treatment.

The tests themselves also must meet several criteria. First, the tests must be valid and reliable. The validity of a screening test indicates the test's ability to distinguish correctly between those who have the disease and those who do not have the disease (Anderson & McFarlane, 1988; Mausner & Kramer, 1985). The validity of a test is measured by determining its sensitivity and specificity.

The sensitivity of a test refers to the test's ability to accurately identify those individuals with the disease or risk factor. As Anderson and McFarlane (1988) state, it is the ability to call a "true positive, positive" (p. 45). The specificity of a test refers to the test's capacity to accurately identify those individuals who do not have the disease. It is the ability to call a "true negative, negative" (Anderson & McFarlane, 1988, p. 45).

The relationship between screening and the true incidence of disease is depicted in Table 3-4. Persons who truly have disease (reading across the top of Table 3-4) can have one of two test results. They may be true positives (actually have the disease) or false-negatives (diseased persons shown to be negative or normal according to test results). Sensitivity, therefore, is the percentage of all individuals with the disease (true positives and false negatives) who test positive (Valanis, 1986).

Similarly, persons who do not have the disease (reading across the bottom of Table 3-4) can have one of two test results. They may be false-positives (found to have the disease on screening when they are actually disease-free) or true-negatives (actually do not have the disease). Specificity, then, is the percentage of disease-free persons (true negatives and false-positives) who are shown to be negative (Valanis, 1986).

The perfect screening test would be a test that is 100% sensitive and 100% specific (Mausner & Kramer, 1985). However, in reality, this does not occur because sensitivity and specificity are usually inversely related. As the sensitivity of a test increases, the specificity of the test decreases. "Ideally, a screening test correctly identifies most of the patients who have the diagnosis (high sensitivity) with a minimum of false-positives (high specificity)," write Matteson and McConnell (1988, p. 73).

Ensuring the validity of a test is complex. It requires a favorable balance of sensitivity and specificity. The sensitivity and specificity of a test change when the cutoff point for an indicator is adjusted. For example, increasing the percentage of weight loss would increase the sensitivity of this indicator to distinguish between malnourished and nourished individuals (Suitor & Crowley, 1984), but label a number of healthy persons malnourished. Lowering the hematocrit and hemoglobin would increase the sensitivity of tests to detect anemia, but also increase the number of false-positive results.

The reliability or precision of a screening test means that the test gives consistent results when the test is performed more than once on the same individual under the same conditions (Mausner & Kramer, 1985). The variations among those performing a screening test, as well as the variation inherent in the method, contribute to inconsistent results. The reliability of a screening test can be improved by training those involved in the screening process and by standardizing the procedure for conducting the test (Anderson & McFarlane, 1988; Valanis, 1986). It is important for the nurse to have a basic understanding of the concepts and princi-

TABLE 3-4
A Grid Illustrating the Relationship Between Screening Test Results and the True Incidence of Disease

	People who do have disease according to the screening test	People who do not have disease according to the screening test
Persons who truly have disease	True-positives	False-negatives
Persons who truly do not have disease	False-positives	True-negatives

Note. Adapted from *Nutrition and Application in Health Promotion* by C. Suitor and M. Crowley, 1984, Philadelphia: Lippincott, p. 311.

ples of screening in order to be more effective as a health educator–screener (Allen, 1986).

Types of Screening

There are five major types of screening with which the nurse may be involved:

1. *Mass screening.* Historically the most common type, mass screening involves testing an entire population for a single condition without consideration of specific risk factors. An example is testing for phenylketonuria (PKU) in all newborn infants.

2. *Selective screening.* This type of screening involves testing a selected group of individuals who are at high risk for a condition. Examples include testing individuals over 40 years of age for glaucoma or for diabetes in obese individuals.

3. *Multiple screening.* Multiple screening refers to testing for two or three potential health problems simultaneously. An example would be vision, hearing, and scoliosis screening of school-age children.

4. *Multiphasic screening.* Multiphasic screening is essentially an extension of multiple screening to include 4 to 10 health problems. Generally, this type of screening is used in well developed health programs such as the Early Periodic Screening, Diagnosis, and Treatment Program (EPSDT). In this program children from birth to 21 years of age are screened periodically for physical growth (height, weight, head circumference), hypertension (blood pressure), anemia (hematocrit), nutritional status, dental status, and developmental progress.

5. *Periodic health examinations.* This type of screening involves testing individuals for a variety of health problems at scheduled intervals during their lives. The frequency and type of examination would vary as the risk to an individual changes over the course of the life cycle. An example would be the standard physical examination applicable to a large population but administered on an individual basis (Allen, 1986).

The Screening Process

Screening is a process requiring a positive working rapport between nurses and other health professionals to whom clients frequently are referred. It is often a nurse who initiates the screening process. Many times, the nurse is also the health professional who selects and administers a number of the screening tools available today (or supervises others who have been trained to administer selected screening tests).

For example, the Denver Developmental Screening Test (DDST) may reveal developmental lags, a height/weight profile may point to an obesity tendency, and nutritional screening may suggest a predisposition for dental caries or anemia, to name a few. The results may support or validate a nursing diagnosis. On the other hand, the test results may warrant referral to other experts in the health-care system for further screening or diagnostic evaluation.

The steps of the screening process are the same

TABLE 3-5
The Screening Process and the Nursing Process Compared

Nursing Process		Screening Process	
Assessment/ Analysis	Assessment ■ Population needs ■ Available screening tools and resources ■ Available referral sources*	Implementation	Implementation ■ Testing using selected tool(s) ■ Checking consistency in test implementation and interpretation ■ Retesting positives according to screening tool guidelines ■ Referral of positive cases
Planning	Planning ■ Population to be screened ■ Tool(s) to be used ■ Notification of target population ■ Facilities, materials, and personnel to implement program ■ Availability, accessibility, and acceptability of referral resources*	Evaluation	Evaluation ■ Effectiveness and efficiency of tool and personnel ■ Client participation and follow-through on referral

*Note: Referral and follow-up options require planning and effort but are an absolute necessity to meet the needs of the population being screened.

as those of the nursing process, with a slightly different focus (Table 3-5). As with all nursing care, a systematic approach is necessary for successful screening.

Selected Examples of Screening

Describing all available screening tools is beyond the scope of this chapter. However, it is essential that the nurse be familiar with the wide variety of screening tools used today. In addition, it is important to recognize that many disorders for which nurses screen are age-related or of particular concern for a specific age group. Therefore, high risk areas may be identified that warrant screening in certain life phases, thereby minimizing exposure to testing that may be inappropriate for a particular age group. A brief summary of life phases and selected health risk areas is provided in Table 3-6. This table is not all-inclusive; it is a guide.

There are a multitude of screening tools available for assessing the general population. Table 3-7 identifies a number of common health problems that should be monitored seriously, along with some of the screening options available to detect each disorder in its early stage. The screening tools in Table 3-7 range from simple questionnaires to highly intricate procedures for which the nurse may need specialized training.

Screening is a unique facet of preventive health care that optimizes use of professional time and money. However, successful programs are contingent upon the nurse's ability to carry out the screening process systematically with careful consideration of the rationale and criteria for screening. To be an appropriate adjunct to total client assessment, screening must be used selectively and must be based upon educated nursing judgment.

Risk appraisal (see chap. 9) is closely related to screening. However, risk appraisal differs from screening in that risk appraisal attempts to estimate an individual's risk for disease in the predisease state. Screening attempts to identify unrecognized or preclinical disease in asymptomatic individuals. Risk appraisal provides clients with a realistic evaluation of health threats to which they are particularly vulnerable prior to the development of signs and symptoms of the disease (Pender, 1987). It is important for health professionals to realize that risk appraisal by itself will not reduce the risks for a given disease or diseases. Risk appraisal must be linked to programs that assist clients in changing their behavior, thereby reducing their risk. We do clients a great disservice by apprising them of

health risks and then not offering a program or resources to help them change (Pender, 1987).

TABLE 3-6
Selected Health Risks Through the Life Span

Life Span Phases	Health Risk Areas
Perinatal period	Toxemia Hypertension Hereditary disorders Anemia Emotional maladaptation
Infancy (0 to 1)	Congenital anomalies Hearing/visual disturbances Hereditary disorders Glucose imbalance
Preschool age (1 to 5)	Hearing, vision, speech, anemia, developmental disturbances
School age (6 to 11)	Hearing and vision disturbances Social maladjustment Dental problems
Adolescence (12 to 17)	Nutritional imbalance Physical activity Drugs Smoking Sexual activity Sexually transmitted disease Pregnancy
Young adulthood (18 to 24)	Nutritional imbalance Hypertension Exercise Sexually transmitted disease Contraception Marriage Pregnancy Family maladjustments
Young middle age (25 to 39)	Hypertension Nutritional imbalance Lack of exercise Parenting difficulties Urinary tract infections Anemia Cervical/breast cancer
Older middle age (40 to 59)	Obesity Stress Alcohol/drug abuse Smoking Marital/parenting difficulties Cancers: Lung, prostate, cervical, uterine, breast
Elderly (60 to 74)	As above, plus possible nutritional imbalance, glaucoma, depression, immobility
Old age (75 and older)	As above plus possible podiatry problems

*All age groups: hypercholesterol levels

TABLE 3-7
Selected Examples of Health Problems and Available Screening Tools for Early Detection

Health Problems to Be Screened	Screening Tools/Measures	Health Problems to Be Screened	Screening Tools/Measures

AIDS	Human Immunodeficiency Virus (HIV); Human T Lymphocytic Virus Type III (HTLV III)	Genitourinary deviations
		  Bacteria
		  Cardiovascular renal disease
			Urinalysis; urine culture, albumin determination; blood pressure

Anemia	Hemoglobin; serum iron	Hematuria	Occultest
Cancer		Hearing impairments	Bell tests; audiometry; tuning fork tests; Denver Audiometric Screening Test (DASE) tympanometry
Breast	Manual examination; mammography		
Cervical/uterine	Pap Smear-cytology; pelvic exam Hemocult	Hydrocephalus	Serial head circumference measures
Colon	Rectal examination; sigmoidoscopy	Lead poisoning	Calorimetric testing
Lung	Smoking history; chest x-ray	Liver damage Alcoholism	Blood transaminase; social history; alcohol consumption history
Oral	Oral examination—inspection	Phenylketonuria	Guthrie test
Cardiac disease		Pulmonary disease	
Arteriosclerosis	Pulse rate; peripheral pulse checks; activity/smoking history; serum cholesterol; family history	Emphysema	Smoking history; chest x-ray; pulmonary function tests; spirometry
		Lung Cancer	(see Cancer)
Hypertension	Blood pressure; diet history; family history	Scoliosis	Visual spine examination/measurements
Developmental deviations	Denver Developmental Screening Test (DDST); Prescreening Developmental Questionnaire (R-PDQ); Development Profile II	Sickle cell anemia	Sickledex test
		Speech impairment	Denver Articulation Screening Examination (DASE)
		Syphillis	Serological tests
		Tuberculosis	Tuberculin test; chest x-ray

Endocrine imbalance
  Diabetes Mellitus
	Blood sugar; Dextrostix/Chemstrips; urine testing	Visual impairments
		  Color blindness
			Snellen Test, Denver Eye Screening Test (DEST);

Growth deviations	Serial height/weight measurements	Glaucoma	Titmus vision tester Color testing (Ishihara plates) Tonometry
Overweight	Anthropometry; height; weight		
Underweight	Anthropometry; height; weight		

Chapter Highlights

■ Gathering information is the foundation of the nursing process.

■ The various types of information collected during assessment (primary and secondary, subjective and objective, current and historical), when combined and interpreted, provide a complete basis on which to plan and implement nursing care.

■ A nurse should collect information in an objective and nonjudgmental manner, respecting the client.

■ The assessment phase involves gathering information, validating it, organizing it into groups, and identifying patterns of health or illness.

■ The nursing history is one of the major assessment tools used by the nurse to identify the status of a client's health.

- The effective and efficient use of physical assessment skills is achieved through regular practice.

- Screening is the process of identifying (rapidly and inexpensively) unrecognized or preclinical disease in apparently healthy, asymptomatic individuals.

- While screening is not diagnostic, it is used to identify persons who probably have a health problem and therefore warrant further, specific diagnostic evaluation.

- Risk appraisal attempts to estimate an individual's risk of disease in the predisease state.

- To be effective, risk appraisal must be linked to programs that assist clients to change their behavior, thereby reducing their risk.

Practice Activities

1. Select two clients. Interview the first client to establish a basis for nursing care before you consult any secondary sources. Before interviewing the second client, consult at least two secondary sources. Compare and contrast the amount and types of information collected from the primary and secondary sources. Which approach do you prefer? Why?

2. For each piece of information, indicate whether it is subjective or objective and the method probably used to collect it.

Headache	Sleeps with two
Hgb 14.0 g	pillows
Numbness	Hiccups
Bluish discoloration of	Stiff neck
nails	Dizziness
Edema	Nausea
BUN 12 mg	Crying
Palpitations	Itching
Sitting without support	

3. Purposefully observe any situation or event for 3 minutes. Record all your observations and determine through which sense(s) the data were perceived.

4. Systematically inspect a client's (or classmate's) arm or leg and record all the information obtained. What approach did you use to ensure that nothing was overlooked?

5. Role-play nurse and client with a student or colleague, and practice inspection, palpation, percussion, and auscultation techniques. Validate findings with an instructor or an experienced clinical nurse.

6. Select a client and identify age-specific health risks. Determine what screening tools or measures would be used to screen for those health problems.

Recommended Readings

Farrell, J. (1980). The human side of assessment. *Nursing '80, 10*(4), 74–75.

McConnell, W. E. (1990). Orderly assessment. *Emergency, 22*(10), 34, 37–38.

Morrison, E. G. (1989). Nursing assessment: What do nurses want to know? *Western Journal of Nursing Research, 11*(4), 469–476.

Nursing (1984). Collecting and documenting patient data. *Nursing '84, 14*(3), 26, 28.

Reichert, A., & Conway, J. (1990). Assessment and diagnosis in one quick step. *RN, 53*(6), 30–31.

Smith, C. E. (1984). With good assessment skills you can conduct a solid framework for patient care. *Nursing '84, 14*(12), 26–31.

References

Alfaro, R. (1986). *Application of nursing process: A step-by-step guide.* Philadelphia: Lippincott.

Allen, P. (1986). Screening. In C. Edelman & C. L. Mandle (Eds.), *Health promotion throughout the lifespan.* St. Louis: Mosby.

American Nurse's Association (1973). *Standards of nursing practice.* Kansas City, MO: Author.

Anderson, E., & McFarlane, J. (1988). *Community as client application of the nursing process.* Philadelphia: Lippincott.

Christensen, P. (1986). Assessment: Data collection for the individual client. In J. Griffith-Kenney & P. Christensen (Eds.) *Nursing process: Application of theories, frameworks, and models.* St. Louis: Mosby.

Gordon, M. (1987). *Nursing diagnoses, process and application.* New York: McGraw-Hill.

Henry, J. (1973). *On shame, vulnerability and other forms of self-destruction.* New York: Vintage.

Hogstel, M. (1987). Teaching students observational skills. *Nursing Outlook 35*(2), 89–91.

Hughes, C., Blackburn, S., & Wargo, M. (1986). On masking among clients. *Topics in Clinical Nursing, 8*(1), 83–90.

Iyer, P., Taptich, B., & Bernocchi-Losey, D. (1986). *Nursing process and nursing diagnosis.* Philadelphia: Saunders.

King, R. C. (1983). Refining your assessment techniques. *RN, 46*, 43–47.

Matteson, M. A., & McConnell, E.S. (1988). *Gerontological nursing.* Philadelphia: Saunders.

Mausner, J., & Kramer, S. (1985). *Epidemiology—An introductory text.* Philadelphia: Saunders.

Pender, N. (1987). *Health promotion in nursing practice.* Norwalk, CT: Appleton and Lange.

Suitor, C., & Crowley, M. (1984). *Nutrition: Principles and applications in health promotion* (2nd Ed.). Philadelphia: Lippincott.

Valanis, B. (1986). *Epidemiology in nursing and health care.* Norwalk, CT: Appleton–Century–Crofts.

Wilson, T., & Jungner, G. (1968). *Principles and practice of screening for disease* (Public Health Paper No. 34). Geneva: World Health Organization.

4

Documentation: Reporting and Recording

OBJECTIVES

Upon completion of this chapter, you should be able to:

■ Delineate the purposes for documenting client information.

■ Compare and contrast the processes of reporting and recording, giving examples of reports and records that may be used to document client information.

■ Explain "charting by exception" and its advantages.

■ Describe the purpose(s), advantages, and disadvantages of the following types of records employed by health agencies to document client information:
1. Traditional health record
2. Problem-oriented record (POR)
3. Nursing assessment forms
4. Flow sheets
5. Computerized records

■ Delineate guidelines for effective reporting and recording:
1. Clarity and legibility
2. Accuracy, objectivity, and specificity
3. Conciseness
4. Completeness and currency
5. Organization and chronology
6. Confidentiality and privacy
7. Legality

■ Effectively report and record nursing assessment information.

Documenting the practice of nursing is an essential aspect of professional nursing care (Grier, 1984; Haller, 1987; Masson, 1990; Morrissey-Ross, 1988). In this age of cost containment, adequate documentation often is a critical factor in determining reimbursement of costs to health-care agencies. As the value of individual services provided to clients is analyzed by the payers for health services, nurses must make certain that their activities are recognized within the health-care industry as essential to achieving desired outcomes of client care. One effective way to achieve such recognition is the accurate and complete documentation of nursing care delivered to a particular client or group of clients. Nurses must assure that reporting and recording of information is accurate, thorough, up-to-date, concise, and done in a way that preserves client privacy and confidentiality.

Documentation is an important component of a complete nursing assessment. Documentation ensures that assessment information obtained from or about a client is communicated appropriately and, when indicated, recorded permanently. Recording may occur while the information is being gathered or after the actual assessment has been completed. The former is often true for information obtained in an interview, with the interviewer recording the client's responses as they are given. However, a summary of the interview may be recorded after it has taken place, with only brief notetaking during the actual interview. Typically, information obtained through clinical appraisal and screening is recorded after the nurse's direct contact with the client.

WHY DOCUMENT?

The delivery of comprehensive, high quality care depends on adequate reporting and recording of information about each client. One of the factors that inhibits careful and systematic documentation of nursing practice, including nursing assessments and diagnoses, is the value system in nursing that emphasizes doing and caring (Morrissey-Ross, 1988). The written documentation of those activities is less valued and often seen as time-consuming and interfering with nursing's "real work." As Morrissey-Ross (1988) notes, "Valuing hands-on care and, simultaneously, holding paperwork in a negative light . . . has led nurses . . . to fall into the trap of seeing charting as an adjunct activity rather than an integral part of care" (p. 364). Documentation requires time, commitment, and effort. Accurate, comprehensive, and timely documentation of nursing assessment data and nursing diagnoses, as

well as actual nursing care—planning, delivery, and outcomes—is important for a number of reasons.

The primary purpose for documenting client care is to communicate accurate and complete information about a client to members of the health team. All health professionals involved in the care of the client depend on an accurate, up-to-date, and comprehensive flow of information. The sharing of information by various members of the health team helps prevent gaps and overlaps in care and, thus, the possibility of serious errors. Information that is documented clearly in a client's record increases the likelihood that explanations and interpretations of the client's behaviors or responses are accurate. Furthermore, when information is documented so all health-care professionals have ready access, clients are less likely to be harassed by repetitious data collection.

In addition to making it easier to communicate information about a client to all members of the team, documentation of nursing care identifies the domain and scope of care for which the nurse is accountable, thus conveying to the client and other health professionals the nurse's various roles and responsibilities. When nurses fail to record their assessments or interventions, not only is important information omitted from the client's record, but nurses' contributions to the client's care and recovery are overlooked and their value diminished. As Masson (1990) points out, documentation may be "the only way to attract an audience and build a constituency for nursing" (p. 196), despite the fact that it is impossible to fully capture the essence of any nurse–client encounter on paper or in an oral report.

Accurate and comprehensive documentation plays an important role in assuring that standards of care are adhered to. Specifically, documentation provides information needed by health agencies to assure they meet accreditation standards and to maintain nursing practice standards. The Joint Commission on Accreditation of Healthcare Organizations (JCAHO) accreditation standards for nursing service include several related to documentation of nursing care (see JCAHO box). Also, the American Nurses Association (ANA) *Standards of Nursing Practice* (1973) reflect the importance accorded the reporting and recording of client data (see ANA box). The standards note that data pertaining to the client's health "must be available for all members of the health-care team." In addition to being accessible, the information also should be retrievable and confidential (ANA, 1973).

Documentation of information pertaining to a

client's care also ensures that health agencies are reimbursed for services delivered. Third-party reimbursement through Medicare, Medicaid, and private insurers depends on providing adequate documentation to assure that care billed has actually been delivered. The prospective payment system, which reimburses hospitals according to diagnostic related groups (DRGs), and stricter home care regulations about which services are covered by Medicare have resulted in increased demands for written justification of care as a basis for reimbursement (Morrissey-Ross, 1988; Omdahl, 1988).

Furthermore, documentation of client information also provides a rich data source for nursing research. Nurse-researchers may use client records to identify researchable nursing problems or to collect data for a particular study. For example, a nurse who wishes to determine which factors contribute to pain relief in a particular client population may wish to refer to client records to document the presence of pain, actions taken to alleviate the pain, and whether the actions achieved the desired outcomes. Without careful recording of this information, the researcher cannot retrieve the data needed for the study. Haller (1987) points out that systematic documentation of practices is essential

for describing clinical nursing phenomena in order to allow researchers to generate data that can be used to develop more complex and extensive clinical investigations. She suggests that more frequent use of standardized data collection forms, including questionnaires and rating scales, contributes to the development of clinical knowledge.

Of particular importance, given the litigious nature of today's society, is the documentation of care for legal purposes. Specifically, the written record ensures that client care is documented for legal purposes. A clear, legible account of care delivered to a particular client and the client's responses to that care affords a high degree of legal protection for the client, the health professionals involved, and the health agency. Written documentation of care serves as a permanent account and legal proof that the client received specific services.

REPORTING

A report is a written or oral relay of information about a client, usually between health professionals. A report provides an account of what is known and relevant about a client. Its primary purpose is to facilitate continuity of care by providing information that can assist in making appropriate decisions about the client's care.

Written reports usually are brief descriptions of specific findings or key information, such as reports of diagnostic tests. An example of a written report is a laboratory report of arterial blood gases. Such written reports usually become part of the client's permanent health record. Another example of a written report is the use of a central log that allows nurses to communicate information that otherwise might be overlooked. For instance, a client's spouse may tell the evening shift nurse that she wishes to be present for a discharge teaching session the next day and plans to visit her husband after lunch. By reporting this information in a central log or notebook, the day shift nurse can plan the teaching session for the spouse's visit. Information reported in a central log may or may not also be recorded in the client's permanent health record, depending on the nature of the information.

Oral reports are short accounts of assessment findings, particular interventions and outcomes, revisions in the plan of care, or a summary of a client's progress. Oral reports increase the efficiency of care providers by reducing the time needed to locate key information in a client's health record (Figure 4-1). The change-of-shift report or notifying the client's physician by telephone of a sudden change in the client's health are examples of oral reports. Consider the following oral report for its efficiency in communicating essential client information:

Tonya Simms is a seven-year-old black female who underwent tonsillectomy and adenoidectomy this morning. She returned to the unit at eleven-fifteen. Her vital signs are stable. Her blood pressure is one-oh-eight over sixty, pulse is ninety and regular, and respirations are twenty-four. Her temperature is ninety-nine point two. There is no evidence of bleeding from the surgical site. Her primary nursing diagnosis is "pain related to surgical incisions." She is taking and retaining sips of clear liquids, but says her throat is sore when she swallows. She has not cried, coughed, or vomited. An ice collar was applied in the recovery room and has just been refilled. Acetaminophen elixir five grains was

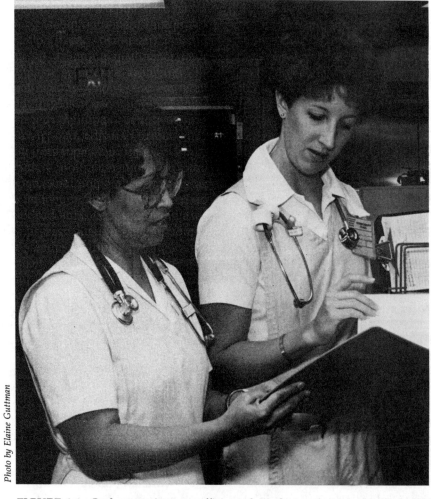

Photo by Elaine Guttman

FIGURE 4-1. Oral reports increase efficiency by reducing the time that would be needed to locate key information in the client's health record. (*Note.* From Servonsky/Opas: *Nursing Management of Children,* © 1987. Boston: Jones and Bartlett Publishers, p. 402.)

administered at two-ten p.m. She has rested, no complaints, since. She should be offered increased amounts of fluids and foods such as jello and popsicles. A clear liquid diet has been ordered for dinner.

When giving an oral report, the nurse must be careful to avoid disclosing information to (or within hearing distance of) people not directly involved in the care of the client. A casual or inappropriate remark made about a client creates potential legal liability for the nurse. It is also unethical to speak about clients in a gossipy or defamatory way when giving oral reports.

Reilly and Stengrevics (1989) recommend putting change-of-shift reports in writing. They note that oral reports are often time-consuming and inefficient. Written reports also minimize legal risks because there is less tendency to engage in casual or gossipy conversation about a client. Written change-of-shift reports have been found to increase staff efficiency and responsiveness to patients (Reilly & Stengrevics, 1989). The quality of nursing notes in the permanent health record also improved. Guidelines for giving oral reports upon change of shift or transfer of clients between units or health agencies are summarized in Table 4-1.

Reporting is an important activity in all types of health-care agencies. The frequency and type of reporting will vary among agencies and is determined by the nature of the client's contact with a particular agency. For example, in a hospital setting, oral and written reports are given frequently throughout the client's stay. On the other hand, a home health nurse may report information about a client to the client's primary care provider less frequently, such as weekly or monthly, depending on the frequency of contact and the client's health.

TABLE 4-1
Guidelines for Oral Reports

Provide essential biographical information for a client (name, age, gender, dates of admission/surgery/delivery, medical diagnosis).

Identify the client's primary nursing diagnoses.

Describe the client's status objectively, with emphasis on any significant changes since the last report. Avoid unsubstantiated or value-laden judgments.

Briefly review the client's plan of care, emphasizing priorities.

Explain any special interventions/treatments or the initiation of new interventions/treatments.

Describe the client's responses to nursing care or medical treatments.

Confirm that those receiving the report understand the information relayed.

RECORDING

Recording is the permanent documentation of a client's health status and progress. There are numerous types of written records used in today's health agencies to document client care. The most commonly used is the health record, sometimes referred to as the medical record or chart.

A client's health record is a permanent legal document containing all information pertinent to a client's health-care management within a particular system, such as a hospital, health department, clinic, physician's office, or home health agency. The written health record provides an ongoing account of the client's health and care and a means for health professionals to communicate and permanently record their assessment findings, diagnoses, plans of care, interventions, and outcomes of care.

Types of Records

The content and organization of health records vary among health agencies and reflect the nature of the agency (e.g., hospital, health department, or skilled nursing facility) and its particular mission (e.g., care-oriented or cure-oriented). Some agencies use an interdisciplinary health record in which all professionals involved in the client's care document their findings, actions, and outcomes in a central place in the record. Others use a traditional type of record, in which each group of health professionals records its information separately. Hospitals tend to employ a traditional record, which isolates medical information from that recorded by other health professionals.

Several of the more commonly used means of recording nursing assessment information about a client are reviewed in the following section. These include the traditional health record, the problem-oriented record, nursing assessment forms, flow sheets, and computerized records.

Traditional Health Record

The traditional health record organizes client information so that each health discipline has its own section or sections in which to record information. Thus, nursing assessment data, the nursing care plan, and narrative nursing notes are separated from the medical history, orders, and progress notes, and from information recorded by members of other health disciplines, such as clinical nutrition, physical therapy, pharmacy, and social services. The advantage of this type of health record is the ease with which information entered by a particular discipline can be located, so that the nursing care plan, the medical care plan, the nutritional plan, and so forth, are clearly identified. Its disadvantage is the possibility, even likelihood, that important information recorded by one professional that has implications for the client's total plan of care may be overlooked by others involved in that care. While nurses typically read the information entered in the client's record by physicians and other health professionals, it is not often that others avail themselves of the information contained in the nursing history or narrative notes.

The traditional health record usually contains the following specific categories of information:

Demographic data

Medical history and examination

Medical orders

Medical progress notes

Nursing assessment (history and clinical appraisal)

Nursing care plan (often kept in the nursing Kardex or a notebook until the client's discharge)

Flow sheets (vital signs, frequent assessments, other measurements)

Narrative nursing notes

Laboratory and other diagnostic reports

Consultation reports

Consent forms

Referrals

Discharge summaries (nursing, medicine, other professions)

The section of the health record that contains narrative nursing notes enables the nurse to describe the client's nursing care and specific responses or outcomes. This traditional format is essentially a log of events that occur during the client's contact with the health-care system. Events, such as information collected, care given, and client responses, are recorded within specific time periods that vary according to the client's health, type of health-care agency, and how significant the event is to the client's care and well-being. In acute care units, a nurse typically records notes about a client once every shift. However, when a client's health changes frequently, such as when a client is critically ill or in the immediate postoperative period, notes may be recorded as often as every hour and usually are supplemented with flow sheets to record frequently obtained measurements (e.g., vital signs or urine output) or frequently administered care (e.g., suctioning). In community-based settings, narrative nursing notes usually are recorded for each contact with the client, which may be weekly, monthly, or less often. A sample of a narrative nursing note is shown in Figure 4-2.

Problem-Oriented Record (POR)

The problem-oriented record (POR) is a structured format for recording client information that emphasizes problems and de-emphasizes the actions of health team members who provide the client's care (Vaughan-Wrobel & Henderson, 1986). POR allows for an interdisciplinary approach to recording because all health team members record their information in a single place and in central progress notes. POR also makes it easier to coordinate the client's care and minimizes the possibility of duplication of services or gaps. Communication among various members of the health team is assured because all use the central plan of care.

The problem-oriented method is similar to the nursing process (Gawlinski & Rasmussen, 1984). It consists of four major components: data base (assessment), problem list (nursing diagnoses), initial plan (goals), and progress notes (interventions and evaluation).

The data base contains all information obtained from or about the client, including history and clinical appraisal, as well as the results of diagnostic tests. The data base then is analyzed to identify problems, and a problem list is formulated. A problem denotes some aspect of the client's health that produces or threatens to produce functional disability, morbidity, or increased risk of mortality.

9/15/91

8:20 a.m. Client reports sharp, continuous abdominal pains for past 10 minutes. Cannot identify any precipitating factors. Lying on right side with legs drawn up. Holding abdomen with hands, and grimacing. Abdomen distended. Bowel sounds absent. Last bowel movement was pre-op. BP 130/92; P 90, regular & bounding; oral T. 99.2. F. N/G tube patent. Change of position to left side provides no relief. Dr. Mitchell notified. Rectal tube inserted. Demerol 50 mg. IM for pain.

N. Robbins, R.N.

8:35 a.m. Passing flatus via rectal tube. Abdomen less distended. Resting on left side in a relaxed posture. States he feels more comfortable, less "crampy." B/P 122/84; P 82, regular & full.

N. Robbins, R.N.

FIGURE 4-2. Sample Narrative Nursing Note.

Thus, the problem list may include diagnoses, either nursing or medical, that relate to physiological, psychosocial, developmental, spiritual, cultural, or environmental needs of the client. Problems are numbered sequentially in chronological order according to the date they are first identified. Each problem retains its original number, even when its priority in the client's plan of care changes. Written entries in the record are numbered according to the problem to which they refer. Once a problem is resolved, the date it is resolved is indicated and a line is drawn through the problem. The complete problem list, containing all active and resolved problems, is used as a table of contents or index to the client's record, which makes for easy retrieval of information.

Once the problem list has been formulated, an initial plan is developed. The initial plan incorporates diagnostic, therapeutic, and educational goals related to each of the problems. For example, a nursing diagnostic goal might state, "Make home visit to assess living facilities"; a therapeutic goal, "Change position every two hours"; and an educational goal, "Teach client to administer regular and NPH insulin." Nursing orders are included in the initial plan and should specify what interventions should be implemented, who is to perform the intervention, and when, or at what intervals, the intervention should occur.

The final portion of the POR includes the progress notes. Progress notes are used to describe changes in the client's condition and to record progress toward resolution of a particular problem. Separate progress notes are written for each problem, although not necessarily for every problem every time an entry is made in the client's POR. However, each time a problem is attended to, a progress note should be recorded for that problem.

The progress notes follow what is known as the SOAP format. SOAP is an acronym for subjective data, objective data, assessment, and plans. Some agencies use an expanded version of SOAP, called SOAPIER. The additional letters represent the implementation, evaluation, and revision of the plan of care. The type of information that should be included in each of these categories is summarized in Figure 4-3.

A modified format for progress notes is the PIE method (Buckley-Womack & Gidney, 1987; Siegrist, 1985). PIE is an acronym for problem, intervention, and evaluation. The PIE format unifies the nursing care plan and nursing notes in a single document and simplifies the documentation of nursing care. This method often is used for hospitalized clients for whom frequent recording of in-

formation is necessary. Daily assessment data are entered on flow sheets kept at the bedside and are not duplicated in the progress notes. A PIE note should be written at least once every 24 hours for each active problem. Sample SOAP and PIE notes are illustrated in Figure 4-4.

Nursing Assessment Forms

Nursing assessment forms are designed for efficient recording of information obtained from or about a client on which the plan of nursing care will be based. The particular format and length will vary with the client population, type of health agency, and the conceptual framework used for practice. A nursing assessment form, which also may be called a nursing admission form, is completed at the time of the client's initial contact with the health agency and focuses on information needed by the nurse to develop the client's nursing care plan. Data are analyzed to formulate nursing diagnoses or problems, which become the focus for developing nursing goals and interventions. The information obtained for the nursing assessment also provides a basis for comparing changes in the client's condition. For instance, while obtaining a nursing history on a 4-year-old child admitted to the hospital for eye surgery, the nurse learns (and records on the admission assessment form) that the child is not a bed-wetter. That night, the child wets the bed. The night nurse refers to the admission data and finds that this is not typical be-

---

S = *Subjective data:* information disclosed by the client or significant others; the client's perceptions, feelings, and life experiences.

O = *Objective data:* observable, measurable behaviors or events; factual information detected by the five senses or measured by instruments.

A = *Assessment:* analysis of subjective and objective data leading to identification of problems or diagnoses; conclusions or impressions of the client's health; clinical judgments.

P = *Plan:* plan of care written as client goals in three areas: diagnostic, therapeutic, educational.

I = *Implementation:* interventions made or actions taken to achieve client goals.

E = *Evaluation:* client's responses to interventions and measurable outcomes of care.

R = *Revision:* modifications in the plan of care based on the evaluation.

FIGURE 4-3. SOAPIER Progress Note Categories.

havior. This information is taken into account in planning the child's subsequent care.

Two formats for obtaining comprehensive nursing assessment data are illustrated in Tables 2-1 and 2-2. Most health-care agencies specify a particular format for recording nursing assessment information.

Flow Sheets

The development and use of flow sheets have made documentation a manageable task for the hospital nurse at bedside. Flow sheets allow the nurse to organize and conveniently and quickly record information in a systematic, standard fashion.

Flow sheets are used to record measurements or observations that must be documented frequently or repeatedly, such as vital signs, personal hygiene measures, intake and output of fluids, diet, activity, treatment measures, and so forth. These data are recorded in tables, graphs, and categories of information that relate to a specific client. Categories not applicable to a particular situation simply can be omitted.

Flow sheets show the client's progress in blocks of time and series of events. They reduce the possibility of error by making it possible to record information on the spot as assessments are made and care is given. Improvement or deterioration in the client's condition can be noted easily and quickly.

Nursing assessment flow sheets often are used for hospitalized clients to record assessment data obtained on a regular basis, such as daily, once each shift, or more frequently. Rather than recording the findings in narrative form, which can be time-consuming, an assessment flow sheet enables the nurse to record assessment data efficiently, concisely, and conveniently. Figure 4-5 illustrates a sample nursing assessment flow sheet.

Computerized Records

Computer technology has dramatically changed the way information is managed in our society. This is no less true for the creation, storage, and retrieval of information about the nursing care of clients in a variety of health-care settings. The widespread use of computers for managing client information requires the practicing nurse to be computer literate (Figure 4-6). Nearly all health-

---

SOAP Notes 10/19/91	PIE Notes 10/19/91
S: 50-year-old housewife with no children at home; states she leads a sedentary life; major daily activity is housework; reports diet with high amounts of refined CHO and fats; states she wants "to lose a few pounds"	P: 1. Altered nutrition: more than body requirements R/T excessive caloric, CHO, & fat intake 2. Activity intolerance r/t sedentary lifestyle
O: WF; ht 5'5" wt 178 lbs.; B/P 130/86, P 86, R 24; 3-minute step test recovery pulse 182; SOB during test	I: Instructed client re: diet and menu planning. Gave client Weight Watchers pamphlet & phone #. Discussed benefits of daily exercise and ways to motivate adherence to plan. Return appt. scheduled 11/23/90.
A: 1. Altered nutrition: more than body requirements R/T excessive caloric, CHO, & fat intake 2. Activity intolerance R/T sedentary lifestyle	E: Client able to explain diet. Planned 3 meals correctly. States she plans to get husband to take daily walks with her "since he needs to lose some weight, too" and this will motivate her to stick with the plan.
P: 1. Client will initiate 1,500 cal. ADA diet immediately. 2. Client will attend weekly Weight Watchers meeting. 3. Client will walk 1/2 mile daily and gradually increase to 2 miles daily by end of 30 days. 4. Client will lose 1–2 lbs./week until goal of 135 lbs. is achieved. 5. Client will achieve 3-min. step test recovery pulse of 150 within 60 days. 6. Client will return to clinic monthly for progress check.	S. Riggs, R.N.
S. Riggs, R.N.	

FIGURE 4-4. Sample SOAP and PIE Notes.

24 HOUR NURSING RECORD DATE_____

NEUROLOGICAL ASSESSMENT: Orientation _____

Level of Consciousness_____Pupils _____

Motor R_____L _____

Sensory R_____L _____

Other Observations _____

_____ ☐ No Problem

EMOTIONAL ASSESSMENT: _____

_____

EENT ASSESSMENT

Ears: Drainage R _____ L _____ Other _____

Eyes: Drainage R_____ L _____Other _____

Nose: _____

Mouth: Lesions_____ Other _____

_____ ☐ No Problem

CARDIOVASCULAR ASSESSMENT: Rhythm _____

Arterial Pulses (P-PRESENT A-ABSENT D-DOPPLER)

Radial R _____ L _____ Dorsalis Pedis R_____ L_____

Venous Temp: Warm Cool Cold Clammy Diaphoretic

VASCULAR CATHETER   SITE   APPEARANCE

_____   _____   _____

_____   _____   _____

_____   _____   _____

Edema _____

Other Observations _____

_____ ☐ No Problem

RESPIRATORY: No Distress SOB Labored

Cough: Productive Non-productive Absent

Breath Sounds: P-PRESENT A-ABSENT D-DIMINISHED

RALES _____

RHONCHI _____

WHEEZES_____

OTHER _____

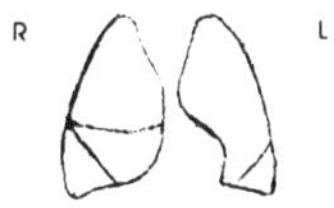

_____☐ No Problem

Airway: Oral Trach ETT (cuff/uncuffed) Nasal O$_2$_____

size _____appearance_____secretions _____

Vent _____ Settings _____

CHEST TUBES   SITE   DRAINAGE   SUCTION

_____   _____   _____   _____

_____   _____   _____   _____

_____   _____   _____   _____

H2O Seal_____ Fluctuations _____ Air Leak _____

GASTROINTESTINAL/ GENITOURINARY ASSESSMENT

Abdomen: Soft Firm Hard Distended _____cm Girth

Bowel Sounds: Normal Hypoactive Hyperactive Absent

NG Tube: SIZE _____ Suction Gravity Clamped

Dobhoff: Feedings _____ Clamped _____

DRAINS   TYPE   SITE   DRAINAGE CHARACTER

_____ _____ _____ _____

_____ _____ _____ _____

_____ _____ _____ _____

Urine: Color _____ Character _____ SP GR _____PH _____

Other_____ Continent Incontinent Condom Cath

Catheter: Size _____ Insertion Date _____ Δ Date _____

Fundus _____Perineum _____

Lochia_____ Breasts _____

Other Observations: _____

_____ ☐ No Problem

SKIN: Normal Pale Cyanotic Jaundice Warm
Cool Dry Moist Flushed Turgor _____

WOUND: SITE   APPEARANCE

_____   _____   _____

_____   _____   _____

_____   _____   _____

_____   _____   _____

Other Observations _____

_____ ☐ No Problem

MUSCULOSKELETAL:	R Arm	L Arm	R Leg	L Leg
Full ROM	_____	_____	_____	_____
Limited ROM	_____	_____	_____	_____
Weakness	_____	_____	_____	_____
Other	_____	_____	_____	_____

TRACTION/DRAIN/CAST: SITE   APPEARANCE

_____   _____   _____

_____   _____   _____

_____   _____   _____

Other Observations _____

_____ ☐ No Problem

SIGNATURE_____TIME _____

RN SIGNATURE_____TIME _____

TIME   RECORD EXCEPTIONS TO ASSESSMENT/INITIAL

_____

_____

_____

_____

_____

_____

_____

_____

_____

_____

_____

_____

_____

_____

_____

_____

_____

_____

_____

_____

_____

_____

_____

_____

_____

FIGURE 4-5. Nursing Assessment Flow Sheet. (*Note.* From Medical University Hospital, Medical University of South Carolina, Charleston, SC. Used with permission.)

CODE: A-NEEDS ASSISTANCE   D-DEPENDENT   I- INDEPENDENT   Date_____

	Activity	0700-1500	1500-2300	2300-0700
H Y G	Bath	I A D	I A D	I A D
	Mouth Care	I A D	I A D	I A D
	Skin care	I A D	I A D	I A D
A C T	Ambulate	I A D	I A D	I A D
	OOB -Chair	I A D	I A D	I A D
	Bedrest/BRP	I A D	I A D	I A D
	Turn/position	I A D	I A D	I A D
	ROM Joints	I A D	I A D	I A D
E L I M	Bathroom	I A D	I A D	I A D
	Bedpan/Urinal	I A D	I A D	I A D
	Catheter	I A D	I A D	I A D
	Ostomy Care	I A D	I A D	I A D
	Diaper Δ			

	Activity	0700-1500	1500-2300	2300-0700
P U L M	Tri Flo	I A D	I A D	I A D
	Deep Breathe	I A D	I A D	I A D
	Cough	I A D	I A D	I A D
	Suction	I A D	I A D	I A D
	Trach Care	I A D	I A D	I A D
S A F E T Y	Siderails Upper			
	Siderails Lower			
	Restraints Type			
	Release time			
I V C A R E	Site			
	Site			
	Site			
	Tubing Change	Yes No	Yes No	Yes No

	TIME	DESCRIPTION
D R S G		
T X		
O T H E R		

N U T R I T I O N	Breakfast I A D	Lunch I A D	Supper I A D
	Type		
	Amount		
	Supplement		

EVALUATION OF PATIENT PROBLEMS/STANDARDS

_____
_____
_____
_____
_____
_____
_____
_____
_____
_____
_____
_____
_____
_____
_____
_____
_____

FIGURE 4-5 (Continued).

care facilities now use computer systems to manage large amounts of complex information, such as laboratory and diagnostic tests, supply inventory and ordering, medication and dietary prescriptions and ordering, patient classification systems, quality assurance monitoring, staffing patterns, and client billing. Programs are available that allow the client's entire health record to be entered, stored, and revised as necessary.

Computer terminals permit data to be entered or retrieved from multiple stations within a health-care agency and even between health-care agencies. Data obtained from the nursing assessment can be entered in the computer and nursing diag-

Signature/Shift	Init.	Signature/Shift	Init.

DATE				WEIGHT			INTAKE						OUTPUT				
TIME	Temp	Pulse	Resp	B/P			Time	PO	IV				Urine	Stool			
							0800										
							0900										
							1000										
							1100										
							1200										
							1300										
							1400										
							1500										
							sub total										
							1600										
							1700										
							1800										
							1900										
							2000										
							2100										
							2200										
							2300										
							sub total										

Time	IV Fluid		Rate		Initial												
						2400											
						0100											
						0200											
						0300											
						0400											
						0500											
						0600											
						0700											
						sub total											
						TOTAL IN						TOTAL OUT					

FIGURE 4-5 (Continued).

noses generated. A computerized yet individualized nursing care plan then may be developed. Computerized records also may be used to record nursing progress notes and to develop discharge planning summaries. Experts project that by the year 2000, voice-activated and handheld computers that the nurse can speak into as information is obtained or as care is delivered will be commonplace (Nornhold, 1990).

The advantages of computerized records for recording and managing client and health-care system information are many. Computerized records

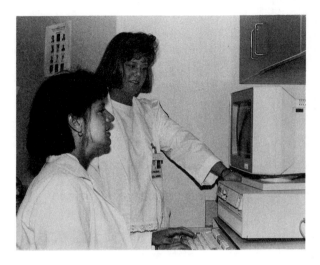

FIGURE 4-6. The widespread use of computers for managing information about clients requires the practicing nurse to be computer literate.

permit integration and ongoing management of client information. For example, once data from the initial assessment are entered, information may be retrieved easily on subsequent contacts with the client, thus eliminating duplication. Such information as demographic data, the client's health history, and previous contacts with health-care providers is readily available during each health visit or hospital admission. Moreover, this information serves as a basis against which current information about the client may be analyzed. Nornhold (1990) predicts that in the future clients will carry their complete health histories and diagnostic tests on laminated wallet-size cards that can be fed into a computer for data retrieval.

Computerized information systems for managing client data are more efficient than traditional, written records because the computer can quickly accept, store, and transmit client information. Once a nurse becomes proficient at using the computer, data can be entered and saved more rapidly than handwritten documentation. This is especially true if computer stations are available at or near where nurse–client contact takes place. Computerized data also can be retrieved more rapidly—within seconds—than data stored in a traditional, written health record.

Computerized records also can reduce errors in documentation. While computers are only as accurate as their users, client information programs typically are designed to reject improperly entered information. Spelling and grammatical errors can be detected and corrected automatically. Computerized information is also easy to read, thus eliminating the possibility of interpreting a handwritten entry, such as a physician's order or nursing progress note, erroneously. Bedside or handheld computers allow the nurse to enter data on the spot, thereby reducing the chance that important information will be forgotten and not recorded.

Perhaps most important, the efficiency of computerized records increases the amount of time available for nurse–client contact and thus enhances the direct delivery of professional nursing care. Computers free the nurse for the person-to-person, nonclerical aspects of nurse–client relationships and assure that clients receive the "high touch" care so essential in our increasingly high tech health-care system.

Charting by Exception

Charting by exception, developed by a group of Milwaukee nurses, is a shorthand method of documenting nursing assessment and interventions (Murphy & Burke, 1990). The practice has several advantages:

- Decreased time is spent charting findings and care
- Significant findings are easily pinpointed
- Pertinent information is entered immediately in the permanent health record
- Documentation is always current
- Standardized forms ensure consistency regardless of caregiver
- Duplication of information is eliminated

Charting by exception requires that clear standards of nursing practice are established and adhered to and flow sheets are used to document ongoing assessments and interventions. Documentation occurs at the hospital bedside, thus minimizing charting time and assuring greater accuracy. With this method, it is not necessary to document routine findings or care because it is assumed that the standards of care have been met unless noted otherwise. Also, findings of ongoing assessments are recorded only if changes have occurred since the previous assessment.

Charting by exception is most useful when documenting ongoing care of clients, particularly those in hospital or home care settings. This method does not take the place of fully documenting the findings of an initial, comprehensive client assessment, including nursing diagnoses.

GUIDELINES FOR EFFECTIVE REPORTING AND RECORDING

Documenting client information is an important part of the nursing assessment, and indeed the entire nursing process, yet too often it is done haphazardly or provides meaningless information. Notes that state, "Slept well," "Ate poorly," or "Refused bath" provide little information. What is mean by "well"? How long did the client sleep? How comfortably? Does the client perceive that her sleep was restful and does she feel ready to meet the challenges of the day?

Failure to report and record client information accurately, clearly, concisely, and objectively can compromise the quality of care. There are several important guidelines that, when followed, will assure that needed information is communicated in ways beneficial to the client, to caregivers, and to the health agency as well. Examples of appropriate and inappropriate documentation of client information that illustrate these guidelines is provided in Table 4-2.

Clarity and Legibility

Information about clients—assessment, care, and outcomes—must be communicated in a way that is readily understandable to all. Correct grammar and spelling are essential. Complete descriptive phrases should be used whenever possible. Slang ("Her recovery has been awesome"), colloquialisms ("He's a right good patient"), labels ("He sure is a mean cuss!"), and clichés ("It takes one to know one") are not appropriate in a written record or oral report.

Commonly accepted abbreviations and symbols can speed the recording process, but should be used carefully and written legibly to prevent misinterpretation. Uncommon or unacceptable abbreviations should be avoided. Most health-care agencies maintain a list of acceptable abbreviations for use in health records. Commonly accepted abbreviations and symbols widely used in the U.S. and Canada are shown in Table 4-3.

Written entries in the health record or on flow sheets should be recorded legibly so they can be read clearly and interpreted correctly by all. Anyone whose script is illegible should print, even if it is more time-consuming. Legibility of client health records offers legal protection for the client, the caregiver, and the health agency. A major advantage of computerized records is their consistent legibility, regardless of who is recording the information.

Accuracy, Objectivity, and Specificity

Information about clients must be accurate and should avoid subjective impressions or opinions. It is best to document objective information that has been obtained through one or more of the five senses or from specific measurements, such as vital signs or blood gases. Subjective information should be clearly identified as such. For example, clients' perceptions, which are important sources of assessment information, should be qualified in such terms as, "Client states he is having sharp pain in his left side," as opposed to, "Client is having sharp pain in his left side."

When recording or reporting, the nurse should avoid interpreting observations or measurements, or making assumptions, particularly when the information is incomplete. Instead of recording, "Client is depressed," the nurse should record the actual observations: "Client has refused to get out of bed today. Lying in bed, staring out the window. States he doesn't feel like eating."

Documentation also should be as specific as possible in order to minimize errors in interpretation. Terms such as "good," "normal," "poorly," "better," and "lengthy" should be avoided. Instead, the nurse should describe as specifically as

---

TABLE 4-2
Reporting and Recording: Appropriate and Inappropriate Examples

Appropriate:
Mother staying with child. Child resting quietly in croup tent. Respirations labored. Visible substernal and intercostal retractions. Frequent hoarse, nonproductive cough. Skin pale and damp. Shows no interest in playing when offered. Refuses fluids. IV infusing 40 ml/h. Mother says child's listlessness "scares" her—"He is usually into everything." Explained to her that child's behavior is typical of acute phase of croup and that his v.s. are stable. Mother says she's relieved.

Inappropriate:
IV is running okay with 180 mill. left to go. Mother is in the room with the child, who is tired and quiet. BP and TPR taken and are normal. Child doesn't want to drink anything. Breathing is poor with retractions. Child is in croup tent and seems to be fine. Mother is afraid of child's cough because it isn't like him. Sheets on bed changed and child's clothing changed.

What errors in documenting client information are illustrated by the *inappropriate* note?

TABLE 4-3
Commonly Accepted Abbreviations and Symbols

Abbreviations and Symbols	Definition	Abbreviations and Symbols	Definition
ā	before	CVP	central venous pressure
$A_1A_2A_3$, etc.	abortus	CXR	chest x-ray
abd.	abdomen	D/C	discontinue; discharge
A.B.G.	arterial blood gas	diff.	differential
ac	before meals	dl	deciliter (100 milliliters)
ACTH	adrenocorticotropic hormone	DNR	do not resuscitate
ADA diet	American Diabetes Association diet	DOA	dead on arrival
ADH	antidiuretic hormone	DOE	dyspnea on exertion
ADL	activities of daily living	DRG	diagnostic related group
ad lib	as desired	Dx.	diagnosis
AFDC	Aid to Families with Dependent Children	ECG or EKG	electrocardiogram
AIDS	acquired immune deficiency syndrome	EDC	estimated date of confinement (due date)
AMA	against medical advice	EEG	electroencephalogram
amt	amount	EENT	eye, ear, nose, and throat
A&O x3	alert and oriented to person, place, and time	EMS	emergency medical service
		ER	emergency room
A/P	anterior/posterior	ESR	erythrocyte sedimentation rate
ARC	AIDS-related complex	ET or ETT	endotracheal tube
ARM (AROM)	artificial rupture of membranes	ETOH	ethyl alcohol
ASA	aspirin	F.	Fahrenheit
ASAP	as soon as possible	FBS	fasting blood sugar
AV	atrioventricular	Fe	iron
A&W	alive and well	FH	family history
ax	axillary	FHT	fetal heart tones
Ba	barium	FSH	follicle-stimulating hormone
BCP	birth control pills	F/U	follow up
BF	black female	FUO	fever of undetermined origin
b.i.d.	twice a day	Fx.	fracture
BM	black male	$G_1G_2G_3$, etc.	primigravida, secundigravida, etc.
B.M.	bowel movement	GI	gastrointestinal
BMI	body mass index	gm	gram
B/P	blood pressure	$G_XP_XA_X$	gravida, para, aborta
BR	bedrest	gr.	grain
BRP	bathroom privileges	gtt.	drop(s)
BS	bowel sounds/breath sounds	GTT	glucose tolerance test
B.S.A.	body surface area	GU	genitourinary
BSE	breast self-examination	Gyn	gynecology
BTL	bilateral tubal ligation	h	hour
BUN	blood urea nitrogen	HA	headache
Bx	biopsy	H.C.	head circumference
c̄	with	HCG	human chorionic gonadotropin
C.	centigrade	Hct.	hematocrit
$C_1C_2C_3$, etc.	first cervical vertebra, second, etc.	HEENT	head, ears, eyes, nose, and throat
Ca	cancer, carcinoma	Hgb (Hg)	hemoglobin
cap	capillary	HIV	human immunodeficiency virus
CAT or CT	computerized axial tomography	HOB	head of bed
C&S	culture and sensitivity	H&P	history and physical
CBC	complete blood count	h.s.	at bedtime
cc	cubic centimeter	ht	height
CC	chief complaint	Hx.	history
CCU	coronary care unit/critical care unit	IgA	immunoglobulin A
CHO	carbohydrate(s)	ICP	intracranial pressure
cm.	centimeter	ICS	intercostal space
CNS	central nervous system	ICU	intensive care unit
c/o	complaining of	IgG	immunoglobin G
CO_2	carbon dioxide	IgM	immunoglobin M
CPR	cardiopulmonary resuscitation	IM	intramuscular
CSF	cerebrospinal fluid	I&O or I/O	intake and output
CT Scan	computerized tomography scan	IPPB	intermittent positive pressure breathing
CVA	costovertebral angle, cerebrovascular accident	IT	intrathecal
		IU	international unit

TABLE 4-3 (Continued)

Abbreviations and Symbols	Definition	Abbreviations and Symbols	Definition
IUD	intrauterine device	P&PD	percussion and postural drainage
IV	intravenous	PO_2	O_2 pressure (arterial blood)
IVP	intravenous pyelogram	POR	problem-oriented record
K+	potassium	PMI	point of maximal impulse
KCl	potassium chloride	post-op	after operation
Kg.	kilogram	pre-op	before operation
KVO	keep vein open	PRM (PROM)	premature rupture of membranes
L.	liter	PRN	as needed
$L_1L_2L_3$, etc.	first lumbar vertebra, second, etc.	pt.	patient
lb.	pound	P.T.	physical therapy
LGA	large for gestational age	PTA	prior to admission
LH	luteinizing hormone	q.	every
liq.	liquid	qd	every day
LLQ	left lower quadrant	q.i.d.	four times a day
LMD	local medical doctor	qh	every hour
LMP	last menstrual period	q2h	every 2 hours
LP	lumbar puncture	q4h	every 4 hours
Lt	left	qhs	every night before bedtime
LUQ	left upper quadrant	qod	every other day
MAP	mean arterial pressure	qt.	quart
mcg	microgram	R	respiration, rectal
mEq	milliequivalents	RBC	red blood cells
mg.	milligram	Rh	Rhesus blood factor
ml	milliliter(s)	RLQ	right lower quadrant
ml/kg	milliliter per kilogram	R/O	rule out
mm	millimeter(s)	ROM	range of motion
mod	moderate	ROS	review of systems
MOM	Milk of Magnesia	r/t	related to
MVA	motor vehicle accident	R.T.	respiratory therapy
Na	sodium	Rt	right
NaCl	sodium chloride	RUQ	right upper quadrant
NAD	no apparent distress	R_x	prescription, treatment
N/G	nasogastric	$\bar{s}$	without
NPO	nothing by mouth	SA	sinoatrial
NS	normal saline	S&A	sugar and acetone (urine)
NT	nasotracheal	SGA	small for gestational age
N/V or N&V	nausea/vomiting	SH	social history
O_2	oxygen	SOB	shortness of breath
OB	obstetrics	S/P	status post
o.d.	right eye	sp. gr.	specific gravity
OOB	out of bed	SQ	subcutaneous
O&P	ova and parasites	SRM (SROM)	spontaneous rupture of membranes
OPD	outpatient department	SSE	soap suds enema
OR	operating room	stat	immediately
o.s.	left eye	STD	sexually transmitted disease
O.T.	occupational therapy	sx	symptom
OTC	over the counter	T	temperature, tablespoon
o.u.	both eyes	$T_1T_2T_3$, etc.	thoracic vertebrae 1, 2, 3, etc.
oz	ounce	tab	tablet
$\bar{p}$	after	tbsp	tablespoonful
P	pulse	t.i.d.	three times a day
$P_1P_2P_3$, etc.	primipara, secundipara, etc.	TLC	total lung capacity
PA	physician assistant	TPN	total parenteral nutrition
pc	after meals	TPR	temperature, pulse, respiration
PCA	patient-controlled analgesia	TSE	testicular self-examination
PCO_2	partial CO_2 pressure (arterial blood)	tsp	teaspoonful
PE	physical examination	UA	urinalysis
PEEP	positive end expiratory pressure	VC	vital capacity (lung)
PERLA	pupils equal and reactive to light and accommodation	VD	venereal disease
		vol.	volume
pH	hydrogen-ion concentration	vs	vital signs
PI	present illness	WBC	white blood count

(continued)

TABLE 4-3 (Continued)

Abbreviations and Symbols	Definition	Abbreviations and Symbols	Definition
w/c	wheelchair	wt	weight
WF	white female	x̄	except for
WM	white male	y.o.	year old
WNL	within normal limits	♂	male
WNWD	well-nourished, well-developed	♀	female

possible the client's behavior or findings. For example, instead of noting the findings of a developmental assessment as "normal," the nurse should report or record the information as "demonstrated age-appropriate abilities in all areas."

Accuracy of recorded information is essential to ensure the legal soundness of the health record. Guidelines related to the legality of documentation are addressed later in this section.

Conciseness

Data should be reported or recorded succinctly. Concise, efficient recording and reporting eliminates irrelevant or unnecessary words and details. Lengthy documentation is inefficient, cumbersome, and often difficult to extract important information from. Furthermore, it is unlikely to be read or listened to by other health team members, with potentially detrimental consequences for the client. However, notes or reports that are too brief may fail to communicate information essential for safe, effective client care or may give the impression that care was incomplete or rushed.

Completeness and Currency

Effective reporting or recording provides enough information to ensure that what is known about a client is complete and up to date. Whether referring to assessment information, nursing diagnoses, the plan of care, or client outcomes, documentation should thoroughly describe the information or client behaviors. For instance, if the client is complaining of abdominal discomfort, the nurse should ascertain and report and record a complete description, including onset, location, severity, precipitating factors, frequency, duration, and factors that aggravate or alleviate the discomfort. When recording an apical pulse, the rate, rhythm, and quality should be noted. Nursing interventions, such as teaching a client or changing a dressing, and the client's response should be fully described.

When assessment data or nursing interventions are not recorded or reported in a timely fashion, the client's care may be compromised. This is particularly true when subsequent judgments or actions depend on all that is known about the client. If such judgments or actions are based on missing information, they can lead to serious errors in care. When changes in a client's condition are not communicated promptly, delays in initiating therapy can occur, sometimes with life-threatening consequences. When a nurse fails to document assessment information that indicates a client lacks knowledge about prescribed medications prior to discharge from the hospital, the client may inadvertently omit a dosage or take more than prescribed.

Organization and Chronology

Documentation of client information should occur in a logical, organized manner. Related information should be clustered together rather than scattered in different parts of the record or reported haphazardly. Also, information should be reported or recorded in orderly sequence so that it flows logically and is easy to follow and comprehend. Moreover, information should be documented as it occurs, in chronological order. For example, a client is experiencing pain. The nurse should record the assessment of the client's pain (objective and subjective data), interventions to relieve the pain, and outcomes—in that order.

Confidentiality and Privacy

The concepts of confidentiality and privacy are of growing concern in this era of computerization. The existence of massive amounts of information about clients is juxtaposed with the problems of disseminating it to appropriate people or agencies while protecting the client's fundamental right to privacy. Superimposed on this complex picture are clients' rights of access to their health records.

Information reported or recorded about a client is considered confidential between the client and the health professionals who provide care. Confidentiality refers to "an express or implied agreement that [health professionals] will not disclose the information received from the [client] to anyone not directly involved in the [client's] care" (Annas, Glantz, & Katz, 1981, p. 171). Nurses, as moral agents, are legally and ethically obliged to adhere to this standard of confidentiality. Thus, a nurse may not disclose to any unauthorized person information about clients or their care. This rule applies to formal releases of information as well as informal disclosures, such as talking about a client in a public place.

Nurses and other health professionals are obligated to safeguard a client's right to privacy and to prevent the release of information unless the client consents to its release, the law requires or allows its release (e.g., health statistics, lawsuits), or the client poses a serious threat to a known third person(s) (Annas et al., 1981). Releasing information that is not disclosed in good faith or with authorization from the client may subject health professionals and health agencies to liability.

Legality

Reports and records are legal documents containing confidential information about clients. Although some health-care professionals may view detailed records as a potential source of liability, the converse is true. An objective, legible, and intelligent account of a client's experience in a health-care setting affords a high degree of protection for the client, the nurse, other health professionals, and the agency. The client's record is a permanent account of care delivered and legal proof that specific services were rendered.

The legal significance of health records is not limited to their use as evidence during malpractice litigation. A well-written record enhances the caregiver's credibility, whereas an incomplete, altered, or misleading record compromises credibility. Courts and juries are likely to regard inconsistencies or omissions in records with suspicion.

There are many other situations in which the medical–legal aspect of client records will be critical to the outcome of a legal action, including: personal injury cases, insurance claims for client reimbursement, workers' compensation cases, will–probate cases in which the client's capacity to execute a will is at issue, and criminal cases in which the victim is injured or dies or in which the criminal defendant's competency is in question.

There are a few instances in which all or part of a health record may be excluded from evidence in a trial, as when the communications in the record are considered privileged. However, client records generally are viewed by the law as competent evidence, provided the information is recorded reasonably concurrently with events, and is not recorded solely in anticipation of a particular legal proceeding.

Standards of Health Records

The standard to be maintained in a health record will be determined primarily by each state's laws and regulations and generally will vary among different health agencies. In general, all client records must comply with prescribed statutes and agency policies. Additionally, hospitals that are accredited by the JCAHO must comply with JCAHO requirements for the content of hospital records. Failure to meet JCAHO standards may result in loss or denial of accreditation by the JCAHO, loss or denial of state licensure, or liability for negligence.

Content of Health Records

Who Should Record. Although there is no universally used or legally dictated system for documentation in health records, documentation is clearly a duty within the realm of nursing practice. For a period of time, nurses' notes were routinely discarded or not considered as competent evidence in legal proceedings. Modern courts, however, recognize nurses' records and impose on nurses the duty of keeping them accurately.

Some institutions employ the practice of proxy charting, in which ancillary personnel are given responsibility for charting all client care, including medications, while signing the name of the person who actually administered the care. This practice is unacceptable for several reasons. First, an unusual occurrence may go unrecorded because the proxy recorder is unable to make the sophisticated judgments required for professional assessments. Also, only the person who actually administers a treatment or medication should chart the occurrence. The only time that signing another's name to a client's record is acceptable is in a situation in which the second person supervises tasks and client care. For example, an R.N. may record nursing care given by an L.P.N. or nursing assistant who works directly under the R.N.'s supervision. Or, an R.N. may cosign an entry written by an L.P.N. or assistant. However, a signature or cosignature carries with it the legal presumption that the (co)signer is accountable for the entry.

What Should Be Recorded. The nurse's account of client care should include routine care, clinical observations, pertinent laboratory data, any change in condition or complaint of the client, treatments and medications administered and the client's responses to them, and health teaching and level of client understanding. Nurses' notes also should document instances of summoning physicians or other health professionals, response to the call, and deviations or omissions from normal procedure or treatment with a full explanation of such.

All entries in the client's health record should indicate the date and time of the event being recorded. Care never should be recorded before it actually is given. If a significant time lapse occurs before an observation or event can be recorded, the actual time a nursing action was carried out or a client's response was noted should be identified. Time should be recorded as a.m. or p.m., or in 24-hour military time.

The reporting of client behavior that may have legal significance (e.g., alcohol or drug intoxication) should focus on clinical observations and facts. Instead of speculations about a client's intoxication, only factual information such as poor motor coordination, slurred speech, or bloodshot eyes, should be recorded. This method of documentation not only allows the nurse to make a valuable clinical assessment but also serves to protect against a potential claim of defamation by a client.

How Data Should Be Recorded. Health records always should be written in indelible ink. Any institutional policy that allows for or encourages rewriting, obliteration of errors, or removal of entries is legally unsound. Correction of errors should be done so that the original entry is identified as an error but is left intact in the record. A commonly used and acceptable method for correcting errors in health records is to draw a single line through the erroneous entry, indicate that it is an error, and initial the entry (Feutz-Harter, 1989). The correct entry should then follow directly. As stated earlier, courts may look upon the concealment of an error or pages missing from a record as an attempted cover-up or as evidence of negligence.

Similarly, addenda to a record may be appropriate should a nurse realize that an important piece of information was omitted originally. The addendum may be out of chronological order but should be entered in the next available blank space in the record. The entry should be headed "Addendum of nurses' notes of (month, day, year, time)." The date and time the nurse entered the addendum also should be noted.

Each new entry should begin on a new line, and lines should be used consecutively to avoid the appearance of gaps in care. A straight line should be drawn through any space that remains on a line

at the end of an entry, following the nurse's initials or signature.

Ownership of Health Records

The general rule concerning ownership of health records is that the record is the physical property of the agency, whereas the information contained therein belongs to the client (Annas et al., 1981). Although there has been a recent trend toward increasing the access of clients to their health records, the procedure still is generally a matter of state law or judicial decision. Additionally, all states provide clients with access to their records in the event of litigation.

Concerns that access to records may harm the client generally are unfounded. Research indicates that the opposite is true; clients who are informed are less anxious about their conditions (Annas et al., 1981). Although family members often desire access to a client's record, in no state do they have the legal right to view it without the client's authorization, unless the client is a minor, in which case the parent or legal guardian may have access.

Clearly, reports and records are considered important evidence in malpractice and negligence cases related to client care. Although this factor should not be the sole motivation for systematic documentation, it does emphasize the importance of being accurate and comprehensive when recording and reporting information about a client.

Chapter Highlights

■ Documenting the practice of nursing, including the nursing assessment and nursing diagnoses, is an essential aspect of professional nursing care.

■ Accurate, comprehensive, and timely documentation of information facilitates coordination and continuity of a client's care, maintains standards required for accreditation, ensures reimbursement for services, provides research data, and affords legal protection for the client, the caregiver, and the health agency.

■ Reporting involves written or oral relay of information about what is known and relevant about a client.

■ Recording is the permanent documentation of a client's health and progress.

■ The content and organization of health records vary among health agencies. Commonly used types of records include the traditional health record, the problem-oriented record (POR), nursing assessment forms, flow sheets, and computerized records.

■ Guidelines for determining the effectiveness of documentation include: clarity, legibility, accuracy, objectivity, specificity, conciseness, completeness, currency, organization, chronology, confidentiality, privacy, and legality.

Practice Activities

1. Observe a change-of-shift report and evaluate the process to determine if the following qualities are reflected: clarity, accuracy, objectivity, specificity, conciseness, completeness, currency, organization, chronology, confidentiality, privacy, and legality.

2. Review nursing notes in a traditional health record or nursing progress notes in a problem-oriented record to determine if the above qualities (plus legibility) are followed. Which are not reflected? Suggest revisions in the notes to increase their effectiveness (according to the above guidelines).

3. Review the health record of a client for whom you are caring in a health agency. Which format is used to record nursing assessment data and nursing care? Which abbreviations are used? Are they acceptable within that health agency?

4. Document the findings of a complete nursing assessment. Exchange your recorded data with one a colleague or classmate has done. Critique each other's documentation, using the guidelines delineated in this chapter for effective recording.

5. Role-play one of the following situations in which an oral report must be given:
   a. A change-of-shift report on a nursing unit.
   b. A report about a client who is being transferred from one nursing unit to another, such as the postanesthesia room to a general hospital unit.
   c. A telephone report to a home health nurse about a client who is being discharged from the hospital.

6. What computerized records are used in your local health agencies? What types of client data are managed by the various computerized information systems? What are some other ways computers can enhance the efficiency and effectiveness of documenting client information?

Recommended Readings

Bergerson, S.R. (1988). Charting with a jury in mind. *Nursing88, 18*(4), 51–56.

Buckley-Womack, C., & Gidney, B. (1987). A new dimension in documentation: The PIE method. *Journal of Neuroscience Nursing, 19,* 256–260.

Feutz-Harter, S. (1989). Documentation principals and pitfalls. *Journal of Nursing Administration, 19*(12), 7–9.

Halloran, E.J. (1988). Computerized nursing assessments. *Nursing and Health Care, 9,* 497–499.

Morrissey-Ross, M. (1988). Documentation: If you haven't written it, you haven't done it. *Nursing Clinics of North America, 23,* 363–371.

Murphy, J., & Burke, L.J. (1990). Charting by exception. *Nursing90, 20,* 65–67.

Reiley, P.J., & Stengrevics, S.S. (1989). Change-of-shift report: Put it in writing! *Nursing Management, 20*(9), 54–56.

Rich, P.L. (1987). Make the most of your charting time. *Nursing87, 17*(5), 68–73.

Richard, J.A. (1988). Congruence between intershift reports and patients' actual conditions. *Image: Journal of Nursing Scholarship, 20*(1), 4–6.

Tapp, R.A. (1990). Inhibitors and facilitators to documentation of nursing practice. *Western Journal of Nursing Research, 12,* 229–240.

References

American Nurses' Association. (1973). *Standards of nursing practice.* Kansas City: Author.

Annas, G.J., Glantz, L.H., & Katz, B.F. (1981). *Rights of doctors, nurses, and allied health professionals.* Cambridge, MA: Ballinger.

Buckley-Womack, C., & Gidney, B. (1987). A new dimension in documentation: The PIE method. *Journal of Neuroscience Nursing, 19,* 256–260.

Feutz-Harter, S. (1989). Documentation principles and pitfalls. *Journal of Nursing Administration, 19*(12), 7–9.

Gawlinski, A. & Rasmussen, S. (1984). Improving documentation through the use of change theory. *Critical Care Focus, 11,* 12–15.

Grier, M.R. (1984). Information processing in nursing practice. In H.H. Werley & J.J. Fitzpatrick (Eds.), *Annual review of nursing research* (vol. 2, pp. 265–287). New York: Springer.

Haller, K.B. (1987). Systematic documentation of practice. *MCN: The American Journal of Maternal-Child Nursing, 12,* 152.

Joint Commission on Accreditation of Healthcare Organizations. (1991). *Accreditation manual for hospitals.* Chicago: Author.

Masson, V. (1990). Nursing the charts. *Nursing and Health Care, 38,* 196.

Morrissey-Ross, M. (1988). Documentation: If you haven't written it, you haven't done it. *Nursing Clinics of North America, 23*(2), 363–371.

Murphy, J., & Burke, L.J. (1990). Charting by exception. *Nursing90, 20*(5), 65–67.

Nornhold, P. (1990). 90 predictions for the '90s. *Nursing90,* 35–41.

Omdahl, D.J. (1988). Changes in Medicare home care forms. *American Journal of Nursing, 88,* 487–489.

Reiley, P.J., & Stengrevics, S.S. (1989). Change-of-shift report: Put it in writing! *Nursing Management, 20*(9), 54–56.

Siegrist, L.M. (1985). The PIE system: Complete planning and documentation of nursing care. *Quality Review Bulletin, 11,* 15–18.

Vaughan-Wrobel, B.D., & Henderson, B.S. (1986). *The problem-oriented system in nursing* (3rd ed.). St. Louis: Mosby.

5

Nursing Diagnosis: Analysis and Synthesis of Assessment Data

CHAPTER OUTLINE

- ▪ Key Concepts
  Analysis of Data   Synthesis of Data
  Diagnostic Reasoning   Clinical Judgment
- ▪ Diagnostic Reasoning Process
  Variables That Influence Diagnostic
  Reasoning   Identifying Cues   Clustering
  Cues   Inferencing and Activating Hypotheses
  Validating Hypotheses   Evaluating
  Hypotheses and Choosing From Alternatives
  Avoiding Diagnostic Errors   Clinical Intuition
  and Diagnostic Reasoning

OBJECTIVES

Upon completion of this chapter, you should be able to:

▪ Differentiate the process and outcome phases of nursing diagnosis, the second step in the nursing process.

▪ Explain factors that have inhibited the development of nurses' diagnostic reasoning abilities.

▪ Define the following key concepts: data analysis, data synthesis, diagnostic reasoning, and clinical judgment.

▪ Explain variables among diagnosticians and environments that influence the diagnostic reasoning process, giving examples of each.

▪ Delineate the phases of the diagnostic reasoning process: identifying cues, clustering cues, inferencing and activating hypotheses, validating hypotheses, and evaluating hypotheses and choosing from alternatives.

▪ Differentiate the diagnostic reasoning abilities of novice and expert nurses.

▪ Suggest ways to avoid diagnostic errors and improve accuracy.

▪ Delineate the role of intuition in the diagnostic reasoning process.

Information collected during the assessment phase of the nursing process is of little value to the nurse or the client unless it is used to make clinical judgments, enhance decision-making, and ultimately, improve client outcomes. Unfortunately, comprehensive information about clients often is obtained only to remain unused on the nursing care plan, in the client's health record, or worse, in the nurse's head. Nurses have a professional, moral, and legal responsibility to make use of the information collected from or about a particular client in order to identify and help resolve the client's health problems or concerns.

After sufficient information has been obtained, the nurse moves to the second phase of the nursing process: nursing diagnosis. This phase consists of two components: data analysis and synthesis, and the formulation of nursing diagnoses for each client. Data analysis and synthesis means reviewing the information critically, analyzing it, and interpreting it. Impressions or conclusions about a client's health and responses to changes in health are formulated. The second component of the diagnosis phase is the identification of one or more nursing diagnoses, or diagnostic statements. A nursing diagnostic statement specifies a problem or the client's response to the problem, including the factors that contribute to the problem/response. Once formulated, nursing diagnoses provide the central focus for nursing care planning.

This chapter focuses on nursing diagnosis as a process involving the analysis and synthesis of data into meaningful patterns. This process has been referred to in the literature as clinical inferencing, diagnostic reasoning, or clinical judgment (Carnevali, 1984; Gordon, 1987; Westfall, Tanner, Putzier, & Padrick, 1986). Thus, the process of nursing diagnosis is an intellectual activity in which the nurse engages to draw conclusions about a client's health or concerns.

Nursing diagnosis is also a product or outcome of the diagnostic process. In this sense, nursing diagnosis is a label for specifying clients' problems and their contributing factors. Nursing diagnosis as the end result of the diagnostic reasoning process is considered in the next chapter. Keep in mind that the separation of nursing diagnosis into diagnostic reasoning and labeling is somewhat artificial (Gordon, 1987). These components are interrelated and overlapping, not discrete, sequential steps. As information is gathered, the nurse continually processes it, trying to fit the many pieces together, and begins to develop preliminary diagnoses of the client's problems. This process often leads the nurse to pursue new or different lines of questioning or data-gathering in order to confirm or rule out various nursing diagnoses. In other words, gathering information does not proceed in linear fashion but in a circular system of feedback and modification to narrow the range of possible explanations or diagnoses. For learning purposes, however, the two components of nursing diagnosis—process and outcome—are considered individually in this and the next chapter to enable thorough study and understanding of each. Understanding enables the nurse to integrate the components for application to clinical practice.

The effectiveness and efficiency of nursing care planning and the achievement of desired outcomes depend on the accurate identification of a client's concerns and problems. The nurse's ability to analyze and synthesize the information obtained from the nursing assessment is the crucial element. The importance of making accurate, valid, and effective clinical judgments cannot be overstated. Failure to pay attention to important pieces of information or to interpret them accurately can compromise the quality of nursing care and, in some cases, lead to life-threatening consequences for clients.

The process of analyzing and synthesizing clinical information is one of reflection and critical thinking. As such, it takes place largely in the nurse's head. Interpretation of nursing assessment data involves mental operations in which the nurse's memory is searched for relevant information in order to connect the various cues in meaningful ways. Interpretation is by and large unseen and traditionally has not been associated with the practice of nursing.

Historically, nursing practice has been characterized by highly visible activity (doing), with primary emphasis on carrying out delegated tasks related to the medical treatment plan (Carnevali, 1984). Until recently, diagnostic reasoning was not considered a necessary skill for nurses nor was it highly valued. Carnevali (1984) notes that this belief "delayed recognition of the distinct perspective from which nurses view phenomena and the areas of expertise in which they were diagnosing implicitly and effectively" (p. 11).

Despite the long-held belief that diagnosis belonged exclusively within the domain of medicine and that nurses did not, could not, or should not diagnose, nurses have, in fact, engaged in diagnostic reasoning for years, probably since Florence Nightingale's time. Only within the last 25 years has the process of nursing diagnosis been recognized explicitly as an essential function of professional nursing practice. We now know that nurses do indeed interpret client information, make clinical judgments about it, and act on the basis of those judgments.

Even today, however, variables within nursing education and nursing practice often inhibit the full development and appreciation of the diagnostic reasoning abilities of nurses and by nurses. For example, heavy workloads in clinical practice diminish the time available for gathering comprehensive information and for critical reflection about its meaning. In nursing education, a great deal of time and energy typically is devoted to designing learning activities related to nursing assessment and diagnosis, yet students rarely are taught how "to make the transition from . . . huge case analyses that demonstrate and foster critical observation and thinking to the rapid, unverbalized thinking and concise, cohesive diagnostic statements that must be the reality in the hectic world of practice" (Carnevali, 1984, p. 16). To develop their diagnostic reasoning abilities, students need time to reflect on the information gathered and to consider a variety of meanings, with assistance from expert nurses or teachers, as a prelude to actual practice situations.

Critical differences exist between beginning and experienced nurses in their abilities to obtain and interpret data and to make valid nursing diag-

noses. Several authors (Benner, 1984; Benner & Wrubel, 1982; Tanner, 1984a) have studied the differences in diagnostic reasoning abilities of novice and expert nurses. The limited knowledge and experiences of novice nurses often lead them to assign inaccurate meanings to cues or to make diagnostic errors. Table 5-1 illustrates these differences.

Students who are novices or advanced beginners cannot be expected to exhibit the high level diagnostic skill that characterizes expert nursing practice. Such skill is acquired as the nurse's knowledge and range of practice experience are expanded. Beginning practitioners need multiple opportunities to observe and interact with experienced nurses as they assess and diagnose. Such mentoring and role modeling for novice nurses is critical if they are to develop and refine their assessment and diagnostic reasoning abilities.

KEY CONCEPTS

Several key concepts provide a framework for understanding the process by which clinical information is interpreted and nursing diagnoses are formulated. These concepts include analysis and

TABLE 5-1
Differences in Diagnostic Reasoning Ability of Novice and Expert Nurses

Factor	Novice	Expert
Perception of cues	May not recognize probable relationship between cues and diagnosis	Recognizes fallibility of cues as indicators of diagnosis
	Observations and inferences are treated equally	Seeks multiple, dependable, and redundant cues to make inferences
	Once probable relationship is recognized, may seek only highly dependable data.	Weighs risk to client before seeking more dependable data
	Little tolerance for uncertainty in diagnosis	High tolerance for uncertainty
Use of experience	Little range and depth of experience	Wide range and greater depth of experience
	Limited experience is used to assign probabilities; chance for bias is great	Experiential sample is more likely to be adequate, reducing chance for bias
Long-term memory	Categories and subcategories are formed but are limited in number and capacity	Hierarchical organization of categories and subcategories to draw upon
	Linkages among categories are few	Complex network of linkages among categories
	Single cues associated with diagnostic categories	Multiple cues and cue patterns cross-referenced to multiple diagnostic categories
	Retrieval often in form of memorized lists triggered by a category label	Retrieval demonstrates complex network, triggered by category label, subcategory cue, or cue pattern (including risk factors as well as actual manifestations)

Note. Adapted from "Factors influencing the diagnostic process" by C.A. Tanner, 1984. In D.L. Carnevali, P.H. Mitchell, N.F. Woods, & C.A. Tanner. *Diagnostic Reasoning in Nursing*, pp. 78–79. Philadelphia: Lippincott. Used with permission.

synthesis of data, diagnostic reasoning, and clinical judgment.

Analysis of Data

Once information has been gathered, the nurse proceeds to analyze all of it. Analysis involves an examination of the various elements of information and how they are related. Analysis also helps to identify missing elements. Consider these essential pieces of information and their relationships:

> Mr. Bell is a 71-year-old white male admitted to the hospital complaining of angina and fatigue. He also complains of shortness of breath on exertion. Mr. Bell is a retired executive who says he feels useless since he was forced by his company to retire last year. He says he smokes two packs of filter cigarettes daily. He has gained 8 lbs. since retirement that he attributes to between-meal snacking and lack of activity. Mr. Bell states he doesn't feel motivated to get out of bed in the morning and that "life just isn't challenging anymore."

The nurse analyzes the information to identify the salient elements. In this case, Mr. Bell's age, recent life change, smoking and activity habits, weight gain, mental status, and symptoms all may be critical pieces of information. Analysis allows the nurse to examine the possible relationships. For example, what is the relationship between Mr. Bell's forced retirement and his physical and mental status, or between his history of smoking and his symptoms? When analyzing, the nurse also should consider what further information is needed to be able to form an accurate and valid opinion about Mr. Bell's responses. For instance, what are Mr. Bell's health, personal, and social histories? What does he value? What does he understand about the relationship between lifestyle and health? It is important to obtain this additional information to gain a complete picture of Mr. Bell's situation to ensure that the nurse's interpretations are both valid and reliable.

The analysis thus focuses on identifying any gaps, supplying missing information, and reviewing the potential relationships. As the amount of information grows, the nurse not only analyzes but also begins to synthesize it.

Synthesis of Data

Synthesis involves pulling the various pieces together to form a coherent whole. It is a reasoning process during which information is evaluated and interpreted and from which patterns emerge. Using the example of Mr. Bell, as information is obtained and analyzed, certain cues begin to fit together and become more relevant. Cues are simply pieces of information that suggest further information is needed or which, when considered in light of all available cues, indicate a pattern or a problem. During synthesis, relevant cues are selected and irrelevant cues are discarded or stored for future reference. The nurse knows which cues are, or may be, relevant because they connect in some way to other available pieces of information. Together they begin to suggest a pattern or a particular concern. For example, Mr. Bell's cues of fatigue, his age, recent retirement, statement of feeling useless, lack of activity, and lack of motivation, when considered in relation to each other, suggest the possibility that Mr. Bell is having difficulty coping with daily life as a result of the recent major change in his lifestyle. When each is considered separately, it can be difficult to get a sense of any particular pattern or problem. For instance, Mr. Bell's age or his forced retirement do not in themselves indicate a problem. Nor does fatigue, which when considered alone suggests numerous possibilities—normal aging, lack of sleep, overexertion, depression, or immunosuppression, among others. When synthesized with the other information available, however, these cues—age, forced retirement, fatigue, statements of feeling useless and unchallenged—suggest a diagnosis of "ineffective coping." Thus, considered together, the cues become relevant and critical contributing factors to an understanding of Mr. Bell's health.

Diagnostic Reasoning

Analysis and synthesis are essential elements of diagnostic reasoning, a complex process that integrates observation, information gathering, and critical thinking, and leads to the identification and categorization of a client's health concerns or problems. The diagnostic reasoning process consists of several phases:

1. identifying cues
2. clustering cues
3. inferencing and activating hypotheses
4. validating hypotheses
5. evaluating hypotheses and choosing from alternatives.

Each of these phases will be considered in depth later in this chapter.

The process of diagnostic reasoning involves the recognition and application of knowledge to clinical situations by classifying and labeling cues. When nurses engage in diagnostic reasoning, their primary focus should be classifying and labeling cues from a nursing perspective and identifying one or more nursing diagnoses for a given client.

Diagnostic reasoning is not a process unique to nursing, however. Other health-care disciplines, such as medicine, social work, clinical nutrition, and physical therapy, engage in diagnostic reasoning. The difference is the content or focus on which the diagnostic reasoning process is brought to bear, not the process itself. In fact, nurses often make tentative medical diagnoses by applying their knowledge of disease and medical treatment to clients' situations. For example, a pulse rate of 124, blood pressure measurement of 84/40, clammy skin, and pallor in an adult client with a traumatic injury may lead the nurse to conclude that the client is in shock, a medical diagnosis. The focus is medicine. The process for reaching this conclusion, however, is the same as that used to identify problems, or nursing diagnoses, that fall within the domain of nursing.

Carnevali (1984) points out that nurses are beginning to value the diagnostic reasoning process within nursing and no longer are willing to simply relabel medical diagnoses as nursing diagnoses—relabeling chronic obstructive lung disease, a medical diagnosis, as impaired gas exchange, a nursing diagnosis. Instead, nurses view nursing diagnosis as an essential component of a client's care that is complementary to medical diagnosis. However, since a portion of nursing practice continues to involve the carrying out of delegated medical functions, nurses must remain clear about the focus of the diagnostic reasoning process (is it nursing or is it medicine?). They also must make judgments about which focus has priority in a particular situation and must acquire "facility in moving between the two discrete discipline-specific perspectives for diagnosis and treatment" (Carnevali, 1984, p. 15).

The diagnostic reasoning process is examined in greater detail later in this chapter. One additional key concept, clinical judgment, is considered first.

Clinical Judgment

Clinical judgment is a term that refers to a conclusion reached by interpreting available information. Clinical judgment is sometimes used synonymously with diagnostic reasoning or nursing diagnosis. Unlike diagnostic reasoning, however, which is a continuous and overlapping process, clinical judgment involves making decisions about the information and choosing among a variety of alternatives or possibilities. Thus, it occurs at certain points throughout the diagnostic reasoning

process. In contrast to nursing diagnosis, clinical judgments are made throughout the diagnostic reasoning process, not just at its conclusion. In the course of collecting and interpreting information about a client, the nurse makes many clinical judgments, but relatively few actual nursing diagnoses. Clinical judgments are formed continually about whether particular pieces of data are relevant, which cues suggest a pattern, what gaps or incongruencies exist in the information, which information requires further validation, what explanations should be considered, and ultimately which diagnoses are chosen.

DIAGNOSTIC REASONING PROCESS

As noted earlier, diagnostic reasoning refers to the thinking processes used to make decisions about client data. Its purpose is to gather, interpret, and make judgments about the complex array of clinical information available for any given client. The process ultimately leads to decisions about what problems, or diagnoses, exist and the formulation of a plan to resolve the diagnoses and achieve desirable outcomes.

Variables That Influence Diagnostic Reasoning

The diagnostic reasoning process is subject to influence by a variety of factors (see Table 5-2), including characteristics of the diagnostician and the environment in which data collection and diagnosis take place (Tanner, 1984a). These variables play an important role in determining what cues the

TABLE 5-2
Factors Influencing the Diagnostic Reasoning Process

Variables Among Diagnosticians
Knowledge and experience
Personal variables
Cultural background and values
Physical and mental status
Intellectual capacity and memory
Philosophy of practice

Variables in Environment
Type and place of setting (acute care, long-term care, clinic, home, school, occupational)
Nature of client population (age, gender, ethnicity/culture, socioeconomic status, common health problems)
Physical environment
Professional role expectations

nurse focuses on and how those cues are interpreted.

Variables Among Diagnosticians

Although there is a core of knowledge common to the practice of nursing, each individual nurse can influence the diagnostic reasoning process and its outcomes. Specifically, the breadth and depth of the nurse's knowledge and experience, personal variables, and philosophy of practice affect the way information is gathered and interpreted.

Researchers have found that accuracy and efficiency of diagnostic reasoning are related to a nurse's knowledge and experience (Benner & Wrubel, 1982; Westfall et al., 1986). Putzier, Padrick, Westfall and Tanner (1985) found that novice nurses have more difficulty synthesizing diagnostic cues than experienced nurses. Beginning nurses may have the necessary theoretical background to grasp a situation, but they lack the clinical practice knowledge needed to rapidly analyze and synthesize diagnostic cues (Benner & Wrubel, 1982). As shown earlier in Table 5-1, as nurses gain experience and expand their clinical knowledge, the rapidity and accuracy of their diagnostic reasoning abilities increase.

There are a number of personal variables that may influence the diagnostic reasoning process as well, including the nurse's cultural background and values, physical and mental status, and intellectual capacity and memory. The nurse's cultural background and values influence what cues are received and how they are interpreted. For example, nurses who have never had any personal experiences with poverty may be so overwhelmed when making a visit to a home that is unkempt, dirty, and crowded, that they are unable to focus attention on the client. A nurse who expresses emotion freely and openly may fail to accurately diagnose pain or grief in a client whose behavior is stoic and unemotional.

Carnevali, Mitchell, Woods and Tanner (1984) note that "the greater the discrepancy between the characteristics of the diagnostician and the [client], the greater the use of stereotypes" (p. 34), which increases the likelihood of diagnostic errors. Socialization and culture are deeply ingrained forces that profoundly influence what cues the nurse looks for, sees, and pays attention to. The nurse may judge a client's behavior as inappropriate or indicative of a problem when the behavior simply is a reflection of socioeconomic forces, another cultural perspective, or different values. Thus, it is critical that nurses learn about other cultures and

gain experience in working with people from different cultural and socioeconomic backgrounds. Such knowledge and experience are needed to minimize the possibility of distorting the collection and interpretation of information.

Another variable that may influence diagnostic reasoning ability is the nurse's mental and physical health at the time information is being collected or interpreted. Fatigue, anxiety, or illness can decrease the nurse's sensitivity to cues, inhibit the capacity for critical thinking, and lead to premature or incorrect nursing diagnoses. Diagnostic reasoning requires high cognitive energy for processing large amounts of data, which often are complex and may have a variety of meanings. When energy is low or anxiety high, the nurse is less able to think carefully and critically, and the diagnostic reasoning process thus may be compromised. For example, nurses who work excessive numbers of hours or days without time off risk making errors in interpreting clinical information.

The acuity of the nurse's vision, hearing, and senses of smell and touch also may affect the collection and interpretation of data. A nurse with a hearing impairment, for example, may misinterpret a client's words or fail to detect subtle changes in breath sounds, unless special devices, such as a hearing aid or amplified stethoscope, are used.

The nurse's intelligence and ability to recall information are additional factors that influence the diagnostic reasoning process. Intellectual capacity and memory are determined by each nurse's inherited characteristics and learning experiences. There is a wide range of individual differences in the ability to assimilate, process, and store information. Each nurse's ability to organize, analyze, synthesize, and express complex diagnostic concepts is influenced by innate intellectual capacity, particularly the ability to store and retrieve information. As Carnevali et al. (1984) note:

> One cannot diagnose what one does not recognize or understand. It is true that some of the discipline content committed to long-term memory, and the . . . system for storage can be assured through . . . education. Still, the analytic, organizational, and language skills, as well as the energy individual clinicians devote to . . . this professional competency . . . are very personal qualities. Hence there are individual differences in diagnostic capabilities despite comparability of training. (p. 32)

Finally, each nurse's personal philosophy of practice can play an important role in how information is gathered, analyzed, and synthesized. The beliefs the nurse holds about people, health, environment, and nursing permeate each nurse–client contact and thus shape the nature of that contact. The process of gathering and interpreting information is governed not only by objective measures but also by the subjectivity both nurse and client bring to their relationship. Consider the following example. Nurse A believes that people are self-determining beings and that the role of the nurse is to support the client's right of self-determination, even when the client's wishes conflict with those of the health team. Nurse B believes that health professionals are best able to determine what is in the client's interest and that responsible clients are those who adhere to prescribed interventions even when they don't fully understand them. The nurses may reach different conclusions about the following situation:

> Sandra Simms is a 37-year-old unmarried white mother of five children. She is 40 pounds overweight and leads a sedentary life. She is unemployed and supports herself and her children on public assistance. She was diagnosed as having insulin dependent diabetes Type II three months ago. During a home visit, the nurse determines that Sandra has not altered her high fat, high carbohydrate diet because "the kids like the way we eat and I don't want to go to the trouble of changing." Her urine sugar and acetone during the visit is 4+/large. She tells the nurse that she has been administering her insulin as prescribed and "that seems to take care of my sugar."

Given their different philosophies, Nurses A and B may reach very different conclusions about this client. Nurse A may conclude that Sandra Simms lacks a full understanding of the nature of her illness and its consequences. Nurse B may decide that Sandra Simms is "noncompliant" and therefore is acting irresponsibly. Each of these conclusions suggests very different goals and nursing interventions.

Variables in Environment

The environment in which nurse–client contact occurs influences data collection and diagnostic reasoning. Specifically, the type and pace of the setting, the nature of the client population, the physical facilities, and professional or bureaucratic role expectations all may affect, either overtly or covertly, the diagnostic reasoning process (Tanner, 1984a).

The type of practice in which nurse–client contact occurs governs the time available to collect and interpret information. In an acute care setting, for example, actual direct contact with clients will be determined by staffing levels and the pace with which information must be gathered and interpreted. Acutely ill clients often are unstable and their responses change rapidly. Thus, they must be monitored frequently, often continuously. Time is of the essence in both obtaining and interpreting information so that decisions are made quickly. The less acutely ill the clients are, the more time a nurse will have to collect data and diagnose. Nurses who work with healthy or chronically ill clients over extended periods of time, as in school, long-term, home, or occupational settings, will have less continuous, direct contact with clients. However, the extended nature of nurse–client contact in these settings allows more time for gathering information and for interpreting it.

The proximity of the client to the nurse also influences diagnostic reasoning. This variable is determined by the physical structure of the setting in which nurse–client contact occurs. In a critical care unit with clients easily visible and accessible virtually around the clock, the nurse is able to gather and process clinical information continually. On a traditional nursing unit, however, the nurse's actual contact with each client is limited both by physical barriers and the client's need for less intensive, less frequent direct nursing care.

Another variable that influences diagnostic reasoning is the nature of the client population the nurse sees regularly. The predominant age, gender, ethnic/cultural orientation, socioeconomic status, and common health problems of a given clientele shape what the nurse decides to look for and how information is interpreted. Particular cues tend to occur with relative frequency in certain client populations, and thus may capture the nurse's attention more readily than cues that occur infrequently. For example, on a cardiology unit, nurses are trained to quickly assess and interpret clients' responses to cardiac dysrhythmias, whereas a nurse in a diabetic clinic may miss cues that indicate a client is experiencing a dysrhythmia. Nurses who do not work with young children regularly may misinterpret their behavioral responses to pain or separation from their parents.

Furthermore, stereotypical behaviors or characteristics may be associated with certain population groups and can influence how those behaviors or characteristics are interpreted. For example, homeless people may have difficulty with hygiene, clothing, food, and shelter because they lack the resources to obtain goods or services. Nurses who work with the homeless on a regular basis may assume that an elderly homeless man who refuses to change clothes or bathe does so because of lack of resources, when the problem really may be his inability to dress or bathe unassisted due to severe arthritis and pain.

The physical facilities of the health-care setting also may directly or indirectly influence the collection and interpretation of clinical information. For example, nurses who work in high tech settings have access to information that may not be so readily available in community settings. Such devices as cardiac monitors, blood gas machines, ventilator readings, and temperature probes supplement the information the nurse can obtain through direct sensing and permit access to internal cues that would be unavailable otherwise. By enlarging the data base, these devices decrease the likelihood of diagnostic error.

Other variables in the physical environment that can influence diagnostic reasoning include lighting, noise, or odors, and furniture arrangements or treatment measures that interfere with access to the client (such as isolation precautions or IV pumps). Lighting, noise, and odors may interfere if they are perceived inaccurately. For example, at night, the nurse may miss a change in the client's skin color if lighting is too dim. On a busy unit, direct contact with clients who are on isolation precautions may be less than it would be otherwise because of the time required to don gown, mask, and gloves. In other words, nurses are less likely to simply drop in to check on a client in isolation and thus may miss important changes in the client's behavior or responses.

Finally, professional and bureaucratic role expectations may exert a powerful influence on data collection and diagnostic reasoning. Role expectations determine the legitimacy of including certain functions within the domain of professional nursing practice, including assessment and diagnosis. Nurses who work in systems that value nursing assessment and diagnosis and that employ adequate numbers of nurses to permit time for these essential nursing activities are able to function as independent professionals. Such systems legitimize and reward the nurse's assessment and diagnostic capabilities by incorporating them in job descriptions, pay scales, and merit recognition. Job descriptions that limit nursing to delegated medical and housekeeping tasks limit the time and motivation for nurses to assess and diagnose and thus assure that the scope and autonomy of nursing practice remains restricted.

Thus, numerous variables play roles in shaping each nurse's diagnostic capability and behavior. In order to minimize bias, Mitchell (1984) suggests that nurses examine their own diagnostic reasoning to become aware of the variables that may be at work. Table 5-3 identifies questions that nurses can ask themselves to enhance their awareness of biases in their diagnostic reasoning.

As noted earlier, the diagnostic reasoning process is characterized by several phases, beginning with identifying cues and concluding with formulating nursing diagnoses. The phases are depicted in Figure 5-1.

Identifying Cues

Cues are pieces of clinical information received through the senses. They are the building blocks of the nursing assessment that eventually lead to formulating nursing diagnoses. Perceptions of cues, and the meanings assigned to them, can vary from person to person. Consider eyewitnesses to auto accidents or criminal events, who often provide varying accounts of the same occurrence. Differences in perception are shaped by a variety of factors, such as sensory functioning, intellectual capacity, context, cultural values, and a host of other variables. Examples of cues include:

- gray hair
- slumped posture
- macular rash on trunk
- pulse rate of 88 beats/min.
- empty IV bag
- house located in high density area

TABLE 5-3
Self-Assessment of Diagnostic Reasoning Biases

What are the common problems in daily living for the clients with whom I work?

How does the setting influence what I notice? Are there certain pieces of information I make certain I obtain before I initiate contact with the client?

How do I make my first contacts? What are the first observations I make? What are the first questions I ask? Do I ask leading questions?

When a client presents a new cue or problem, what are the first causes that come to mind? How many other causes do I usually consider? How does this shape the kind of information I seek next?

How do I avoid premature closure of data-gathering? Do I have a system to avoid jumping to conclusions?

Do my interpretations fit all that is known about the situation? Have I made sure to validate my inferences?

Do the diagnoses I make follow logically from the available information? If I find myself making a diagnosis without careful deliberation, can I back up and make the intuitive diagnosis explicit?

Note. Adapted from "Clinical examples: A comparison" by P.H. Mitchell, 1984. In D.L. Carnevali, P.H. Mitchell, N.F. Woods, & C.A. Tanner. *Diagnostic Reasoning in Nursing,* pp. 177–178. Philadelphia: Lippincott. Used with permission.

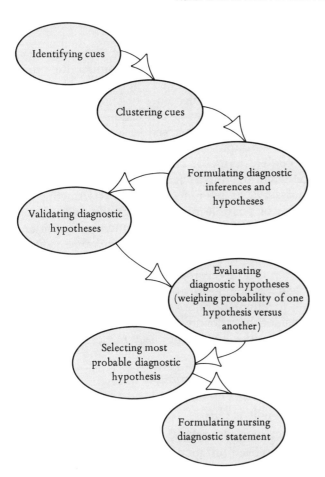

FIGURE 5-1. Phases of Diagnostic Reasoning Process.

Cues come from the entire field of available information. The data field has been referred to as the "search field" because the clinician must search and select from all available data those cues that are relevant (Tanner, 1984b). When people encounter new situations, they try to "narrow the search field, reduce its complexity, and . . . define it in such a way that their information-processing capacity can handle it" (Tanner, 1984b, p. 83).

The nurse begins to attend to relevant cues within seconds of initiating contact with the client. For example, upon entering a client's hospital room, the nurse's senses immediately begin to work, noting the client's appearance, sounds and smells in the room, the physical environment, and so forth. Among those cues that draw attention, some stand out as more salient. For instance, the nurse is more likely to notice fresh blood or drainage on a client's hospital gown than an empty water pitcher.

The nurse may encounter some cues prior to initial contact with a client. For instance, information available through reports and client records will yield cues that help the nurse begin to narrow

the search. Tanner (1984) calls these cues pre-encounter data. Pre-encounter data also may include expectations the nurse has formed by virtue of working in a particular setting or with a particular client population. These expectations exert a powerful influence on which cues the nurse looks for, attends to, and uses to make clinical decisions. The ability to detect and evaluate the vast array of available cues depends on the many factors discussed earlier that influence diagnostic reasoning.

Types of Cues

Gordon (1987) points out that cues may be categorized or labeled in several ways. Cues may be valid–invalid, reliable–unreliable, relevant–irrelevant, subjective–objective, current–historical, and diagnostic–supporting.

In Chapter 3, the differences between subjective and objective cues (data) and between current and historical cues are discussed. A cue is considered valid if it represents reality and accurately reflects the actual properties of what is being diagnosed. Bright red fluid on an abdominal dressing is a valid cue for fluid volume deficit *if* the fluid is blood. If the fluid is red ink or cherry Koolaid, then the cue is an invalid indicator for the diagnosis.

Reliable cues are dependable indicators or accurate measurements of a client's responses to actual or potential health alterations. Direct measurements, such as blood pressure readings or fluid output, and first-hand observations, such as developmental screening test results or clinical appraisal of musculoskeletal functioning, yield highly reliable cues. Such cues are considered more reliable than a client's report of fluid intake or developmental capabilities. The validity and reliability of isolated cues increase as the number of cues that fit the potential diagnosis also increase. Using the earlier example of bright red fluid on an abdominal dressing, the validity and reliability of this cue increase if the following additional cues also are present: pallor, pulse rate 96 beats/min., thready, blood pressure 86/40, and clammy skin. Together these cues suggest a diagnosis of "fluid volume deficit." However, if the client's pulse and blood pressure are within expected limits and the client's skin is warm and dry, the cue "bright red fluid on abdominal dressing" cannot be considered valid or reliable for this nursing diagnosis.

Relevant cues are those that contribute critical and essential information. Examples of relevant cues for the nursing diagnosis of "potential for trauma" are boldfaced in the following client situation:

Mr. Clarence Jameson is an **83-year-old** white-haired, black male who appears undernourished. His posture is stooped and he **limps**. He **lives alone** in a **second story** apartment in a **high-crime neighborhood**. Mr. Jameson is **three days post cataract surgery**. He uses a **walker** due to **right side muscle weakness**.

The cues of *black, male, undernourished, white-haired, stooped,* and *apartment-dwelling* are not relevant to this particular diagnosis. The boldfaced cues are relevant because they place Mr. Jameson at risk for trauma.

Relevant cues often are also valid and reliable. The ability to focus on relevant information and discard irrelevant data increases the efficiency, ease, and accuracy of the diagnostic reasoning process.

Cues also may be diagnostic or supporting. Diagnostic cues are specific characteristics of a particular diagnosis that permit the nurse to discriminate one diagnosis from another. For example, "bladder distention" and "sensation of bladder fullness" are diagnostic cues for urinary retention because they are unique and specific to this diagnosis. Supporting cues provide additional evidence to support diagnostic cues, but are not specific to the diagnosis itself. In the case of urinary retention, "dribbling of urine" and "nocturia" are supporting cues because they also may be indicators of other diagnoses, such as incontinence.

While acquiring cues (data collection), the nurse is confronted with many pieces of information. The sheer number of cues encountered during any clinical situation, as well as their complexity, require the nurse to organize the information in order to retain it in short-term memory. Information can be organized in a variety of ways. Use of a particular nursing assessment framework, such as functional health patterns (Gordon), behavioral systems (Johnson), self-care requisites (Orem), or adaptive modes (Roy), among others, provides an effective means of categorizing the huge amounts of information obtained during the nursing assessment.

Regardless of the framework used, the ultimate goal of assessing a client's health is to determine the client's nursing diagnoses. Thus, nursing diagnoses serve as a critical guide during the diagnostic reasoning process. Certain cues will fit certain diagnoses and not fit others. Many cues suggest more than one diagnostic possibility. In order to remember the sheer amount and variety of data obtained during the nursing assessment, the nurse must develop the ability to "chunk" or cluster the information.

Clustering Cues

To make sense of the vast array of data available to the nurse in any nurse–client encounter, the nurse must learn to group related information. How does the nurse know which cues fit together to form a pattern? Such knowledge is acquired through formal education and in practice.

The grouping of related data often is referred to as cue clustering or chunking. As information is gathered, the nurse begins to sort it into categories that serve as reference points in narrowing the realm of possible nursing diagnoses. Clustering must occur if the nurse is to remember important pieces of data. Chunking allows the nurse to store information in short-term memory until the information can be recorded, analyzed, or understood when missing information is collected.

To illustrate how clustering facilitates recall, consider the following list of cues obtained from a 32-year-old client in her last trimester of pregnancy:

Sleeps 6 hours per night

3+ edema of ankles

Weight 142 lbs.

Resting pulse rate 90 beats/min.

Employed full-time as a secretary

Exercise limited to activities of daily living

Nocturia X 2 nightly

Caloric intake 2,200 calories in 4 food groups daily

Complaining of fatigue

Eats fast foods or convenience foods for breakfast & lunch

Shortness of breath with minimal exertion or when reclining

To retain this information in working memory, the nurse must organize it in some way. Using the categories of activity/exercise, sleep, and nutrition/fluids, the data can be clustered as follows:

Activity/Exercise

Resting pulse rate 90 beats/min.

Employed full-time as a secretary

Exercise limited to activities of daily living

Complaining of fatigue

Shortness of breath with minimal exertion or when reclining

Sleep

Sleeps 6 hours per night

Nocturia 2 X nightly

Complaining of fatigue

Nutrition/Fluids

3+ edema of ankles

Weight 142 lbs.

Caloric intake 2,200 calories in 4 food groups daily

Eats fast food or convenience foods for breakfast & lunch

Note that "complaining of fatigue" is clustered in both activity/exercise and sleep categories. The nurse has yet to determine whether the client's fatigue is related to her lack of sleep or lack of sufficient activity/exercise. Further information is needed to make this determination.

Thus, as the nurse assesses the client, the data are analyzed in light of all available information to determine whether they suggest a pattern or simply reflect an isolated behavior or symptom. As more and more cues are accumulated, patterns begin to emerge. In the above example, the cue "sleeps 6 hours per night" doesn't provide much information in and of itself. However, the additional cues of "nocturia X 2 nightly" and "complaining of fatigue," considered in light of the first cue and the nurse's knowledge of the effects of late pregnancy on sleep patterns, suggest a diagnosis of "sleep pattern disturbance."

Failure to cluster cues as information is gathered increases the likelihood that important pieces of information will be ignored or lost during the diagnostic reasoning process. Cue clustering and recognition of patterns allow the nurse to begin formulating diagnostic hypotheses or inferences.

Inferencing and Activating Hypotheses

As cues are clustered and begin to form patterns, they trigger the development of tentative hypotheses or inferences.

Inferences are the interpretations the nurse makes about the data gathered during the assessment. An inference is a clinical judgment formed by the nurse about the meaning of each cluster of clinical data. That is, what hypotheses do the data or data clusters suggest? Though it is sometimes necessary to infer on the basis of incomplete information, every attempt should be made to formulate inferences that are supported or confirmed by adequate information.

The ability to distinguish cues (data) from inferences is a critical nursing skill. Cues in and of themselves do not have meaning. A nurse assigns meaning to cues through inference. This process involves explaining or interpreting the cues based on what is known about a given client's situation. Gordon (1987) points out that inferences "are created in the mind of the diagnostician," whereas cues are available for others to sense (see, hear, touch, smell) and validate. The following examples clarify the important difference between cues and inferences:

Cues (data)	*Inference (interpretation)*
1. Pulse rate of 110 beats/min. in a 50-year-old male lying in bed.	1. Rapid pulse rate.
2. Weight 190 lb., height 5 ft. 6 in. Protuding abdomen.	2. Client is obese.
3. Fists clenched. Shouting obscenities. Pacing.	3. Client is angry.
4. 18-year-old client with diabetes diagnosed 2 days ago. Eyes filled with tears. Sitting slumped in a chair. Unshaven. No eye contact with the nurse. States, "What's the use? I'll never be able to learn to give myself this stuff."	4. Client is coping ineffectively with change in health.

In each of the preceding examples, single cues are grouped together to make the inference. Using multiple cues to make inferences increases the likelihood of an accurate inference. The last example illustrates this point. If only a single cue—"eyes filled with tears"—were considered, the nurse might have inferred that the client was in pain, had a foreign body in his eye, or was lonely. The use of multiple cues, or a cue cluster, increases the accuracy of the nurse's inference.

There are varying degrees of inferences. Some inferences are concrete and simple; others abstract and more complex. In the first two examples, the inferences are fairly straightforward in light of the cues available to the nurse. The inferences are based on scientific knowledge and require minimal interpretation. In the last two examples, however, the inferences are more abstract and thus more subject to error. Since greater interpretation is involved, the possibility of inaccuracy or diversity of interpretation increases. In the third example, consider the possibility that the client is an actor who is rehearsing lines for a scene in a play.

The thought process the nurse uses to make inferences may be based on inductive or deductive reasoning. With inductive inferences, the thought process moves from the particular to the general; generalizations are developed from a set of observations or facts. For example, the nurse may observe that two diabetic clients are fearful about administering their own insulin. The nurse infers that most people with diabetes are somewhat fearful about insulin administration. This inference is inductive, since the nurse's thought process moves from two particular clients to the general population of diabetic clients. With deductive inferences, the thought process moves in the opposite direction, from the general to the specific. For example, from the study of death and dying and experience in caring for clients who are dying, the nurse knows that the usual initial response to a diagnosis of terminal illness is shock and disbelief. As the nurse prepares to care for a client recently diagnosed as having inoperable lung cancer, the nurse may draw the inference that the client is experiencing shock and disbelief. This inference is deductive, since the thought process moves from generalized knowledge regarding death and dying to the anticipated response of an individual client.

The inference process takes the nurse one step beyond data collection and, therefore, allows some margin of error. The nurse must use inferences with caution and must remember that inferences are highly subjective and should not be treated as fact. Any two nurses may make different inferences based on the same data. Little and Carnevali (1976) point out that:

> Inferencing . . . depends on information that has been *screened* by the sense organs, which may or may not be transmitting accurate signals, and second, *processed* by a brain where the input can be modified by attention, previous experience, knowledge, the language available for description, to say nothing of being modified by the beholder's value system as well. (p. 56)

On the other hand, nurses *must* infer. Cautions about the accuracy of inferences should not be interpreted as a case against making them. Collecting data is not an end in itself; ultimately, nurses must use data to provide safe and effective nursing care. Making inferences is a crucial intermediate step between data collection and nursing action.

Formulating inferences quickly leads to activating one or more diagnostic hypotheses. This process results from early recognition of cue patterns as data are gathered and enables the nurse to process the large amounts of information obtained during each encounter with the client (Tanner,

1984b). Diagnostic hypotheses are well-developed inferences that go beyond interpretation to suggest potential nursing diagnoses. For example, irritability may indicate several diagnostic hypotheses: ineffective coping, fatigue, sleep pattern disturbance, or acid-base disturbance. Each of these diagnostic hypotheses may or may not be supported by other data. As the nurse collects additional information, the range of potential diagnoses narrows. If, in addition to irritability, the client expresses lack of motivation and energy to accomplish routine activities, difficulty concentrating on tasks, and excessive sleeping, the likelihood of a diagnosis of fatigue increases and the probability of other diagnoses decreases. Once diagnostic hypotheses are activated and the possibilities are narrowed, it is important to test or validate them against available data.

Validating Hypotheses

Once diagnostic hypotheses have been formulated, the nurse seeks to confirm or rule out each one. The outcome may be confirmation of the accuracy of the hypothesis or its elimination from further consideration. Generally speaking, validation involves systematic, focused collection of additional information that supports or eliminates the hypothesis.

Whenever possible, the client should serve as the primary source for validation. Frequently, nurses may validate their interpretations simply by checking perceptions with the client. For example, the following conversation might occur:

CLIENT IN CLINIC: (Pacing the waiting room): How much longer until it is my turn?

NURSE, VALIDATING: The doctor will see you next. I notice that you can't sit still, Mrs. W. You seem anxious about seeing Dr. S.

CLIENT: Yes, I am. The doctor told me he would tell me the results of the tests today.

In this instance, the nurse validated a hypothesis of anxiety by sharing it with the client. During the exchange, the client also provided some additional information on which subsequent nursing interventions can be based. The nurse now knows that the client is anxious specifically about her test results.

In some instances, the hypothesis cannot be confirmed by talking with the client. For example, small children or comatose clients may not be able to confirm diagnostic hypotheses. Many hypotheses about physiological status—hyperthermia or fluid volume deficit for example—cannot be validated by the client. In such instances, diagnostic tools often are helpful. For example, the hypothesis of hyperthermia might be confirmed by measuring the client's temperature. In another instance, a nurse may infer that a client who reports dizziness when getting out of bed for the first time since surgery is experiencing orthostatic hypotension. A blood pressure reading may validate this hypothesis.

Reference to established defining characteristics for a particular diagnosis can aid in its confirmation or elimination. Defining characteristics have been developed for each of the approved nursing diagnoses accepted by the North American Nursing Diagnosis Association (NANDA, see chap. 6). Thus, if a nurse hypothesizes that a parent is experiencing parental role conflict based on the parent's stated feelings of helplessness and inadequacy in caring for her hospitalized child, reference to the defining characteristics will indicate that these behaviors do indeed support a diagnosis of "parental role conflict."

Other health-care professionals may assist with validation by agreeing with the hypothesis. Using other professionals as references for validating impressions or hypotheses is known as consensual validation. Suppose a nurse infers that a client is depressed, basing the hypothesis on many cues. If other nurses, the client's physician, and the physical therapist agree, their consensus adds credence to the hypothesis and increases the likelihood of its validity.

Reference to an authoritative source such as an expert practitioner, textbook, or periodical is another means of validating a diagnostic hypothesis. If a nurse infers that a year-old client who is not walking unassisted has a developmental delay, checking an authoritative source on child development will negate this hypothesis. Using research reports is an excellent way to validate diagnostic hypotheses, provided the subjects and clinical situations are congruent with the client's.

When it is impractical or impossible to consult the literature or other health-care professionals, a nurse can always test the hypothesis for consistency with all else that is known about the situation. If all cues are compatible with the hypothesis, the likelihood that the hypothesis is correct increases.

Any of the foregoing validation methods may be used alone or in combination to confirm hypotheses. The importance of validation cannot be overstressed, for its purpose is to prevent error, misinterpretation, or bias from influencing the data. Using an invalid diagnosis as a basis for planning nursing care can lead to interventions that are ineffective, inefficient, or even harmful.

Evaluating Hypotheses and Choosing From Alternatives

Evaluating the diagnostic hypotheses for a particular client is the final task in the diagnostic reasoning process. Evaluating a hypothesis involves weighing the probability of one diagnosis against other potential or probable diagnoses. As a nurse attempts to validate a particular diagnosis, each new piece of information is factored into the total picture and either may increase or decrease the probability that the diagnosis is correct.

Tanner (1984b) notes that the ability to evaluate diagnostic hypotheses effectively depends on the nurse's grasp of the connection between individual cues and each hypothesis, and the ability to search for and recognize cues that confirm or rule out a particular hypothesis. These abilities are related to the nurse's level of knowledge and experience. Thus, novices are less adept than experienced nurses at evaluating the likelihood of one hypothesis vis-à-vis another. In particular, novices are more likely to complete the evaluation of alternative hypotheses prematurely, thus increasing the probability of diagnostic error. Table 5-4 delineates differences between novice and expert nurses in using various diagnostic strategies, including hypothesis evaluation.

While engaged in the diagnostic reasoning process, the nurse should remain continually aware of alternative explanations for the information gathered. Even when a particular diagnostic hypothesis seems obvious, it is important to remain receptive to other possibilities to increase the likelihood of accuracy. The ability to remain open to alternative explanations for particular sets of data increases with experience. Expert nurses are more likely to be willing to tolerate the uncertainty involved in considering a variety of alternative diagnostic hypotheses because they (1) have a larger number of sample experiences from which to draw, (2) are able to search memory stores more efficiently and thoroughly, (3) are less likely to be swayed by a single piece of confirming data, and (4) are aware of the risks associated with premature acceptance of a particular hypothesis (Tanner, 1984a).

Consideration of all potential hypotheses increases the probability of accuracy. As alternatives are evaluated and ruled in or out, the nurse nar-

TABLE 5-4
Diagnostic Strategies: The Novice and the Expert

Phase of Diagnostic Process	Novice	Expert
Narrowing the Search Field	1. Stereotypes on basis of pre-encounter information	1. Uses pre-encounter data to expedite early directed data search; validates data in presenting situation
	2. Uses general systematic search; relies on memory of past experiences to narrow search field	2. Begins with general systematic search to avoid premature narrowing
	3. Looks for data that confirm pre-encounter influence	3. Looks for data which differ from pre-encounter expectations.
	4. May miss patterns in cues	4. Recognizes patterns in cues
	5. Does not realize full information value from cues to narrow search field	5. Extracts maximum information from cues to narrow search field
Hypothesis Activation	1. Uses single cues to trigger hypotheses	1. Uses cue patterns/clusters as triggers for hypotheses
	2. Hypotheses are very global or very specific; level of specificity may not fit data	2. Seeks hypotheses at level of abstraction necessary to explain as much of the data as possible
	3. May ignore or forget cues that do not fit hypothesis	3. Holds in reserve for later exploration cues that cannot be "chunked" into the hypotheses activated
Information-Seeking	1. Uses hypothesis testing to a limited degree	1. Uses hypothesis testing efficiently and more thoroughly than novice
	2. Usually uses routine general questioning strategy when stumped	2. Uses routine questioning strategy when stumped and as a means to avoid premature closure
	3. Uses cue characterization or data-driven searches as primary approach	3. Uses cue characterization as a means to test or refine hypotheses
	4. Has difficulty shifting focus of search and strategy	4. Can shift focus and strategy with great facility
	5. May be uncomfortable validating with client	5. Validates with client
Hypothesis Evaluation	1. Uses recency of experience and availability to assess likelihood of hypothesis	1. Uses more reliable sample (wide range of experience) to increase likelihood of hypothesis
	2. Nonselective in data obtained	2. Uses data with greatest information
	3. Tends to gather either too much or too little data depending on initial probability	3. Efficient in data gathering and hypothesis evaluation
	4. Underestimates value of disconfirming data and overestimates value of confirming data	4. Information value less influenced by confirming/disconfirming nature
	5. Tendency toward premature closure on favored hypothesis	5. Recognizes the importance of avoiding premature closure

Note. From "Factors influencing the diagnostic process" by C.A. Tanner, 1984. In D.L. Carnevali, P.H. Mitchell, N.F. Woods, & C.A. Tanner. *Diagnostic Reasoning in Nursing*, pp. 99–101. Philadelphia: Lippincott. Reprinted with permission.

rows the range of potential diagnoses. Drawing from knowledge and experience, the nurse then chooses the most probable hypothesis that is supported by all that is known about the client.

Considering alternative hypotheses for particular data sets reduces the likelihood of interpreting the information in a biased or habitual way. Gordon (1987) notes that the tendency to rely solely on habit and experience may lead either to very accurate hypotheses in most instances, based on their high probability of occurrence in a given client population or clinical setting, or lead to errors because there always are clients who deviate from the norm.

Avoiding Diagnostic Errors

There are two types of diagnostic errors: those that fail to diagnose an existing or potential problem (underdiagnosing) and those that diagnose a problem that does not exist (overdiagnosing). Both can result in harm to clients.

Diagnostic errors can occur at any step of the diagnostic reasoning process. Important data may be missed while collecting information and identifying cues, or irrelevant data may be considered important. When data collection is haphazard and disorganized, the nurse's ability to process the information is impaired. Key pieces of information may be lost. Tanner (1984b) believes "the best predictor of diagnostic accuracy is thoroughness of data collection" (p. 102). However, data collection also must be systematic and guided by a framework for organizing the information if thoroughness is to be of value.

Variables that influence data collection that may result in errors include the nurse's knowledge and experience, personal biases, cognitive ability, and the context in which data collection takes place. These variables also may lead to errors in interpretation. If cues are interpreted erroneously, the nurse is likely to formulate inaccurate diagnostic hypotheses. For example, nurses may attribute certain characteristics—"All women in labor experience pain"—to a particular population of clients, which may lead to a diagnosis of "pain related to uterine contractions" for all women in labor despite the absence of confirming data for some women.

Premature acceptance of a diagnostic hypothesis can occur when a nurse forms a judgment on the basis of incomplete or insufficient information. Consider the case of parents who fail to visit their hospitalized child. The nurse formulates a diagnostic hypothesis of "altered parenting." However, the parents may have an excellent relationship with their child, yet simply lack transportation to the hospital and trust that their child is being well cared for by hospital staff.

Some nurses may be so concerned about making diagnostic errors, however, that they are fearful of formulating hypotheses even when the data are sufficient to support a particular hypothesis. While it is desirable to be as certain as possible when formulating diagnostic hypotheses, there is nearly always some uncertainty in the process. The nurse must attempt to collect sufficient data to formulate the best judgment possible while remaining open to further information that can help confirm or eliminate that judgment. The inability or unwillingness to take a stand can be as detrimental to clients as making stereotypical and premature diagnoses.

When alternative hypotheses are not considered and evaluated, a variety of problems can occur. Aspinall and Tanner (1981) point out the likelihood that the nurse may:

- fail to consider the correct diagnosis while forming an initial hypothesis,

- neglect to consider all available data because the focus was narrowed too soon,

- overvalue the probability of one hypothesis because it is familiar and comfortable, or

- accept an inaccurate hypothesis because of speed, bias, or inaccurate assumptions.

A number of safeguards may be employed to avoid diagnostic errors. Tanner (1984b) offers several suggestions for improving diagnostic accuracy, which are outlined in Table 5-5.

Clinical Intuition and Diagnostic Reasoning

Although much emphasis in this chapter and in the nursing literature has been placed on ensuring the accuracy of diagnostic hypotheses through careful and deliberate data collection, interpretation, validation, and hypothesis evaluation, the diagnostic reasoning process is never entirely objective and quantifiable. In recent years, increasing attention has been paid to the important role intuition plays in diagnostic reasoning and clinical decision-making (Benner, 1984; Rew, 1988; Young, 1987).

Intuition may be defined as a subjective gut feeling or hypothesis based on incomplete, insufficient, or uncertain information, but that nevertheless exerts a strong influence on a nurse's decisions and actions. Young (1987) refers to clinical intuition as "a process whereby the nurse knows something about a [client] that cannot be verbalized, that is verbalized with difficulty, or for which the source of knowledge cannot be determined" (p. 52). An expert nurse's intuitive knowledge of a client or clinical situation leads to clinical judgments and nursing actions that, more often than not, are shown to be accurate (Benner, 1984).

The phenomenon of clinical intuition is widely accepted and experienced among expert nurses and is embodied in their diagnostic reasoning skills. Young (1987) studied the intuitive experiences of 41 nurses in a variety of settings. She

TABLE 5-5
Strategies to Improve Diagnostic Reasoning Accuracy

Remember that cues are less-than-perfect indicators of the diagnosis, not the same as the diagnosis.

Be cautious when separating observations from inferences. It is easy for us to leap from a fact to a conclusion (inferential leap), without ever knowing we did it.

When you observe a sign or symptom, don't settle for the first explanation that comes to mind. Always look for competing diagnoses.

Try to consider two to three diagnoses at one time. When you get additional information, consider each diagnosis in light of the new information. Check to be sure that competing diagnoses have been ruled out, or can wait until you've tried some competing interventions.

Follow up on each cue. Explore its characteristics, watching carefully for the influence of biases or your favored hypothesis on the kind of questions you ask.

Validate both your observations and your inferences with your client.

As you narrow the range of diagnostic possibilities, go back and evaluate what data led you to favor one diagnosis and begin to rule out others.

> Are the data reliable and dependable indicators of your diagnosis?
>
> Was your diagnosis influenced by a recent experience or dramatic event?
>
> Are the diagnostic possibilities reminiscent of another client situation? And if so, is the client you recall representative of a larger group of clients?

Be cautious of premature closure. Remember the information we obtain from a client and the observations we make are determined largely by what we think the diagnostic possibilities are. Don't abandon routine general questioning too quickly. While focused data collection is efficient, failure to uncover problems in daily living can come from a premature narrowing of the search field.

Be tentative in your diagnosis. There is seldom a time when all uncertainty can be removed. The final diagnosis is at best a conjecture. The process of collaborative diagnosis with the client may in itself be therapeutic. It may assist the client to sufficiently mobilize resources such that no further intervention is needed.

Be confident in your reasoning skills and your ability to draw accurate inferences. As a nurse, you have finely tuned observation skills and a vast storehouse of knowledge. Belief in your own ability, coupled with an open, inquisitive mind, go a long way toward effective problem-solving.

Note. From "Factors influencing the diagnostic process" by C.A. Tanner, 1984. In D.L. Carnevali, P.H. Mitchell, N.F. Woods, & C.A. Tanner. *Diagnostic Reasoning in Nursing*, pp. 102–103. Philadelphia: Lippincott.

found that subjectivity is a common element in nurse–client relationships and that this subjectivity influences the nurse's intuitive judgments. Because the nurse–client relationship is intensely personal, intimate, and often subjective, the information needed to formulate accurate diagnoses cannot be derived exclusively from facts. Thus, the diagnostic reasoning process is at once objective and subjective, deliberative and intuitive.

Clinical intuition is developed through direct experience with clients and is influenced by the nurse's receptivity to such feelings, the nurse's energy level, and the nurse's self-confidence (Young, 1987). Expert nurses have been shown to have more highly developed clinical intuition, to be able to provide detailed descriptions of their decision-making based on intuition, and to trust their intuitive judgments when compared with novice practitioners (Benner, 1984; Rew, 1988; Schraeder & Fischer, 1987; Young, 1987).

It is important for nurses to acknowledge their intuitive feelings and thoughts about a particular client's situation and to take them into account when formulating diagnostic hypotheses. There is increasing recognition that clinical intuition is a valid basis for making and acting on clinical judgments.

Chapter Highlights

- The second phase of the nursing process, nursing diagnosis, consists of two components: data analysis and synthesis, and the formulation of nursing diagnoses.

- The process of analyzing and synthesizing assessment data involves reflection and critical thinking about what the data mean in order to formulate and evaluate diagnostic hypotheses.

- Data analysis is the examination of information collected in order to identify any gaps and to determine the relationships among the various pieces of data. Synthesis involves pulling the data together to form patterns or a coherent whole.

- Diagnostic reasoning is a process that involves interpreting the data to identify and categorize a client's health concerns or problems. The process consists of identifying and clustering cues, inferencing and activating hypotheses, validating hypotheses, evaluating hypotheses, and choosing from alternative hypotheses.

■ Numerous variables influence diagnostic reasoning, including characteristics of the diagnostician and of the environment in which nurse–client interaction occurs.

■ There are significant differences in the diagnostic reasoning abilities of novice and expert nurses, based on their knowledge, experience, role performance, and self-confidence.

■ There are two types of diagnostic errors: those that fail to diagnose an existing or potential problem (underdiagnosing) and those that diagnose a nonexistent problem (overdiagnosing). Both can result in harm to clients.

■ Diagnostic reasoning is both deliberative and intuitive.

■ Clinical intuition is a subjectively derived hypothesis about a client's situation that cannot be described objectively but that forms the basis for many clinical decisions. Clinical intuition is most highly developed in expert nurses.

Practice Activities

1. For each of the following inferences, identify at least five cues that support, or validate, the inference:

obese	depressed
elderly	angry
frightened	pregnant

2. Study Figures 5-2 and 5-3. Write a paragraph that describes what you see in each. Review what you have written to determine whether you have included only cues (observable facts) or if you also have formulated inferences about the meaning of the cues. What diagnostic hypotheses are suggested by the cues? What strategies could you use to validate your hypotheses? Compare your writ-

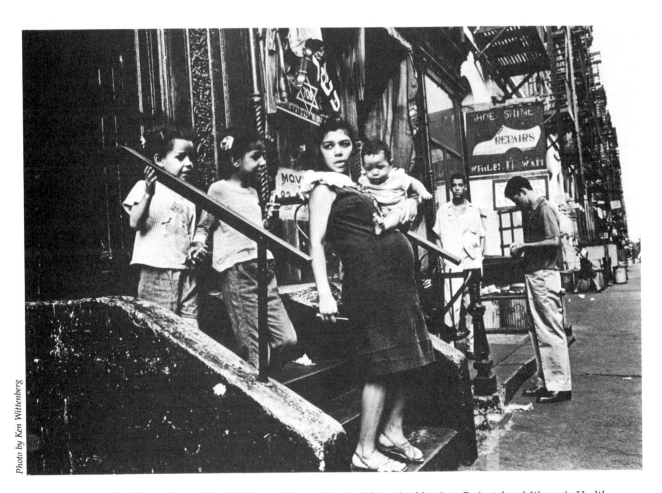

Photo by Ken Wittenberg

FIGURE 5-2. (*Note.* From Auvershine/Enriquez: *Comprehensive Maternity Nursing: Perinatal and Women's Health,* Second Edition, © 1990. Boston: Jones and Bartlett Publishers, p. 822.)

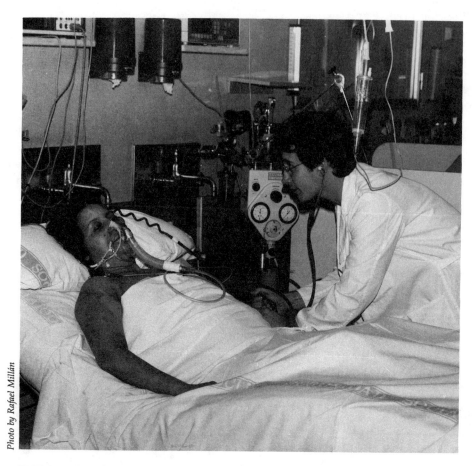

Photo by Rafael Millán

FIGURE 5-3. (*Note.* From Lee/Estes: *The Nation's Health*, Third Edition, © 1990. Boston: Jones and Bartlett Publishers, p. 336.)

ten paragraphs and diagnostic hypotheses with those of a classmate or colleague. What degree (high, moderate, low) of consensual validation did you achieve?

3. Cluster the following information using a framework of your choice (e.g., the framework presented in this text, functional health patterns, adaptive modes, self-care requisites, etc.):

Hospitalized for coronary artery bypass

Smokes two packs of cigarettes daily

Recently widowed

Expresses concern about recovery time and desire to "get back to work so I don't lose my job"

Drinks 7 to 8 cups of regular coffee daily

Height 5'10", weight 210 lbs.

Eats fast foods or frozen prepared foods

Does not exercise

Blood pressure 150/100

Pacing in room evening before surgery

Jokingly says, "Maybe it's time for me to join my wife"

What tentative diagnostic hypotheses are suggested? What additional information is needed to confirm or eliminate these hypotheses? What strategies could be employed to avoid making a diagnostic error?

Recommended Readings

Benner, P.A. & Tanner, C.A. (1987). Clinical judgment: How expert nurses use intuition. *American Journal of Nursing, 87,* 23–31.

Derdiarian, A. (1988). A valid profession needs valid diagnoses. *Nursing and Health Care, 9,* 137–140.

Fredette, S.L. (1988). Common diagnostic errors. *Nurse Educator, 13*(3), 31–35.

McPhee, A. (1987). Can't tell facts from inferences? Ask Van Gogh. *Nurse Educator, 12*(3), 43–44.

Rew, L. (1988). Intuition in decision-making. *Image: The Journal of Nursing Scholarship, 20,* 150–154.

Tanner, C.A., Padrick, K.P., Westfall, U.E., & Putzier, D.J. (1987). Diagnostic reasoning strategies of nurses and nursing students. *Nursing Research, 36,* 358–363.

Westfall, U.E., Tanner, C.A., Putzier, D., & Padrick, K.P. (1986). Activating clinical inferences: A component of diagnostic reasoning in nursing. *Research in Nursing and Health, 9,* 269–277.

Young, C.E. (1987). Intuition and nursing process. *Holistic Nursing Practice, 1*(3), 52–62.

References

Aspinall, M.J. & Tanner, C.A. (1981). *Decision making for patient care: Applying the nursing process.* New York: Appleton-Century-Crofts.

Benner, P. (1984). *From novice to expert.* Reading, MA: Addison-Wesley.

Benner, P. & Wrubel, J. (1982). Skilled clinical knowledge: The value of perceptual awareness. *Nurse Educator, 7,* 11–13.

Carnevali, D.L. (1984). Nursing diagnosis: An evolutionary view. *Topics in Clinical Nursing, 6,* 10–20.

Carnevali, D.L., Mitchell, P.H., Woods, N.F., & Tanner, C.A. (1984). *Diagnostic reasoning in nursing.* Philadelphia: Lippincott.

Gordon, M. (1987). *Nursing diagnosis: Process and application* (2nd ed.). New York: McGraw–Hill.

Little, D.E. & Carnevali, D.L. (1976). *Nursing care planning* (2nd ed.). Philadelphia: Lippincott.

Mitchell, P.H. (1984). Clinical examples: A comparison. In D.L. Carnevali, P.H. Mitchell, N.F. Woods, & C.A. Tanner (Eds.), *Diagnostic reasoning in nursing* (pp. 175–178). Philadelphia: Lippincott.

Putzier, D.J., Padrick, K., Westfall, U.E., & Tanner, C.A. (1985). Diagnostic reasoning in critical care nursing. *Heart and Lung, 14,* 430–437.

Rew, L. (1988). Intuition in decision-making. *Image: Journal of Nursing Scholarship, 20,* 150–154.

Schraeder, B.D., & Fischer, D.K. (1987). Using intuitive knowledge in the neonatal intensive care nursery. *Holistic Nursing Practice, 1*(3), 45–51.

Tanner, C.A. (1984a). Factors influencing the diagnostic reasoning process. In D.L. Carnevali, P.H. Mitchell, N.F. Woods, & C.A. Tanner (Eds.), *Diagnostic reasoning in nursing* (pp. 61–82). Philadelphia: Lippincott.

Tanner, C.A. (1984b). Diagnostic problem-solving strategies. In D.L. Carnevali, P.H. Mitchell, N.F. Woods, & C.A. Tanner (Eds.), *Diagnostic reasoning in nursing* (pp. 83–104). Philadelphia: Lippincott.

Westfall, U.E., Tanner, C.A., Putzier, D., & Padrick, K.P. (1986). Activating clinical inferences: A component of diagnostic reasoning in nursing. *Research in Nursing and Health, 9,* 269–277.

Young, C.E. (1987). Intuition and nursing process. *Holistic Nursing Practice, 1*(3), 52–62.

6

Nursing Diagnosis:
The Diagnostic Statement

CHAPTER OUTLINE

- Historical and Contemporary Perspectives
- Key Characteristics of a Nursing Diagnosis
- Advantages of Nursing Diagnosis
- Limitations of Nursing Diagnosis
- Nursing Diagnosis versus Medical Diagnosis
- Formulating the Nursing Diagnostic Statement
- Clients' Perceptions and Relativity of Nursing Diagnoses

OBJECTIVES

Upon completion of this chapter, you should be able to:

- Define the following terms: taxonomy, nursing diagnosis, defining characteristics, and related factors.

- Trace the historical development of nursing diagnosis as a separate and distinct phase of the nursing process.

- Trace the historical development of the North American Nursing Diagnosis Association's (NANDA) classification system of nursing diagnoses.

- Explain the relationships among the four essential characteristics of nursing practice, the phases of the nursing process, and the American Nurses Association's *Standards of Nursing Practice.*

- Delineate the key characteristics of a nursing diagnosis.

- Explain the advantages and limitations of nursing diagnosis for nursing practice and for the profession.

- Differentiate nursing diagnosis and medical diagnosis, citing examples of each.

- Explain how the related factors that form the second part of the diagnostic statement individualize a nursing diagnosis.

- Formulate valid and appropriate nursing diagnoses using the accepted two-part format.

- Explain how a client's perceptions and contextual variables may influence the validity of a nursing diagnosis.

Nursing diagnosis is a critical step in the nursing process; it depends on an accurate and comprehensive nursing assessment and forms the basis for nursing care planning. The process of analyzing the data obtained from the nursing assessment is delineated in the previous chapter. Nursing diagnosis, the end product of the nursing assessment, refers to the actual statement formulated to describe the client's responses and the related factors, or *etiology*, that contribute to the responses.

The *American Heritage Dictionary* defines *diagnosis* as "an analysis of the nature of something; the conclusion reached by such analysis." Although the term *diagnosis* long has been equated with the practice of medicine, the dictionary definition illustrates the generic nature of the term and the need to provide an appropriate modifier to reflect the type of diagnosis being made. For example, educators diagnose learning problems, auto mechanics diagnose car malfunctions, physicians diagnose disease, and nurses diagnose persons' responses to health problems.

A nursing diagnosis is a statement of an important nursing activity, which communicates to other professionals and the public the unique and critical functions that nurses contribute to health care. This activity delineates clearly the domain of nursing practice, specifically those aspects of health care that nurses are uniquely qualified and capable of treating. Although nursing diagnosis continues to be the subject of much debate, it unquestionably has influenced the way nursing care is perceived and delivered. Over the past four decades, nursing diagnosis has evolved from its early rejection by the profession to wide acceptance and use, despite its limitations.

HISTORICAL AND CONTEMPORARY PERSPECTIVES

The term *nursing diagnosis* first appeared in the literature in the 1950s when Fry (1953) suggested that creative and individualized nursing care planning depends on the formulation of nursing diagnoses. In 1955, however, the American Nurses Association (ANA) rejected this novel idea that nursing as an activity includes "acts of diagnosis or prescription of therapeutic or corrective measures." The ANA's stance inhibited further exploration and development of nursing diagnosis for a number of years.

Several articles on nursing diagnosis were published in the 1960s, emphasizing the importance of nursing diagnosis to nursing practice. Several authors offered specific definitions of the term nursing diagnosis:

A careful investigation of the facts to determine the nature of a nursing problem (Chambers, 1962, p. 102)

A conclusion based on scientific determination of an individual's nursing needs, resulting from critical analysis of his [or her] behavior, the nature of his [or her] illness, and numerous other factors which affect his [or her] condition (Komorita, 1963, p. 84)

A statement of a conclusion resulting from a recognition of a pattern derived from nursing investigation of a patient (Durand & Prince, 1966, p. 50)

An evaluation, within the framework of current knowledge, of the patient's condition as a person, including physical, physiologic, and behavioral aspects (Rothberg, 1967, p. 1041)

All these authors encouraged the use of nursing diagnosis as an essential basis for nursing care planning.

In 1973, two significant events stimulated further efforts within the profession to incorporate nursing diagnosis as a critical component of the nursing process. The publication of the ANA document, *Standards of Nursing Practice* (1973), stipulated explicitly in Standard II that "Nursing diagnoses are derived from health status data." This document made clear that health assessment information should be compared to norms as a means of identifying a client's capabilities and limitations, which then become the basis for formulating the client's nursing care plan.

Perhaps more significant were the efforts of Gebbie and Lavin (1974), who in 1973 organized the First National Conference on Classification of Nursing Diagnoses. The purpose of the conference, which was attended by 100 nurses, was to "initiate the process of preparing an organized, logical, comprehensive system for classifying those health problems or health states diagnosed by nurses and treated by means of nursing intervention" (Gebbie & Lavin, 1975, p. 1). Although 100 nursing diagnoses were proposed, participants could not agree on a classification system and recognized the need for further work. Thus, a series of conferences was launched with the express purpose of defining "a standard nomenclature for describing health problems amenable to treatment by nurses, and a beginning theoretical framework for placing the terms into a taxonomy" (Kim & Moritz, 1982, p. xvii). A *taxonomy* is a framework for classifying and organizing nursing diagnoses according to a hierarchy of categories.

During the 1970s the nursing literature on nursing diagnosis increased dramatically. Mundinger and Jauron (1975) added a significant component to the definition of nursing diagnosis by suggesting that a nursing diagnosis should "identify essential factors related to the unhealthful response" (p. 97). They maintained that delineation of the causative or contributory factors is needed to provide direction for specific nursing interventions. A nursing diagnosis of "impaired skin integrity" does not help the nurse target specific interventions since the etiology is unknown. When the diagnosis includes the etiology, for example, impaired skin integrity "related to prolonged bedrest" or impaired skin integrity "related to acne," the nurse has much clearer information for planning appropriate nursing interventions, which would be quite different in each of these instances.

In 1976, Gordon further expanded the definition of nursing diagnosis to include those problems (or clients' responses) that nurses "by virtue of their education and experience are capable and licensed to treat" (p. 1299). Thus, Gordon recognized explicitly that nursing diagnoses encompass only those problems that fall within the domain of independent nursing practice and for which nurses are uniquely qualified to intervene.

Since 1973, the conferences on nursing diagnosis classification have been held every two years, most recently in 1990. In 1982, conference members formalized their organization and adopted the name North American Nursing Diagnosis Association (NANDA). Under its bylaws, the group assumes responsibility for further development and refinement of the taxonomy for nursing diagnoses, reviews newly proposed diagnoses through its Diagnosis Review Committee, and accepts diagnostic labels for clinical testing by majority vote of NANDA's members.

Over the years, the classification system has undergone several revisions. In 1986, all approved nursing diagnoses were placed within a classification framework of nine human response patterns referred to as Level One of the NANDA taxonomy. The nine human response patterns are: exchanging, communicating, relating, valuing, choosing, moving, perceiving, knowing, and feeling. Level Two consists of subcategories that identify specific human patterns and behaviors within each particular human response pattern. The taxonomy levels are described in Table 6-1. In place of the previous alphabetical listing of diagnoses, a NANDA committee developed a hierarchical classification scheme (taxonomy) for existing diagnoses; this system was endorsed by the membership and given the title *NANDA Taxonomy I*. Within this scheme, nursing diagnoses are arranged according to their level of abstraction. For example, altered role performance is the higher, or broader, diagnostic category for the more specific diagnoses of

TABLE 6-1

NANDA Taxonomy I Revised (1990)—Levels One and Two*

1. **EXCHANGING:** Mutual giving and receiving
    1.1. Nutrition
    1.2. Physical regulation
    1.3. Elimination
    1.4. Circulation
    1.5. Oxygenation
    1.6. Physical integrity
2. **COMMUNICATING:** Sending messages
    2.1 Communications
3. **RELATING:** Establishing bonds with others
    3.1. Socialization
    3.2. Role
    3.3. Sexuality patterns
4. **VALUING:** Assigning relative worth
    4.1. Spiritual state
    4.2. Meaningfulness
5. **CHOOSING:** Selection of alternatives
    5.1. Coping
    5.2. Participation
    5.3. Judgment
    5.4. Health-seeking behaviors
6. **MOVING:** Activity
    6.1. Activity
    6.2. Rest
    6.3. Recreation
    6.4. Activities of daily living
    6.5. Self-care
    6.6. Growth and development
7. **PERCEIVING:** Reception of information
    7.1. Self-concept
    7.2. Sensory-perception
    7.3. Attention
8. **KNOWING:** Meaning associated with information
    8.1. Knowing
    8.2. Thought processes
9. **FEELING:** Subjective awareness of information
    9.1. Comfort
    9.2. Emotional integrity
    9.3. Emotional state

*Level One—Human response patterns; Level Two—Subcategories of human patterns and behaviors.

parental role conflict, altered parenting, potential altered parenting, and sexual dysfunction.

In 1988, *Taxonomy I Revised* was accepted. In 1990, further revisions of the *Taxonomy I Revised* were made. The most recently approved taxonomy (1990) consists of 99 diagnoses, including 2 new diagnoses. Changes also were made in 15 diagnostic labels for consistency. The *Taxonomy I Revised* (1990) is presented in Table 6-2.

In November 1988, NANDA representatives met with ANA to prepare the taxonomy for coding to enable its inclusion in the World Health Organization's 10th Revision of the International Classifi-

TABLE 6-2
NANDA Approved Nursing Diagnoses—Taxonomy I
Revised (1990)

This list represents the NANDA approved nursing diagnoses for clinical use and testing (1990). Changes have been made in 15 labels for consistency.

PATTERN 1: EXCHANGING

1.1.2.1	Altered Nutrition: More than body requirements
1.1.2.2	Altered Nutrition: Less than body requirements
1.1.2.3	Altered Nutrition: Potential for more than body requirements
1.2.1.1	Potential for Infection
1.2.2.1	Potential Altered Body Temperature
1.2.2.2	Hypothermia
1.2.2.3	Hyperthermia
1.2.2.4	Ineffective Thermoregulation
1.2.3.1	Dysreflexia
*1.3.1.1	Constipation
1.3.1.1.1	Perceived Constipation
1.3.1.1.2	Colonic Constipation
*1.3.1.2	Diarrhea
*1.3.1.3	Bowel Incontinence
1.3.2	Altered Urinary Elimination
1.3.2.1.1	Stress Incontinence
1.3.2.1.2	Reflex Incontinence
1.3.2.1.3	Urge Incontinence
1.3.2.1.4	Functional Incontinence
1.3.2.1.5	Total Incontinence
1.3.2.2	Urinary Retention
*1.4.1.1	Altered (Specify Type) Tissue Perfusion (Renal, cerebral, cardiopulmonary, gastrointestinal, peripheral)
1.4.1.2.1	Fluid Volume Excess
1.4.1.2.2.1	Fluid Volume Deficit
1.4.1.2.2.2	Potential Fluid Volume Deficit
*1.4.2.1	Decreased Cardiac Output
1.5.1.1	Impaired Gas Exchange
1.5.1.2	Ineffective Airway Clearance
1.5.1.3	Ineffective Breathing Pattern
1.6.1	Potential for Injury
1.6.1.1	Potential for Suffocation
1.6.1.2	Potential for Poisoning
1.6.1.3	Potential for Trauma
1.6.1.4	Potential for Aspiration
1.6.1.5	Potential for Disuse Syndrome
#1.6.2	Altered Protection
1.6.2.1	Impaired Tissue Integrity
*1.6.2.1.1	Altered Oral Mucous Membrane
1.6.2.1.2.1	Impaired Skin Integrity
1.6.2.1.2.2	Potential Impaired Skin Integrity

PATTERN 2: COMMUNICATING

2.1.1.1	Impaired Verbal Communication

PATTERN 3: RELATING

3.1.1	Impaired Social Interaction
3.1.2	Social Isolation
*3.2.1	Altered Role Performance
3.2.1.1.1	Altered Parenting
3.2.1.1.2	Potential Altered Parenting
3.2.1.2.1	Sexual Dysfunction
3.2.2	Altered Family Processes
3.2.3.1	Parental Role Conflict
3.3	Altered Sexuality Patterns

PATTERN 4: VALUING

4.1.1	Spiritual Distress (distress of the human spirit)

PATTERN 5: CHOOSING

5.1.1.1	Ineffective Individual Coping
5.1.1.1.1	Impaired Adjustment
5.1.1.1.2	Defensive Coping
5.1.1.1.3	Ineffective Denial
5.1.2.1.1	Ineffective Family Coping: Disabling
5.1.2.1.2	Ineffective Family Coping: Compromised
5.1.2.2	Family Coping: Potential for Growth
5.2.1.1	Noncompliance (Specify)
5.3.1.1	Decisional Conflict (Specify)
5.4	Health Seeking Behaviors (Specify)

PATTERN 6: MOVING

6.1.1.1	Impaired Physical Mobility
6.1.1.2	Activity Intolerance
6.1.1.2.1	Fatigue
6.1.1.3	Potential Activity Intolerance
6.2.1	Sleep Pattern Disturbance
6.3.1.1	Diversional Activity Deficit
6.4.1.1	Impaired Home Maintenance Management
6.4.2	Altered Health Maintenance
*6.5.1	Feeding Self Care Deficit
6.5.1.1	Impaired Swallowing
6.5.1.2	Ineffective Breastfeeding
#6.5.1.3	Effective Breastfeeding
*6.5.2	Bathing/Hygiene Self Care Deficit
*6.5.3	Dressing/Grooming Self Care Deficit
*6.5.4	Toileting Self Care Deficit
6.6	Altered Growth and Development

PATTERN 7: PERCEIVING

*7.1.1	Body Image Disturbance
*7.1.2	Self Esteem Disturbance
7.1.2.1	Chronic Low Self Esteem
7.1.2.2	Situational Low Self Esteem
*7.1.3	Personal Identity Disturbance
7.2	Sensory/Perceptual Alterations (Specify) (Visual, auditory, kinesthetic, gustatory, tactile, olfactory)
7.2.1.1	Unilateral Neglect
7.3.1	Hopelessness
7.3.2	Powerlessness

PATTERN 8: KNOWING

8.1.1	Knowledge Deficit (Specify)
8.3	Altered Thought Processes

(continued)

TABLE 6-2 (Continued)

PATTERN 9:	FEELING
*9.1.1	Pain
9.1.1.1	Chronic Pain
9.2.1.1	Dysfunctional Grieving
9.2.1.2	Anticipatory Grieving
9.2.2	Potential for Violence: Self-directed or directed at others
9.2.3	Post-Trauma Response
9.2.3.1	Rape-Trauma Syndrome
9.2.3.1.1	Rape-Trauma Syndrome: Compound Reaction
9.2.3.1.2	Rape-Trauma Syndrome: Silent Reaction
9.3.1	Anxiety
9.3.2	Fear

#New diagnostic categories approved 1990
*Categories with modified label terminology
Note. From North American Nursing Diagnosis Association. (1990). *Taxonomy I: Revised 1990*, St. Louis: Author, pp. 6–8.

cation of Diseases (ICD–10). Review of *Taxonomy I Revised* for coding resulted in some minor changes to increase specificity, such as replacement of the word "potential" with "risk." If the coding system is accepted for inclusion in ICD–10, *Taxonomy I Revised* (or its successor) will become a computerized system for categorizing nursing care of clients based on their nursing diagnoses. Such a system also would facilitate quality assurance review, determination of staffing workloads, and cost reimbursement for specific nursing services.

Work on the *Taxonomy I Revised* continues. A number of issues must be addressed in refining it: the varying levels of abstraction, the possibility of including diagnoses that focus on clients' strengths, and the development of a working definition of nursing diagnosis (NANDA, 1988). NANDA views the current development of the nursing diagnosis taxonomy as a beginning, despite the many advances since 1973. Given that it has taken the field of medicine more than 150 years to develop its highly sophisticated classification system, it is not surprising that nursing still has a way to go before a highly developed and workable taxonomy is in place.

The incorporation of nursing diagnosis as an accepted, valid, and valuable nursing activity is given further support in the ANA publication, *Nursing: A Social Policy Statement* (1980). In this document, nursing is defined as "the diagnosis and treatment of human responses to actual or potential health problems" (p. 9). Four essential characteristics of nursing practice are described: the *phenomena* of interest to nurses: the "human re-

sponses to actual or potential health problems;" *theory*, which encompasses the knowledge needed to understand nursing phenomena as a basis for making clinical judgments; *actions*, which are nursing behaviors aimed at promoting health, preventing illness, and restoring function; and *effects*, which refer to the outcomes that occur as a result of nursing actions. The *Social Policy Statement* also delineates nursing diagnosis as a separate and distinct step in the nursing process and provides an illustration of the relationship of the essential characteristics to the phases of the nursing process and the *Standards of Nursing Practice* (see chap. 1).

KEY CHARACTERISTICS OF A NURSING DIAGNOSIS

Despite changes as the concept of nursing diagnosis has developed and been refined, there is common agreement about its characteristics. A nursing diagnosis:

> Is a concluding statement that results from identification of a pattern derived from clinical cues;
>
> Describes a client's responses to actual or potential health problems for which the professional nurse is qualified and licensed to intervene;
>
> Is based on subjective and objective clinical data that can be confirmed;
>
> Is based upon conceptual, scientific, or clinical knowledge the nurse uses to make clinical nursing judgments; and,
>
> Involves analytical and synthetic thinking about the meaning of available clinical data.

During the 1980s, in addition to the ongoing work of the NANDA membership, nursing diagno-

---

American Nurses Association Standards of Practice

STANDARD II.

Nursing diagnoses are derived from health status data.

STANDARD III.

The plan of nursing care includes goals derived from the nursing diagnoses.

Note. From *Standards of Nursing Practice*, American Nurses' Association, 1973, Kansas City, MO: Author. Used with permission.

sis gained widespread acceptance in nursing education and practice. Clinical nursing textbooks incorporated nursing diagnosis as an essential step in the nursing process, and a number of textbooks devoted solely to the topic of nursing diagnosis were published (Carnevali, Mitchell, Woods, & Tanner, 1984; Carpenito, 1984, 1991; Gordon, 1982a, 1987; McFarland & McFarlane, 1989; Taptich, Iyer & Bernocchi-Losey, 1989). Also, numerous articles debating the advantages and limitations of nursing diagnosis appeared (Baretich & Anderson, 1987; Maas, 1986; Martens, 1986; Popkess-Vawter & Pinnell, 1987; Porter, 1986; Shamansky & Yanni, 1983), and practicing nurses began to develop nursing care plans using nursing diagnoses as the primary focus (Smaldone, Greenberg & Perez, 1988; Vandenbosch, Bentley, Jones & Blake, 1986). Nursing diagnosis also became the focus of a number of studies (Anderson & Briggs, 1988; Halloran, 1985; Turkoski, 1988).

In response to the acceptance of nursing diagnosis as an integral part of the nursing process, over the last two decades many states have revised their nurse practice acts to explicitly or implicitly include nursing diagnosis as a unique function of the registered nurse. Today, most nurse practice acts prescribe nursing diagnosis as an activity within the legal scope of nursing practice, and some even mandate its use.

Because of widespread acceptance and use, it is essential that today's nurse be familiar with nursing diagnoses and the process for deriving diagnoses from clinical data. It is also important that nurses remain aware of the advantages and limitations of nursing diagnosis for clinical practice and for the profession so they may use nursing diagnoses in effective and appropriate ways.

ADVANTAGES OF NURSING DIAGNOSIS

As the process and nomenclature of nursing diagnosis have gained acceptance and become increasingly familiar to nurses and other health professionals, the reasons for incorporating nursing diagnosis as a routine phase of the nursing process have become more evident. One of the primary advantages is that nursing diagnosis *helps nurses define the domain and scope of their practice*. It is especially important in today's competitive health-care market that nurses communicate to others, particularly health-care consumers, what specific and unique services they provide. Walker (1986) notes that without nursing diagnosis, the significance of a client's behavior may be lost or incorrect

interpretations of nursing phenomena may be made. She suggests that nursing diagnosis *provides a way for nurses to communicate in a common language about a client's responses* and to help nurses and others see that their work involves unique and distinct services that are beyond and different from medically dependent nursing actions.

Halloran (1985) studied nursing workload in relation to both medical diagnosis related groups (DRGs) and nursing diagnoses and found that nursing diagnoses were twice as likely to be effective predictors of nursing time than were medical diagnoses. For example, the nursing diagnosis category "impaired physical mobility" was a better predictor of the amount of nursing time than the medical diagnosis, "hip fracture." Halloran concludes that nursing diagnoses provide a more valid basis for defining what nurses do and for reimbursement of nursing costs.

Nursing care planning also is facilitated by the use of nursing diagnoses. Traditionally, standardized nursing care plans were developed with medical diagnoses as the focus. Unfortunately, nurses have been slow to overcome their identification with the medical model.

Vandenbosch and colleagues (1986) point to the pitfalls of using medical diagnoses as guides to nursing care. These authors developed standard nursing care plans focused on nursing diagnoses. They discovered that nursing staff found the new format helpful in ensuring comprehensive nursing care, individualizing care, and focusing care planning on nursing activities rather than medical interventions. Moreover, staff satisfaction was increased and time spent writing care plans was decreased.

By helping define the unique domain of nursing practice, nursing diagnosis also *enables nurses to delineate and develop the body of knowledge that is an essential underpinning of all nursing activity*. The discipline's theory-building and research efforts may be enhanced by organizing nursing knowledge around nursing diagnostic categories (Maas, 1986). Use of nursing diagnoses would ensure collaboration of the discipline's researchers and practitioners toward the common goal of developing nursing's body of knowledge. Nurse researchers and theorists often are involved in suggesting new diagnostic labels based on their conceptual and scientific understanding of nursing phenomena. Practicing nurses provide valuable suggestions in the development of defining characteristics and related factors for each diagnosis, and then try out those diagnoses that have been accepted for clinical testing. Outcomes of clinical testing lead to further refinement of the taxonomy.

The use of a standard system for classifying nursing knowledge *facilitates nursing research by making storage and retrieval of data much easier.* For example, a nurse may wish to study the effectiveness of different nursing interventions for pregnant women during labor who have the nursing diagnosis of "pain related to uterine muscle contractions." Use of a single diagnostic label to catalog nursing studies of this human response may facilitate further development and testing of this area of nursing knowledge.

Maas (1986) and Warren (1983) identify a number of other advantages of nursing diagnosis for professional nursing practice, for effective nursing administration, and for the profession. These include:

Facilitating the development of nurse autonomy and accountability by delineating clearly the phenomena that comprise the scope of nursing practice.

Promoting nurses' control of their practice by expanding decision-making opportunities, thereby increasing job satisfaction and retention.

Developing a common language for communicating within the profession and with others about nursing phenomena.

Increasing nursing's power and influence within the health-care system through use of a system for classifying nursing phenomena, achieved by consensus.

Providing an organized structure for developing outcome standards to measure effectiveness of nursing care, resulting in meaningful and relevant quality assurance review.

Providing a framework for developing staff education programs and facilitating staff development.

Ensuring a valid means of determining the costs of nursing care and creating specifications for staffing (size, workload, mix).

Standardizing nursing information to enable the development of computerized nursing information systems that will be essential as nursing moves toward the 21st century.

The development and use of nursing diagnostic labels, while beneficial for the profession in many respects, has been criticized on a number of counts. Given its relative youth, it is not surprising that limitations exist. It is important that nurses are aware of the limitations and continue to address

them as the classification system is further developed, tested, and refined.

LIMITATIONS OF NURSING DIAGNOSIS

One of the most commonly cited limitations of nursing diagnosis is the cumbersome language developed to categorize nursing phenomena (Shamansky & Yanni, 1983). For example, the diagnostic label of "altered nutrition: less than body requirements" is considered by some to be lengthy and awkward. Why not say instead "inadequate caloric intake" or "inadequate intake of iron"? The NANDA conferences work on improving the clarity and conciseness of nursing diagnoses. For instance, the nursing diagnosis of "bowel elimination, alterations in: constipation" has been revised to state simply "constipation." It is important that nursing diagnoses communicate clearly the client's problem or response, not only so nurses can converse with each other but also so they may make themselves clear to other health professionals and to the clients they serve.

Shamansky and Yanni (1983) also point out other pitfalls of nursing diagnosis, including the possibility of limiting nursing to the boundaries defined by the taxonomy, applying premature labels to clients that may inhibit the dynamic flow of nursing observations and interpretations, and stereotyping clients.

Some authors have criticized specific diagnoses as inappropriate terms for the phenomena they are intended to describe. For example, Jenny (1987) proposes dropping the diagnosis "knowledge deficit" from the taxonomy because it does not adhere to the criteria used for acceptance, namely, appropriate conceptual focus, necessary attributes, theoretical validity, and clinical utility. Instead, she suggests that knowledge deficit is a related factor or defining characteristic, not a diagnostic label per se. Edel (1985) criticizes the inclusion of the diagnosis "noncompliance," believing that its use creates a superior–subordinate power relationship between nurse and client and detracts from efforts to determine the underlying cause of the behavior.

Another major criticism frequently levied against nursing diagnosis is its failure to account for client strengths (Martens, 1986; Popkess-Vawter & Pinnell, 1987; Stolte, 1986). Critics argue that focusing exclusively on a client's problems limits the scope of nursing practice and fails to take into account assessment data that form the basis for promoting health and preventing illness. They maintain that diagnosis of a client's strengths should be an essential part of a client's nursing care. However, others (Baretich & Anderson, 1987;

Gordon, 1982b) counter that while it is important to assess a client's strengths to help people overcome health problems, phrasing strengths as positive diagnostic statements provides no clues for nursing interventions. These authors note that even nursing interventions aimed at health promotion or illness prevention imply a problem or deficiency that should be addressed with an appropriate diagnostic label. For example, risk is flagged by the diagnosis "potential for trauma," which may be related to the client's age or lack of knowledge or a sensory-perceptual alteration. Phrasing a client's strength as "avoidance of injury related to accurate knowledge of risk and methods of prevention" does not help the nurse decide what interventions are necessary. Baretich and Anderson (1987) point out that nursing diagnoses are not the same as assessment summaries. The nurse must indeed make clinical judgments (assessment summaries) about data that indicate a client's strengths and capitalize on these strengths when planning nursing care. But Baretich and Anderson (1987) also assert that nursing diagnoses should be reserved for problems or the taxonomy will become forced and artificial.

In addition to the above-mentioned criticisms, Fawcett (1986) argues that the current taxonomy is logically incongruent since no consistent conceptual perspective has been delineated, resulting in "a confusing array of terms and a logically suspect mix of perspectives of nursing phenomena" (p. 399). In a similar vein, Porter (1986) notes that the nine categories of patterns of human responses are used inappropriately as distinct, mutually exclusive entities when, in fact, they overlap conceptually. She also points out that some diagnoses are used both as diagnostic labels as well as a group name for more specific diagnoses. For example, the diagnosis "potential for injury" is both a diagnostic label and a group name for the diagnoses of potential for suffocation, potential for poisoning, and potential for trauma.

Turkoski (1988) reviewed articles on nursing diagnosis published between 1950 and 1985 and concludes that nursing has not yet achieved consensus on the definition, purpose, and application of nursing diagnosis in practice. She also notes that medical labels and language frequently are used to describe the defining characteristics or related factors. Gordon (1982b) shares this concern. Gordon believes that several of the accepted diagnoses, including impaired gas exchange, altered tissue perfusion, and decreased cardiac output are not within the domain of independent nursing practice and are disguised medical diagnoses. Kim (1983) disagrees and suggests that these diagnoses require interdependent and collaborative nursing interventions that critical care nurses are qualified to carry out.

Rather than citing fundamental concerns about the nature or usefulness of nursing diagnosis, some authors have focused on problems in applying nursing diagnosis to clinical practice. Pendleton (1986) notes that nurses frequently make the mistake of applying diagnostic labels without performing a careful nursing assessment. For example, a nurse may assume that a client who has had a mastectomy is experiencing a change in body image and thus apply the label "body image disturbance." However, in the absence of a careful assessment of a client's own response to this event, the nursing diagnosis is invalid. Pendleton points out that nurses often make the mistake of assuming the related factors, but emphasizes that data must support both the choice of the diagnostic label as well as the related factors that are identified. When the nurse lacks adequate data, a tentative diagnosis may be modified by the term "possible" (Carpenito, 1984; Pendleton, 1986), such as "possible body image disturbance related to loss of breast." Further data should be collected to confirm or eliminate a tentative diagnosis.

A study conducted by Anderson and Briggs (1988) reveals that nurses often do apply nursing diagnoses and identify etiologies without adequate supporting information. Moreover, the researchers found that nurses frequently use medical diagnoses as etiological factors, which is problematic since nurses are not qualified and licensed to treat medical diagnoses independently.

Despite the limitations noted above, nursing diagnosis has proved useful for delineating the domain of independent nursing practice. The incorporation of nursing diagnosis in nursing curricula and nursing practice has gained almost universal acceptance. Nurses must continue to work together to strengthen the taxonomy and address and overcome the limitations that interfere with its full acceptance. It is especially important for nurses to understand the distinctions between nursing diagnosis and medical diagnosis. The two complement rather than compete with each other, and both are essential aspects of comprehensive health care for a client.

NURSING DIAGNOSIS VERSUS MEDICAL DIAGNOSIS

How does a nursing diagnosis differ from a medical one? In essence, a medical diagnosis is disease-focused and constant, regardless of how well or ill the client may be at any given time. For example, a client with a medical diagnosis of "diabetes mellitus" retains the diagnosis whether managing well at home or acutely ill and hospitalized. While additional medical diagnoses may be made when the client is experiencing complications, such as "ketoacidosis" or "decubitus ulcer, left heel," the primary diagnosis remains unchanged.

Conversely, a nursing diagnosis describes a client's *responses* to alterations in health and thus changes as the client's responses change. For instance, the nursing diagnoses for a 55-year-old woman undergoing hysterectomy may be several:

1. Pain related to surgical incision,

2. Ineffective breathing pattern related to effects of general anesthesia,

3. Fear related to diagnosis of uterine cancer,

4. Ineffective family coping related to temporary family role changes.

As the client recovers from surgery, diagnoses 1 and 2 are likely to be resolved. Also, as she is discharged to home and resumes her usual roles and activities, diagnosis 4 should be resolved. Diagnosis 3 may be a continuing concern, depending on the prognosis, further treatment, and the client's coping patterns. It is also possible that new nursing diagnoses may arise over time, especially if the client's cancer metastasizes.

This example illustrates how a client with a single medical diagnosis of uterine cancer (hysterectomy) is likely to have multiple, varied nursing diagnoses that change as the client's responses to the health problem and its treatment change. Nursing diagnoses tend to be dynamic, and they must be modified in response to changes in the client. Failure to revise a client's nursing diagnoses, and the nursing care plan, ignores the dynamic and fluid nature of the human being and may compromise the quality of nursing care.

Nurses do, however, carry out many interventions dictated by the medical plan of care. Nurses also may make independent judgments about medical care—for instance, deciding when a client needs medication prescribed for pain, regulation of intravenous fluid therapy, or irrigation of a clogged nasogastric tube. In these instances, though, the nurse does not prescribe the interventions since they are aimed at treating the client's medical diagnoses. Carpenito (1984) points out that despite the fact that nurses may draw medical conclusions based on the nursing assessment, such as identifying signs of hypovolemic shock or the presence of angina, such conclusions should not be labeled nursing diagnoses. And attempts to rename medical diagnoses with nursing terminology ("decreased cardiac output" instead of "congestive heart failure," for example) "muddies the waters and fails to describe an independent nursing domain" (Carpenito, 1984, p. 1418).

Nursing diagnoses encompass those problems for which the nurse has the knowledge and legal authority to prescribe interventions. The nursing care plan should be guided by a client's nursing diagnoses, not by medical diagnoses. While it may be necessary to include medical regimens that the nurse is responsible for implementing, such as medication administration, IV therapy, dressing changes, and suctioning, they should not be the primary focus of the nursing care plan. The nursing care plan should be developed with nursing diagnoses as the basis for prescribing independent nursing interventions.

FORMULATING THE NURSING DIAGNOSTIC STATEMENT

Once information has been obtained, interpreted, clustered, and validated, the nurse is ready to make a clinical judgment about the presence or absence of a client's responses to problems that are amenable to nursing intervention. Diagnosis involves searching the clinical data for relationships or patterns, clustering the data that seem to be related, and hypothesizing one or more nursing diagnoses.

A nursing diagnosis should be clear and concise, yet contain enough information to suggest nursing goals, interventions, and desired outcomes. Thus, it should readily communicate to others the client's responses or problems that are amenable to nursing intervention.

A nursing diagnostic statement is composed of two parts: the problem (diagnostic label) and its etiology (related factors). The two parts of the statement are connected by the phrase "related to."

The first part of any nursing diagnosis should clearly identify the specific problem. The problem may be qualified by a modifying phrase, such as "altered," "potential," "ineffective," or "impaired." Most important, there should be sufficient nursing assessment data to support the diagnosis.

Generally, the diagnostic label should be selected from the most recent NANDA-approved taxonomy. However, the taxonomy is not exhaustive, and there may be situations in which the approved diagnoses do not accurately or adequately describe the problem. In such cases, the nurse may have to create a diagnostic label to fit the situation, making sure, however, that it is a problem for which nurses are qualified and licensed to intervene.

When selecting a diagnostic label, the nurse should compare the information obtained from the nursing assessment with the definition and the defining characteristics for the selected nursing diagnosis. The defining characteristics are "observable signs and symptoms that are present when the . . . problem is present" (Gordon, 1982b, p. 340) and provide a means for validating the diagnostic label. For example, consider the following nursing assessment data:

> Eight-year-old white male; weight above the 95th percentile; height at the 50th percentile; diet history reveals daily caloric intake of 3,000+ calories; engages in minimal physical activity; prefers to watch TV and play videogames; mother describes him as "in the cupboard or refrigerator" every hour.

Based on the data, the nurse identifies the nursing diagnosis of "altered nutrition: more than body requirements." The definition and defining characteristics listed below for this diagnosis indicate that the appropriate diagnosis has been selected.

> *Definition:* The state in which the individual consumes more than adequate nutritional intake in relation to metabolic demands.
> *Defining Characteristics:*
> Weight 10–20% over ideal for height and frame
> Measured food consumption exceeds recommendations for activity level, age, and sex
> Reported or observed dysfunctional eating patterns
> Sedentary activity level

The second part of the diagnostic statement should identify the factors that are causing or contributing to the problem. These are the "related factors" and help the nurse tailor interventions for the individual client. Related factors may reflect physiological, psychological, sociocultural, or environmental etiologies that are causing or contributing to the client's response(s). Examples of related factors are categorized in Table 6-3. It is essential that sufficient information exists to support the second part of the diagnostic statement. Without such data, interventions may be misguided and fail to address the underlying cause, in which case the nursing diagnosis likely will not be resolved.

In the case of the 8-year-old boy, the related factors contributing to his nutritional excess may be numerous:

Lack of physical exercise

Eating as a comfort measure/substitute gratification

TABLE 6-3
Examples of Related Factors for Nursing Diagnoses

Physiological
Aging
Malnutrition
Prolonged bed rest
Pain or discomfort
Fatigue
Inadequate fluid intake

Psychological
Anxiety
Fear
Recent retirement
Loss of significant other
Values conflict
Effects of chronic illness

Sociocultural
Inadequate support systems
Social isolation
Religious or cultural values
Limited financial resources
Language barrier

Environmental
Health-care environment
Architectural barriers
Lack of privacy
Noxious stimuli (light, noise, odors)
Restrictive devices (IV lines, cast, traction, restraints)

Learned eating behaviors

Decreased metabolic need

Ethnic and cultural values

Negative body image

Feelings of boredom, depression, frustration

An accurate and comprehensive nursing assessment is needed to provide clues to the related factors appropriate in this case.

Once the related factors have been identified, the diagnostic statement is complete. The following statements are examples of correctly worded nursing diagnoses, assuming of course there is sufficient information from the nursing assessment to support both parts of each statement:

Potential for infection related to burn wounds

Ineffective breathing pattern related to abdominal pain

Spiritual distress related to death of spouse

Altered growth and development related to effects of physical disability

In some instances, there may be more than one related factor contributing to a problem. All related factors can and should be specified in order to provide sufficient guidance for nursing care planning. For example,

> Ineffective breathing pattern related to effects of general anesthesia, chest incisional pain, and bed rest.

Occasionally, the etiology will be unknown even though there is sufficient information to support the selection of a diagnostic label. The nurse may write the diagnosis as, for example, "sleep pattern disturbance related to unknown factors," while continuing to collect data to determine the etiology.

Because the second part of the diagnostic statement helps to suggest nursing interventions to alleviate the problem or prevent a problem from occurring, it is essential that specific contributing factors be identified. Most diagnoses have numerous possible etiologies, so accuracy and precision are important. For instance, a diagnosis of constipation may be related to any of the following factors:

> Inadequate dietary fiber and fluids
> Pregnancy
> Immobility
> Physical changes associated with aging
> Chronic use of laxatives

Identification of effective and appropriate nursing interventions will depend upon which related factor is contributing to the problem.

Guidelines and helpful hints for writing nursing diagnoses are outlined in Table 6-4. These are followed by the complete *NANDA Taxonomy I* (1990), classified according to the nine human response patterns. This section, which is color-edged for easy reference, includes all 99 currently approved nursing diagnoses, their definitions, defining characteristics, and related factors.

CLIENTS' PERCEPTIONS AND RELATIVITY OF NURSING DIAGNOSES

Once nursing diagnoses for a client have been developed, the nurse should, whenever possible, share them with the client. The nurse should explain the nursing diagnoses that have been identified as the basis for the client's nursing care plan. The purpose of seeking a client's input is to ensure that the nursing care plan addresses the client's unique responses to actual or potential health problems. The client may provide further information that validates or refutes a particular diagnosis.

(*Text continues on page 171.*)

TABLE 6-4
Guidelines for Writing Nursing Diagnoses

State the diagnosis and related factors in terms that suggest interventions within the scope of nursing practice.

Appropriate: Diarrhea related to ingestion of contaminated formula

Inappropriate: Salmonella poisoning secondary to contaminated formula, or
Diarrhea related to salmonella poisoning

State the diagnosis as a response rather than a need.

Appropriate: Altered oral mucous membrane related to inadequate oral hygiene

Inappropriate: Needs mouth care

Use the phrase "related to" instead of "due to" or "caused by" to connect the two parts of the diagnostic statement.

Appropriate: Impaired skin integrity related to prolonged bed rest

Inappropriate: Impaired skin integrity due to (or caused by) prolonged bed rest

Avoid value-laden terms when phrasing the diagnosis.

Appropriate: Impaired home maintenance management related to lack of motivation

Inappropriate: Impaired home maintenance management related to laziness

Avoid reversing the diagnosis and the related factors.

Appropriate: Ineffective breathing pattern related to decreased lung expansion

Inappropriate: Decreased lung expansion related to ineffective breathing pattern

Ensure that the parts of the statement are not redundant.

Appropriate: Body image disturbance related to loss of right leg

Inappropriate: Body image disturbance related to altered perception of body integrity

Avoid using a medical diagnosis as the related factor.

Appropriate: Altered growth and development related to effects of physical disability

Inappropriate: Altered growth and development related to cerebral palsy

Write the diagnosis in clear and concise terms.

Appropriate: Hopelessness related to loss of job and home

Inappropriate: Hopelessness related to loss of self-esteem in response to being fired from job and mortgage foreclosure

NANDA Taxonomy I Revised (1990)

1.1.2.1 ALTERED NUTRITION: MORE THAN BODY REQUIREMENTS (1975)

DEFINITION

The state in which an individual is experiencing an intake of nutrients which exceeds metabolic needs.

DEFINING CHARACTERISTICS:

Weight 10% over ideal for height and frame; *weight 20% over ideal for height and frame; *triceps skin fold greater than 15 mm in men, 25 mm in women; sedentary activity level; reported or observed dysfunctional eating pattern: pairing food with other activities; concentrating food intake at the end of day; eating in response to external cues such as time of day, social situation; eating in response to internal cues other than hunger, e.g., anxiety.

RELATED FACTORS:

Excessive intake in relation to metabolic need.

*Critical

1.1.2.2 ALTERED NUTRITION: LESS THAN BODY REQUIREMENTS (1975)

DEFINITION:

The state in which an individual experiences an intake of nutrients insufficient to meet metabolic needs.

DEFINING CHARACTERISTICS:

Loss of weight with adequate food intake; body weight 20% or more under ideal; reported inadequate food intake less than RDA (recommended daily allowance); weakness of muscles required for swallowing or mastication; reported or evidence of lack of food; aversion to eating; reported altered taste sensation; satiety immediately after ingesting food; abdominal pain with or without pathology; sore, inflamed buccal cavity; capillary fragility; abdominal cramping; diarrhea and/or steatorrhea; hyperactive bowel sounds; lack of interest in food; perceived inability to ingest food; pale conjunctival and mucous membranes; poor muscle tone; excessive loss of hair; lack of information, misinformation; misconceptions.

RELATED FACTORS:

Inability to ingest or digest food or absorb nutrients due to biological, psychological, or economic factors.

Note: From *Taxonomy I Revised—1990,* North American Nursing Diagnosis Association, 1990, pp. 10–108. St. Louis: NANDA.

1.1.2.3 ALTERED NUTRITION: POTENTIAL FOR MORE THAN BODY REQUIREMENTS (1980)

DEFINITION:

The state in which an individual is at risk of experiencing an intake of nutrients which exceeds metabolic needs.

DEFINING CHARACTERISTICS:

Presence of risk factors such as:

*Reported or observed obesity in one or both parents; *rapid transition across growth percentiles in infants or children; reported use of solid food as major food source before 5 months of age; observed use of food as reward or comfort measure; reported or observed higher baseline weight at beginning of each pregnancy; dysfunctional eating patterns: pairing food with other activities; concentrating food intake at end of day; eating in response to external cues such as time of day, social situation; eating in response to internal cues other than hunger such as anxiety.

RELATED FACTORS:

See risk.

*Critical

120

1.2.1.1 POTENTIAL FOR INFECTION (1986)

DEFINITION:

The state in which an individual is at increased risk for being invaded by pathogenic organisms.

DEFINING CHARACTERISTICS:

Presence of risk factors such as:

Inadequate primary defenses (broken skin, traumatized tissue, decrease in ciliary action, stasis of body fluids, change in pH secretions, altered peristalsis); inadequate secondary defenses (e.g., decreased hemoglobin, leukopenia, suppressed inflammatory response) and immunosuppression; inadequate acquired immunity; tissue destruction and increased environmental exposure; chronic disease; invasive procedures; malnutrition; pharmaceutical agents; trauma; rupture of amniotic membranes; insufficient knowledge to avoid exposure to pathogens.

RELATED FACTORS:

See risk factors.

1.2.2.1 POTENTIAL ALTERED BODY TEMPERATURE (1986)

DEFINITION:

The state in which the individual is at risk for failure to maintain body temperature within normal range.

DEFINING CHARACTERISTICS:

Presence of risk factors such as:

Extremes of age; extremes of weight; exposure to cold/cool or warm/hot environments; dehydration; inactivity or vigorous activity; medications causing vasoconstriction/vasodilation; altered metabolic rate; sedation; inappropriate clothing for environmental temperature; illness or trauma affecting temperature regulation.

RELATED FACTORS:

See risk factors.

1.2.2.2 HYPOTHERMIA (1986, 1988R)

DEFINITION:

The state in which an individual's body temperature is reduced below normal range.

DEFINING CHARACTERISTICS:

Major:

Reduction in body temperature below normal range; shivering (mild); cool skin; pallor (moderate).

Minor:

Slow capillary refill; tachycardia; cyanotic nail beds; hypertension; piloerection.

RELATED FACTORS:

Exposure to cool or cold environment; illness or trauma; damage to hypothalamus; inability or decreased ability to shiver; malnutrition; inadequate clothing; consumption of alcohol; medications causing vasodilation; evaporation from skin in cool environment; decreased metabolic rate, inactivity; aging.

121

1.2.2.3 HYPERTHERMIA (1986)

DEFINITION:

A state in which an individual's body temperature is elevated above his/her normal range.

DEFINING CHARACTERISTICS:

Major:

Increase in body temperature above normal range.

Minor:

Flushed skin, warm to touch, increased respiratory rate, tachycardia, seizures/convulsions.

RELATED FACTORS:

Exposure to hot environment; vigorous activity; medications/anesthesia; inappropriate clothing: increased metabolic rate; illness or trauma; dehydration; inability or decreased ability to perspire.

1.2.2.4 INEFFECTIVE THERMOREGULATION (1986)

DEFINITION:

The state in which the individual's temperature fluctuates between hypothermia and hyperthermia.

DEFINING CHARACTERISTICS:

Major:

Fluctuations in body temperature above or below the normal range. See also major and minor characteristics present in hypothermia and hyperthermia.

RELATED FACTORS:

Trauma or illness; immaturity; aging; fluctuating environmental temperature.

122

1.2.3.1 DYSREFLEXIA (1988)

DEFINITION:

The state in which an individual with a spinal cord injury at T7 or above experiences a life threatening uninhibited sympathetic response of the nervous system to a noxious stimulus.

DEFINING CHARACTERISTICS:

Major: Individual with spinal cord injury (T7 or above) with:

Paroxysmal hypertension (sudden periodic elevated blood pressure where systolic pressure is over 140 mmHg and diastolic is above 90 mmHg); bradycardia or tachycardia (pulse rate of less than 60 or over 100 beats per minute); diaphoresis (above the injury); red splotches on skin (above the injury); pallor (below the injury); headache (a diffuse pain in different portions of the head and not confined to any nerve distribution area).

Minor:

Chilling; conjunctival congestion; Horner's Syndrome (contraction of the pupil, partial ptosis of the eyelid, enophthalmos and sometimes loss of sweating over the affected side of the face); paresthesia; pilomotor reflex (gooseflesh formation when skin is cooled); blurred vision; chest pain; metallic taste in mouth; nasal congestion.

RELATED FACTORS:

Bladder distention; bowel distention; skin irritation; lack of patient and care giver knowledge.

1.3.1.1 CONSTIPATION (1975)

DEFINITION:

A state in which an individual experiences a change in normal bowel habits characterized by a decrease in frequency and/or passage of hard dry stools.

DEFINING CHARACTERISTICS:

Decreased activity level; frequency less than usual pattern; hard formed stools; palpable mass; reported feeling of pressure in rectum; reported feeling of rectal fullness; straining at stool.

OTHER POSSIBLE CHARACTERISTICS:

Abdominal pain; appetite impairment; back pain; headache; interference with daily living; use of laxatives.

RELATED FACTORS:

To be developed.

1.3.1.1.1 PERCEIVED CONSTIPATION (1988)

DEFINITION:

The state in which an individual makes a self-diagnosis of constipation and ensures a daily bowel movement through abuse of laxatives, enemas, and suppositories.

DEFINING CHARACTERISTICS:

Major:

Expectation of a daily bowel movement with the resulting overuse of laxatives, enemas, and suppositories; expected passage of stool at same time every day.

RELATED FACTORS:

Cultural/family health beliefs; faulty appraisal; impaired thought processes.

1.3.1.1.2 COLONIC CONSTIPATION (1988)

DEFINITION:

The state in which an individual's pattern of elimination is characterized by hard, dry stool which results from a delay in passage of food residue.

DEFINING CHARACTERISTICS:

Major:

Decreased frequency; hard, dry stool; straining at stool; painful defecation; abdominal distention; palpable mass.

Minor:

Rectal pressure; headache, appetite impairment; abdominal pain.

RELATED FACTORS:

Less than adequate fluid intake; less than adequate dietary intake; less than adequate fiber; less than adequate physical activity; immobility; lack of privacy; emotional disturbances; chronic use of medication and enemas; stress; change in daily routine; metabolic problems, e.g., hypothyroidism, hypocalcemia, hypokalemia.

1.3.1.2 DIARRHEA (1975)

DEFINITION:

A state in which an individual experiences a change in normal bowel habits characterized by the frequent passage of loose, fluid, unformed stools.

DEFINING CHARACTERISTICS:

Abdominal pain; cramping; increased frequency; increased frequency of bowel sounds; loose liquid stools; urgency.

OTHER POSSIBLE CHARACTERISTICS:

Change in color.

RELATED FACTORS:

To be developed.

1.3.1.3 BOWEL INCONTINENCE (1975)

DEFINITION:

A state in which an individual experiences a change in normal bowel habits characterized by involuntary passage of stool.

DEFINING CHARACTERISTICS:

Involuntary passage of stool.

RELATED FACTORS:

To be developed.

1.3.2   ALTERED URINARY ELIMINATION (1973)

DEFINITION:

The state in which the individual experiences a disturbance in urine elimination.

DEFINING CHARACTERISTICS:

Dysuria; frequency; hesitancy; incontinence; nocturia; retention; urgency.

RELATED FACTORS:

Multiple causality, including: anatomical obstruction, sensory motor impairment, urinary tract infection.

1.3.2.1.1   STRESS INCONTINENCE (1986)

DEFINITION:

The state in which an individual experiences a loss of urine of less than 50 ml occurring with increased abdominal pressure.

DEFINING CHARACTERISTICS:

Major:

Reported or observed dribbling with increased abdominal pressure.

Minor:

Urinary urgency; urinary frequency (more often than every 2 hours).

RELATED FACTORS:

Degenerative changes in pelvic muscles and structural supports associated with increased age; high intra-abdominal pressure (e.g., obesity, gravid uterus); incompetent bladder outlet; overdistention between voidings; weak pelvic muscles and structural supports.

1.3.2.1.2 REFLEX INCONTINENCE (1986)

DEFINITION:

The state in which an individual experiences an involuntary loss of urine, occurring at somewhat predictable intervals when a specific bladder volume is reached.

DEFINING CHARACTERISTICS:

Major:

No awareness of bladder filling; no urge to void or feelings of bladder fullness; uninhabited bladder contraction/spasm at regular intervals.

RELATED FACTORS:

Neurological impairment (e.g., spinal cord lesion which interferes with conduction of cerebral messages above the level of the reflex arc).

1.3.2.1.3 URGE INCONTINENCE (1986)

DEFINITION:

The state in which an individual experiences involuntary passage of urine occurring soon after a strong sense of urgency to void.

DEFINING CHARACTERISTICS:

Major:

Urinary urgency; frequency (voiding more often than every two hours); bladder contracture/spasm.

Minor:

Nocturia (more than two times per night); voiding in small amounts (less than 100 cc) or in large amounts (more than 550 cc); inability to reach toilet in time.

RELATED FACTORS:

Decreased bladder capacity (e.g., history of PID, abdominal surgeries, indwelling urinary catheter); irritation of bladder stretch receptors causing spasm (e.g., bladder infection); alcohol; caffeine; increased fluids; increased urine concentration; overdistention of bladder.

1.3.2.1.4 FUNCTIONAL INCONTINENCE (1986)

DEFINITION:

The state in which an individual experiences an involuntary, unpredictable passage of urine.

DEFINING CHARACTERISTICS:

Major:

Urge to void or bladder contractions sufficiently strong to result in loss of urine before reaching an appropriate receptacle.

RELATED FACTORS:

Altered environment; sensory, cognitive, or mobility deficits.

1.3.2.1.5 TOTAL INCONTINENCE (1986)

DEFINITION:

The state in which an individual experiences a continuous and unpredictable loss of urine.

DEFINING CHARACTERISTICS:

Major:

Constant flow of urine occurs at unpredictable times without distention or uninhibited bladder contractions/spasm; unsuccessful incontinence refractory treatments; nocturia.

Minor:

Lack of perineal or bladder filling awareness; unawareness of incontinence.

RELATED FACTORS:

Neuropathy preventing transmission of reflex indicating bladder fullness; neurological dysfunction causing triggering of micturition at unpredictable times; independent contraction of detrusor reflex due to surgery; trauma or disease affecting spinal cord nerves; anatomic (fistula).

1.3.2.2 URINARY RETENTION (1986)

DEFINITION:

The state in which the individual experiences incomplete emptying of the bladder.

DEFINING CHARACTERISTICS:

Major:

Bladder distention; small, frequent voiding or absence of urine output.

Minor:

Sensation of bladder fullness; dribbling; residual urine; dysuria; overflow incontinence.

RELATED FACTORS:

High urethral pressure caused by weak detrusor; inhibition of reflex arc; strong sphincter; blockage.

129

1.4.1.1 ALTERED TISSUE PERFUSION (SPECIFY TYPE) (RENAL, CEREBRAL, CARDIOPULMONARY, GASTROINTESTINAL, PERIPHERAL)++ (1980)

DEFINITION:

The state in which an individual experiences a decrease in nutrition and oxygenation at the cellular level due to a deficit in capillary blood supply.

DEFINING CHARACTERISTICS:

	Chances that characteristics will be present in given diagnosis.	Estimated sensitivities and specificities. Chances that characteristic will not be explained by any other diagnosis.
Skin temperature, cold extremities	High	Low
Skin color dependent blue or purple	Moderate	High
*Pale on elevation, color does not return on lowering of leg	High	High
*Diminished arterial pulsations	High	High
Skin quality: shining	High	Low
Lack of lanugo	High	Moderate
Round scars covered with atrophied skin		
Gangrene	Low	High
Slow-growing, dry brittle nails	High	Moderate
Claudication	Moderate	High

1.4.1.2.1 FLUID VOLUME EXCESS (1982)

DEFINITION:

The state in which an individual experiences increased fluid retention and edema.

DEFINING CHARACTERISTICS:

Edema; effusion; anasarca; weight gain; shortness of breath, orthopnea; intake greater than output; S/3 heart sound; pulmonary congestion (chest x-ray); abnormal breath sounds, rales (crackles); change in respiratory pattern; change in mental status; decreased hemoglobin and hematocrit; blood pressure changes; central venous pressure changes; pulmonary artery pressure changes; jugular vein distension; positive hepatojugular reflex; oliguria; specific gravity changes; azotemia; altered electrolytes; restlessness and anxiety.

RELATED FACTORS:

Compromised regulatory mechanism; excess fluid intake; excess sodium intake.

1.4.1.1 (continued)

	Chances that characteristics will be present in given diagnosis.	Estimated sensitivities and specificities. Chances that characteristic will not be explained by any other diagnosis.
Blood pressure changes in extremities		
Bruits	Moderate	Moderate
Slow healing of lesions	High	Low

RELATED FACTORS:

Interruption of flow, arterial; interruption of flow, venous; exchange problems; hypovolemia; hypervolemia.

++Further work and development are required for the subcomponents, specifically cerebral, renal, and gastrointestinal

*Critical

130

1.4.1.2.2.1 FLUID VOLUME DEFICIT (1978)

DEFINITION:

The state in which an individual experiences vascular, cellular, or intracellular dehydration.

DEFINING CHARACTERISTICS:

Change in urine output; change in urine concentration; sudden weight loss or gain; decreased venous filling; hemoconcentration; change in serum sodium.

OTHER POSSIBLE CHARACTERISTICS:

Hypotension; thirst; increased pulse rate; decreased skin turgor; decreased pulse volume/pressure; change in mental state; increased body temperature; dry skin; dry mucous membranes; weakness.

RELATED FACTORS:

Active fluid volume loss; failure of regulatory mechanisms.

1.4.1.2.2.2 POTENTIAL FLUID VOLUME DEFICIT (1978)

DEFINITION:

The state in which an individual is at risk of experiencing vascular, cellular, or intracellular dehydration.

DEFINING CHARACTERISTICS:

Presence of risk factors such as:

Extremes of age; extremes of weight; excessive losses through normal routes, e.g., diarrhea; loss of fluid through abnormal routes, e.g. indwelling tubes; deviations affecting access to or intake or absorption of fluids, e.g., physical immobility; factors influencing fluids needs, e.g., Hypermetabolic state; knowledge deficiency related to fluid volume; medications, e.g., diuretics.

RELATED FACTORS:

See risk factors.

1.4.2.1 DECREASED CARDIAC OUTPUT (1975)

DEFINITION:

A state in which the blood pumped by an individual's heart is sufficiently reduced that it is inadequate to meet the needs of the body's tissues.

DEFINING CHARACTERISTICS:

Variations in blood pressure readings; arrhythmias; fatigue; jugular vein distention; color changes, skin and mucous membranes; oliguria; decreased peripheral pulses; cold clammy skin; rales; dyspnea, orthopnea; restlessness.

OTHER POSSIBLE CHARACTERISTICS:

Change in mental status; shortness of breath; syncope; vertigo; edema; cough; frothy sputum; gallop rhythm; weakness.

RELATED FACTORS:

To be developed.

1.5.1.1 IMPAIRED GAS EXCHANGE (1980)

DEFINITION:

The state in which the individual experiences a decreased passage of oxygen and/or carbon dioxide between the alveoli of the lungs and the vascular system.

DEFINING CHARACTERISTICS:

Confusion; somnolence; restlessness; irritability; inability to move secretions; hypercapnea; hypoxia.

RELATED FACTORS:

Ventilation perfusion imbalance.

1.5.1.2 INEFFECTIVE AIRWAY CLEARANCE (1980)

DEFINITION:

A state in which an individual is unable to clear secretions or obstructions from the respiratory tract to maintain airway patency.

DEFINING CHARACTERISTICS:

Abnormal breath sounds (rales [crackles], rhonchi [wheezes]); changes in rate or depth of respiration; tachypnea; cough, effective/ineffective, with or without sputum; cyanosis; dyspnea.

RELATED FACTORS:

Decreased energy/fatigue; tracheobronchial infection, obstruction, secretion; perceptual/cognitive impairment; trauma.

1.5.1.3 INEFFECTIVE BREATHING PATTERN (1980)

DEFINITION:

The state in which an individual's inhalation and/or exhalation pattern does not enable adequate pulmonary inflation or emptying.

DEFINING CHARACTERISTICS:

Dyspnea, shortness of breath, tachypnea, fremitus, abnormal arterial blood gas, cyanosis, cough, nasal flaring, respiratory depth changes, assumption of 3-point position, pursed-lip breathing/prolonged expiratory phase, increased anteroposterior diameter, use of accessory muscles, altered chest excursion.

RELATED FACTORS:

Neuromuscular impairment; pain, musculoskeletal impairment; perception/cognitive impairment; anxiety; decreased energy/fatigue.

1.6.1 POTENTIAL FOR INJURY (1978)

DEFINITION:

A state in which the individual is at risk of injury as a result of environmental conditions interacting with the individual's adaptive and defensive resources.

DEFINING CHARACTERISTICS:

Presence of risk factors such as:

Internal: Biochemical, regulatory function: sensory dysfunction, integrative dysfunction, effector dysfunction; tissue hypoxia; malnutrition; immune/autoimmune; abnormal blood profile; leukocytosis/leukopenia; altered clotting factors; thrombocytopenia; sickle cell, Thalassemia; decreased hemoglobin; physical: broken skin, altered mobility; developmental age: physiological, psychosocial; psychological: affective, orientation.

External: Biological: immunization level of community, microorganisms; chemical: pollutants, poisons, drugs, pharmaceutical agents, alcohol, caffeine, nicotine, preservatives, cosmetics and dyes; nutrients: vitamins, food types; physical: design, structure, and arrangement of community, building, and/or equipment; mode of transport/transportation; people/provider: nosocomial agents; staffing patterns: cognitive, affective, and psychomotor factors.

RELATED FACTORS:

See risk factors.

1.6.1.1 POTENTIAL FOR SUFFOCATION (1980)

DEFINITION:

Accentuated risk of accidental suffocation (inadequate air available for inhalation).

DEFINING CHARACTERISTICS:

Presence of risk factors such as:

Internal (individual): reduced olfactory sensation; reduced motor abilities; lack of safety education; lack of safety precautions; cognitive or emotional difficulties; disease or injury process.

External (environmental): pillow placed in an infant's crib; propped bottle placed in an infant's crib; vehicle warming in closed garage; children playing with plastic bags or inserting small objects into their mouths or noses; discarded or unused refrigerators or freezers without removed doors; children left unattended in bathtubs or pools; household gas leaks; smoking in bed; use of fuel-burning heaters not vented to outside; low-strung clothesline; pacifier hung around infant's head; person who eats large mouthfuls of food.

RELATED FACTORS:

See risk factors.

1.6.1.2 POTENTIAL FOR POISONING (1980)

DEFINITION:

Accentuated risk of accidental exposure to or ingestion of drugs or dangerous products in doses sufficient to cause poisoning.

DEFINING CHARACTERISTICS:

Presence of risk factors such as:

Internal (individual): reduced vision; verbalization of occupational setting without adequate safeguards; lack of safety or drug education; lack of proper precaution; cognitive or emotional difficulties; insufficient finances.

External (environmental): large supplies of drugs in house; medicines stored in unlocked cabinets accessible to children or confused persons; dangerous products placed or stored within the reach of children or confused persons; availability of illicit drugs potentially contaminated by poisonous additives; flaking, peeling paint or plaster in presence of young children; chemical contamination of food and water; unprotected contact with heavy metals or chemicals; paint, lacquer, etc., in poorly ventilated areas or without effective protection; presence of poisonous vegetation; presence of atmospheric pollutants.

RELATED FACTORS:

See risk factors.

1.6.1.3 POTENTIAL FOR TRAUMA (1980)

DEFINITION:

Accentuated risk of accidental tissue injury, e.g., wound, burn, fracture.

DEFINING CHARACTERISTICS:

Presence of risk factors such as:

Internal (individual): weakness; poor vision; balancing difficulties; reduced temperature and/or tactile sensation; reduced large or small muscle coordination; reduced hand-eye coordination; lack of safety education; lack of safety precautions; insufficient finances to purchase safety equipment or effect repairs; cognitive or emotional difficulties; history of previous trauma.

External (environmental): slippery floors, e.g., wet or highly waxed; snow or ice collected on stairs, walkways; unanchored rugs; bathtub without hand grip or antislip equipment; use of unsteady ladders or chairs; entering unlighted rooms; unsturdy or absent stair rails; unanchored electric wires; litter or liquid spills on floors or stairways; high beds; children playing without gates at the top of the stairs; obstructed passageways; unsafe window protection in homes with young children; inappropriate call-for-aid mechanisms for bed-resting client; pot handles facing toward front of stove; bathing in very hot water, e.g., unsupervised bathing of young children; potential igniting gas leaks; delayed lighting of gas burner or oven; experimenting with chemicals or gasoline; unscreened fires or heaters; wearing plastic apron or flowing clothes around open flame; children playing with matches, candles, cigarettes; inadequately stored combustibles or corrosives, e.g., matches, oily rags, lye; highly flammable children's toys or clothing; overloaded fuse boxes; contact with rapidly moving machinery, industrial belts, or pulleys; sliding on coarse bed linen or struggling within bed restraints; faulty electrical plugs, frayed wires, or defective appliances; contact with acids or alkalis; playing with fire-

135

1.6.1.3 (continued)

works or gunpowder; contact with intense cold; overexposure to sun, sun lamps, radiotherapy; use of cracked dishware or glasses; knives stored uncovered; guns or ammunition stored unlocked; large icicles hanging from the roof; exposure to dangerous machinery; children playing with sharp-edged toys; high crime neighborhood and vulnerable clients; driving a mechanically unsafe vehicle; driving after partaking of alcoholic beverages or drugs; driving at excessive speeds; driving without necessary visual aids; children riding in the front seat in car; smoking in bed or near oxygen; overloaded electrical outlets; grease waste collected on stoves; use of thin or worn potholders or misuse of necessary headgear for motorized cyclists or young children carried on adult bicycles; unsafe road or road-crossing conditions; play or work near vehicle pathways, e.g., driveways, laneways, railroad tracks; nonuse or misuse of seat restraints.

RELATED FACTORS:

See risk factors.

1.6.1.4 POTENTIAL FOR ASPIRATION (1988)

DEFINITION:

The state in which an individual is at risk for entry of gastrointestinal secretions, oropharyngeal secretions, or solids or fluids into tracheobronchial passages.

DEFINING CHARACTERISTICS:

Presence of risk factors such as:

Reduced level of consciousness; depressed cough and gag reflexes; presence of tracheostomy or endotracheal tube; incomplete lower esophageal sphincter; gastrointestinal tubes; tube feedings; medication administration; situations hindering elevation of upper body; increased intragastric pressure; increased gastric residual; decreased gastrointestinal motility; delayed gastric emptying; impaired swallowing; facial/oral/neck surgery or trauma; wired jaws.

RELATED FACTORS:

See risk factors.

1.6.1.5 POTENTIAL FOR DISUSE SYNDROME (1988)

DEFINITION:

A state in which an individual is at risk for deterioration of body systems as the result of prescribed or unavoidable musculoskeletal inactivity.*

DEFINING CHARACTERISTICS:

Presence of risk factors such as:

Paralysis; mechanical immobilization; prescribed immobilization; severe pain; altered level of consciousness.

RELATED FACTORS:

See risk factors.

*Complications from immobility can include pressure ulcer, constipation, stasis of pulmonary secretions, thrombosis, urinary tract infection/retention, decreased strength/endurance, orthostatic hypotension, decreased range of joint motion, disorientation, body image disturbance and powerlessness.

137

1.6.2 ALTERED PROTECTION (1990)

DEFINITION:

The state in which an individual experiences a decrease in the ability to guard the self from internal or external threats such as illness or injury.

DEFINING CHARACTERISTICS:

Major:

Deficient immunity; impaired healing; altered clotting; maladaptive stress response; neuro-sensory alteration.

Minor:

Chilling; perspiring; dyspnea; cough; itching; restlessness; insomnia; fatigue; anorexia; weakness; immobility; disorientation; pressure sores.

RELATED FACTORS:

Extremes of age; inadequate nutrition; alcohol abuse; abnormal blood profiles (leukopenia, thrombocytopenia, anemia, coagulation); drug therapies (antineoplastic, corticosteroid, immune, anticoagulant, thrombolytic); treatments (surgery, radiation) and diseases such as cancer and immune disorders.

1.6.2.1 IMPAIRED TISSUE INTEGRITY (1986)

DEFINITION:

A state in which an individual experiences damage to mucous membrane, corneal, integumentary, or subcutaneous tissue.

DEFINING CHARACTERISTICS:

Major:

Damaged or destroyed tissue (cornea, mucous membrane, integumentary, or subcutaneous).

RELATED FACTORS:

Altered circulation; nutritional deficit/excess; fluid deficit/excess; knowledge deficit; impaired physical mobility; irritants, chemical (including body excretions, secretions, medications); thermal (temperature extremes); mechanical (pressure, shear, friction); radiation (including therapeutic radiation).

1.6.2.1.1 ALTERED ORAL MUCOUS MEMBRANE (1982)

DEFINITION:

The state in which an individual experiences disruptions in the tissue layers of the oral cavity.

DEFINING CHARACTERISTICS:

Oral pain/discomfort; coated tongue; xerostomia (dry mouth); stomatitis; oral lesions or ulcers; lack of or decreased salivation; leukoplakia; edema; hyperemia; oral plaque; desquamation; vesicles; hemorrhagic gingivitis, carious teeth; halitosis.

RELATED FACTORS:

Pathological conditions—oral cavity (radiation to head or neck); dehydration; trauma (chemical, e.g., acidic foods, drugs, noxious agents, alcohol; mechanical, e.g., ill-fitting dentures, braces, tubes [endotracheal/nasogastric], surgery in oral cavity); NPO for more than 24 hours; ineffective oral hygiene; mouth breathing; malnutrition; infection; lack of or decreased salivation; medication.

1.6.2.1.2.1 IMPAIRED SKIN INTEGRITY (1975)

DEFINITION:

A state in which the individual's skin is adversely altered.

DEFINING CHARACTERISTICS:

Disruption of skin surface; destruction of skin layers; invasion of body structures.

RELATED FACTORS:

External (environmental): hyper- or hypothermia; chemical substance; mechanical factors (shearing forces, pressure, restraint); radiation; physical immobilization; humidity.

Internal (somatic): medication; altered nutritional state (obesity, emaciation); altered metabolic state; altered circulation; altered sensation; altered pigmentation; skeletal prominence; developmental factors; immunological deficit; alterations in turgor (change in elasticity).

1.6.2.1.2.2 POTENTIAL IMPAIRED SKIN INTEGRITY (1975)

DEFINITION:

A state in which the individual's skin is at risk of being adversely altered.

DEFINING CHARACTERISTICS:

Presence of risk factors such as:

External (environmental): hypo- or hyperthermia; chemical substance; mechanical factors (shearing forces, pressure, restraint); radiation; physical immobilization; excretions/secretions; humidity.

Internal (somatic): medication; alterations in nutritional state (obesity, emaciation); altered metabolic state; altered circulation; altered sensation; altered pigmentation; skeletal prominence; developmental factors; alterations in skin turgor (change in elasticity); psychogenic; immunologic.

RELATED FACTORS:

See risk factors.

2.1.1.1 IMPAIRED VERBAL COMMUNICATION (1973)

DEFINITION:

The state in which an individual experiences a decreased or absent ability to use or understand language in human interaction.

DEFINING CHARACTERISTICS:

*Unable to speak dominant language; *speaks or verbalizes with difficulty; *does not or cannot speak; stuttering; slurring; difficulty forming words or sentences; difficulty expressing thought verbally; inappropriate verbalization; dyspnea; disorientation.

RELATED FACTORS:

Decrease in circulation to brain; brain tumor; physical barrier (tracheostomy, intubation); anatomical defect, cleft palate; psychological barriers (psychosis, lack of stimuli); cultural difference; developmental or age related.

*Critical

3.1.1 IMPAIRED SOCIAL INTERACTION (1986)

DEFINITION:

The state in which an individual participates in an insufficient or excessive quantity or ineffective quality of social exchange.

DEFINING CHARACTERISTICS:

Major:

Verbalized or observed discomfort in social situations; verbalized or observed inability to receive or communicate a satisfying sense of belonging, caring, interest, or shared history; observed use of unsuccessful social interaction behaviors; dysfunctional interaction with peers, family and/or others.

Minor:

Family report of change of style or pattern of interaction.

RELATED FACTORS:

Knowledge/skill deficit about ways to enhance mutuality; communication barriers; self-concept disturbance; absence of available significant others or peers; limited physical mobility; therapeutic isolation; sociocultural dissonance; environmental barriers; altered thought processes.

3.1.2 SOCIAL ISOLATION (1982)

DEFINITION:

Aloneness experienced by the individual and perceived as imposed by others and as a negative or threatened state.

DEFINING CHARACTERISTICS:

Objective: *absence of supportive significant other(s) [family, friends, group]; sad dull affect; inappropriate or immature interests/activities for development age/stage; uncommunicative, withdrawn, no eye contact; preoccupation with own thoughts, repetitive meaningless actions; projects hostility in voice, behavior; seeks to be alone, or exists in a subculture; evidence of physical/mental handicap or altered state of wellness; shows behavior unaccepted by dominant cultural group.

Subjective: *expresses feelings of aloneness imposed by others; *expresses feelings of rejection; experiences feelings of difference from others; inadequacy in or absence of significant purpose in life; inability to meet expectations of others; insecurity in public; expresses values acceptable to the subculture but unacceptable to the dominant cultural group; expresses interests inappropriate to the developmental age/stage.

RELATED FACTORS:

Factors contributing to the absence of satisfying personal relationships, such as: delay in accomplishing developmental tasks; immature interests; alterations in physical appearance; alterations in mental status; unaccepted social behavior; unaccepted social values; altered state of wellness; inadequate personal resources; inability to engage in satisfying personal relationships.

*Critical

141

3.2.1 ALTERED ROLE PERFORMANCE (1978)

DEFINITION:

Disruption in the way one perceives one's role performance.

DEFINING CHARACTERISTICS:

Change in self-perception of role; denial of role; change in others' perception of role; conflict in roles; change in physical capacity to resume role; lack of knowledge of role; change in usual patterns of responsibility.

RELATED FACTORS:

To be developed.

3.2.1.1.1 ALTERED PARENTING (1978)

DEFINITION:

The state in which a nurturing figure(s) experiences an inability to create an environment which promotes the optimum growth and development of another human being.[+]

DEFINING CHARACTERISTICS:

Abandonment; runaway; verbalization, cannot control child; incidence of physical and psychological trauma; lack of parental attachment behaviors; inappropriate visual, tactile, auditory stimulation; negative identification of infant/child's characteristics; negative attachment of meanings to infant/child's characteristics; constant verbalization of disappointment in gender or physical characteristics of the infant/child; verbalization of resentment toward the infant/child; verbalization of role inadequacy; *inattentive to infant/child needs; verbal disgust at body functions of infant/child; noncompliance with health appointments for self and/or infant/child; *inappropriate caretaking behavior (toilet training, sleep/rest, feeding); inappropriate or inconsistent discipline practices; frequent accidents; frequent illness; growth and development lag in the child; *history of child abuse or abandonment by primary caretaker; verbalizes desire to have child call him/herself by first name versus traditional cultural tendencies; child receives care from multiple caretakers without consideration for the needs of the infant/child; compulsively seeking role approval from others.

RELATED FACTORS:

Lack of available role model; ineffective role model; physical and psychosocial abuse of nurturing figure; lack of support between/from significant other(s); unmet social/emotional maturation needs of parenting figures; interruption in bonding process, i.e., maternal, paternal, other; unrealistic expectation for self, infant, partner; perceived threat to own survival, physical and emotional; mental and/or physi-

142

3.2.1.1.1 (continued)

cal illness; presence of stress (financial, legal, recent crisis, cultural [mores]); lack of knowledge; limited cognitive functioning; lack of role identity; lack of inappropriate response of child to relationship; multiple pregnancies.

[+]It is important to state as a preface to this diagnosis that adjustment to parenting in general is a normal maturational process that elicits nursing behaviors of prevention of potential problems and health promotion.

*Critical

3.2.1.1.2 POTENTIAL ALTERED PARENTING (1978)

DEFINITION:

The state in which a nurturing figure(s) is at risk to experience an inability [to create an] environment which promotes the optimum growth and development of another human being.[+]

DEFINING CHARACTERISTICS:

Presence of risk factors such as:

Lack of parental attachment behaviors; inappropriate visual, tactile, auditory stimulation; negative identification of infant/child's characteristics; negative attachment of meanings to infant/child's characteristics; constant verbalization of disappointment in gender or physical characteristics of the infant/child; verbalization of resentment towards the infant/child; verbalization of role inadequacy; *inattentive to infant/child's needs; verbal disgust at body functions of infant/child; noncompliance with health appointments for self and/or infant/child; *inappropriate caretaking behaviors (toilet training, sleep/rest, feeding); inappropriate or inconsistent discipline practices; frequent accidents; frequent illness; growth and development lag in the child; +history of child abuse or abandonment by primary caretaker; verbalizes desire to have child call him/herself by first name versus traditional cultural tendencies; child receives care from multiple caretakers without consideration for the needs of the infant/child; compulsively seeking role approval from others.

RELATED FACTORS:

Lack of available role model; ineffective role model; physical and psychosocial abuse of nurturing figure; lack of support between/from significant other(s); unmet social/emotional maturation needs of parenting figures; interruption in bonding process, i.e., maternal, paternal, other; unrealistic expectation for self, infant, partner; perceived threat to own survival, physical and emotional; mental and/or physical illness; presence of stress (financial, legal, recent crisis, cultural

3.2.1.1.2 (continued)

[mores]); lack of knowledge; limited cognitive functioning; lack of role identity; lack or inappropriate response of child to relationship; multiple pregnancies.

+It is important to state as a preface to this diagnosis that adjustment to parenting in general is a normal maturational process that elicits nursing behaviors of prevention of potential problems and health promotion.

*Critical

3.2.1.2.1 SEXUAL DYSFUNCTION (1980)

DEFINITION:

The state in which an individual experiences a change in sexual function that is viewed as unsatisfying, unrewarding, inadequate.

DEFINING CHARACTERISTICS:

Verbalization of problem; alterations in achieving perceived sex role; actual or perceived limitation imposed by disease and/or therapy; conflicts involving values; alteration in achieving sexual satisfaction; inability to achieve desired satisfaction; seeking confirmation of desirability; alteration in relationship with significant other; change of interest in self and others.

RELATED FACTORS:

Biopsychosocial alteration of sexuality; ineffectual or absent role models; physical abuse; psychosocial abuse, e.g., harmful relationships; vulnerability; values conflict; lack of privacy; lack of significant other; altered body structure or function (pregnancy; recent childbirth, drugs, surgery, anomalies, disease process, trauma, radiation); misinformation or lack of knowledge.

144

3.2.2 ALTERED FAMILY PROCESSES (1982)

DEFINITION:

The state in which a family that normally functions effectively experiences a dysfunction.

DEFINING CHARACTERISTICS:

Family system unable to meet physical needs of its members; family system unable to meet emotional needs of its members; family system unable to meet spiritual needs of its members; parents do not demonstrate respect for each other's views on child-rearing practices; inability to express/accept wide range of feelings; inability to express/accept feelings of members; family unable to meet security needs of its members; inability of the family members to relate to each other for mutual growth and maturation; family uninvolved in community activities; inability to accept/receive help appropriately; rigidity in function and roles; a family not demonstrating respect for individuality and autonomy of its members; family unable to adapt to change/deal with traumatic experience constructively; family failing to accomplish current/past developmental task; unhealthy family decision-making process; failure to send and receive clear messages; inappropriate boundary maintenance; inappropriate/poorly communicated family rules, rituals, symbols; unexamined family myths; inappropriate level and direction of energy.

RELATED FACTORS:

Situation transition and/or crises; developmental transition and/or crisis.

3.2.3.1 PARENTAL ROLE CONFLICT (1988)

DEFINITION:

The state in which a parent experiences role confusion and conflict in response to crisis.

DEFINING CHARACTERISTICS:

Major:

Parent(s) expresses concerns/feelings of inadequacy to provide for child's physical and emotional needs during hospitalization or in the home; demonstrated disruption in care taking routines; parent(s) express concerns about changes in parental role, family functioning, family communication, family health.

Minor:

Expresses concern about perceived loss of control over decisions relating to their child; reluctant to participate in usual caretaking activities even with encouragement and support; verbalize, demonstrate feelings of guilt, anger, fear, anxiety and/or frustrations about effect of child's illness on family process.

RELATED FACTORS:

Separation from child due to chronic illness; intimidation with invasive or restrictive modalities (e.g., isolation, intubation) specialized care centers, policies; home care of a child with special needs (e.g. apnea monitoring, postural drainage, hyperalimentation); change in marital status; interruptions of family life due to home care regimen (treatments, caregivers, lack of respite).

3.3 ALTERED SEXUALITY PATTERNS (1986)

DEFINITION:

The state in which an individual expresses concern regarding his/her sexuality.

DEFINING CHARACTERISTICS:

Major:

Reported difficulties, limitations, or changes in sexual behaviors or activities.

RELATED FACTORS:

Knowledge/skill deficit about alternative responses to health-related transitions, altered body function or structure, illness or medical [treatments]; lack of significant other; ineffective or absent role models; conflicts with sexual orientation or variant preferences; fear of pregnancy or of acquiring a sexually transmitted disease; impaired relationship with a significant other.

4.1.1 SPIRITUAL DISTRESS (DISTRESS OF THE HUMAN SPIRIT) (1978)

DEFINITION:

Disruption in the life principle which pervades a person's entire being and which integrates and transcends one's biological and psychosocial nature.

DEFINING CHARACTERISTICS:

*Expresses concern with meaning of life/death and/or belief systems; anger toward God; questions meaning of suffering; verbalizes inner conflict about beliefs; verbalizes concern about relationship with deity; questions meaning of own existence; unable to participate in usual religious practices; seeks spiritual assistance; questions moral/ethical implications of therapeutic regimen; gallows humor; displacement of anger toward religious representatives; description of nightmares/sleep disturbances; alteration in behavior/mood evidenced by anger, crying, withdrawal, preoccupation, anxiety, hostility, apathy, and so forth.

RELATED FACTORS:

Separation from religious/cultural ties; challenged belief and value system, e.g., due to moral/ethical implications of therapy, due to intense suffering.

*Critical

146

5.1.1.1 INEFFECTIVE INDIVIDUAL COPING (1978)

DEFINITION:

Impairment of adaptive behaviors and problem-solving abilities of a person in meeting life's demands and roles.

DEFINING CHARACTERISTICS:

*Verbalization of inability to cope or inability to ask for help; inability to meet role expectations; inability to meet basic needs; *inability to problem-solve; alteration in societal participation; destructive behavior toward self or others; inappropriate use of defense mechanisms; change in usual communication patterns; verbal manipulation; high illness rate; high rate of accidents.

RELATED FACTORS:

Situational crises; maturational crises; personal vulnerability.

*Critical

5.1.1.1 IMPAIRED ADJUSTMENT (1986)

DEFINITION:

The state in which the individual is unable to modify his/her life style/behavior in a manner consistent with a change in health status.

DEFINING CHARACTERISTICS:

Major:

Verbalization of non-acceptance of health status change: non-existent or unsuccessful ability to be involved in problem-solving or goal-setting.

Minor:

Lack of movement toward independence; extended period of shock, disbelief, or anger regarding health status change; lack of future-oriented thinking.

RELATED FACTORS:

Disability requiring change in life style; inadequate support systems; impaired cognition; sensory overload; assault to self-esteem; altered locus of control; incomplete grieving.

147

5.1.1.2 DEFENSIVE COPING (1988)

DEFINITION:

The state in which an individual repeatedly projects falsely positive self evaluation based on a self protective pattern which defends against underlying perceived threats to positive self regard.

DEFINING CHARACTERISTICS:

Major:

Denial of obvious problems/weaknesses; projection of blame/responsibility; rationalizes failures; hypersensitive to slight/criticism; grandiosity.

Minor:

Superior attitude toward others; difficulty establishing/maintaining relationships; hostile laughter or ridicule of others; difficulty in reality testing [of] perceptions; lack of follow through or participation in treatment or therapy.

5.1.1.1.3 INEFFECTIVE DENIAL (1988)

DEFINITION:

The state of a conscious or unconscious attempt to disavow the knowledge or meaning of an event to reduce anxiety/fear to the detriment of health.

DEFINING CHARACTERISTICS:

Major:

Delays seeking or refuses health care attention to the detriment of health; does not perceive personal relevance of symptoms or danger.

Minor:

Uses home remedies (self-treatment) to relieve symptoms; does not admit fear of death or invalidism; minimizes symptoms; displaces source of symptoms to other organs; unable to admit impact of disease on life pattern; makes dismissive gestures or comments when speaking of distressing events; displaces fear of impact of the condition; displays inappropriate affect.

5.1.2.1.1 INEFFECTIVE FAMILY COPING: DISABLING (1980)

DEFINITION:

Behavior of significant person (family member or other primary person) that disables his or her own capacities and the client's capacities to effectively address tasks essential to either person's adaptation to the health challenge.

DEFINING CHARACTERISTICS:

Neglectful care of the client in regard to basic human needs and/or illness treatment; distortion of reality regarding the client's health problem, including extreme denial about its existence or severity; intolerance; rejection; abandonment; desertion; carrying on usual routines, disregarding client's needs; psychosomaticism; taking on illness signs of client; decisions and actions by family which are detrimental to economic or social well-being; agitation, depression, aggression, hostility; impaired restructuring of a meaningful life for self, impaired individualization, prolonged over-concern for client; neglectful relationships with other family members; client's development of helpless, inactive dependence.

RELATED FACTORS:

Significant person with chronically unexpressed feelings of guilt, anxiety, hostility, despair, etc.; dissonant discrepancy of coping styles for dealing with adaptive tasks by the significant person and client or among significant people; highly ambivalent family relationships; arbitrary handling of family's resistance to treatment, which tends to solidify defensiveness as it fails to deal adequately with underlying anxiety.

5.1.2.1.2 INEFFECTIVE FAMILY COPING: COMPROMISED (1980)

DEFINITION:

A usually supportive primary person (family member or close friend) is providing insufficient, ineffective, or compromised support, comfort, assistance, or encouragement which may be needed by the client to manage or master adaptive tasks related to his or her health challenge.

DEFINING CHARACTERISTICS:

Subjective: Client expresses or confirms a concern or complaint about significant other's response to his or her health problem; significant person describes preoccupation with personal reaction, (e.g., fear, anticipatory grief, guilt, anxiety, to client's illness, disability, or to other situational or developmental crises); significant person describes or confirms an inadequate understanding or knowledge base which interferes with effective assistive or supportive behaviors.

Objective: Significant person attempts assistive or supportive behaviors with less than satisfactory results; significant person withdraws or enters into limited or temporary personal communication with the client at the time of need; significant person displays protective behavior disproportionate (too little or too much) to the client's abilities or need for autonomy.

RELATED FACTORS:

Inadequate or incorrect information or understanding by a primary person; temporary preoccupation by a significant person who is trying to manage emotional conflicts and personal suffering and is unable to perceive or act effectively in regard to client's needs; temporary family disorganization and role changes; other situational or developmental crises or situations the significant person may be facing; little support provided by client, in turn, for primary person; prolonged disease or disability progression that exhausts supportive capacity of significant people.

5.1.2.2 FAMILY COPING: POTENTIAL FOR GROWTH (1980)

DEFINITION:

Effective managing of adaptive tasks by family member involved with the client's health challenge, who now is exhibiting desire and readiness for enhanced health and growth in regard to self and in relation to the client.

DEFINING CHARACTERISTICS:

Family member attempting to describe growth impact of crisis on his or her own values, priorities, goal, or relationships; family member moving in direction of health-promoting and enriching life-style which supports and monitors maturational processes, audits and negotiates treatment programs, and generally chooses experiences which optimize wellness; individual expressing interest in making contact on a one-to-one basis or on a mutual-aid group basis with another person who has experienced a similar situation.

RELATED FACTORS:

Needs sufficiently gratified and adaptive tasks effectively addressed to enable goals of self-actualization to surface.

5.2.1.1 NONCOMPLIANCE (SPECIFY) (1973)

DEFINITION:

A person's informed decision not to adhere to a therapeutic recommendation.

DEFINING CHARACTERISTICS:

*Behavior indicative of failure to adhere (by direct observation or by statements of patient or significant others); objective tests (physiological measures, detection of markers); evidence of development of complications; evidence of exacerbation of symptoms; failure to keep appointments; failure to progress.

RELATED FACTORS:

Patient value system: health beliefs, cultural influences, spiritual values; client-provider relationships.

*Critical

5.3.1.1 DECISIONAL CONFLICT (SPECIFY) (1988)

DEFINITION:

The state of uncertainty about course of action to be taken when choice among competing actions involves risk, loss, or challenge to personal life values.

DEFINING CHARACTERISTICS:

Major:

Verbalized uncertainty about choices; verbalization of undesired consequences of alternative actions being considered; vacillation between alternative choices; delayed decision making.

Minor:

Verbalized feeling of distress while attempting a decision; self-focusing; physical signs of distress or tension (increased heart rate, increased muscle tension, restlessness, etc.); questioning personal values and beliefs while attempting a decision.

RELATED FACTORS:

Unclear personal values/beliefs; perceived threat to value system; lack of experience or interference with decision making; lack of relevant information; support system deficit; multiple or divergent sources of information.

5.4 HEALTH SEEKING BEHAVIORS (SPECIFY) (1988)

DEFINITION:

A state in which an individual in stable health is actively seeking ways to alter personal health habits, and/or the environment in order to move toward a higher level of health.*

DEFINING CHARACTERISTICS:

Major:

Expressed or observed desire to seek a higher level of wellness.

Minor:

Expressed or observed desire for increased control of health practice; expression of concern about current environmental conditions on health status; stated or observed unfamiliarity with wellness community resources; demonstrated or observed lack of knowledge in health promotion behaviors.

*Stable health status is defined as age appropriate illness prevention measures achieved, client reports good or excellent health, and signs and symptoms of disease, if present, are controlled.

151

6.1.1.1 IMPAIRED PHYSICAL MOBILITY+ (1973)

DEFINITION:

A state in which the individual experiences a limitation of ability for independent physical movement.

DEFINING CHARACTERISTICS:

Inability to purposefully move within the physical environment, including bed mobility, transfer, and ambulation; reluctance to attempt movement; limited range of motion; decreased muscle strength, control and/or mass; imposed restrictions of movement, including mechanical, medical protocol; impaired coordination.

RELATED FACTORS:

Intolerance to activity/decreased strength and endurance; pain/discomfort; perceptual/cognitive impairment; neuromuscular impairment; musculoskeletal impairment; depression/severe anxiety.

+SUGGESTED FUNCTIONAL LEVEL CLASSIFICATION

0 = Completely independent.

1 = Requires use of equipment or device.

2 = Requires help from another person, for assistance, supervision, or teaching.

3 = Requires help from another person and equipment device.

4 = Dependent, does not participate in activity.

Code adapted from E. Jones, et al. *Patient Classification for Long-Term Care: Users' Manual,* HEW, Publication No. HRA-74-3107, November 1974.

6.1.1.2 ACTIVITY INTOLERANCE (1982)

DEFINITION:

A state in which an individual has insufficient physiological or psychological energy to endure or complete required or desired daily activities.

DEFINING CHARACTERISTICS:

*Verbal report of fatigue or weakness; abnormal heart rate or blood pressure response to activity; exertional discomfort or dyspnea; electrocardiographic changes reflecting arrhythmias or ischemia.

RELATED FACTORS:

Bed rest/immobility; generalized weakness; sedentary life-style; imbalance between oxygen supply/demand.

*Critical

152

6.1.1.2.1 FATIGUE (1988)

DEFINITION:

An overwhelming sustained sense of exhaustion and decreased capacity for physical and mental work.

DEFINING CHARACTERISTICS:

Major:

Verbalization of an unremitting and overwhelming lack of energy; inability to maintain usual routines.

Minor:

Perceived need for additional energy to accomplish routine tasks; increase in physical complaints; emotionally labile or irritable; impaired ability to concentrate; decreased performance; lethargic or listless; disinterest in surroundings/introspection; decreased libido; accident prone.

RELATED FACTORS:

Decreased/increased metabolic energy production; overwhelming psychological or emotional demands; increased energy requirements to perform activity of daily living; excessive social and/or role demands; states of discomfort; altered body chemistry (e.g. medications, drug withdrawal, chemotherapy).

6.1.1.3 POTENTIAL ACTIVITY INTOLERANCE (1982)

DEFINITION:

A state in which an individual is at risk of experiencing insufficient physiological or psychological energy to endure or complete required or desired daily activities.

DEFINING CHARACTERISTICS:

Presence of risk factors such as:

History of previous intolerance; deconditioned status; presence of circulatory/respiratory problems; inexperience with the activity.

RELATED FACTORS:

See risk factors.

6.2.1 SLEEP PATTERN DISTURBANCE (1980)

DEFINITION:

Disruption of sleep time causes discomfort or interference with desired life-style.

DEFINING CHARACTERISTICS:

*Verbal complaints of difficulty falling asleep; *awakening earlier or later than desired; *interrupted sleep; *verbal complaints of not feeling well-rested; changes in behavior and performance (increasing irritability, restlessness, disorientation, lethargy, listlessness); physical signs (mild fleeting nystagmus, slight hand tremor, ptosis of eyelid, expressionless face, dark circles under eyes, frequent yawning, changes in posture); thick speech with mispronunciation and incorrect words.

RELATED FACTORS:

Sensory alterations; internal (illness, psychological stress); external (environmental changes, social cues).

*Critical

6.3.1.1 DIVERSIONAL ACTIVITY DEFICIT (1980)

DEFINITION:

The state in which an individual experiences a decreased stimulation from or interest or engagement in recreational or leisure activities.

DEFINING CHARACTERISTICS:

Patient's statements regarding: boredom, wish there was something to do, to read, etc.; usual hobbies cannot be undertaken in hospital.

RELATED FACTORS:

Environmental lack of diversional activity, as in: long-term hospitalization, frequent lengthy treatments.

6.4.1.1 IMPAIRED HOME MAINTENANCE MANAGEMENT (1980)

DEFINITION:

Inability to independently maintain a safe growth-promoting immediate environment.

DEFINING CHARACTERISTICS:

Subjective: *Household members express difficulty in maintaining their home in a comfortable fashion; *household requests assistance with home maintenance; *household members describe outstanding debts or financial crises.

Objective: Disorderly surroundings; *unwashed or unavailable cooking equipment, clothes, or linen; *accumulation of dirt, food wastes, or hygienic wastes; offensive odors; inappropriate household temperature; *overtaxed family members, e.g., exhausted, anxious; lack of necessary equipment or aids; presence of vermin or rodents; *repeated hygienic disorders, infestations, or infections.

RELATED FACTORS:

Individual/family member disease or injury; insufficient family organization or planning; insufficient finances; unfamiliarity with neighborhood resources; impaired cognitive or emotional functioning; lack of knowledge; lack of role modeling; inadequate support systems.

*Critical

154

6.4.2 ALTERED HEALTH MAINTENANCE (1982)

DEFINITION:

Inability to identify, manage, and/or seek out help to maintain health.

DEFINING CHARACTERISTICS:

Demonstrated lack of knowledge regarding basic health practices; demonstrated lack of adaptive behaviors to internal/external environmental changes; reported or observed inability to take responsibility for meeting basic health practices in any or all functional pattern areas; history of lack of health seeking behavior; expressed interest in improving health behaviors; reported or observed lack of equipment, financial and/or other resources; reported or observed impairment of personal support systems.

RELATED FACTORS:

Lack of, or significant alteration in communication skills (written, verbal and/or gestural); lack of ability to make deliberate and thoughtful judgments; perceptual/cognitive impairment (complete/partial lack of gross and/or fine motor skills); ineffective individual coping; dysfunctional grieving; unachieved developmental tasks; ineffective family coping; disabling spiritual distress; lack of material resources.

6.5.1 FEEDING SELF CARE DEFICIT + (1980)

DEFINITION:

A state in which the individual experiences an impaired ability to perform or complete feeding activities for oneself.

DEFINING CHARACTERISTICS:

Inability to bring food from a receptacle to the mouth.

RELATED FACTORS:

Intolerance to activity, decreased strength and endurance; pain, discomfort; perceptual or cognitive impairment; neuromuscular impairment; musculoskeletal impairment; depression, severe anxiety.

+See suggested Functional Level Classification under diagnosis 6.1.1.1 Impaired Physical Mobility.

155

6.5.1.1 IMPAIRED SWALLOWING (1986)

DEFINITION:

The state in which an individual has decreased ability to voluntarily pass fluids and/or solids from the mouth to the stomach.

DEFINING CHARACTERISTICS:

Major:

Observed evidence of difficulty in swallowing, e.g., stasis of food in oral cavity, coughing/choking.

Minor:

Evidence of aspiration.

RELATED FACTORS:

Neuromuscular impairment (e.g., decreased or absent gag reflex, decreased strength or excursion of muscles involved in mastication, perceptual impairment, facial paralysis); mechanical obstruction (e.g., edema, tracheostomy tube, tumor); fatigue; limited awareness; reddened, irritated oropharyngeal cavity.

6.5.1.2 INEFFECTIVE BREASTFEEDING (1988)

DEFINITION:

The state in which a mother, infant, or child experience dissatisfaction or difficulty with the breastfeeding process.

DEFINING CHARACTERISTICS:

Major:

Unsatisfactory breastfeeding process.

Minor:

Actual or perceived inadequate milk supply; infant inability to attach on to maternal breast correctly; no observable signs of oxytocin release; observable signs of inadequate infant intake; nonsustained suckling at the breast; insufficient emptying of each breast per feeding; persistence of sore nipples beyond the first week of breastfeeding; insufficient opportunity for suckling at the breast; infant exhibiting fussiness and crying within the first hour after breastfeeding; unresponsive to other comfort measures; infant arching and crying at the breast; resisting latching on.

RELATED FACTORS:

Prematurity; infant anomaly; maternal breast anomaly; previous breast surgery; previous history of breastfeeding failure; infant receiving supplemental feedings with artificial nipple; poor infant sucking reflex; nonsupportive partner/family; knowledge deficit; interruption in breastfeeding; maternal anxiety or ambivalence.

6.5.1.3 EFFECTIVE BREASTFEEDING (1990)

DEFINITION:

The state in which a mother-infant dyad/family exhibits adequate proficiency and satisfaction with breastfeeding process.

DEFINING CHARACTERISTICS:

Major:

Mother able to position infant at breast to promote a successful latch-on response; infant is content after feeding; regular and sustained suckling/swallowing at the breast; appropriate infant weight patterns for age; effective mother/infant communication patterns (infant cues, maternal interpretation and response).

Minor:

Signs and/or symptoms of oxytocin release (let down or milk ejection reflex); adequate infant elimination patterns for age; eagerness of infant to nurse; maternal verbalization of satisfaction with the breastfeeding process.

RELATED FACTORS:

Basic breastfeeding knowledge; normal breast structure; normal infant oral structure; infant gestational age greater than 34 weeks; support sources; maternal confidence.

6.5.2 BATHING/HYGIENE SELF CARE DEFICIT+ (1980)

DEFINITION:

A state in which the individual experiences an impaired ability to perform or complete bathing/hygiene activities for oneself.

DEFINING CHARACTERISTICS:

*Inability to wash body or body parts; inability to obtain or get to water source; inability to regulate temperature or flow.

RELATED FACTORS:

Intolerance to activity, decreased strength and endurance; pain, discomfort; perceptual or cognitive impairment; neuromuscular impairment; musculoskeletal impairment; depression, severe anxiety.

+See suggested Functional Level Classification under diagnosis 6.1.1.1 Impaired Physical Mobility.

*Critical

157

6.5.3 DRESSING/GROOMING SELF CARE DEFICIT+ (1980)

DEFINITION:

A state in which the individual experiences an impaired ability to perform or complete dressing and grooming activities for oneself.

DEFINING CHARACTERISTICS:

*Impaired ability to put on or take off necessary items of clothing; impaired ability to obtain or replace articles of clothing; impaired ability to fasten clothing; inability to maintain appearance at a satisfactory level.

RELATED FACTORS:

Intolerance to activity, decreased strength and endurance; pain, discomfort; perceptual or cognitive impairment; neuromuscular impairment; musculoskeletal impairment; depression, severe anxiety.

+See suggested Functional Level Classification under diagnosis 6.1.1.1 Impaired Physical Mobility

*Critical

6.5.4 TOILETING SELF CARE DEFICIT+ (1980)

DEFINITION:

A state in which the individual experiences an impaired ability to perform or complete toileting activities for oneself.

DEFINING CHARACTERISTICS:

*Unable to get to toilet or commode; *unable to sit on or rise from toilet or commode; *unable to manipulate clothing for toileting; *unable to carry out proper toilet hygiene; unable to flush toilet or commode.

RELATED FACTORS:

Impaired transfer ability; impaired mobility status; intolerance to activity, decreased strength and endurance; pain, discomfort; perceptual or cognitive impairment; neuromuscular impairment; musculoskeletal impairment; depression, severe anxiety.

+See suggested Functional Level Classification under diagnosis 6.1.1.1 Impaired Physical Mobility

*Critical

6.6 ALTERED GROWTH AND DEVELOPMENT (1986)

DEFINITION:

The state in which an individual demonstrates deviations in norms from his/her age group.

DEFINING CHARACTERISTICS:

Major:

Delay or difficulty in performing skills (motor, social, or expressive) typical of age group; altered physical growth; inability to perform self-care or self-control activities appropriate for age.

Minor:

Flat affect; listlessness, decreased responses.

RELATED FACTORS:

Inadequate caretaking; indifference, inconsistent responsiveness, multiple caretakers; separation from significant others; environmental and stimulation deficiencies; effects of physical disability; prescribed dependence.

159

7.1.1 BODY IMAGE DISTURBANCE (1973)

DEFINITION:

Disruption in the way one perceives one's body image.

DEFINING CHARACTERISTICS:

A or B must be present to justify the diagnosis of Body Image Disturbance *A = verbal response to actual or perceived change in structure and/or function; *B = non-verbal response to actual or perceived change in structure and/or function. The following clinical manifestations may be used to validate the presence of A or B.

Objective: Missing body part; actual change in structure and/or function; not looking at body part; not touching body part; hiding or overexposing body part (intentional or unintentional); trauma to non-functioning part; change in social involvement; change in ability to estimate spatial relationship of body to environment.

Subjective: Verbalization of: change in life-style; fear of rejection or of reaction by others; focus on past strength, function, or appearance; negative feelings about body; and feelings of helplessness, hopelessness, or powerlessness; preoccupation with change or loss; emphasis on remaining strengths, heightened achievement; extension of body boundary to incorporate environmental objects; personalization of part or loss by name; depersonalization of part or loss by impersonal pronouns; refusal to verify actual change.

RELATED FACTORS:

Biophysical; cognitive/perceptual; psychosocial; cultural or spiritual.

*Critical

7.1.2 SELF ESTEEM DISTURBANCE (1978, 1988R)

DEFINITION:

Negative self evaluation/feelings about self or self capabilities, which may be directly or indirectly expressed.

DEFINING CHARACTERISTICS:

Self negating verbalization; expressions of shame/guilt; evaluates self as unable to deal with events; rationalizes away/rejects positive feedback and exaggerates negative feedback about self; hesitant to try new things/situations; denial of problems obvious to others; projection of blame/responsibility for problems; rationalizing personal failures; hypersensitive to slight or criticism; grandiosity.

7.1.2.1 CHRONIC LOW SELF ESTEEM (1988)

DEFINITION:

Long standing negative self evaluation/feelings about self or self capabilities.

DEFINING CHARACTERISTICS:

Major: long standing or chronic:

Self negating verbalization; expressions of shame/guilt; evaluates self as unable to deal with events; rationalizes away/rejects positive feedback and exaggerates negative feedback about self; hesitant to try new things/situations.

Minor:

Frequent lack of success in work or other life events; overly conforming; dependent on others opinions; lack of eye contact; nonassertive/passive; indecisive; excessively seeks reassurance.

7.1.2.2 SITUATIONAL LOW SELF ESTEEM (1988)

DEFINITION:

Negative self evaluation/feelings about self which develop in response to a loss or change in an individual who previously had a positive self evaluation.

DEFINING CHARACTERISTICS:

Major:

Episodic occurrence of negative self appraisal in response to life events in a person with a previous positive self evaluation; verbalization of negative feelings about the self (helplessness, uselessness).

Minor:

Self negating verbalizations; expressions of shame/guilt; evaluates self as unable to handle situations/events; difficulty making decisions.

7.1.3 PERSONAL IDENTITY DISTURBANCE (1978)

DEFINITION:

Inability to distinguish between self and nonself.

DEFINING CHARACTERISTICS:

To be developed.

7.2 SENSORY/PERCEPTUAL ALTERATIONS (SPECIFY) (VISUAL, AUDITORY, KINESTHETIC, GUSTATORY, TACTILE, OLFACTORY) (1978, 1980R)

DEFINITION:

A state in which an individual experiences a change in the amount or patterning of oncoming stimuli accompanied by a diminished, exaggerated, distorted or impaired response to such stimuli.

DEFINING CHARACTERISTICS:

Disoriented in time, in place, or with persons; altered abstraction; altered conceptualization; change in problem-solving abilities; reported or measured change in sensory acuity; change in behavior pattern; anxiety; apathy; change in usual response to stimuli; indication of body-image alteration; restlessness; irritability; altered communication patterns.

OTHER POSSIBLE CHARACTERISTICS:

Complaints of fatigue; alteration in posture; change in muscular tension; inappropriate responses; hallucinations.

RELATED FACTORS:

Altered environmental stimuli, excessive or insufficient; altered sensory reception, transmission and/or integration; chemical alterations, endogenous (electrolyte), exogenous (drugs, etc.); psychological stress.

7.2.1.1 UNILATERAL NEGLECT (1986)

DEFINITION:

A state in which an individual is perceptually unaware of and inattentive to one side of the body.

DEFINING CHARACTERISTICS:

Major:

Consistent inattention to stimuli on an affected side.

Minor:

Inadequate self-care, positioning and/or safety precautions in regard to the affected side; does not look toward affected side; leaves food on plate on the affected side.

RELATED FACTORS:

Effects of disturbed perceptual abilities, e.g., hemianopsia; one-sided blindness; neurologic illness or trauma.

7.3.1 HOPELESSNESS (1986)

DEFINITION:

A subjective state in which an individual sees limited or no alternatives or personal choices available and is unable to mobilize energy on own behalf.

DEFINING CHARACTERISTICS:

Major:

Passivity, decreased verbalization; decreased affect; verbal cues (despondent content, "I can't," sighing).

Minor:

Lack of initiative; decreased response to stimuli; decreased affect; turning away from speaker; closing eyes; shrugging in response to speaker; decreased appetite; increased/decreased sleep; lack of involvement in care/passively allowing care.

RELATED FACTORS:

Prolonged activity restriction creating isolation; failing or deteriorating physiological condition; long-term stress; abandonment; lost belief in transcendent values/God.

163

7.3.2 POWERLESSNESS (1982)

DEFINITION:

Perception that one's own action will not significantly affect an outcome; a perceived lack of control over a current situation or immediate happening.

DEFINING CHARACTERISTICS:

Severe: Verbal expressions of having no control or influence over situation; verbal expressions of having no control or influence over outcome; verbal expressions of having no control over self-care; depression over physical deterioration which occurs despite patient compliance with regimens; apathy.

Moderate: Nonparticipation in care or decision-making when opportunities are provided; expressions of dissatisfaction and frustration over inability to perform previous tasks and/or activities; does not monitor progress; expression of doubt regarding role performance; reluctance to express true feelings; fearing alienation from care givers; passivity; inability to seek information regarding care; dependence on others that may result in irritability, resentment, anger, and guilt; does not defend self-care practices when challenged.

Low: Expressions of uncertainty about fluctuating energy levels; passivity.

RELATED FACTORS:

Health care environment; interpersonal interaction; illness-related regimen; life-style of helplessness.

8.1.1 KNOWLEDGE DEFICIT (SPECIFY) (1980)

[DEFINITION:

The state in which an individual lacks specific knowledge or skills that affect ability to maintain health.]

DEFINING CHARACTERISTICS:

Verbalization of the problem; inaccurate follow-through of instruction; inaccurate performance of test; inappropriate or exaggerated behaviors, e.g., hysterical, hostile, agitated, apathetic.

RELATED FACTORS:

Lack of exposure; lack of recall; information misinterpretation; cognitive limitation; lack of interest in learning; unfamiliarity with information resources.

8.3 ALTERED THOUGHT PROCESSES (1973)

DEFINITION:

A state in which an individual experiences a disruption in cognitive operations and activities.

DEFINING CHARACTERISTICS:

Inaccurate interpretation of environment; cognitive dissonance; distractibility; memory deficit/problems; egocentricity; hyper- or hypo-vigilance.

OTHER POSSIBLE CHARACTERISTICS:

Inappropriate nonreality-based thinking.

RELATED FACTORS:

To be developed.

9.1.1 PAIN (1978)

DEFINITION:

A state in which an individual experiences and reports the presence of severe discomfort or an uncomfortable sensation.

DEFINING CHARACTERISTICS:

Subjective: Communication (verbal or coded) of pain descriptors.

Objective: Guarding behavior, protective; self-focusing; narrowed focus (altered time perception, withdrawal from social contact, impaired thought process); distraction behavior (moaning, crying, pacing, seeking out other people and/or activities, restlessness); facial mask of pain (eyes lack luster, "beaten look," fixed or scattered movement, grimace); alteration in muscle tone (may span from listless to rigid); autonomic responses not seen in chronic stable pain (diaphoresis, blood pressure and pulse change, pupillary dilation, increased or decreased respiratory rate).

RELATED FACTORS:

Injury agents (biological, chemical, physical, psychological).

9.1.1.1 CHRONIC PAIN (1986)

DEFINITION:

A state in which the individual experiences pain that continues for more than six months in duration.

DEFINING CHARACTERISTICS:

Major:

Verbal report or observed evidence of pain experienced for more than 6 months.

Minor:

Fear of re-injury; physical and social withdrawal; altered ability to continue previous activities; anorexia; weight changes; changes in sleep patterns; facial mask; guarded movement.

RELATED FACTORS:

Chronic physical/psychosocial disability.

165

NANDA TAXONOMY

9.2.1.1 DYSFUNCTIONAL GRIEVING (1980)

[DEFINITION:

The state in which an individual experiences an exaggerated response to an actual or potential loss of person, relationship, object, or functional abilities.]

DEFINING CHARACTERISTICS:

Verbal expression of distress at loss; denial of loss; expression of guilt; expression of unresolved issues; anger; sadness; crying; difficulty in expressing loss; alterations in: eating habits, sleep patterns, dream patterns, activity level, libido; idealization of lost object; reliving of past experiences; interference with life functioning; developmental regression; labile affect; alterations in concentration and/or pursuits of tasks.

RELATED FACTORS:

Actual or perceived object loss (object is used in the broadest sense); objects may include: people, possessions, a job, status, home, ideals, parts and processes of the body.

9.2.1.2 ANTICIPATORY GRIEVING (1980)

[DEFINITION:

The state in which an individual experiences a predisposition to violent, destructive acts directed toward self or others.]

DEFINING CHARACTERISTICS:

Potential loss of significant object; expression of distress at potential loss; denial of potential loss; guilt; anger; sorrow; choked feelings; changes in eating habits; alterations in sleep patterns; alterations in activity level; altered libido; altered communication patterns.

RELATED FACTORS:

[Actual or potential loss of significant other, health status, social status, or valued object.]

9.2.2 POTENTIAL FOR VIOLENCE: SELF-DIRECTED OR DIRECTED AT OTHERS (1980)

DEFINITION:

A state in which an individual experiences behaviors that can be physically harmful either to the self or others.

DEFINING CHARACTERISTICS:

Presence of risk factors such as:

Body language: clenched fists, tense facial expression, rigid posture, tautness indicating effort to control; hostile threatening verbalizations: boasting to or prior abuse of others; increased motor activity: pacing, excitement, irritability, agitation; overt and aggressive acts: goal-directed destruction of objects in environment; possession of destructive means (gun, knife, weapon); rage; self-destructive behavior, active aggressive suicidal acts; suspicion of others, paranoid ideation, delusions, hallucinations; substance abuse/withdrawal.

OTHER POSSIBLE CHARACTERISTICS:

Increasing anxiety levels; fear of self or others; inability to verbalize feelings; repetition of verbalizations: continued complaints, requests, and demands; anger; provocative behavior: argumentative, dissatisfied, overreactive, hypersensitive; vulnerable self-esteem; depression (specifically active, aggressive, suicidal acts).

RELATED FACTORS:

Antisocial character; battered women; catatonic excitement; child abuse; manic excitement; organic brain syndrome; panic states; rage reactions; suicidal behavior; temporal lobe epilepsy; toxic reactions to medication.

167

9.2.3 POST-TRAUMA RESPONSE (1986)

DEFINITION:

The state of an individual experiencing a sustained painful response to an overwhelming traumatic event(s).

DEFINING CHARACTERISTICS:

Major:

Re-experience of the traumatic event which may be identified in cognitive, affective, and/or sensory motor activities (flashbacks, intrusive thoughts, repetitive dreams or nightmares, excessive verbalization of the traumatic event, verbalization of survival guilt or guilt about behavior required for survival).

Minor:

Psychic/emotional numbness (impaired interpretation of reality, confusion, dissociation or amnesia, vagueness about traumatic event, constricted affect); altered life-style (self-destructiveness, such as substance abuse, suicide attempt or other acting out behavior, difficulty with interpersonal relationship, development of phobia regarding trauma, poor impulse control/irritability and explosiveness).

RELATED FACTORS:

Disasters, wars, epidemics, rape, assault, torture, catastrophic illness or accident.

9.2.3.1 RAPE-TRAUMA SYNDROME (1980)

DEFINITION:

Forced, violent sexual penetration against the victim's will and consent. The trauma syndrome that develops from this attack or attempted attack includes an acute phase of disorganization of the victim's life-style and a long-term process of reorganization of life-style.**

DEFINING CHARACTERISTICS:

Acute phase: Emotional reactions (anger, embarrassment, fear of physical violence and death, humiliation, revenge, self-blame); multiple physical symptoms (gastrointestinal irritability, genitourinary discomfort, muscle tension, sleep pattern disturbance).

Long-term phase: Changes in life-style (change in residence; dealing with repetitive nightmares and phobias; seeking family support; seeking social network support).

**This syndrome includes the following three subcomponents: Rape-trauma, Compound reaction, and Silent reaction. In this text, each appears as a separate diagnosis.

9.2.3.1.1 RAPE-TRAUMA SYNDROME: COMPOUND REACTION (1980)

DEFINITION:

Forced, violent sexual penetration against the victim's will and consent. The trauma syndrome that develops from this attack or attempted attack includes an acute phase of disorganization of the victim's life-style and a long-term process of reorganization of life-style.**

DEFINING CHARACTERISTICS:

Acute phase: Emotional reaction (anger, embarrassment, fear of physical violence and death, humiliation, revenge, self-blame); multiple physical symptoms (gastrointestinal irritability, genitourinary discomfort, muscle tension, sleep pattern disturbance); reactivated symptoms of such previous conditions, i.e., physical illness, psychiatric illness; reliance on alcohol and/or drugs.

Long-term phase: Change in life-style (changes in residence; dealing with repetitive nightmares and phobias; seeking family support; seeking social network support).

**This syndrome includes the following three subcomponents: Rape-trauma, Compound reaction, and Silent reaction. In this text, each appears as a separate diagnosis.

9.2.3.1.2 RAPE-TRAUMA SYNDROME: SILENT REACTION (1980)

DEFINITION:

Forced, violent sexual penetration against the victim's will and consent. The trauma syndrome that develops from this attack or attempted attack includes an acute phase of disorganization of the victim's life-style and a long-term process of reorganization of life-style.**

DEFINING CHARACTERISTICS:

Abrupt changes in relationships with men; increase in nightmares; increased anxiety during interview, i.e., blocking of associations, long periods of silence, minor stuttering, physical distress; pronounced changes in sexual behavior; no verbalization of the occurrence of rape; sudden onset of phobic reactions.

**This syndrome includes the following three subcomponents: Rape-trauma, Compound reaction, and Silent reaction. In this text, each appears as a separate diagnosis.

169

9.3.1 ANXIETY (1973, 1982R)

DEFINITION:

A vague uneasy feeling whose source is often nonspecific or unknown to the individual.

DEFINING CHARACTERISTICS:

Subjective: Increased tension; apprehension; painful and persistent increased helplessness; uncertainty; fearful; scared; regretful; overexcited; rattled; distressed; jittery; feelings of inadequacy; shakiness; fear of unspecific consequences; expressed concerns re change in life events; worried; anxious.

Objective: *Sympathetic stimulation—cardiovascular excitation, superficial vasoconstriction, pupil dilation; restlessness; insomnia; glancing about; poor eye contact; trembling/hand tremors; extraneous movement (foot shuffling, hand/arm movements); facial tension; voice quivering; focus "self"; increased wariness; increased perspiration.

RELATED FACTORS:

Unconscious conflict about essential values/goals of life; threat to self-concept; threat of death; threat to or change in health status; threat to or change in role functioning; threat to or change in environment; threat to or change in interaction patterns; situational/maturational crises; interpersonal transmission/contagion; unmet needs.

*Critical

9.3.2 FEAR (1980)

DEFINITION:

Feeling of dread related to an identifiable source which the person validates.

DEFINING CHARACTERISTICS:

Ability to identify object of fear.

RELATED FACTORS:

To be developed.

In any event, congruence of the nurse's and client's perceptions of the client's health is essential for establishing and achieving desired outcomes.

Nursing diagnoses are not absolute labels that apply to all situations with similar characteristics. Instead, they acquire meaning within a particular context and become relevant only when they fit a particular client's situation. Nurses and clients bring their unique perspectives to any nurse–client relationship. Their perspectives are shaped by a host of variables, including education, ethnic/cultural background, gender, age, and life experiences.

Occasionally, a nurse may formulate a diagnosis that on evidence appears to be valid: a diagnosis of "chronic low self-esteem" based on observations of passive behavior, lack of eye contact, and chronic underemployment. It may be, however, that the client is satisfied with work and comes from a culture that teaches deference (passivity, avoidance of eye contact) to authority figures, including health-care professionals. The nurse should avoid making attributions about client behaviors without considering variables and the particular context in which they are observed.

In summary, nursing diagnosis provides a means for categorizing a client's problems in order to give clearer direction to nursing care planning. Nursing diagnoses are not meant to be rigid formulations, however; therefore, the nurse should remain continually aware of the influence of situational or contextual variables in collecting, interpreting, and validating information.

Chapter Highlights

■ Nursing diagnosis is a critical phase in the nursing process; it depends on an accurate and comprehensive nursing assessment and forms the basis for nursing care planning.

■ A nursing diagnosis is a concise statement of a human response to actual or potential health problems and is based on subjective and objective clinical information that can be confirmed.

■ Nursing diagnoses may encompass the developmental, family/cultural, psychosocial, and physiological dimensions of the client.

■ Nursing diagnosis helps define clearly the domain and scope of nursing practice.

■ Nursing diagnoses include a client's responses or problems for which the professional nurse has the knowledge and legal authority to prescribe interventions.

■ The NANDA classification system for categorizing nursing diagnoses is widely accepted for clinical use, but is still evolving.

■ The current *Taxonomy I Revised* (1990) includes 99 diagnoses, organized within a framework of nine human response patterns (exchanging, communicating, relating, valuing, choosing, moving, perceiving, knowing, feeling) and accompanied by defining characteristics and related factors.

■ The nursing diagnostic statement consists of two parts: the specific response or problem *and* the related or etiological factors.

■ Nursing diagnoses are meaningful and relevant only when they fit each client's unique situation.

Practice Activities

1. Obtain a copy of the nurse practice act in your state. Is nursing diagnosis implied or explicitly stated as a responsibility of the professional nurse? What are the implications for a practicing registered nurse?

2. Review the nursing records (care plans, nurses' notes, discharge summaries) in one or more clinical agencies. Are nursing diagnoses reflected? If so, do they use the appropriate format and terminology? To what extent do they suggest client goals/objectives and nursing interventions?

3. Using an actual or sample nursing history, formulate nursing diagnoses. Ask a colleague or classmate to use the same nursing history to do the same. Compare your diagnoses with those of your colleague or classmate. Collaborate to achieve a mutually agreed upon set of nursing diagnoses for the sample history.

4. Several of the *Taxonomy I Revised* (1990) nursing diagnoses do not indicate related factors. Working alone or in small groups, generate at least three related factors for each of the following diagnoses:

> Diarrhea (p. 125)
> Altered role performance (p. 141)
> Self-esteem disturbance (p. 161)
> Altered thought processes (p. 164)

Recommended Readings

Anderson, J.E., & Briggs, L.L. (1988). Nursing diagnosis: A study of quality and supportive evidence. *Image: Journal of Nursing Scholarship, 20,* 141–144.

Baretich, D.M., & Anderson, L.B. (1987). Should we diagnose strengths? No: Stick to the problems. *American Journal of Nursing, 87,* 1211–1212.

Carpenito, L.J. (1984). Is the problem a nursing diagnosis? *American Journal of Nursing, 84,* 1418–1419.

Edel, M.K. (1985). Noncompliance: An appropriate nursing diagnosis? *Nursing Outlook, 33,* 183–185.

Gordon, M. (1985). Nursing diagnosis. In H.H. Werley & J.J. Fitzpatrick (Eds.), *Annual review of nursing research* (Vol. 3, pp. 127–146). New York: Springer.

Jenny, J.L. (1987). Knowledge deficit: Not a nursing diagnosis. *Image: Journal of Nursing Scholarship, 19,* 184–185.

Jenny, J. (1989). Classifying nursing diagnoses: A self-care approach. *Nursing and Health Care, 10,* 83–88.

Levin, R.F., Krainovitch, B.C., Bahrenburg, E., & Mitchell, C.A. (1989). Diagnostic content validity of nursing diagnoses. *Image: Journal of Nursing Scholarship, 21,* 40–44.

Popkess-Vawter, S. & Pinnell, N. (1987). Should we diagnose strengths? Yes: Accentuate the positive. *American Journal of Nursing, 87,* 1211, 1216.

Roberts, S.L. (1990). Achieving professional autonomy through nursing diagnosis and nursing DRG's. *Nursing Administration Quarterly, 14*(4), 54–60.

Vandenbosch, T.M., Bentley, C.L., Jones, K.A. & Blake, D. (1986). Tailoring care plans to nursing diagnoses. *American Journal of Nursing, 86,* 313–314.

Warren, J. (1983). Accountability and nursing diagnosis. *Journal of Nursing Administration, 13,* 34–37.

References

American Nurses Association. (1955). *Model practice act of 1955.* New York: Author.

American Nurses Association. (1973). *Standards of nursing practice.* Kansas City: Author.

American Nurses Association. (1980). *Nursing: A social policy statement.* Kansas City: Author.

Anderson, J.E., & Briggs, L.L. (1988). Nursing diagnosis: A study of quality and supportive evidence. *Image: Journal of Nursing Scholarship, 20,* 141–144.

Baretich, D.M., & Anderson, L.B. (1987). Should we diagnose strengths? No: Stick to the problems. *American Journal of Nursing, 87,* 1211–1212.

Carnevali, D.L., Mitchell, P.H., Woods, N.F., & Tanner, C.A. (1984). *Diagnostic reasoning in nursing.* Philadelphia: Lippincott.

Carpenito, L.J. (1991). *Nursing diagnosis: Application to clinical practice* (4th ed.). Philadelphia: Lippincott.

Carpenito, L.J. (1984). Is the problem a nursing diagnosis? *American Journal of Nursing, 85,* 458.

Chambers, W. (1962). Nursing diagnosis. *American Journal of Nursing, 53,* 301–302.

Durand, M., & Prince, R. (1966). Nursing diagnosis: Process and decision. *Nursing Forum, 5,* 50.

Edel, M.K. (1985). Noncompliance: An appropriate nursing diagnosis? *Nursing Outlook, 33,* 183–185.

Fawcett, J. (1986). Guest editorial: Conceptual models of nursing, nursing diagnosis, and nursing theory development. *Western Journal of Nursing Research, 8,* 397–399.

Fitzpatrick, J.J. et al. (1989). Translating nursing diagnosis into ICD code. *American Journal of Nursing, 89,* 493–495.

Fry, V.S. (1953). The creative approach to nursing. *American Journal of Nursing, 53,* 301–302.

Gebbie, K., & Lavin, M.A. (1974). Classifying nursing diagnoses. *American Journal of Nursing, 74,* 250–253.

Gebbie, K., & Lavin, M.A. (1975). *Classification of nursing diagnoses.* St. Louis: Mosby.

Gordon, M. (1976). Nursing diagnosis and the diagnostic process. *American Journal of Nursing, 76,* 1298–1300.

Gordon, M. (1982a). *Nursing diagnosis: Process and application.* New York: McGraw–Hill.

Gordon, M. (1982b). Conceptual issues in nursing diagnosis. In N. Chaska (Ed.), *The nursing profession: A time to speak* (pp. 551–562). New York: McGraw–Hill.

Gordon, M. (1987). *Nursing diagnosis: Process and application* (2nd ed.). New York: McGraw-Hill.

Halloran, E.J. (1985). Nursing workload, medical diagnosis related groups, and nursing diagnoses. *Research in Nursing and Health, 8,* 421–433.

Jenny, J.L. (1987). Knowledge deficit: Not a nursing diagnosis. *Image: Journal of Nursing Scholarship, 19,* 184–185.

Kim, M.J. (1983). Nursing diagnoses in critical care. *Dimensions of Critical Care Nursing, 2,* 5.

Kim, M.J., & Moritz, D.A. (1982). *Classification of nursing diagnoses: Proceedings of the 3rd and 4th national conferences.* New York: McGraw–Hill.

Komorita, N.I. (1963). Nursing diagnosis. *American Journal of Nursing, 63,* 83–85.

Maas, M.L. (1986). Nursing diagnoses in a professional model of nursing: Keystone for effective nursing administration. *Journal of Nursing Administration, 16,* 39–42.

Martens, K. (1986). Let's diagnose strengths, not just problems. *American Journal of Nursing, 86,* 192–193.

McFarland, G.K., & McFarlane, E.A. (1989). *Nursing diagnosis and intervention: Planning for patient care.* St. Louis: Mosby.

Mundinger, M.O. & Jauron, G.D. (1975). Developing a nursing diagnosis. *Nursing Outlook, 23,* 94–98.

North American Nursing Diagnosis Association. (1988). NANDA approved diagnostic categories. *Nursing Diagnosis Newsletter, 15*(1), 1–3.

Pendleton, S.H. (1986). Clarification or obfuscation? *American Journal of Nursing, 86,* 944.

Popkess-Vawter, S., & Pinnell, N. (1987). Should we diagnose strengths? Yes: Accentuate the positive. *American Journal of Nursing, 87,* 1211, 1216.

Porter, E.J. (1986). Critical analysis of NANDA nursing diagnosis Taxonomy I. *Image: Journal of Nursing Scholarship, 18*, 136–139.

Rothberg, J.S. (1967). Why nursing diagnosis? *American Journal of Nursing, 67*, 1041–1042.

Shamansky, S.L., & Yanni, C.R. (1983). In opposition to nursing diagnosis: A minority opinion. *Image: Journal of Nursing Scholarship, 15*, 47–50.

Smaldone, A., Greenberg, C., & Perez, P.W. (1988). Nursing diagnosis: Translate please! *American Journal of Nursing, 88*, 363.

Stolte, K. (1986). A complementary view of nursing diagnosis. *Public Health Nursing, 3*, 23–28.

Taptich, B.J., Iyer, P.W., & Bernocchi-Losey, D. (1989). *Nursing diagnosis and care planning.* Philadelphia: Saunders.

Turkoski, B.B. (1988). Nursing diagnosis in print, 1950–1985. *Nursing Outlook, 36*, 142–144.

Vandenbosch, T.M., Bentley, C.L., Jones, K.A., & Blake, D. (1986). Tailoring care plans to nursing diagnoses. *American Journal of Nursing, 86*, 313–314.

Walker, L. (1986). Nursing diagnoses and interventions: New tools to define nursing's unique role. *Nursing and Health Care, 7*, 323–326.

Warren, J. (1983). Accountability and nursing diagnosis. *Journal of Nursing Administration, 13*, 34–37.

PART
II

7

Family Assessment

OBJECTIVES

Upon completion of this chapter, you should be able to:

■ Define "family."

■ Describe variations in family constellations.

■ Describe major concepts and theoretical approaches to family assessment.

■ Delineate the various dimensions of family assessment.

■ Use selected tools and approaches to family assessment.

■ Formulate valid and appropriate nursing diagnoses based on family assessment information.

As the basic social unit of society, the family is a powerful force that shapes its members' behaviors and interactions within the larger society. The importance of the family to the physiological and psychological health of its members cannot be overstated. Families serve to meet the basic needs of individuals for food, shelter, love, belonging, and cultural orientation. A family influences the formation of identity and self-esteem in its members, factors that are critical to an individual's success (or failure) in life.

Every client the nurse encounters in clinical practice belongs to some type of family constellation. Failure to consider the importance of the family to a client's health and well-being or, conversely, the impact of an alteration in the family member's health on the family unit may lead to missed nursing diagnoses and less than optimal outcomes of nursing intervention. Consider the following situation: A 4-year-old girl is diagnosed with cystic fibrosis. The child's illness is likely to have a major impact on the family's lifestyle as well as its self-image and values. In turn, the family's ability to cope emotionally with this crisis, to provide the necessary daily physical care for the child, to secure needed financial resources, and to continue to promote the child's normal developmental progress can greatly influence the course of the child's illness and, ultimately, the length and quality of her life.

The family is the individual's link to a cultural group and the larger society. Ideally, the family buffers the individual from the stresses and demands of the more complex social structure, while also transmitting the expectations of the social structure to the individual in a way that is consistent with the family's values.

PURPOSES OF FAMILY ASSESSMENT

To achieve a clear understanding of an individual client, the nurse must gain an appreciation of the client's family—its structure, its functions, and especially the roles of the client within the family network. There are a number of reasons why the client's family should be assessed as part of a comprehensive nursing assessment.

First, there is a strong relationship between an individual client's health and the health of the family as a whole. The family plays a crucial role in shaping the individual's health beliefs and health practices. Knowledge of these is important to gain an understanding of the client's and family's values toward health, since values significantly influence the client's and family's health practices.

Second, any alteration in an individual client's health will, at least to some extent, affect other family members and the functioning of the entire family unit. Therefore, it is important to assess family parameters to determine the impact of the client's health, especially a change in health, on family functioning.

Third, because family members depend heavily on the family unit for support and care, knowledge of the client's family helps the nurse determine the ability of the family to meet the basic needs of its members, including its ability to help an ill member regain functioning capacities.

Finally, collection of family data yields information that allows the nurse to assess the health of the family as a whole. This is important to detect any interferences with family functioning. Although families usually come to the nurse's attention because an individual member seeks health care, the nurse may find that it is the family unit, rather than the individual client per se, that has a problem. Family dysfunction must be addressed if the individual client's health is to be restored. In many instances, it is not enough to treat the individual client; the family as a whole must become the focus of nursing intervention. This is often true when an individual client suffers a psychosocial disturbance, such as anorexia nervosa or child abuse. It also may be true when there is a disturbance in physiological functioning, such as obesity or hypertension in all family members. Careful assessment of the family can help determine whether the health problem is an individual or family one.

KNOWLEDGE NEEDED FOR FAMILY ASSESSMENT

The family is the primary social group in the life of every person. The family is a reference group for its members and profoundly affects their values and outlook. Even when people seem to reject family values, the rejection itself is an indication of the strength of family influence. The family is also the social group that, when joined with other families, becomes part of a community. A family can function only as long as it manages to satisfy some important needs and expectations of its members. A community can function only as long as its norms are upheld by a majority of its families.

Definitions of Family

Although families are the basic units of society, there are variations in their composition and in the nature of their interactions. Minuchin (1986) notes that the family is not a statistical entity conforming to standard patterns, but a dynamic configuration reflecting individual preferences and social trends. No family is an island, for every family must interact with larger social organizations. All interactions between a family and society are reciprocal; thus, families are both cause and consequence of social change. As individual and social needs change, so do the structures (compositions) and functions (transactions and interactions) of families.

The family unit formed by a male, a female, and their offspring comprises the nuclear family. While the nuclear family may not have been the earliest family structure, it is probably the most prominent in Western society, even today. Despite variations in contemporary families, the traditional nuclear family generally is considered the ideal. In premodern times, Western mothers and young children needed help in order to survive. This prolonged dependence strengthened attachments between males and females, encouraged the formation of nuclear families, and led to the development of communities. Nature dictated reproductive pairing between men and women; rigorous living conditions dictated task pairing between men and women. Thus, the reproductive pair became the working pair, with each partner contributing to the well-being of the other. Gradually tasks were differentiated according to gender, with men hunting and fishing and women cultivating and gathering. Tasks were assigned to growing children according to gender and ability, so economic survival and the socialization of children were among the earliest family functions. Today, however, children's developmental needs are often met within the context of the single-parent family (see Figure 7-1).

One of the most significant developments in modern life is the disappearance of the family as a cooperative working unit. The economic centrality of the family has been replaced by vast agencies for production and distribution of goods (see Figure 7-2). These agencies have the power to transfer workers from one place to another, and they regard the individual rather than the family as the basic working unit. This means that geographic mobility of today's families is directed by impersonal, external forces. Workers often commute great distances between home and the workplace and must relocate their families far from familiar people and places. This creates high levels of tension within the family, as members come to rely on each other in new ways. Having lost touch with extended families and old friends, the mobile families of today turn inward for companionship and security. The intense involvement of family members may

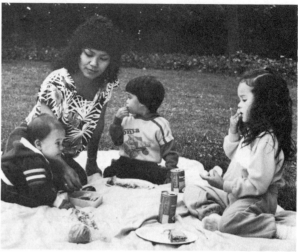

FIGURE 7-1. Most single parents are able to meet the developmental needs of individual family members. (*Note.* From Servonsky/Opas: *Nursing Management of Children,* © 1987. Boston: Jones and Bartlett Publishers, p. 290.)

be useful for a time but eventually proves detrimental, especially if family members have unrealistic expectations of one another (Astrachan, 1986). The proliferation of dual career families does not signify a return to the family as a paired or cooperative working unit, for dual career partners usually pursue paths that are individualistic rather than familial.

There is disagreement in many circles as to what constitutes a family, partly because "family" is an emotionally charged word that means different things to different people. For years nuclear and extended families were defined by two criteria: consanguinity (blood ties) and legality (marriage and adoption). Nuclear and extended families meeting these criteria still exist in great numbers, but so do single-parent families, step-parent families, foster parent families, and cohabiting individuals who may be heterosexual or homosexual. In addition, there are arrangements by which a residence is shared by a group of people, unrelated by blood or marriage, who consider themselves a family. At one time such communal living was organized mostly by young people, but recently many senior citizens have pooled their resources and find communal life practical and rewarding.

A recent census report notes that only 27 percent of the nation's households now consist of two parents living with their children, down from 40 percent in 1970 (Lewin, 1990). In 1989, the New York Court of Appeals ruled that for rent control purposes, a homosexual couple who had lived to-

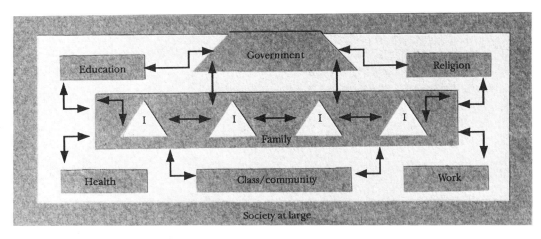

FIGURE 7-2. Forces Operating on a Family and Its Members. (*Note.* From Davies/Janosik: *Mental Health and Psychiatric Nursing: A Caring Approach*, © 1991. Boston: Jones and Bartlett Publishers.)

gether for a decade or more constitutes a family. The ruling states that protection from eviction depends not on legal distinctions or genetic history but on the reality of family life. According to the ruling, family life is defined through exclusive and lasting relationships and by the emotional commitment of the participants. In 1989 the same court affirmed the right of four unrelated people to live together in a single family zone and said that barring them was unconstitutional (Lewin, 1990) (see boxed insert).

There are a number of explanations for the diversity of modern families. High divorce rates, the tendency of divorced people to marry again, the decisions of unmarried mothers to keep their children, the popularity of cohabitation without marriage, and the increased acceptance of homosexual liaisons have contributed to family diversity. Regardless of the forms that contemporary families take, the variations are the result of a search for personal fulfillment. Legal rights gradually are being granted to untraditional families, and this contributes to their continued presence, although untraditional families make some people uneasy. Without taking sides, it is important to recognize that variations demonstrate that families are active, responsive systems operating within the larger social order. In actuality, family diversity shows how deeply and reciprocally families react to changes in the social climate (Frazer, 1985).

Variations in family composition include

Natural or biological family: Family into which an individual is born or is related to by consanguinity

Adoptive family: Family to which an individual belongs by means of legal adoption

Foster family: Family in which an individual is reared or cared for over an extended period without being legally adopted

Family of origin: Family into which an individual was born or enters at a very early age

Nuclear family: Family created by a marital or ongoing relationship between two heterosexual partners and their offspring, if any

Family of procreation: Family created by two individuals establishing a relationship into which children are born

---

Legalizing Family Diversity

- Los Angeles and Berkeley, California, and Madison, Wisconsin grant sick leave to municipal employees to care for "a domestic partner."

- Ithaca, New York; Madison, Wisconsin; and West Hollywood, California, permit all residents to register domestic partnerships with municipal clerks.

- Seattle, Washington enacted a law giving benefits to "partners" of city employees.

- The American Psychological Association, along with a few municipal and private employers, offers health insurance to domestic partners of their members and/or employees. However, the Internal Revenue Service ruled that the cost of health insurance premiums is taxable income for the domestic partner.

- New York's highest court ruled that a gay or lesbian couple was legally considered a family under municipal rent control laws.

Note. From Lewin, T. (1990, September 21). Suit over death benefit asks, What is a family? *The New York Times*, p. B7. Copyright © 1990 by The New York Times Company. Reprinted by permission.

Extended family: Family group that includes one or more nuclear families plus other individuals related by blood or marriage

Intact family: Family that includes two parents and their natural or adopted children living in one household

Single-parent family: Family consisting of children and one parent, either father or mother, living in one household

Step-parent family: Family created by the remarriage of one or both parents; this family may include children of the current marriage as well as children from the previous marriages of one or both spouses.

Theoretical Approaches to Family Assessment

Clinicians and researchers working with schizophrenic persons in the 1950s found that certain patterns seemed to differentiate functional from dysfunctional families. The nature of certain interactions seemed to aggravate the problems of the schizophrenic member, shorten periods of remission, and lengthen episodes of relapse. Soon clinicians and researchers in psychiatric and other fields realized that family patterns identified in work with schizophrenic persons also were present in families for which no one had a diagnosed psychiatric illness. From these beginnings family theory and family therapy emerged.

Family theory begins with the premise that the problems of most individuals originate, are worsened, or are relieved through interactions taking place within the family. The individual is an interdependent part of the family; therefore, family assessment is a means of understanding the actions and reactions of the individual. In family therapy, the family itself is considered the client. Family therapy per se is rarely within the grasp of a generalist nurse, but family assessment and family-centered care are within the scope of any nurse who has completed a basic nursing program and acquired adequate communication skills. This assumes that the nurse has sufficient education in individual and family development and the ability to recognize actual or potential deviations. If a nurse has the skill and experience to offer more than family assessment, interventions should deal with social and environmental modification rather than intrapersonal change. Qualifications for family-centered care and family therapy are described in the boxed insert.

Family-centered nursing is discussed philosophically in some nursing programs without benefit of a strong theoretical foundation. While most nurses agree that families should be included in health-care measures, some of them act in ways that make families feel like onlookers or intruders. In doing so, nurses overlook a rich source of information and cooperation. Perhaps families would

---

Family-Centered Care and Family Therapy Qualifications

Family-Centered Care

Graduates of basic nursing programs, preferably holders of baccalaureate degrees

Generalist practitioners with proven skills in interviewing and assessment of families, using a family assessment tool

Generalist practitioners with proven ability to recognize normal, adaptive family patterns and offer reinforcement

Generalist practitioners who can recognize and assess maladaptive family patterns and make appropriate referrals when indicated

Generalist nurses who use supervisory and consultation services of nurse specialists in offering care

Family Therapy

Graduates of master's programs in nursing or doctoral programs in nursing or another relevant field, such as psychology, education, or human services

Specialists with experience and preparation in a particular field of nursing, such as psychiatric nursing, pediatric nursing, or gerontological nursing

Specialists who can differentiate normal, adaptive family patterns from maladaptive alterations and intervene accordingly

Specialists who can intervene with adaptive and maladaptive family patterns, using positive and negative feedback integrated by means of a viable therapeutic approach

Specialists with sufficient knowledge of family theory to use theoretical constructs to assess and conceptualize family dynamics in offering care

Note. From Janosik/Davies: *Psychiatric-Mental Health Nursing* (2nd ed.), © 1989. Boston: Jones and Bartlett Publishers, p. 646.

feel less excluded if nurses had more knowledge of family dynamics based on concepts and theories relevant to the clinical situation. Because family theory is relatively new and because pioneers in the field worked independently for a number of years, there is some overlap in the various theories. One path to understanding various family theories is to identify the major theories and explain their basic concepts. Familiarity with various theories and concepts helps nurses acquire terminology for describing their observations of families and for sharing them with colleagues. In moving toward family assessment, a nurse may begin by using a single theoretical approach and drawing upon others as needed.

Nurses working with individual clients soon realize that their efforts can be enhanced or sabotaged by the family. In the absence of family assessment, the behaviors of an individual client can be very puzzling. Nurses searching for answers find themselves wondering about the impact of family dynamics on the client. They ask themselves why some families always are fighting while others preserve peace at the expense of progress. They see that some families cope in adverse situations while others cannot cope even in the most favorable circumstances. Along the same lines, nurses ask why some tranquil, apparently well-adjusted families cannot make decisions, while some quarrelsome, contentious families manage to reach a consensus on what needs to be done. These are complex questions, but the search for answers is part of comprehensive health assessment and requires some knowledge of family theory. An assessment that looks only at the individual is incomplete.

Several theoretical approaches have been proposed to explain aspects of family life and their impact on family members.

Family Development

Family development theory uses a life cycle perspective. Families are perceived as changing from day to day and year to year. An important contributor to family development theory is Evelyn Duvall (1977) who suggests that families proceed through a series of developmental stages that parallel the developmental stages of the individual's life cycle. Each developmental stage of the family is characterized by a set of developmental tasks the family must master if it is to remain healthy.

Duvall identifies eight core developmental tasks that are common to American families:

1. Providing shelter, food, clothing, and health care for its members.

2. Meeting family costs and allocating such resources as time, space, and facilities according to each member's needs.

3. Determining who does what in the support, management, and care of the home and its members.

4. Ensuring each member's socialization through the internalization of increasingly mature roles in the family and beyond.

5. Establishing ways of interacting, communicating, and expressing affection, aggression, or sexuality, within limits acceptable to society.

6. Bearing (or adopting) and rearing children; incorporating and releasing family members appropriately.

7. Relating to school, church, work, community life; establishing policies for including in-laws, relatives, guests, friends, mass media.

8. Maintaining morale and motivation, rewarding achievements, meeting personal and family crises, setting attainable goals, and developing family loyalties and values.

Duvall (1977) has formulated an eight-stage family life cycle similar to the eight-stage model of individual development presented by Erikson (1963). The stages and critical tasks of the two models are shown in Table 7-1.

Duvall divides family development into two broad phases: expanding family life and contracting family life (Figure 7-3). The expanding period begins with the marital dyad and lasts until children are grown and launched. Contraction begins when the first child leaves home and ends with the death of the surviving spouse.

By comparing the eight stages of the family life cycle with the eight stages of the individual life cycle, it is possible to identify potential hazards to family development. According to Erikson (1963), each critical task is related to preceding tasks; there is a time of "ascendence" when a critical task can be accomplished best. The time of ascendence is determined by physical and psychological influences on an individual and by cultural expectations. Some families have difficulty integrating the individual tasks of all members into the developmental progression of the family. For example, the critical task of an adolescent is to establish identity. This requires a degree of separation from parents and other family members. The separation may be opposed by parents unwilling to exchange the characteristics of a teenage family for those of a launching family. Reluctance to move to the next family life stage also may be seen in couples who

TABLE 7-1
Comparison of Family Stages and Tasks with
Individual Stages and Tasks

Duvall's Family Stages and Critical Tasks	Erikson's Stages and Critical Tasks
Marital stage: Establishing a marriage	Trust versus mistrust
Childbearing stage: Adjusting to parenthood and maintaining a home	Autonomy versus shame and doubt
Preschool stage: Nurturing children	Initiative versus guilt
School-age stage: Socializing and educating children	Industry versus inferiority
Teenage stage: Balancing teenagers' freedom and responsibility	Identity versus role confusion
Launching stage: Releasing children as young adults; developing postparental interests	Intimacy versus isolation
Middle-aged stage: Reestablishing the marital dyad; maintaining links with older and younger generations	Generativity versus stagnation
Aging stage: Adjusting to retirement, aging, loneliness, and death	Ego integrity versus despair

resist moving from the carefree life of a marital dyad to the responsibilities of a childbearing family. Unless a couple can accept parenthood, their children may be impeded in moving toward trust and autonomy, the first two individual tasks identified by Erikson (1963).

Hymovich and Chamberlin (1980) have adapted Duvall's framework to identify five core developmental tasks:

1. Meeting the basic physical needs of the family.

2. Assisting each family member to develop his or her individual potential.

3. Providing emotional support and communicating effectively with all family members.

4. Maintaining and adapting family organization and management to meet changing needs.

5. Functioning in the community.

These five developmental tasks are common to all functionally healthy families, regardless of the type of family structure. Thus, they can be used as a framework for assessing the developmental

progress and growth of traditional and untraditional family types. Hymovich and Chamberlin's (1980) family assessment framework is presented in a later section of this chapter.

When families are inflexible, the critical tasks of individual members may be difficult to accomplish. Nurses using developmental theory can note the life cycle stage of a family and assess the progress being made by individual members in critical tasks. If individual progress is slow, it may be possible to discern the cause and assess its impact. Sometimes raising family awareness of the importance of stage-appropriate behavior is enough to lower impediments to progress.

The traditional family life cycle with stages of expansion and contraction is not followed by those who experience stages of estrangement, separation, divorce, single parenthood, remarriage, and stepparenthood. Transitional stages occur between the end of one marriage and the beginning of another, and complicated family structures challenge the concepts of family developmental theory. Even so, it is possible to determine with some accuracy the critical tasks that family members should be accomplishing and the current life cycle tasks that a family should be addressing.

Carter and McGoldrick (1980) assert that family development is more than the current relationships between people who happen to be connected by ties of blood, marriage, or commitment. Beyond the individual life stages of its members, the family shares in interdependent tasks and emotional changes over time. Not all individuals and families move easily from one transitional stage to the next. Some members of a family move willingly, even eagerly, to the next life stage cycle while others cling to customary behaviors that are no longer needed or appropriate. In addition to the changing needs of individuals within the family, the entry or departure of any member, whether through natural development, divorce, birth, death, or abandonment, creates further stress.

Family Systems

In many respects, a family is a system of interdependent components. A system consists of two or more connected elements that form an organized whole and interact with one another. A system, therefore, is a goal-directed unit composed of interdependent, interacting parts that endure over a period of time.

From this perspective, the family is viewed as a system made up of a group of closely interrelated and interdependent individuals who function in an integrated fashion. In healthy families, the

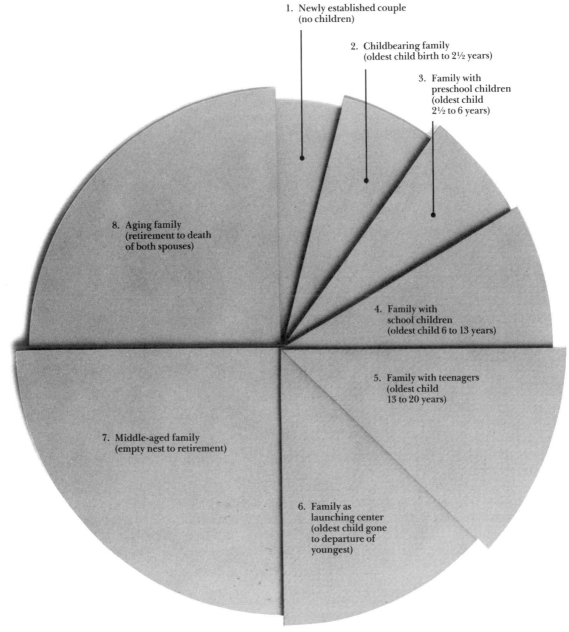

FIGURE 7-3. Phases, Stages, and Critical Family Life Cycle Tasks. (*Note.* From Davies/Janosik: *Mental Health and Psychiatric Nursing: A Caring Approach*, © 1991. Boston: Jones and Bartlett Publishers, p. 413.)

members share common goals and interact with one another in ways that preserve the stability of the family system. A family is considered to be an open system because it interacts with the community and society of which it is a part. The family does this by exchanging information, materials, and energy (in the forms of work and play) with its community, its cultural group, and the society as a whole. For example, adults in the family engage in productive work outside the family system. By doing so, they contribute to the functioning of the community and the society of which it is a part. In turn, the family receives inputs from the external environment, such as cultural norms, food and water, and health care, which are necessary for family maintenance and growth.

Change in any part of the family system affects the functioning of the entire family. Thus, hospitalization of a family member is likely to disrupt family functioning, at least temporarily. In addition, disruptions in the functioning of the family system, such as those caused by divorce, unemployment, or poverty, will in turn affect its individual members.

Family members are separated from each other and from the external environment by boundaries.

Boundaries surround individual members and also surround groups of members who form subsystems. In many families parents constitute one subsystem and children another, or females may form one subsystem and males another. It is possible for one family member to be part of several subsystems. Depending on the characteristics of boundaries between the family and the external environment, a family system may be open, closed, or somewhere in between. Energy in the form of tension within the family maintains the interdependence of members. All families generate some tension because of emotional connections among members. Excessive internal tension strains the family system. Boundaries therefore must be permeable enough to permit some discharge of tension among members and across boundaries surrounding the whole family.

Because the family is an open system, its boundaries are relatively flexible to allow for changes. Boundary flexibility makes it possible for the family to adapt to changes in its internal or external environments as well as changes in the family system itself, such as those resulting from birth, marriage, divorce, or death. However, if external boundaries are too weak and easily penetrated, family life may become unstable. An example of weak family boundaries occurs in upwardly mobile families who promptly discard old customs and immediately copy the customs of a higher socioeconomic group, even when it is impractical. Conversely, impenetrable boundaries prevent the transmission of information that might help the family cope. An example of this is seen in immigrant families in which parents resist all influence from mainstream society and preserve old habits despite opposition from their children.

Feedback is another systems concept applicable to family assessment. Through feedback the family transmits output to the environment in the form of emotional and behavioral responses. The external environment, by means of community, school, and church, reacts by sending responses (input) to the family. Sometimes feedback is informal, consisting of covert approval or disapproval of family actions. A family that does not meet community standards in caring for its home or children might become the subject of gossip or censure. More formal feedback might come in the form of complaints from the children's teachers or in a summons from the local police. Feedback is a continuous process of positive and negative exchange between families and the external environment.

Feedback takes place inside the family between individual members and subgroups. Feedback is not a series of linear events but a circular process in which all elements of a system and the immediate environment act upon one another. In circular feedback the actions of A affect the actions of B and C. Thereupon B and C react with each other and with A, who initiated the circular events. The circular pattern is shown in Figure 7-4.

By balancing what it gives and takes from its subsystems and the external environment, the family maintains a relative stability—not a static stability but a dynamic stability that allows for continual modifications in response to changes that occur in the family systems hierarchy. For example, the family must adapt its functioning when a new family member joins the household (e.g., through birth, marriage, adoptions, or a change in living arrangements). A family may or may not be able to maintain stability depending on its resources and adaptive capacity. For example, the birth of a baby with multiple birth defects poses a crisis for the family. If the family does not have the resources for coping with this threat to the family system, family disorganization or instability may result.

In order to preserve stability, the family system must grow and develop in response to change. By doing so the family system becomes more complex and differentiated. Lewis and associates (1976) describe the healthy family system as a "viable system characterized by complexity of structure; a highly flexible organization capable and tolerant of internal changes; and an openness with the outer environment that results in a continual flow of a wide variety of information, experience, and input into the family" (p. 10).

An advantage of adopting a systems approach to family assessment is the avoidance of blame. If the family represents a system in which parents, children, extended family members, and the community all influence one another reciprocally, then interactions are a shared responsibility. Since systems theory contends that alterations in one part of a family lead to alterations in all parts, nurses should be able to see family strengths as well as weaknesses (see boxed insert). Examining the quality of family boundaries and the presence of subgroups explains the origin of some forms of family dysfunction. Functional families with protective but permeable boundaries can adjust to changes within the family and in the outside environment. Dysfunctional families with impermeable boundaries tend to oppose change and growth. Such families strive to maintain the status quo regardless of the cost to individual members and ultimately to the family itself.

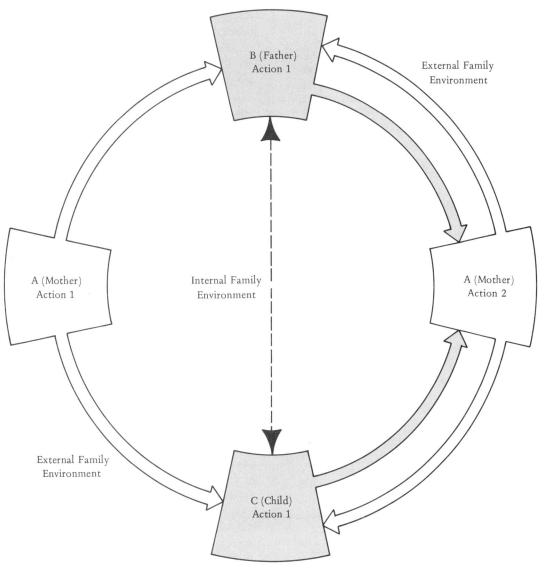

The action of A influences the actions of B and C, who then interact with each other and with A, who initiated the circular feedback. The actions of A, B, and C are influenced by forces within the family and in the external environment.

FIGURE 7-4. Diagram of Circular Feedback. (*Note.* From Davies/Janosik: *Mental Health and Psychiatric Nursing: A Caring Approach,* © 1991. Boston: Jones and Bartlett Publishers, p. 521.)

Family Structure

Every family is organized along structural lines that show relationships among family members. Family structure refers not only to the composition of the family but to the relative positions of members. In all families there are patterns regarding how, when, and with whom various members interact. These patterns relate to the placement of members and determine family function because members know what interactions are acceptable. Family subsystems, as previously noted, are divisions based on age, gender, and other natural divisions. Families begin with a marital dyad that

becomes the parental subsystem after children arrive. Children constitute the sibling subsystem, and in some families there may be more than one sibling subsystem. Within families there may be alliances and coalitions. These are divisions based not on natural divisions, but on the emotional needs of family members. Because they originate in irrational sources, alliances and coalitions are less likely to be functional than subgroup structures.

The foremost exponent of structural family theory is Minuchin (1974), whose work is compatible with systems theory. Minuchin believes that sub-

Basic Assumptions of Family Systems Theory

Living organisms are organized in a hierarchy where complex, higher level systems emerge from simpler, lower level systems. Every system is contained within boundaries that are more or less penetrable. Individuals are part of family systems that are organized into larger systems such as the community. Within families, various members are organized into subgroups.

A change in one family member or subgroup causes changes in other family members and subgroups. If any family member becomes dysfunctional for any reason, there is a shift that affects everyone in the family. Restoration of function to an impaired member also creates a shift. Families that coped well with the dysfunction of a member must readjust to allow the improved person to function more adaptively.

Family equilibrium is not static but involves constant search for balance among internal and external forces impinging on families.

Family interactions are circular not linear. Exploring circular patterns means that there is no search for a victim or culprit and no single truth to be uncovered. What is more important is the impact of various forces on family members and their interpretations of events.

Families have the ability to monitor themselves internally and externally, regulating interactions between members and with external systems by means of positive and negative feedback. Feedback is merely a response to events and actions. Positive feedback tends to increase or maintain whatever is happening; negative feedback tends to modify or decrease whatever is happening.

systems enable the family to differentiate and carry out various functions. He says that family boundaries should be clearly defined but not weak or rigid. Rigid boundaries interfere with family relatedness and cause members to suffer isolation or disengagement from one another. On the other hand, weak or diffuse boundaries create a sense of involvement and enmeshment between members, so that autonomy, mastery, and individuation are sacrificed. In disengaged families there is an attitude of indifference; in enmeshed families there is intrusiveness and interference. Functional families usually fall somewhere between disengagement and enmeshment. Any stress on an enmeshed family causes overreaction, often expressed by excessive solicitude and emotionalism. In a disengaged family, stress may temporarily increase interactions between members but concern is

rarely expressed, and help is neither requested nor offered.

Family Function

Family structure refers to how a family is organized; family function refers to how a family operates: What does the family do for its members and for the community and society of which it is a part? Certain critical functions characterize families. Two ways of categorizing family functions are suggested by Friedman (1986) and Roberts (1983). These views of family functions are compared in the boxed insert.

Structure and function are interdependent and influence each other in many ways. For example, in families where there are male and female subsystems, tasks are likely to be differentiated according to gender. In functional families where most of the needs of members are being met, natural family boundaries are maintained, and the parental subsystem is comprised of two partners with strong ties to one another. Closeness between the partners is a structural concept that contributes to effective family functioning. In a sense, boundaries enforce rules about subsystems, including who belongs in the system and how subsystems interact with other subsystems. Boundaries also monitor exchanges of information and interaction between the family and larger social systems in the community. Extremely rigid boundaries inhibit exchanges between family members or across subsystems. This means there is little caring in the family because members disengage from each other. At the other extreme, families with diffuse boundaries are characterized by excessive involvement and intrusiveness. Thus, boundaries maintain balance in the family and promote adaptation to change unless they are overly rigid or diffuse. Boundaries also regulate exchanges of energy and information according to the family's ability to cope. In stressful situations, families may be able to tolerate little interaction with the surrounding environment and inhibit participation from outside sources, as in the immediate aftermath of the death of a family member. When there is illness in a family, however, help from outside sources may be needed. When boundaries are too rigid, the family may not receive needed help simply because the extent of need is not communicated outside the family.

Functional aspects of family life are the focus of Murray Bowen (1971;1974;1976) whose work centers on the emotional life of families. Among Bowen's concepts related to family function are the nuclear family emotional system, differentiation of

Family Functions

Friedman[1]

1. **Affective function:** Personality development; meeting the emotional needs of family members.
2. **Socialization function:** Socializing children to assume adult roles; transmission of cultural customs, beliefs, and values.
3. **Reproductive function:** Ensuring the survival of the species by producing new offspring.
4. **Family coping function:** Helping members and the family as a whole deal with developmental and environmental stressors; adapting to internal and external changes to ensure stability of the family.
5. **Economic function:** Meeting the economic requirements of the family; providing adequate income (money and resources).
6. **Providing physical necessities:** Making sure the family has adequate food, clothing, shelter, safety, and health care.

Roberts[2]

1. **Management function:** Decision-making patterns in the family concerning the use of power, distribution of resources, establishment of rules, economic support, negotiation with systems outside the family, and planning for the future.
2. **Boundary function:** Maintaining clear distinctions between individual family members, among the family's subsystems (such as parents and children), and between the family and other systems (such as schools, church, employer, and social organizations).
3. **Communication function:** Sharing of ideas, feelings, needs; ways family members interact with each other (verbally and nonverbally).
4. **Emotional-supportive function:** Providing for healthy emotional development of family members.
5. **Socialization function:** Teaching appropriate social behavior within the norms of the family's cultural reference group; role assignment and adapting to role changes.

[1]Friedman, M.M. (1986). *Family nursing: Theory and assessment* (2nd ed.). Norwalk, CT: Appleton-Century-Crofts, p. 53.
[2]Roberts, F.B. (1983). An interaction model for family assessment. In I.W. Clements & F.B. Roberts (Eds.), *Family health: A theoretical approach to nursing care* (pp. 199–203). New York: Wiley.

self, multigenerational transmission, and family constellation.

Nuclear Family Emotional System. In some families the members do not see themselves as separate individuals but as people emotionally joined or fused together. The result of family fusion is that members do not think, speak, or act for themselves. Thoughts, words, and actions are not individualized; even feelings are not attributed to a single member but are experienced by everyone. This sharing causes a fused or undifferentiated ego, which makes it hard for members to identify clearly what they think and how they feel. Confusion develops between what an individual member thinks or feels and what other family members think and feel. When thoughts and feelings always are shared and never individualized, family events are confusing and distorted. This confusion and distortion further hinders the ability of individual members and of the whole family to handle problems.

When deep attachment to the family of origin persists after an adult has formed a new family, problems may arise. Prolonged attachment to the

original family can be a source of contention between marital partners and threaten their relationship. "Emotional cutoff" is a term used to describe the healthy detachment from the family of origin that should develop when a new family is established. It is not necessary to break all connection with the original family nor abandon it. What is needed is for adults forming a new family to be autonomous without feeling anxious and disloyal to their respective families of origin.

Differentiation of Self. In some respects self-differentiation is similar to emotional cutoff, but is a broader concept. Self-differentiation does not bar interaction with the original family, but indicates that adults who have left home are ruled by rational rather than emotional forces. Bowen (1974) differentiates between "the solid self" and "the pseudo-self" and proposes a differentiation-of-self scale with the solid self at one extreme and the pseudo-self at the other extreme (Figure 7-5). One's place on the scale is determined by one's tendencies to act according to principles of logic and reason. According to Bowen, one's degree of self-differentiation is not fixed but may move in

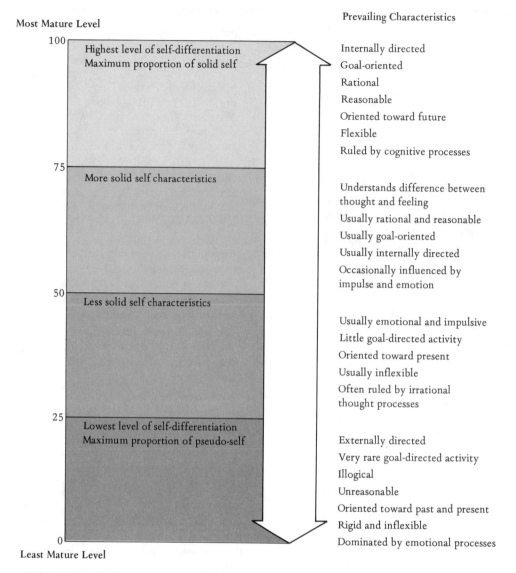

FIGURE 7-5. Differentiation-of-Self Scale. (*Note.* From Bowen, M. [1974]. Toward the differentiation of self in one's family of origin. In F. Andres & J. Loria (Eds.), *Georgetown family symposia: Collection of papers.* Washington, DC: Georgetown University Press.)

either direction over the course of the life cycle. He also notes that people at similar points on the self-differentiation scale tend to form relationships and marry each other.

Multigenerational Transmission. Multigenerational transmission is the means by which certain family values, attitudes, and behaviors persist across generations. Multigenerational transmission helps explain the devotion of certain families to specific occupations or pursuits, such as politics or music. Bowen (1974) connects intergenerational transmission to self-differentiation, explaining that families can move toward or away from self-differentiation from one generation to another. After several generations of decreasing self-differentia-

tion in families, dysfunctional patterns become dominant. Eventually the psychological development of some family members is so impaired that they are at risk for psychiatric disorders of one kind or another.

Multigenerational transmission is a useful concept for practitioners trying to understand the durability of family value systems. For instance, a man raised in very poor circumstances may continue to behave in a miserly fashion toward his wife and children long after he is financially secure. In other families there may be a tradition that members are expected to enter a particular profession, such as medicine or the ministry. Such expectations may lead to dissension and even the expulsion of members who reject family values.

Individuals who reach mature levels of self-differentiation are more likely to be guided by personal rather than family ambitions.

Family Constellation. It is generally accepted that sibling rank and order in the family have an effect on achievement and personality. Toman (1976) suggests that sibling position, gender differences, and family configurations influence the personality traits and social tendencies of children. In addition to only child or one of twins, Toman lists these significant family positions:

Oldest brother of brother(s)

Youngest brother of brother(s)

Oldest brother of sister(s)

Youngest brother of sister(s)

Oldest sister of sister(s)

Youngest sister of sister(s)

Oldest sister of brother(s)

Youngest sister of brother(s)

The concept of family constellation makes certain assumptions about behavior and personality development. One assumption is that oldest siblings tend to be more directive and responsible, whereas youngest siblings tend to be more dependent and willing to take direction. Family constellation is a very broad concept and one that should be applied with care. As part of a provisional assessment it may be useful, but it does not take into account relevant family history. Therefore, assumptions should be validated in order to note exceptions to generalizations about sibling positions and family constellation (Hoopes & Harper, 1987).

Family Communication

Family interactions and transactions are carried on by means of communication patterns. In using communication patterns to assess families, the nurse should observe the communication process, noting how messages are sent, received, validated, and answered. The process of communication (how messages are transmitted) is just as important as the content (what messages are transmitted).

Communication consists of a message and response. It is impossible not to respond to a message, but the response need not be verbal. Silence is a response to a message, as is failure to answer a letter or the ring of a phone. Such behavioral responses actually transmit a strong emotional or cognitive message. In most families, communication patterns are entrenched and durable. For instance, in some families children rarely make direct requests of the father but use the mother as an intermediary.

Family communication, like family boundaries, should be clear, consistent, and specific.

Healthy interaction patterns are characterized by open and honest communication among family members. Members feel free to express their individual needs, emotions, and opinions. Individual differences in family members are accepted and their imperfections are tolerated. Self-esteem of family members is likely to be high in these families because individual members are seen as important contributors to family health and stability.

Functionally healthy families also provide opportunities for members to interact as subsystems within the family (for example, siblings are allowed to share secrets without being expected to disclose them to the entire family, and parents are able to maintain their identity as marital partners separate from their parenting roles). Members also are encouraged to interact with others outside the family system, such as participating in community and school activities, without disruption to family stability. At the same time, however, members are expected to interact with the family unit in ways that fulfill their role expectations and obligations. Thus, a balance must be maintained between individual and family needs to ensure smooth family functioning.

Dysfunctional communication fails to validate meanings, omits connecting sentences, accuses rather than questions, and uses global words like "always" or "never" when disputing issues. When family members generalize, digress, blame, or appease, the message recipient becomes confused or angry, and problems escalate. Most families sometimes engage in dysfunctional communication patterns, partly because they are outside the awareness of family members.

Family Roles

Within the family network, individual family members are assigned or achieve certain rights and responsibilities that define their roles. Each role is defined by a set of acceptable behaviors determined by social and cultural norms. Thus, there is a set of accepted behaviors for the various family roles, such as parent, spouse, child, sibling, in-law, and grandparent.

Acceptance and enactment of socially acceptable role behaviors are necessary for successful family functioning. According to Friedman (1986), adequate role performance is essential not only to individual functioning but to family functioning, since family functions are fulfilled through various individual and family roles.

Generally, each family member occupies a number of clearly defined formal roles such as husband, parent, daughter, economic provider, housekeeper, or sexual partner. Formal roles vary according to age, gender, and the type of family structure. For example, a toddler in a small, traditional, nuclear family would have few formal roles: son or daughter, perhaps sister or brother, and grandson or granddaughter. The wife in the same family might have many roles in addition to that of spouse: mother, in-law (to her husband's family), daughter (to her own parents), and perhaps sister, aunt, and so on in the extended family. She would also have occupational roles (housekeeper, economic provider) assigned within the family and by societal expectations. The older a person becomes, and the larger the family, the more formal roles the individual assumes. Formal roles are explicit, but family members also may assume a variety of informal roles to meet the family's emotional needs. These informal roles strongly influence family communication patterns.

Informal roles generally contribute to family stability, although some informal roles may interfere with family equilibrium. For example, the family member who constantly criticizes other family members or dominates the family at the expense of individual members' autonomy precipitates family instability. Informal roles are based less on age and gender of family members and more on their individual personality attributes.

Informal roles often are learned through socialization. As children observe their parents, other adults in the family, and siblings, they begin to imitate those behaviors that they perceive as successful. For instance, they may learn that playing a martyr role elicits attention and solicitous behavior from their parents.

Informal roles usually are more difficult to assess than formal roles, especially when the nurse does not know the family well. Assessment of informal roles is often possible only after the nurse has worked with the family for a period of time. Much depends, of course, on the family's willingness to disclose information concerning family role behavior.

Maturation, readiness, aptitude, and experience are factors that affect adequate role performance. These considerations are sometimes overlooked in single-parent families, dual-career families, and families where the partners are not in agreement concerning role expectations. Men who have grown up in traditional families of origin where tasks were assigned on the basis of gender differentiation may cling to familiar patterns in households where both partners hold jobs outside the home.

Contemporary changes in society have greatly influenced traditional nuclear family roles, including sex-role behavior of husband and wife. Parents now are sharing childrearing and housekeeping responsibilities. They often share breadwinning responsibilities as well. Even with these changes, though, the father's primary role is still seen as that of financial provider and the mother's as childrearing and housekeeping. Families in which these roles are completely reversed are the exception rather than the rule.

Family role changes may be precipitated by temporary or permanent changes in family structure. For example, as new family members are added, such as a new baby or an aging parent, the family must adjust its formal and informal roles. Illness and hospitalization of a family member will necessitate some shifting of family role responsibilities. When a 41-year-old mother of three children was diagnosed as having multiple sclerosis, her husband and two older children adapted their roles to share some responsibilities that had formerly belonged solely to the mother, such as grocery shopping, chauffeuring children to social activities, cooking, and housecleaning. Although the mother continued to do as much as she could, she was confined to a wheelchair and adjustment of roles was necessary to maintain family stability. Healthy families with adequate resources and support available to them are able to cope with such role transitions and role changes without undue harm to family functioning.

Family Power

Power refers to the ability of some family members to influence or control the behavior of other family members. Certain family roles determine the locus of power in some family interactions (for example, parents are expected to have power in their relationships with their children). It is the way in which power is exercised that concerns the nurse when assessing the family power structure. By observing family interactions and interviewing family members, the nurse tries to determine what kinds of power are used by family members, how the power is used, and whether one family member dominates or the power is shared among family members.

Friedman (1986) has developed a continuum for identifying the power dimensions of a family (Figure 7-6). Friedman (1986) describes family power on a continuum ranging from chaotic (leaderless) to egalitarian syncretic and autonomic (decisions and power are shared) to dominance (power

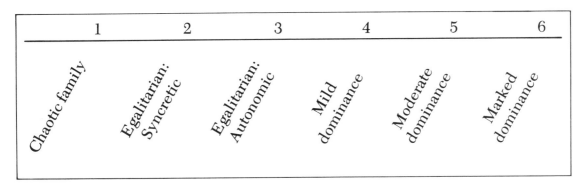

FIGURE 7-6. The Family Power Continuum. The chaotic family (1) refers to a leaderless family, wherein no member has adequate power to make decisions effectively. In egalitarian syncretic and autonomic families (2–3), decisions and power are shared. In the syncretic form, the decisions are made together; in the autonomic form, they are made independently. Dominance or power (4–6) ranges from marked, where there is practically absolute control by an individiual and no negotiation, to mild, where there is a tendency for dominance and submissiveness but most decisions are reached through respectful, mutual negotiation. (*Note.* Reprinted with permission. M.M. Friedman [1986]. *Family nursing: Theory and assessment* [2nd ed.]. New York: Appleton-Century-Crofts, p. 148.)

ranges from mild dominance where decisions are made through some negotiation to marked dominance with one family member exerting absolute control).

FAMILY STRESS AND CRISIS

Functional families manage to be flexible and consistent. Consistency is shown by adherence to agreed upon family rules and priorities. Flexibility is shown by sharing and delegating family responsibilities as needs and circumstances change. Dysfunctional families may be divided into marginal families in which appropriate role enactment is attempted even though family resources are barely adequate for daily life, and disorganized families in which appropriate role enactment really is not attempted. Marginal families manage to maintain minimum levels of functioning when no excessive stressors are present, but suffer serious disruption when demands on the family exceed resources. Illness, unemployment, death, or natural disasters are among the stressors that threaten the fragile balance of marginal families.

The disorganized family engages in deficient and inappropriate role enactment even in ordinary circumstances. The disorganized family is well known to community agencies, for in these crisis-prone families, disequilibrium is chronic and commonplace. A significant factor in the role enactment of disorganized families is substance abuse by one or more family members. Substance abuse, especially alcoholism, is not only a problem

in itself but contributes to spouse and child neglect and abuse.

Socioeconomic class differences influence the behavior and lifestyle of families and therefore should be part of the assessment process. It is hard to consign families to a particular socioeconomic class without being somewhat arbitrary. While a number of indicators are used to determine socioeconomic class, indices frequently employed include education, occupation, and income. Absolute dividing points are less reliable than comparative ones, since the region in which a family lives or the stage of a family's life cycle are variables affecting lifestyle and class designation. A family living on a modest income in San Francisco where the cost of living is high, and a family living in a rural Midwest town where the cost of living is low probably would have very different standards. On the same income living in the rural town would mean affluence, while residing in San Francisco could mean substandard living. Frequently, the family's opinion of its lifestyle and socioeconomic class is the most influential measure of its relative rank. A young couple just finishing college might have the same limited income as a retired laborer and his sickly wife. Yet, the upward vision of the young couple and the downward view of the elderly couple cause them to adopt very different perspectives and lifestyles. Education is also an important indicator of the class to which families believe they belong, regardless of income.

Families often have problems when each parent has originated in a different class or when they are moving as a family from one socioeconomic class to another. Values held by one parent but not the other may lead to disagreements about child rearing and family activities. Even though they hold the same values, upwardly and downwardly mobile couples may feel lonely and alienated as their lifestyles change, and their habits no longer coincide either with those of old neighbors or with those of newer neighbors. This becomes extremely problematic when parents and children within a family disagree on what is important, even when both parents are in accord.

Changes of any kind always produce additional family stress. Even ordinary life situations, such as birth, marriage, death, illness, changing residence, and starting school, introduce stress into family life. The impact of these stressors on the family depends on the nature of the event, how the family perceives the event, and the family's internal and external resources for coping with the event. The number of stressors the family must cope with simultaneously is also a factor. The combined impact of an employment change, move to a new state, and the birth of a first baby within a short period of time is likely to be more stressful than if the family must cope with only one of these.

Families with clearly defined roles for family members, open communication patterns, and available support systems (emotional, social, financial) are more likely to cope effectively with stressors than a disorganized family.

Stressors may be categorized as situational or developmental (maturational). Situational stressors occur as a result of unanticipated or unplanned events that threaten the family's equilibrium. Examples of situational stressors are family illness, separation or divorce, unemployment, relocation, natural or man-made disasters, and the birth of a child with a defect.

Developmental stressors are part of the normal process of growth and development that occur as an individual family member or the family as a whole moves from one developmental stage to another. Developmental stressors also may be associated with the achievement of developmental tasks, such as weaning, toilet training, establishing a clear gender identity, school success or failure, choosing a career, and retirement. Family developmental stressors include adapting to the addition of a new family member, childrearing, and elective family decisions to relocate. Whether developmental stressors occur as a result of individual or family developmental changes, the family as a whole usually is affected.

Neuman (1983) describes three types of family stressors:

Intrafamily: Stressors that occur as a result of interactions among family members, that is, within the family unit.

Interfamily: Stressors resulting from family interactions with the immediate or direct external environment.

Extrafamily: Stressors caused by forces in the larger environment.

An example of an intrafamily stressor is marital discord or a disturbance in parent–child interaction. Interfamily stressors include disagreements with the family's landlord, or discord with the school that the children in the family attend. Barriers to adequate health care are also interfamily stressors. Extrafamily stressors are caused by the larger social and political environments, such as massive funding cuts in government social programs or monetary inflation.

When the stressors impinging on a family intensify or exceed the family's usual coping abilities, they may precipitate a family crisis. In order for a crisis to develop, several conditions must be present. First, a precipitating event must intrude on an individual, family, or community, causing a distressing state of tension. Second, the people feeling the tension respond by using customary coping measures to handle the situation. If the coping efforts are adequate, tension is reduced, and a state of crisis is avoided. If coping measures are unsuccessful, however, the people involved enter a state of uncomfortable disequilibrium known as *crisis*. During the crisis period people experience emotional, cognitive, and behavioral distortions that further reduce their coping ability.

Crisis is a phenonemon that combines danger with opportunity for growth. When customary coping methods fail, people search for alternatives with varying success. In the search, some individuals and families discover new coping strategies, which then are available to them in the future. A crisis is less urgent than an emergency, which requires an immediate response. Marrying, divorcing, and relocating are not in themselves crises or emergencies. It is the *perception* of an event that propels people into crisis, depending on their reactions to rising tension levels.

All crises are of limited duration. At the end of that time tension, distortion, and disequilibrium lessen. Whether coping has been effective or not, the crisis abates. However, new crises may be superimposed on resolving or resolved crises, activating a new crisis response. Although crisis is limited, it has long-term consequences in that coping skills may improve, remain unchanged, or worsen. Changes in coping ability influence how people will respond to future crises.

Every family reacts to health problems in its own way, exhibiting different strengths and weaknesses in responding to the stress caused by illness or change. The ages of family members and the stage of the family life cycle greatly affect a family's coping skills. Families differ also in their willingness to recognize and respond to acute and chronic health problems. Their responses are influenced by ethnic, class, and idiosyncratic factors. Families with sufficient income and insurance are likely to seek professional assistance for health problems. Such families are apt to be sensitive to changes in the health of members and to deal with early warning signs. At the other extreme are marginal families, who regard health as the ability to work and ignore warning signs until a family member no longer is able to function. Procrastination in getting help should be viewed in the context of a family's limited resources. Many marginal and disorganized families ignore health problems as long as possible because they consider the health-care system to be harsh and uncaring. There are individuals in every socioeconomic class who see illness as a personal weakness and fiercely reject the idea of being sick. The realistic and symbolic meaning of illness greatly determines people's responses to any health problem, acute, chronic, or terminal (see chap. 8).

Strong kinship and community ties can be very valuable to families dealing with any health problem. However, in our mobile, pluralistic society neighborhood connections may be tenuous, and extended family groups may be separated by great distances. Community groups try to extend help once given by relatives and neighbors, but families may not know what is available. The disorganized family is more likely to be known by community agencies. The marginal family is less visible but may suffer greater stress. Solving the everyday problems of buying food, paying rent, and clothing its members may consume all the resources of the marginal family. Investigation of a family's knowledge of and access to aid from relatives, neighbors, and community programs should be part of a comprehensive family assessment.

Even families that enjoy high incomes, live in congenial surroundings, and lead stable, satisfying lives occasionally find themselves at the mercy of culturally or environmentally induced stressors. An example of stress beyond the control of most families is unemployment. Losing a job reminds the worker and the family that life is uncertain and security elusive. Family conflict is a by-product of unemployment and prolonged economic deprivation (Powers, 1986). Marital dissension is more common, and parents find it harder to deal with their children.

Unemployment alters the roles in families when the primary provider is affected and other members assume the provider's role. Being unable to support one's family makes workers blame themselves for earlier decisions. They wish they had moved somewhere else or obtained more education or chosen another occupation. The guilt and depression of the unemployed worker is another source of stress for the entire family. Role shifts in families mean different things to different family members, and the forcible role shifts introduced by economic factors seldom are welcome, even in families that regroup and continue to manage. Here, as in other aspects of family assessment, role theory provides an objective way of exploring family dynamics.

Environmental stress may originate in the housing conditions in which a family lives or in more pervasive conditions, such as widespread pollution or catastrophes affecting many families. When crises affect a whole community rather than one or two families, the terms *catastrophe* and *disaster* are used. The equilibrium of a community is important to its families; when community equilibrium is disturbed, the social and physical resources of families are tested to the utmost. The suddenness of a disaster and the inexperience of families in coping with the event may alter the outcomes. People who live where landslides, hurricanes, or floods occur learn to take preventive and restorative steps. The same is true of arid regions where fire is a constant danger. However, when a disaster comes without warning to an area never before affected, the consequences can be devastating.

Disaster conditions disrupt roles that have been established over a lifetime. In ordinary circumstances role performance is distributed among family, job, and social responsibilities. In times of disaster people often must choose to enact one set of responsibilities at the expense of others. The result is uncertainty and role conflict, as people struggle to balance family obligations with community needs. Stress rises in the family when such central figures as parents are no longer able to protect and care for dependents. In the aftermath of a disaster, families should be kept together if at all possible. Powers (1986) reports that being separated from their families and evacuated from London in World War II was more detrimental to children than remaining and enduring air raids. Powers also reports that police and fire personnel tend to continue their accustomed duties during a disaster, but their efforts are enhanced when they know their own families are safe.

During a disaster, young children tend to regress and cling to parents or a favorite possession. Adolescents may become withdrawn, tearful, or angry. Encouraging younger family members to perform tasks that are useful but not very demanding encourages age-appropriate behavior. There always are some people who cannot deal with disaster as a limited crisis. Instead of gradually recovering, they relive events in the form of nightmares, flashbacks, or endless rumination. This is a form of post-traumatic stress disorder that aggravates the problems of other family members. For such people, more than crisis intervention may be needed to help the family reorganize itself.

In assessing any crisis situation a first step is exploring the meaning of the crisis to those who are involved. Often the symbolic meaning of the crisis far outweighs the reality. Cognitive, emotional, and behavioral distortions are characteristic of people in crisis, and the extent of distortion must be explored. By tracing the sequence of events before a crisis, by asking what happened, to whom, and what remedies have been tried, the nurse begins to understand the meaning of the situation for those who are overwhelmed by it. While assessing the real proportions of the crisis, the nurse should accept the validity of a client's experience.

FAMILY ASSESSMENT: APPROACHES AND TOOLS

Because individual and family health influence each other, clients must be assessed within the context of their family systems. A fundamental aspect of any family assessment is an assessment of the cultural background of the particular family. As the primary social group in the life of the individual, the family preserves and transmits culture. The nurse's ability to understand the family's cultural orientation is established through an assessment of the family's cultural background (Friedman, 1990). To assist the nurse in assessing family culture, Friedman (1990) provides some valuable guidelines (Table 7-2). Several of the ques-

TABLE 7-2
Cultural Assessment Guidelines

Assessment Criteria	Questions
Ethnic/racial identity	Does the family identify itself as belonging to a certain ethnic or racial group? Are the parents both from the same cultural background?
Place of birth	Where were the parents and children born? If born in the U.S., where were the parents' parents born? If born out of the U.S., how many years have parents lived in the U.S.?
Geographic mobility	Where have the parents lived? When did they move to their present residence?
Languages spoken	What language(s) is/are spoken in the home and by whom? What language is preferred when speaking with outsiders?
Family's religion	What is the family's religion? Are both parents from the same religious background? How actively involved is the family in religion-based activities and practices?
Ethnic group affiliation	What are the characteristics of the family's social network? Are friends and associations all from the family's ethnic group? Are recreational, educational, and other social activities within the ethnic reference group or the wider community? To what extent does the family use services and shop within the family's neighborhood or within the wider community?
Neighborhood affiliation	What are the characteristics of the family's neighborhood? Is it ethnically heterogeneous or homogeneous?
Dietary habits and dress	What are the family's dietary habits and dress? Are the family's home decorations, art, and religious objects from the family's ethnic background?
Use of folk systems	To what extent does the family use folk healing practices or practitioners?
Acceptance by community	To what extent is the family affected by discrimination?

Other cultural questions can easily be incorporated into each of the family assessment areas, such as within family roles, because culture is one of the primary modifying factors of family patterns.
Note. From Friedman, M. (1990). Transcultural family nursing: Application to Latino and Black families. *Journal of Pediatric Nursing, 5*(3), 214–222.

tions provide basic identifying information about the family. The remaining questions can be used within the context of any of the theoretical approaches discussed in this chapter. These guidelines assist the nurse in determining a family's cultural orientation.

To facilitate the family assessment, mutual trust and respect between the nurse and family is essential. The relationship must be open and honest. Active listening is especially important.

Prior to visiting, the nurse should telephone the family to arrange the time and explain the purpose of the visit. If the family does not have a telephone, the nurse can write a note or attempt to make contact with the family during a visit to the health agency in order to arrange a home visit.

In a hospital setting, family members are to some degree a captive audience if they are in attendance during a family member's hospital stay. When family members visit, the nurse should attempt to establish a relationship with them and use the opportunity to gather information.

Interviewing family members can elicit valuable information about family structure, communication, roles, and power. Family structure, or constellation, is the most easily assessed. Most families are willing to describe their family constellation. Occasionally, however, families will be reluctant to divulge that certain members are part of the family or reside with the family, particularly if there are concerns about legal entanglements. For example, a woman who is receiving Aid to Families with Dependent Children (AFDC) may be unwilling to acknowledge a live-in boyfriend for fear her payments may be cut off.

Assessment of family communication is an important part of the family assessment, as are family roles, which have a profound influence on family interaction patterns (Figure 7-7). Assessing family decision-making provides clues to who exercises the greatest power within the family unit. Suggested interview questions for each of these areas are outlined in Table 7-3.

It is especially important to assess the effect of a client's illness and hospitalization on family members. The following questions are helpful in ascertaining this information:

Who are the client's family members (their ages, roles, and relationships)? How has the client's illness and hospitalization altered family roles and relationships?

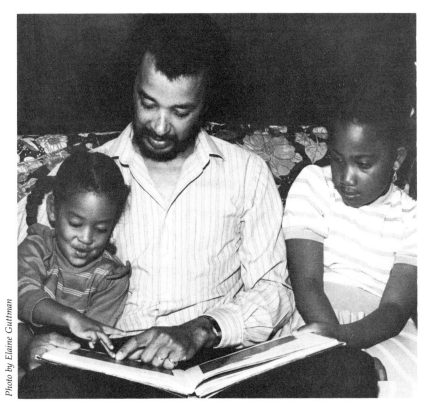

Photo by Elaine Guttman

FIGURE 7-7. Family interaction patterns should be assessed for strengths and problems in communication. (*Note.* From Servonsky/Opas: *Nursing Management of Children,* © 1987. Boston: Jones and Bartlett Publishers, p. 230.)

TABLE 7-3
Family Assessment Interview Questions

Family Structure

Who are the family members (ages, gender, race/ethnicity, educational level, occupation/school)?

Family Communication Patterns

Are messages clearly and directly expressed, or are they vague, ambiguous, and indirectly stated?

Do family members listen to one another?

Do they show interest in one another's activities, concerns, problems?

Is there mutual sharing of information or does one member dominate?

Are information exchanges open, honest, calm, and caring, or are they aggressive, angry, hurtful, and suspicious?

Are verbal messages consistent with nonverbal behaviors, and vice versa?

What factors may be interfering with effective family communication?

Family Roles

What formal and informal roles do individual family members occupy?

Are family members fulfilling their role expectations?

Are there any role conflicts at the present time (such as an adolescent who wants more freedom without increased responsibility, or a working mother who needs but is not receiving any assistance with child care or household responsibilities from her spouse)? How has the family managed previous role conflicts? What is the family doing to resolve current role conflicts?

Have there been any recent changes in the family that have necessitated role changes? How is the family adapting to these shifts in role?

Family Decision-Making

Which family members make what decisions? For example, who decides what major purchases the family makes? Who decides where the family resides? Who makes decisions concerning childrearing practices? Concerning health care?

What process is used to make important family decisions? For example, are all family members consulted, do the adults collaborate, or does a single family member control the decision-making?

If there is a disagreement over family decisions, whose decision is the final one?

Are family members satisfied with the family's decision-making process?

Which family members are most significant to the client?

What is the family's understanding of the client's illness, treatments, reason for hospitalization?

What special needs does the family have while the client is ill or hospitalized? How are they managing?

What concerns does the family have?

What sources of support and assistance are available to the family during the client's hospitalization?

Answers to these interview questions can assist the nurse in identifying potential or actual interferences with family status and functioning while the client is ill or hospitalized. Resources then can be identified for helping the family adapt to or cope with these problems, whether temporary or permanent.

Assessing Family Development

Hymovich and Chamberlin (1980) suggest an outline of useful information the nurse can obtain by interviewing family members to determine achievement of family developmental tasks. Their framework is presented in Table 7-4. The nurse can interpret the findings to identify progress and potential problems in family development as a basis for selecting appropriate nursing interventions to facilitate healthy family development. For example, parents who suppress the expression of such feelings as affection, fear, or anger inhibit family members' ability to provide emotional support and communicate openly and effectively with each other.

Assessing Family Function

A number of approaches have been developed to assess family functioning, including the Family Function Index (Pless & Satterwhite, 1973), the Feetham Family Functioning Survey (Roberts & Feetham, 1982), the Family APGAR (Smilkstein, 1978), and the Family Function Checklist (Roberts, 1983).

The Family Function Index (Pless & Satterwhite, 1973) is designed for use by clinicians to assess husband-wife perceptions of a number of dimensions of family functioning, such as communication, decision making, and marital satisfaction. The index requires the spouse to respond to a series of items using a Likert scale from 1 (husband always) to 3 (husband and wife exactly the same) to 5 (wife always).

The Feetham Family Functioning Survey (1982), designed for use with families who have children, was developed originally to measure the effect of a child's disability (myelodysplasia) on

TABLE 7-4
Assessment of Family Developmental Tasks

Task	Useful information
Meeting the basic physical needs of the family	Family satisfaction with: housing, food, clothing, health, community, health care, financial situation Resources available, used, needed Seek and accept help when needed
Assisting each family member to develop his or her individual potential	Satisfaction with accomplishment of developmental tasks Extent to which each family member is accomplishing his or her individual developmental tasks Parental understanding of needs of each family member Availability of resources needed for each family member to accomplish tasks Adaptation of approaches to developmental level of each member Extent to which each member's tasks support or conflict with those of others
Providing emotional support and communicating effectively with all family members	Satisfaction with relationships Relationship between family members Communication patterns Decision-making patterns Expression and sharing of feelings Stability of marriage (e.g., spouse abuse) Relationships with extended family Individual family member's temperament, personality, cognitive level, self-concept How individual needs for affection, acceptance, and encouragement are met
Maintaining and adapting family organization and management to meet changing needs	Satisfaction with organization and management Daily schedule Role of each family member Strengths and weaknesses in organization and management Role flexibility Availability of external supports Policies for including others in family (e.g., friends, neighbors, relatives)
Functioning in the community	Satisfaction with community involvement Leisure activities outside home Organizations belong to, (e.g., PTA, volunteer, parents groups) Use of community resources (e.g., day care, baby-sitting) Availability of community resources Satisfaction with available resources

Note. From Hymovich, D. P., & Chamberlin, R. (1980). *Child and family development.* New York: McGraw-Hill, 1980, pp. 78–79. Copyright © 1980 by McGraw-Hill Book Company. Reprinted with permission.

family functioning. Additional testing has confirmed its validity for use with families of healthy children, families of children with health problems, families with adult children, and single-parent families. Feetham recommends that the instrument's use be confined to research purposes until clinical validity is established (S.L. Feetham, personal communication, July 11, 1991). However, it may be used clinically to provide family profile information (Feetham & Humenick, 1982).

The Feetham Family Functioning Survey consists of a series of 25 items for which the parent is asked to answer three questions each (see Figure 7-8). The survey also includes two open-ended questions, "What is most *difficult* for you now?"

and "What is most *helpful* for you now?" A family functioning discrepancy score is calculated to determine the discrepancy between what *is* and what the parent believes *should be*. If the parent identifies an item with a high discrepancy score (a large difference between what is and what should be) as very important, further assessment and intervention may be indicated.

The Family APGAR is an easy-to-administer screening questionnaire designed to assess the functional status of nuclear or alternative lifestyle families (Smilkstein, 1978). The Family APGAR has been shown to be a valid and reliable tool to measure satisfaction with family functioning (Smilkstein, Ashworth, & Montano, 1982). The

The amount of time you spend with your spouse.

   a. How much is there now?

Little   Much

1   2   3   4   5   6   7

   b. How much should there be?

Little   Much

1   2   3   4   5   6   7

   c. How important is this to you?

Little   Much

1   2   3   4   5   6   7

The amount of help from relatives with family tasks such as care of children, house repairs, household chores, etc. *(do not include spouse)*.

   a. How much is there now?

Little   Much

1   2   3   4   5   6   7

   b. How much should there be?

Little   Much

1   2   3   4   5   6   7

   c. How important is this to you?

Little   Much

1   2   3   4   5   6   7

FIGURE 7-8. Sample Items from the Feetham Family Functioning Survey. (*Note.* From Feetham, S.L. [1983]. *Feetham Family Functioning Survey.* Washington, DC: Children's Hospital National Medical Center. The complete survey instrument may be obtained for $7.50 from Suzanne Feetham, PH.D., R.N., F.A.A.N., Children's Hospital National Medical Center, 111 Michigan Avenue, N.W., Washington, DC 20010.)

five areas of family function that are assessed include:

> **A**daptation: the utilization of intra- and extrafamilial resources for problem solving when family equilibrium is stressed during a crisis.
>
> **P**artnership: the sharing of decision making and nurturing responsibilities by family members.
>
> **G**rowth: the physical and emotional maturation and self-fulfillment that are achieved by family members through mutual support and guidance.
>
> **A**ffection: the caring or loving relationship that exists among family members.
>
> **R**esolve: the commitment to devote time to other members of the family for physical and emotional nurturing. It also usually involves a decision to share wealth and space. (Smilkstein, 1978, p. 1232)

The Family APGAR elicits a family member's satisfaction with each of the dimensions of family functioning by asking five simple questions (see Figure 7-9). The results are scored as follows: "Almost al-

ways"—2 points; "Some of the time"—1 point; "Hardly ever"—0 points. The scores for the five items are totaled, and they are interpreted as follows:

> A score of 8 to 10 suggests a highly functional family.
>
> A score of 4 to 7 suggests a moderately dysfunctional family.
>
> A score of 0 to 3 suggests a severely dysfunctional family. (Smilkstein, 1978, p. 1234)

Responses to Part II of the questionnaire can be used to identify supportive relationships within the family and the strengths and weaknesses of family interaction patterns.

Roberts (1983) proposes an interaction model for assessing family function. Client needs are assessed in five categories—management function, boundary function, communication function, emotional-supportive function, and socialization function—according to four levels of need (see Figure 7-10). A family's level of need for each of the five family functions may be assessed using the Family Function Checklist illustrated in Figure 7-10 (Roberts, 1983). The results of the assessment should be used as a basis for determining appropriate nursing responses, or interventions, within each category.

Assessing Family Strengths

There is a tendency to label families seeking professional help as dysfunctional. While a family may be dysfunctional in some respects, every family has strengths that can be mobilized once they are identified. The concept of family strengths has been defined as "the factors or forces that contribute to family unity and solidarity and that foster the development of the potentials inherent within the family" (Otto, 1973, p. 87). Assessment of family strengths emphasizes the family's capabilities, especially the family's resources, both inner and external, for solving problems and coping with family stress and crisis.

According to a framework developed by Otto, assessment of strengths of a family should include, but not be limited to:

> *Physical, emotional, and spiritual needs of the family.* How does the family meet members' qualitative and quantitative needs such as food, shelter, safety, privacy, and clothing? How does it meet emotional and spiritual needs?
>
> *Childrearing practices and discipline.* Is parental responsibility shared equally? Do parents re-

spect each other and their children? Do they foster child self-discipline?

Communication. What functional and dysfunctional interaction patterns are present? What about open, honest verbal expression? Sensitive listening? Consensual decision-making?

Support, security, and encouragement. Does the family promote feelings of security? Does it offer emotional, moral, physical, financial, and other support? Do members receive encouragement, commendation, praise, and recognition? Are family activities balanced?

Growth-producing experiences internal and external to the family. Are interpersonal relationships developed and maintained within the family network? With friends? In the community? With the larger society? Such relationships indicate the maturity of the family.

Responsible involvement in community relationships. Do family members assume responsible positions in schools, in religious or ethical groups, in social, political, and cultural organizations? Do they discuss and share opinions and beliefs about issues and developments on local, state, and national levels? Do parents encourage the involvement of children in these activities? These factors contribute to family unity and growth.

Growing with and through children. Is self-actualization in children and adults being fostered through mutual sharing and open communication?

Self-help and acceptance of help. Does the family give help to its members? Does it accept help from friends, neighbors, agencies, and health professionals when needed? Ability to give and receive help indicates that the family has the potential to solve its own problems.

Flexible family roles and functions. Are family members able and willing to shift roles and functions to fill the void left by an absent member?

The following questions have been designed to help us better understand you and your family. You should feel free to ask questions about any item in the questionnaire.

The space for comments should be used when you wish to give additional information, or if you wish to discuss the way the question applies to your family. Please try to answer all questions.

For each question, check only one box.

	Almost always	Some of the time	Hardly ever
I am satisfied that I can turn to my family* for help when something is troubling me. Comments:			
I am satisfied with the way my family talks over things with me and shares problems with me. Comments:			
I am satisfied that my family accepts and supports my wishes to take on new activities or directions. Comments:			
I am satisfied with the way my family expresses affection and responds to my emotions, such as anger, sorrow, or love. Comments:			
I am satisfied with the way my family and I share time together. Comments:			

*"Family" is the individual(s) with whom you usually live. If you live alone, consider family as those with whom you now have the strongest emotional ties.

FIGURE 7-9. The Family APGAR. (*Note.* From Smilkstein, G. (1986). *Instructions for use of The Family APGAR: A family function screening questionnaire.* Seattle, WA: Author.)

Who lives in your home?* List by relationship
(e.g., spouse, significant other,** child or friend).

RELATIONSHIP	AGE	SEX

Please check below the column that best describes
how you now get along with each member of the
family listed.

WELL	FAIRLY	POORLY

If you don't live with your own family, please list
below the individuals to whom you turn for help
most frequently. List by relationship (e.g., family
member, friend, associate at work, or neighbor).

RELATIONSHIP	AGE	SEX

Please check the column below that best describes
how you now get along with each person listed.

WELL	FAIRLY	POORLY

* Home. If you have established your own family, consider home to be the place where you live with your
  spouse, children, or significant other; otherwise, consider home as your place of origin, e.g., the place where
  your parents or those who raised you live.

** "Significant other" is the partner you live with in a physically and emotionally nurturing relationship, but to
   whom you are not married.

FIGURE 7-9 (Continued).

Respect for individuality. Are parents and children recognized as individuals who deserve mutual respect and who have needs and emotions to be considered?

Coping with crisis. Does the family draw together during situational or maturational crises (such as birth of a baby, illness or death of a family member, unemployment)?

Unity, loyalty, and cooperation. Do family members demonstrate loyalty to one another and to the family unit? Does the family demonstrate cooperative, productive relationships that enhance family unity and maintain family traditions?

The 12 categories of family strengths should be considered as dynamic, fluid, interrelated factors that change according to a family's developmental level. Together, the strengths provide a picture of a functional family. However, in some instances certain strengths may become a family limitation if they prevent the family from engaging in solving problems. For example, too much time devoted to community relationships may reduce the time parents have to deal with the emotional and social needs of children. Thus, the parameters also must be assessed for flexibility in adapting to change to meet family needs.

The foregoing framework is a guide for consistent, continuous, concrete assessment of family strengths for solving problems. The nurse should consider current family strengths, the family's awareness of its strengths and resources, potential untapped strengths and resources, methods of assisting the family to develop and use its strengths, and the family's awareness of its strengths and resources after nursing intervention. By being aware of existing and potential strengths, the nurse can encourage the family to capitalize on them in problem situations.

Client Family _____ Date of Assessment _____

Family Functions	Observed Behavior	Assessed Need Level (I-IV)	Suggested Nursing Responses
I. Management Function A. Use of power for all family members			
B. Rule making clear, accepted			
C. Fiscal support adequate			
D. Successful negotiations with extrafamilial systems			
E. Future planing present			
II. Boundary Function A. Clear individual boundaries			
B. Clear generational boundaries			
C. Clear family boundaries			
III. Communication Function A. Straight messages			
B. No manipulation			
C. Expression of positive and negative feelings safely			
IV. Emotional-Supportive Function A. Mutual positive regard			
B. Deals with conflict			
C. Uses resources for all family members			
D. Allows growth for all family members			
V. Socialization Function A. Children growing and developing in a healthy pattern			
B. Mutual negotiation of roles by age and ability			
C. Parents feeling good about parenting			
D. Spouses happy with each other's role behavior			

Need Levels

Level I: Current needs being met; no behaviors likely to lead to future problems.

Level II: Behaviors likely to lead to future problems; some needs recognized by nurse but not by client.

Level III: Current needs not being met.

Level IV: Unmet needs threaten survival.

Nursing Responses

Level I: *Prospective* (anticipatory guidance)

Level II: *Educative–Facilitative* (health education, support)

Level III: *Collaborative* (mutual problem-solving, shared responsibility for health actions)

Level IV: *Protective* (intervening on behalf of family, doing for family until family can assume collaborative or higher level of responsibility for its members)

FIGURE 7-10. Family Function Checklist. (Copyright 1982, Florence B. Roberts. Printed with permission).

Assessing Family Coping

Families use a variety of coping strategies to help them confront and resolve the problems they face. Members' individual personalities, as well as cultural values, influence the selection and use of particular coping mechanisms. Most individuals learn strategies for coping with stress and crisis within the context of their families. Children observe how their parents and other family members react when faced with stress or crisis and selectively mimic those behaviors. Throughout life, people develop a repertoire of coping strategies that they draw upon in times of crisis. Depending on the nature and intensity of the problem, family members may sit down together, talk about it, and negotiate a resolution, or they may withdraw from one another. Temporary withdrawal from a family problem may be a constructive strategy in some instances, such as potentially abusive or violent family situations. Healthy families often cope by confronting family problems head on; the problem is identified, alternatives are generated, and a course of action is selected and implemented.

Our society and many of its cultural subgroups have rituals for helping families deal with certain developmental and situational crises. For example, the ritual of a funeral with its many activities is intended to help families cope with the loss of a loved one. The bat mitzvah (for girls) and the bar mitzvah (for boys) is designed to ease the transition of Jewish adolescents from childhood to adulthood.

The nurse can assess family coping strategies by asking the family members how they usually handle a problem when it arises. Is the family usually able to resolve problems satisfactorily? Does the family have a preventive approach to handling stressors, or do members usually wait until problems reach crisis proportions before seeking relief? Does the family have faith in its ability to confront and deal with problems (active problem-solving) or is their attitude one of helplessness and hopelessness?

When families are experiencing a crisis, the nurse can observe family behaviors, including role changes and interaction patterns, to assess how the family is coping with the crisis. For example, a 36-year-old husband and father of two school-age sons suddenly abandons his family. The situation results in a personal crisis for each of the family members and for the family as a whole. In this instance, the nurse should focus on the meaning of the crisis for the family and ways the family is coping. What behaviors do family members exhibit (such as crying, sleeplessness, school problems)? What role changes have occurred? How have family communication patterns and parent–child interaction been affected? What support systems are available to the family? Are they helpful? What positive steps has the family taken to resolve the crisis? For example, has the mother sought family counseling for herself and her children?

One of the most important aspects of assessing family coping involves looking at the family's use of resources during times of crisis or as a means of reducing stress. Resources may include use of emotional support systems, such as close extended-family members, or seeking assistance from community agencies. What resources are available to the family? Does the family actively seek assistance? Are they willing to accept help when it is offered? Families who make use of the resources available to them, whether emotional, financial, or social, are more likely to cope in functionally healthy ways.

Family Mapping

Structural family theorists use a technique called family mapping to assess certain family characteristics. The family map demonstrates the spatial and organizational relationships of family members. Distant relationships between a mother and father can be shown on a family map, as can erosion of natural subsystems when a selected child is given a position in the parental subsystem that rightfully belongs to a mother or father. Family mapping is an assessment tool that organizes information into a working hypothesis of positions, subgroups, and alliances within a family system. Its usefulness is illustrated in the clinical example depicted in the boxed insert.

Integrated Family Systems Assessment

An integrated family systems assessment (see Table 7-5) uses concepts from the various theoretical approaches presented in this chapter and looks at the family as an interdependent system. Since no single theoretical approach is adequate for assessing a family, an integrated or eclectic approach is preferable. In this way a family can be assessed from several vantage points. The focus of the nurse is expanded to include elements that might otherwise be overlooked. Assessment questions are included to guide the observations of the nurse and obtain relevant information.

NURSING DIAGNOSES RELATED TO FAMILY

Information from the family assessment should be analyzed to identify actual or potential nursing diagnoses related to family functioning. Problems

Family Mapping: A Case Example

Rosalie was a teenage mother who chose not to marry the father of her child. Because Rosalie wanted to finish high school, she lived at home and relinquished the care of her baby to her mother. Rosalie was a good student who was eager to return to school and to resume some of the social activities she had enjoyed before the birth of the baby. At the same time she was dismayed to find that her mother took full charge of the infant, making all decisions and indicating to Rosalie that the girl was incapable of taking proper care of the baby. Rosalie had expected that having a baby would make her more mature and independent. Instead she discovered that both she and her baby were being treated as children. The conflict between Rosalie and her mother over the baby became evident to the nurse in charge of the well baby clinic where the health of the infant was supervised. Aware of the struggle, the nurse began to deal with Rosalie's mixed feelings about motherhood and with the reluctance of the older woman to accept her proper place as grandmother and relate to Rosalie as the baby's mother.

When Rosalie brought the baby to the clinic, the nurse tried to reinforce her confidence in handling the baby. At the same time the nurse acknowledged the contribution that Rosalie's own mother was making. Because the grandmother had moved into the position of mother to her granddaughter as well as to Rosalie, positions in the family were confused. Generational boundaries were unclear because the grandmother related to the baby in a way that excluded Rosalie, who needed help in order to finish high school but resented the price her mother exacted. It became the objective of the clinic nurse to define responsibilities in the family in order to reduce conflict. In attempting this the nurse supported the contributions of the grandmother as teacher and adviser for Rosalie. The nurse also encouraged Rosalie to perform mothering tasks while seeking guidance and support from her mother. The nurse's interventions produced some structural changes in the family that are illustrated in the accompanying family maps.

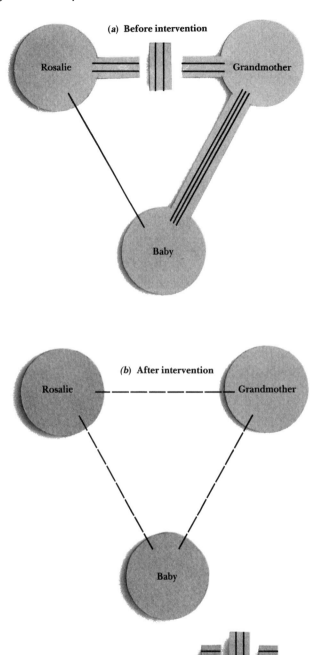

Note. From Davies/Janosik: *Mental Health and Psychiatric Nursing: A Caring Approach,* © 1991. Boston: Jones and Bartlett Publishers, p. 528.

TABLE 7-5
Integrated Family Systems Assessment

Contributing Theory	Focus	Assessment Questions
1. Family Development	Tasks and Transitions	What is the family's life cycle stage? What are family members' life cycle tasks at this time?
2. Family Structure	Positions and Boundaries	What subgroups, alliances, and coalitions exist in the family? Are family positions based on natural boundaries and differences?
3. Family Function	Roles and Behaviors	What roles are present in the family? How are roles assigned and enacted? Does family role enactment limit or exploit any member? Which family member has the most to gain or lose by changed behaviors and role enactment?
4. Family Roles & Relationships	Individuation, Interdependence, Attachment, Separation	Do family attachments permit members' individuation and growth? Is separation encouraged, tolerated, or thwarted? What attributes of members are highly valued in the family? Conformity? Creativity? Self-expression? What is the prevailing emotional climate in the family? Who is the most powerful family member? Who is the least powerful family member?
5. Family Communication	Verbal Messages Nonverbal Messages	Are verbal messages direct and specific? What nonverbal messages are sent? Are verbal and nonverbal messages congruent? Is there a family spokesperson? Whose messages are unheard or disregarded?
6. Family Learning	Stimulus and Response Conditioning Rewards	What functional behaviors are rewarded in the family? What dysfunctional behaviors are rewarded in the family?

may affect family development, interaction, or coping.

Selected nursing diagnoses related to family functioning are listed in Table 7-6. These nursing diagnoses are categorized in the North American Nursing Diagnosis Association (NANDA) Taxonomy I (1990) under the human response patterns of "relating" or "choosing." However, the definitions and defining characteristics for most of these diagnoses reflect a focus on the individual client or individual family member, rather than the family unit or system. For example, the diagnosis "ineffective family coping: compromised" is defined as the lack of support by a family member or primary

support person needed by the client to adapt effectively to a particular health problem. However, since the entire family system is affected by a change in one of its family members, as with acute or chronic illness, this diagnosis may be applied appropriately to the entire family system.

The nursing diagnosis "family coping: potential for growth" may be indicated for families that demonstrate healthy development and functioning and are able to support the maturational and health-promoting behaviors of their members. Such families usually require minimal nursing intervention, with the exception of guidance and support.

"Altered family processes" is a diagnostic label that can be used to identify disrupted family functioning, whether temporary or long-standing. Families who are unable to meet their members' needs, who demonstrate ineffective or inappropriate interaction patterns, or who resist role changes as the family moves from one developmental stage to another may warrant this diagnosis.

When a family is unable to meet the basic needs of its members or responds in ways that are detrimental to its members, the nursing diagnosis of "ineffective family coping: disabling" may be indicated. This diagnosis may result from such factors as unresolved hostility or guilt, extreme defensiveness, or highly ambivalent family relationships.

When family roles change, particularly when the changes are precipitous, a family may experience "altered role performance." For example, loss of employment by the family's primary breadwinner may result in major changes in role perceptions and ability to fulfill needed family roles.

"Parental role conflict" results when a parent experiences disruption or confusion related to parental role performance, usually in response to a crisis, such as hospitalization of a child or change in parental role due to divorce or death of the spouse.

"Decisional conflict" may occur within a family when there is uncertainty about choices the family must make, such as whether to move to a new locale or seek available social services. Families who must make difficult decisions about terminating medical treatment for a dying family member may experience severe decisional conflict, particularly when there is disagreement among family members about the acceptable course of action.

Once family nursing diagnoses have been formulated, the nurse should collaborate with the family to plan a course of action for resolving the diagnoses. Because of the complex dynamics of family functioning and interaction, these diagnoses often require the nurse to sustain contact with the family over a period of weeks, months, or sometimes years in order to achieve resolution.

TABLE 7-6
Nursing Diagnoses Related to Family Functioning

Family coping: potential for growth related to stage of family development or changes in family structure or function

Altered family processes related to situational or developmental crises

Ineffective family coping: compromised related to family disorganization, developmental transitions, situational crises, or prolonged illness or disability

Ineffective family coping: disabling related to chronic guilt or anxiety, highly ambivalent family relationships, or family defensiveness

Altered role performance related to change in family role responsibilities or inability to assume responsibilities associated with new family roles (e.g., parenthood)

Parental role conflict related to prolonged hospitalization of child, or divorce from or death of spouse

Decisional conflict related to multiple or different sources of information, threat to family value system, or lack of social support

Chapter Highlights

- The family is the primary social group that transmits the values and expectations of the family's cultural group and society to its members.

- Families are active, responsive systems operating within the larger social order. As individual and societal needs change, so do the structures and functions of families.

- Today's families reflect many diverse constellations, including biological, adoptive, foster, nuclear, single-parent, step-parent, and extended families.

- Several theoretical approaches are used to explain family dynamics, including theories of family development, family systems, family structure and function, family communication, family roles, and family power. Each of these approaches provides a different perspective for viewing families.

- Every family responds to stress and crisis, including health problems, in its own way, exhibiting different strengths and weaknesses and its unique coping strategies.

- Because individual and family health influence each other, clients should be assessed within the context of their family system.

- Interviewing and observation are the primary ways the nurse collects information about family structure, communication patterns, roles, decision making, stressors, and coping.

- Occasionally, a specially designed tool for assessing family development or functioning is warranted to augment the information obtained through interview and observation.

■ Information from the family assessment should be analyzed to identify actual or potential nursing diagnoses related to family functioning.

Practice Activities

1. Compare and contrast the various theoretical approaches to family assessment. What are the advantages and disadvantages of each approach? Which do you prefer? Why?

2. Using the guidelines for assessing family culture presented in Table 7-2, assess two families from different cultural groups. Record your findings. What conclusions can you draw?

3. Using Table 7-3 as a guide, assess at least one family. Record your findings. What conclusions can you draw? What nursing diagnoses are suggested?

4. Assess at least one family using the Family APGAR (Figure 7-9) or the Family Function Checklist (Figure 7-10). What conclusions can you draw? What nursing responses are indicated?

5. Using Otto's framework for assessing family strengths, assess at least one family system. What strengths does the family possess? To what extent is the family able to identify its strengths? What strategies can be employed to help the family develop and use its strengths?

6. Using the family mapping example, identify potential nursing diagnoses. Develop a plan of care related to each nursing diagnosis.

Recommended Readings

Beutler, I.F., Burr, W.R., & Bahr, K.S. (1989). The family realm: Theoretical contributions for understanding its uniqueness. *Journal of Marriage and the Family, 51*(3), 805–815.

Dubowitz, H., Newberger, C.M., Melnicoe, L.H., & Newberger, E.H. (1988). The changing American family. *Pediatric Clinics of North America, 35,* 1291–1311.

Friedman, M.M. (1990). Transcultural family nursing: Application to Latino and Black families. *Journal of Pediatric Nursing, 5*(3), 214–222.

Fsife, B.L. (1985). A model for predicting the adaptation of families to a medical crisis: An analysis of role integration. *Image: Journal of Nursing Scholarship, 17,* 108–112.

Mancini, J.A., & Orthner, D.K. (1988). The context and consequences of family change. *Family Relations, 37*(4), 363–366.

McLanahan, S., & Booth, K. (1989). Mother-only families: Problems, prospects, and politics. *Journal of Marriage and the Family, 51*(3), 557–580.

Speer, J., & Sachs, B. (1985). Selecting the appropriate family assessment tool. *Pediatric Nursing, 11,* 349–355.

Staples, R. (1985). Changes in Black family structure: The conflict between family ideology and structural conditions. *Journal of Marriage and the Family, 47,* 1005–1013.

Sund, K., & Ostwald, S.K. (1985). Dual-earner families' stress levels and personal and lifestyle-related variables. *Nursing Research, 34,* 357–361.

Tschann, J., Johnston, J.R., Kline, M., & Wallerstein, J.S. (1990). Family process and children's functioning during divorce. *Journal of Marriage and the Family, 51,* 431–444.

Weinberg, T.S. (1985). Single fatherhood: How is it different? *Pediatric Nursing, 11,* 173–175.

References

Astrachan, A. (1986). *How men feel: Their response to women's demands for independence, equality, and power.* New York: Anchor/Doubleday.

Bowen, M. (1971). The use of family therapy in clinical practice. In J. Haley (Ed.), *Changing families,* (pp. 159–192). New York: Grune & Stratton.

Bowen, M. (1974). Toward the differentiation of self in one's family of origin. In F. Andres & J. Loria (Eds.), *Georgetown family symposia: Collection of selected papers,* (pp. 77–102). Washington, DC: Georgetown University Press.

Bowen, M. (1976). Theory in the practice of psychotherapy. In P. Guerin (Ed.), *Family therapy,* (pp. 42–90). New York: Gardner.

Carter, E.A., & McGoldrick, M. (1980). *The family life cycle.* New York: Gardner.

Davies, J.L. & Janosik, E.H. (1990). *Mental health and psychiatric nursing: A caring approach.* Boston: Jones & Bartlett.

Duvall, E.M. (1977). *Marriage and family development.* Philadelphia: Lippincott.

Erikson, E.H. (1963). *Childhood and society.* New York: Norton.

Feetham, S.L. & Humenick, S.S. (1982). The Feetham Family Functioning Survey. In S.S. Humenick (Ed.), *Analysis of current assessment strategies in the health care of young children and childbearing families* (pp. 259–268). Norwalk, CT: Appleton-Century-Crofts.

Frazer, A. (1985). *The weaker vessel.* New York: Random/Vintage.

Friedman, M.M. (1986). *Family nursing: Theory and assessment* (2nd ed.). Norwalk, CT: Appleton-Century-Crofts.

Friedman, M.M. (1990). Transcultural family nursing:

Application to Latino and Black families. *Journal of Pediatric Nursing, 5*(3), 214–222.

Hoopes, M.M., & Harper, J.H. (1987). *Birth order, roles, and sibling patterns in individual and family therapy.* Rockville, MD: Aspen.

Hymovich, D.P., & Chamberlin, R. (1980). *Child and family development.* New York: McGraw-Hill.

Lewin, T. (1990, September 21). Suit over death benefits asks, What is a family? *The New York Times,* p. B7.

Lewis, J.M., Beavers, W.R., Gossett, J.T., & Phillips, V.A. (1976). *No single thread.* New York: Brunner/Mazel.

Minuchin, S. (1974). *Families and family therapy.* Cambridge, MA: Harvard University Press.

Minuchin, S. (1986). Beyond benign neglect. *Journal of Review and Commentary on Mental Health, 1*(4), 6–10.

Neuman, B. (1983). Family intervention using the Betty Neuman health care systems model. In I.W. Clements & F.B. Roberts (Eds.), *Family health: A theoretical approach to nursing care* (pp. 239–254). New York: Wiley Medical.

Otto, H. (1973). A framework for assessing family strengths. In A. Reinhardt & M. Quinn (Eds.), *Family-centered community nursing* (pp. 87–93). St. Louis: Mosby.

Pless, I.B., & Satterwhite, B. (1973). A measure of family functioning and its application. *Social Science and Medicine, 7,* 613–621.

Powers, K.A. (1986). Communities in crisis: Disasters and unemployment. In E.H. Janosik (Ed.), *Crisis counseling: A contemporary approach.* Boston: Jones & Bartlett.

Roberts, C.S., & Feetham, S.L. (1982). Assessing family functioning across three areas of relationships. *Nursing Research, 31*(4), 231–235.

Roberts, F.B. (1983). In I.W. Clements & F.B. Roberts (Eds.), *Family health: A theoretical approach to nursing care* (pp. 189–204). New York: Wiley Medical.

Smilkstein, G. (1978). The family APGAR: A proposal for a family function test and its use by physicians. *The Journal of Family Practice, 6*(6), 1231–1240.

Toman, W. (1976). *Family constellation.* New York: Basic.

8

Cultural Assessment

CHAPTER OUTLINE

- The Nature of Culture
  Culture Is Learned   Culture Is Shared
  Culture Is Integrated   Culture Contains
  Both Ideal and Real Components   What
  Culture Is Not
- The Importance of Cultural Variables in
  Nursing Assessment
  Ethnocentrism and Cultural Relativity
- Values, Beliefs, and Customs
  Values   Beliefs   Customs
- Cultural Assessment and Nursing Diagnosis

OBJECTIVES

Upon completion of this chapter, you should be
able to:

- Explain the concept of culture.
- Describe why cultural factors are an essential
  part of the nursing assessment.
- Differentiate the concepts of ethnocentrism
  and cultural relativity.
- Compare and contrast values of selected cultural groups.
- Discuss ethnic variations in communication
  patterns, dietary habits, kinship systems, religious practices, and illness behaviors.
- Assess clients' cultural beliefs and behaviors.
- Explain the relationship between cultural variables and nursing diagnoses.

Sensitivity to cultural variables is a requisite for accurate nursing assessment in multi-ethnic situations. In all nursing settings the potential for misunderstanding is accentuated when the health provider and client are from different ethnic or cultural groups. These misunderstandings most often arise from nurse–client differences in values, beliefs, and customs. Knowledge of the nature of culture is crucial in understanding these variables, including the ways in which cultural groups vary in their values, beliefs, customs, and behaviors (see Figure 8-1).

THE NATURE OF CULTURE

Culture is the total lifeways of a human group. It consists of learned patterns of values, beliefs, customs, and behaviors that are shared by a group of interacting individuals. More than unique material objects, culture is a set of rules or standards for behavior. Knowledge of certain characteristics of culture facilitates the nurse's understanding of cultural influences on clients' behaviors.

Culture Is Learned

Culture is not transmitted biologically; it does not rely on genetic inheritance. Although all humans have basic biological needs (such as nutrients, reproduction, safety, and health), they respond to these biological needs in culturally prescribed ways. For example, every individual has a biological need for sleep, but culture determines the patterns of behavioral responses to this need, including the place, facilities, and with whom one sleeps.

Culture is acquired by experience. The process whereby culture is transmitted from one generation to the next is called *enculturation*. It may be acquired formally through education, or it may be learned informally by observing the behaviors of various individuals within the culture. By watch-

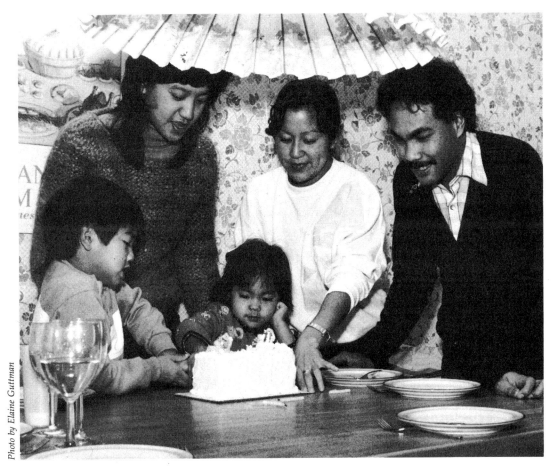

Photo by Elaine Guttman

FIGURE 8-1. By knowing the scope of cultural variations, nurses are able to provide more culturally sensitive approaches to health care. (*Note*. From Servonsky/Opas: *Nursing Management of Children*, © 1987. Boston: Jones and Bartlett Publishers, p. 70.)

ing different people, modeling their behavior, and noting the reactions of others to this behavior, we learn what is appropriate and acceptable. We also learn that patterns of appropriateness depend on a number of factors, including one's age and sex. For example, behaviors that are tolerated or even promoted in young children, such as public nudity or sleeping in church, typically are not acceptable for adults. Similarly, cultures differentiate masculine from feminine behaviors.

Culture Is Shared

By sharing a common culture, members of a group can predict one another's actions and react accordingly, although individual behavior is not necessarily representative of the culture. Culture defines dominant patterns of values, attitudes, beliefs, and behaviors, but does not determine all the behaviors in any group. Variation from the dominant culture always occurs. A variation that is exhibited by a single person is called *individualism*. Depending on how the group interprets individualistic behavior, the person may be labeled eccentric or deviant. However, when a whole group of individuals within a society has shared values, beliefs, and behaviors different from those of the dominant society, that group is referred to as a *subculture* or *ethnic group*.

Simply exhibiting the same characteristics does not make a group a cultural group, however. A frequently misunderstood issue is what exactly constitutes a cultural group. Currently there is a tendency to see cultural groups in more places than they rightly belong. A class of people does not share a culture simply because they have some common characteristics. Culture connotes shared beliefs, norms, values, and patterns of behavior that are learned through socialization.

For example, some have promoted the idea that the elderly population in the United States constitutes a subculture. This is an inappropriate application of the term, based on the erroneous practice of observing life patterns, such as living on fixed incomes, that only superficially indicate homogeneity. These characteristics are not representative of an aged subculture; they are merely features dictated by such specific life circumstances as mandatory retirement laws and declining physical integrity. Similarly, a socioeconomic class, such as those living below the poverty level, is not a cultural group.

Culture Is Universal

Because cultures must fulfill certain common functions, they resemble one another in basic domains.

Universal aspects of culture include patterns of communication, kinship, education, diet, religion, art, politics, economics, and health. Because these categories are so closely interrelated, it is difficult to study only one aspect of culture. The tendency for all aspects of a culture to function as an interrelated whole is called *integration*.

Culture Contains Both Ideal and Real Components

Every society has ideal cultural patterns that represent what most members of the society say they ought to do in a particular situation. Such ideal patterns, or norms, may be enforced through legal or social means. For example, there are laws governing marriage and divorce, and there are social norms that prescribe how an individual should act toward the elderly. However, real behavior may differ from either of these types of norms and still be acceptable. There often is a gap between ideal and real patterns of behavior.

What Culture Is Not

Cultural features do not refer to racial or biological characteristics. Cultural affiliation differs from race, although both are important parameters to assess. Remember that culture concerns shared values, beliefs, and patterns of behavior of a group of people. Racial identity has to do with biophysiologic differences among population groups. Race refers to biologically inherited characteristics that are transmitted genetically and may be observed in such physical traits as skin color, blood groups, and hair texture.

Cultures are not immutable. Although cultures are integrated, they are not static. Cultures are dynamic entities. However, all aspects of a culture do not change at the same time. Changes in technology or in economic systems often precede changes in family relationships or political organization. For example, the shift from an agrarian to an industrial economy brought about major changes in American culture and its subgroups. As American society has become more industrialized and mobile, the importance of the extended family has diminished, with increased reliance of individuals on a relatively small nucleus of immediate family members and friends.

Cultural characteristics are not changed easily. Although some cultural habits and behaviors are malleable, other characteristics, such as values, are acquired early and are much more stable. Culture is not concerned simply with matters of individual preference but is ingrained in an individual. Consequently, cultural characteristics may be difficult to alter.

Cultures are not deterministic; they do not automatically determine individual values, beliefs, or behaviors. Individuals within all groups may differ in their values, beliefs, or behaviors. Thus, it is essential not to prejudge or form stereotypes of individuals on the basis of their cultural affiliations. All individuals from one culture are not the same. In the United States there is a dominant core value that advocates equality. However, from it arose the "melting pot" myth that declares all Americans have a common culture. This misguided notion precludes sensitive understanding of individuals' cultures and subcultures.

Culture is not something that belongs only to others. Individuals tend to view their own behaviors as being objective and correct, so many people harbor the misconception that only other people are culturally different. Because culture is so deeply embedded, it is difficult to ascertain its influence on values, attitudes, and behavior. It is critical that nurses remember that all people, including themselves, are the products of their own culture and, therefore, influenced by it.

THE IMPORTANCE OF CULTURAL VARIABLES IN NURSING ASSESSMENT

Health care involves contact between two or more individuals: provider and client. Each comes to an encounter with preconceived notions that include attitudes, beliefs, and expectations for patterns of behavior. The health-care situation can, therefore, be approached from two perspectives: that of the provider and that of the recipient.

Because the United States is a pluralistic society, nurses in most clinical settings work with clients from a number of different cultural groups. Because values, beliefs, and customs directly influence health, nurses must understand the cultures of the clients for whom they provide care. Consideration of cultural factors decreases misunderstandings and frustrations between the nurse and the client and increases the client's satisfaction and acceptance of health-care recommendations.

Nursing's claim of concern for the total person mandates inclusion of the cultural dimension. As Clark (1978) points out:

> Ignorance of cultural differences can indeed pose serious problems in diagnosis and treatment, for without such knowledge we will alienate the individual and run the risk of making recommendations which will be ignored. Only if the cultural dimensions are considered, can we claim that we are practicing holistic or comprehensive health care. (p. vii)

To be accepted, health care must be provided in ways that the client considers appropriate and acceptable. Nurses who understand specific factors that influence the behaviors of a particular cultural group are in a better position to meet the needs of people from that group. Considering cultural variables enhances a nurse's understanding of a client's behavior and the client's perception of the nurse and leads to a more realistic treatment plan and mutually respectful nurse–client relationship.

Cultural anthropology suggests cues to look for when collecting assessment information. The definitions of health and illness, the range of available choices, and the selection of health practitioners are variables determined largely by cultural factors. The more that is known about a client and the client's culture, the more accurately the nurse can assess the influence of these variables on the client's health and behavior. A culturally aware nurse can anticipate variations in clients' dietary practices, their responses to authority, and beliefs about what causes illness and how it should be treated. Thus, the nurse may anticipate what will be acceptable or unacceptable to a particular client, including alternative sources of health care in the client's own culture.

Finally, by understanding cultural factors, nurses may realize that their own values and preconceptions can impede their effectiveness. They, in turn, may come to more completely understand themselves and their relationships with colleagues. Culture is not something that only other people have.

However, a caution is in order. The nurse should remember that cultural affiliation may provide clues to assessment, but only as a background variable. Each client should be approached as a unique individual. It is essential not to overgeneralize or stereotype individuals according to their cultural or ethnic affiliations. Each ethnic group has members who are more or less acculturated to the dominant society. Rates of acculturation differ among individuals in a variety of ways. The degree to which any one individual in a subculture adheres to the traditional culture depends on a number of factors, including age, sex, education, and generation. For example, Tripp-Reimer (1983) found that among four generations of Greek immigrants in an Ohio city, the group's ethnicity remained culturally distinct even though it was politically, economically, and geographically integrated into the larger metropolitan community. However, the retention of specific cultural traits varied dramatically by generation. Even though some cultural traits (religion, food, language) remained strong, there was a wider variation in the retention of folk medicine and folk-healing practices. In the first generation virtually all community members both knew and used a practice known as "the evil eye." However, among members of the fourth generation, only half knew of this tradition and none used it. This study illustrates the importance of not assuming that traditional behaviors will be retained by individuals with strong ethnic affiliations.

Ethnocentrism and Cultural Relativity

Ethnocentrism and cultural relativity denote the perspectives from which cultural characteristics are interpreted. For example, an ethnocentric nurse judges the behaviors of clients of a different culture with the standards of the nurse's own culture. A nurse who understands cultural relativity attempts to place the behavior of culturally different clients within the context of the clients' own cultures.

Ethnocentrism flows logically from the process of early acculturation and characterizes the way many individuals feel about their own culture, whether they verbalize their feelings or not. Saunders (1954) notes that ethnocentrism generally is understood as "the universal tendency of human beings to think that their ways of thinking, acting, and believing are the only right, proper, and natural ones, and to regard the beliefs and practices of other people, particularly if they differ greatly, as strange, bizarre or unenlightened" (p. 237).

On the other hand, a perspective of cultural relativity holds that judgments are based on experience, and experience is interpreted by individuals in terms of their own acculturation. Thus, nurses are culturally biased observers, influenced by the perspectives of their own ethnic or social culture, and the subcultures of nursing and health care. By using a relativist perspective, however, nurses try to accept or understand the behaviors of culturally different clients in their own contexts.

Sometimes stereotyping is done unconsciously, simply because nurses interpret clients' behaviors with their own value systems. For example, the Appalachian poor tend to have large families (Tripp-Reimer, 1982). A nurse from another culture who sees this as a negative characteristic might say, "They do it just to get more welfare" or "They're uneducated—you can't teach them about birth control." In this case, the nurse is judging Appalachians from the perspective of his or her own culture. On the other hand, a nurse who is familiar with the values of the Appalachian poor is more likely to understand the cultural reasons for large families and might say, "Appalachians value their children as the most important part of their lives" or "Having many children offers security for the future" (in a group that generally is without retirement programs). This example illustrates the difference between culturally relativistic and ethnocentric perspectives. Nurses must be careful to interpret a client's behavior in the context of the client's culture.

As health-care professionals, nurses need to be careful not to stereotype individuals on any basis. Nursing care must be personalized and individualized. By knowing the scope of cultural variations, nurses can provide approaches to health care that are culturally sensitive. However, if cultural plurality is seen as a menu, accurate assessment of a culturally different individual will be unlikely. This approach is sometimes evidenced in lists of "characteristics" of African-Americans, Mexican-Americans, native Americans, Asians, and others. Cultural information is presented as if cultural traits are held uniformly and are static. The underlying assumption is that if only the "right" formula were known, then appropriate nursing interventions could be planned. But the cultural background of the client should be used only to provide contextual cues to the nurse. Given these cultural cues, the nurse can conduct an individualized assessment and establish a personalized nursing care plan.

VALUES, BELIEFS, AND CUSTOMS

Anthropologists often see culture as being stratified, or having layers, as illustrated in Figure 8-2. The uppermost tier consists of customs. This layer is easiest to describe because it can be identified through overt behaviors. The middle layer is beliefs. The bottom tier, representing values, is the least apparent and the most difficult to assess.

Values, beliefs, and customs are mechanisms for ordering human experience and behavior. Through them, group members share orientations to life situations.

Values

Cultural values give meaning and direction to life. Values are at the bottom of Figure 8-2 because they are the foundation for beliefs, attitudes, and behaviors. Values are acquired early in childhood during the socialization process. Because this is largely an unconscious process, individuals generally are unaware that they are either teaching or learning values. Because of this abstract and basic

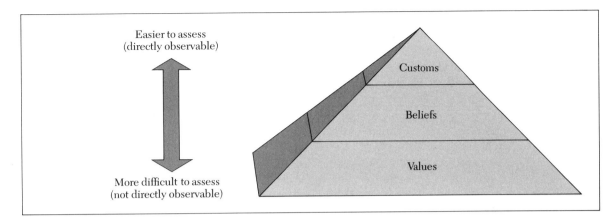

FIGURE 8-2 Cultural Strata.

quality, values are at once difficult to assess and to alter.

A culture's value system includes goals that individuals should pursue and indicates the ways in which people should behave. Values tell individuals internally what they ought to do in certain situations, such as respecting authority, or contributing to family and society by holding a productive job.

Values are not just preferences but also formulations of what is desirable. They guide actions by framing an individual's perspective, by establishing a hierarchy of needs and goals, and by limiting alternatives. Because values generally are deeply ingrained, individuals often respond to situations without being aware that values are guiding their choice of actions, and their presence generally can be inferred only through analysis of behavior.

Cultural Variations in Values

A variety of approaches has been used to compare the values of different cultural groups. One of the most common approaches is to simply describe the dominant values of a specific group. For example, Noshpitz (1979) studied the values of Jewish Americans. He reported that Jewish childrearing practices strongly emphasize dependency rather than autonomy. He also found that the culture demands literacy and that the religion is especially geared to complex cognitive forms. Noshpitz concluded, then, that two major vocational ideals (to be a great scholar or a business person) were dominant values incorporated early in the ideal ego formation for a Jewish child.

A second basic approach is to contrast several dimensions of the value systems of two or more groups. Table 8-1, an example of this approach, compares dominant native American and Anglo-American values.

A third approach to cultural values is to compare a few dimensions of several cultures. The classic method of approaching value systems in this way was developed by Kluckhohn and Strodtbeck (1961) and concerns dominant and variant value orientations. They developed a pattern of domi-

TABLE 8-1
Comparison of Native American and
Anglo-American Values

Native American Values	Anglo-American Values
1. Respect for elders	1. Premium on youth and young adulthood
2. Reticence	2. Openness and verbosity
3. Humility	3. Competitiveness
4. Giving and sharing	4. Thriftiness and property acquisition
5. Giving human characteristics to animals and nature	5. Scientific objectivity
6. Strong spiritual beliefs	6. Rationalistic attitudes
7. Individual is responsible for group	7. Individual responsible for self
8. Group decisions by consensus; internal conflict resolved or action not taken	8. Group decisions by majority; internal conflict continues and may provide new direction
9. Appeal to tradition as final authority (supported by spiritual beliefs)	9. Appeal to power as final authority (supported by pragmatism, efficiency, and sometimes abstract ideals)
10. Inborn characteristics unchangeable	10. Malleability and changeability of humans (especially children)

nant value orientations that presents the various ways a social group may choose to perceive and structure certain human problems. These authors note that although in all cultures some members will hold value orientations that vary from those of the rest of their group, there are dominant value orientations that can be identified for each cultural group. Kluckhohn and Strodtbeck organized various problems with which all societies must cope. Specifically, they considered the way humans organize their thinking about time, personal activity, interpersonal relations, and the relationship of the individual to nature.

Time Orientation. Time, or temporal orientation, may be broken into three point ranges: past, present, and future. All societies must deal in all three, but they differ in their emphasis. For example, some cultural groups, such as Anglo-Americans, value the future more than the past. Other cultural groups, including southern blacks, Mexican-Americans, Appalachians, native Americans, and Puerto Ricans, are present-oriented. Asian cultures tend to value the past.

Activity Orientation. Activity orientation identifies whether a given culture is oriented primarily toward doing (achievement) or being. Anglo-Americans have been characterized as achievement-oriented. People are valued for their accomplishments, not for their inherent existence. In societies with a being orientation, such as native Americans, Mexican-Americans, and Asians, people are valued for their existence, not for their accomplishments. The being pattern is typical of lineage societies in which a person is valued as a link in a chain of continuity between generations.

Relational Orientation. This orientation distinguishes among interpersonal patterns and is concerned with how the society sets goals for its individual members. Goal-setting is described as collateral, lineal, or individualistic.

When the collateral principle is dominant, primary importance is ascribed to the goals and welfare of the laterally extended group, such as siblings or members of the same age set. Collectivist societies such as the Soviet Union and Israel typically demonstrate a collateral orientation. In these societies the goals of the individual are subordinated to the goals of the group, and the group maintains responsibility for all its members.

When the lineal mode is dominant, group goals and group welfare have primary importance. With lineal orientation, however, one of the important goals is continuity through time. Continuity of the group and line of succession for positions within the group are crucial issues. Kinship is the basis for nearly all societies with an emphasis on lineality. Most often, the group traces its descent through the male line, with authority resting with the eldest male. In China before the Maoist revolution, lineage was the primary mechanism of social structure. Lineality fulfills the functions of education, economic production, discipline, religion, and social programs (caring for the destitute, old, and infirm). In this kind of society, filial piety is more important than spousal relationships or individualism.

When an individualistic principle is dominant, individual goals have primacy over the goals of specific collateral or lineal groups. Each person's responsibility to and place within the total society are defined by autonomous goals. The United States, like most other developed Western cultures, emphasizes the individual. People are held individually responsible for their behavior and are judged on the basis of their work. Religion is largely a personal matter (rather than a structured group experience), and work is not closely tied to the individual's extended family.

Orientation to Nature. The orientation of the individual to nature focuses on whether the individual dominates nature, lives in harmony with nature, or is subjugated to nature.

The United States contains diverse ethnic populations and, therefore, exhibits greater heterogeneity than most other Western cultures. Because it is ethnically diverse, the United States does not exhibit a uniform dominant value system. Although a dominant value system can be identified for middle class Americans of European descent, members of American subcultural groups may have dominant value orientations that vary considerably from those of mainstream America.

Typically, Anglo-Americans exhibit a dominant orientation to nature as evidenced by attempts to predict and control natural events. Native Americans and Asians emphasize the need to achieve harmony with nature, whereas southern blacks, Appalachians, and Mexican-Americans tend to perceive themselves as subjugated to nature.

Relationship of Values to Health Care

Health behaviors generally are consistent with cultural values. To illustrate this point, consider the influence of two different value orientations on health behaviors.

The white, middle class American approaches time from a future orientation. An example of future orientation is the practice of deferring gratification and emphasizing the importance of extended education. In regard to health, middle class Americans tend to emphasize promoting health and preventing illness. In addition, they tend to structure time rigidly. On the other hand, cultural groups that are present-oriented often exhibit a crisis orientation rather than a preventive approach to health.

In their relational orientation values, middle class Americans tend to be individualistic. They stress individual fulfillment and personal achievement. Individuals set their own goals, make their own choices in seeking health care, and personally decide whether to follow a prescribed program. In contrast, among Southeast Asians, the lineal mode is dominant. The family is the unit of primary importance and the individual is subordinate to it. The crux of family loyalty is filial piety, which teaches children to honor their parents. The importance of lineal orientation can be seen in the health setting when one family member escorts another to a clinic, physician's office, or hospital. In many cases it is the relatives who must be convinced that the person should accept treatment. In addition, family members may expect to stay with the client throughout a course of treatment or hospitalization.

A related area has to do with ideas or values promoting family responsibility versus individualism. This is an important consideration in the dependency that may accompany serious or chronic illnesses. If the group values autonomy, then the dependency that can accompany illness may contribute to a client's anxiety. However, when there is more of an emphasis on family orientation, as among southern blacks or the Amish, then dependency is more acceptable. In family-oriented groups, relatives often assume responsibility for caring for an ill person in the home, even at considerable personal cost and inconvenience.

Assessing Values

Because they are generally held at an unconscious level, values are not directly observable but must be inferred from behavior. It is often difficult to verbalize values, and people seldom are aware that values are directly influencing their behavior.

Because nurses rarely need to assess a client's values directly, no assessment tools are presented here. However, a number of excellent sources are available for this purpose (Sue, 1981; Pederson, Lonner & Draguns, 1976).

Nurses, however, should recognize that their own values are important factors in transcultural understanding. Nurses need to seriously consider their own values as they relate to the nursing care they deliver. Specifically, values held by nurses may influence health care in the following ways. Values

- help determine how individuals define their health problems,

- are instrumental in establishing priorities of health problems,

- help determine what actions individuals take in response to their perceived health problems, and

- influence the criteria individuals use to determine whether they have achieved their health goals.

Nurses who wish to evaluate their personal values may refer to those sources cited above and, additionally, Bonaparte (1979) and Ruiz (1981).

Beliefs

Beliefs include knowledge, opinions, and faith about various aspects of the world. This section focuses on beliefs related to illness.

Defining Illness

How one defines illness is part of one's belief system and largely is determined by one's culture. The distinctions between the concepts of disease and illness are becoming more clearly defined. Diseases are abnormalities in the structure and function of body organs and systems and thus are a problem of biological malfunctioning. Illness, on the other hand, encompasses the subjective experiences of the individual who is sick, including the way in which the illness is perceived and experienced by the individual and the social group.

Whether people consider themselves well or ill is largely a matter of cultural definition. A person with obvious or detectable pathology may not come to the attention of a scientific health-care professional for three major reasons: the condition may be

- ignored,
- undetected, or
- attributed to nonscientific causes.

Many chronic illnesses such as hypertension, diabetes, and renal or respiratory problems may not have symptoms that are readily identifiable by nonprofessionals. These "hidden" diseases are detectable only by laboratory tests or with such specialized equipment as sphygmomanometers, x-rays, or bronchoscopes. Often, especially among groups that do not emphasize prevention, illnesses are not identified because they are not detected. For instance, among low income Appalachians, unless the individual loses the capacity to function in activities of daily living, traditional health care generally is not sought (Hansen & Resick, 1990).

Illnesses that are attributed to nonscientific causes generally are termed *folk illnesses*. If a group identifies a condition as a folk illness, members may not seek professional health care because it is considered inappropriate. Professionals are not considered knowledgeable about the treatment of folk illnesses. In such instances, assistance is sought from a folk practitioner. For convenience, folk conditions may be divided into two major categories: naturalistic and personalistic illnesses.

Naturalistic illnesses are caused by impersonal factors, entities with no regard for the individual. Generally, naturalistic illnesses are based on equilibrium. When the balance is disturbed, illness results. Examples of equilibrium theories are common throughout the world. Two of the most prevalent are the yin and yang of the Chinese and the hot/cold model of Mexican-Americans.

Among most traditional Chinese, health is based on the balance of yin and yang forces. Yin forces are characterized as cold, weak, female, and small. Yang forces are characterized as hot, strong, male, and large. An excessive biological or psychological state—childbirth or adolescent "acting-out" behavior—is a yang illness. A deficiency, such as tuberculosis or the Koro syndrome (male fears his penis will shrivel, indicating he is losing too much yang), results in a yin illness. Treatment for yin and yang conditions is based on the "principle of opposition." Yin illnesses are treated by yang foods, medications, or techniques. Yang illnesses, on the other hand, are treated by yin foods, medications, and techniques. Examples of cold or yin treatments are acupuncture, herbal teas, and vegetables. One example of hot or yang treatments is moxibustion: An incense cone is placed on the skin, usually the wrist or head, and burned. Foods that are spicy or high in protein or fat content also are yang treatments.

The application of these treatments can be seen in an example from a clinical setting. Many Southeast Asians traditionally believe that during childbirth the mother dissipates considerable heat from her body. To restore balance she should be fed yang foods. Therefore, such a woman should eat spicy and protein-rich foods after delivery and should reject vegetables. In addition, it is believed that walking and bathing is dangerous soon after delivery because the pores are open and the mother is more susceptible to the cold, or yin, forces. Nurses who work with a postpartum woman from the Vietnamese culture, for example, need to be sensitive to her beliefs and allow her family to bring her spicy foods. In addition, a protein-rich diet should be ordered for her.

There is a similar belief common among Spanish-speaking groups. Working with a Mexican-American group, Clark (1970) identified diseases of hot and cold imbalance. The theory can be traced to the Hippocratic model of pathology that the Spanish brought to the New World in the sixteenth century. According to this model, a disproportion of hot or cold will lead to illness. Examples of hot/cold illnesses among Mexican-Americans are found in Table 8-2. Cold illnesses generally are caused by an intrusion of coldness into a part of the body. An excess of warmth makes the body vulnerable to cold. Hot illnesses, in contrast, often are generated within the body itself. The heat warms the individual by being displaced from the center of the body toward the surfaces.

As with yin and yang, hot and cold illnesses are treated by the principle of opposition. Hot conditions such as epistaxis (nosebleed) are treated by cold therapies such as giving a cool bath or feeding the person "cold" foods. For example, Mexican-Americans who hold to the hot/cold theory believe that infants are especially vulnerable to a cold stomach. Consequently, they generally do not give them large quantities of such cold foods as melons, citrus, or carrots. Examples of hot/cold food classifications among Mexican-Americans are found in Table 8-3.

Personalistic illnesses result from punishment or aggression directed at an individual. Two personalistic folk beliefs are the evil eye and witchcraft.

A pervasive personalistic folk illness known throughout Mediterranean and Spanish-speaking cultures is the evil eye (*mal de ojo*). The evil eye usually is caused unintentionally and may result simply from envy and admiration. A common example is for a woman to compliment another's child. The woman's envy or admiration alone may cast the

TABLE 8-2
Hot and Cold Illnesses (Mexican-American)

Hot Illnesses	Cold Illnesses
Skin rashes	Chest pain
Fever	Earache
Sore throat	Colic
Kidney diseases	Teething
	Abdominal pain

TABLE 8-3
Hot and Cold Foods (Mexican-American)

Hot Foods	Cold Foods
Fish, pork, turkey	Beef, lamb, rabbit
Goat's milk	Human and cow's milk
Garlic, onions, chile peppers, white beans	Tomatoes, spinach, green beans, beets, cabbage, carrots, oranges, red beans
Bread, potatoes, rice	Oatmeal, lentils, corn tortillas

eye unintentionally. The child later may feel lethargic, have a headache, or be irritable. If the parents bring the child to a clinic they may explain the child's illness as being caused by the eye. Nurses and other professionals should be sensitive to these cultural beliefs and should not laugh or ridicule the family for them.

Cultural groups vary in ways they use to determine whether the eye has been cast. Among Greeks, to detect if the eye (*matiasma*) has been cast, one puts drops of oil into a glass of water. If the oil disperses, then the eye has been cast. Among Mexican-Americans, casting of the eye (*mal de ojo*) is detected by rubbing a raw egg in the shell over the abdomen of the affected individual. The egg then is broken into a glass of water. If the egg assumes a sunny-side-up position, the eye has been cast. The glass containing the egg then may be placed under the affected individual's bed overnight to draw energy out of the eye.

Groups that believe in the evil eye also have general methods for protecting against it. For example, Greek children may wear a *phylacto*, which is blessed wood or incense. Children also may wear gold crosses or blue beads, which are said to reflect the eye. Among Mexican-Americans, tiny spiders may be embroidered on the dresses of young girls to defray the effects of admiration. Additionally, after complimenting a child, the Mexican-American admirer may touch the child lightly on the head, again to thwart any unintentional effects of envy.

Belief in witchcraft as a cause of illness also falls into the personalistic category. Snow (1978) found evidence of this belief among Puerto Ricans, Haitians, and American blacks. He estimated that one third of the black clients treated in southern psychiatric centers believe they are victims of witchcraft. Among blacks, the terms commonly used to describe such occurrences include roots, root work, witchcraft, voodoo, hoodoo, a fix, a hex, or mojo. Regardless of the term used, Snow points out that the common theme is that someone has done something to cause another person illness, injury, or death. Among people who believe in this type of witchcraft, a recurring theme is that animals are in the body or wriggling in the stomach. Because of the fear of adulterated food, there is often anxiety about eating in the homes of other individuals. Snow (1978) notes that witchcraft beliefs are an extreme example of distrust and cites a survey of a federal low income housing project in St. Louis where 91 percent of black respondents agreed with the statement, "It's not good to let your friends know everything about your life because they may take advantage of you" (pp. 86–87). They believed, for example, that friends might have the "root doctor" (also known as the "root worker") "take away their luck."

Among people who believe in personalistic causes of illness, traditional health care may not be sought immediately when a serious problem develops. In these instances, clients likely will seek assistance from a person trained in the use of folk treatments. If the condition abates, it may never come to the attention of a health professional. Common folk illnesses in Spanish-speaking and African-American cultures are described in Table 8-4.

Assessing Belief Systems

A variety of methods can be used to assess the belief system of a client. An excellent assessment model has been developed by Kleinman, Eisenberg, and Good (1978). Using their explanatory model, the nurse may assess a client's beliefs with a series of questions that attempt to elicit beliefs about illnesses (cause, severity, underlying pathology, impact on daily living), preferred methods of treatment, expected outcomes, and fears related to the illnesses. The explanatory model for assessing health beliefs is presented in Table 8-5.

Binn (1980) used this model to understand how ethnic clients perceive problems of hypertension. She points out that questions from the explanatory model elicit information from the perspective of the client on etiology, onset of symptoms, pathophysiology, and the course of the treatment. This information is highly useful to the nurse in understanding how clients perceive and interpret their responses. In addition, these questions assist in identifying cues that indicate cultural influences. Because these questions can be adapted to any health or illness situation to elicit the belief system of the client, they constitute an important tool for nursing assessment.

TABLE 8-4
Folk Illnesses in Spanish-Speaking and African-American Cultures

Culture	Folk Illness	Etiology	Behaviors	Practitioner	Treatment
Hispanic	*Susto* (fright)	An individual experiences a stressful event at some time prior to the onset of symptoms. The stressor may vary from death of a significant person to a child's nightmare to inability to adequately fulfill social-role responsibility. Children are more susceptible to *susto*. It is believed that the soul or spirit leaves the body.	Restlessness during sleep Anorexia Depression Listlessness Disinterest in personal appearance	*Curandero* or *Espiritualista* (*Espiritista*)	A ceremony is performed using branches from a sweet pepper tree and a candle. Motions by the ill person and the curer are performed that form a cross. Three Ave Marias or credos (Apostles' Creed) are said.
	Empacho	Bolus of undigested food adheres to the stomach or wall of intestine. The cause may be the food itself, or it may be due to eating when one is not hungry or when one is stressed.	Stomach pain Diarrhea Vomiting Anorexia	Family member *Sabador* *Curandero*	Massage of the stomach or back until a popping sound is heard. A laxative may be given.
	Caida de la Mollera (Fallen fontanel)	Trauma—a fall or blow to the head or the rapid dislodging of a nipple from an infant's mouth causes the fontanel to be sucked into the palate.	Inability to suckle Irritability Vomiting Diarrhea Sunken fontanel	Family member *Curandero*	One or more of these practitioners insert a finger into the child's mouth and push the palate back into place. Hold the child by the ankles with the top of the head just touching a pan of tepid water for a minute or two. Apply a poultice of soap shavings to the fontanel. Administer herb tea.
	Mal de ojo (Evil eye)	A disease of magical origin cast by a person who is jealous or envious of another person or something the person owns. The evil eye is cast by the envious person's vision upon the subject thereby heating the blood and	Fever Diarrhea Vomiting Crying without apparent cause	*Curandero* *Brujo*	Passing an unbroken egg over the body or rubbing the body with the egg to draw the heat (fever) from the body. Prayers such as the Our Father or Hail Mary may be said simultaneously with the passing of the egg. The egg is then

TABLE 8-4 (Continued)

Culture	Folk Illness	Etiology	Behaviors	Practitioner	Treatment
		producing symptoms. Usually a beautiful child is envied or admired but is not touched by the admirer and the evil eye can be inflicted. The admirer may not be aware of the damage done. If the child is admired and then touched by that person the evil eye is not inflicted.			broken in a bowl, placed under the head of the bed and left there all night. By morning if the egg is almost cooked from the heat of the body, this is a sign that the sick person had *mal de ojo*.
	Mal Puesto (evil)	Illness caused by a hex put on by a *brujo*, witch, or *currandero*, or other person knowledgeable about witchcraft.	Vary considerably Strange behavioral changes Labile emotions Convulsions	*Curandero Brujo*	Varies, depending on the hex.
Black	High blood (too much blood)	Diet very high in red meat and rich food. Belief that high blood causes stroke.	Weakness, paralysis, vertigo, or other behaviors related to stroke	Family member or friend of Spiritualist or self (the latter does this after referring to a Zodiac almanac)	Take internally lemon juice, vinegar, epsom salts, or other astringent food to sweat out the excess blood. Treatment varies depending on what is appropriate for each person according to the Zodiac almanac.
	Low blood (not enough blood . . .)	Too many astringent foods, too harsh a treatment for high blood. Remaining on high blood-pressure medication for too long.	Fatigue Weakness	Same as for high blood	Eat rich red meat, raw beets. Stop taking treatment for high blood. Consult the Zodiac almanac.
	Thin blood (predisposition to illness)	Occurs in women, children, or old people. Blood is very thin until puberty and [again in] . . . old age . . .	Greater susceptibility to illness	Individual	Individual should exercise caution in cold weather by wearing warm clothing or by staying indoors.
	Rash appearing on a child after birth (no specific disease name—the concept is that of body defilement)	Impurities within the body coming out. The body is being defiled and will therefore produce skin rashes.	Rash anywhere on the body; may be accompanied by fever	Family member	Catnip tea as a laxative or other commercial laxative. The quantity and kind depend on the age of the individual.

(continued)

TABLE 8-4 (Continued)

Culture	Folk Illness	Etiology	Behaviors	Practitioner	Treatment
	Diseases of witchcraft, hex or conjuring	Envy and sexual conflict are the most frequent causes of having someone hex another person.	Unusual behavior not normal for the person Sudden death Symptoms related to poisoning (i.e., foul taste, fall off [weight loss], nausea, vomiting) A crawling sensation on the skin or in the stomach Psychotic behavior	Voodoo Priest(ess) Spiritualist	*Conja* is the help given to the conjured person. Treatment varies depending on the spell cast.

Note. From Hautman, M.A. (1979). Folk health and illness beliefs. *The Nurse Practitioner: The American Journal of Primary Health Care,* 4(4), 27. Copyright 1979 The Nurse Practitioner: The American Journal of Primary Health Care. Reprinted by permission.

Customs

In the cultural pyramid, customs and behaviors are the uppermost tier. This layer is easiest to assess—the nurse can identify customs through observation and direct questioning. However, cultural differences in customs easily can lead to misunderstandings if they are ignored. In an act as apparently obvious as determining the age of a child, differences in customs are crucial. For example, for most Southeast Asian and Chinese children, age is calculated roughly from conception. Consequently, most children are considered to be one year of age when they are born. They then gain another year at

every new year, or Tet. A child born just before Tet would shortly be 2 years old by Vietnamese counting but less than 2 months old by Western counting. These different calculations have obvious implications for the nursing assessment.

Customs related to health include dietary practices, communication patterns, family interactions, religious practices, and specific health practices. Assessment of a client's health-related customs is essential to providing comprehensive and culturally sensitive care.

Dietary Practices

No human society deals rationally with the food available in its environment. No society determines diet solely on the basis of availability and nutritional value of food materials. Food is always culturally defined. A plant that may be classified as food in one group may be considered inedible by another. The pig is not a food item in Moslem or some Jewish groups, and cattle are not considered food by Hindus. All societies ignore certain nutritional plants or animals in their environments. Thus, food is primarily a matter of cultural definition.

Food patterns are a particularly crucial area for assessment. An individual's culture defines what is considered food. Within this range of culturally approved items, an individual's diet depends on a host of economic, religious, and psychological factors and personal preferences. Because food tradi-

TABLE 8-5
Explanatory Model for Assessing Health Beliefs

1. What do you think caused your problem?
2. Why do you think it started when it did?
3. What does your sickness do to you? How does it work?
4. How severe is your sickness? Will it have a long or short duration?
5. What kind of treatment do you think you should receive?
6. What are the most important results you hope to receive from this treatment?
7. What are the chief problems your sickness has caused you?
8. What do you fear most about your sickness?

tions are among the last ethnic customs to change, and because of the ethnic diversity in American society, clients' dietary practices may vary dramatically from those of the nurse. It is essential for the nurse to respect the food habits and preferences of all clients.

A number of areas are particularly important for nutritional assessment of culturally distinct clients:

Identification of food items

Methods of food preparation

Additional ingredients (spices, condiments, additives)

Timing and frequency of meals

Food considered harmful or beneficial to health

Types of Foods. Every cultural group has an accepted standard of food practices. These dietary habits have developed over many generations and have a variety of emotional, family, symbolic, and religious meanings. For example, guidelines for the Orthodox Jewish diet are derived from the Old Testament. Kosher foods may be natural or processed. Natural kosher foods include grains, fruits, vegetables, and teas. Processed kosher foods are meats, fruits, vegetables, and fish. Processed kosher foods must be slaughtered in accordance with specified ritual patterns that are overseen by a rabbi. Only animals that have uncloven hoofs (cattle, sheep, etc.) and chew a cud may be eaten; animals with cloven hoofs (pigs) are forbidden. In addition, only fish with scales or fins (salmon, tuna, sturgeon, herring, etc.) can be used; shellfish (e.g., shrimp, lobster, scallops, oysters, clams, etc.) are taboo. Milk and meat may not be eaten at the same meal, and separate plates and cooking utensils must be kept for dairy and meat foods. For example, an Orthodox Jew will not eat meat prepared in butter or with a cream sauce nor put milk into coffee when served with a meat course. The Jewish dietary laws or *kashruth* are observed by many members of the Jewish faith. The extent to which the laws are followed is partly dependent on the specific Jewish subgroup to which the client belongs: Orthodox, Conservative, or Reform (progressing from most to least strict).

Food Preparation. In addition to what food is eaten, the methods of food preparation also merit special attention when taking a diet history. While some methods may remove nutrients (e.g., overcooking vegetables), other methods may increase the available nutrients. For example, soaking corn tortillas in lime water adds calcium to the diet.

Condiments/Additives. The ingredients used in cooking constitute another crucial area for dietary assessment. Asian clients should be asked about use of soy and MSG (monosodium glutamate) in addition to salt since these substances have a very high sodium content. Clients should be asked about specific ingredients if the foods are not familiar to the nurse. For example, most nurses are familiar with Italian lasagna, but they may not be familiar with pastichio, which is a comparable Greek dish.

Meal Time and Frequency. In addition to learning what is eaten and how it is prepared, it is important to determine the timing and frequency of meals. The nurse should not assume that everyone eats three meals a day with the largest meal in the evening. For example, Latin Americans customarily have a midmorning coffee, whereas the British enjoy the late afternoon tea. At these times, food items usually are served, too.

The timing of meals varies in American society. In the eastern part of the United States, dinner at 8 p.m. is common, while in the Midwest, dinner may be served as early as 5 p.m., and in Mediterranean cultural groups as late as 10 p.m. It is important to clarify the client's meaning of the terms "dinner" and "supper." Some cultural groups eat "dinner" at midday and "supper," a light meal, in the evening. A frequently missed area of assessment concerns the timing of medications and treatments. Clients may be told to take a medication before or after meals, with the nurse assuming a typical breakfast, lunch, and dinner pattern. The timing and frequency of a client's meals should be noted in the health record and on the nursing care plan.

Food and Its Relationship to Health. All cultural groups consider certain nutrients to have health-promoting qualities. Chicken soup and high doses of Vitamin C are well known among Americans. Other common examples include the previously discussed hot and cold foods of Mexican-Americans and Asian-Americans. Among most American ethnic groups, special situations such as illness, pregnancy, infancy, and childhood, are associated with special diets. Some foods are considered health-promoting and others dangerous.

In addition to exploring these general areas, the following specific questions should be addressed when assessing the diet of clients to determine cultural differences in food habits:

■ What times during the day do you usually eat?

- How many meals do you eat in a typical day?
- What circumstances increase your appetite?
- What takes your appetite away?
- What foods do you like most?
- What foods do you like least?
- What foods can you not eat because of your religious customs, personal beliefs, or health reasons?
- What seasonings do you regularly use in preparing foods?

Assessing acceptance of a prescribed therapeutic diet may pose difficulties if nurses are unfamiliar with ethnic foods. To augment the nurse's assessment skills, dietary exchange lists are available for the major ethnic groups, such as Asians, Mexican-Americans, and Orthodox, Conservative, and Reform branches of Judaism. Sample ethnic food exchanges are included in Table 18-9 (see chapter 18).

Finally, when assessing dietary practices of ethnic clients, all types of untoward reactions to food should be noted. It is important to identify the offending food as well as the nature of the response, because this may be important in other areas of assessment. For example, a true food allergy may present as an urticarial reaction to egg consumption. This response has very different assessment implications from a hemolytic crisis after a person with Mediterranean glucose–6–phosphate dehydrogenase (G–6–PD) deficiency consumes fava or broad beans, or from the bloating, flatulence, diarrhea, and cramping experienced when a person with lactase deficiency consumes a threshold quantity of milk.

Communication Patterns

Culturally defined communication styles may cause misunderstandings when the nurse and client are from different cultural groups. Brownlee (1978) is particularly helpful in identifying techniques for assessing cultural styles of communication. She points out that methods of persuasion and explanation may differ among cultures. A variety of styles may be used, including logical explanations, proverbs, or debates.

Verbal communication patterns differ among cultural groups in a variety of dimensions. The first is the tempo or the speed of communication, which tends to differ in various regions of the United States. For instance, northerners generally speak more rapidly than do individuals from the South. These differences in tempo are also impor-

tant among ethnic groups. We may find that an individual who is used to speaking rapidly may stereotype a slow-speaking interviewer as ignorant or unsure. On the other hand, an individual who typically speaks slowly may characterize a fast-speaker as brusque and impersonal.

The meaning of silence also may vary considerably among cultures. To some groups, silence is quite uncomfortable, and attempts are made to fill every gap in the conversation. Among native Americans and Asians, however, silence often is considered essential. A person should fully consider what another has said before giving a response. Thus, data collection may take longer when the client needs to pause and reflect about what is being asked. The nurse should be sensitive to and respect the client's need for silence.

A second area of communication assessment concerns topics that may be taboo. Among some groups, naming a recently deceased relative is inappropriate. It may also be considered unseemly for a male or an unmarried young female to ask a woman questions regarding sexuality or childbirth. In other groups, finances are topics only family members should discuss; it may be inappropriate to give outsiders information about the financial condition of the family. Clients should retain the right to not disclose information they believe is inappropriate to share. At the same time, the nurse may use the nursing assessment interview as an opportunity to help clients understand how such information is helpful in addressing the client's health concerns and needs, providing the information is obtained and used with sensitivity and concern for the client's privacy.

Proper forms of address may vary among regional or ethnic groups. In the South, it is proper to address a stranger by the titles Mr. or Mrs. or Miss. Southeast Asian forms of address also differ. Among Southeast Asians and Chinese, the family name appears first, with the second name referring to the given name of the individual, for example, Ngoc (family name) Li (given name). However, many immigrants change their names to Western syntax. Clients from Japanese, Korean, and Asian Indian cultures use the same name order as English speakers. The nurse should ascertain at the beginning of the assessment interview the client's family name (surname) and given name, and how the client prefers to be addressed.

Communicating emotions and feelings is another area strongly influenced by culture. Many Southeast Asians emphasize self-control because they believe it is one's duty to maintain an even temper. Emotions usually are kept to oneself, and expressions of disagreement that might irritate or offend are avoided. Hostility usually is not expressed toward people who are considered superior, such as parents, elders, teachers, or health professionals. A client's smile or "yes" may not necessarily indicate understanding, agreement, or compliance as much as it indicates unwillingness to be disrespectful or impolite. Therefore, an authoritarian or direct approach by the nurse may elicit only token verbal agreement from the Southeast Asian client.

Even when English is the common language of client and nurse, verbal communication may be misunderstood because of important colloquial differences. For example, among Appalachians, the phrase "I don't care to" means "I would like to." A person who is "ill" is a person who is bad-tempered, and "running-off" means diarrhea. Although these colloquial differences may engender only minor misunderstandings, other differences can have serious clinical implications. For example, one of the major concerns of people who practice folk medicine is the state of the blood. The blood may be characterized as thick or thin, good or bad, high or low. One of these, high and low blood, is seen as the measure of blood volume. Variations in high or low blood can be regulated through diet. If high blood symptoms occur (headache, vision problems, palpitations, or dizziness) certain foods are omitted and others are prescribed. A clinical problem may arise if an Appalachian client is told he has high blood pressure, because he may interpret this as having "high blood" (volume). This is potentially harmful because the folk prescription for treating high blood or "bringing it down" is to drink the brine from pickles or olives, which is very high in sodium.

When language differences are great, a translator may be necessary. Kay (1979) suggests the following guidelines for using a translator, which can be applied to the nursing assessment interview:

- Look at the [client]. (Talk to the [client]. Do not carry on the conversation with the translator.)
- When the translator is not a member of the health profession, keep language free of technical words.
- Maintain a simple sentence structure and speak sentence by sentence, having each translated individually.
- Do not assume that the meaning has been translated without distortion. Anticipate misunderstandings.
- Get "back translation" to determine misunderstandings. Ask the [client] to repeat what you said, with the translator facilitating.
- Whenever possible, talk to the translator ahead of time to give the translator time to think through the information and determine the best way of conveying it to the [client]. (p. 97)

Nonverbal communication patterns also may cause misunderstandings between the client and the nurse. Members of many ethnic groups such as Appalachians, native Americans, and Southeast Asians may try to avoid direct eye contact. In these groups, members may consider direct eye contact impolite and thus will avert their eyes during an interview. This behavior may be misinterpreted by the nurse as disinterest, dishonesty, or low self-esteem.

The meaning and appropriateness of body contact is another nonverbal form of communication that varies among ethnic groups. Groups differ in how, when, and where to touch other individuals. In addition, some groups use touch to communicate feelings, whereas others perceive touch as an invasion of privacy. For example, individuals of Mediterranean descent are more likely to use intimate touching behaviors, such as hugging and kissing, in public than are Americans descended from northern Europeans. Similarly, desired physical proximity may vary so that some interviewers prefer to sit very close to the client, while the client wishes to have a more respectful distance between them. In other cases the client prefers to sit closer for more intimate personal communication while the interviewer wishes to remain more formal. The nurse should be sensitive to cues that indicate the client's need for closer proximity or greater distance. At the same time, nurses need to be aware of their own responses to close physical proximity and touching, in order to avoid misunderstanding.

When using written material, it is important to remember that many individuals, even if they are literate, may not be literate in English. Others who have learned to speak English well may not be able to read it. Those who are native English speakers may never have learned the written language. Chapter 12 provides guidelines for assessing client literacy.

Polacca's (1973) study of Navajos elucidates a number of issues just discussed. She noted that Navajos usually are not direct in expressing a difference of opinion. To indicate a disagreement, they may use ridicule or teasing about an entirely different topic. In other instances, people may leave the room or may start paying attention to something else. Sometimes when a difference of opinion exists, the Navajo may tell a story or fable to show the non-Navajo what the people are thinking and feeling. Polacco points out that the use of "maybe" is an English word and not a concept that is readily known to the Navajo. They may interpret "maybe" as meaning a promise that will not be kept, and the nurse who uses it may engender distrust.

Family Structure and Relationships

Although its form varies among different ethnic groups, the concept of family is universal. The family constitutes perhaps the most important social context within which illness occurs and is resolved. It consequently serves as a primary unit in health care.

The family frequently is involved in defining whether a member is ill, in selection of lay consultants or professional practitioners, in adherence to prescribed therapy, and in determining whether long-term care for chronic illnesses can be provided in the home.

In groups with a greater emphasis on the family (for example, among Amish or African-Americans), dependency is more accepted than it is in the dominant American society. Family members may consider it their responsibility to care for an ill person in the home. An investigation of residential preferences of ethnic groups of European descent found wide variation (Tripp-Reimer & Schrock, 1982). For example, when asked where they would prefer to live if they were bedfast, a majority of Amish preferred to reside with a relative, with the remainder wishing to stay in their own home with assistance. However, in a comparable sample of Czech-Americans, three-fourths wished to reside in a care facility or a retirement center, with virtually none wishing to reside with a relative if they were bedfast.

The process of becoming a client and using various health services encompasses decisions and events involving the interaction of family, friends, and professional providers of care. The role the family plays in the process varies over time, depending upon the nature of the condition (acute, chronic, or terminal), its perceived severity, the degree of familial concern, as well as the member affected. The family is involved in every stage of a member's illness, from diagnosis through treatment and rehabilitation, or death (Tripp-Reimer & Lauer, 1987).

The way in which a family is affected by a member's illness is mediated by a number of important factors such as the person's role and status within the family, and the extent of social, material, and professional support available to the family. When families have a high degree of ethnic affiliation, these patterns may vary dramatically. The ethnic group defines culturally prescribed beliefs and behaviors for the family.

The structure and organization of the family varies widely among American ethnic groups. In highlighting the structure of certain traditional ethnic groups, it is important to remember that nuclear families, isolated individuals, and extended families exist in all ethnic groups as do male-dominated, female-dominated, and egalitarian families. While it is possible to characterize the dominant, ideal, or modal family type within particular traditional ethnic groups, it is more important to be aware of the variation that may occur in family organization and structure.

Defining Family Members. The identification of the specific individuals who constitute the family is a crucial area of assessment (see chap. 7). Family composition will influence what support is likely to be available, how health decisions are likely to be made, availability of people to care for an ill family member, and even who has visitation rights. A good example of differing familial compositions emerges when examining kinship systems. Among some native Americans, first cousins are treated as siblings and some children may have more than two sets of grandparents. Similarly, acquired kin such as godparents or co-parents are highly important in many families of southern Mediterranean origin (e.g., Greek and Italian). Such kin may be actively involved in the family, particularly with regard to children. It is critical, therefore, to understand that family members may be broadly defined and do not necessarily conform to nuclear or legal boundaries.

Extended versus Nuclear Families. The family structure that generally is thought to be most characteristic of American society is a nuclear family consisting of parents and their young children. Yet, other patterns may be modal for certain other ethnic groups. For example, the Amish perceive the family as a religious or social unit. A typical Amish residential pattern consists of a large family farmhouse with an adjacent *Grossdaadi Haus*, or grandparent house. The elder parents retire to this smaller unit when they confer farming rights on one of their children. Similarly, many immigrants tend to live in extended three- or four-generation family clusters (particularly when elders are not as fluent in English as younger family members).

Male- or Female-based Families. Labeling a family as patriarchal or matriarchal (male- or female-headed) is more subtle than is often recognized. While the Italian-American family has been described as patriarchal, this is somewhat misleading, because it implies that the power is held by the male members of the family. In actuality, the Italian mother usually is the center of the family and has a great deal of power in internal matters. Similarly, while Mexican-American women may appear outwardly subservient to wishes of males, they tend to hold the position of primacy in household matters and are the basis of the family's internal support system.

Contrary to some notions about the black family, most research indicates that an egalitarian pattern typifies black families. In most two-parent black families, husbands are actively involved in decision-making and the performance of household tasks. Conversely, most wives, while strong, are not dominant matriarchs, but share with their husbands the making of family decisions. Staples (1976) contends that the myth of black matriarchy has been reinforced by the failure of many students of black family life to distinguish between the terms *dominant* and *strong*. While black women have needed to be strong for the black family to survive, they have not necessarily been dominant.

Matriarchal or female-based forms of family organization are common among many groups of native Americans, including the Navajo, Hopi, Crow, Mohawk, Seneca, Creek, and Seminole. However, again this is not as clear-cut as some believe. For example, among the Hopi, while men join the households of their wives and provide for the family economically, they retain ritual, individual, and disciplinary roles in their household of origin. Thus, they may make decisions for their sisters' children.

Interdependence versus Autonomy. The extended family is the central, most durable, and influential social institution of groups from the Mediterranean. Families make spontaneous visits and intergenerational contact almost daily. Children often live with their parents until they marry and maintain close contact with parents after marriage. During illness, they tend to rely heavily on other people instead of trying to cope alone.

Lock (1983) points out that the Japanese tend to value the maintenance of harmony of the social group over the individual. For nurses reared in families of European descent, it may be difficult to acknowledge the value that the goals of the group take precedence over individual needs and autonomy. This contrasts dramatically with Americans of Scandinavian descent who place high value on individualism and autonomy and who tend to be much less interdependent in their responses to health and illness.

Family Decision-making. All the features influencing the structure and organization of the family affect patterns of decision-making regarding health matters. Frequently, the decision of whether a sick person should seek health care or be hospitalized is not solely an individual decision but is one shared by the family. For example, among many Navajo, the decision to enter a hospital often is reached only after a family conference. A woman and her husband alone may not be free to exercise their discretion in this regard. Similarly, for many traditional Southeast Asian clients, their relatives more than they are the ones to be convinced before a therapeutic program can be initiated or continued. It is common for Appalachians to ask the grandmother about the advisability of seeking or accepting health care and for Mexican-Americans to ask the father or grandmother. In these instances, decisions regarding health care are not so much the responsibility of the individual as they are of the family or senior family members. The subordination of the individual to the family should not be assessed as detrimental or irrational. There are important reasons for group decisions in cases dealing with medical treatment. Illness is more than a biological disorder; it may disrupt the social and economic order of the family. Only when the family accepts the client's condition as a legitimate illness can the client be excused from role responsibilities. Because an illness may affect the entire family, it is only logical that the family should participate in the decisions related to care and treatment.

Religious Practices

The role of religion in an ethnic group will depend on a number of variables too detailed to explore here. However, Brownlee (1978) offers extensive guidelines for a more complete assessment. In brief, religion may affect the practice of health care in all its phases. Most groups have religious rituals or ceremonies that mark stages in the life cycle, including birth, entrance to adulthood, marriage, and death. Religious dictates often influence dietary or food habits, at least during special ceremonial times. Religious rituals, such as circumcision of Jewish infants or the ghost dance among the Plains Indians, may be associated indirectly with the health of the client. Beliefs associated with religion, such as interpreting illness as a punishment from God or viewing the health professional as the instrument of God, also may have implications for assessment when working with ethnically diverse clients. However, other religions, such as Christian Science (which prescribes avoidance of traditional health-care practitioners) and Jehovah's Witnesses (which prohibits blood transfusions) have a more direct influence on the health and health behaviors of their members.

Family Customs Specifically Related to Health

In general, it can be said that individuals learn about health-care behaviors from their adult family members. These activities related to seeking health care and maintaining health are nested within the family and are linked closely to the family's ethnic community. Common medical beliefs and practices of various cultural groups are summarized in Table 8-6.

There are a number of reasons why clients' medical behaviors reflect ethnically distinct customs. Home remedies and folk healers are familiar to the client and generally treat illness in a manner that is meaningful and understandable to the client and family. In such instances, the family is intimately involved in the determination of both a diagnosis and the proper course of therapy, thus increasing the family's and client's sense of control. Also, folk healers are able to relate more personally to the client and family, using familiar language and asking about things that are important to them.

Home Remedies. Patterns of self-care vary among ethnic groups. One area in which this variation is seen is in the use of home remedies. Self-

TABLE 8-6
Examples of Some Beliefs and Practices of Different Cultural Groups

	Native American	Latino/Chicano	Asian	African-American
Views of health	Holistic view: spiritual forces give life and health	Holistic view: as a state of equilibrium; children may wear amulets for protection	Seen as a balance of energy, called yin and yang	Health means being able to work productively, being in a state of harmony with others in the universe
Views of illness	Tied into religion	Has spiritual, social ramifications; good or "natural" diseases due to imbalance; "supernatural" diseases due to satanic forces	Seen as an imbalance of energy	Seen as a state of incapacitation, sense of disharmony, lack of communication
Resource person for treatment	Healing specialists, herbalists, diagnosticians	*Curanderos*, other types of healers	Healers, herbalists	Older woman with experience; the caregiver must develop a healing relationship with the ill person
Treatments	Herbs; sweat baths; a family conference if necessary to decide if a family member enters a hospital (Navajo)	Folk medicine; prayers; herbs; hot-cold foods and fluids to offset specific illnesses classified as derived from "hot" or "cold" causes	Herbs; nutrition; meditation; spiritual healing; massage; acupressure; acupuncture; hot-cold foods and fluids to counteract illnesses; moxibustion	Religious healing; folk remedies; herb teas; poultices
Views of children's health risks	Fear of strangers coming close to infants; fear of "witching" infant (Navajo)	If a stranger lavishes attention on but fails to touch a child, the child may develop "evil eye"; i.e., diarrhea, vomiting		A stout child is admired

Note. From Servonsky/Opas: *Nursing Management of Children,* © 1987. Boston: Jones and Bartlett Publishers, p. 293.

prescribing and treatment often are identified with minor illnesses, such as hot tea and dry toast to calm a stomach flu. However, the practice may be clinically complex as well. Home remedies are usually the only ones available to treat health problems, such as the evil eye, that are not recognized by the biomedically dominated health-care system.

Often home remedies are the first level of care that a client uses to treat an illness. Not only may they be effective, but they are usually less costly. Folk treatments are known to the client's family and social network. Therefore, support for home prescriptions, both the knowledge and the provision of the product, is readily available.

It is not unusual to find folk therapies used concurrently with traditional forms of medical treatment. One example of the importance of assessing home remedies was presented in the discussion of colloquial differences in Appalachia. Another example of the importance of nurses assessing and understanding home remedies concerns the practice of *cao gio* (dermabrasion) among the Vietnamese. Problems of misdiagnosis may occur because of the nurse's lack of familiarity with Vietnamese folk medicine practices. The Vietnamese lay practice of cao gio is a home treatment for such minor ailments as fever, chills, and headaches. In this procedure, oil is applied to the back and chest with cotton. The oil is massaged into the skin until the skin is warm. Then, with firm strokes, the edge of a coin is used to produce purpura or petechiae. This treatment has led to the misdiagnosis of child abuse by health providers unfamiliar with the practice.

Although the use of home remedies may be positive, there are associated risks. Home remedies may delay the client's seeking traditional medical care that could rapidly and effectively alleviate an illness. In these situations, the client should be appraised of available treatment options with appropriate, culturally sensitive counseling. Health practitioners always should be cautious in such situations and recognize they are imposing their own cultural values on the situation, values the client may or may not hold.

Finally, there are instances in which home remedies have been found to be hazardous to health. *Empacho* is an Hispanic folk illness of infants. Some clinicians in the United States have analyzed samples of the home treatments used for this folk illness (*azarcon* and *greta*) and have found that they may contain high levels of lead oxide, resulting in lead poisoning of these infants (Trotter, 1985).

Choice of Practitioners. The choice of a health provider, including both traditional health professionals and folk practitioners, is influenced by one's family and, ultimately, ethnic heritage. In many ethnic groups, folk practitioners may be used separately or in combination with health professionals. For example, among Mexican-Americans, there is a variety of folk health specialists, including *curandero* (male) or *curandera* (female) who have special spiritual healing powers, a *partera* or midwife, a *sobador* who massages and sets bones, and an *albolario* who specializes in removing hexes. In a large traditional Mexican-American community, a number of these folk practitioners as well as traditional health professionals may be available to clients. The choice of health professionals versus folk practitioners depends on a variety of factors, including the severity of illness. Dramatic problems such as a broken arm or loss of consciousness usually are given emergency treatment in a traditional health-care setting. Chronic problems that are not readily ameliorated by health professionals, and problems that are characterized as folk illnesses (colds, flu, chronic pain) may more often be treated by folk practitioners.

Specific Illness Behaviors. A number of investigators have studied illness behaviors cross-culturally. For example, Zola (1979) studied the differences in symptoms that bring clients to physicians. By comparing diagnostically matched clients from different ethnic groups, he found distinct cultural patterns of response to symptoms and to definitions of illness. Even with the same pathologic condition, Italian-American patients presented a significantly wider assortment of bodily dysfunctions than did the Irish-Americans. Irish-American clients tended to deny pain as a feature of their disorder and tended to see a physician only after they had received the approval of others who urged their visit. Italian-Americans tended to seek medical attention after their symptoms interfered with social or personal relations or when they were experiencing a situational or interpersonal crisis. In contrast, Anglo-American clients came for help only after their disorders interfered with specific vocational or physical activities. Zola concluded that patterns of seeking health care and critical symptoms for entry into a health-care system vary widely among cultural groups.

The expression and interpretation of pain also varies dramatically among ethnic groups. Although people in all groups tend to have about the same neurophysiologic threshold of pain, the way that people perceive, react to, and express pain differs. These behaviors depend, among other things, on whether the culture values or censors the display of emotional response to injury or pain. If clients do not report discomfort from pain, it may mean that the cultural group values stoicism. For example, native Americans and Asian maternity clients tend to be more stoic in their expressions of pain during childbirth than do maternity clients of Mediterranean descent.

In a classic study, Zborowski (1969) investigated the pain responses of Jewish, Italian, and elderly Americans. He found that elderly Americans attempt to be stoic in their reactions to pain ("to take pain like a man, not to cry"). Italian-Americans tend to be concerned with the immediacy of pain and are disturbed by the actual pain sensation. They were most expressive in their reactions to pain. Jewish Americans also tend to be expressive but focus more on the symptomatic meaning of pain: what the pain means in relation to their health and the future welfare of the family.

When assessing clients' responses to pain, then, it is important to know what the baseline of pain expression is for various cultural groups. Otherwise, individuals who freely express pain may receive excessive medication and those who are stoic may be undermedicated for pain.

A format for assessing family cultural values and health-care practices is provided in Table 8-7.

CULTURAL ASSESSMENT AND NURSING DIAGNOSIS

Because culture pervades all domains of life, there are no nursing diagnoses specific to cultural areas. Virtually any behavioral category of nursing diagnosis can have a cultural etiology. For example, language differences may result in a diagnosis of "impaired verbal communication." Defining a

TABLE 8-7
Assessment of Family Cultural Values and Practices Related to Health Care

Cultural Factor	Assessment Questions
Language	What is the first language of the family?
	If English is not spoken, is there a family member or friend who can speak for the others?
	Is an interpreter necessary? Should language cards be used? (These cards are pictures with appropriate statements or questions in a specified foreign language.)
Diet	Does the family have cultural food preferences?
	Are any foods forbidden by the family's cultural or religious beliefs?
	Is there special etiquette surrounding eating practices (for example, a practice that eating is done only in privacy)?
	Is special preparation of foods required?
	Are there special foods for certain occasions?
	What are the customary mealtimes in the family's culture?
Health and illness beliefs	How are health and illness described in the family's culture? Do all family members hold these beliefs?
	What are the family's beliefs about the causes of illness (e.g., punishment for sin, an imbalance of the body system)?
	Whom does the family respect as a health practitioner (e.g., a physician, public health nurse, grandmother, *curandero*, spiritualist, herbalist, acupuncturist)?
	What are the usual remedies used by the family for illness (e.g., home remedies, over-the-counter medications, herbs, prayers, prescription drugs)?
	What are the family's customs and beliefs related to death?
Family relationships	Are there religious practices surrounding birth, illness, and death? What are they?
	How is the birth of a child received in the family?
	What are the family's goals for the child? What approach does the family take to help the child reach those goals?
	What health care practices for the child's welfare does the family value? Are there cultural objections to any practices (e.g., immunizations, dental care, teaching of hygiene and other self-care practices)?
	From what source does the family derive its greatest support (e.g., extended family, religion, friends)?
	What role does the extended family play?
	What are the major values of the family (e.g., education, wealth, spiritual life, sports)?

Note. From Servonsky/Opas: *Nursing Management of Children,* © 1987. Boston: Jones and Bartlett Publishers, p. 294.

health problem as a folk illness may result in an inappropriate diagnosis of "noncompliance" with prescribed scientific therapy. Because cultural variables may be the dominant etiological factor in any behavioral category of nursing diagnosis, they merit careful assessment and consideration. The following case examples illustrate the importance of incorporating cultural variables in nursing assessment, diagnosis, and care planning.

Case Illustration A: Mrs. Theresa Ruiz is a 34-year-old who moved to New York City from Puerto Rico three years ago. She was admitted to the hospital 10 days ago with severe abdominal pain and fever, and subsequently underwent an emergency appendectomy and received medical treatment for peritonitis.

Although Mrs. Ruiz was friendly and cooperative with the nursing staff preoperatively, after surgery she became highly anxious and withdrew. Rather than walking and visiting with other clients as she did preoperatively, she sat in her bed with the curtains drawn and cried intermittently.

Mrs. Ruiz's primary nurse developed an effective relationship with Mrs. Ruiz while obtaining the nursing history upon admission. The nurse learned that Mrs. Ruiz's mother-in-law convinced her that she was a victim of a neighbor's *envidia* (envy) and that her physical ailments were only beginning. In conducting the initial assessment, the nurse learned that Mrs. Ruiz practices the religion *espiritism* and belongs to a *centro* in her neighborhood. The nurse diagnosed Mrs. Ruiz's response to her illness as "spiritual distress" and intervened by making arrangements, with Mrs. Ruiz's permission, for the head medium at the *centro* to come to the hospital to perform *despojo* (exorcism). Mrs. Ruiz regained her previous demeanor the day after the ritual was performed and recovered uneventfully.

Case Illustration B: Lee Tran is a 4-year-old boy who was born in the United States to parents who were Vietnamese refugees. During his preschool physical, he was examined by a nurse in a general pediatric clinic. The nurse observed that Lee Tran had multiple bruises around his neck and that his back and abdomen appeared to have been whipped with a belt. The nurse quickly identified a nursing diagnosis of "altered parenting" and reported the findings to the clinic staff prior to filing a report of child abuse with the department of social services. However, while discussing the diagnosis with the staff, another clinic nurse pointed out that dermabrasion (cao gio) is a common Vietnamese folk practice used to cure respiratory illnesses. The nurse further explained that pinch-

ing around the neck area often is done to allow the "wind" causing the illness to escape from the body. Additional information gathered from the family indicated that, indeed, Lee Tran recently had suffered a severe respiratory illness and had been treated with antibiotics at a different clinic. In addition to administering the prescribed antibiotics, the family also treated Lee Tran with herbal remedies and dermabrasion. The nurse determined the diagnosis of "altered parenting" was inaccurate and did not file a report of child abuse.

Chapter Highlights

▪ Culture consists of learned patterns of values, beliefs, customs, and behaviors that are shared by a group of interacting persons.

▪ Careful cultural assessment is crucial to minimize misunderstandings that arise from nurse–client differences in values, beliefs, and customs.

▪ Cultural awareness provides cues for more in-depth assessment of particular aspects for individual clients.

▪ A nurse should carefully avoid stereotyping individuals on the basis of their ethnic affiliation because there is wide variation in adherence to traditional cultural ways.

▪ Clients should be assessed from a culturally relativist perspective: within the context of their own cultural norms. The nurse should resist the inclination to judge a client's behaviors from the perspective of the nurse's own culture.

▪ Cultural values generally are unconscious and, therefore, are difficult to assess. Cultural beliefs and customs may be more easily assessed through interview, and in the case of the latter, observation of behavior.

▪ Cultural definitions of health and illness may be highly complex and differ dramatically among cultural groups.

▪ Cultural assessment should include eliciting information from clients regarding patterns of communication, family structure and relations, religious practices, dietary habits, health beliefs, health care practices, and responses to illness.

▪ A complete cultural assessment rarely is indicated in most clinical situations. However, the nurse must be aware of and sensitive to cultural differences that may affect nurse–client relationships and the client's responses to health care. Cultural assessment should be tailored to those areas of clinical concern.

■ Cultural variables may be the dominant etiological factor for any given nursing diagnosis and thus merit careful assessment and consideration.

Practice Activities

1. Interview at least one client from a different ethnic group. Assess the client's belief system using Table 8-5. How do the data collected differ from your initial perceptions of the client?

2. Interview an elderly member of your family and another elderly person. Determine their ethnic heritages. Ask them to describe home remedies they used when they were young and those they use now.

3. Ask a friend from a different ethnic group to keep a 24-hour diet history during an important cultural or religious holiday. Compare and contrast the diet with your own on the same holiday.

4. Identify the major religious or cultural groups in your community. Select one different from your own and interview a leader from the group to determine: a) dietary practices and restrictions, and b) beliefs or rituals surrounding birth, infancy, adolescence, marriage, old age, death, and illness.

Recommended Readings

Ailinger, R. (1988). Folk beliefs about high blood pressure in Hispanic immigrants. *Western Journal of Nursing Research, 10,* 629–636.

Anderson, J.M. (1990). Health care across cultures. *Nursing Outlook, 38,* 136–139.

Geissler, E.M. (1991). Transcultural nursing and nursing diagnoses. *Nursing and Health Care, 12,* 109–192, 203.

Giger, J.N., & Davidhizer, R. (1990). Transcultural nursing assessment: A method for advancing nursing practice. *International Nursing Review, 37,* 199–202.

Hansen, M.M., & Resick, L.K. (1990). Health beliefs, health care, and rural Appalachian subcultures from an ethnographic perspective. *Family and Community Health, 13*(1), 1–10.

Kirkpatrick, S. & Cobb, A. (1990). Health beliefs related to diarrhea in Haitian children: Building transcultural nursing knowledge. *Journal of Transcultural Nursing, 1*(2), 2–12.

Lipson, J. & Meleis, A. (1985). Culturally appropriate care: The case of immigrants. *Topics in Clinical Nursing, 9,* 469–78.

Martin, M.E., & Henry, M. (1989). Cultural relativity and poverty. *Public Health Nursing, 6*(1), 28–34.

Phillips, S., & Lobar, S.L. (1990). Literature summary of some Navajo child health beliefs and rearing practices within a transcultural nursing framework. *Journal of Transcultural Nursing, 1*(2), 13–20.

Roberson, M. (1985). The influence of religious beliefs on health choices of Afro-Americans. *Topics in Clinical Nursing, 7*(3), 57–63.

Young, C.K., Camilleri, D.D., McElmurry, B.J., & Ohlson, V.M. (1988). Folk medicine in the health practice of Hmong refugees. *Western Journal of Nursing Research, 10*(5), 647–660.

References

Biermann, J., & Toohey, B. (1974). *The diabetes question and answer book.* Los Angeles: Sherbourne.

Binn, M. (1980). Using the explanatory model to understand ethnomedical perceptions of hypertension. *Transcultural Nursing Care, 5,* 60–78.

Bonaparte, B. (1979). Ego defensiveness, open–closed mindedness, and nurses' attitudes toward culturally different patients. *Nursing Research, 28,* 166–172.

Brownlee, A. (1978). *Community, culture, and care.* St. Louis: Mosby.

Clark, A. (1978). *Culture, childbearing and health professionals.* Philadelphia: Davis.

Clark, M. (1970). *Health in the Mexican-American culture.* Los Angeles: University of California Press.

Foster, G. (1976). Disease etiologies in non-western medical systems. *American Anthropologist, 78,* 773–782.

Hansen, M.M., & Resick, L.K. (1990). Health beliefs, health care, and rural Appalachian subcultures from an ethnographic perspective. *Family and Community Health, 13*(1), 1–10.

Kay, R. (1979). Personal communication. Cited in J. Freebairn & K. Gwinup (Eds.), *Cultural diversity and nursing practice: Instructor's manual* (p. 97). Irvin, CA: Concept Media.

Kleinman, A., Eisenberg, L., & Good, G. (1978). Culture, illness, and care: Clinical lessons from anthropological and cross-cultural research. *Annals of Internal Medicine, 88,* 256–257.

Kluckhohn, F., & Strodtbeck, F. (1961). *Variations in value orientations.* New York: Row, Peterson.

Lock, M. (1983). Japanese response to social change: Making the strange familiar. *Western Journal of Medicine, 139,* 829–834.

Noshpitz, J. (1979). The Jewish child. In J. Noshpitz (Ed.), *The basic handbook of child psychiatry* (pp. 276–282). New York: Basic.

Pederson, P., Lonner, W., & Draguns, J. (1976). *Counseling across cultures.* Honolulu: University Press of Hawaii.

Polacca, K. (1973). Ways of working with Navajos who have not learned the white man's ways. In A.

Reinhardt & M. Quinn (Eds.), *Family centered community nursing.* St. Louis: Mosby.

Ruiz, M. (1981). Open–closed mindedness, intolerance of ambiguity, and nursing faculty attitudes toward culturally different patients. *Nursing Research, 30,* 177–181.

Saunders, L. (1954). *Cultural differences and medical care.* New York: Russell Sage.

Snow, L. (1978). Folk medical beliefs and their implications for care of patients. *Annals of Internal Medicine, 88,* 85.

Staples, R. (1976). The black American family. In C. Mendel & R. Hakerstein (Eds.), *Ethnic families in America* (pp. 221–247). New York: Elsevier.

Sue, D. (1981). *Counseling the culturally different: Theory and practice.* New York: Wiley Interscience.

Tripp-Reimer, T. (1982). Barriers to health care: Perceptual variations of Appalachian clients by Appalachian and non-Appalachian health care professionals. *Western Journal of Nursing Research, 4,* 179–191.

Tripp-Reimer, T. (1983). Retention of a folk health practice (Matiasma) among four generations of urban Greek immigrants. *Nursing Research, 32,* 97–101.

Tripp-Reimer, R., & Lauer, G. (1987). Ethnic considerations for families with chronic illness. In L. Wright & M. Leahey (Eds.), *Families and chronic illness* (pp. 77–100). Philadelphia: Springhouse.

Tripp-Reimer, T., & Schrock, M. (1982). Residential patterns and preferences of ethnic aged: Implications for transcultural nursing. In C.N. Uhl & J. Uhl (Eds.), *1982 Proceedings of the 7th Annual Transcultural Nursing Society* (pp. 144–157). Salt Lake City: Transcultural Nursing Society.

Trotter, R. (1985). Greta and Azarcon: A survey of episodic lead poisoning from a folk remedy. *Human Organization, 44*(1), 64–72.

Tung, T. (1972). The family and the management of mental health problems in Vietnam. In W. Lebra (Ed.), *Transcultural research in mental health* (p. 108). Honolulu: University Press of Hawaii.

Whitaker, J. (1976). *Guidelines for primary health care in rural Alaska.* (U.S. DHEW Publication No. 017-026-00049-6). Washington, DC: U.S. Government Printing Office.

Zola, I. (1979). Culture and symptoms: An analysis of patients' presenting complaints. In R. Spector (Ed.), *Cultural diversity in health and illness.* New York: Appleton-Century-Crofts.

Zborowski, M. (1969). *People in pain.* San Francisco: Jossey-Bass.

9

Environmental Assessment

CHAPTER OUTLINE

- Person–Environment–Health Relationship
  Ecological System   Epidemiological
  Framework
- Parameters of Environmental Assessment
  Biological Environment   Physical
  Environment   Socioeconomic Environment
- Components of Environmental Assessment
- Selected Tools for Assessing the Client's
  Environment
  Home Screening Questionnaire (HSQ)
  Assessment of Home Safety for the Elderly
- Assessment of Health Risk
  Health Risk Appraisal (HRA)   Health Risk
  Appraisal/Lifestyle Assessment Tools
- Environmental Assessment and Nursing
  Diagnosis

OBJECTIVES

Upon completion of this chapter, you should be able to:

- Describe the relationship of person, environment, and health.

- Use an epidemiologic framework as the basis for environmental assessment.

- Delineate the various components of biological, physical, and socioeconomic environments that affect human health.

- Explain the potential effects, both positive and negative, of biological, physical, and socioeconomic environments on human health.

- Delineate the parameters for assessing the various environments in which people live: home, work or school, and health care.

- Describe the goals, purposes, advantages, and limitations of health risk appraisal.

- Conduct a comprehensive environmental assessment of clients throughout the lifespan, including health risk/lifestyle appraisal.

- Explain the role of environmental data in formulating nursing diagnoses.

People are embedded in the environments in which they live, work, and play. Thus, their behavior cannot be understood apart from the environmental context in which it occurs. The forces and influences within the environment that influence human behavior and health comprise a critical dimension of a comprehensive nursing assessment.

The environment consists of all those factors that affect human life and health, and encompasses a number of parameters: physical, biological, cognitive, spiritual, social, cultural, aesthetic, political, economic, legal, ethical, and technological. Each influences human behavior, individually and collectively. Environmental forces may be internal ones, such as cellular growth, carcinogens, inflammation, communicable diseases, and biochemical and neurohormonal substances, or external forces, such as air, water, noise, climate, toxic chemicals, physical space, architectural design, social contacts, and the communities in which people live.

The relationship between people and their environments is not linear. Instead, it is like a double helix, each influencing and receiving from the other in a system of continuous feedback. This person–environment relationship often is referred to as *reciprocity*.

Historically, nurses have been concerned with the impact of the environment on a person's health. The concept of environment was first introduced to nursing by Florence Nightingale and was the cornerstone of her theory of nursing. She postulated that elements of the physical environment, most notably pure air, pure water, sanitation, hygiene, and light, in conjunction with proper diet, are essential for reducing the incidence of disease. She also recognized the impact of modifying the environment according to clients' responses to their illnesses:

> The thing which strikes the experienced observer most forcibly is this, that symptoms or suffering generally considered to be inevitable and incident to the disease are very often not symptoms of disease at all, but of something quite different—of want of fresh air, or of light or of warmth, or of quiet, or of cleanliness, or of punctuality and care in the administration of diet, of each or all of these. (Nightingale, 1859, p. 5)

Since Nightingale's time, the role that environment plays in human health has received increasing attention from nursing and other disciplines. Nightingale was primarily concerned about the immediate environment in caring for the sick. Nurses today, however, are concerned with the care of people in the context of broader environments, including family, community, and culture. Also, greater emphasis is being placed on the relationship of the environment to wellness and health promotion in addition to the traditional focus on illness.

Many nursing interventions are aimed at enhancing, modifying, minimizing, or eliminating environmental forces. Examples include fostering a child's development by teaching parents age-appropriate learning activities, modifying the home environment for a physically disabled person to increase ease of daily living, eliminating risk of premature death through smoking cessation programs, or educating the public about specific environmental hazards, such as toxic wastes and food additives.

As discussed in Chapter 1, environment is one of the four concepts central to nursing's philosophy. Most nursing theories and conceptual models incorporate environment as a major concept. Several theorists, most notably Rogers (1970) and Parse (1981), focus on environment–person interaction as the core of their models. Generally, theorists view the role of the nurse as managing the relationship of the client and the environment to promote or restore health. The nurse is seen as a regulator, modifier, and monitor of the environment.

Because the environment dramatically affects quality of life and individual health, it is a critical aspect of a comprehensive nursing assessment. Without careful attention to environmental influences, a nurse may miss important data and thereby misdiagnose a client's unique problems or misdirect nursing interventions to resolve them. Thus, assessment of the environment will help the nurse:

- Determine actual or potential environmental hazards
- Identify aspects of the environment that may be used or strengthened to promote or maintain a client's health, and
- Provide clients with feedback about elements in their environments that should be changed to reduce health risks and prevent illness.

An understanding of the complex interactions between people and their environments helps focus the nurse's assessment of a client's environment for strengths and for potential or actual health hazards.

PERSON–ENVIRONMENT–HEALTH RELATIONSHIP

The interdependence of humans and their environments has been long recognized and has received increasing attention in the latter part of the twentieth century as manipulation of the environment and the resulting noxious effects become more evident. The effects of air and water pollutants, toxic substances, hazardous wastes, radiation, and noise on human health and well-being have been the subject of much political debate and legislative action (Abelson, 1984). Although some attention was paid to pollution control in the early part of this century, since 1965 major legislative efforts have targeted environmental hazards. These efforts include the Clean Air and Solid Waste Disposal Act (1965), the Clean Water Restoration Act (1966), the Pesticides Control Act (1972), the Resource Conservation and Recovery Act (1974), and the Toxic Substances Control Act (1976). In addition, the Environmental Protection Agency (EPA) was created in 1970 to coordinate and administer federal efforts to protect and restore environmental resources.

Environmental standards have been established to regulate production, control, and disposal of many substances that pose risks to the environment and to human health. However, the benefits and advantages, whether real or perceived, gained by technological and biochemical advances sometimes outweigh the risks or at least cause the public to accept at some level the risks inherent in such advances (Lave, 1981). Willingness to accept or tolerate environmental risk may be motivated by psychological, social, or economic reasons. For example, coal miners risk health and safety to provide economic support for their families. The American public consumes billions of dollars worth of medications, tobacco, and alcohol for the perceived psychological benefits, despite known risks. Other examples of products that carry significant risks but use of which is tolerated and even encouraged because of their benefits include automobiles, pesticides, barbecue grills, and some food additives.

Much attention has been paid in recent years to studying the effects of environmental forces, including human manipulation of the environment, on biophysiological and psychosocial health (Figure 9-1). Advances in biomedical technology have altered daily lifestyles and the public's perceptions of health care dramatically. For instance, modern appliances and contraceptive control have freed

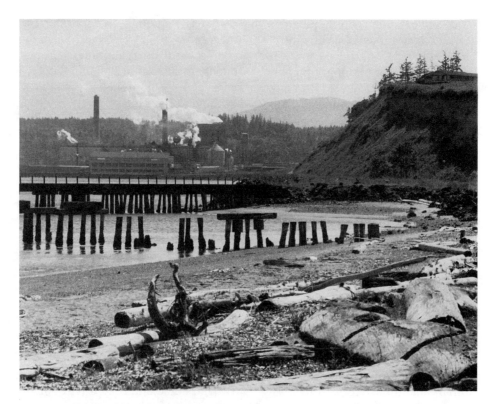

FIGURE 9-1. The effects of air and water pollutants, toxic substances, hazardous wastes, radiation, and noise on human health and well-being have been the subject of much political debate and legislative action.

women to develop interests beyond home and childbearing. The success of kidney dialysis and renal transplants has changed the public's view of such interventions from a privilege to a health-care right.

The impact of political, legal, and economic forces on the environment cannot be overstated. These forces in turn affect the quality of the environments in which people live. When gathering information for a nursing assessment, the nurse should be ever mindful of environmental influences on the client's health and attempt to determine what actual or potential environmental supports as well as hazards exist.

The relationship of health to the environment is illustrated graphically in Figure 9-2. Using this grid, one can predict health according to various person–environment interactions. For example, a healthy 4-year-old whose environment is favorable (i.e., proper food, clothing, and shelter, appropriate developmental stimulation, loving and caring parents) would tend toward "high level wellness." Another 4-year-old who lives in an unfavorable environment (i.e., homeless, inadequate clothing to keep warm, diet high in starch and low in protein, lack of appropriate developmental stimulation, and tired and distressed parents) may be said, in the absence of overt health problems, to have "emergent high level wellness." Such a child also may be said to be at greater risk for illness than the child living in the more favorable environment.

Studies of morbidity and mortality provide strong evidence that environment plays a promi-

nent role in health (MMWR, 1981; NCHS, 1985; Silverberg, 1985). It has been estimated that as much as 50% of U.S. mortality is due to unhealthy behavior or lifestyle, such as smoking, failure to use seat belts, or consumption of a high-fat diet; 20% due to environmental factors, such as pollution and toxic chemicals; 20% due to human biological factors (genetic constitution); and 10% to inadequacies in health care (*Healthy People*, 1979). Thus, nearly all causes of death in the United States relate in some way to environmental forces, whether naturally occurring or imposed by humans.

Ecological System

Humanity and the external environment are changing continuously, one adapting to the other. This interrelationship is termed the ecological system or *ecosystem*. Of particular concern to ecologists, who study the environment and its effects on people, is how people and their biological, physical, and sociocultural environments interact and are mediated by each individual's physiological and cognitive–perceptual characteristics. Figure 9-3 illustrates this relationship. The dotted line around the person indicates that matter, energy, and information are exchanged continually with the various environments.

Ideally a balance exists between people and their environments, with relatively equal exchange occurring, although the balance is never static; rather, it is homeostatic.

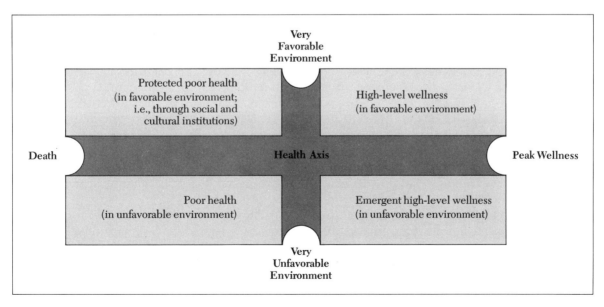

FIGURE 9-2. The Relationship of Health and Environment. (*Note.* From Dunn, H. "High-level Wellness for Man and Society," *American Journal of Public Health, 49,* 788 [June 1959]. Reprinted with permission.)

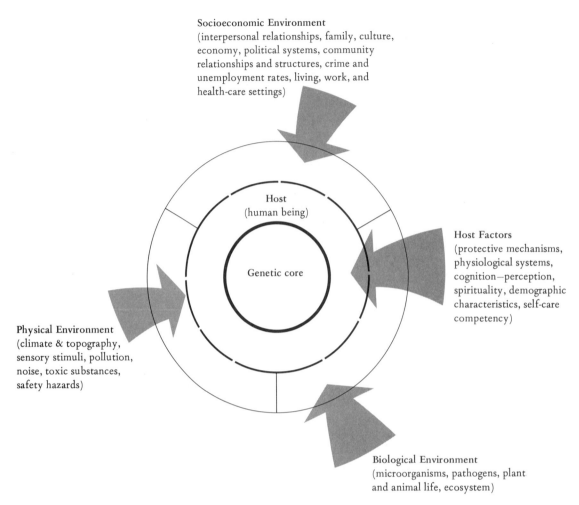

FIGURE 9-3. Interaction of Person and Environment.

Although homeostasis ideally involves a growth response, this may not necessarily result. *Adaptation* is a positive response to the environment and favors survival. *Tolerance*, on the other hand, eventually leads to diminished capacity.

Variations in the exchange between person and environment occur, but within defined limits. These limits are determined by the nature of the person–environment interchange. The limits of neurochemical regulation, such as blood pH, are narrow and sensitive to minute changes in the internal environment, whereas the acceptable limits for social interaction between two people are wide and allow for much greater variation. Typically, variations in person–environment interchange are predictable, whether they are governed by physiological regulatory mechanisms, cognitive factors, or social norms.

Biological rhythms are one example of predictable variations. Circadian rhythms are of particular relevance. Circadian rhythms are bodily changes, such as body temperature variation and sleep–

wake cycles, that occur in humans approximately every 24 hours and are influenced by internal regulatory mechanisms as well as external cues (Mason, 1988; Luce, 1970). External cues that influence the period, timing, and intensity of cyclic variations include light, temperature, sound, pattern of daily activities, and social cues. For instance, Czeisler and colleagues (1987) found that bright lights have a profound influence on wakefulness independent of the individual's biological sleep–wake cycle. Synchronization of the various daily biological rhythms and the environment is essential to optimal health (Luce, 1970).

The body's various physiological processes operate on several different biological rhythms (e.g., cycles of a few hours, days, or months). When a person's biological rhythms become dysrhythmic (out of synchrony with the environment), it may take as long as two weeks for all processes to return to their usual pattern. A number of environmental forces may alter a person's biological rhythms, such as jet travel across different time zones, rotating shifts at work, surgery and anesthesia, some medications, sensory overload or deprivation, or unfamiliar environments (Moore-Ede, Sulzman, & Fuller, 1982).

Humans adapt to environmental circumstances in a number of ways. They may try to change their perceptions of environmental circumstances or to alter the way they cope with these conditions. For example, a person in a traffic jam may decide that it is not useful to become frustrated (perception) and may decide instead to listen to a relaxing song on the radio (coping). If the person feels stressed by the traffic jam and worries about getting somewhere on time, a "fight or flight" response will occur. If the person merely tolerates such situations repeatedly, instead of adapting, "burnout" of physiological and psychological systems is likely to happen.

Another mode of adapting to the environment is to manipulate it to better meet human needs. Technological advances are an example of this type of environmental manipulation. From such early developments as the wheel to such technically sophisticated devices as dynamos and computers, humans have made the environment work for them. In the course of these developments, numerous artificial pollutants (or artificially induced pollutants) have become part of the environment responsible for deleterious health conditions.

People can adapt to a vast range of environmental circumstances, but there are certain limits beyond which they cannot adapt without specific intervention. Humans cannot endure extremes of temperature, water and food supply, or physical injury without specific measures to assist adaptation. Also, a person in poor health has a diminished capacity for adapting to environmental extremes. For example, a person under stress has decreased immunologic functions with which to combat microbial invasion. An individual in a critical care unit who is attached to several monitors and subjected to invasive treatments (e.g., intravenous therapy, nasogastric suction) is unable to manipulate the environment to cope with sensory overload.

Certain individual characteristics influence adaptive capacity. Among these is the age of the person. The very young and the elderly have limited adaptive capabilities. Because an infant's nervous system is immature and because the infant lacks experience, it cannot evaluate the external environment and its situation to meet its needs. The elderly have difficulty coping with the multiple stressors common at their stage of life because their sensory capacities are decreased, their musculoskeletal functioning is impaired, and one or more chronic diseases usually are present.

Exposure to the environment occurs through a number of routes, such as eating, drinking, breathing, and penetration of the skin. For example, an individual may be exposed to residual levels of antibiotics in meat, Nutrasweet in diet drinks, and carbon monoxide and lead from automobile exhaust—all while eating at an outdoor restaurant near the noise of a busy street!

Perception of the environment is modulated by the cerebral cortex. Perception of the same situation often varies remarkably from one person to another, as studies of eyewitness accounts have demonstrated graphically. These variations result from the attributes each person brings to the situation, such as past experiences, cultural biases, the values attached to the event, and such physical characteristics as the integrity of the sensory system and the individual's overall health.

Thus, many factors influence the individual's adaptive responses to changing environmental circumstances.

Epidemiological Framework

The epidemiological approach to assessing a client's environment is useful because it takes into account the interaction of the client and the environment as it contributes to health. Although epidemiology most often refers to the study of the incidence distribution and control of disease or injury within population groups, it is also useful for examining the potential risk for health problems in specific populations for designing and implementing strategies that promote health and prevent illness.

Epidemiology is concerned with three interacting variables that together form the "epidemiologic triangle." These variables are the *agent*, the *host*, and the *environment*. The agent is a substance or force that may cause a specific illness or injury. It is the primary cause, without which illness or injury would not occur. However, the agent must find a host and an environment conducive to its invasion or action. The host is a person who may be infected or affected by the agent, resulting in disease or injury to the host. The environment consists of all external factors that either contribute to or interfere with host–agent interaction.

The interaction of agent–host–environment depends on the specific characteristics of each. These characteristics are depicted in Table 9-1, with examples of specific factors that may contribute to the occurrence of disease or injury. To illustrate the agent–host–environment interaction, consider the incidence of falls in the elderly. The elderly person (host) may have certain characteristics, such as im-

TABLE 9-1
Agent, Host, and Environmental Factors That Contribute to the Prevalence of Illness and Injury

Category	Examples
Agent	
Biological	Microorganisms, allergens, vitamins, proteins, fats, cholesterol
Chemical	Medications, poisons, toxic chemical wastes, insecticides
Physical	Radiation, safety hazards, mechanical devices
Host	
Hereditary factors	Genes, chromosomes, family history
Age, developmental level	
Gender	
Racial/ethnic group	
Health	Nutritional state, physiologic functioning, immunologic response (hypersensitivity, immunization history, previous infection), presence of disease
Lifestyle factors	Shelter, hygiene, education/ occupation, leisure, social support, interpersonal relationships, type and frequency of unhealthful behaviors (smoking, alcohol, drugs, sedentary lifestyle), health-promoting behaviors (balanced diet, auto seatbelt use, adequate sleep, regular exercise)
Environment	
Biological	Disease carriers, food sources, ecosystem
Physical	Climate, topography, sensory stimuli; exposure to toxic substances, safety hazards; natural or man-made disasters (earthquakes, floods, tornadoes, hurricanes, nuclear plant leaks)
Socioeconomic	Population density, social isolation; family, culture; political and economic systems; organizational milieu; community structures and relationships; crime and unemployment rates; health-care resources; human assistance programs

paired vision, decreased muscular agility, and slowed response time, all of which increase susceptibility to accidental injury. The agent may be a wet bathroom floor, poorly fitting shoes, or an un-secured rug. The environment may include such factors as inadequate lighting, stairs, or inadequate finances to install handrails. The interaction of agent, host, and environment may result in a fall and subsequent injury. If a fall causes an elderly person to sustain a fractured hip, the fracture itself becomes a new agent that may cause further injury or illness, depending on its interaction with the host and the environment. Host characteristics in this instance may include the person's nutritional and immunological status, stress and coping responses, and the presence or absence of other illness. Access to adequate and affordable health care, family support, and medical technology are examples of positive environmental factors that can influence host–agent interaction and lead to favorable outcomes for the client.

Because of the strong connections among the agent, host, and environment, a comprehensive nursing assessment should include attention to all three. The focus of this chapter, however, is devoted primarily to assessing characteristics of the environment for factors that may influence agent–host interaction, although agent and host characteristics cannot be ignored. Certain agents and the host are brought together by the environment, which in turn influences their particular characteristics and interrelationships. The environment thus may be seen as a variable intervening between agent and host.

PARAMETERS OF ENVIRONMENTAL ASSESSMENT

The three major environmental parameters that influence agent–host interaction and, ultimately, health status may be categorized as *biological, physical,* and *socioeconomic.* These environmental parameters should be included in a comprehensive nursing assessment of any client because of the significant role that environmental factors play in health. These parameters are summarized in Table 9-2. The nurse should keep in mind that these parameters affect the client's home, community, work, school, and health-care environments. Each of these settings may contribute to or interfere with a client's health and well-being and thus should not be overlooked.

Biological Environment

Millions of microorganisms inhabit the environment in which humans live. Most of these probably are not harmful to people, and many are in fact helpful. Microorganisms (agents) that cause disease in people are called pathogens. Some diseases

TABLE 9-2
Parameters of the Environment Related to Health

Biological Environment

　Microorganisms, pathogens
　Plant and animal life
　Ecosystem
　Health risk factors (exposure, susceptibility to disease; hereditary predisposition)
　Specific protection from disease (immunizations, isolation precautions, waste disposal, refrigeration, water treatment, personal hygiene practices)

Physical Environment

　Climate and topography
　Sensory stimuli
　Pollution, noise, toxic substances
　Physical facilities (architecture, access, space, condition)
　Safety hazards (e.g., electrical, chemical, traffic/vehicle, architectural obstacles)
　Personal health habits (diet, use of seatbelts, substance use/abuse, exercise)

Socioeconomic Environment

　Social network (interpersonal relationships, family, community organizations, self-help groups, religious affiliations)
　Social control
　Locus of control
　Territoriality (space, privacy, crowding vs. isolation)
　Economy (cost/standard of living, personal income, unemployment rates, government vs. private resources)
　Services (educational and health facilities, police and fire protection, social and economic welfare services)

that result from pathogens include measles, mumps, chickenpox, and herpes.

Pathogenic biological agents include bacteria, viruses, fungi, rickettsiae, yeasts, molds, and protozoa. Some biologic agents are more virulent than others; they cause pathogenesis more easily than others, or they are more likely to cause a disease of greater severity. The host may or may not become ill as a result of the biologic agent's infestation. A carrier is a host who harbors the infectious agent within the body but does not become ill. Carriers may, however, spread the microorganisms to other people so that they become ill. An example is that of the chronic dialysis patient who may be a carrier of hepatitis and does not become ill with the disease, but unknowingly spreads it to the dialysis staff by way of bodily secretions, fluids, and mists. The staff so infected may develop acute, and occasionally chronic, clinical cases of hepatitis.

Conditions within the environment are usually more or less favorable to such factors as:

The development of the pathogen in the first place (this includes development of varying degrees of virulence and resistance).

The spread of the pathogen to the host.

The development of disease in the host.

The course of the disease in the host (i.e., whether the host recovers or dies, and the various potential complications during the course of the disease).

A common example of environmental conditions that favor pathogenesis is malaria. Because malarial pathogens develop in anopheles mosquitoes, anopheles mosquitoes are a necessary part of the life cycle of the malarial parasite. Swamps, dumps, and pools of stagnant water are breeding grounds for mosquitoes; they are environmental conditions favorable to the development of the pathogenic organism, which is transmitted to the host by a vector (the mosquito). Malaria is endemic (normally present) to tropical and subtropical areas such as Africa, Southeast Asia, and Central and South America.

In the example given, a relationship called the *chain of infection* has been implied. This term refers to the sequence of events that takes place when pathogenesis occurs. The chain of infection is depicted in Figure 9-4.

The impact of the biological environment on a client's health is influenced by several factors. These include exposure to disease, susceptibility, and hereditary predisposition, as well as specific measures to avert disease, such as immunizations, appropriate use of isolation precautions, water treatment, proper disposal of wastes, and personal hygiene practices (e.g., bathing, handwashing, dental care). Risk appraisal and risk reduction are discussed more thoroughly later in this chapter.

Physical Environment

The physical environment consists of the macroenvironment, the ambient environment, and the personal environment (Figure 9-5). These categories are not mutually exclusive. They overlap considerably.

Macroenvironment refers to the elements in the physical world in which humans live. This aspect of the physical environment includes noise and vibration; air, water, and soil pollution; climate; and topography. Noise is unwanted or undesirable sound that arouses, distresses, or overloads the senses. Loud noise, especially if it is continuous, interferes with social interaction and decreases

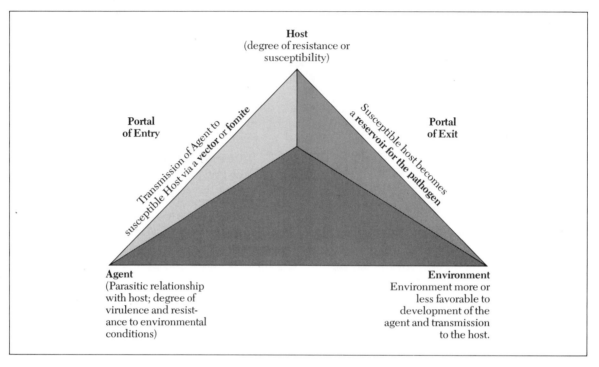

FIGURE 9-4. The Chain of Infection. (*Note. From Preventive Medicine for the Doctor in His Community*, 3rd ed., by H.R. Leavell and E.G. Clark. Copyright © 1965 by McGraw-Hill Book Company. Reprinted by permission.)

sensitivity to others. It also may engender angry and aggressive responses to people or situations. Noise may affect health adversely (e.g., with temporary or permanent hearing impairment). The type and intensity of noise, proximity to the individual, length of exposure, and person's age and health affect the degree of actual or potential damage to hearing. The EPA has identified sounds above 55 decibels as potentially harmful to human hearing. Common machinery with decibel levels greater than 55 include vacuum cleaners, auto-

matic dishwashers, lawnmowers, heavy farm equipment, jet engines, motorcycles, heavy traffic, loud stereo music, and live rock and rap music. Hot weather may create discomfort or distress and has been linked to higher crime rates (Harries & Stadler, 1983). Thus, the macroenvironment has a major effect on human health and functioning.

The *ambient environment* refers to elements present in the areas in which humans live, work, and play. Examples include the design and layout of living spaces and work or school settings as well

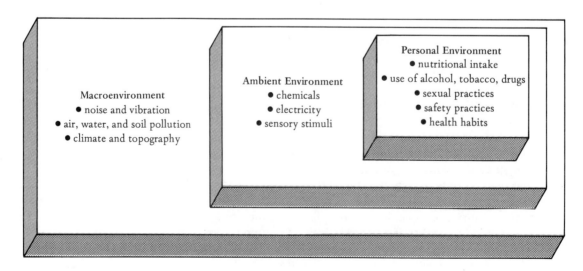

FIGURE 9-5. Components of the Physical Environment.

as architectural design and accessibility. For instance, the appearance and arrangement of a room can have a profound impact on productivity and on interpersonal behavior (Sundstrom, 1986) (Figure 9-6). Rooms with seating arrangements within personal distance (1½ to 4 feet apart) and facing each other tend to encourage interaction, whereas those with seats arranged in rows or at social distance (4 to 12 feet apart) tend to discourage interaction. Conference rooms and dining halls are examples of the former; large classrooms, clinic waiting rooms, and airport waiting areas illustrate the latter.

Architecture may increase or interfere with accessibility to a home, work, or school. Much attention has been paid in recent years to overcoming architectural barriers for disabled people when designing new buildings or renovating old ones. Less obvious but as important is the influence of architecture, esthetics, and residential planning. For example, easy access to essential services, such as grocery and drug stores, schools, public transportation, and health-care facilities; adequate lighting (natural and artificial) in homes and offices; and aesthetically pleasing recreational environments may enhance health and well-being. Conversely, difficult access, harsh or inadequate lighting, and deteriorating recreational areas may affect people's health and daily functioning adversely.

The *personal environment* encompasses those components of daily living within a person's immediate control and influenced by personal choice. The personal environment is determined by such factors as an individual's nutritional intake, smoking or substance abuse, health habits, and safety practices.

The physical environment is a source of stress. Stress may be beneficial or harmful and can result from necessary sensory stimulation or overstimulation. For example, sensory stimulation provides variety in daily life and can motivate people to greater productivity and satisfaction when available in the quality and quantity judged pleasing and meaningful by the individual. Conversely, too much sensory stimulation, or "environmental overload," can result in confusion, agitation, paranoia, and hallucinations. Insufficiently meaningful sensory stimulation can have similar consequences, including disorientation, faulty perception, impaired reasoning and memory, and hallucinations.

Overstimulation may cause irritation, hypersensitivity, or toxicity. Certain colors, sounds, and smells may be a nuisance (irritation) and, if present on a daily basis, a major stressor. Exposure to dusts, pollens, molds, and food additives can result in hypersensitivity in predisposed individuals. Some environmental substances can be toxic (lethal) to humans in very small amounts (e.g., botulism) or in larger amounts than the body can tolerate (e.g., radiation).

Socioeconomic Environment

The socioeconomic environment encompasses the network of people and organizations with whom the individual interacts directly and indirectly. This

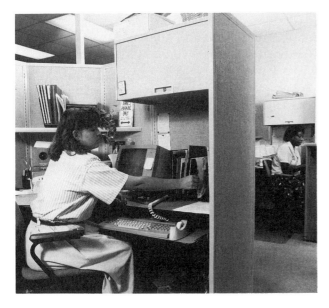
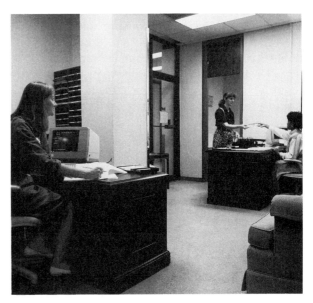

FIGURE 9-6. The design and layout of work space can have a profound impact on productivity and interpersonal behavior.

network includes family members, friends, co-workers, teachers, merchants, work superiors, schools, churches, and various administrative networks. It also includes the social, political, and economic systems of the community and the larger society, because what happens in these systems sooner or later affects the individual to some degree. For example, widespread unemployment or high crime rates in a community have a direct bearing on an individual's lifestyle.

Although it is easy to understand the importance of the social environment to a client's behavior, values, and needs, there are still no clear-cut criteria for delineating a "good" or "bad" social milieu. Various studies have, however, described characteristics of social networks as well as variables within the individual and the physical environment that mediate the influence of the social environment on the individual. These parameters include the individual's social network, perceived social control, and economic status.

Social Network

An individual's social network consists of people with whom the person has some kind of relationship—from the most intimate to quite distant. The people who compose this network may or may not have relationships among themselves.

What functions do social networks serve? Human beings have a lifelong need for social support or attachment. For infants, forming strong bonds with another constitutes the primary developmental task of establishing a sense of trust. Acceptance within one's peer group is crucial to the maintenance of self-esteem during adolescence, and formation of an intimate relationship with another person is vital during young adulthood. Recent studies have shown that mentor relationships assist with healthy adult development. Disengagement theory proposes that one of the tasks of older adults is letting go of earlier relationships. Social networks, then, contribute to healthy development throughout life.

Shrock (1980) points out that healthy development is fostered when a person's social network appropriately provides both affective and instrumental support. *Affective support* is emotional; it helps people develop feelings of belonging and positive self-esteem. *Instrumental support* helps people accomplish tangible goals, such as sharing goods and services within a community. Neighbors often provide one another with this kind of support.

Many types of social support—including family support, community organizations, religious affiliations, and self-help groups—are both effective and instrumental. For example, self-help groups such as Weight Watchers and Alcoholics Anonymous assist people to achieve specific goals while also enhancing their self-worth and sense of shared support.

Recent research suggests that social support is a critical factor for good health (Dimond & Jones, 1982; Hubbard, Muhlenkamp, & Brown, 1984; Muhlenkamp & Sayles, 1986; Norbeck, 1981). Social support buffers the effects of stress on individual health and coping by altering a person's perception of a stressful event, by helping a person develop effective coping strategies, and by mediating the individual's response to distress (House & Kahn, 1985). Thus, attention to the client's social network can provide important clues to health and behavior (Figure 9-7).

Perceived Social Control

The degree of control that individuals believe they exercise over their lives and their environment is an important aspect to consider when assessing the socioeconomic environment. Two concepts that have special relevance for this assessment are locus of control and territorial behavior.

Locus of Control. Rotter (1966) theorizes that a major variable in how people interact with the environment is the extent to which they believe that what happens to them is the result of their own efforts and actions or is due to chance. People who believe they exert a strong influence over the shape and direction of their lives are said to have an *internal locus of control.* Those who believe that luck, fate, chance, or powerful others control their lives

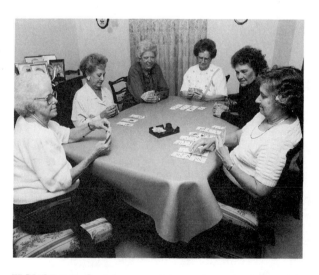

FIGURE 9-7. Social support is an important factor in human health.

have an *external locus of control*. Rotter and his colleagues have developed a personality scale of "internal versus external control"; the scale is composed of sets of statements from which subjects must make a choice (for example, "I can control my own fate" versus "Much that happens to me is probably a matter of luck").

Collins (1974) suggests that internal versus external locus of control depends largely on whether the individual lives in a world that is easy or hard, just or unjust, predictable or unpredictable, and politically responsive or unresponsive. Collins's theory may be used to explain why people reared in poverty, those from minority groups, and victims of abuse or oppression often exhibit behaviors that indicate an external locus of control. If individuals perceive their world as difficult, unjust, unpredictable, and politically unresponsive to their needs, they are less likely to believe that they control their own fate or have the power to change the course of their lives.

The degree of control that people believe they have over their lives may influence greatly their responses to illness, hospitalization, and health-care professionals. For instance, clients who exhibit an internal locus of control usually take a more active role in their health-care practices because they believe their actions do, in fact, make a difference to health and well-being. When confronted with a serious illness, they are more likely to have a positive attitude about its outcome and to take actions to increase the likelihood of success or at least cope with the illness in a positive way. Conversely, clients with an external locus of control often say that what they do makes little or no difference to the outcomes of illness or health care, and their behaviors reflect this belief.

Locus of control is closely related to an individual's motivation, achievement, success, ability to delay gratification, and ability to cope with and adapt to stress and change. Locus of control of health (beliefs about influences that affect health) may be linked to preventive measures. When people believe they can influence their health and improve it, rather than leaving it to chance or fate, they may be more likely to initiate health-promoting behaviors (Zindler-Wernet & Weiss, 1987). Many variables influence locus of control, including family and cultural beliefs and norms as well as the individual's unique life experiences.

Territorial Behavior. People interact with their environments within the context of space. Space includes not only the physical space that one's body and possessions occupy but also dimensions of personal and interpersonal space. Territorial behavior may be defined as the behavior an individual displays toward his or her personal and interpersonal space, or territory, particularly behavior that is used to defend the territory. Territorial behavior is learned within the context of one's family and culture. Some cultural or family groups staunchly defend their territories by not allowing outsiders to "invade" their territory physically, emotionally, or socially. For example, a family might protect its territory by not allowing a nurse to make a home visit or by refusing to disclose personal family information.

The degree of territorial behavior an individual or group exhibits seems to be related to the degree of security they perceive they have in their environment, and the degree of control they exercise. The less secure they feel, or the greater the perceived threat to their territory, the more territorial behaviors they will manifest.

To an extent, an individual's age may be correlated with manifestations of territorial behavior. Young children, especially toddlers and preschoolers, tend to be very possessive of their bodies and their belongings. They often become quite resistive during assessment or nursing intervention procedures, particularly ones that are invasive, such as temperature-taking or an otoscopic examination. This characteristic behavior is related to the fact that young children are just beginning to be aware of their bodies and of themselves as distinct beings. Any perceived threat to their body wholeness or their possessions (which they see as extensions of themselves) may cause them to retreat or to try to defend themselves physically.

All humans exhibit territorial behaviors to some extent. Having a home and allotted space within the home (such as a bedroom or bed), a personal office or work space, a desk and locker at school, or an assigned bed or room in a hospital or long-term care facility helps an individual maintain a sense of security and control in these environments.

Territoriality is an especially important concept in the care of clients in health-care settings because it is often perceived as the territory of the workers rather than the clients. People who are ill are vulnerable to threats to their territory because they have less energy with which to defend themselves and their space. Ill clients may expend a great deal of energy protecting themselves in such situations, leaving less energy to deal with the physiological and emotional demands imposed by the illness itself.

Unfortunately, blatant invasion of a client's territory is common in health-care settings. Staff often talk about clients to others in their presence, enter and leave their rooms without asking permission, and institute treatments or procedures without first explaining and preparing the client. Staff often are unaware of how their behaviors, which they take for granted, may threaten a client's sense of security and control.

It is important to assess clients for behaviors that may indicate their attempts to protect their physical, personal, and interpersonal space or territory. This is true whether the client is at home, at work or school, or in a health-care setting such as a clinic or hospital. For example,

Does the client have his or her own space

- At home: does the client have his or her own bed or room, a particular place at the dinner table, a favorite chair?
- At work: does the client have a personal work space, desk, place to keep belongings?
- In the hospital: Does the client have the same room and bed assignment from admission to discharge whenever possible?

To what extent is the client's privacy and modesty respected?

Is the client allowed to keep personal possessions while hospitalized (own pajamas, robe, or clothes, attachment objects)?

Altman's (1975) theory that maintenance of a desired level of privacy is a basic need that influences much of human behavior provides support for the concept of territoriality. Altman suggests that variations of personal space and territorial mechanisms are the means by which individuals maintain privacy and control. Crowding or social isolation occurs when these mechanisms are inef-

fective. Figure 9-8 illustrates the relationships of privacy, personal space, and territory that may result in crowding or social isolation.

Economic Environment

The client's economic status is an important facet of the socioeconomic environment. Having an income adequate to meet living expenses provides people with a sense of control and security. Economic status has been correlated with health; people in lower income groups are generally at greater risk for developing health problems. They may lack the financial resources to gain access to food, warm shelter, clothing, and health care, and they face additional stressors in trying to meet their basic human needs. People in middle and upper income brackets also may face economic stress as a result of pressures to get ahead, overspending, or the threat of unemployment in a tight job market. Elderly people often face financial pressures if they live on fixed incomes in an inflationary economy.

Assessing the client's economic status is an important part of the environmental assessment, but inquiries concerning personal income may be perceived as invasive by some clients. It may be more helpful to ask the client about level of satisfaction with current income and whether the client is experiencing any financial distress. If so, the nurse should identify sources of economic stress, their degree of severity, and how the client is managing (or planning to manage) the problem. More important, the nurse should ascertain the client's perception of the impact of economic distress on health and well-being. Is it interfering with daily functioning, such as sleeping and eating, or with interpersonal relationships or job performance?

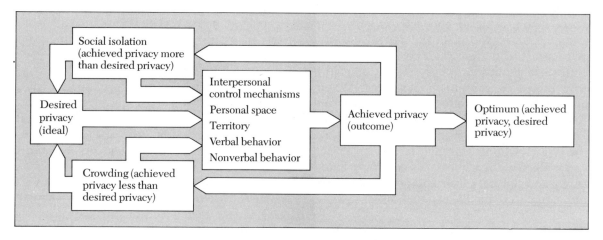

FIGURE 9-8. Overview of Relationships of Privacy, Personal Space, Territory, and Crowding. (*Note.* Adapted from *The Environment and Social Behavior,* by I. Altman. Copyright © 1975 by Wadsworth Publishing Company [Copyright © 1981 by Irwin Altman]. Reprinted by permission.)

The client's income should be evaluated in relation to local cost-of-living standards. An annual income of $30,000 may provide a decent standard of living in some locales, whereas in others it would be inadequate to meet expenses, depending on family size, availability of affordable housing, and transportation costs. The community's unemployment rates and human assistance programs also influence the quality of the economic environment, and should be assessed.

It is particularly important to ascertain the client's ability to pay for health care. Health-care facilities may be available, but if the client cannot afford to pay or is inadequately insured or uninsured, accessibility to needed services will be hampered.

Socioeconomic Services

The availability of and accessibility to services in the community are crucial factors to assess since lack of adequate resources or failure to use them may be detrimental to the client. Factors that influence the quality of socioeconomic services include the economic base of the community, government funding of services, private (e.g., business or philanthropic) support, and personnel qualifications and attributes. Use of services may depend on a variety of factors, including a client's beliefs and values (see chap. 8), the public images of various services, and accessibility (e.g., affordability, proximity, days/hours service is available, and transportation).

Attention should be given to determining the quality, accessibility, and acceptability of such socioeconomic services as schools, day care for children, elders, and others with special needs, health-care facilities and services, police and fire protection, recreational facilities, and social and economic welfare agencies. A community's ability to provide adequate socioeconomic services can reduce crime, drug use, homelessness, and illiteracy, thereby improving the health, safety, and well-being of all its residents.

COMPONENTS OF ENVIRONMENTAL ASSESSMENT

Every person spends each day in a variety of environments. Each person's environment encompasses the Earth on which we all live, a specific geographic location in which he or she exists at any given point in time, and the unique contexts of home, work, school, or play, which vary from person to person. Thus, there are some components of the environment that everyone shares, such as the changing ozone layer of the Earth, and some specific to each individual, such as the place in which one sleeps. Each environment plays a role in individual health and well-being. The relative influence of each depends on a number of factors. These include the amount of time the person spends in the specific environment each day, the individual's perception of the environment as a positive, neutral, or negative influence, and the supports or hazards that exist and enhance or interfere with the person's health and well-being. For example, an infant who spends most of her waking hours in a playpen with little or no stimulation may be safe from physical injury but unable to explore and learn from the environment beyond.

Because the environment is so inextricably connected with health and well-being, it is essential to ascertain in what kinds of environments a client lives, works, and plays in order to assess whether they are supportive, potentially detrimental, or clearly hazardous. Typically, a nurse collects information about two major environments in which clients spend the greatest part of their daily lives: the home environment, which includes the surrounding neighborhood and community, and the work, school, or day care environment. In addition, because so much nurse–client contact takes place in health-care settings away from the client's home, work, or school environment, the nurse should be cognizant of factors in the health-care environment that contribute to or interfere with a client's well-being. For example, when assessing a 4-year-old girl who attends a full-day preschool program, the nurse should gather information about the child's home, neighborhood, and school environments. If a 45-year-old male factory worker is hospitalized with hypertension, it would be important to assess aspects of the client's home, work, and hospital environments to determine their previous, current, and potential effects on the client's health.

Nurses working in a hospital setting also should collect information about the hospitalized client's home to plan appropriately for the client's discharge. Nursing care delivered in day care centers, schools, and the workplace should reflect an understanding of the ways in which those settings influence clients' health, especially because people spend many of their waking hours in one or more of these places.

Environmental data should be collected and evaluated from the perspective of the client's age. How a client responds to outside influences depends largely on the maturity and integrity of that individual's physiological and psychological coping mechanisms, as well as the individual's needs in relation to growth and development. Generally, the very young and the very old are more vulnerable to alterations in environmental conditions. For example, newborns and the aged have difficulty coping with extremes in temperature. In newborns, thermoregulatory mechanisms are incompletely developed. In the aged, the efficiency of those same mechanisms is diminished.

A major developmental task of adulthood is involvement in some kind of satisfying productive work. The safety of the work environment and the extent to which work is a source of satisfaction or anxiety are major concerns at this stage.

Occupational safety regulations, such as standards of the federal Occupational Safety & Health Administration (OSHA), and surveillance systems for monitoring health risks in the workplace are important aspects of a comprehensive assessment of a client's work environment (Froines, Dellenbaugh, & Wegman, 1986).

Because children spend such a large portion of their lives in school, the quality of their school environment should be assessed. Attention to the physical environment, biological hazards, and cognitive/social influences is essential. Increasing numbers of children spend extended hours in afterschool programs or as latchkey children. Assessment of the afterschool environment as it contributes to or inhibits the child's physical safety and mental health should not be neglected.

Assessment of specific clients in each type of setting (home and neighborhood, school or work, and health care) is determined by the particular advantages or hazards that those settings pose for individuals of different ages. Tables 9-3, 9-4, and 9-5 illustrate assessment parameters of biophysiological and socioeconomic assessment in various settings. These parameters are not all-inclusive; rather, they are intended as guides that may be adapted to a particular client's situation.

SELECTED TOOLS FOR ASSESSING THE CLIENT'S ENVIRONMENT

Generally speaking, Tables 9-3, 9-4, and 9-5 provide an adequate and comprehensive guide for assessing a client's environment. Occasionally, however, it may be helpful to assess a specific component of the environment, such as locus of control, social support, or particular environmental hazards (e.g., noise or pollution), or to use an assessment tool that is age-specific, in order to gain a more complete picture of the variables influencing a client's health. Two tools selected for inclusion in

this chapter represent situation-specific types of environmental assessment: the "Home Screening Questionnaire" (Coons, Gay, Fandal, Ker, & Frankenburg, 1981; see Figures 9-9 and 9-10) for its potential to aid in early detection of environmental problems that may contribute to developmental delays in childhood, and Burnside's (1988) guide to "Assessment of Home Safety for the Elderly" (see Figure 9-11), the purpose of which is to detect hazards in the home environment of elderly persons. These assessment tools are relatively easy to administer, are cost-effective, and provide information for a more comprehensive assessment of the client's environment.

Home Screening Questionnaire (HSQ)

The Home Screening Questionnaire (HSQ) was developed to assess the adequacy of a child's home environment for promoting optimal development (Coons et al., 1981). The tool is designed to screen the home environment of low income children under age 6 who are from American, English-speaking homes. The sample population on which the HSQ was standardized included children of black and Hispanic as well as Anglo origins. There are two versions of the questionnaire—one for children under age 3 (0–3 HSQ) and one for children aged 3 to 6 (3–6 HSQ).

The purpose of the HSQ is to detect children who are at risk for developmental delays and later school problems as a result of the environment's failure to support their optimal development. The tool is based on the assumption that the home environment can support or inhibit a child's development, depending on the quality and quantity of social, emotional, and cognitive supports.

The HSQ is based on Caldwell's (1970, 1975) more extensive Home Observation Measurement of the Environment (H.O.M.E.). The H.O.M.E. requires that a trained interviewer visit the home to complete the inventory, which is both costly and time-consuming. Conversely, the HSQ may be completed by a parent in a health care or school setting. The HSQ specifically targets children of poverty because it has been determined that the H.O.M.E., on which the HSQ is based, does not yield reliable information in middle and upper income populations.

The HSQ, written at a fourth grade reading level, consists of multiple choice, fill-in-the-blank, and yes/no questions, plus a toy inventory checklist. If the parent is unable to read the items, the interviewer may ask them of the parent and record the answers. Upon completion, the HSQ is scored

TABLE 9-3
Critical Assessment Parameters of Home/Neighborhood/Community Environment

I. Physical-biological environment

Pollutants/allergens/noise

Is the home dusty? Is mildew or mold present?

Sources of dust? How is dust controlled?

Are there pets in the household? Does child sleep with stuffed animals?

Is home air-conditioned or is there an air filtration system?

Does client have food allergies? Other allergies? What are the symptoms? How are they controlled?

Is there smoke from cigarettes, cigars, pipes?

Sources of water supply? Are there potentially harmful chemical additives in the water?

City sewer or septic tank? Any sanitation problems?

Are pools or lakes for swimming properly maintained?

What is noise level in household (e.g., loud stereo or TV)? In neighborhood?

Climate/susceptibility to pathogens

How is home heated? Ventilated?

Is income adequate to pay heating bills?

Are there means for cooling the home during extremely hot weather (air conditioning, fans)?

Is climate temperate? What are seasonal variations in temperature? Is climate dry, humid, rainy?

Is the community at risk for natural or manmade disasters (e.g., floods, mudslides, tornadoes, hurricanes, earthquakes, nuclear power plant leaks)?

Does the altitude pose any health risks?

Are home and neighborhood free of infestation and breeding grounds?

Is there adequate refrigeration to prevent food spoilage?

Is home sufficiently clean to prevent infestations?

Are hygiene practices (handwashing, dishwashing, laundry, trash disposal) adequate to minimize cross-contamination?

Are immunizations current for all family members?

Have elderly family members received flu immunizations?

Does individual avoid exposure to others with communicable diseases?

Does sexually active person use "safe sex" practices?

Physical safety

Are electrical outlets plugged or covered? Are electrical cords in safe condition, tucked behind furniture or under rugs? Are outlets not overloaded?

Are electric lights, appliances, equipment in safe condition? Are they used safely?

Are smoke detectors and fire extinguishers present and in working condition? Is fireplace or woodstove protected?

Is home painted with lead-free paint? Are there other hazardous sources of lead in the home or neighborhood?

Are chemicals such as cleaning products, paints, or gasoline stored safely (and out of reach of inquisitive children)?

Is house adequately ventilated (especially when using paints, solvents, oven cleaners)?

Are medications properly labeled and stored (and out of reach of young children)?

Is there any evidence of substance abuse (alcohol, prescription or street drugs, glue or gasoline sniffing)?

Is client familiar with medications (dosage, frequency, side effects, drug interactions)?

Are there traffic hazards (is the home on a busy street)? Are there safe play areas? Do individual and family members observe safe driving/passenger practices (auto safety belts or child car restraints, crash helmet on motorcycle, not driving while drinking or taking certain medications)?

Do physical facilities of the home present any obstacles or hazards (number of rooms, stairs, plumbing, refrigeration, furniture)?

Is home/neighborhood in safe condition (no broken stairs, loose rugs, broken glass on playgrounds and sidewalks)?

II. Socioeconomic environment

Social environment

Are family relationships supportive and stable?

To what extent is individual involved in family and community activities? In what ways?

How does individual relate to authority?

What is geographic proximity to extended family? To friends? To community resources (e.g., grocery stores, retail businesses, schools)?

Are social activities age-appropriate (see chaps. 10 and 11)?

Are social relationships satisfying and stable? Is there evidence of social isolation or loneliness?

Is there adequate space in the home and neighborhood for personal needs and privacy?

Are there feelings of esteem and pride in the home/neighborhood/community? How are these exhibited?

Does individual express feelings of being "in control" of his or her life (within realistic limits imposed by age and other limitations)? Or does individual express feelings of powerlessness, helplessness, and hopelessness?

Does environment provide age-appropriate stimulation? Is it pleasant to live in?

What services (health, social, religious, educational)

(continued)

TABLE 9-3 (Continued)

does the community offer? Are they accessible? Acceptable?

What is crime rate in the neighborhood/community?

What precautions does client exercise (does not go out alone at night, locks on doors and windows, neighborhood "crime watch")?

Economic environment

Sources of income? Is income adequate to meet living expenses?

Is there financial stress in the home (unemployed family member, overspending) or community (widespread unemployment, inadequate funds for human services)?

to determine whether the child's home environment is "suspect" or "nonsuspect." If suspect, a more thorough evaluation of the home environment with a tool such as the H.O.M.E. is indicated. Coons et al. (1981) recommend that the HSQ be used in conjunction with the Denver II, a developmental screening test [see chap. 10] to detect developmental problems that may result from the home environment as well as those that may be due to biological or genetic insults.

Sample questions from both versions of the HSQ are presented in Figures 9-9 and 9-10. The administration and scoring of the questionnaire

should be followed carefully to ensure its validity and reliability (Coons et al., 1981).

It is important to remember that the HSQ is designed to *screen* the child's home environment. It does not predict future development or diagnose developmental problems that stem from inadequacies in the home environment. More in-depth evaluation is indicated if the results of the HSQ are suspect. If the nurse decides to administer the HSQ, it is important to assure that follow-up evaluation is available before proceeding. Intervention programs to help parents modify the home environment also should be available. There is little

TABLE 9-4
Critical Assessment Parameters of Work, School, or Day Care Environment

1. Physical-biological environment

What allergens or irritants are present (dusts, mists, chemicals, fumes, asbestos)? What pollutants (smoke, auto exhaust, water)?

Do particular safety hazards exist (radiation, high noise levels, heavy machinery, extremes of heat or cold, electrical)?

Are safety rules understood and adhered to or enforced?

Are protective measures used (safety glasses, protective clothing)?

For children in schools or day care centers: Are play areas fenced? Is play equipment age-appropriate and safe? Are children adequately supervised?

Is the school/work environment clean, free of debris and unsafe clutter? Is the environment pleasant, comfortable (temperature, lighting), stimulating, and conducive to learning or working?

What is the incidence of communicable diseases? What measures are used to control the incidence and minimize the spread of disease (e.g., strict handwashing, proper food handling, required immunizations, illness policies)?

What eating facilities are provided or available nearby? Are foods nutritionally adequate?

II. Socioeconomic environment

Does client have a network of supportive relationships within the work, school, or day care environment?

How does client describe relationships with coworkers,

friends, classmates, teachers, supervisors?

Do physical facilities encourage socialization? How does environment provide for social and health needs (e.g., fitness center, jogging track, lounges, play areas, health programs, health professional on site)?

What are formal and informal rules for behavior in the work or school environment? How are infringements handled?

Does client have adequate work or play space? Is the work or school environment crowded? Is client able to personalize work or school space?

Does client express pride and positive esteem about work or school?

Is work or school routine rigidly structured, reasonably predictable yet flexible, or unstructured? Is client happy or dissatisfied with this?

Does client have appropriate opportunities for participating in policy setting and decision making?

How many hours per week does client spend at work or in school? What hours of the day does the client work or go to school?

Is client satisfied with income/wages? What is benefit package (health insurance, retirement)?

What is cost of school or day care? What is cost of extras (extracurricular activities, supplies, transportation, meals)? Is family or individual able to meet these expenses?

What are the economic, social, and political influences affecting the work or school environment?

TABLE 9-5
Critical Assessment Parameters of the Health-Care Environment

I. Physical-biological environment

Is the temperature appropriate to the setting (for example, is the newborn nursery adequately warm, are the exam rooms in a health maintenance clinic warm)?

Are noise levels monitored? Are unpleasant or irritating noises kept to a minimum? Are there pleasant sounds (e.g., soft music)?

Is the setting clean and free of clutter?

Is equipment properly maintained (clean and in working order)?

Are unpleasant odors controlled?

Are unnecessary x-rays avoided? Are proper precautions used during x-rays (e.g., lead apron)?

Are handwashing techniques and isolation procedures strictly adhered to? Are "universal precautions" observed? Are aseptic techniques used correctly and appropriately?

Are dressings and soiled materials properly disposed of?

Are procedures and policies written and available to staff? Are clients informed of policies/procedures that pertain directly to them (e.g., isolation procedures, no tub baths after abdominal or perineal surgery)?

Is electrical equipment properly maintained and used (e.g., grounding)? Do personnel observe safety precautions related to electrical equipment?

Are safety precautions consistently used (e.g., side rails up when appropriate according to client's age or condition, no smoking when oxygen in use, floor spills wiped up, ID band checked prior to administering medications or IV fluids, supplies and medications locked up or stored appropriately)?

II. Socioeconomic environment

Are visiting policies flexible and appropriate for client population (e.g., rooming-in or 24-hour visiting for parents of a hospitalized child, provisions for a family member to be with client during examination if desired)?

Is client allowed (encouraged) to have family members or significant others present?

Are family and significant others considered in assessment and planning of nursing care?

Is client in a private room or with other clients? What is the quality of interaction among clients in the same room or on the same unit?

Is the environment pleasant with appropriate types and amounts of sensory stimuli (colors, pictures, music, TV or radio, telephone)?

Is the client allowed to keep personal belongings? Is there space for keeping belongings? Is client allowed to keep the same bed and room assignment while in the hospital or long-term care facility?

Are the client's privacy and modesty protected and respected? To what extent is the client allowed to participate in decision making concerning activities and routines (bath times, diet selection)?

Is the unit or clinic adequately staffed?

Are the facilities and personnel adequate for meeting the client's basic needs (hygiene, nutrition, elimination, safety, sleep/rest, comfort, activity)?

Are unit or clinic routines reasonable, consistent, yet flexible enough to provide for individual needs? Are routines explained to client?

Is the institutional budget adequate for providing for client needs?

How will client meet health-care expenses (private insurance, Medicare, Medicaid, private pay, other)? Does the client (or family) have any concerns about this?

---

point in administering the HSQ if such services are not available and accessible, since the results may instill anxiety in the parent, who then has no recourse to assistive services.

Assessment of Home Safety for the Elderly

Because the elderly are at particular risk for injury from hazards in their homes, special assessment may be indicated. Many characteristics of the elderly place them at risk for accidental injury. These characteristics include decreased sensory acuity (all senses), slowed response time, diminished sense of balance, decreased pain perception and pain response, and diminished mobility. Special attention to the home environment is indicated to ensure that potential hazards are identified and corrected.

Burnside (1988) has presented an easy guide for assessing the home environment of the elderly person for safety hazards. This tool is presented in Figure 9-11. "No" answers to any of the items indicate a potential safety hazard that should be further investigated and corrected.

ASSESSMENT OF HEALTH RISK

Throughout life, the environment poses potential health risks as well as advantages. In fact, the environment is identified by the *Surgeon General's Report* (*Healthy People*, 1979) as a major source of risk that may adversely affect health and well-being. Air pollution, toxic wastes, pathogenic microorganisms, food additives, natural disasters, and traffic hazards are examples of environmental risks that

How often do you and your child see relatives?

_____ never

_____ at least once a year

_____ at least 6 times a year

_____ at least once a month

_____ at least once a week

About how many hours each day does your child spend in a playpen, jumpchair, infant swing, or infant seat?

_____ none

_____ up to 1 hour

_____ 1 to 3 hours

_____ more than three hours

Does the father (or other adult male) provide some caregiving (such as babysitting, feeding, putting to bed, etc.) for the child? YES NO If yes, how often?

_____ at least once a month

_____ at least once a week

_____ at least 3 or 4 times a week

_____ every day

*Available from Denver Developmental Materials, Inc., P.O. Box 6919, Denver, CO 80206–0919.

FIGURE 9-9 Sample Items from the Home Screening Questionnaire, Birth to age 3 (0–3) HSQ)* (*Note.* From Home Screening Questionnaires, By William K. Frankenburg, M.D. Reprinted by permission.)

How often does someone get a chance to read stories to your child?

_____ hardly ever

_____ at least once a week

_____ at least 3 times a week

_____ at least 5 times a week

How often does someone get a chance to take your child out of the house for an outing (shopping, park, zoo, restaurant, museum, car trip, library, etc.)?

_____ at least 6 times a year

_____ at least once a month

_____ at least twice a month

_____ at least once a week

What would you do if your child got angry and hit you?

_____ hit him/her to show it hurts

_____ send him/her to his/her room

_____ spank him/her

_____ talk to him/her

_____ ignore it

*Available from Denver Developmental Materials, Inc., P.O. Box 6919, Denver, CO 80206–0919.

FIGURE 9-10 Sample Items from the Home Screening Questionnaire 3 to 6 Years (3–6 HSQ)* (*Note.* From Home Screening Questionnaires, by William K. Frankenburg, M.D. Reprinted by permission.)

threaten health and life. At the same time, the environment provides life-enhancing and life-sustaining benefits, such as sunshine, water, natural foods, oxygen, and aesthetically pleasing scenery.

The Surgeon General's Report identifies two health risk categories: biological factors, such as age, gender, race, and family history, and behavioral factors, including lifestyle and health habits. Lifestyle includes diet, exercise, sleep, use of harmful substances, and use or non-use of seatbelts. Health habits refer to frequency of checkups, health practices such as monthly breast self-exam, and access to affordable, quality health care.

Although individuals have little control over their biological makeup, many other risks can be reduced or eliminated altogether. Over the past two decades, much public and professional emphasis has been placed on strategies that minimize health risks associated with the environment and with individual lifestyles and health habits.

Beginning in the early 1970s, health risk appraisal and risk reduction became a major focus in health care. Skyrocketing health-care costs, knowledge gleaned from several major epidemiological

studies, and the public's attention to health sparked the self-health movement and resulted in a proliferation of improvement programs. Such efforts include commercial and voluntary weight management programs, smoking cessation clinics, aerobics classes, and numerous self-help groups, such as Weight Watchers, Recovery, and Mothers Against Drunk Driving (MADD). The health, auto, and life insurance industries also now provide incentives for people to reduce health risks, such as lower premiums for non-smokers and those who use seatbelts, as a way to contain costs.

The proliferation of risk appraisal and reduction programs was prompted by several epidemiological studies that yielded data that indicate certain factors increase the risk of disease and death. The Framingham Heart Study and the Alameda County Study identified specific risks associated with certain diseases. For example, the Framingham study found that people with hypertension, a high serum cholesterol level, a low level of exercise, and who smoked were more likely to have heart disease (Shurtleff, 1970).

The Alameda County Study investigated the

1. Throughout the interior there are several common features which should be checked for safety. For example:
   a. Are scatter rugs firmly anchored with rubber backing?
   b. Are electrical cords in good repair, especially a heating pad?
   c. Light, heat, and ventilation
      (1) Is there adequate night lighting?
      (2) Are stairways continually illuminated?
      (3) Is temperature within comfortable range (70–75°F)?
      (4) Is the heater vented properly?
      (5) Is there cross ventilation?
   d. Is furniture sturdy enough to give support?
   e. Is there a minimum of clutter, allowing enough room for easy mobility as well as less fire hazard?
   f. Are emergency telephone numbers posted in a handy place and easily read, such as doctor, fire department, ambulance, paramedics, nearest relative?
   g. If the client has limited vision, does phone have enlarged dial?
2. The kitchen can be evaluated for the following:
   a. Stove, refrigerator, and sink
      (1) Is the stove free of grease and flammable

objects?
      (2) Is baking soda available in case of fire?
      (3) Are matches used or is there a pilot light?
      (4) Is the refrigerator working properly?
      (5) Is the sink draining well?
   b. Is food being stored properly?
   c. Is trash taken out daily?
   d. Is there a sturdy stepping stool in evidence?
   e. Are there skid-proof mats on the floor?
3. In the bathroom, are safety measures observed?
   a. Are handrails beside the tub and toilet?
   b. Are skid-proof mats in the bathtub and/or shower?
   c. Are electrical outlets a safe distance from the tub?
4. Outside the home, points to consider include:
   a. Walks and stairs
      (1) Are sidewalks even and free of cracks and debris?*
      (2) Are stairs in good repair?
      (3) Are the top and bottom stairs painted white or a bright contrasting color to improve visibility?
      (4) Are handrails securely fastened?
   b. Are screens on doors and windows in good repair?
   c. Is there an alternate exit for the house?

*Reworded from the original.

FIGURE 9-11 Assessment of Home Safety for the Elderly (*Note.* From Remnet, Valerie L.: The home assessment. In Burnside, Irene Mortenson, editor: *Nursing and the aged,* ed. 2, New York, 1981 McGraw-Hill Book Co.; copyright by Mosby-Year Book, Inc., St. Louis. Reprinted with permission.)

---

relationship between physical health and self-health practices in the general population (Belloc & Breslow, 1972). This study was based on the assumption that host resistance/susceptibility to disease is affected by behaviors that alter the host's internal and external environments. Belloc and Breslow (1972) and Belloc (1973) report significant correlations between certain lifestyles and physical health and mortality rates. Specifically, seven health practices (see boxed insert) were shown to be significant predictors of longevity: sleeping 7 to 8 hours each night, eating breakfast regularly, maintaining body weight within recommended limits for height and body frame, snacking infrequently between meals, exercising actively, using alcohol moderately, and not smoking (Belloc and Breslow, 1972).

In a follow-up study of the same population, Wiley and Camacho (1980) report that dietary factors (eating breakfast, not snacking between meals) were no longer significant predictors of mortality. However, the relationship between the remaining lifestyle practices and physical health continued to

be significant. Wiley and Camacho also report that the predicted effect of these practices (not smoking, moderate alcohol consumption, regular physical activity, 7–8 hours of sleep per night, and weight in relation to height) on health is stable re-

---

Seven Healthy Practices

Sleeping 7 to 8 hours each night
Eating breakfast regularly*
Snacking infrequently between meals*
Maintaining body weight within recommended limits for height and body frame
Exercising actively
Using alcohol moderately
Not smoking

*Not shown to be significant in follow-up study
Note. From Belloc, N.B., & Breslow, L. (1972). The relationship of physical health status and health practices. *Preventive Medicine, 1,* 420–421; and Wiley, J.A., & Camacho, T.C. (1980). Life-style and future health: Evidence from the Alameda County Study. *Preventive Medicine, 9,* 1–21.

gardless of a client's income or educational level. A limitation of the Alameda County Study, however, is its all-white sample, which prohibits translation to non-white populations.

Health Risk Appraisal (HRA)

Health risk appraisal (HRA), also referred to as health hazard appraisal (HHA), examines an individual's health practices and lifestyle in order to identify risks potentially harmful to health. The findings then may be used to counsel clients about their health risks and help them change their lifestyle and health habits to reduce the risk of disease, injury, and premature death.

Caution about the use of health risk appraisal, however, is in order. Health risk appraisal should not be undertaken without appropriate teaching, counseling, and support to ensure adequate follow-up. Health risk appraisal, in and of itself, is not likely to be beneficial and may even be harmful to the client unless it is part of a specific plan for promoting health and reducing risk. For example, Fielding (1982) cites a situation in which "several competitive hard driving sedentary men started exercising at an unhealthful rate," which was attributed to their misinterpretation of the meaning of their computed health age.

In order to be successful, health risk appraisal should be a beginning step in identifying a client's lifestyle and health habits that leads to a specific program of reducing risk and promoting health, with monitoring of changes over time. It can be difficult to change and even more difficult to maintain changes in lifestyle. A plan for changing a client's behaviors must be individually tailored to meet the client's needs and must be acceptable to the client, affordable, and possible. For instance, designing a plan that requires a mother of preschool children whose family income is limited to join a daytime, structured, relatively expensive aerobics class that does not provide childcare facilities would be doomed to failure. More acceptable, affordable, and possible would be an in-home plan for aerobic exercise using a commercial audiocassette or videocassette, or a daily televised exercise program.

Goals of Health Risk Appraisal

The primary goal of health risk appraisal is to prevent or reduce the risk of disease. A secondary goal is early detection of health problems before they compromise a client's lifestyle and daily functioning. Health risk appraisal is predicated on current scientific knowledge, which correlates certain risk factors, such as genetic makeup, daily habits, and environmental hazards, with disease and mortal-

ity. Because health risks compromise the quality and possibly the longevity of life, it is important to ascertain a client's health risks and to recommend a plan for modifying lifestyle or health habits (Figure 9-12).

Wildavsky (1977) estimates that only 10% of the variability in health risks can be ameliorated by specific interventions, such as medications, surgery, or technological devices. The majority of interventions that reduce the risk of disease and injury are self-help behaviors: those that clients must implement or change. For example, regular exercise, weight management, use of seat belts, stress reduction techniques, and avoiding harmful substances are behaviors that people must undertake themselves. Although health professionals can provide information to increase clients' knowledge and understanding of health risks and advise ways to change risky behaviors, ultimately it is up to individuals to eliminate or reduce potentially harmful behaviors from their daily lives.

The purposes of health risk appraisal are to assess an individual's risk of morbidity and mortality, and to motivate changes in the individual's health practices and lifestyle to reduce the risk. Doerr and Hutchins (1981) point out that health risk appraisal, unlike screening for the presence of disease, emphasizes the time prior to the onset of disease or injury in order to prevent its occurrence (see Figure 9-13). Thus, health risk appraisal is a primary prevention tool, whereas screening focuses on secondary prevention, specific detection of disease prior to the onset of symptoms for early intervention, and prevention of further sequelae.

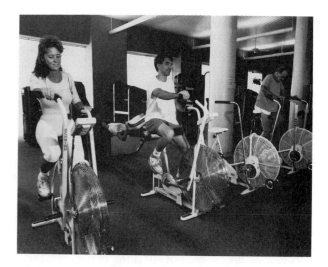

FIGURE 9-12. Lifestyle can increase or reduce a person's health risks and thus is important to identify as part of a comprehensive nursing assessment.

Advantages of HRA

Health risk appraisal has several advantages for clients and health professionals. HRA is a convenient and simple method of assessing a client's health risks. Health risk appraisal can be a useful adjunct to the health history and clinical examination, highlighting behaviors that predispose people to certain health risks. The results of health risk appraisal provide clear direction to professionals for teaching and counseling.

A major advantage of health risk appraisal is the possibility that it will enhance clients' awareness of unhealthy behaviors and lifestyles that place them at risk for disease and injury (Bartlett, Pegues, Shaffer, & Crump, 1983). Such awareness may serve as a motivator for reducing or eliminating risk by making clients more receptive to change. The nurse then can capitalize on the client's receptivity and work with the client to design specific risk reductions or refer the client to an established program.

In addition, health risk appraisals increase clients' receptivity to health counseling (Fielding, 1982), reinforce positive health practices (Fielding, 1982; Schultz, 1984), and (ideally) motivate clients to reduce or eliminate unhealthy ones (Doerr & Hutchins, 1981; Schultz, 1984). Fielding (1982) recommends the use of HRA to help clients track their progress (or failure to progress) in reducing health risks over a period of time.

Wagner, Beery, Schoenbach, and Graham (1982) suggest there are compelling social, political, and economic reasons for the widespread use of HRAs. These authors point out that HRA

1. provides a helpful focus for counseling people about their health and behavior,

2. can be easily and efficiently administered to large numbers of clients at relatively low expense,

3. reflects society's fascination with the trappings of modern science because of its reference to empirical studies, quantitative data, and computerized results,

4. fits the conventional wisdom about the role lifestyle plays in causing disease, and implies hope that people can change their destinies, and

5. can be easily and profitably marketed by commercial firms.

Despite these advantages and the widespread acceptance and use of HRA, the process is not without limitations and has been criticized on several counts.

Limitations and Criticisms of HRA

The limitations of HRA relate to the instruments themselves as well as the ways in which they are used. Limitations include

1. their questionable validity and reliability,

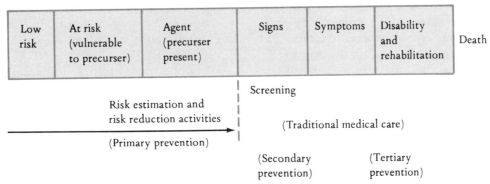

FIGURE 9-13. Relationship of Health Risk Appraisal to the Natural History of Disease. (*Note.* From Doerr, B.T., & Hutchins, E.B. Health risk appraisal: Process, problems, and prospects. Copyright 1981 American Journal of Nursing Company. Reprinted from *Nursing Research*, 1981, 30, p. 299. Used with permission. All rights reserved.)

2. the lack of adequate scientific evidence to support risk predictions,

3. the discrepancy among various HRAs with regard to which health risks are measured,

4. the limited attention to risks other than lifestyle practices, such as environmental hazards, availability and accessibility of health care, social inequities, and public policy, and

5. failure to identify a client's strengths.

(Doerr & Hutchins, 1981; Fielding, 1982; Sacks, Krushat, & Newman, 1980; Vogt, 1981; Wagner et al., 1982).

Major criticisms of the reliability and validity of HRAs revolve around their overreliance on what the client says, problems with risk calculations and risk projections, use of nonrigorous statistical analyses, the scarcity of epidemiological data for some risks (e.g., homicide, suicide), and HRA's dependence on data extrapolated primarily from studies of white, middle class, middle-aged, self-selected subjects (Acquista, Wachtel, Gomes, Saizillo, & Stockman, 1988; Sacks et al., 1980; Wagner et al., 1982).

Limitations in the actual use or administration of HRAs include (1) the potential for error in measuring specific health characteristics, such as blood pressure or serum cholesterol, (2) failure to identify certain risks, which may create a sense of complacency in clients, (3) potential physical or psychological risks to the client, such as anxiety, depression, hypochondriasis, excessive dieting or exercise, and unnecessary expense, (4) the possibility of misinterpretation or overinterpretation of the data (for example, interpreting longevity score as forecasting the client's year of death), and (5) failure, in numerous instances, to link risk appraisal with established health promotion and risk reduction programs (Fielding, 1982; Vogt, 1981; Wagner et al., 1982).

In addition, most HRAs require that the client be able to read and write, thus limiting their use with illiterate populations. Understanding numerical data and risk projections generated by most HRAs requires clients to have a higher than average educational level (Wagner et al., 1982). Others have criticized HRAs on the grounds that they create a "blame the victim" mentality, especially when risk factors are beyond the client's control, such as family history, age, race, or gender.

Despite these limitations and criticisms, sufficient evidence exists to suggest that health risk appraisal can be a valuable part of a comprehensive health assessment (Doerr & Hutchins, 1981; Schultz, 1984). While there is little definitive evidence to indicate that health risk appraisal is suc-

cessful in leading to improved lifestyle practices and health habits, HRA does appear to be a useful means for assessing a client's health risks and increasing a client's awareness (Wagner et al., 1982; Schultz, 1984). It is essential, however, that the findings of health risk appraisal become not an end, but rather a means of assisting nurses and other health professionals in counseling clients about their health risks and strategies for improving lifestyle and health practices. Health risk appraisal itself cannot reduce health risks or prompt changes in a client's behavior. Instead, HRAs can complement the nurse's own assessment skills, enhance the information about a client, and help clients implement specific risk reduction strategies as part of an overall program.

Health Risk Appraisal/Lifestyle Assessment Tools

The first HRA tool was developed by Robbins and Hall (1970) and marketed as "Health Hazard Appraisal." It was based on 20 years of statistical data and developed for use by physicians. Its appearance sparked the interest of other professionals and commercial groups. Since then, at least 29 HRA inventories have been developed, many of which have a broader focus and include such categories as health knowledge, daily stressors, and coping abilities, in addition to health history and health practices (National Health Information Clearinghouse, 1981).

Variations in length, scoring, target audience, and cost are great (Fielding, 1982). HRAs vary in length from fewer than 20 questions to several hundred items. Some are self-scored, others computer-analyzed, and still others must be scored by professionals. The majority of HRAs are designed for middle-aged, healthy adults, although a few target school-age children, teens, and young adults. Cost ranges from no charge to more than $50 per appraisal.

Selection of a particular health risk appraisal or lifestyle assessment tool depends on a number of factors. The purpose of doing a health risk appraisal should be the primary basis for choosing a tool. For example, is the purpose to detect a client's risk for one or more specific diseases or to evaluate lifestyle behaviors that may be preventing a client from reaching a higher level of health? Different tools fulfill different purposes. Therefore, the nurse should select a tool to fit the specific client's situation.

Once a health risk appraisal or lifestyle assessment is chosen, the nurse should take care to administer it exactly as directed in order to obtain reliable results. The nurse should ascertain whether responses reflect the client's typical lifestyle since circumstances and lifestyle practices often vary over time, and may even change day to day. Findings and their interpretation should be shared with the client as part of the complete nursing assessment.

It is especially important that information obtained from health risk appraisal or lifestyle assessment be interpreted within the context of what is known about all dimensions of the client's health and functioning. The client's family, community, and cultural context are what make the information meaningful and provide the basis for developing an individualized plan for reducing health risks and improving habits. As noted earlier, health risk appraisal should not be carried out as an isolated activity, but rather should be integrated with appropriate health promotion and health maintenance follow-up (Fielding, 1982; Doerr & Hutchins, 1981; Pender, 1987; Schultz, 1984; Wagner et al., 1982).

Figures 9-14 and 9-15 illustrate sample lifestyle assessment tools, with scoring guidelines. These

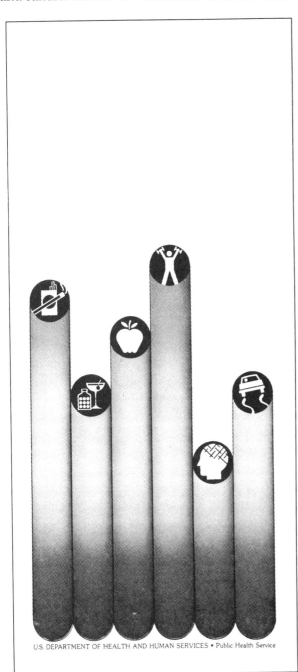

U.S. DEPARTMENT OF HEALTH AND HUMAN SERVICES • Public Health Service

How This Booklet Can Help You

All of us want good health. But, many of us do not know how to be as healthy as possible. Good health is not a matter of luck or fate. You have to work at it.

Good health depends on a combination of things . . . the environment in which you live and work . . . the personal traits you have inherited . . . the care you receive from doctors and hospitals . . . and the personal behaviors or habits that you perform daily, usually without much thought. All of these work together to affect your health. Many of us rely too much on doctors to keep us healthy, and we often fail to see the importance of actions we can take ourselves to look and feel healthy. You may be surprised to know that by taking action individually and collectively, you can begin to change parts of your world which may be harmful to your health.

Every day you are exposed to potential risks to good health. Pollution in the air you breathe and unsafe highways are two examples. These are risks that you, as an individual, can't do much about. Improving the quality of the environment usually requires the effort of concerned citizens working together for a healthier community.

There are, however, risks that you can control: risks stemming from your personal behaviors and habits. These behaviors are known as your lifestyle. Health experts now describe lifestyle as one of the most important factors affecting health. In fact, it is estimated that as many as seven of the ten leading causes of death in the United States could be reduced through common sense changes in lifestyle.

That's what the brief test contained in this booklet is all about. The few minutes you take to complete it may actually help you add years to your life! How? Well to start, it will enable you to identify aspects of your present lifestyle that are risky to your health. Then it will encourage you to take steps to eliminate or minimize the risks you identify. All in all, it will help you begin to change your present lifestyle into a new HEALTHSTYLE. If you do, it's possible that you may feel better, look better, and live longer too.

FIGURE 9-14. DHHS Health Style Self-Test Booklet. (*Note.* From United States Department of Health and Human Services, Office of Disease Prevention and Health Promotion. [1981]. *Health Style: A Self-Test.* [DHHS Pub. No. PHS 81-50155]. Washington, DC: U.S. Government Printing Office. May be ordered at no charge.)

Before You Take the Test

This is not a pass-fail test. Its purpose is simply to tell you how well you are doing to stay healthy. The behaviors covered in the test are recommended for most Americans. Some of them may not apply to persons with certain chronic diseases or handicaps. Such persons may require special instructions from their physician or other health professional.

You will find that the test has six sections: smoking, alcohol and drugs, nutrition, exercise and fitness, stress control, and safety. Complete one section at a time by circling the number corresponding to the answer that best describes your behavior (2 for "Almost Always", 1 for "Sometimes", and 0 for "Almost Never"). Then add the numbers you have circled to determine your score for that section. Write the score on the line provided at the end of each section. The highest score you can get for each section is 10.

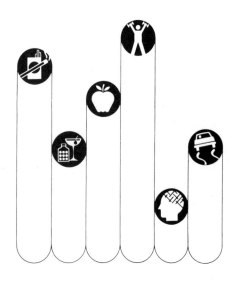

A Test for Better Health

	Almost Always	Sometimes	Almost Never

If you never smoke, enter a score of 10 for this section and go to the next section on *Alcohol and Drugs.*

	Almost Always	Sometimes	Almost Never
1. I avoid smoking cigarettes.	2	1	0
2. I smoke only low tar and nicotine cigarettes *or* I smoke a pipe or cigars.	2	1	0

Smoking Score: _____

	Almost Always	Sometimes	Almost Never
1. I avoid drinking alcoholic beverages *or* I drink no more than 1 or 2 drinks a day.	4	1	0
2. I avoid using alcohol or other drugs (especially illegal drugs) as a way of handling stressful situations or the problems in my life.	2	1	0
3. I am careful not to drink alcohol when taking certain medicines (for example, medicine for sleeping, pain, colds, and allergies).	2	1	0
4. I read and follow the label directions when using prescribed and over-the-counter drugs.	2	1	0

Alcohol and Drugs Score: _____

FIGURE 9-14 (Continued)

Eating Habits

	Almost Always	Sometimes	Almost Never
1. I eat a variety of foods each day, such as fruits and vegetables, whole grain breads and cereals, lean meats, dairy products, dry peas and beans, and nuts and seeds.	4	1	0
2. I limit the amount of fat, saturated fat, and cholesterol I eat (including fat on meats, eggs, butter, cream, shortenings, and organ meats such as liver).	2	1	0
3. I limit the amount of salt I eat by cooking with only small amounts, not adding salt at the table, and avoiding salty snacks.	2	1	0
4. I avoid eating too much sugar (especially frequent snacks of sticky candy or soft drinks).	2	1	0

Eating Habits Score: _____

Exercise/Fitness

	Almost Always	Sometimes	Almost Never
1. I maintain a desired weight, avoiding overweight and underweight.	3	1	0
2. I do vigorous exercises for 15-30 minutes at least 3 times a week (examples include running, swimming, brisk walking).	3	1	0
3. I do exercises that enhance my muscle tone for 15-30 minutes at least 3 times a week (examples include yoga and calisthenics).	2	1	0
4. I use part of my leisure time participating in individual, family, or team activities that increase my level of fitness (such as gardening, bowling, golf, and baseball).	2	1	0

Exercise/Fitness Score: _____

Stress Control

	Almost Always	Sometimes	Almost Never
1. I have a job or do other work that I enjoy.	2	1	0
2. I find it easy to relax and express my feelings freely.	2	1	0
3. I recognize early, and prepare for, events or situations likely to be stressful for me.	2	1	0
4. I have close friends, relatives, or others whom I can talk to about personal matters and call on for help when needed.	2	1	0
5. I participate in group activities (such as church and community organizations) or hobbies that I enjoy.	2	1	0

Stress Control Score: _____

Safety

	Almost Always	Sometimes	Almost Never
1. I wear a seat belt while riding in a car.	2	1	0
2. I avoid driving while under the influence of alcohol and other drugs.	2	1	0
3. I obey traffic rules and the speed limit when driving.	2	1	0
4. I am careful when using potentially harmful products or substances (such as household cleaners, poisons, and electrical devices).	2	1	0
5. I avoid smoking in bed.	2	1	0

Safety Score: _____

FIGURE 9-14 (Continued)

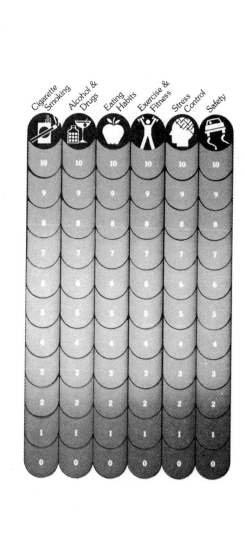

What Your Scores Mean to YOU

Scores of 9 and 10

Excellent! Your answers show that you are aware of the importance of this area to your health. More importantly, you are putting your knowledge to work for you by practicing good health habits. As long as you continue to do so, this area should not pose a serious health risk. It's likely that you are setting an example for your family and friends to follow. Since you got a very high score on this part of the test, you may want to consider other areas where your scores indicate room for improvement.

Scores of 6 to 8

Your health practices in this area are good, but there is room for improvement. Look again at the items you answered with a "Sometimes" or "Almost Never". What changes can you make to improve your score? Even a small change can often help you achieve better health.

Scores of 3 to 5

Your health risks are showing! Would you like more information about the risks you are facing and about why it is important for you to change these behaviors. Perhaps you need help in deciding how to successfully make the changes you desire. In either case, help is available. See the last page of this booklet.

Scores of 0 to 2

Obviously, you were concerned enough about your health to take the test, but your answers show that you may be taking serious and unnecessary risks with your health. Perhaps you are not aware of the risks and what to do about them. You can easily get the information and help you need to improve, if you wish. A source of contact appears on the last page. The next step is up to you.

FIGURE 9-14 (Continued)

YOU Can Start Right Now!

In the test you just completed were numerous suggestions to help you reduce your risk of disease and premature death. Here are some of the most significant:

 Avoid cigarettes. Cigarette smoking is the single most important preventable cause of illness and early death. It is especially risky for pregnant women and their unborn babies. Persons who stop smoking reduce their risk of getting heart disease and cancer. So if you're a cigarette smoker, think twice about lighting that next cigarette. If you choose to continue smoking, try decreasing the number of cigarettes you smoke and switching to a low tar and nicotine brand.

 Follow sensible drinking habits. Alcohol produces changes in mood and behavior. Most people who drink are able to control their intake of alcohol and to avoid undesired, and often harmful, effects. Heavy, regular use of alcohol can lead to cirrhosis of the liver, a leading cause of death. Also, statistics clearly show that mixing drinking and driving is often the cause of fatal or crippling accidents. So if you drink, do it wisely and in moderation.

 Use care in taking drugs. Today's greater use of drugs—both legal and illegal—is one of our most serious health risks. Even some drugs prescribed by your doctor can be dangerous if taken when drinking alcohol or before driving. Excessive or continued use of tranquilizers (or "pep pills") can cause physical and mental problems. Using or experimenting with illicit drugs such as marijuana, heroin, cocaine, and PCP may lead to a number of damaging effects or even death.

 Eat sensibly. Overweight individuals are at greater risk for diabetes, gall bladder disease, and high blood pressure. So it makes good sense to maintain proper weight. But good eating habits also mean holding down the amount of fat (especially saturated fat), cholesterol, sugar and salt in your diet. If you must snack, try nibbling on fresh fruits and vegetables. You'll feel better—and look better, too.

 Exercise regularly. Almost everyone can benefit from exercise—and there's some form of exercise almost everyone can do. (If you have any doubt, check first with your doctor.) Usually, as little as 15-30 minutes of vigorous exercise three times a week will help you have a healthier heart, eliminate excess weight, tone up sagging muscles, and sleep better. Think how much difference all these improvements could make in the way you feel!

 Learn to handle stress. Stress is a normal part of living; everyone faces it to some degree. The causes of stress can be good or bad, desirable or undesirable (such as a promotion on the job or the loss of a spouse). Properly handled, stress need not be a problem. But unhealthy responses to stress—such as driving too fast or erratically, drinking too much, or prolonged anger or grief—can cause a variety of physical and mental problems. Even on a very busy day, find a few minutes to slow down and relax. Talking over a problem with someone you trust can often help you find a satisfactory solution. Learn to distinguish between things that are "worth fighting about" and things that are less important.

Be safety conscious. Think "safety first" at home, at work, at school, at play, and on the highway. Buckle seat belts and obey traffic rules. Keep poisons and weapons out of the reach of children, and keep emergency numbers by your telephone. When the unexpected happens, you'll be prepared.

FIGURE 9-14 (Continued)

Where Do You Go From Here?

Start by asking yourself a few frank questions:
Am I really doing all I can to be as healthy as possible? What steps can I take to feel better? Am I willing to begin now? If you scored low in one or more sections of the test, decide what changes you want to make for improvement. You might pick that aspect of your lifestyle where you feel you have the best chance for success and tackle that one first. Once you have improved your score there, go on to other areas.

If you already have tried to change your health habits (to stop smoking or exercise regularly, for example) don't be discouraged if you haven't yet succeeded. The difficulty you have encountered may be due to influences you've never really thought about—such as advertising—or to a lack of support and encouragement. Understanding these influences is an important step toward changing the way they affect you.

There's Help Available. In addition to personal actions you can take on your own, there are community programs and groups (such as the YMCA or the local chapter of the American Heart Association) that can assist you and your family to make the changes you want to make. If you want to know more about these groups or about health risks contact your local health department or mail in the card contained in this booklet. There's a lot you can do to stay healthy or to improve your health—and there are organizations that can help you. Start a new HEALTHSTYLE today!

FIGURE 9-14 (Continued)

tools were chosen for inclusion here because they are easy to understand, simple to administer, and can be self-administered, scored, and interpreted. In addition, "Health Style: A Self Test" (Figure 9-14) provides recommendations for changes in lifestyle and health practices and suggests resources for follow-up.

ENVIRONMENTAL ASSESSMENT AND NURSING DIAGNOSIS

Data obtained from environmental assessment may indicate an actual or potential problem that contributes to a client's risk. Typically, environmental factors play an etiological role in clients' health responses. For example, noise in the environment may contribute to a sensory–perceptual alteration or sleep pattern disturbance; unsafe working conditions or a client's failure to use seatbelts may result in potential for injury. Because of the strong link between the environment and health, the client's identified problems or health responses are frequently related to internal or external environmental factors. Therefore, environmental information often is specified as the second part of the nursing diagnostic statement (the "related factors" portion of the statement).

Numerous factors in the environment may contribute to a client's specific responses to actual or potential health problems. Thus, lifestyle and health habits can contribute to actual or potential nursing diagnoses. Examples of environmental or lifestyle factors (in italics) related to specific nursing diagnoses include:

Altered nutrition: potential for more than body requirements related to *sedentary lifestyle* or *family/cultural eating patterns*

Hypothermia related to *exposure to cold environment*

Potential for trauma related to *smoking in bed* or *hot bath water* or *dangerous machinery*

Potential for infection related to *improper waste disposal*

Impaired tissue integrity related to *effects of therapeutic radiation*

Self-care deficit: bathing/hygiene related to *skeletal traction*

Altered growth and development related to *environmental deprivation*

Powerlessness related to *health-care environment* or *social isolation*

Post-trauma response related to *effects of natural disaster* or *military combat*

Identifying environmental or lifestyle factors that compromise a client's health provides a focus for developing a plan of care to eliminate or reduce risks in the environment. The nurse's role is to support the interaction of the client and the environment in ways that promote or restore health, or assist the client to die peacefully. Nursing actions may involve regulating, modifying, and monitor-

Your Lifestyle Profile

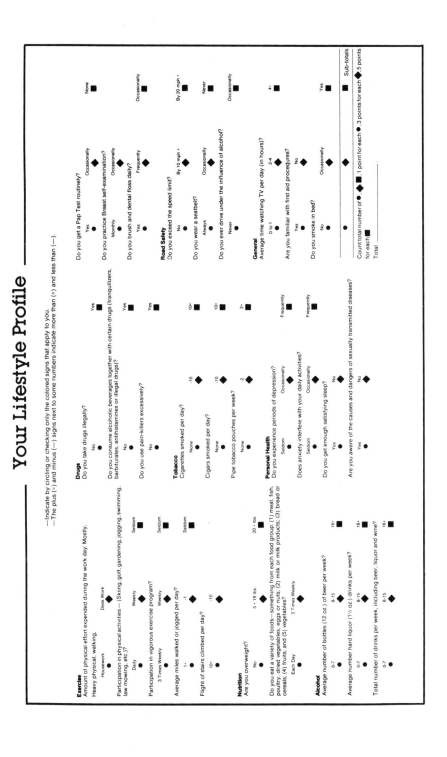

—Indicate by circling or checking only the colored signs that apply to you.
—The plus (+) and minus (—) signs next to some numbers indicate more than (+) and less than (—).

How To Calculate Your Score:

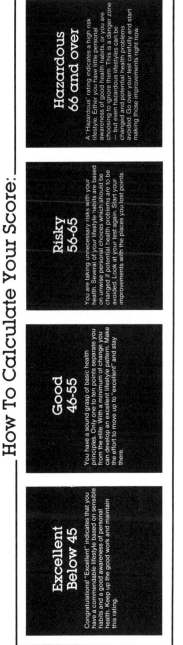

FIGURE 9-15. Operation Lifestyle: Your Lifestyle Profile. (*Note.* Reprinted with permission from Georgia Department of Human Resources, 1984.)

ing the environment in order to take advantage of environmental supports and reduce or eliminate environmental hazards.

The importance of the environment to a client's health cannot be overstated. Comprehensive assessment of the environment is essential in order to gain a complete picture of the context and lifestyle within which people conduct their lives. Once supportive or detrimental environmental forces have been identified and nursing diagnoses formulated, nursing care may be geared toward making the environment more favorable, or helping clients to do so.

Chapter Highlights

■ The relationship between people and their environments is like that of a double helix, each influencing and receiving from the other in a system of continuous feedback.

■ Human behavior cannot be understood outside of the environmental context in which it occurs. Therefore, the environment constitutes a critical dimension of a comprehensive nursing assessment.

■ Human environments are both internal and external and encompass numerous parameters: physical, biological, cognitive, spiritual, social, cultural, aesthetic, political, economic, legal, ethical, and technological.

■ Nearly all causes of morbidity and mortality relate in some way to naturally occurring or manufactured environmental forces.

■ The balance between people and their environments is homeostatic. People's abilities to adapt to variations in their environments are determined by a variety of factors, including age, physical and mental health, culture, and the use of assistive measures.

■ The epidemiological framework provides a basis for assessing the environment because it takes into account three variables, agent, host, and environment, which interact to produce positive or negative health outcomes.

■ Human environments consist of three major components: biological, physical, and socioeconomic. Each component of the various environments in which a client lives, works, and plays should be assessed.

■ The nurse should assess the client's home environment; work, school, or day care environment; and, when appropriate, health-care setting environment, in order to determine whether they are supportive, potentially detrimental, or hazardous to the client's health.

■ Health risk appraisal is a process that examines an individual's health practices and lifestyle in order to identify potentially harmful risk factors. The health risk appraisal has both advantages and limitations.

■ The findings of health risk appraisal must be interpreted within the context of what is known about all dimensions of the client's health and functioning, and should lead to a specific program of risk reduction and health promotion, with periodic monitoring over time.

■ Findings from environmental assessment often provide the information needed to formulate the second part of the nursing diagnostic statement, since environmental factors nearly always are related to the client's identified problems or health responses.

Practice Activities

1. Conduct an assessment of your own home–neighborhood–community environments and your work or school environment, using Tables 9-3 and 9-4 as guides. What advantages or supports are present? What actual or potential health hazards can you identify? Formulate nursing diagnoses based on your assessment findings. What modifications in your environments are indicated?

2. Assess the environment of one or more of the following clients, using Tables 9-3, 9-4, or 9-5 as guides:

    a. an infant or young child at home.
    b. a child in a day care or school setting.
    c. a hospitalized client.
    d. an elderly client in a long-term care facility.
    e. an adult client in a work/occupational setting.
    f. a client in a walk-in clinic or physician's office.

What environmental supports are present? What actual or potential health hazards can you identify? Formulate appropriate nursing diagnoses based on your assessment findings. Develop a plan of care, including evaluation outcomes.

3. Using Figure 9-11, assess the home of an elderly

person. Summarize your findings. What nursing diagnoses can you formulate? What interventions are indicated?

4. Assess your own lifestyle using "Health Style: A Self Test" (Figure 9-14) or "Your Lifestyle Profile" (Figure 9-15), and calculate your health risk score. What do the findings suggest about your lifestyle? Develop a plan to improve your lifestyle score, including goals, actions, and outcome measures.

5. Using a nursing history you have obtained or the sample history in Chapter 25, identify environmental factors that should be considered when analyzing the information. What environmental factors contribute to the nursing diagnoses suggested at the end of Chapter 25?

Recommended Readings

Bradley, R.H., & Caldwell, B.M. (1988). Using the H.O.M.E. Inventory to assess the family environment. *Pediatric Nursing, 14*, 97–102.

Doerr, B.T., & Hutchins, E.B. (1981). Health risk appraisal: Process, problems, and prospects for nursing practice and research. *Nursing Research, 30*, 299–306.

Mason, D.J. (1988). Circadian rhythms of body temperature and activation and the well-being of older women. *Nursing Research, 37*, 276–281.

Muhlenkamp, A.F., & Sayles, J.A. (1986). Self-esteem, social support, and positive health practices. *Nursing Research, 35*, 334–338.

Norbeck, J. (1981). Social support: A model for clinical application and research. *Advances in Nursing Science, 3*, 43–59.

Riffle, K.L., Yoho, J., & Sams, J. (1989). Health-promoting behaviors, perceived social support, and self-reported health of Appalachian elderly. *Public Health Nursing, 6*, 204–211.

Ross, S.O., & Krieger, J.N. (1989). The latest studies on occupational exposure to HIV. *American Journal of Nursing, 89*, 1424–1425.

Schultz, C.M.S. (1984). Lifestyle assessment: A tool for practice. *Nursing Clinics of North America, 19*, 271–281.

Smith, M.J. (1986). Human–environment process: A test of Rogers' principle of integrality. *Advances in Nursing Science, 9*, 21–28.

Stevens, P.E. (1989). A critical social reconceptualization of environment in nursing: Implications for methodology. *Advances in Nursing Science, 11*(4), 56–68.

Tynan, C., & Cardea, J.M. (1987). Home health hazard assessment. *Journal of Gerontological Nursing, 13*(10), 25–28.

References

Zindler-Wernet, P., & Weiss, S.J. (1987). Health locus of control and preventative health behavior. *Western Journal of Nursing Research, 9*(2), 160–179.

Abelson, P.H. (1984). Environmental risk management. *Science, 226*, 30.

Acquista, V.W., Wachtel, T.J., Gomes, C.I., Salzillo, M., & Stockman, M. (1988). Home-based health risk appraisal and screening program. *Journal of Community Health, 13*, 43–52.

Altman, I. (1975). *The environment and social behavior.* Monterey, CA: Brooks/Cole.

Bartlett, E.E., Pegues, H.U., Shaffer, C.R., & Crump, W. (1983). Health hazard appraisal in a family practice center: An exploratory study. *Journal of Community Health, 9*(2), 135–144.

Belloc, N.B. (1973). Relationships of health practices and mortality. *Preventative Medicine, 2*, 67–81.

Belloc, N.B., & Breslow, L. (1972). The relationship of physical health status and health practices. *Preventative Medicine, 1*, 409–421.

Burnside, I. (1988). *Nursing and the aged: A self-care approach* (3rd ed.). New York: McGraw–Hill.

Caldwell, B.M. (1970). *Instruction manual for infants: (Home Observation and Measurement of the Environment).* Little Rock, AR: Center for Child Development.

Caldwell, B.M. (1975). *Instruction manual—Preschool version. (Home Observation and Measurement of the Environment).* Little Rock, AR: Center for Child Development.

Collins, B.E. (1974). Four components of the Rotter internal–external scale: Belief in a difficult world, a just world, a predictable world, and a politically responsive world. *Journal of Personality and Social Psychology, 29*, 381–391.

Coons, C.E., Gay, E.C., Fandal, A.W., Kerr, C., & Frankenburg, W.K. (1981). *The Home Screening Questionnaire.* Denver: J.F.K. Child Development Center.

Czeisler, C.A., Allan, J.S., Strogatz, S.H., Ronda, J.M., Sanchez, R., Rios, D., Freitag, W.O., Richardson, G.S., & Kronauer, R.E. (1987). Bright light resets the human circadian pacemaker independent of the time of the sleep–wake cycle. *Science, 233*, 667–671.

Dimond, M., & Jones, S.L. (1982). Social support: A review and theoretical integration. In P.L. Chinn (Ed.), *Advances in nursing theory development* (pp. 235–249). Rockville, MD: Aspen Systems.

Doerr, B.T., & Hutchins, E.B. (1981). Health risk appraisal: Process, problems, and prospects for nursing practice and research. *Nursing Research, 30*, 299–306.

Farr, L.A., Campbell-Grossman, C., & Mack, J.M.

(1988). Circadian disruption and surgical recovery. *Nursing Research, 37,* 170–175.

Fielding, J.E., (1982). Appraising the health of health risk appraisal. *American Journal of Public Health, 72,* 337–340.

Froines, J.R., Dellenbaugh, C.A., & Wegman, D.H. (1986). Occupational health surveillance: A means to identify work-related risks. *American Journal of Public Health, 76,* 1089–1096.

Harries, K.D., & Stadler, S.J. (1983). Determinism revisited: Assault and heat stress in Dallas, 1980. *Environment and Behavior, 15,* 235–256.

Healthy people: The Surgeon General's report on health promotion and disease prevention. (1979). PHS (Pub. No. 79–55071.) Washington, DC: U.S. Department of Health and Human Services.

House, J.S., & Kahn, R.L. (1985). Measures and concepts of social support. In S. Cohen & L. Syme (Eds.), *Social support and health* (pp. 83–108). New York: Academic.

Hubbard, P., Muhlenkamp, A.F., & Brown, N. (1984). The relationship between social support and self-care practices. *Nursing Research, 33,* 266–270.

Lave, L.B. (1981). Balancing economics and health in setting environmental standards. *Annual Review of Public Health, 2,* 183–200.

Luce, G. (1970). *Biological rhythms in psychiatry and medicine.* (Pub. No. PHS 70-2088). Washington, DC: U.S. Department of Health, Education, & Welfare.

Mason, D.J. (1988). Circadian rhythms of body temperature and activation and the well-being of older women. *Nursing Research, 37,* 276–281.

Moore-Ede, M., Sulzman, F., & Fuller, C. (1982). *The clocks that time us.* Cambridge, MA: Harvard University Press.

Muhlenkamp, A.F., & Sayles, J.A. (1986). Self-esteem, social support, and positive health practices. *Nursing Research, 35,* 334–338.

National Center for Health Statistics (1985, September 20). *Monthly vital statistics report, 34* (supplement).

National Information Clearinghouse. (1981). *Health risk appraisals: An inventory.* (DHHS Pub. No. 81-50163). Washington, DC: Office of Health Information, Health Promotion, and Physical Fitness and Sports Medicine.

Nightingale, F. (1859). *Notes on nursing: What it is and what it is not.* London: Harrison.

Norbeck, J. (1981). Social support: A model for clinical application and research. *Advances in Nursing Science, 3,* 43–59.

Parse, R.R. (1981). *Man–living–health: A theory of nursing.* New York: Wiley.

Pender, N.J. (1987). *Health promotion in nursing practice.* (2nd ed.). Norwalk, CT: Appleton & Lange.

Robbins, L.C., & Hall, J.H. (1970). *How to practice prospective medicine.* Indianapolis: Methodist Hospital of Indiana.

Rogers, M.E. (1970). *An introduction to the theoretical basis of nursing.* Philadelphia: Davis.

Rotter, J. (1966). Generalized expectancies for internal vs. external control of reinforcement. *Psychological Monographs, 80,* 601–603.

Sacks, J.J., Krushat, W.M., & Newman, J. (1980). Reliability of health hazard appraisal. *American Journal of Public Health, 70,* 730–732.

Schultz, C.M. (1984). Lifestyle assessment: A tool for practice. *Nursing Clinics of North America, 19*(2), 271–281.

Shurtleff, D. (1970). Some characteristics related to incidence of cardiovascular disease and death: Framingham study, a 16-year followup. In W.B. Kannel & T. Gordon (Eds.), *The Framingham study.* Washington, DC: U.S. Government Printing Office.

Shrock, M.M. (1980). *Holistic assessment of the healthy aged.* New York: Wiley.

Silverberg, E. (1985). Cancer statistics. *CA, 35,* 19–35.

Staff. (1981). *Morbidity and mortality weekly reports, 30,* 305–307. Atlanta: U.S. Centers for Disease Control.

Sundstrom, E. (1986). Privacy in the office. In J. Wineman (Ed.), *Behavioral issues in office design* (pp. 177–201). New York: Van Nostrand Reinhold.

Vogt, T.M. (1981). Risk assessment and health hazard appraisal. *Annual Review of Public Health, 2,* 31–47.

Wagner, E., Beery, W.L., Schoenbach, V.S., & Graham, R.M. (1982). An assessment of health hazard/health risk appraisal. *American Journal of Public Health, 72,* 347–352.

Wildavsky, A. (1977). Doing better and feeling worse: The political pathology of health policy. *Daedalus, 106,* 105.

Wiley, J.A., & Camacho, T.C. (1980). Life-style and future health: Evidence from the Alameda County study. *Preventive Medicine, 9,* 1–21.

Zindler-Wernet, P., & Weiss, S.J. (1987). Health locus of control and preventive behavior. *Western Journal of Nursing Research, 9*(2), 160–179.

PART III

Developmental Assessment

10

Developmental Assessment of the Child

OBJECTIVES

Upon completion of this chapter, you should be able to:

■ Delineate the rationale for periodic assessment of a child's development.

■ Use knowledge of developmental concepts, principles, and theories as a guide for assessing a child's development from birth through adolescence.

■ Describe the three essential components of developmental assessment—developmental history, clinical appraisal, and screening.

■ Delineate self-care behaviors appropriate to a child's developmental level.

■ Select appropriate tools for screening a child's developmental status.

■ Trace the development of children's concepts of health and their health knowledge from preschool through adolescence.

■ Describe children's health knowledge and health concerns at various developmental levels.

■ Analyze children's health practices, including factors that promote responsibility for their own health.

■ Conduct a comprehensive developmental assessment of selected children from birth through adolescence.

■ Analyze developmental data to formulate valid and appropriate nursing diagnoses.

Developmental progress throughout the lifespan can provide major clues to a person's overall health. Positive forces in a person's genetic makeup or the environment may enhance developmental outcomes. Conversely, adverse maturational or environmental factors may interfere with normal developmental processes and cause delays. Periodic monitoring of development permits a nurse to affirm that an individual is developing appropriately for age or to detect potential problems that may require intervention.

Developmental assessment provides a systematic means for appraising a person's developmental abilities and capabilities in a number of areas—physical, motor, language, cognitive, social, and self-care. Such appraisals are particularly important in children because of the rapid developmental changes that occur in early childhood. Undetected problems in a child's development can lead to lifelong disabilities. The specific reasons for assessing a particular child's development vary with the child's age, health, and the setting in which the child is seen.

One important reason for collecting data about a child's development is to provide an ongoing record of the child's developmental achievement and progress. Such a record allows the nurse to compare the child's current level and rate of development with the child's previous development (longitudinal comparison). The nurse also can use the data to compare the child with other children of the same age (cross-sectional comparison) to determine if the child is functioning within the expected range of developmental achievements for her or his age.

A second purpose of developmental assessment is to detect potential delays in development that may require further assessment and intervention. The early identification of potential problems can lead to appropriate interventions aimed at preventing, or at least minimizing, long-term impairments.

A third reason for assessing children's development is to provide anticipatory guidance to parents about ways they can promote their child's continued development. The nurse can alert parents about what to expect in terms of the child's future development while offering specific suggestions of ways parents can foster the child's progress.

Finally, the nurse can use the developmental appraisal to guide interactions with children that are appropriate for the child's developmental level. This is especially important for structuring health teaching for children. Explanation of a procedure, for example, should be geared to the child's level of understanding. By being aware of children's cognitive abilities, a nurse can better understand and deal appropriately with their responses to various health-care situations.

There are a number of parameters that should be included in a comprehensive developmental assessment. Parameters that should be assessed during any contact with a child will depend on the nature and frequency of the contact as well as the nurse's previous knowledge of the child (or lack of it). The three major parameters for assessment are the developmental history, clinical observation, and developmental screening, when the latter is indicated.

KNOWLEDGE NEEDED TO ASSESS CHILDREN'S DEVELOPMENT

Developmental assessment should not be carried out haphazardly. It should proceed systematically, guided by knowledge of certain concepts, principles, and theories that help the nurse organize the collection of developmental information in a logical and meaningful way. This knowledge also is helpful for correlating developmental concepts and theories with age-related characteristics for a workable whole, which gives structure and direction to the developmental assessment.

Developmental assessment builds on theoretical knowledge derived from the large body of literature in child development. The principles and theories of child development provide a basis for understanding human behavior along the age continuum and give the nurse a framework for collecting developmental information from clients in a variety of health-care settings.

Growth and development are dynamic processes that ebb and flow throughout the lifespan. They are dynamic in that they interact with and are influenced continuously by each other and by the environment (Lerner, 1978). They ebb and flow in that changes in growth and development are more noticeable during some developmental periods, such as early childhood, than they are in others, such as middle adulthood.

Concepts and Principles of Development

The terms *growth* and *development* refer to two dimensions of an interactive process. Growth is defined typically as *quantitative* changes in physical size and structure, whereas development refers to *qualitative* changes in function. These two dimensions are closely interrelated since physical growth often paves the way for changes in function. For instance, complete myelinization of the child's bowel and bladder tracts enables the child to become toilet-trained.

Knowledge of the concepts and principles that govern human growth and development helps a nurse understand the maturational sequence of developmental patterns, which are especially noticeable in children. These concepts and principles serve only as general guidelines, however. Each child is unique, and specific behaviors and abilities reflect the interactive influences of the child's own maturity and environment.

Three key concepts provide a basis for understanding the various principles of development. One particularly important developmental concept is *maturation:* the inborn, genetically transmitted capacity for development. The maturational sequence of development has been well documented by a number of noted individuals (Gesell & Ilg, 1949; Ilg & Ames, 1960). Erikson (1963) defines maturation as the emergence of skill according to a predetermined capacity. According to this theory, an individual is born with a finite, or predetermined, developmental potential. Maturation, however, is influenced by *learning*, a second essential concept. Thus, the actual development of skills or capacities in the child is brought about by the interaction of the child and the environment, not by genetic endowment alone. The child's potential for optimal development depends to a great extent on the kinds of enrichment opportunities provided. For example, an infant cannot pull to a standing position until physiological maturation of the spinal nerve tracts makes standing possible. Maturation alone, though, will not result in the infant's learning to stand. The infant must be stimulated, guided, and reinforced while attempting to acquire this new skill.

The extent to which maturation (heredity, nature) and learning (environment, nurture) contribute to development continues to be a subject of debate among developmental theorists. A summary of this debate may be found in Table 10-1. It is important to keep in mind that people are complex, multidimensional beings whose development is influenced by a host of interactive forces. Children both shape and are shaped by their environments, and it is usually difficult to distinguish cause and effect (Lerner, 1978).

A third, closely related concept is *critical periods*, which are best defined as sensitive periods during which a child is most ready to learn a new developmental task. Critical periods for acquiring new skills are determined by a child's maturational readiness. Once a child is maturationally ready to learn a new skill, the environment must be developmentally appropriate for nurturing and stimulating mastery of the skill. If the child is not given opportunities to practice and master a new skill during its critical period, the skill may not be learned as well or as completely after the sensitive period has passed.

The concept of critical periods is perhaps best noted in the first trimester of pregnancy, a crucial time for development of body organs. Any interference with development during this critical period can lead to irreversible changes in structure and function. The critical periods for psychosocial and cognitive development are less specific, but they do appear to exist. Perhaps the most familiar critical period in psychosocial development is the period of attachment, or "bonding," which occurs between parent and child during the newborn period and early infancy. An example of a critical period in cognitive development is the acquisition of language skills. Although this critical period is less well defined than that for bonding, children who receive inadequate stimulation and reinforcement for learning language during the first two years of life may never overcome the deficit, re-

TABLE 10-1
Summary of Nature–Nurture Issue

	Nature	Nurture
Basic Influences	Biological variables—both genetic and nongenetic	Psychological environment and social–cultural milieu
Developmental Approach	Organismic theory: Individual is active agent of own development	Mechanistic theory: Individual reacts but does not initiate
Developmental Tempo	Development in stages— qualitative leaps	Continuous development
Salient Processes	Maturation	Experience
Driving Force	Ontogenesis	Operant responses

Note. From Hayes, J.S. (1987). Theories of child development. In Servonsky/Opas: *Nursing Management of Children,* © 1987. Boston: Jones and Bartlett Publishers, p. 233.

gardless of later attempts to make up for lost opportunities. The concept of critical periods also is evident in stage theories of development, which suggest that a child must master a particular task or tasks during each developmental stage to move successfully to the next.

The major principles that govern the emergence and unfolding of developmental progress in the child are discussed below.

Development Is Directional

Human development follows a threefold directional pattern: *cephalocaudal*, *proximodistal*, and *general-to-specific*. (Figure 10-1).

The cephalocaudal pattern describes the progression of development from head to toe. This pattern, or flow, is most easily seen in the embryonic and fetal stages of life when an organism's skull and brain develop in advance of the trunk, tail, and limbs. Other examples can be seen in the infant's ability to control head and neck muscles before arm and leg muscles and to sit alone before learning to stand alone.

Proximodistal development refers to the tendency for development to proceed from the central axis of the body (trunk) to the periphery (extremities). A child will achieve gross arm control before learning to manipulate the hand and fingers. Even within the central nervous system, development proceeds in a proximodistal direction, as evidenced by the presence of brain stem activity (breathing, sucking, and other primitive reflexes) before higher cortical activities (reasoning and thinking) emerge.

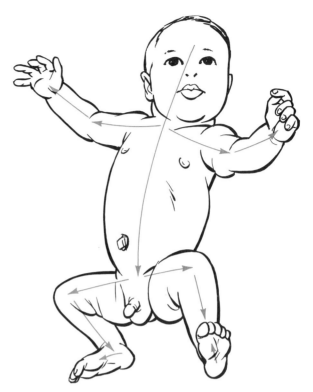

FIGURE 10-1. Directional Flow of Development (Cephalocaudal, Proximodistal).

The third directional principle, general-to-specific, is also known as *differentiation*. As children develop, their behaviors and responses become increasingly more refined and differentiated. A newborn infant, for example, responds to a pinprick of the foot in a generalized, undifferentiated way, whereas a similar stimulus will evoke a more specific response in an older child (withdrawal of the foot that was pricked). Large muscle functions such as throwing and running develop in advance of the skills needed to write with a pencil or hop on one foot.

Development Is Sequential

A child's growth and development follow an orderly, predictable, and generally universal sequence. For instance, it is characteristic of all children to experience periods of rapid growth and change in infancy and early adolescence. Children learn to talk and walk, develop hand–eye coordination, lose their primary teeth, and acquire secondary sex characteristics according to a predictable timetable common to the human species.

Principles of Human Development

Development follows a threefold directional pattern: *cephalocaudal* (head to toe), *proximodistal* (from center of body outward), and *general-to-specific* (increasing refinement and differentiation).

Development is *sequential*.

The rate of development is *uniquely individual*.

Development is *asynchronous*.

Development is *cyclical*.

Development becomes *increasingly complex and integrated*.

All aspects of development are *interrelated*.

Development Is Individual

Each child has a unique pattern of emerging abilities. Although the sequence of development is predictable for all children, the rate at which a particular child achieves the various milestones is highly individual. For example, all infants must learn to sit unsupported before they can learn to walk. One infant may learn to sit alone at 5 months of age, whereas another may be unable to do so until 8 months of age. Both, however, fall within the normal developmental range for achieving this skill. Individuality also is reflected in the fact that some children excel in a particular area of development, such as physical prowess, whereas others are advanced in language or social skills.

Many factors influence the child's unique pattern of development, including the child's gender, race, culture, family characteristics, and physical and social environments. For instance, Asian children as a group are smaller in stature than Caucasian or black children. Within a group of Asian children, though, there exists a wide range of individual variation in size. These differences among children of varying racial and cultural backgrounds must be considered when comparing them with norms derived from racially or culturally different groups.

Development Is Asynchronous

During the different developmental phases, the focus of growth and development shifts. Physically, the various body regions and subsystems develop at different rates and times. For example, growth of lymphatic tissue peaks in the early school years, but the reproductive system matures rapidly during early adolescence. The principle of asynchronous development helps explain the distinguishing physical characteristics of the different age groups, such as the wide stance of the toddler and the typical facial features of the early school-age child.

In addition, as the focus of development changes, a particular skill tends to assume primary importance as the child learns to master it. Thus, progress in speech development may slow while the child's energies are devoted to learning bowel and bladder control.

Development Is Cyclical

Throughout childhood, development tends to occur in cycles of accelerated and decelerated growth. This principle explains the rapid growth periods that occur during infancy and early adolescence. It also accounts for the slower growth periods of the preschool and school-age years, as well as the leveling off of the growth rate in young adulthood. Cycles in personality also have been proposed (Ilg, Ames, & Baker, 1960). Table 10-2 depicts cyclical variations that occur throughout childhood.

Development Becomes Increasingly Complex and Integrated

As children grow and develop, they acquire new skills and behaviors that qualitatively change who they are. Skill acquisition is not simply cumulative. Rather, each new ability is integrated with those previously learned to enable the child to master more complex and difficult functions. The infant first must learn to coordinate sucking and swallowing and later combine them with more advanced lip and tongue movements, as well as grasping, hand–eye and hand–mouth coordination in order to feed itself. A more refined grasp, an increasing variety of foods, and the addition of social and cultural cues result in eating becoming a complex physiological, psychological, and sociocultural behavior (Figure 10-2).

TABLE 10-2
Alternation of Stages of Equilibrium and Disequilibrium in Child Behavior

Stages of Child Behavior				
First Cycle	Second Cycle	Third Cycle	General	Quality
Age	Age	Age	Personality Trends	of the Age
2	5	10	Smooth, consolidated	Better
2½	5½–6	11	Breaking up	Worse
3	6½	12	Rounded, balanced	Better
3½	7	13	Inwardized	Worse
4	8	14	Vigorous, expansive	Better
4½	9	15	Inwardized–outwardized, troubled, "neurotic"	Worse
5	10	16	Smooth, consolidated	Better

Note. Adapted from Ilg, F.L., Ames, L.B., & Baker, S.M. (1981). *Child behavior* (rev. ed.). New York: Harper & Row, p. 14. Reprinted by permission.

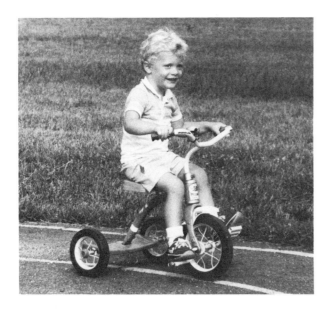

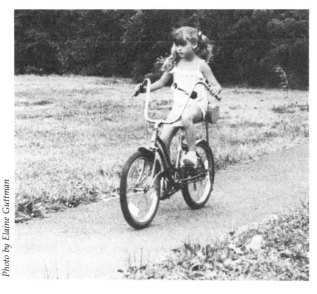

FIGURE 10-2. Previously learned abilities become integrated with new and more complex ones. Riding a bicycle is a complex function that requires a child to integrate skills acquired from tricycle pedaling. (*Note.* From Servonsky/Opas: *Nursing Management of Children,* © 1987. Boston: Jones and Bartlett Publishers, p. 315.)

All Aspects of Development Are Interrelated

Although the various dimensions of development often are separated for purposes of study, it is essential to remember that they are intricately interwoven and interrelated. Children and adults grow and develop as whole beings. Physical, emotional, social, and cognitive development occur simultaneously and interrelatedly. Factors that promote or inhibit development in one area also will affect other

areas. A toddler whose exploration of the environment is curtailed because of a body cast probably will exhibit delays in language and social development, as well as in motor development. An infant whose special need for love and sensory stimulation is neglected is likely also to be delayed in physical and cognitive development.

Knowledge of these developmental principles provides a useful framework for assessing a child's developmental progress. For example, as the nurse assesses the development of a 3-year-old, the following questions can serve as a guide.

> Is the child beginning to show evidence of developing more refined motor skills such as copying a circle (differentiation)?
>
> Has the child's achievement of developmental milestones followed the directional flow of development (cephalocaudal, proximodistal) and occurred in the expected sequence?
>
> Is the child showing consistent progress in all areas of development (interrelatedness)?
>
> What factors should be considered in assessing the individuality of this child (race, culture, gender, social environment, family characteristics)?

By considering developmental data in relation to these principles, the nurse can determine whether the child is developing appropriately for age or has a potential delay in development that requires further evaluation.

Theories of Human Development

Developmental theories provide useful explanations for interpreting human behaviors along a continuum. They also provide a framework for organizing data or facts about children and give meaning to those facts. Thus, theories provide a practical guide for understanding a child's development and behavior and can be used as a basis for assessing a child (Thomas, 1985).

There are numerous theories of human development. Some explain behavior from a maturation perspective (Gesell & Ilg, 1949; Lorenz, 1937; Sheldon, 1942), others from a learning perspective (Bandura, 1977; Skinner, 1945). Still other theorists (Erikson, 1963; Havighurst, 1972; Kohlberg, 1968; Piaget, 1963) attribute behavior and personality to an interaction of varying degrees of maturation and learning. Each of the major theorists, however, explains development from a single perspective, such as biological maturation, cognitive development, moral development, or psychosocial development. None explains the full range of human development, although each contributes to an understanding of the whole. Therefore, a synthesis of the various theories is necessary to achieve a useful perspective for understanding and assessing the complexity of a particular child's developmental status. Developmental theories do not, however, account for each child's individuality. They serve as guides rather than rules or axioms.

Several of the more widely accepted theories are known as stage theories of development. These theories describe development as a sequential series of defined stages, each of which builds on the previous one and serves as a foundation for subsequent stages. Changes in development are seen to occur in steps with each period characterized by distinct behaviors common to individuals in the particular developmental stage. Prominent stage theories include Erikson's psychosocial theory (1963), Piaget's cognitive theory (1963), Havighurst's developmental tasks theory (1972), and Kohlberg's theory of moral development (1968).

By contrast, other theorists suggest that development occurs in a continuous, gradual fashion in barely perceptible increments. Such perspectives include Skinner's theory of operant conditioning (1945) and Bandura's theory of social learning (1977).

Psychosocial Theory

Development is viewed from a psychosocial perspective by Erik Erikson (1963). His theory evolved from Freud's psychosexual theory. Erikson is known especially for his "eight stages of man," which describe a sequence of core conflicts that occur from birth to senescence. Each developmental stage—infancy, adolescence, middle adulthood—is characterized by a central conflict that the individual resolves favorably or unfavorably. Favorable resolution of each conflict lays a solid foundation for subsequent stages, whereas failure to resolve a conflict satisfactorily may interfere with later development. It must be pointed out, though, that at each stage the individual is left with both positive and negative aspects of the conflict.

Erikson's first five stages are outlined in Table 10-3. These stages are especially significant for the nurse who is concerned with assessing the development of children. The three subsequent stages

TABLE 10-3
Erikson's Theory of Psychosocial Development (First Five Stages)

Stage/Age Range	Core Conflict	Significant People	Description of Positive Resolution
Infancy— birth to 1 year	Trust vs. mistrust	Mother, father, primary caregiver	When infants' needs are met consistently and with a degree of predictability, they develop a sense of trust, a feeling that the world is a dependable and secure place.
Toddlerhood— 1 to 3 years	Autonomy vs. shame and doubt	Parents	Children discover their world and their ability to explore and manipulate the environment. They assert independence (autonomy) in the face of parental control and develop a sense of will.
Preschool period— 3 to 6 years	Initiative vs. guilt	Parents, siblings	Children move toward increasing independence from their parents and begin to assert themselves in the larger world outside the home. They involve themselves in mastering new tasks and acquiring new skills and capacities.
School-age period— 6 to 12 years	Industry vs. inferiority	Peers, family, teachers	Children work hard to be successful at what they do. Belonging to and gaining the approval of the peer group is especially important.
Adolescence— 12 to 18+ years	Identity vs. identity diffusion	Peers, significant adults other than parents (coach, teacher)	Children move toward becoming adults and achieving emancipation from parents. They struggle to find their place in society, establish career goals, deal with their sexuality, and give consideration to the problems of a complex world.

that pertain to adult development are discussed in Chapter 11.

Cognitive Theory

Jean Piaget (1896–1980) was a Swiss psychologist whose theory of cognitive development has been one of the most influential in developmental psychology in recent years. Piaget's theory, like Erikson's, is a stage theory, but it focuses on the changes that occur in thinking as children develop.

Central to an understanding of Piaget's theory are the concepts of assimilation and accommodation. *Assimilation* is the taking in of information that is consistent with what the individual already knows. For example, 5-month-old Aaron sees his bottle. He assimilates this information because he knows his bottle from previous experience. Assimilation is knowledge-based thinking that becomes more efficient with experience. Aaron's parents decide to introduce him to a cup. Because this is new and unfamiliar, Aaron does not know what to do with his cup. He must accommodate the new object through trial and error. *Accommodation* involves physical adaptation (Aaron alters the way he uses his mouth) and mental adaptation (he now knows what to do when he sees his cup). Piaget suggests that assimilation and accommodation are lifelong processes that foster the individual's ongoing adaptation to the environment.

Piaget delineates four stages of cognitive development. The first stage, the *sensorimotor period*, generally spans the first 2 years of life.[1] During this stage the infant slowly progresses from being a reflexive organism to being capable of intentional, goal-oriented behavior. This change is accomplished by assimilation and accommodation as a result of direct interactions with the environment. The infant responds to sensory perceptions with motor activity, becoming more coordinated with each interaction. Thus, a series of simple reflexes evolves to a system of coordinated actions and thoughts. For example, as infants begin to visualize objects within their reach, they progress through a complex sequence of sensory–motor processes, the outcome of which is their ability to grasp the objects they see.

An important accomplishment of the sensorimotor period involves learning *object permanence*, the ability to retain a mental image of objects when they are out of sight. This begins to occur around 8 months of age. Before this age, an object hidden from view ceases to exist for the child. As children learn object permanence, they begin to search for objects out of their sight. Object permanence helps children gain a less centralized view of their world and begin to see others as separate and distinct from themselves.

Another important concept of the sensorimotor period is *egocentrism*, the inability to see things from another's point of view. Egocentrism is characteristic of infants and young children. They believe their thoughts and feelings are held by others around them and that others perceive things the way they do. Children eventually learn that their thoughts and feelings are their own and that they have a singular, separate self with a distinct perspective of the world. This process of differentiation is known as *decentering* and occurs during the second stage of cognitive development.

Piaget's second stage, the *preoperational period*, lasts from approximately age 2 to age 7, and is characterized by tremendous advances in language ability, physical coordination, and perceptual awareness. The preoperational period is a time for refining skills that emerged during the sensorimotor stage.

Language development is characterized by vast increases in vocabulary and improvements in grammar and syntax (sentence structure). Physical ability also improves. Hand–eye coordination is perfected, and the sensorimotor system works as a coordinated whole. This increase in sensory and motor development enables the child to become more perceptually aware of the environment.

However, children in the early preoperational period believe things are as they perceive them to be, even when their perceptions distort reality. As a result, they have difficulty differentiating between fantasy and reality. This explains why young preschoolers see monsters and ghosts in the dark instead of the furniture and shadows that are actually there.

Piaget's classic example of perceptual change is the phenomenon of conservation. *Conservation* is the ability to understand that the quantity of something remains the same even when its appearance is altered. For example, water is poured from a tall, thin glass into a short, wide one. Early preoperational children perceive a change in quantity, although none actually occurs, and thus conclude that the tall glass has more water. Later preoperational children realize that although the amount of water appears to be different, the actual quantity is the same. This ability to "conserve" indicates a more complex, logical thought process.

---

[1]Age parameters for each stage are flexible and vary from child to child and culture to culture.

Children in the preoperational stage of cognitive development have only a vague concept of time. Although they are able to distinguish past, present, and future, they cannot yet grasp refined differences in time (days, weeks, hours). The preoperational child may use "yesterday" to mean anything from two hours ago to two months ago.

In addition, children in the preoperational period have an immature concept of cause and effect. For instance, they do not understand the causes of illness, frequently believing illness results from doing bad things or thinking bad thoughts. Thus, a child who lies to her mother and is admitted to the hospital the following week for a tonsillectomy may believe that hospitalization and surgery are punishments for telling lies. Remnants of such beliefs often persist into adult years even when more abstract thought processes have been established.

Between the ages of 7 and 11, Piaget considers the child to be in the *period of concrete operations*. Children in this period are less egocentric and gradually learn to see things from another's point of view. They also begin to understand cause and effect and have a fairly well developed concept of time, including clock time and historical time.

The ability to classify and categorize objects according to a variety of characteristics such as shape, color, or function emerges during this stage. Children in the concrete operations period are able to think more logically and can understand rules and reasoning.

Thought processes, however, are not fully developed in the 7- to 11-year-old, as illustrated by the difficulty they have dealing with possibilities versus reality. Children in the concrete operations period fail to see the benefit of considering potential events or alternatives; they are concerned only with things as they actually happen. As children near the end of this stage, they overcome their cognitive limitations and move into Piaget's final stage of cognitive development, *formal operations*. Piaget suggests that during this stage, the child gradually becomes capable of abstract, systematic thinking and no longer has to rely on concrete visual images. At this age children are able to think about the future. They can consider several different approaches and potential outcomes to solving a problem. They learn to think and reason beyond their own world and their own values. In essence, by age 15 or so, adolescents think like adults.

Moral Development Theory

One aspect of cognitive development that Piaget studied was the development of judgment and moral reasoning in the child. More recently, Lawrence Kohlberg (1968) has elaborated on Piaget's model of development with a theory that focuses on the reasoning and logic underlying an individual's choice of action when presented with a moral dilemma. It should be emphasized that it is not the choice per se that is the crucial indicator of moral reasoning ability, but the *reason* the individual gives for choosing a particular course of action. Kohlberg suggests that people proceed through three levels, or six stages, of moral development. Progression through these levels closely approximates the child's progression through Piaget's stages of cognitive development. Thus, it seems the acquisition of moral values is linked intimately to an individual's cognitive complexity. It is also important to note that moral development is strongly influenced by the individual's life experiences, relationships, the family's values, and the values of the cultural group and society. Table 10-4 outlines Kohlberg's stages of moral development.

Gilligan (1982) points out that Kohlberg's theory of moral development reflects a masculine perspective because the subjects from which he derived his theory were males. Gilligan (1982) argues that women's moral development is concerned with responsibilities (to others and to society) rather than with rights and rules as Kohlberg emphasized. Moral development in women thus is tied closely to relationships and to the uniqueness of each context in which moral decisions are made (Gilligan, 1982). Therefore, Kohlberg's theory should be viewed with caution when applied to the moral development of women.

Developmental Tasks Theory

Robert J. Havighurst's theory of developmental tasks (1972) evolved from the work of several child psychologists and educators. Havighurst defines a developmental task as,

> . . . a task which arises at or about a certain period in the life of an individual, successful achievement of which leads to . . . happiness and to success with later tasks, while failure leads to unhappiness in the individual, disapproval by the society, and difficulty with later tasks. (p. 2)

Tasks for the various developmental stages are determined by (1) physical maturation, (2) social and cultural pressures, and (3) values and aspirations of the person. Some tasks, such as learning to walk, arise from biological maturation, common across cultures, whereas others are unique to a particular culture or society. Havighurst's tasks are

TABLE 10-4
Kohlberg's Stages of Moral Development

Level	Stage
Preconventional Level (4 to 10 years) Rules and expectations are external	Stage 1: Obedience–Punishment Orientation Child obeys to avoid punishment Stage 2: Naive Hedonistic–Instrumental Orientation (Bargaining Stage) Child's motivations are rewards and benefits
Conventional Level (10 to 13 years) Rules and expectations are internalized	Stage 3: Good Boy or Good Girl Orientation Motivation is to win approval and avoid disapproval especially by peer group; rules are extremely important Stage 4: Law and Order Orientation Person literally accepts society's conventions and rules
Postconventional Level (13 years to adulthood) Self is differentiated from rules and expectations of others, and own self-chosen principles are defined	Stage 5: Social-Contract Orientation Purpose of law is seen to preserve human rights, and if it is unjust, one must change the law, but one must still follow the existing laws Stage 6: Universal Ethical Principle Orientation There is an internal set of ideas that, if violated, result in guilt and self-condemnation

Note. From Hayes, J.S. (1987). Theories of child development. In Servonsky/Opas: *Nursing Management of Children* © 1987. Boston: Jones and Bartlett Publishers, p. 237. Compiled from Kohlberg, L. (1968). The child as a moral philosopher. *Psychology Today*, 2(4), 25–30.

based on middle class American cultural norms and should be interpreted with caution for people from other cultural or socioeconomic groups. Havighurst's tasks for childhood and adolescence are presented in Table 10-5.

Learning Theories

Learning theories, also known as stimulus–response (S–R) theory or behavioral learning theory, are based on the premise that all behavior is learned. Behaviorists believe individuals are born blank slates and that environmental influences shape their behavior.

Unlike stage theories, learning theories explain developmental progress as a consequence of environmental forces. Learning, as explained by Skinner (1945, 1974), is a process involving stimuli and responses. Stimuli, such as cold, light, or a parent's voice and touch, evoke responses that are rewarded, ignored, or punished. Responses that are rewarded or bring pleasure to the individual are repeated and become part of the individual's behavioral repertoire. Responses that are ignored or punished tend not to be repeated. It is important to note, however, that punishment itself may serve as a reward in that the person is receiving attention, however negative it may be.

Behavioral learning theorists are concerned only with observable behaviors and the associations the individual makes between stimuli and responses. Learning theorists reject, or at least are not interested in, the internal mechanisms that may underlie emotions, thoughts, or attitudes.

Another somewhat modified learning theory is social learning. Social learning theory, proposed by Albert Bandura (1977), presents a model for continuous human development that helps explain both individual characteristics based on a person's learning history and similarities among people related to the influence of culture. Most human behavior leads to consequences that either maintain or change the probability of similar behavior in the future. Learning can occur through a variety of experiences, including directly experiencing the consequences of behavior, watching what happens to others, or listening to or reading about how specific cues, behaviors, and consequences are related (vicarious learning). People learn relationships between such stimuli as behaviors and feelings. They learn to discriminate between stimulus events based on differing consequences for the same behavior (e.g., smoking at home or on the job) and to generalize across situations by responding to variations in stimuli in a similar manner (e.g., friendly response to all customers, no matter how the customers approach the salesperson).

People influence and change their environ-

TABLE 10-5
Havighurst's Developmental Tasks

Tasks of Infancy and Early Childhood (birth to 6 years)
1. Learning to walk
2. Learning to take solid foods
3. Learning to talk
4. Learning to control the elimination of body wastes
5. Learning sex differences and sexual modesty
6. Forming concepts and learning language to describe social and physical reality
7. Getting ready to read
8. Learning to distinguish right and wrong and beginning to develop a conscience

Tasks of Middle Childhood (6–12 years)
1. Learning physical skills necessary for ordinary games.
2. Building wholesome attitudes toward oneself as a growing organism
3. Learning to get along with age mates
4. Learning appropriate masculine or feminine social role
5. Developing fundamental skills in reading, writing, and calculating

6. Developing concepts necessary for everyday living
7. Developing conscience, morality, and a scale of values
8. Achieving personal independence
9. Developing attitudes toward social groups and institutions

Tasks of Adolescence (12–18 years)
1. Achieving new and more mature relations with age mates of both sexes
2. Achieving a masculine or feminine social role
3. Accepting one's physique and using the body effectively
4. Achieving emotional independence of parents and other adults
5. Preparing for marriage and family life
6. Preparing for an economic career
7. Acquiring a set of values and an ethical system as a guide to behavior—developing an ideology
8. Desiring and achieving socially responsible behavior

Note. From Havighurst, R. (1972). *Developmental tasks and education* (3rd ed.), New York: Longman, Inc. Copyright © 1972 by Longman, Inc. Reprinted by permission of Longman, Inc., New York.

ment and are modified by it. People are neither free agents who can become whatever they choose nor powerless objects controlled by environmental factors. Human behavior is the result of a continuous reciprocal interaction of cognitive, behavioral, and environmental determinants. Bandura calls this *reciprocal determinism.*

Social learning is influenced by (1) modeling; (2) reinforcing, punishing, or ignoring a person's behavior directly or that of a model vicariously; and (3) instruction about rules and other persuasive communications that the person is to use in certain situations (self-management techniques). Whether social learning occurs depends on many interrelated processes (attention, memory, interaction, motor processes, motivation, modeling, social reinforcement).

Bandura argues that much of human behavior is self-regulated by self-produced reinforcement or punishment. Standards for self-reinforcement are learned by children through direct instruction and by observing others. These standards play a major role in shaping the self-concept and how a person responds to and evaluates his or her own behavior. How two people respond to the same situation (e.g., a grade in a course) may differ greatly because of the different standards they have set for their performances and the self-management techniques they use (Bandura, 1977).

In summary, it is essential to remember that theories of human development are useful guides, but should be used with caution when making clinical judgments about the appropriateness of a particular behavior. Many factors influence an individual's development and behavior, and there is reason to believe that currently accepted theories may provide biased views of life cycle development (Gilligan, 1982). This notion is discussed more fully in Chapter 11.

GENERAL CONSIDERATIONS IN DEVELOPMENTAL ASSESSMENT

Generally, there are three components, or steps, in assessing development of children. These include obtaining a developmental history, clinically observing the child's behavior to validate the subjective information gathered in the history, and, if indicated, screening the child for developmental delays. Child–parent interaction should also be assessed. The nature of the parent–child relationship has been shown clearly to influence a child's development.

In most instances, interview and observation provide the information needed to affirm that the child's developmental progress is within the expected range. However, when the objective information collected via observation contradicts the subjective data obtained in the interview, or if the information indicates the child may be at risk for developmental delay, then developmental screening with a carefully chosen screening tool may be indicated.

The frequency with which developmental assessment should be done depends on the age of the child. Generally speaking, the younger the child, the more frequently developmental progress should be assessed, because there is an inverse relationship between the age of the child and the pace of development: the younger the child, the faster the pace of development. Therefore, during infancy, developmental progress should be assessed ideally at least every two months. During the second year, every six months is recommended, and after age 2, annual assessments should be made. Most health-care agencies adopt a recommended schedule of preventive health care for children and include developmental assessment as part of the total health assessment for each visit.

The importance of the setting in which developmental assessment is done and its potential effect on a child's behavior cannot be emphasized enough. Children who are frightened or anxious, who see nothing familiar or comforting in the health-care environment, are unlikely to relax enough to permit an accurate assessment of their developmental capabilities. A child who is usually very talkative at home may be reluctant to speak in the health-care setting, making it difficult for the nurse to validate, for example, the parents' report that the child's speech and language are developing normally.

It is especially important to remember that developmental assessment of an ill or hospitalized child may yield questionable or even false findings. Children who are ill and confined to a health facility, especially if separated from their parents, often regress. In such circumstances, the child's behavior is unlikely to reflect the child's typical behavior when feeling well and in a more familiar setting. This is not to say the nurse should avoid assessing an ill or hospitalized child's development, but simply to recommend caution in drawing conclusions based upon what may be incomplete or invalid information about a child's current developmental abilities.

The environment, whether clinic, hospital room, or physician's office, can be modified easily to create a climate that promotes a feeling of security for the child and thus facilitates the assessment. Bright colors, pictures on the walls, child-size furniture, and age-appropriate toys and activities all help a child relax. While the nurse is interviewing the parent, the child can be encouraged to play with available materials. As the child becomes involved with play, the nurse can observe some of the child's developmental skills.

Play materials also provide a means for communicating with children. Asking a child to draw a picture and then tell about it allows the nurse to assess the child's verbal abilities. A puppet or doll "interviewing" a young child may be more successful in eliciting responses than direct questioning by the nurse.

It is crucial to remember that the child is always the *primary* source of data even though much, or most, of the information is obtained from the parent. Because very young children cannot participate in the interview, it will be necessary for parents to provide information relative to the child's developmental history and current achievements. However, this does not negate the importance of validating or supplementing this information with direct observations of the child.

THE DEVELOPMENTAL HISTORY

A large part of the developmental assessment is done via interview. The developmental history is the major interviewing tool the nurse uses to gather information about a child's developmental achievements or concerns parents may have. Information about the child's earlier development and the parents' perceptions of the child's current level of functioning is helpful in determining whether the child's development is within the expected range.

It is essential to remember that children's development does not occur in isolation from their social, cultural, or temporal contexts. Many variables play a role in shaping a child's development, including genetic potential, parent–child interaction, sociocultural resources, and other factors. A number of studies, for instance, have shown a relationship between such parent variables as maternal age, parents' knowledge of child development, parental life change, and social support, and a child's developmental outcomes (Becker, 1987; Bee, Hammond, Eyres, Barnard, & Snyder, 1986; Mercer, Hackley, & Bostrom, 1984; Simkins, 1984). Schraeder, Rappaport, and Courtwright (1987) found that almost half (49%) of the variance in preschool cognitive development could be attributed to environmental factors. The multiple variables that influence development should be kept in mind when obtaining a developmental history.

Because young children have a limited ability

to provide accurate information about their past development, parents are usually the major source of information. Depending on their cognitive development and language skills, however, preschool children may participate actively in the assessment interview (Figure 10-3). They often can respond to questions about their age, their favorite foods, who their family members are, and what they like to do. Their responses provide information about their mental status, speech, and social responsiveness. Parents, of course, may need to validate the accuracy of the information the child provides. Most important, such interaction with a young child helps to secure the child's trust and cooperation and teaches the child that nurses are helpful people.

If other significant people care for the child on a regular basis, such as grandparents, other relatives, schoolteachers, or staff in day care centers, it may be necessary to ask them to supplement the developmental history obtained from the parents. This becomes necessary only when the parents are unable to provide the needed information or if the information given by the parents is questionable.

Children over age 7 can and should be included as active participants in the interview by directing appropriate questions to them; an example is, "Tell me what kinds of things you do in gym class at school." With children over the age of 10 or 11, the nurse may wish to spend a few minutes alone with the child, since there may be areas of

question or concern about which the child is hesitant to talk in the parents' presence.

The developmental history should begin with a review of the parents' general health. Usually this information is obtained as part of the general health history. The nurse should collect information about the mother's health and care during her pregnancy with the child, including the course of the mother's labor and delivery and the child's neonatal period. The child's postnatal developmental history provides data about the child's accomplishment of significant milestones in motor, language, and personal–social skills. If problems occurred during the prenatal, perinatal, or postnatal period, this information may alert the nurse to a child who is at risk for developmental delay.

Learning self-care skills such as feeding, dressing, and independent toileting, and accepting responsibility for self-management are major tasks of childhood. Therefore, the nurse should ascertain the child's self-care competencies as part of the developmental history. Sample questions pertaining to self-care are provided in Table 10-6.

The parents' perceptions of the child's current level of functioning also should be assessed. The nurse can review age-appropriate tasks and ask the parents to indicate whether the child is performing them. Table 10-7 may be used as a guide in formulating these questions. For example, the nurse can ask the parent(s) of a 15-month-old:

"Does Beth stand alone? Walk alone?"

"Does she drink from a cup?"

"Does she name objects?"

"How does she express her needs or desires?"

"How does Beth respond when you leave her with a familiar person?"

"With an unfamiliar one?"

"Has Beth shown any interest in potty training?"

Such questioning allows the nurse to assess the parents' knowledge of the child's developmental progress.

Parents also should be asked what concerns they have about their child's development. Are they satisfied with the child's developmental progress? Do they wish the child would advance more rapidly? The competitive nature of today's world often leads parents to push their children to acquire skills that are beyond the child's current capabilities or for which the timing is developmentally inappropriate. Examples include teaching a toddler to read or enrolling a child in a structured

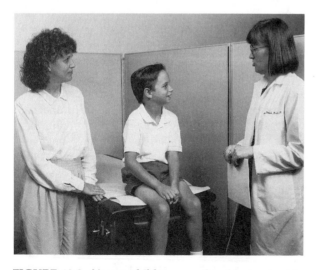

FIGURE 10-3. Young children may be able to provide information for the developmental history by answering simple questions about their favorite activities, who their family members are, and what they usually eat.

learning environment before age 5 or 6. Several authors (Meyrowitz, 1985; Postman, 1982; Rosemond, 1981) have taken issue with exposing children to experiences that are inappropriate for their age. These authors suggest that parents often act out of their own needs for esteem and prestige rather than the child's developmental needs. Critics note that such experiences actually may be detrimental to the child (McCall, 1981), or at least not of any particular benefit since early differences tend to disappear with age (Rosemond, 1981).

The nurse also should query parents about any specific developmental concerns they have or problems they have noted, such as fears, school difficulties, or perceived problems with skill acquisition. Because a child's potential development depends to a large extent on the support and nurturing provided by significant people, an assessment of the child's relationships with family members and significant others (e.g., peers, teachers) is also an important part of the total developmental assessment. Table 10-6 presents a suggested format for the developmental history, with sample questions.

Another important part of the developmental history involves collecting information about the child's home and school environments and their adequacy in promoting or inhibiting the child's development. Questions should be asked about the child's home and neighborhood as well as the availability of toys, books, and other play materials. Assessment of the environment is covered thoroughly in Chapter 9.

TABLE 10-6
The Developmental History—Child

Child's name, birth date, current age (years, months)

Perinatal History (Children Under Age 3 or Those with a History of Developmental Problems)
Maternal history:
Gravida, para, aborta (with this child)
Prenatal care (month began, frequency, nutritional patterns, history of smoking/alcohol/drug use, medications, illness)
Labor and delivery (length of labor, analgesia, anesthesia, type of delivery, complications)
Neonatal history:
Weeks gestation; birth weight and length; APGAR scores; length of hospital stay
Neonatal problems (hyperbilirubinemia, congenital abnormalities, blood incompatibility, respiratory distress, infection)

Postnatal Development (Significant Milestones)
Feeding (methods, problems)
Significant milestones:
Motor (age at which infant rolled over, sat alone, walked alone, achieved bowel and bladder control)
Language (age at which child said first word, used first sentences)
Personal/social (age at which child smiled responsively, was shy with strangers, began eating with fingers, separated easily from mother, learned to dress self)

Parent History
Parents' ages at child's birth
Parents' educational level; parents' work/career patterns: perceived impact on child and parents; parents' source(s) of information about child care and development
Recent critical events or life changes (changes in residence or income, divorce, death of family member); parents' perception of impact on child and family

What parents like most about child; what they would like to change about child
Parents' style of childrearing and discipline (what parents expect of child, e.g., achievements, level of responsibility, etc.; how parents handle child's misbehavior)
Parents' concerns about child's development or any noted problems; parental stressors related to childrearing

Child History
Parents' perceptions of child's current level of functioning (in comparison with other children of same age)
NOTE: The parent can be asked specific questions appropriate to the child's age, i.e., specific capabilities in motor, language/cognition, and personal/social areas of development (see Table 10-7).
Description of child's typical day (schedule, activities)
Child's interactions with others (parents, siblings, peers, teachers): frequency of interaction, activities with others, any problems in interpersonal relationships
School performance and problems (grades K through 12)

Self-Care Responsibility
Extent to which the parent encourages the child to do things for himself/herself (appropriate to child's age), e.g., feeding, dressing, toileting, preparation for bedtime, personal hygiene, self-control
Decisions the child makes without assistance (e.g., spending allowance money, choosing clothes, choosing recreational activities and friends, bedtime)
Household responsibilities the child manages.
Effectiveness, efficiency, and reliability of the child about these responsibilities
Child's ability to manage time (goal setting, planning ahead, completion of assigned tasks on time)

CLINICAL APPRAISAL

Although the developmental history provides much of the information for the developmental assessment, the history depends on the parents' recall ability and is therefore highly subjective (Byrne, Blackman, & Smith, 1986). Thus, it is important that the history be supplemented with objective data. Direct observation of the child's abilities is the most reliable and objective means of assessing developmental achievements (Figure 10-4). Specifically, the nurse should observe the child's gross and fine motor skills, speech and language abilities, and the child's interactions with people and objects in the environment. These observations provide clues about how well the child is adapting and what tools or techniques the child uses to deal with the world.

Table 10-7, which outlines the expected behaviors and abilities of children and adolescents from 1 month to 18 years of age, can be used as a guide for

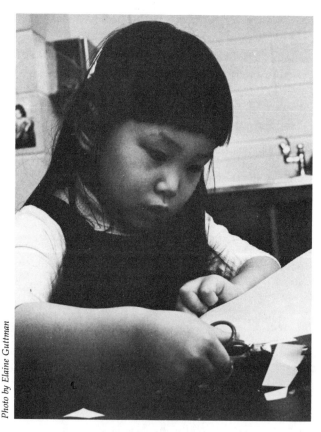

FIGURE 10-4. Observation of the child's abilities, such as the fine motor skills needed for using scissors, is the most reliable way to assess developmental achievements. (*Note.* From Servonsky/Opas: *Nursing Management of Children,* © 1987. Boston: Jones and Bartlett Publishers, p. 241.)

Photo by Elaine Guttman

identifying what age-appropriate characteristics the nurse should look for, including self-care abilities.

The nurse may wish to have the child demonstrate a few selected skills. For example, a 4-year-old may be asked to copy a square, identify three colors, and hop on one foot.

The nurse's observations should be recorded as part of the data base. In addition to noting skills the child exhibits, a description of the child's interaction with the parent (voice tones, verbal interchange, eye contact, touching) and how the child responds to unfamiliar people and objects in the health-care setting should be included.

Again, the nurse should be cautious about drawing conclusions about a child's development based on a single contact, without considering the possible effects of the health-care setting on the child's behavior. The nurse should ask the parent if the observed behavior is typical of the child's behavior at home or school. If the child is too shy or frightened to participate in the assessment willingly, a visit to the child's home or school to validate impressions may be indicated, particularly if there is some concern about the child's developmental progress.

DEVELOPMENTAL SCREENING

The developmental history combined with observation generally will yield enough information for the nurse to formulate valid impressions of a child's developmental status. Sometimes, however, developmental screening with a standardized tool may be indicated, especially if a child seems to be exhibiting a delay in one or more areas of development or if the parent expresses concern.

Factors that place children at particular risk of developmental delays are delineated in Table 10-8. A child whose history yields one or more of these indicators should be screened with an appropriate tool as a routine part of regular health visits.

The general purposes of screening are discussed in Chapter 2 along with criteria for selecting conditions to be screened. It is important to remember that developmental screening tools are not diagnostic, nor can they predict a child's future developmental capabilities. They also may have other limitations. In particular, developmental screening tools may be time-consuming to administer and may not take into account racial, social, or cultural differences among children (Frankenburg, Dick, & Carland, 1975).

When screening for developmental problems,

TABLE 10-7
Developmental Milestones

Age	Physical	Motor/adaptation	Language/cognition	Socialization
Birth to 1 month	Gains between 5 and 7 ounces weekly through the first 6 months Grows about 1 inch monthly through the first 6 months Breathes through nose only Head circumference exceeds chest circumference Strong primitive reflexes Doll's eye and dance reflex diminishing Heart rate: 120–140/min. Respiratory rate: 30–60/min.	Distinct head lag in ventral suspension and sitting position Raises head briefly and turns head while lying prone Makes crawling movements in prone position Back is rounded when propped in sitting position Keeps hands tightly fisted Grasps but instantly drops objects placed in hand	Is in the first stage of the sensorimotor phase, use of reflexes Behaves reflexively Is totally self-centered Tolerates minimal frustration Quiets in response to a human voice Cries to show displeasure Makes contented sounds while feeding Makes small throaty sounds	Eyes follow dangling object to midline Observes faces and bright objects in line of vision Gazes indefinitely at surroundings Smiles vaguely
2 months	Posterior fontanel closes Crawling reflex vanishes Moro and tonic neck reflexes diminishing	No head lag in ventral suspension Minimal head lag in sitting position Raises head nearly 45° while lying prone Back remains rounded when propped in sitting position Turns from side to back Moves arms and legs energetically Hands often open Brings hand to mouth Touches but does not grasp objects Holds rattle briefly	Is in the second stage of the sensorimotor phase, primary circular reactions, which persists until 4 months of age. During this time the infant increasingly acts voluntarily rather than reflexively; begins to separate self from others; engages in activities for pleasure, not results; combines visual and sucking schema; i.e., opens mouth at sight of breast or bottle Seeks attention through differentiated crying Coos Vocalizes in response to familiar voices Utters single vowel sounds such as "ah," "eh"	Eyes follow dangling object past midline Eyes follow moving person Alert facial expression Smiles in response to human voice
3 months	Weighs 12–13 lb Grasp reflex diminishing Landau reflex appears (infant's legs draw reflexively up	Head remains erect but bobs in sitting position Raises head and shoulders 45°–90° when lying prone	Cries less Vocalizes frequently when spoken to Utters two-syllable vowel sounds Chuckles, babbles,	Eyes follow objects 180° Recognizes mother and familiar objects Responds to parents' presence

(continued)

TABLE 10-7 (Continued)

Age	Physical	Motor/adaptation	Language/cognition	Socialization
	against body when suspended in horizontal prone position with head flexed against trunk)	and supports weight on forearms Back is rounded in propped sitting position Plays with fingers and hands	and squeals with pleasure Enjoys making sounds Repeats sounds	Notices surroundings
4 months	Weighs 13–14 lb Begins to drool Tonic neck, Moro, and Perez reflexes vanish. (Perez reflex—infant prone on a firm surface cries, flexes extremities, and raises head and pelvis when thumb is pressed along spine from sacrum to neck. Lordosis of the spine, urination, and defecation also may occur)	Holds head consistently erect when pulled to sitting position Raises head and chest 90° when lying prone Back is straighter in propped sitting position Supports some weight on legs when held in standing position Grasps objects put in hand Clasps hands together Reaches for but overshoots objects	Is in the third stage of the sensorimotor phase—secondary circular reactions, which persist until 8 months of age. During this time the infant assimilates new objects such as toys into established patterns; i.e., touches, sucks, drops a stuffed animal; acts intentionally rather than repetitively to achieve a goal; i.e., tugs on a string to obtain an object; repeats actions that result in new experiences; i.e., infant accidentally hits a ball, ball rolls, infant repeats action to determine if ball will move again Vocalizes according to mood changes Includes some consonant sounds such as "m," "p," "b" Laughs aloud Is "talkative"	Enjoys being with people Attends closely to unfamiliar stimuli Smiles responsively Invites social interactions by smiling
5 months	Birth weight doubles Signs of tooth eruption may appear—lower central incisors first Breathes through mouth when nose is obstructed	Balances head in sitting position Raises head when pulled to sitting position Raises self on extended arms Rolls from side to side and from prone to supine Sits with back straight with minimal support Grasps objects voluntarily	Stops crying in response to music Intersperses vowel and consonant sounds	Smiles at mirror image Begins to differentiate strangers from significant people Enjoys being played with Responds negatively to removal of a toy

TABLE 10-7 (Continued)

Age	Physical	Motor/adaptation	Language/cognition	Socialization
		Carries objects directly to mouth Plays with toes and puts in mouth		
6 months	Gains 3 to 5 ounces weekly through the second six months Grows about ½ inch monthly through the second six months of life May begin teething	Raises head spontaneously when supine Rolls completely from prone to prone Sits supported in high chair Supports most of weight when held erect Bounces briefly on feet when held standing Grasps and manipulates small objects Can hold own bottle Transfers object from hand to hand	"Talks" to mirror image Tries to mimic sounds Enjoys sound of own vocalization Single-syllable babbling increases	Extends arms to be held Fears strangers Imitates actions of others Makes known specific likes and dislikes Waves arms and legs when frustrated
7 months	Upper central incisors may erupt	Sits unsupported using hands as props Rolls more easily from supine to prone Feeds self cracker using only one hand	"Talks" while others are talking—vocalizes impatience Makes four distinct vowel sounds	Increasingly fears strangers Frets when mother leaves Enjoys peek-a-boo Fluctuates easily between laughing and crying
8–9 months	Regular bowel and bladder patterns emerge Upper lateral incisors may erupt Plantar reflex vanishes Parachute reflex appears	Sits steadily unsupported Leans forward to reach an object Crawls along floor Stands while holding onto an object Uses crude pincer grasp Shows marked preference in use of one hand over the other	Is in the fourth stage of the sensorimotor phase, coordination and application of secondary schemata to new situations, which persists until 12 months of age. During this time the infant recognizes anticipatory signs: e.g., cries when mother dons coat; behaves intentionally; e.g., turns head away from disliked foods; searches for absent objects; e.g., toy under a blanket "Shouts" for attention Babbles in two syllables; e.g., "mama," "a-la," "a-ba" "Listens" to conversations Responds to simple verbal commands; e.g., "No!"	Fears loss of mother Fears being alone at bedtime; may protest bedtime

(continued)

TABLE 10-7 (Continued)

Age	Physical	Motor/adaptation	Language/cognition	Socialization
10–11 months	Neck-righting reflex vanishes Body-righting reflex appears Lower lateral incisors may erupt	Sits unsupported indefinitely Pulls self into sitting and standing positions Crawls on hands and knees Cruises awkwardly around furniture Isolates fingers and demonstrates crude release Uses handle to raise cup Uses delicate pincer grasp	Speaks one word besides mama and dada Says mama and dada with comprehension Mimics speech sounds Responds to name	Extends toys to others Repeats actions that elicit a response from others Dislikes restrictions Delights in achievement of a task Waves bye-bye Plays pat-a-cake
12 months	Birth weight triples: 21 to 22 pounds Birth length increases by 50%: 30 inches Head and chest circumference are approximately equal Anterior fontanel is nearly closed Has six to eight teeth Landau reflex is diminishing Babinski reflex vanishes Drooling is decreasing	Stands alone briefly Cruises well Walks with one hand held Holds a crayon Releases objects from hand at will Turns pages of a book, several at once Increasingly practices locomotion skills	Is in the fifth stage of the sensorimotor phase—tertiary circular reactions—which persists until 18 months of age. During this time, the infant experiments to discover how objects behave and how they can be manipulated; e.g., repeatedly drops a block to observe deviations that occur each time; begins determining alternate ways of achieving an end; e.g., goes around a table to find a ball that has rolled underneath the table Speaks two words Mimics animal sounds Obeys simple commands; e.g., "Give me the toy" Understands the meaning of several words Recognizes some objects by name	Shows emotions; e.g., love, anger, fear Fears unfamiliar situations Will leave mother's side to explore in familiar surroundings
15 months		Assumes standing position without aid Kneels unsupported Stands and walks alone Builds a two-block tower	Speaks 4–6 words Uses jargon Knows own name Names known objects or pictures Touches pictures in a book	Hugs and kisses parents Tolerates some separation from mother Has temper tantrums Imitates parents Indicates wet diaper

TABLE 10-7 (Continued)

Age	Physical	Motor/adaptation	Language/cognition	Socialization
		Drinks from a cup Scribbles spontaneously	Vocalizes needs	
18 months	Anterior fontanel closes Abdomen protrudes Appetite decreases as growth needs lessen Urinary and anal sphincter control emerges	Walks upstairs with one hand held Runs awkwardly Climbs Pushes and pulls toys Builds a three–four block tower Uses a spoon without spilling Turns book pages several at a time Squats to recover objects or while playing	Is in the sixth stage of the sensorimotor phase—invention of new means through mental combinations—which persists until 24 months of age. During this time the infant solves problems by combining mental images as opposed to trial and error experimentation; mimics and retains characteristics of models; i.e., parents; is egocentric Speaks 6–10 words Points to familiar objects and at least one body part Uses phrases containing nouns and adjectives	Has temper tantrums more frequently May attach to security object; e.g., blanket Increasingly imitates parents Begins to understand ownership May regulate bowel movements Enjoys solitary play or observing others' activities
21 months		Walks upstairs alone Walks downstairs with one hand held Runs fairly well Builds five–six block tower	Speaks 15–20 words Combines 2 or 3 words Points to at least three body parts	Pulls on people to attract their attention Helps with very simple tasks in the home; e.g., dusting
24 months	Weighs 26–28 lb. Is 32–33 inches tall Has about 16 temporary teeth Chest circumference is greater than head circumference Physiological systems with exception of reproductive and endocrine are mature Respiratory rate averages 26–28 breaths/minute Heart rate averages 100 beats/minute Blood pressure averages 99 mm Hg systolic and 64 mm Hg diastolic	Walks upstairs alone Retains balance while picking up an object Claps hands Builds five–seven block tower Turns pages singly Turns door knob to open doors Drinks well from a small cup held in one hand	Is in the preconceptual stage of preoperational period; persists until 4 years of age. During this time the toddler believes inanimate objects possess life and consciousness; possesses an immature concept of causality; i.e., must be disciplined immediately after the event or is unsure about the reason for discipline; uses play as a primary means of adaptation Has a 300-word vocabulary Uses personal pronouns Talks continuously	Has fewer temper tantrums Has an increased attention span Engages in parallel play Helps to undress self Pulls on simple garments Does not share belongings Asks for help reluctantly

(continued)

TABLE 10-7 (Continued)

Age	Physical	Motor/adaptation	Language/cognition	Socialization
			Verbalizes need for food, drink, and toileting Refers to self by name	
30 months	Birth weight is quadrupled Has a complete set of 20 temporary teeth May attain bowel and bladder control during the day	Walks on tiptoe Jumps in place with both feet Tries to stand on one foot Builds a nine-block tower Throws a large ball about 4 feet Rides a kiddie car or tricycle Holds crayon with fingers, not fist Copies vertical and horizontal lines	Uses plurals Uses correct pronoun in reference to self Names one color Names familiar objects when asked Responds to simple questions	Separates more readily from mother Knows own sex Recognizes some sex differences Attends to own toilet needs except for wiping Helps put toys away
3 years	Between 3 and 5 years of age the child gains 4–6 pounds annually, grows 2–2½ inches annually; has an average respiratory rate of 20; has an average pulse rate between 90 and 110; has an average blood pressure of 85 mm Hg systolic and 60 mm Hg diastolic	Walks backward Jumps from bottom step Rides a tricycle or "big wheel" cycle Builds a 9–10 block tower Feeds self with little spilling Pours liquid from a pitcher Washes hands May brush teeth Strings large beads Copies a circle	Has a 900-word vocabulary Constructs 3–4 word sentences Begins to comprehend the concept of time (past, present, future)	Separates easily from parents for short periods Notices family relationships and sex role functions Tries to please parents Engages in parallel and associative play Begins learning simple games Enjoys being read to Helps dress self
4 years	(See 3 years)	Hops on one foot Throws a ball overhand Dresses self partially Copies drawings of a cross and square Draws a person with 2–4 parts other than the head	Is in the intuitive thought stage of the preoperational period—persists until 7 years of age. During this time the child verbalizes thought processes; is less egocentric and more aware of others; can consider only one idea at a time; considers only parts of the whole, not the whole itself Has a 1500-word vocabulary Constructs 4–5 word sentences Questions continuously Understands simple analogies Counts to 3	Is independent Rebels at excessive parental expectations May show feelings of sibling rivalry Exaggerates, brags, and tattles May be impatient and selfish Prefers playmates to solitary play May have an imaginary playmate Cooperates in play

TABLE 10-7 (Continued)

Age	Physical	Motor/adaptation	Language/cognition	Socialization
			Repeats four numbers Knows own age Names one or more colors Identifies the longer of two lines	
5 years	(See 3 years)	Skips on alternate feet Hops well Roller-skates on four wheels Jumps rope Puts away toys neatly Hits a nail with a hammer Dresses and undresses without aid Ties shoelaces Copies a drawing of a triangle Draws a person with six parts Prints first name	Has a 2100-word vocabulary Constructs 6–8 word sentences Knows colors Questions the meaning of words Begins questioning beliefs of parents Begins seeing things from others' perspective (emotionally) Understands increasingly time and conservation of numbers Identifies dimes, nickels, and pennies Counts ten coins Knows address and phone number	Relies on parents for security and reassurance Identifies strongly with parent of the same sex Gets along well with parents Rebels less than 4-year-old Tries to live by the rules Plays cooperatively; rigidly adheres to rules, but may cheat to win Provides total self-care; e.g., bathing, dressing Is increasingly responsible for own actions
6 years	Weighs 48 pounds Is 46 inches tall First permanent teeth, central mandibular incisors, erupt	Uses a table knife for spreading Ties a bow Washes hands at appropriate times Brushes own hair Makes simple clay figures Enjoys table games Walks steadily on chalk mark Rides two-wheel bicycle	Is in the first grade Enjoys school Enjoys reading Is increasingly aware of time Differentiates between morning and afternoon, days of week, months of year, seasons Able to assemble simple jigsaw puzzles	Mimics adult behavior Has an increasing need to socialize with children of the same age Enjoys rough play May be jealous of younger sibling Has emotional outbursts Is easily hurt by criticism Knows simple table manners
7 years	Grows 2–2½ inches annually Weighs 49–50 lb Is 47–49 inches tall Permanent mandibular incisors and maxillary central incisors erupt	Plays hopscotch Cuts meat with a table knife Copies a diamond	Is in the period of concrete operations, which persists until 11 years of age. During this time the child mentally performs actions without carrying out the behaviors; classifies objects according to characteristics such as size, shape, and color; recognizes that others may	Takes an increasingly active part in the family group Plays mostly with children of the same sex Participates in group play Likes being alone, can entertain self with reading, games, drawing, other quiet play

(continued)

TABLE 10-7 (Continued)

Age	Physical	Motor/adaptation	Language/cognition	Socialization
			view things from a perspective different than child's own Is in the second grade Recognizes the absence of certain parts in pictures Reads a clock to the nearest quarter hour Is able to solve simple crossword puzzles and mazes	
8–9 years	Continues growing 2–2½ inches annually Is 51–55 inches tall Mandibular cuspids and maxillary incisors erupt	Bathes without aid Assists with routine household chores; e.g., dusting, washing dishes Uses common tools and household utensils Explores the neighborhood alone or with friends	Is proud of accomplishment in school Enjoys reading Fully comprehends time Classifies objects Is in the 3rd–4th grade	Gets along with family members Prefers certain friends Begins to play with children of the opposite sex Enjoys competition and game playing Is well behaved
10–12 years	Growth in height slows Weighs 71–100 lb Is 55–60 inches tall Remaining permanent teeth erupt Pubescent changes may begin Contours of girls soften	Cares for pets Creates drawings and paintings Makes useful articles; e.g., potholders	Is in the period of formal operations. During this time, the child begins thinking abstractly; e.g., develops and tests hypotheses; is able to reason beyond own concrete world and beliefs Is in the 5th–7th grade Reads for enjoyment or to obtain information Writes letters to friends or relatives	Loves and respects both parents Tries to please parents, but increasingly influenced by peer group Continues to need friends Uses the telephone May stay alone at home for several hours Attends successfully to own needs and those of children left in care
13–15 years	Girls grow 2–8 inches and gain 15–55 lb Boys grow 4–12 inches and gain 15–65 lb Often appears physically awkward Menses begins (mean age of 12 years) Nocturnal emissions occur in boys Secondary sex characteristics mature	May abandon childhood hobbies Performs routine chores on own initiative	Uses hypothetical-deductive reasoning Manipulates more than two categories of variables simultaneously	Is less involved in family affairs May increasingly criticize parents Accepts criticism or advice reluctantly Values peers increasingly Belongs to a peer group Develops crushes Begins dating Strives for independence but continues to desire dependence

TABLE 10-7 (Continued)

Age	Physical	Motor/adaptation	Language/cognition	Socialization
16–18 years	Growth in height ceases Wisdom teeth begin to erupt Physically resembles an adult	Coordination improves Drives a car	Gains much intellectual maturity Questions established moral views Views the world from a relativistic perspective	Is increasingly concerned with physical appearance Continues to have conflicts with parents Devotes majority of time to peer group activities Supports peer group members Experiments with adultlike roles; e.g., part-time jobs, babysitting May adopt many of the values and ideas of peer group Is attaining emotional independence Plans for the future May experiment with smoking, alcohol, sexual behavior Consolidates sex-role identity Indulges in petting May be sexually active

the nurse should avoid the temptation to use the results to assign a child a developmental age. The most the nurse can say about the findings of developmental screening is that they are an estimate of the child's current abilities compared with the average. Even if the findings are abnormal, the nurse knows only that the child *may* have a potential problem or delay, in which case the child should be referred for further testing.

Developmental screening tools are useful in alerting the nurse or other health professionals to the possibility that a health problem or developmental delay exists. Early detection and treatment of such problems are crucial if the child's maximum potential is to be realized.

There are numerous standardized tools for screening children's development. Some of these tools screen for delays in one particular area of development, such as speech, while others screen for potential developmental delays in multiple areas (language, motor, social).

Most developmental screening tools are de-signed for use with infants and preschool children because development progresses rapidly in these age groups and periodic screening is of utmost importance. Fewer tools are available for screening development in children over 6 years of age.

Four of the more widely used developmental screening tools are discussed in this chapter: the Denver II, the Revised Prescreening Developmental Questionnaire (R–PDQ), the Developmental Profile II, and the Goodenough-Harris Draw-a-Person Test. The first two are the well-known Denver tests developed at the University of Colorado Medical Center for use with infants and preschool children. The Developmental Profile II can be used to screen development of children from birth to 9 years of age in five areas, while the Goodenough-Harris Draw-a-Person Test screens children's intellectual development from 3 to 10 years of age. Many other tools are available, and the interested reader is encouraged to seek them out. Castiglia & Petrini (1985) provide an excellent guide for selecting an appropriate developmental screening tool.

TABLE 10-8
Children at Risk for Developmental Problems

Those with history of:

- Maternal infectious disease, smoking, alcohol or drug abuse, exposure to hazardous substances (chemicals, radiation, toxic waste) during pregnancy
- Intrapartal fetal distress or complicated labor and delivery
- Genetic or chromosomal disorders
- Low birth weight (small for gestational age or prematurity)
- Neonatal hyperbilirubinemia, Rh or ABO incompatibility, respiratory distress syndrome, sepsis, hypoglycemia
- Chronic illness (e.g., cardiac disease, cystic fibrosis, bowel disorders)
- Serious acute illness (e.g., meningitis or recurrent otitis media) or accidental injury (e.g., head trauma)
- Dysfunctional social environment (family violence, frequent family crises or life-change events [loss of family members—divorce, death, abandonment], dysfunctional parenting practices, poverty)

Denver II[2]

The Denver Developmental Screening Test (DDST) is a standardized tool that screens for developmental problems in children from birth to age 6 years. The DDST has been used widely since it first was published in 1967.

Over the years, a number of concerns have been raised about the appropriateness of the DDST. For example, Fleming (1981) concluded that the test is not fully sensitive to a child's previous history, socioeconomic status, cultural context, and individual variations. Miller, Onotera, and Deinard (1984) evaluated the use of the DDST with Southeast Asian immigrant children and found that responses to certain items reflect social and cultural differences. For instance, the game of pat-a-cake does not exist in Hmong, Laotian, or Vietnamese cultures. Plurals are not part of Asian languages; therefore, when Asian children were shown two blocks and asked what they were, their response was "two block," thus distinguishing one block from more than one block (Miller et al., 1984).

In response to these and other concerns, the DDST underwent revision and restandardization and was released in 1990 as the Denver II (Franken-

[2]Screening manual, test kit, scoring forms, and training videotape are available from Denver Developmental Materials, Inc., P.O. Box 6919, Denver, CO 80206.

burg et al., 1990a). Like the DDST, the Denver II is designed to screen for developmental problems in children from birth to six years of age. Three purposes have been identified for administering the Denver II:

1. Screening apparently healthy children for developmental problems.

2. Validating intuitive concerns about a child's development with an objective test.

3. Monitoring high risk children, such as low birthweight infants, for developmental problems.

The Denver II is *not* an intelligence test and should not be used to predict developmental ability or to identify diagnostic labels, such as learning disability or language disorder.

Restandardization of the Denver II involved a more representative sample of the national child population. The characteristics of the sample population are as follows:

- *Gender:* 50% females, 50% males
- *Residence:* 70% urban, 16% semirural, 14% rural
- *Maternal education:* 30% less than 12 years, 34% 12 years, 36% more than 12 years
- *Racial group:* 17% Black, 28% Hispanic, 54% Anglo, 1% other (Asian, Native American, etc.).

The Denver II includes 125 items, 20 more than the DDST. Most of the new items are in the language category. Like the DDST, The Denver II arranges the items in four areas:

- *Personal–Social:* getting along with people and caring for personal needs.
- *Fine Motor–Adaptive:* eye–hand coordination, manipulation of small objects, and problem-solving.
- *Language:* hearing, understanding, and using language.
- *Gross Motor:* sitting, walking, jumping, and overall large muscle movement (Frankenburg et al., 1990b, p. 1).

Unlike the DDST, the Denver II includes five "Test Behavior" descriptors to rate the child's behavior during the test. This rating reflects the screener's subjective impression of the child's overall behavior. Behavior ratings are as follows:

- *Complies with examiner's requests:* complies, usually complies, rarely complies
- *Alertness, interest in surroundings:* alert, somewhat disinterested, seriously disinterested

■ *Fearfulness* (unusual for age-peers): none, somewhat fearful, very fearful

■ *Attention span* (age-appropriate): attentive, somewhat distractable, very distractable (Frankenburg et al., 1990a, p. 2).

A major advantage of the Denver II is that it is relatively simple to use and requires a minimum amount of time to administer. Generally, the Denver II involves tasks that the child must demonstrate in the presence of the screener. Certain items, though, allow the child to receive credit if the parent has observed the child performing the task, so both child and parent must be present during testing. However, fewer items may be scored by report on the Denver II (31%) than on the original DDST (48%).

The Denver II test form has items arranged in four sectors (see Figure 10-5). The age scales across the top of the scoring form coincide with the American Academy of Pediatrics' recommended ages for periodic checkups for healthy children. A detailed instruction manual accompanies the test kit and scoring sheets and should be used by those not thoroughly familiar with the tool. Failure to use the exact materials and protocol may reduce test reliability.

The child's name, birth date, and testing date should be recorded at the top of the test form. The child's age is calculated, and an age line is drawn on the test form to determine the items to be tested. Children under 2 who were born more than two weeks prematurely should have the age line adjusted as instructed in the screening manual.

The examiner should explain to the parent that the Denver II is being administered to assess the child's development and that the child is not expected to pass all items (Figure 10-6). Further, the parent should be told the test is not an IQ test.

The number of items to be tested will vary with the age and abilities of the child, as well as (1) the time available for testing, and (2) the purpose of administering the test. All children should be tested on all items in each sector intersected by the age line, plus at least three items in each sector immediately to the left of the age line. If the child fails any item, additional items to the left of the age line should be tested until the child is able to pass at least three items in each sector. In order to determine the developmental strengths of children who are successful on the tested items, additional items to the right of the age line should be administered until at least three failures in each sector are recorded.

Frankenburg et al. (1990a) recommend presenting the items in an organized way that takes into account the responsiveness of the individual child. They provide general guidelines for administering the Denver II test items (see boxed insert).

Each item is scored "P" for pass, "F" for fail, "N.O." for no prior opportunity to perform the item, or "R" for refusal to attempt the item. Upon completion of testing, individual items are interpreted as follows:

■ "Advanced" items: "Pass" on an item that falls completely to the right of the child's age line.

■ "Normal" items: "Fail" or "Refusal" on an item that falls completely to the right of the child's age line, *or* "Pass," "Fail," or "Refusal" on an item on which the child's age line falls between the 25th and 75th percentiles.

■ "Caution" items: "Fail" or "Refusal" on an item on which the age line falls between the 75th and 90th percentiles.

■ "Delayed" items: "Fail" or "Refusal" on an item that falls completely to the left of the age line.

The overall Denver II test results are interpreted according to the chart in Figure 10-7. Complete instructions for administration and scoring of the Denver II are provided in the Denver II Screening Manual, available commercially.

Revised Prescreening Developmental Questionnaire (R–PDQ)[3]

The Denver R-PDQ[4] is a parent-administered, prescreening questionnaire designed to identify children from birth to 6 years of age who should be screened more thoroughly with the Denver II. The R-PDQ is designed to achieve three goals: (1) to make parents more aware of the development of their children, (2) to document the developmental progress of individual children in a systematic manner, and (3) to facilitate early identification of children whose development may be delayed.

The 105-item questionnaire, written at the sixth-grade reading level, is divided into four color-coded forms [see Figure 10-8] that are available for use: 0–9 months (orange), 9–24 months (purple), 2–4 years (gold), and 4–6 years (white). The appropriate age form is selected, and the child's exact age

---

[3]This section is reprinted from Servonsky, J. and Opas, S.R. (Eds.). (1987). *Nursing management of children* (pp. 130–132). Boston: Jones & Bartlett.

[4]The R-PDQ can be obtained from Denver Developmental Materials, Inc., P.O. Box 6919, Denver, CO 80206.

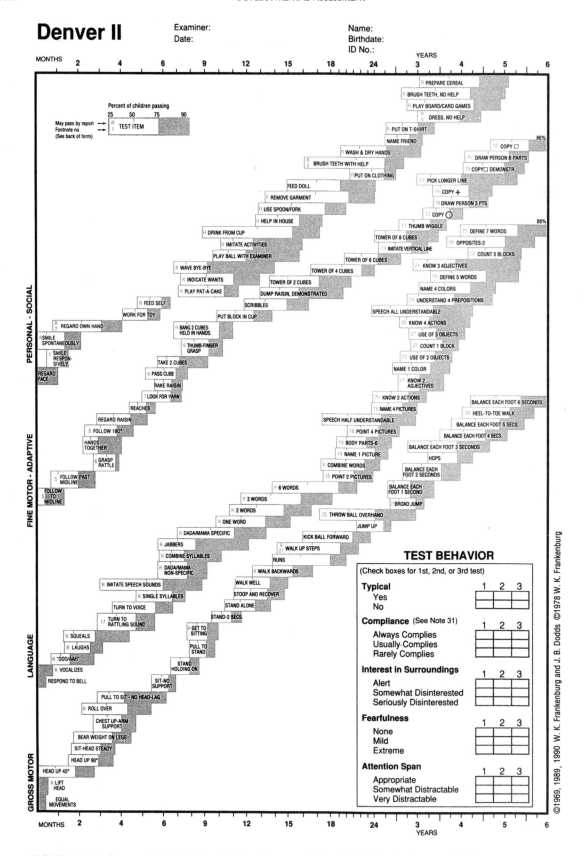

FIGURE 10-5. Denver II. (*Note*. Reprinted with permission, W.K. Frankenburg, 1990.)

DIRECTIONS FOR ADMINISTRATION

1. Try to get child to smile by smiling, talking or waving. Do not touch him/her.
2. Child must stare at hand several seconds.
3. Parent may help guide toothbrush and put toothpaste on brush.
4. Child does not have to be able to tie shoes or button/zip in the back.
5. Move yarn slowly in an arc from one side to the other, about 8" above child's face.
6. Pass if child grasps rattle when it is touched to the backs or tips of fingers.
7. Pass if child tries to see where yarn went. Yarn should be dropped quickly from sight from tester's hand without arm movement.
8. Child must transfer cube from hand to hand without help of body, mouth, or table.
9. Pass if child picks up raisin with any part of thumb and finger.
10. Line can vary only 30 degrees or less from tester's line. $|/$
11. Make a fist with thumb pointing upward and wiggle only the thumb. Pass if child imitates and does not move any fingers other than the thumb.

         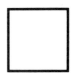

12. Pass any enclosed form. Fail continuous round motions.
13. Which line is longer? (Not bigger.) Turn paper upside down and repeat. (pass 3 of 3 or 5 of 6)
14. Pass any lines crossing near midpoint.
15. Have child copy first. If failed, demonstrate.

When giving items 12, 14, and 15, do not name the forms. Do not demonstrate 12 and 14.

16. When scoring, each pair (2 arms, 2 legs, etc.) counts as one part.
17. Place one cube in cup and shake gently near child's ear, but out of sight. Repeat for other ear.
18. Point to picture and have child name it. (No credit is given for sounds only.)
    If less than 4 pictures are named correctly, have child point to picture as each is named by tester.

   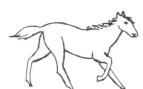   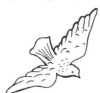   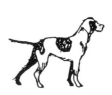   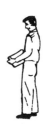

19. Using doll, tell child: Show me the nose, eyes, ears, mouth, hands, feet, tummy, hair. Pass 6 of 8.
20. Using pictures, ask child: Which one flies?... says meow?... talks?... barks?... gallops? Pass 2 of 5, 4 of 5.
21. Ask child: What do you do when you are cold?... tired?... hungry? Pass 2 of 3, 3 of 3.
22. Ask child: What do you do with a cup? What is a chair used for? What is a pencil used for?
    Action words must be included in answers.
23. Pass if child correctly places <u>and</u> says how many blocks are on paper. (1, 5).
24. Tell child: Put block **on** table; **under** table; **in front of** me, **behind** me. Pass 4 of 4.
    (Do not help child by pointing, moving head or eyes.)
25. Ask child: What is a ball?... lake?... desk?... house?... banana?... curtain?... fence?... ceiling? Pass if defined in terms of use, shape, what it is made of, or general category (such as banana is fruit, not just yellow). Pass 5 of 8, 7 of 8.
26. Ask child: If a horse is big, a mouse is __? If fire is hot, ice is __? If the sun shines during the day, the moon shines during the __? Pass 2 of 3.
27. Child may use wall or rail only, not person. May not crawl.
28. Child must throw ball overhand 3 feet to within arm's reach of tester.
29. Child must perform standing broad jump over width of test sheet (8 1/2 inches).
30. Tell child to walk forward, ∞∞∞∞→ heel within 1 inch of toe. Tester may demonstrate.
    Child must walk 4 consecutive steps.
31. In the second year, half of normal children are non-compliant.

OBSERVATIONS:

FIGURE 10-5 (Continued)

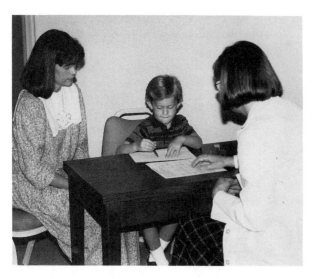

FIGURE 10-6. The nurse should administer the Denver II in the parent's presence. This child is copying a square.

is converted to an R–PDQ age. The parent is instructed to continue answering R–PDQ questions until a total of three "no" responses is recorded (they need not be consecutive), or until all questions on both sides of the form are answered.

To interpret the form requires the identification of delays. A *delay* is any item passed by 90% of children at an younger age (by even one day) than the child being screened. Ages at which 90% of children in the Denver sample passed the items are indicated in parentheses in the "For Office Use" column. These ages are shown in months and weeks up to 24 months (for example, "20–2" indi-

cates 20 months, 2 weeks) and in years and months after 24 months (for example, "3y–6" indicates 3 years, 6 months).

It is recommended that children without delays on initial R–PDQ screening be given activities to promote their development. Children scoring one delay should be rescreened with the R–PDQ one month later, and given activities to promote their development. If upon rescreening one or more delays are recorded, the child should be rescreened with the more lengthy Denver II. If upon initial screening with the R–PDQ, the child has two or more delays it is important to confirm the delays and then to refer the child for the Denver II (see Table 10-9).

For ease in interpreting R–PDQ results to a child's caregiver, each item has been given the same title as the corresponding Denver II item. The

---

Guidelines for Administering the Denver II

Items that require less active participation by the child should be administered first, generally in the following order: personal–social, fine motor–adaptive, language, gross motor.

Tasks that the child should be able to perform easily (i.e., those to the left of the age line) should be administered first to ensure the child's initial success and increase the child's interest and cooperation.

Items that require the same text kit materials, such as blocks or ball, should be administered consecutively to maximize the flow of the testing session.

For infants, items that require the infant to be lying down should be administered sequentially.

The examiner always should be alert to the child's behavior and score any relevant behavior (for example, "Indicates wants" to parent or "Stands holding on" while examiner is interviewing parent).

Normal:
- No Delays and a maximum of 1 Caution.
- Conduct routine rescreening of next well-child visit.

Abnormal:
- 2 or more Delays.
- Refer for diagnostic evaluation.

Questionable:
- One Delay and/or 2 or more Cautions.
- Offer the parent suggestions on improving the child's knowledge or skills in delay or caution areas, and rescreen in 3 months or at the next well-child visit, whichever comes first. If upon rescreen the child's score is again Questionable or has become Abnormal, refer for diagnostic evaluation.

Untestable:
- Interpret depending on the number of Refusals that would be Delays or Cautions if scored as failures.
- If the test would be Abnormal, rescreen in two to three weeks. If the rescreen is also Untestable or Abnormal, refer for diagnostic evaluation. If return for rescreen is unlikely, refer directly for diagnostic evaluation.
- If the test would be Questionable, follow-up is the same as for Questionable above.

Referral Criteria:
- While initial referral criteria might be those listed above, the final criteria for referral must be determined locally on the basis of everything one knows about the child and local eligibility criteria for various types of services.

FIGURE 10-7. Denver II Test Interpretation. (*Note:* Reprinted with permission, W.K. Frankenburg, 1990)

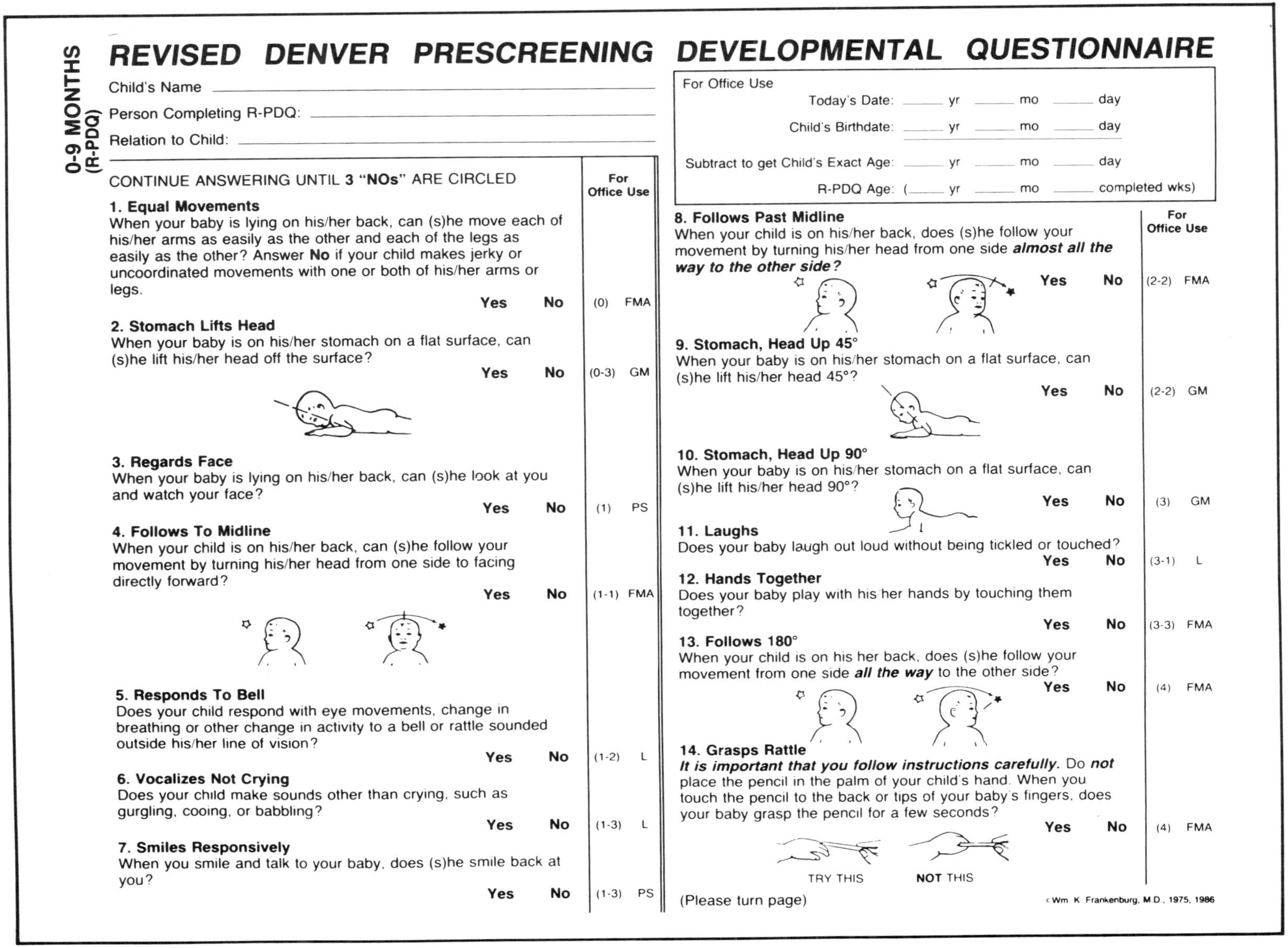

0-9 MONTHS (R-PDQ)

REVISED DENVER PRESCREENING DEVELOPMENTAL QUESTIONNAIRE

Child's Name _____

Person Completing R-PDQ: _____

Relation to Child: _____

For Office Use

Today's Date: _____ yr _____ mo _____ day

Child's Birthdate: _____ yr _____ mo _____ day

Subtract to get Child's Exact Age: _____ yr _____ mo _____ day

R-PDQ Age: _____ yr _____ mo _____ completed wks)

CONTINUE ANSWERING UNTIL 3 "NOs" ARE CIRCLED

		For Office Use

1. Equal Movements
When your baby is lying on his/her back, can (s)he move each of his/her arms as easily as the other and each of the legs as easily as the other? Answer **No** if your child makes jerky or uncoordinated movements with one or both of his/her arms or legs.
    Yes   No   (0) FMA

2. Stomach Lifts Head
When your baby is on his/her stomach on a flat surface, can (s)he lift his/her head off the surface?
    Yes   No   (0-3) GM

3. Regards Face
When your baby is lying on his/her back, can (s)he look at you and watch your face?
    Yes   No   (1) PS

4. Follows To Midline
When your child is on his/her back, can (s)he follow your movement by turning his/her head from one side to facing directly forward?
    Yes   No   (1-1) FMA

5. Responds To Bell
Does your child respond with eye movements, change in breathing or other change in activity to a bell or rattle sounded outside his/her line of vision?
    Yes   No   (1-2) L

6. Vocalizes Not Crying
Does your child make sounds other than crying, such as gurgling, cooing, or babbling?
    Yes   No   (1-3) L

7. Smiles Responsively
When you smile and talk to your baby, does (s)he smile back at you?
    Yes   No   (1-3) PS

8. Follows Past Midline
When your child is on his/her back, does (s)he follow your movement by turning his/her head from one side *almost all the way to the other side?*
    Yes   No   (2-2) FMA

9. Stomach, Head Up 45°
When your baby is on his/her stomach on a flat surface, can (s)he lift his/her head 45°?
    Yes   No   (2-2) GM

10. Stomach, Head Up 90°
When your baby is on his/her stomach on a flat surface, can (s)he lift his/her head 90°?
    Yes   No   (3) GM

11. Laughs
Does your baby laugh out loud without being tickled or touched?
    Yes   No   (3-1) L

12. Hands Together
Does your baby play with his her hands by touching them together?
    Yes   No   (3-3) FMA

13. Follows 180°
When your child is on his her back, does (s)he follow your movement from one side *all the way* to the other side?
    Yes   No   (4) FMA

14. Grasps Rattle
It is important that you follow instructions carefully. Do *not* place the pencil in the palm of your child's hand. When you touch the pencil to the back or tips of your baby's fingers, does your baby grasp the pencil for a few seconds?
    Yes   No   (4) FMA

TRY THIS   NOT THIS

(Please turn page)

© Wm. K. Frankenburg, M.D., 1975, 1986

FIGURE 10-8. Revised Prescreening Developmental Questionnaire (R-PDQ). (*Note.* Reprinted with permission, W.K. Frankenburg, University of Colorado Medical Center, Denver, 1975, 1986.)

TABLE 10-9
Summary of R–PDQ Interpretation

Initial Screening	Follow-Up
0 delays	No rescreening necessary. Suggest age-appropriate activities.
1 delay	Rescreen with R-PDQ 1 month later. If one or more delays on rescreening, refer for Denver II.
2 delays	Refer for Denver II. Suggest age-appropriate activities.

name of the sector where the item is located on the Denver II is shown in the "For Office Use" column of the R–PDQ as follows: PS (Personal–Social), FMA (Fine Motor–Adaptive), L (Language), and GM (Gross Motor).

If the R–PDQ is administered at regular intervals, it provides an ongoing record of the child's developmental progress. Most parents enjoy completing the questionnaire because it enhances their awareness of their child's development. Use of the R–PDQ therefore is an excellent means of introducing parents to activities they may undertake with their child to promote the child's development. Although the PDQ has been the subject of some criticism, it remains a useful tool for screening.

Developmental Profile II[5]

The Developmental Profile II is a reliable inventory that assesses children's development from birth to age 9 on five scales: physical, self-help, social, academic, and communication. Alpern, Boll, and Shearer (1980) state that the tool is equally valid for use with boys and girls, black and white children from all social classes. The authors do not mention its use with other racial groups. A description of the skills assessed in each of the five areas appears in Table 10-10.

The Developmental Profile II is administered in a structured interview with the child's parent or another person who knows the child well. It consists of 217 items divided among the five scales. Within each scale the items are arranged according to age levels. Approximately 30 minutes is required to administer the test. Sample questions from each scale appear in Table 10-11. The test yields a developmental age for the child on each scale. The nurse must remember, though, that this "developmental

age" is simply an estimate of the child's current level of development. The Developmental Profile II manual includes tables for each of the scales that indicate when delays should be considered significant, requiring more comprehensive evaluation.

Goodenough-Harris Draw-a-Person Test

The Goodenough-Harris Draw-a-Person Test provides a very simple method of assessing children's intellectual development from 3 to 10 years of age. The child is given a pencil, eraser, and paper, and is asked to "draw a person, any person you wish." If necessary, the child is urged to "draw the best person you can." The child then should be left alone and allowed as much time as needed to complete the picture.

The picture is scored by assigning the child a base age of 3 years if a circle is drawn. For each additional detail, the child is given credit for 3 months. For example, the drawing in Figure 10-9 yields a base age of 3 years plus 36 months (12 details) for a mental age of 6 years. This mental age can be compared to the child's chronological age, in this case 5 years, 8 months, to give an indication of whether the child's mental functioning is average, advanced, or delayed. The complete list of criteria used in scoring is presented in Table 10-12.

In summary, developmental screening with a standardized tool usually is indicated only when the developmental history and observation of the child lead the nurse to suspect a delay in the child's developmental progress. However, there may be instances when the nurse may appropriately use developmental screening tools to determine, for example, a child's readiness to enter school. Use of standardized screening tools often is helpful in validating the nurse's initial assessment of a child's development and can lead to early detection of potential problems that may require further evaluation and intervention.

ASSESSING CHILD–PARENT INTERACTION

Interviewing parents about their parenting practices should be part of any child health assessment. This should include assessment of discipline styles and the parents' perceptions of the quality of their interactions with their child. Reassuring parents of the normality and universality of childrearing problems may facilitate open discussion and sharing. For example, during the interview the nurse might say to the parents of a 14-year-old, "Many parents feel very exasperated and frustrated with their children at this age. What problems or con-

---

[5]Manual and scoring forms are available from Psychological Development Publications, P.O. Box 3198, Aspen, CO 81611.

TABLE 10-10
Developmental Profile II Scales

Physical age	This scale measures physical development by determining abilities with tasks requiring large and small muscle coordination, strength, stamina, flexibility, and sequential control skills.		in which the child relates to friends, relatives, and various adults exemplifies the skills that measure functional performance in the social situation.
Self-help age	This scale measures the ability to cope independently with the environment and measures the child's skills with tasks such as eating, dressing, and working. This scale assesses the degree to which children are capable of responsibly caring for themselves and others.	Academic age	This scale measures intellectual abilities by assessing, at the younger preschool level, the development of skills prerequisite to scholastic functioning and, at older preschool and school-age levels, actual academic achievement.
Social age	This scale measures interpersonal relationship abilities. The child's emotional needs for people, as well as the manner	Communication age	This scale measures expressive and receptive communication skills with both verbal and nonverbal language. The use and understanding of spoken, written, and gesture languages are assessed by this scale.

Note. From Alpern, G.D., Boll, T.J., and Shearer, M.S. *Developmental Profile II Manual.* Copyright © 1980 by Psychological Development Publications, 1980, Aspen, Colorado. Reprinted with permission.

cerns are you having?" The nurse can follow this with a question about the parents' perceptions of how they are managing any childrearing problems.

Older children and adolescents should be given an opportunity to meet privately with the nurse to discuss their perceptions of their relationships with their parents and other family members such as siblings. The nurse then can compare the parents' and child's perceptions for consistency. This can help pinpoint communication problems.

Baumrind (1971) has identified four styles of parenting: authoritarian, authoritative, permissive, and harmonious. These styles can be used as a framework for assessing a particular parent's style of exercising parental authority. The nurse should keep in mind that parental styles are influenced by numerous factors, such as the parent's personality, temperament, and educational level, the child's age and temperament (see chap. 12), and the family's social class and cultural values (see chap. 8).

Authoritarian parents tend to exercise strict control over their children's behavior. They expect unquestioning obedience and respect. These parents rely on external controls to manage the child's behavior. For example, disobedience is immediately and negatively reinforced through withdrawal of privileges or physical punishment.

Authoritative parents use a more democratic childrearing approach. They establish clear and consistent limits of acceptable behavior, but emphasize helping the child learn inner control by teaching the child there are social consequences for certain behaviors. These parents take time to explain to their children what is and is not acceptable behavior, including their rationale. Both positive and negative reinforcers are used: praise and granting privileges or withdrawal of privileges and use of "time-out."

Permissive parents rarely demand that their child develop behavioral controls. Misbehavior is ignored or at least tolerated, although permissive parents often express a helpless anger over their seeming lack of control. These children tend to rule the roost and often develop socially unacceptable behaviors for getting what they want.

Harmonious parents emphasize reason and harmony. They rarely exercise overt control of the child, but the child senses who is in charge and generally conforms to the parents' standards of behavior. Harmonious parents tend to be egalitarian to the extent that they recognize their child's developmental abilities and unique personality. Baumrind (1971) found that these parents try to "create an environment in which all family mem-

TABLE 10-11
Developmental Profile II Sample Questions

Physical Scale: 2½ to 3 years (toddler III: 31–36 months)

P16.   Does the child use scissors with one hand to cut paper or cloth? The other hand can be used to hold the paper or cloth, or the material can be held for the child. The child must be able to use the scissors to cut rather than to merely tear.

P17.   Can the child hop forward on one foot without support for a distance of at least five feet?

P18.   Does the child usually walk upstairs and downstairs by placing only one foot on each stair? S/he may use a railing or wall but this should not be necessary for ordinary support or balance.

Self-Help Scale: 8 years (primary-elementary III: 91–102 months)

S-H 34.   Does the child usually decide what to wear? This includes choosing the proper kinds of clothes for school, dress-up occasions and outer clothing appropriate for the weather.

S-H 35.   Does the child have at least *two* jobs of taking care of her/his own room and clothes? Washing and ironing clothes, shining shoes, cleaning, or dusting furniture or making a bed are examples of chores that pass. Needing to be reminded to do the chores is allowed.

S-H 36.   Does the child manage money well enough that s/he is allowed to buy some things without asking or telling adults?

Social Scale: 4 years (preschooler II: 43–54 months)

S 22.   Does the child draw a person so that an adult could tell what was drawn? It need not be a whole person but there should be a head and a body or a head and eyes, nose, or mouth which any adult could recognize.

S 23.   Is the child allowed to play in her/his own neighborhood without being watched by an adult? This does not mean the child is allowed to cross the street alone.

S 24.   Does the child know and use (though not always) the terms "thank you," "please," and "you're welcome" at the right times?

Academic Scale: 9 years (upper elementary I: 103–115 months)

A 33.   Can the child multiply through the sixth table with only a few errors? For example, the child will know the answers to six times nine, five times eight, four times three, etc.

A 34.   Does the child know by memory at least three telephone numbers or mailing addresses which s/he is able to use?

Communication Scale: second ½ year (infant I: 7–12 months)

C 4.   Does the child sometimes imitate spoken "words" such as "da-da" or "ma-ma"? The child may not know what these words mean.

C 5.   Does the child use motions or gestures as a way of talking; e.g., shaking head "no," or holding out arms to be picked up?

C 6.   Does the child answer an adult's words with gestures such as waving "bye-bye" when an adult says good-bye, shaking the head up and down for "yes" or side to side for "no."

Note. From Alpern, G.D., Boll, T.J., and Shearer, M.S. *Developmental Profile II Manual.* Copyright © 1980 by Psychological Development Publications. 1980, Aspen, Colorado. Reprinted with permission.

bers [can] operate from the same vantage point, one in which the recognized differences in power [do] not put the child at a disadvantage" (p. 99).

These categorical styles should be used as a loose framework for assessing child–parent interaction rather than as definitive labels. Although one style is likely to predominate, parents often use a combination of styles, depending upon the child's age and temperament and the particular situation. For example, parents may tend toward authoritarian methods with an inquisitive, active 2-year-old but adjust their style to an authoritative one as the child grows and becomes more capable of self-management. Parents may use quite different parenting styles with their individual children, especially if there are major differences in their ages and temperaments.

Some situations necessitate strict parental control, such as those in which a child's safety is in jeopardy. Other times parents may alter their usual parenting style to accommodate different social environments, such as a grocery store, the home of a friend, or when grandparents are visiting. Such adaptations also are likely to occur when parents and child are in a health-care situation such as a clinic or hospital. Frequently, a child's illness or hospitalization will cause parents to suspend the usual behavioral limits they impose on the child. Because this can be disruptive and can threaten the security of the ill child, the nurse should make an

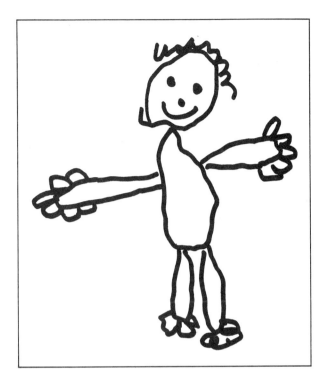

FIGURE 10-9. Drawing by Jason (5 years, 8 months) yields a mental age of 6 years.

effort to assess the impact of the child's illness or hospitalization on the parent's usual style of parenting.

Although observation is a useful means of assessing styles of parent–child interaction, the nurse should be careful to consider the context in which the behavior occurs when interpreting its meaning. Which parenting style is predominant? Is it used consistently or does it vary according to situation? Does the parent report strict adherence to one parenting style for all children in the family or is there some flexibility to allow for the needs of each individual child? What concerns do parents express about the methods they use? Many parents, especially those who are better educated and widely read on the subject of child care, will seek confirmation from the nurse that they are doing the right thing.

Other questions the nurse can use to guide the assessment of parenting styles include:

How do parents communicate rules and the limits of acceptable behavior to the child?

Do the adults agree on childrearing practices (style of parenting, handling of misbehavior)?

Are the rules and limits appropriate for the

TABLE 10-12
Goodenough-Harris Draw-a-Person Test Scoring Criteria

1. Head present	24. Correct number of fingers
2. Legs present	25. Fingers in two dimensions, length greater than breadth, angle subtended not greater than 180°
3. Arms present	26. Opposition of thumbs shown
4. Trunk present	27. Hands shown distinct from fingers and arms
5. Trunk longer than broad	28. Arm joints shown (elbow or shoulder or both)
6. Shoulder indicated	29. Head in proportion
7. Both arms and legs attached to trunk	30. Arms in proportion
8. Legs and arms attached to trunk at proper level	31. Legs in proportion
9. Neck present	32. Feet in proportion
10. Outline of neck continuous with that of head and trunk or both	33. Arms and legs in two dimensions
11. Eyes present	34. Heel shown
12. Nose present	35. Lines somewhat controlled
13. Mouth present	36. Lines well controlled
14. Both nose and mouth in two dimensions; two lips shown	37. Head outline well controlled
15. Nostrils indicated	38. Trunk outline well controlled
16. Hair shown	39. Outline of arms and legs well controlled
17. Hair on more than circumference of head, nontransparent, better than scribble	40. Outline of features well controlled
18. Clothing present	41. Ears present
19. Two articles of clothing, nontransparent	42. Ears present in correct position
20. Entire clothing with sleeves and trousers shown, nontransparent	43. Eyebrows or lashes present
21. Four or more articles of clothing definitely indicated	44. Pupil shown
22. Costume complete without incongruities	45. Proportion of eyes correct
23. Fingers shown	46. Glance directed to front in profile drawing
	47. Both chin and forehead shown
	48. Projection of chin shown
	49. Profile with not more than one error
	50. Correct profile

child's developmental level (or are they too strict or too lenient)?

Are limits, once established, clearly and consistently reinforced? In what ways?

Older children and adolescents can be asked about the limits that their parents have established for their behavior. It is important also to elicit children's feelings about these limits and what they do if they disagree with their parents' rules. For example, do they talk to their parents about it, quietly accept it, or secretly disobey?

It is especially important to note whether the lines of communication between child and parent are open. Does the child feel free to express feelings, including negative ones, without fear of punishment? Do parents *listen* to what the child is saying? Are parents and child respectful of one another's viewpoints even when they differ? Are rules and limits reevaluated and modified to allow for increasing self-reliance appropriate to the child's developmental level?

Dual career parenting, in which both parents are employed outside the home, may have a significant impact on child–parent interaction. Dilemmas that confront dual career parents and that influence their childrearing practices include obtaining adequate child care; such personal stressors as the energy demanded for balancing family and career responsibilities, lack of social support, and parental guilt over relinquishing child care responsibilities to others; conflicts related to work schedules and parental role responsibilities; and attitudes of coworkers (Kutzner & Toussie-Weingarten, 1984).

The nurse can assess the impact of dual career parenting on a child's development by incorporating the following questions into the parent interview:

What are the arrangements for child care? How satisfied are the parent(s) with the arrangements?

How does the child respond to child care arrangements? How do the parents' handle negative responses?

How do the parents' work schedules and demands influence their childrearing responsibilities and practices?

To what extent are child care, household management, and decision-making responsibilities shared (by parents, by child)?

What degree of support do the parent(s) receive from others (family members, coworkers, friends) related to their childrearing responsibilities, practices, and stressors?

How do the parent(s) resolve conflicts related to the dual demands of childrearing and career?

CHILDREN'S HEALTH KNOWLEDGE AND HEALTH BEHAVIORS

Evidence suggests that in the early preschool period, children begin to develop an awareness of health and activities that contribute to staying healthy (Dielman, Leech, Becker, Rosenstock, & Horvath, 1980; Natapoff, 1982). The inquisitiveness that characterizes the preschooler extends to curiosity about health and illness. Health-related ideas become paramount, however, when the child begins formal schooling.

Factors that influence children's knowledge of health and their health behaviors include parental knowledge and family health practices, school health education classes, the child's own experiences with health (e.g., child health maintenance, immunizations, illness, and medication), encounters with people who are experiencing illness or who have disabilities, and the media (television, radio, newspapers, magazines).

Natapoff (1982) studied the relationship of children's concepts of health to their age, using a Piagetian developmental framework. She found that young children view health in a positive way, unrelated to illness, whereas older children view health and illness as associated concepts. Table 10-13 outlines children's concepts of development by age.

Queen (personal communication, May, 1986) outlines behaviors that are characteristic of healthy children. These include: (1) acceptance of responsibility for their own health, (2) consideration of alternatives to various lifestyle practices, (3) clarification of health values, (4) development of skills for coping with peer pressure, (5) learning how to handle health emergencies, (6) coping effectively with apprehensions related to health personnel, facilities, and procedures, and (7) developing a positive concept of self responsible for their own health and able to make health-related decisions appropriate to their ages and experiences. In order to assess whether a particular child possesses these characteristics, Barleben (1987) has developed an inventory to assess children's health behaviors in five areas: responsibility, nutritional awareness, physical activity, stress management, and sensitivity to environmental hazards (see Table 10-14). This inventory can be administered to school-age children and adolescents to assess their health practices. The findings of this assessment can help the nurse identify behaviors that place the child at risk for future health problems.

TABLE 10-13
A Comparison of Cognitive Development and Concept of Health by Age

Age[1]	Cognitive Development[2]	Concept of Health
Below 7 or 8	*Preoperational* Egocentric Intuitive Cannot consider whole and part simultaneously Present oriented	Health is doing desired activities and feeling good. Concrete and sometimes unrelated practices are considered part of health. Does not consider cause and effect.
7 or 8–10	*Concrete Operational* Cause and effect considered Conservation develops (can consider original and changed state) Reversibility develops (thinking processes can take place in opposite directions) Can think through a chain of events. Classifies objects and concrete ideas into a hierarchical arrangement	Health is being able to perform desired activities. Understands cause and effect—action and health status are related. Believes it is possible to be part healthy and part not healthy. Can reverse from health to sickness and back to health.
Above 10 or 11	*Formal Operational* Future oriented Can formulate hypotheses Can consider abstractions Deductive reasoning develops	Health is performing desired activities. Mental health considered by many. Health is long-term, sickness is short-term. Future health considered.

[1]Ages vary but sequence is invariant.
[2]Based on theories of Jean Piaget.

Note. From Natapoff, J.N. (1982). A developmental analysis of children's ideas of health. *Health Education Quarterly, 9*(2 & 3), 34/130–45/141. © 1982 John Wiley & Sons, Inc. Reprinted by permission of John Wiley & Sons, Inc.

Byler, Lewis & Totman (1969) conducted a mass survey of 5,000 students in grades K through 12. They found that children are interested in learning about their bodies (structure and function), nutrition, exercise, safety and first aid, mental health, fears, peer relations, relations with parents, sexuality, disease, alcohol, drugs, and smoking. Common concerns by age group are presented in Table 10-15. Part of the developmental assessment should include asking children what they think it means to be healthy, what concerns they have about their health, and what they want to learn about health-related topics.

Results of the assessment of children's health knowledge and health practices can serve as a basis for identifying a child's need for instruction and models in a particular area or for interventions that will encourage the child to engage in healthy behaviors. Children whose behaviors indicate a potential health risk, such as overeating, smoking, using drugs or alcohol, or inability to manage stress, may need special interventions, such as behavior modification or self-management techniques, or to be referred for special assistance.

NURSING DIAGNOSES RELATED TO CHILDREN'S DEVELOPMENT

As developmental information is collected through interview, clinical observation, and developmental screening, the nurse begins to identify relevant information and formulate inferences and diagnostic hypotheses. Comparison of tentative diagnostic hypotheses with the defining characteristics of selected nursing diagnoses approved by the North American Nursing Diagnosis Association (NANDA) helps determine the validity of the nurse's impressions.

Perhaps the most significant nursing diagnosis related to development is "altered growth and development." Delays in achieving developmental milestones appropriate to the child's chronological age are defining characteristics that support this diagnosis. Related factors may include environmental deprivation, lack of opportunities for learning new skills, multiple caretakers, prolonged hospitalization, lack of parental knowledge about child development, or the effects of chronic illness or disability.

TABLE 10-14
Wellness Inventory for Children

Self-Responsibility	Always	Some-times	Never
I can do something to stay healthy.			
I can make myself well again.			
I need a doctor when I have a cold.			
When I am sick I can't do anything about it.			
My health is important to me.			
Sometimes it's nice to be sick.			
Other people make me well.			
If it's meant to be, I'll get sick.			
If I'm sick, it's bad luck.			
If I'm well, it's good luck.			
I am responsible for being healthy.			
I can prevent my being ill.			
I pay attention to my body's signals.			
I have no worries about my health.			
I am scared of getting sick.			
I am sick a lot.		.	
I am usually well.			

Nutritional Awareness	Always	Some-times	Never
I know the basic four food groups.			
I eat three meals a day.			
I snack on wholesome food.			
I avoid adding salt.			
I peel skin off fish, poultry.			
I eat fresh foods as much as possible.			
I can cook one meal for myself.			
I know that TV ads promote foods that are not healthy.			

Nutritional Awareness Continued	Always	Some-times	Never
I do not go to a fast-food restaurant more than once a week, if that much.			
I brush my teeth at least two times a day.			
I floss my teeth at least once a day.			
I overeat.			
I drink 2% fat milk at meals (if milk is tolerated).			
I usually eat meals with my family (except when at school) in a relaxed environment.			
I avoid food with preservatives.			
I know what foods contain caffeine.			
I know when I have too much sugar.			
I take drugstore medicine often.			

Physical Activity	Always	Some-times	Never
I can count my pulse at the wrist for one minute.			
I select proper shoes for walking or running.			
I select appropriate clothing for playing sports or jogging.			
I know the ideal weight range for my height.			
I can describe warm-up exercises to do before engaging in sports.			
I exercise regularly four times a week for thirty minutes.			
Because I don't exercise regularly now, I plan to begin a progressive schedule of exercise.			
I do cooling-down exercises.			
I plan to exercise when convenient and when I'm rested.			

(continued on next page)

TABLE 10-14 (Continued)

Physical Activity Continued	Always	Some-times	Never
I get at least seven hours of sleep per night.			
I eat properly before and after exercise.			
I drink sufficient liquid in hot weather.			
I know how to avoid injuries in exercise and sports.			
I wear protection as required.			
I can handle a minor muscle ache or strain myself.			
I know how to win and how to lose in competitive sports.			
I enjoy exercise.			
I feel better after exercising.			
I watch less than two hours of TV per day.			

Stress Management	Always	Some-times	Never
I know why I'm feeling happy.			
I know why I'm feeling frustrated.			
I try to talk with my parents.			
I usually like my brothers and sisters.			
I know what makes me nervous in school.			
I can plan my time for: chores school play			
I am usually on time.			
I know what I like about myself.			
I know what I don't like about myself.			
I can think of ways I want to change.			
I feel I'm in charge of my life.			
My opinion is listened to at home.			

Stress Management Continued	Always	Some-times	Never
I have a friend or a group of friends.			
When I have a conflict with someone, I try to talk about it.			
When I am depressed, I know what makes me feel better.			
I have some hobbies.			
I can listen to another person's opinion.			
I can take responsibility for my actions.			
I usually finish things I start.			
I get encouragement and support from: parents friends teachers relatives			
I get understanding when I am upset.			
I give support to my: parents friends brothers sisters			

Environmental Sensitivity	Always	Some-times	Never
I know that smoking is hazardous to my health.			
I do not smoke.			
I do not take candy from strangers.			
I do not accept a ride in a car from a stranger.			
I ride my bike with traffic.			
I know hand signals for turning and stopping.			
I use hand signals when riding a bike.			
I do not listen to stereo with headphones for longer than one hour per day.			
I cross at crosswalks and with the light.			

(continued on next page)

TABLE 10-14 (Continued)

Environmental Sensitivity Continued	Always	Some-times	Never	Environmental Sensitivity Continued	Always	Some-times	Never
I wear a seatbelt in the car.				Our family has guns in the home.			
I wear a helmet when riding a motorcycle.				I am home alone after school.			
I am careful not to leave toys on stairs.				I wear sunscreen when appropriate.			
I play with BB guns.							

Note. From Barleben, S.S. (1987). Promotion of health in the child. In Servonsky/Opas: *Nursing Management of Children,* ©1987. Boston: Jones and Bartlett Publishers, 119–121.

Although "self-care deficit" is specified in the NANDA-approved taxonomy, its application to children who are experiencing developmental delays is probably not appropriate. The more appropriate diagnosis for children who are experiencing delays in self-reliance is "altered growth and development" related to, for example, effects of physical disability or mental retardation.

When problems related to child–parent interaction are reflected in the parents' childrearing behaviors, a diagnosis of "altered parenting" (actual or potential) may be indicated. Defining characteristics may include inappropriate caretaking behaviors, inappropriate or inconsistent discipline practices (overprotective or overpermissive), frequent illness or injury of the child, inattention to the child's needs, or lack of parental attachment behaviors. Altered parenting also may occur when the parents and child are separated from each other for long periods of time, such as occurs with low birthweight infants who may spend their first months of life in a special care hospital nursery. Other related factors include lack of knowledge about childrearing, unmet developmental needs of the parent(s), or family stressors. Early detection of altered parenting practices and initiation of appropriate interventions is essential to enhance optimal development.

When a child exhibits a socially inappropriate behavioral pattern, whether at home, school, or in public, a nursing diagnosis of "impaired social interaction" may be indicated. Observation of the child's interactions with others, particularly family members and peers, is useful in validating this diagnosis. Difficulty in relating to others in a social context may reflect a child's lack of experience with social situations, failure of the child's parents to teach or show appropriate social behavior, or a self-esteem disturbance.

Children who express concern about their health, interest in learning more about health, and a desire to engage in healthy lifestyle behaviors may warrant a nursing diagnosis of "health-seeking behaviors." Factors that may contribute to this diagnosis include sufficient cognitive maturity, health education opportunities, and appropriate modeling of good health practices by the child's parents and significant others (e.g., sports heroes, older siblings, coaches).

A diagnosis of "altered health maintenance" reflects a child's decreased ability or unwillingness to take responsibility for meeting basic health

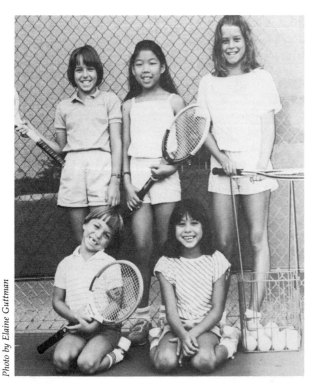

Photo by Elaine Guttman

FIGURE 10-10. Physical fitness and activity are an important part of how children learn to lead healthy lives. (*Note.* From Servonsky/Opas: *Nursing Management of Children,* © 1987. Boston: Jones and Bartlett Publishers, p. 326.)

TABLE 10-15
Health Concerns by Age Group

Young School-Age Child (5 to 8 years of age)
Body structure and function—external appearance, growth, familiar behaviors (sneezing, choking, running, seeing, hearing), what the body looks like inside
Proper food habits, exercise
Safety, injuries
Fears, protection from harmful events
Handling difficult situations (fights with friends or siblings, family discord, embarrassment)
Sexuality (where babies come from, gender differences)
Diseases (those common in children; those they hear about on television, such as AIDS, cancer, heart disease)

Older School-Age Child (9 to 12 years of age)
Body structure and function—intricate details, terminology, onset of secondary sex characteristics
Nutrition—requirements, effects on health, hazards (sugar, salt, cholesterol)
Physical fitness
Safety—prevention of accidents, first aid, CPR
Concern for others who are different (disabled or retarded persons)
Fears (being alone, unfamiliar events and situations, being different, being laughed at)
Relationships with friends
Interactions with parents; family discord
Sexuality—reproductive structure and function, gender

differences, menstruation, pregnancy, sexually transmitted diseases, contraception, relationships with opposite sex, handling feelings of sexuality and love
Disease—communicability, infectious disease, common ailments, AIDS, cancer, heart disease
Alcohol, drugs, and smoking—effects, hazards

Adolescent (13+ years of age)
Body structure and function—scientific terminology, differences in male–female development, mental function
Nutrition—improved appearance, muscle development, weight control
Physical fitness; sports activities
Safety; driver education; first aid and CPR
Self-understanding; handling life problems
Stress management
Values clarification
Relationships with others
Identity and independence; self-responsibility
Mental illness
Sexuality—accurate and complete knowledge of human sexual function; decision-making (sexual relations, contraception, safe sex); preparation for marriage and family life
Disease—communicable diseases, STDs, common ailments, cancer, heart disease, AIDS
Alcohol, drugs, smoking—effects, hazards, alcoholism, addiction

---

needs, such as nutrition, sleep, exercise, or safety, appropriate to the child's developmental capabilities. As children acquire health knowledge and learn to enhance and maintain optimal health and well-being, their ability to take responsibility for their own health increases. Factors that may contribute to a child's inability or unwillingness to assume this responsibility include lack of knowledge, self-esteem disturbance, lack of motivation, lack of support systems or appropriate role models, or cultural values. Table 10-16 summarizes common nursing diagnoses related to child development.

Chapter Highlights

■ Development should be assessed as part of a comprehensive nursing assessment of children from birth through adolescence.

■ The purposes of developmental assessment include provision of an ongoing record of the child's progress, early detection of potential developmental delays, guidance for parents about ways to promote optimal development, and direction for

nurse–child interaction appropriate for the child's developmental level.

■ The three major components of a comprehensive developmental assessment include the de-

TABLE 10-16
Nursing Diagnoses Related to Children's Development

Altered growth and development related to lack of opportunities for acquiring new skills, lack of parental knowledge about child development, prolonged hospitalization, or the effects of chronic illness or disability

Health-seeking behaviors related to health education or appropriate modeling of good health practices by parents and significant others

Altered health maintenance related to knowledge deficit, self-esteem disturbance, lack of motivation, lack of appropriate role models, or cultural values

Altered parenting related to prolonged separation from child, lack of knowledge about childrearing, unmet developmental needs of parent(s), or family stressors

Impaired social interaction related to lack of appropriate role models, lack of experience with social situations, or self-esteem disturbance

velopmental history, clinical observation, and developmental screening.

■ Developmental assessment should be based on knowledge of developmental concepts, principles, and theories, which provide a framework for assessing systematically a child's development and progress.

■ Many variables influence the content and process of the developmental assessment, including the age of the child, social and cultural factors, the child's health, the setting in which the assessment is done, and the nurse–child–parent relationship.

■ The developmental history and clinical observation usually provide adequate information on which to base clinical judgments about a child's developmental progress.

■ Developmental screening may be indicated if the nurse suspects a delay, wishes to validate initial impressions, or identifies a concern on the part of the parent.

■ Developmental screening tools provide an estimate of a child's current abilities. They are not diagnostic, nor can they predict developmental potential. Therefore, screening tools should be used with caution.

■ The developmental assessment should include an assessment of child–parent interaction, including parenting style, child–parent communication, and the child's and parent's perceptions of the quality of interaction.

■ Children's concepts of health and illness should be assessed, as should their health concerns, desires for health-related information, and health-care practices, including responsibility for staying healthy.

■ Findings of the developmental assessment should be analyzed carefully as a basis for formulating nursing diagnoses.

■ Identified developmental problems should be more thoroughly evaluated by the nurse, or the child should be referred for intervention in order to prevent or minimize problems.

Practice Activities

1. Observe one or several groups of children (on a playground, at a day care center or school, in an infant stimulation program) and identify examples of behaviors or characteristics that illustrate the following principles of development:

    a. development is directional (cephalocaudal, proximodistal, general-to-specific)
    b. development is sequential
    c. development is individual
    d. development is asynchronous
    e. development is cyclical
    f. all aspects of development are interrelated

Share your observations in a group discussion with your peers, and identify implications of these developmental principles for nursing.

2. Assess the development of three children: an infant, a preschooler, and a school-age child or adolescent, using the developmental history (Table 10-6) and direct observation. Identify the purposes for doing each developmental assessment. Document and record your findings systematically. Formulate appropriate nursing diagnoses.

3. Administer at least one of the following screening tests to at least two different children, using the established guidelines: Revised Prescreening Development Questionnaire (R–PDQ), Denver II, Developmental Profile II. Explain the rationale for selecting the tests you choose to administer. Interpret and score the results. What conclusions can you draw? Share your findings with the child's parents.

4. Administer the Goodenough-Harris Draw-a-Person Test to three children between the ages of 3 and 10. Score their drawings, using the criteria presented in Table 10-12. Interpret the results and share the findings with each child's parents.

5. Familiarize yourself with at least one other developmental screening tool. What are its advantages and disadvantages?

6. In a public setting such as a day care center, park, shopping mall, sports event, or health-care setting, observe interactions between a parent (or parents) and child. Describe your observations and draw conclusions about parenting style, child–parent communication, factors that may be influencing the interaction in that particular setting, and the quality of child–parent interaction. Why should caution be used in interpreting child–parent interaction?

7. Ask at least one preschooler, one school-age child, and one adolescent the following questions:

    What is health? What does it mean to be healthy?
    What things do you do to stay healthy?
    What worries do you have about your health?
    What would you like to learn about your body? About health? About illness?

If possible, administer the Wellness Inventory (Table 10-14). Summarize your findings, and compare responses across age groups. What conclusions can you draw? What are the nursing implications?

Recommended Readings

Becker, P.T. (1987). Sensitivity to infant development and behavior: A comparison of adolescent and adult single mothers. *Research in Nursing and Health, 10,* 119–127.

Bee, H.L., Hammond, M.A., Eyres, S.J., Bernard, K.E., & Snyder, C. (1986). The impact of parental life change on the early development of children. *Research in Nursing and Health, 9,* 65–74.

Byrne, J., Backman, J., & Smith, I. (1986). Developmental assessment: The clinical use and validity of parental report. *Journal of Pediatric Psychology, 11*(4), 549–559.

Castiglia, P.T., & Petrini, M.A. (1985). Selecting a developmental screening tool. *Pediatric Nursing, 11*(1), 8–17.

Fleming, J.W. (1981). An evaluation of the use of the Denver Developmental Screening Test. *Nursing Research, 30*(5), 290–293.

Kutzner, S.K., & Toussie-Weingarten, C. (1984). Working parents: The dilemma of childrearing and career. *Topics in Clinical Nursing, 6,* 30–37.

Natapoff, J.N. (1978). Children's views of health: A developmental study. *American Journal of Public Health, 10,* 995–1000.

Olade, R.A. (1984). Evaluation of the Denver Developmental Screening Test as applied to African children. *Nursing Research, 33,* 204–207.

Pontius, S.L. (1982). Practical Piaget: Helping children understand. *American Journal of Nursing, 82*(1), 114–117.

Sande, D.R., & Billingsley, C.S. (1985). Language development in infants and toddlers. *Nurse Practitioner, 10*(9), 39–47.

Schrader, B.D., Rappaport, J., & Courtwright, L. (1987). Preschool development of very low birthweight infants. *Image: Journal of Nursing Scholarship, 19*(4), 174–178.

Steele, S.M. (1988). Assessing developmental delays in preschool children. *Journal of Pediatric Health Care, 2*(3), 141–145.

References

Alpern, G.D., Boll, T.J., & Shearer, M.S. (1980). *The Developmental Profile II Manual.* Aspen, CO: Psychological Development Publications.

Bandura, A. (1977). *Social learning theory.* Englewood Cliffs, NJ: Prentice-Hall.

Barleben, S.S. (1987). Promotion of health in the child. In J. Servonsky & S.R. Opas (Eds.), *Nursing management of children* (pp. 110–175). Boston: Jones & Bartlett.

Baumrind, D. (1971). Current patterns of parental authority. *Developmental Monographs, 1,* 1–103.

Becker, P.T. (1987). Sensitivity to infant development and behavior: A comparison of adolescent and adult single mothers. *Research in Nursing and Health, 10,* 119–127.

Bee, H.L., Hammond, M.A., Eyres, S.J., Barnard, K.E., & Snyder, C. (1986). The impact of parental life change on the early development of children. *Research in Nursing and Health, 9,* 65–74.

Byler, R., Lewis, G., & Totman, R. (1969). *Teach us what we want to know.* New York: Mental Health Materials Center.

Byrne, J.M., Blackman, J.E., & Smith, I.M. (1986). Developmental assessment: The clinical use of validity of parental report. *Journal of Pediatric Psychology, 11,* 549–559.

Castiglia, P.T., & Petrini, M.A. (1985). Selecting a developmental screening tool. *Pediatric Nursing, 11*(1), 8–17.

Dielman, T.E., Leech, S.L., Becker, M.H., Rosenstock, I.M., & Horvath, W.J. (1980). Dimensions of children's health beliefs. *Health Education Quarterly, 7*(3), 219–238.

Erikson, E.H. (1963). *Childhood and society* (2nd ed.). New York: Knopf.

Fleming, J. (1981). An evaluation of the use of the Denver Developmental Screening Test. *Nursing Research, 30,* 290–293.

Frankenburg, W.K., Dick, N.P., & Carland, J. (1975). Development of preschool-aged children of different social and ethnic groups: Implications for developmental screening. *Journal of Pediatrics, 87,* 125–132.

Frankenburg, W.K., Dodds, J., Archer, P., Bresnick, B., Mascha, P., Edelman, N., & Shapiro, H. (1990a). *Denver II technical manual.* Denver: Denver Developmental Materials.

Frankenburg, W.K., Dodds, J., Archer, P., Bresnick, B., Mascha, P., Edelman, N., & Shapiro, H. (1990b). *Denver II screening manual.* Denver: Denver Developmental Materials.

Gesell, A., & Ilg, F.L. (1949). *Child development: An introduction to the study of human growth.* New York: Harper & Row.

Gilligan, C. (1982). *In a different voice: Psychological theory and women's development.* Cambridge, MA: Harvard University Press.

Havighurst, R.J. (1972). *Developmental tasks and education* (3rd ed.). New York: David McKay.

Ilg, F.L. & Ames, L.B. (1960). *The Gesell Institute's child behavior.* Boston: Dell.

Kohlberg, L. (1968). The child as moral philosopher. *Psychology Today, 2*(4), 25–30.

Kutzner, S.K., & Toussie-Weingarten, C. (1984). Working parents: The dilemma of childrearing and career. *Topics in Clinical Nursing, 6,* 30–37.

Lerner, R.M. (1978). Nature, nurture, and dynamic interactionism. *Human Development, 21,* 1–20.

Lorenz, K. (1937). The companion in the bird's world. *Auk, 54,* 245–273.

McCall, R.B. (1981). Nature–nurture and the two realms of development: A proposed integration with respect to mental development. *Child Development, 52,* 1–12.

Mercer, R.T., Hackley, K.C., & Bostrom, A. (1984). Adolescent motherhood: Comparison of outcome with older mothers. *Journal of Adolescent Health Care, 5,* 7–13.

Meyrowitz, J. (1985). *No sense of place.* New York: Oxford.

Miller, V., Onotera, R.T., & Deinard, A.S. (1984). Denver Developmental Screening Test: Cultural variations in Southeast Asian children. *Pediatrics, 104,* 481–482.

Natapoff, J.N. (1978). Children's views of health: A developmental study. *American Journal of Public Health, 86,* 995–1000.

Natapoff, J.N. (1982). A developmental analysis of children's ideas of health. *Health Education Quarterly, 9,* 34/130–45/141.

Piaget, J. (1963). *The origins of intelligence in children* (2nd ed.). New York: Norton.

Postman, N. (1982). *The disappearance of childhood.* New York: Delacorte.

Rosemond, J.K. (1981). *Parent power.* New York: Pocket Books.

Schraeder, B.D., Rappaport, J., & Courtwright, L. (1987). Preschool development of very low birth weight infants. *Image: The Journal of Nursing Scholarship, 19,* 174–178.

Sheldon, W.H. (1942). *Varieties of physique.* New York: Harper & Row.

Simkins, L. (1984). Consequences of teenage pregnancy and motherhood. *Adolescence, 19,* 39–54.

Skinner, B.F. (1945). Baby in a box. In B.F. Skinner (Ed.), *Cumulative record: A selection of papers* (3rd ed.). New York: Appleton-Century-Crofts.

Skinner, B.F. (1974). *About behaviorism.* New York: Knopf.

Thomas, R.M. (1985). *Comparing theories of child development* (2nd ed.). Belmont, CA: Wadsworth.

Developmental Assessment
of the Adult

OBJECTIVES

Upon completion of this chapter, you should be
able to:

■ Discuss the purposes of assessing the developmental status of adults.

■ Describe the normal aging process.

■ Apply four developmental theories to describe
adult development.

■ Evaluate the influence of social and cultural
norms on adult development.

■ Conduct a comprehensive developmental assessment of selected young, middle-aged, and
elderly adults.

■ Describe adults' health knowledge and health
practices as adults progress from young adulthood through old age.

■ Analyze developmental information to formulate appropriate nursing diagnoses.

Adults, like children, change in patterned ways. However, development is less predictable and less dependent on physical change than in childhood. Assessment of developmental progress in adulthood is essential for understanding the adult client's physical and psychosocial status and the social milieu in which the client lives and interacts. Much of adult development is related to cultural expectations for adult behaviors (Neugarten, 1976).

Knowledge of adult development helps nurses anticipate responses to stress and illness. Developmental information also highlights areas of special competence and deficiencies in the adult client's life experiences. The information gained from a developmental assessment enables the nurse to make accurate, individualized nursing diagnoses about a client's developmental progress (McWeeny, 1988).

In addition, awareness of normal developmental patterns assists nurses in helping clients prepare themselves for change. Guidance may help adults more realistically gauge opportunities for the future, recognize dilemmas, and prepare to resolve or cope with them. Discussion of normal development helps people better understand their own experience, their coping strategies, and their strengths and limitations.

Adult assessment parameters help the nurse understand normal aging changes that occur with adult development. Table 11-1 has been divided into early adulthood, early middle age, late middle age, and old age and presents specific characteristics of development at each age. There is some overlap in the range of expected behaviors during these adult years. Type and rate of change are determined by a variety of factors, including heredity, lifetime health habits, and disease processes. This table is intended as a guide to normal changes over the adult life span based on current knowledge of physiology, developmental psychology, and the influence of social norms. Included are the broad categories of physiological changes, sensory and cognitive changes, and psychosocial expectations and transitions. Sensory and cognitive changes are grouped together because observable cognitive behavior is dependent upon the functioning of the sensory system. Clinical assessment of these changes is important and is discussed more fully in Chapter 24. Differences between men and women are included where appropriate.

KNOWLEDGE NEEDED TO ASSESS ADULT DEVELOPMENT

Knowledge needed to assess adult development is multifaceted, and includes various theoretical per-spectives. The numerous theories of adult development provide the nurse with a useful assessment framework.

Theories of Adult Development

Theories of adult development are relatively new compared to those that explain child development. Adults change more slowly than children, and individual adults and their lifestyles vary more than children. Despite variations, commonalities can be discerned in physical changes, psychological experiences, and social roles and expectations. Interest in adulthood and adult developmental concerns is on the rise because people are living longer and the percentage of older people in the population is increasing. Important theories of adult development include psychosocial theories, developmental tasks theory, adaptation theory, and life transition theories.

Psychosocial Theory

Erik Erikson (1963) was one of the first psychologists to describe adult development. According to Erikson, adult development is based on successful resolution of basic psychosocial conflicts. Adulthood begins when young people have resolved the adolescent crisis of identity versus role confusion and have determined who they are and who they are likely to become. These young adults then face the developmental crisis of intimacy versus isolation. Intimacy, in addition to sexuality and procreation, implies a reciprocal commitment to a partner, mutual trust, and an ability to care about the partner's wishes, needs, and aspirations without fear of sacrificing one's own sense of identity in the process. The counterdevelopmental crisis is a sense of isolation from others characterized by avoidance of intimate relationships and failure to achieve a shared identity with others in one's social group or a sense of intimate connection to the larger society.

The crisis facing the mature adult is that of generativity versus stagnation, or self-absorption. Generative adults are productive and creative. They guide the next generation within and beyond the family and show a desire to make the world a better place. Generativity involves joining society in supporting child care and education initiatives, promoting the arts and humanities, and assuming civic and political responsibilities. The adult who avoids responsibility for guiding the next generation risks becoming stagnant and self-absorbed and estranged from participation in community life. Such persons are concerned only with pro-

TABLE 11-1
Adult Developmental Characteristics

Stage	Physical changes	Sensory-cognitive changes	Psychosocial expectations
Early adulthood (ages 18–30)	Peak physical status for height, strength, speed of response, efficiency and endurance; affected by nutrition, climate, exercise, and hereditary factors. Wisdom teeth erupt and may need care Optimal time for pregnancy Skin begins to lose moisture Peak sexual development	Highest scores on intelligence tests Capacities for new learning, abstraction, and creativity at peak	Style and pattern of life established Mate selection and marriage Birth of children and parenting Making commitments to self and others Establishment of self-concept as an adult Achievement-oriented Move from dependency to responsibility Role adjustment
Early middle age (ages 30–50)	Skin loses elasticity and becomes coarser, thinner, dryer, and more easily bruised and cracked; healing occurs more slowly Changes in hair—grayness, receding hairline in men; women may notice more facial hair. Bone mass decreases Muscle mass may decrease depending on level of exercise Joints stiffen and muscles lose resiliency; connective tissue loses flexibility, becomes weaker, and loses water. Endurance declines; may notice decline in manual dexterity Decrease in gastric secretions and deterioration of chemical components of gastric secretions, especially for men Cardiovascular changes; hypertrophy of left ventricle, hardening of heart muscle; decreased rhythm and tone if lifestyle is sedentary Menopause: degenerative changes of ovaries due to decrease in estrogen and progesterone	Tendency toward farsightedness Gradual slowing of reactions Gradual loss of hearing acuity, especially high tones Brain cell loss begins, usually without noticeable symptoms	Re-evaluation of current lifestyle and value system Modeling for younger generation Involvement in institutions of society Working way up career ladder Parenting Responsible for children and aging parents Adjustment to changes in body image
Late middle age (ages 50–65)	Increase in body fat distribution around abdomen and hips Change in skeleton, some loss in height Endocrine changes: increased anti-inflammatory hormone,	Visual acuity decreased due to lens changes in accommodation and convergency. Glasses may be needed. Diameter of pupils decreases so brighter lighting necessary; recovery from glare and adaptation to dark take longer.	Concern for health increases Grandparenthood Ability to separate—last child leaves home Retirement planning; establishment of avocation and leisure time activities

(continued)

TABLE 11-1 Continued

Stage	Physical changes	Sensory-cognitive changes	Psychosocial expectations
	decreased ability to respond to stress due to decreased hormonal, blood sugar, and acid-base regulating mechanisms Decreased tolerance of heat and cold Decreased muscle mass Increased fat mass Decreased peripheral circulation Cardiac status dependent on activity; heart may begin to lose tone, decrease rate, and show rhythm changes; atria stiffer; left ventricular hypertrophy Renal function decline due to gradual decrease in number of functioning nephrons Further decline in gastric secretions may cause food intolerances Atrophy of female vagina, uterus, and breasts following menopause Further loss of teeth may require dental care and changes in food intake	Hearing loss, especially of high tones, related to environmental noise level. Some decrease in sensitivity of taste buds and sensitivity to smell Decreased sensitivity and decreased tolerance of pain More hesitant to respond; uses strategy rather than speed; less risk-taking Decrease in central nervous system integration; response to stressors slower	Re-establishment as a couple Religious-spiritual interests may increase Coming to terms with accomplishments and potentials Valuing wisdom over physical powers Flexibility in emotional relationships
Old age (60–death)	Wrinkling due to infolding of epithelium; loss of fat layers on limbs and face, making bones more prominent; changes in pigmentation; thinning of hair which is also less oily; decreased perspiration Posture becomes one of general flexion; shrinkage of intervertebral disks leads to shortening of body and thoracic bowing Decrease in muscle mass, decalcification of bones, stiffening of joints Decrease in homeostatic mechanisms, fluid and electrolyte balance, hormonal regulation, glucose utilization, antibody formation; decreased ability to tolerate stresses, including drugs Renal function decreases; more time needed for filtering	Cognitive functioning depends greatly on earlier cognitive abilities and on general health and involvement in society; motivation is an important component of performance; important information remembered; encoding may change Learning may be slower or more difficult; best when self-paced; seeks irrelevant and redundant information; less organized. Cautiousness due to discomfort with uncertainty; fear of failure may be interpreted as rigidity Drop in performance before death Less efficiency in receiving, processing, and responding to stimuli due to decreased electrical stimulation rate, quantity of neurotransmitter, and	Retirement Grieving death of friends or spouse Agreeable relationships Mobility Stimulation of mind and body Comfort of mind and body Involvement in society Introspection and life review Acceptance of death Relocation Decreased autonomy Decreased self-esteem

TABLE 11-1 Continued

Stage	Physical changes	Sensory-cognitive changes	Psychosocial expectations
	due to decreased renal blood flow; urine more dilute; may experience increased frequency due to decreased bladder muscle tone	less oxygen to brain Stronger stimulation needed for all senses to experience sensation	
	Men may experience urinary problems due to prostatic hypertrophy; testes smaller and less firm	Reaction time increases; decrease in ability to respond to multiple stimuli	
	GI tract: decreased motility and absorption rate; decreased saliva production; tooth loss may be due to bone and gum resorption	Decreased sense of balance Decreased pain perception and response	
	Cardiovascular: increase in peripheral resistance with resultant increase in systolic blood pressure due to arteriosclerosis; inefficiency of heart muscle and valves; decrease in cardiac output and reserve; decreased ability to respond to stress	Cataracts; decreased color vision and depth perception Paresthesias in extremities; decreased sensitivity to light touch and vibration Less deep sleep; more easily aroused	
	Pulmonary: increased rigidity of airways causes decrease in maximal breathing capacity and vital capacity; decrease in gaseous exchange; decreased respiratory rate, oxygen uptake, and expired carbon dioxide; decreased ciliary effectiveness and cough reflex causes increased susceptibility to lower respiratory tract infections		

moting their own welfare, often at the expense of others or society at large.

The final crisis faced in adulthood is integrity versus despair. People who age successfully achieve integrity. Integrated people are satisfied with their accomplishments and the way they have lived their lives. They accept death more easily as the end of a meaningful and productive life. Persons who fail to resolve the final developmental crisis become despairing. They often harbor regrets about their lives, become depressed, and are fearful of death. Table 11-2 summarizes Erikson's stages of adult development.

Developmental Tasks Theory

Robert J. Havighurst's concept of developmental tasks (1972) was influenced heavily by Erikson's

work, and is described in Chapter 10. Early adulthood encompasses a number of developmental tasks—establishing living arrangements separate from parents, beginning a career, selecting a mate, starting a family, and becoming active in civic affairs. It is also a time of life when individuals are making a transition from an age-graded to a social status society. In the middle years, from age 30 to 60, people reach their peak influence in society and also respond to demands for responsible participation in social institutions. The tasks of later life (age 60 to death) involve a decrease in active involvement in social institutions and a realignment of priorities. During the middle and late years, adjustment to physiological changes in oneself and others becomes important for successful mastery of the developmental tasks. Table 11-3 lists

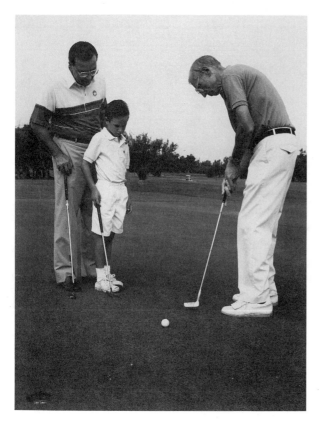

FIGURE 11-1. Generative adults are productive and guide the next generation within and beyond the family.

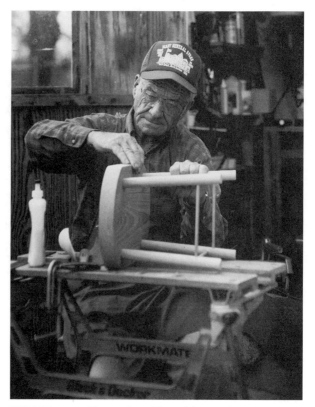

FIGURE 11-2. The tasks of later life involve a decrease in active involvement in social institutions and a realignment of priorities.

Havighurst's developmental tasks during early adulthood, middle age, and later maturity. Tasks of childhood are discussed in Chapter 10.

Joanne Stevenson (1977), a nurse theorist and researcher, has adapted developmental tasks theory to reflect current lifestyles and a positive perspective of development throughout adulthood. Stevenson views developmental tasks as processes through which people progress at their own pace in unique ways. She delineates four stages of adulthood—*young adulthood, core middle years, new middle years*, and *late adulthood*—and identifies tasks for each. Stages overlap, and there are many ways adults can achieve the tasks within each stage.

Stevenson's unique contribution to adult developmental theory is her characterization of middle adulthood as *middlescence*. She subdivides middlescence into two stages: middlescence I (core middle years) and middlescence II (new middle years). This division more accurately represents today's healthy aging population. The core middle years refer to people age 30 to 50, while the new middle years refer to those who are 50 to 70 years old. People who are 50 years old do not consider themselves elderly and, on average, have another

quarter century or more yet to live (Karp, 1988). Thus, theories of adult development must now incorporate this extended middle age period of life.

Stevenson proposes four areas of life experience that adults are concerned with: *family life and parenting, work and recreation, social involvement and community responsibility*, and *personal maturity*. Specific developmental tasks surrounding these areas of life and the major developmental objective for each of Stevenson's adult stages are identified in Table 11-4. According to Stevenson, these tasks and objectives may be used as standards for personal growth, ideal statements to guide adults in moving from stage to stage, and ways to evaluate developmental progress through the adult years.

Adaptation Theory

Bernice Neugarten (1976) views development as age-appropriate adaptation to social expectations and norms. Healthy adaptation is determined within the context of three dimensions of time: *historical time, life time* (chronological age), and *social time*, all of which are interwoven. She points out that the historical setting in which development occurs determines what is appropriate at various ages

TABLE 11-2
Erikson's Stages of Adult Development

Young adulthood: 18–30	Intimacy vs. Isolation	Mate, friends	Young adults are able to involve themselves in loving and intimate relationships with others. They are concerned with building their careers. Community welfare becomes important during this stage.
Middle adulthood: 30–65	Generativity vs. self-absorption	Mate, children, friends	People in middle adulthood are settled in their careers and devote themselves to parenting and guiding the next generation. The future welfare of the family and community are of paramount importance.
Senescence: 65–death	Integrity vs. despair	Mate, friends	This stage is seen as a time of wisdom and positive reflection on life. The elderly engage in leisure activity and continue to be concerned about the future of society.

Age ranges are approximate.

TABLE 11-3
Havighurst's Adult Developmental Tasks

Tasks of early adulthood (18–30):

1. Selecting a mate.
2. Learning to live with a partner.
3. Starting a family.
4. Rearing children.
5. Managing a home.
6. Getting started in an occupation.
7. Taking on civic responsibility.
8. Finding a congenial social group.

Tasks of middle age (30–60):

1. Assisting teenaged children to become responsible and happy adults.
2. Achieving adult social and civic responsibility.
3. Reaching and maintaining satisfactory performance in one's occupational career.
4. Developing adult leisure time activities.
5. Relating oneself to one's spouse as a person.
6. Accepting and adjusting to physiological changes of middle age.
7. Adjusting to aging parents.

Tasks of later maturity (60–death):

1. Adjusting to decreasing physical strength and health.
2. Adjusting to retirement and reduced income.
3. Adjusting to death of spouse [or partner].
4. Establishing an explicit affiliation with one's age group (elder of society).
5. Adopting and adapting social roles in a flexible way.
6. Establishing satisfactory physical living arrangements.

Age ranges are approximate.

Note. From Havighurst, R.J. (1972). *Developmental tasks and education* (3rd ed.). New York: Longman.

of development. For example, a young man who reached young adulthood during the Vietnam War era had to adapt to very different social forces and expectations than one who became a young adult during the 1980s.

Social time is defined by the relationship between historical time and life time. As Neugarten points out:

> Every society is age-graded, and every society has a system of social expectations regarding age-appropriate behavior. There exists a socially prescribed timetable for the ordering of major life events: a time in the lifespan when men and women are expected to marry, a time to raise children, a time to retire. The social change that occurs with the passage of historical time creates alterations in the rhythm and timing of the life cycle, leading in turn to changes in age norms and in expectations regarding age-appropriate behavior. (p. 16)

This helps explain Stevenson's (1977) motivation to redefine "middle age," which is different now from what it was 50 or 100 years ago.

Neugarten notes that most people expect certain life events such as parenthood, retirement, widowhood, and so forth to occur at predictable times ("on-time") in the life cycle, and prepare themselves accordingly. Stressors are created when events occur out of sequence ("off-time") in the life cycle. Thus, it is the *timing* of life events, rather than the events themselves, that influence development in positive or potentially detrimental ways. For example, first-time pregnancy during the twenties and early thirties is on-time, whereas its occurrence in the forties is off-time and may precipitate a

TABLE 11-4
Stevenson's Developmental Tasks for the Four Stages of Adulthood

Developmental tasks of young adulthood or youth (18–30):

Major Objective: Achieve relative independence from parental figures and a sense of emotional, sociocultural, and economic responsibility for one's life.

1. Advancing self-development and the enactment of appropriate roles and positions in society.
2. Initiating the development of a personal style of life.
3. Adjusting to heterosexual marital relationship or to a variant companionship style.
4. Developing parenting behaviors for biological offspring or in the broader framework of social parenting (adopting, involvement with children through coaching, scouting, etc.).
5. Integrating personal values with career development and socioeconomic constraints.

Developmental tasks for middlescence I, the core of the middle years (30–50):

Major Objectives: (1) Assume responsibility for growth and development of self and of major institutions of society; (2) provide help for younger and older generations without trying to control them.

1. Developing socioeconomic consolidation.
2. Evaluating one's occupation or career in light of a personal value system.
3. Helping younger people to become integrated human beings (biological and social parenting, becoming mentors).
4. Enhancing or redeveloping intimacy with spouse or most significant other.
5. Developing a few deep friendships.
6. Helping aging persons progress through the later years.
7. Assuming responsible positions in occupational, social, and civic activities, organizations, and communities.
8. Maintaining and improving the home and other forms of property.
9. Using leisure time in satisfying and creative ways.
10. Adjusting to biological or personal system changes that occur.

Developmental tasks of middlescence II, the new middle years (50–70):

Major Objective: Assume primary responsibility for the continued survival and enhancement of the nation.

1. Maintaining flexible views in occupational, civic, political, religious, and social positions.
2. Keeping current on relevant scientific, political, and cultural change.
3. Developing mutually supportive (interdependent) relationships with grown offspring and other members of the younger generation.
4. Re-evaluating and enhancing the relationship with spouse or most significant other or adjusting to their loss.
5. Helping aged parents or other relatives progress through the last stage of life.
6. Deriving satisfaction from increased availability of leisure time.
7. Preparing for retirement and planning another career when feasible.
8. Adapting self and behavior to signals of accelerated aging processes.

Developmental tasks of late adulthood (70+):

Major Objective: Assume responsibility for sharing the wisdom of age, reviewing life, and putting affairs in order.

1. Pursuing a second or third career, new interest, hobbies, and/or community activities that fulfill some heretofore untapped inner resource or otherwise enhance the self-image and maintain worth in society.
2. Learning new skills that are well removed from prior learning or at least do not produce cognitive dissonance or interference with prior learning.
3. Sharing wisdom accrued from the past with individuals, groups, communities, and nations.
4. Evaluating the totality of past life and putting successes and failures into perspective.
5. Progressing through the stages of grief, death, and dying with significant others and with oneself.

Note. From Stevenson, J.S. (1977). *Issues and crises during middlescence.* New York: Appleton-Century-Crofts.

developmental crisis. Death of a spouse is usually a crisis event in young adulthood but an anticipated event in late adulthood.

Life Transition Theories

Other theorists have proposed that the life transitions that occur in adulthood provide a useful framework for explaining adult development. Roger Gould (1972) and Daniel Levinson (1978) both studied patterns of adult life by examining de-

velopmental transitions and the abilities of adults to cope with these transitions. Their work focused on men and not until the late seventies did Gail Sheehy (1976) and Carol Gilligan (1982) study life transitions and adult development of women.

Gould, a psychoanalyst, suggests that transformation is the central concept of adult development. He believes people have an innate drive to grow and change. By studying both healthy, middle-class, educated men and women and psychiatric patients he identified general themes for the transformations that take place during the adult life span (Gould, 1972). Table 11-5 maps Gould's themes.

Levinson, a psychologist, (1978) describes several developmental periods and transition crises requiring a reassessment of one's life. Levinson's theory considers the development of values, skills, and motives in terms of individual personality, role expectations of groups and institutions, and the adaptation of the individual to specific events and expectations. Adult development is seen as an evolving process of mutual interaction of the self and the world. Family and work are the central components of adult life. Career choice and work influence the choice of one's associates, life goals, and social roles, as well as the adoption of ethical standards and values, the use of intellectual capacities, and the development of self-concept. Responses to life's events are greatly influenced by

TABLE 11-5
Gould's Themes for Adult Transformations

Years	Themes
20's	Work is based on values and fantasies developed during childhood. People try to establish themselves as adults and master what they are supposed to be as defined by others.
Early 30s	Adults begin to question what life is about and whether they are doing the right thing. They seek information about the fit of their inner needs and work. They express a desire to be accepted "as I am" and make an attempt to accept children as they are. There is a strong identification with family, but marital happiness decreases.
35–43	Continued questioning, along with increasing awareness of time limitations. Men become more affective, sensitive, less aggressive, and more interested in social relationships than power. Women become more independent, and less sentimental. People begin to express concern for their health.
43–50	Adults become more resigned to finite time. May be competitive with children. There is increased interest in spouse, friends, and social activities. Authenticity and generativity are organizing themes of transformation.
50–60	Mellowing and decreased negativeness. Realization of mortality and concern for health. Less responsibility and concern for children.

Note. From Gould, R.L. (1972). The phases of adult life: A study in developmental psychology. *American Journal of Psychiatry, 129*(5), 521–531.

relationships within people's families and work (Levinson, 1980). Levinson's work is particularly noted for its identification of a midlife transition, often referred to as "midlife crisis." For most people, the midlife transition occurs in the early forties. During the midlife transition, people critically evaluate their life structures and question what they have done with their lives and what they want to do with the time remaining. The midlife transition often involves major life changes such as career change, divorce, or relocation. Table 11-6 outlines Levinson's eras and periods of development.

Gail Sheehy (1976) was one of the writers to look at adult female transitions in her book *Passages*. Women's development in the adult years is divided roughly into 10-year increments (see Table 11-7). Sheehy calls the 20s "trying" as women leave the safety of home behind and begin to look for the perfect career and the perfect partner. In the 30s illusions are shaken and women either must break or deepen life's commitments. At 40, the dreams of youth demand reassessment; age 50 arrives with positive outcomes for those who find a renewal of purpose.

Several years later, Sheehy published another book, *Pathfinders* (1981), and continued the work begun in *Passages*, this time including men as well as women. She expanded her developmental stages to age 80. Sheehy questions the reasons certain people navigate a successful passage through adulthood while others slip backward. Her research led to identification of 10 hallmarks of well-being (Table 11-8). Sheehy states that the first requirement for well-being is to confront a crossroad and emerge from the completed passage with renewed strength and expanded potential. Women who do not experience well-being often describe themselves as feeling trapped, and unable to navigate the passage through adulthood successfully.

Gilligan (1982) asserts that most developmental theories are fraught with gender bias. As she notes, nearly all theories of human development have been proposed by men or based on models developed by male theorists. Therefore, they offer interpretations of life cycle phenomena from a male perspective and fail to account for differences between the sexes. For example, Gilligan (1982) suggests that Erikson's stages of identity and intimacy are sequentially inappropriate for women. Women's identity is embedded in relationships and their need to be intimate with others. Men seek emancipation from relationships in order to achieve ego identity as defined by Erikson. Men thus become independent while women remain interdependent, according to Gilligan. These differ-

TABLE 11-6
Levinson's Eras and Periods of Adult Development

Eras and Periods	Characteristics
Preadulthood: birth–22	Rapid biological, psychological, and social growth resulting in capabilities for living independently.
Early adulthood: age 17–45	Peak years biologically; establishing a niche in family, career, and society; conflict between inner ambitions and demands of society.
Transition	Search for independence; make and test career and lifestyle choices; modify relationships with family and institutions.
Entering the adult world	New home base; exploration and commitment to adult roles.
Age 30 transition	Evaluation of lifestyle, values, family, and career.
Settling down	Rebuild life structure to realize dreams; become a person in own right; upward striving.
Middle adulthood: age 40–60	Dominant generation, responsible for own work and the development of those younger; biological capacities beginning to wane.
Midlife transition	Critical examination of current life structure; recognition of time limitations: "What have I done with my life?" "What do I want?"; implement modifications of lifestyle (May involve career change, divorce, relocation); integration of polarities of: young/old, destruction/creation, masculine/feminine.
Entering middle adulthood	Restablization after transition.
Age 50 transition	Reassessment; often more of a crisis if midlife went smoothly.
Culmination of middle adulthood	Work toward major goals; exert leadership on society.
Late adulthood: age 60–death	Not studied by Levinson.

Note. From Levinson, D.J. (1980). Toward a conception of the adult life crisis. In N.J. Smelser & E.H. Erikson (Eds.), *Themes of work and love in adulthood.* Cambridge, MA: Harvard University Press.

ences in development influence the moral choices people make. Gilligan points out that men tend to resolve moral dilemmas on the basis of what is fair and just, as determined by their understanding of societal rights and rules. Women, on the other hand, base moral decisions on their understanding of their responsibility to and relationships with others.

In summary, use of developmental theories as frameworks for assessing adult development should take into account the client's chronological age, gender, social and cultural contexts, and life events ("on-time" or "off-time"). The nurse can use developmental information to make inferences about clients' special competencies, deficiencies in experience, relationships, lifestyle, expectations of development of disease, and responses to illness and caregivers. Anticipatory guidance or other nursing interventions can be designed to promote development and foster successful aging.

The Aging Process

For such social reasons as eligibility for retirement and Social Security pensions, old age begins somewhere between 60 and 65. However, the majority of older adults are vigorous and completely independent. Only 5% of people over 65 live in institutions. About 20% have some disabilities that interfere with their ability to move about freely; the rest are quite active (Gioella & Bevil, 1985).

At present there are roughly 29.8 million Americans over age 65, accounting for 12.3 percent of the population. By 2030, there will be about 66 million older persons, two and one-half times their number in 1980. If current fertility and immigration levels remain stable, the only age group to experience significant growth in the next century will be those past age 55 (American Association of Retired Persons, 1988).

The aging of the population is the result of de-

TABLE 11-7
Sheehy's Passages for Adult Women

Trying 20s	Leave home
Catch 30s	Illusions shaken
Forlorn 40s	Reassess dreams
Refreshed 50s	Renew purpose
Selective 60s	Choose carefully
Thoughtful 70s	Reflect on life
Proud-to-be 80s	I made it, I'm here

Note. From *Passages* by Gail Sheehy. Copyright © 1974, 1976 by Gail Sheehy. Used by permission of the publisher, Dutton, an imprint of New American Library, a division of Penguin Books USA Inc.

TABLE 11-8
Sheehy's Ten Hallmarks of Well-Being

1. My life has meaning and direction.
2. I have handled important transitions in a creative way.
3. I rarely feel disappointed by life.
4. I have attained several important long-term goals.
5. I am pleased with my personal growth and development.
6. I am in love, mutually.
7. I have many friends.
8. I am a cheerful person.
9. I am not sensitive to criticism.
10. I have no major fears.

Note. From *Pathfinders* by Gail Sheehy. Copyright © 1981 by Gail Sheehy. Used by permission of the publisher, Dutton, an imprint of New American Library, a division of Penguin Books USA Inc.

clining birth and mortality rates. Life expectancy for a person born in 1940 is 64 years. The older population itself is getting older. In 1987 the 65–74 age group (17.7 million) was eight times larger than in 1900 but the 75–84 group (9.3 million) was 12 times larger and the 85+ group (2.9 million) was 23 times larger ([AARP], 1988).

Aging is a normal phase of development and should be considered as such. The way people age is influenced by heredity and lifestyle. Physical and mental changes occur with aging and are considered normal. Most of the physical aging changes are addressed in Chapter 24. Mental aging changes, including those that affect the developmental assessment, are addressed in this chapter.

Physiological Aging

Several theories have been proposed to explain the reasons people age and eventually die. Although none of the theories has been proved, several theories offer promising explanations of the aging process.

Walford (1983) suggests that there are two major categories into which theories of biological aging can be divided: *programmed theories* and *damage theories.* Programmed theories emphasize that aging is controlled by genetic mechanisms; cells contain a genetic clock that controls the speed of metabolic processes and the number of cell divisions possible. Damage theories focus on the destruction of body cells and organs over time; aging results from the accumulation of cell damage caused by such forces as metabolic processes and environmental hazards (radiation, pollutants, substance abuse, etc.).

Table 11-9 briefly describes current theories of physiological aging. None of these theories has been proved to be the sole explanation for why people age. Most likely, several aging mechanisms

are responsible for the aging process and ultimately death.

Cognitive Aging

Older persons process information differently from younger individuals, but it is not yet known which

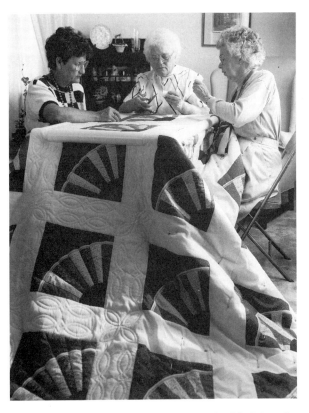

FIGURE 11-3. Women's identity is embedded in relationships and their need to be intimate with others.

TABLE 11-9
Theories of Physiological Aging

Programmed Theories

Maximum Life Span: The human species has its own characteristic maximum life span that is genetically programmed. Aging and death are maturational changes like puberty and menopause.

Endocrine Theory: The human genetic code controls hormonal changes which cause the body to age and ultimately die.

Immune System Theory: The genetically-controlled immune system is less effective in detecting and counteracting foreign substances, such as infectious agents and cancer cells.

Autoimmune Theory: The genetically-controlled immune system is less effective in differentiating normal cells from foreign substances, and produces antibodies that attack normal cells, causing age-related changes in normal body cells.

Damage Theories

Stress-Adaptation Theory: Aging results from cellular loss and degeneration as a result of lifelong attempts to maintain homeostasis. Cells and organs become less able to adapt to internal and external stressors, and eventually can no longer sustain life.

DNA Repair Theory: DNA is progressively damaged throughout life by metabolic processes and environmental forces, becoming less able to repair damaged cells. Cellular dysfunction and eventual death result.

Cross-Link Theory: Chemical reactions create cross links between collagen molecules, interfering with normal cellular functioning, and causing stiffness and degeneration of collagen tissue.

Free Radical Theory: Unstable free radicals (pieces of molecules that result from oxygen metabolism) accumulate, causing damage and degeneration of cells and organs.

age differences are specific adaptive changes in strategy and which changes are due to irreversible neurological deficits. The results of research concerning age-related changes in intelligence and cognition may be flawed. Most studies have been conducted by younger people using tasks that are familiar to young people, such as intelligence tests. It is likely that tests for elderly persons should involve familiar tasks based on cognitive abilities used in the day-to-day activities of older adults. In other words, poor performance on standardized intelligence tests may be due to obsolescence of knowledge rather than decline of abilities. Norms for standardized tests cannot be applied to the elderly because otherwise healthy, well-functioning older people often show test patterns that suggest brain damage.

Understanding of the process of aging is best gained through longitudinal research; that is, by following one group of people through the life span. In this way, differences in life experiences based on the culture in which the people developed are eliminated. Recent longitudinal studies have consistently found that the following cognitive and intellectual functions do decline with age:

Older persons are less able to perform tasks that require the individual to perform mental manipulation at the same time items are stored or recalled. This deficit may be related to problems with processing the information (i.e., coding it) or with memory.

The elderly tend to organize material to be stored in memory less than younger persons do, so recall is weaker.

The elderly have inconsistent recall; that is, they sometimes forget. Forgetting may be related to faulty retrieval of the information rather than loss of memory, to lack of organization, to disuse, to interference from previous learning, to internal or external stimuli, to changed cues and expectations as the culture changes, to physiological changes, or to a combination of these factors.

Speed of response and perceptual integration begin to decline in the seventies. This decline affects both motor and sensory responses and is probably due to neurobiological changes in the central nervous system. For this reason cognitive tests should be untimed.

Recent research indicates that decline in intellectual functions is a normal part of aging, but may occur later, be smaller in magnitude, and affect fewer functions than previously thought. Function does seem to decline rapidly in the few years before death. Mental function tests conducted at age 73 in subjects who died at 75 show much lower results than tests administered at 73 to subjects who died at 90. This phenomenon is known as terminal drop. Even slight alterations in health can seriously affect intellectual functioning.

Psychosocial Aging

Interest in how people respond to becoming old has led to formulation of several psychosocial theories of aging. *Disengagement theory* states that aging involves a mutual withdrawal, or disengagement, between the person and others in the social system. Older individuals find this releases them from societal pressures, and the disengagement of elders allows younger persons to take over the functional roles in society. *Activity theory* states that the optimal way to grow old is to stay active and manage to resist diminishing the parameters of one's world. For example, a small group of elderly widows named themselves the "Crazy Eighties," involving themselves in community activities as well as enrolling in courses at the local university. One member explained, "If we didn't stay so busy, we'd fall apart in a week."

As roles change, the person finds substitute activities. *Continuity theory* states that behavior in old age is a result of habits, commitments, preferences, and personalities of individuals. How a person adapts and responds to the changes of aging depends on the individual's personality, previous experience, and previous coping strategies. The response may be either to disengage, to continue being active, or some modification in between (Yurick et al., 1984). A 74-year-old retired printer spends most of his time at home reading or engaging in spirited political debates with his elderly neighbor. Another 74-year-old retiree who spent 45 years working in the busy garment district of New York City rarely spends an evening alone, preferring to invite friends for dinner or to join in the active social life of his condominium community. It is obviously difficult to stereotype the elderly just as

it is difficult to stereotype 30 year olds.

Using continuity theory, Neugarten (1968) describes specific personality patterns, including responses to aging. Some of these patterns contribute to successful aging, and some do not (see Table 11-10).

The Final Stage: Death

The final stage of human growth and development is death. It is the inevitable outcome of life and an integral part of human existence. The prospect of death sets limits on the time for development and provides impetus for people to be productive. It is hard for people to die, because dying means giving up what they know on Earth. Concern about dying often focuses on fear of prolonged illness, pain, and loss of social role and dignity. Older people fear becoming a burden to others more than they fear death. Religious beliefs often play a major role in an individual's reaction to anticipated death and should be part of the assessment.

Grief and death confront everyone. However, for the older adult, grief and dying become more immediate realities. For many older people the loss of their loved ones has a greater psychological impact than the thought of their own impending death (Dimond, 1981). Thus, knowledge of the grieving process is helpful in understanding people who have suffered loss (Dessonville-Hill, 1988). Lindemann (1944) studied the grieving process and identified the ways people act when they grieve. Often grief is misunderstood by health-care providers as depression or confusion. To avoid misdiagnosis, providers must recognize the characteristics of grief (Dessonville-Hill, Thompson, & Gallagher, 1988).

Lindemann identifies five classes of symptoms of normal grieving: somatic distress, preoccupation with the deceased's image, guilt, hostility, and altered activity patterns. Specific behaviors for each category are delineated in Table 11-11. Ebersole and Hess (1985) describe stages of grief that are helpful to the practitioner working with the grieving client. In addition, specific interventions are identified for each stage. The practicing nurse who recognizes the symptoms can help the grieving individual work through grief using the stages and interventions presented in Table 11-12.

Elizabeth Kübler-Ross (1975), a psychiatrist who worked with dying people for many years, developed a stage theory of dying that may help nurses assess persons who are dying. Her stages of dying describe individual adjustment to the knowledge of impending death. The stages also may apply to other situations involving loss, such as loss of health in those experiencing illness, loss

---

TABLE 11-10
Aging Personality Patterns

1. **Integrated**—functions well with a complex inner life and a competent ego.
   a. **Reorganizer**—competent with a wide variety of activities (volunteer). (**Age Successfully**)
   b. **Focused**—competent, but more selective in activities (golfer). (**Age Successfully**)
   c. **Disengaged**—competent and choosing a low activity level (rocking chair). (**Age Successfully**)
2. **Armored-Defended**—strives, with high defense against anxiety.
   a. **Holding on**—aging constitutes a threat. "I'll work till I drop." (**Age Successfully**)
   b. **Constricted**—defends self against aging and preoccupied with losses. (**Age Poorly**)
3. **Passive-Dependent**—demonstrates recurrent needs.
   a. **Succor-seeking**—strong dependency needs and seeks support from others. (**Ages successfully if support system is available**)
   b. **Apathetic**—passivity is a striking feature of personality (man allows wife to talk for him). (**Age Poorly**)
4. **Disorganized**—gross defects in psychological functioning. (**Age Poorly**)

Note. Adapted from Neugarten B., Havighurst, R., & Tobin, S. (1968). "Personality and patterns of aging." In B. Neugarten (Ed.), *Middle age and aging.* Chicago: The University of Chicago Press.

TABLE 11-11
Lindemann's Symptoms of Grief

1. Somatic Distress.
 a. Occurs in waves lasting from 20 minutes to one hour.
 b. Deep, sighing respirations especially when discussing grief.
 c. Lack of strength.
 d. Loss of appetite and sense of taste.
 e. Tightness in throat.
 f. Choking sensation accompanied by shortness of breath.

2. Preoccupation with image of deceased.
 a. Similar to daydreaming.
 b. May mistake others for deceased person.
 c. May be oblivious to surroundings.
 d. Slight sense of unreality.
 e. Fear that he or she is becoming insane.

3. Feelings of guilt.
 a. Accuses self of negligence.
 b. Exaggerates existence and importance of negative thoughts, feelings, and actions toward deceased.
 c. Views self as having failing deceased, "If I had only . . ."

4. Feelings of hostility.
 a. Irritability, anger, and loss of warmth towards others.
 b. May attempt to handle feelings of hostility in formalized and stiff manner.

5. Loss of patterns of conduct.
 a. Inability to initiate or maintain organized patterns of activity.
 b. Restlessness with aimless movements.
 c. Loss of zest, tasks and activities are carried on as though with great effort.
 d. Activities formally carried on in company of deceased have lost their significance.
 e. May become strongly dependent on whoever stimulates him or her to activity.

Note. From Lindemann, E. (1944). Symptomatology and management of adult grief. *American Journal of Psychiatry, 101,* 141–148. Copyright 1944, The American Psychiatric Association. Reprinted by permission.

TABLE 11-12
Stages of Successful Grieving

Stage One: Reactionary (first few weeks)
 Early responses of disbelief, anger, indecision, detachment, and inability to communicate in a logical, sustained manner are common. Searching for loved one, visions, hallucinations, and depersonalization may be experienced.
 Intervention: Support, validate, be available, listen to talk about loved one, reduce expectations.

Stage Two: Withdrawal (first few months)
 Depression, apathy, physiological vulnerability occur; movement and cognition are slowed; insomnia, unpredictable waves of grief, sighing, and anorexia occur.
 Intervention: Protect against suicide and involve in support groups.

Stage Three: Recuperation (second 6 months)
 Periods of depression are interspersed with characteristic capability. Feelings of personal control begin to return.
 Intervention: Support accustomed lifestyle patterns that sustain and assist person to explore new possibilities.

Stage Four: Exploration (second year)
 Individual begins new ventures, testing suitability of new roles; anniversaries of holidays, birthdays, and date of death may be especially difficult.
 Intervention: Prepare individual for reactions during anniversaries and holidays. Encourage and support new trial roles.

Stage Five: Integration (fifth year)
 Individual will feel fully integrated into new and satisfying roles if grief has been resolved in a healthy manner.
 Intervention: Assist individual to recognize and share own pattern of growth.

Note. Adapted from Ebersole, Priscilla, and Patricia Hess: *Toward healthy aging,* ed. 3, St. Louis: The C.V. Mosby Co.

of a job, or loss of a home. Not all people pass through all stages, and for some the progression may not be sequential. For example, a person may revert to denial after expressing anger or bargaining, or may display a combination of behaviors. The reader should consider Kübler-Ross's stages only an aid in understanding the dying person and not a proven course of events. Most people express hope for possible cure in all stages. Table 11-13 describes Kübler-Ross's five stages of grief or loss.

Adult Maturation

As demonstrated by the theories of adult development, people can anticipate specific events as they become older. Many factors affect adult maturation. Timing of biological changes is influenced by heredity, environmental and psychosocial stressors, and health habits. Psychosocial development is influenced by social, religious, legal, and cultural factors. Loss of status and objects, relocation, and retirement can affect a successful passage through life (McCracken, 1987). Reactive depression in the elderly often is a response to difficult passages and losses, but can be eased by the nurse (Lum, 1988). There is wide variation in development among adults of the same chronological age.

Superimposed on these developmental changes are situational aspects that require coping. An event becomes a crisis when the available coping strate-

TABLE 11-13
Kübler-Ross's Stages of Coping with Dying or Loss

Denial	"No, not me." Response to overwhelming anxiety is refusal to accept the diagnosis or loss. Person may accuse the health professional of incompetence and may refuse treatment and continue life as before.
Anger	"Why me?" Person acknowledges prognosis and realizes he or she won't finish what had been planned for life. Angry at health professionals, God or fate, family, anyone who is healthy, or anyone who may perceive them as dying. May be hard to live with and care for.
Bargaining	"If you let me live I will . . ." Bargains with God or others to postpone death or change severity of diagnosis. May promise to change life or cooperate or be stoic if given more time to live.
Depression	"I'm losing everything." Person expresses sorrow about losing everything and everyone he or she loves. May feel hopelessness, shame, or guilt for past deeds.
Acceptance	"Death is coming." Person is tired and weak, detaches self from people and the world, except for one or two significant people. Tends to be silent, uninterested in the world and people in it, and may seem devoid of feeling.

Note. Adapted from Kübler-Ross, E. (1975). *Death: The Final Stage of Growth.* Copyright © by Elisabeth Kübler-Ross. Reprinted by permission of Simon & Schuster, Inc.

gies of an individual fail to meet the requirements of a current problem or situation (Greenberg, 1983). Normal developmental changes may result in smooth transitions or crises, depending on how they are perceived and how people use their coping strategies. The same is true of situational events. For example, the aging of a parent is a common event for most people. Aging and illness, such as Alzheimer's disease, superimpose a situational challenge on that developmental event, with the event more likely to become a crisis.

Defining the meaning of an event that results in crisis depends on a variety of factors. These factors include the characteristics of the individual; gender and sex role identification, chronological, age life stage, state of health, race, ethnicity and culture, socioeconomic status, values, and previous experience with similar events (Fuller & Larson, 1980). Second, perception of a life event is important. Perceptions include role gain or loss, positive or negative effect, expected or unexpected

event, sudden or gradual timing of the event, and whether the event is permanent or temporary. Retirement often is described as a major event that may affect emotional health (Daly & Futrell, 1989). Admission to a nursing home is another potentially traumatic event (Brooke, 1989), as is diagnosis of chronic or terminal illness. Finally, individual and personal characteristics are important. These characteristics may include self-concept, relationships with family and friends, institutional supports, and the physical environment. Each of them affects the individual's ability to adjust to life changes.

THE DEVELOPMENTAL HISTORY

The developmental history is the major tool for assessing adult development, and should be incorporated with the nursing interview (Table 11-14). It is important to recognize that much of developmental information overlaps with other areas of the nursing assessment. For example, the ability of the client to relate thoughts clearly and logically and demonstrate appropriate affect and congruence between verbal and nonverbal behavior is an indicator of mental status. On the other hand, information provided about friendships, marriage, and family life reflect intrapersonal and interpersonal areas of assessment.

In obtaining the developmental history, the nurse should consider the social, cultural, and temporal contexts of adult development. Assessing adults' perceptions of their own development is important, as opposed to just comparing individuals to standard theories or a table of characteristics. For example, a 25-year-old woman raised in a very strict religious home may have little or no experience with loving and intimate relationships and not perceive this to be a problem. In fact, the young women indicates that she believes intimacy is for marriage and has many friends who share this belief. If the nurse fails to consider the woman's perceptions and her social context, the nurse might conclude that the woman has a problem with the issue of intimacy.

The frequency and extent to which developmental assessment is done depends on the client situation and the purpose for obtaining this type of information. Usually, a complete developmental history is not obtained routinely on every client unless indicated. However, multiple areas of the assessment process contribute developmental information. Aspects of development that are important to assess in every client include significant life events, physical changes and their impact on the ability to function, life style, value system (importance placed on matters such as concern for one's

TABLE 11-14
The Developmental History

Significant Life Events:

Childhood

Nature of the relationship with parents or guardians

Presence of siblings and the nature of the relationship

Loss of important person(s) or things

Major illness, hospitalization(s)

School attendance and feelings about school

Influence of church

Adolescence

Important people especially close to you

Involvement in school, church, and community activities

Achievements and successes

Work experiences

Feelings of attraction toward another person

Feelings about sexual identity and sexual activities

Earlier Adulthood

Career choice and responsibilities

Relationship with significant other, marriage, children

Satisfaction with intimate relationship(s)

Divorce, separation, widowhood

Achievements and successes

Major illness, hospitalizations

Leisure activities

Physical Changes:

General Health

Major illnesses, hospitalizations
Preventive health practices

Health Status of Each Body System

Recent changes, problems
Impact of changes/problems on ability to function
Ability to manage changes/problems

Sensory-Cognitive Changes:

Health Status of the Special Senses (vision, hearing, taste, smell, touch/proprioception)

Recent changes, problems
Impact of changes/problems on ability to function
Ability to manage changes/problems

Cognitive Function (thought processes, memory, reaction time, learning)

Recent changes problems
Impact of changes/problems on ability to function
Ability to manage changes/problems

Psychosocial Expectations:

Established life style
Independence
Role responsibilities
Commitment made to self and others
Accomplishment of career goals
Involvement in institutions in society
Involvement in leisure activities
Ability to cope with failures and accomplishments
Adjustment to changes in body image
Ability to cope with illness, disability
Concern for younger generation
Retirement planning
Acceptance of death

---

health, success, relationships, family life, involvement in institutions of society), role responsibilities, life satisfaction, and expectations for the future. Many of these aspects are gleaned only when the nurse and the client have an ongoing relationship.

There are a number of situations in which it is important to obtain a complete developmental history. One is when an adult makes a change in health care providers and is not known to those delivering care. Obtaining a complete history is also helpful when an adult experiences a major crisis. The loss of personal health, for example, may require substantial changes in life style. Developmental information is important for understanding the client's functioning now and how the client can be helped to manage change. A significant life event such as the birth of a child may result in an

individual's inability to cope effectively with parenting. A developmental history may provide clues about the adult's childhood and the parenting behavior modeled by the parents or identify current life stresses affecting the individual's ability to cope. While much of what is gathered in other areas of assessment relates to development, the developmental history per se should be confined to the following: significant life events (childhood, adolescence, earlier adulthood), physical changes or problems, sensory-cognitive changes or problems, and psychosocial expectations.

Significant life events refer to social milestones that individuals have experienced in childhood, adolescence, and earlier adulthood. Educational achievements, puberty, death of a parent or sibling, marriage, divorce, birth of a child, career choice, athletic or artistic accomplishments, and relocation to a retirement home are examples of significant life events. In assessing this area, the nurse explores major life events from the perspective of their significance and meaning for the client.

For example, as the nurse explores significant events in childhood, the nurse can determine how the individual felt about school. Was it a happy place? Did the client meet with success or repeated obstacles that eventually would lower self-esteem? Was the client motivated in school? Did the client achieve? Maybe the client never completed school because of a need to work in the fields during harvest time. The inability to complete even grade school can be a lifetime regret for some older people, who imagine themselves inferior because of the lack of education.

Changes in physical and sensory-cognitive functions occur over the lifespan. The developmental characteristics listed in Table 11-1 are a useful guide for evaluating several of the major components of the developmental history. In obtaining developmental information, the nurse considers what is characteristic for a specific stage of adult development. Physical and sensory-cognitive changes or problems are noted and their impact on the client's ability to function is explored. For example, changes in sensory perception, particularly vision, commonly occur with aging. The impact on the client's life may be significant. Older adults have difficulty with glare, visual acuity, and depth perception. Because of these physical changes, an older adult may restrict driving to only the daytime hours out of concern for personal safety and eliminate or curtail evening social activities. The client may feel a sense of isolation and dependence as a result of the impact of these physical changes.

Psychosocial expectations are developmental markers or tasks appropriate to specific stages of adult development (Table 11-1). The ability to have meaningful relationships is an important developmental task. Relationships throughout a lifetime certainly affect adult relationships. The presence of brothers and sisters may have contributed to an adult's ability to be comfortable with other people. If the client was an only child, abused, neglected, or just too often alone, he or she may have difficulty establishing relationships. As the person moves through adolescence, relationships with those outside the family become important. Did the client have a love relationship? Was the client ever rejected, or have all relationships been positive? The patterns and adaptations of relationships established in childhood contribute to the client's persona in adulthood.

The use of Haight's Life Review and Experienc-

ing Form (1988), depicted in Table 11-15, may serve as a helpful developmental assessment tool. It is an expansion of the significant life events portion of the developmental history and would be appropriate for use with clients, especially during times of change, crisis, death, and grief. This form is presented here in its entirety. The nurse may use the complete form or select questions appropriate for the client situation.

Life Review

The life review first was described by Robert Butler (1963) as a naturally occurring process often instigated by crisis or impending death. In a life review, the person takes stock of life. If the assessment is positive, the individual moves on and puts things in perspective. If the life review is not positive, the person may be stuck in despair or depression. While published research has mainly indicated its usefulness with older clients (Haight, 1988), life review can be used with other client populations such as children, adolescents, and young adults. The nature of the client situation would determine its appropriateness. Also, the nurse may need to modify the questions to fit the client situation.

Haight (1988) uses a structured form of life review as a nursing intervention for increasing life satisfaction and psychological well-being. As the individual describes childhood, adolescence, and adulthood, the nurse can assess the number, type, and severity of traumatic events in the client's life. While listening to the life story the nurse also can assess coping abilities, outlook on life, and personality patterns. The nurse can tell whether the client is satisfied with life up to that point. If the client is not satisfied, the life review may be therapeutic.

CLINICAL APPRAISAL

The developmental history will generally provide sufficient information on which to draw conclusions about the appropriateness of the adult client's developmental progress. Throughout the interview, however, the nurse should be alert to the client's verbal and nonverbal behaviors, which can help confirm what the client says. For example, if a 50-year-old client denies any problems with movement, yet winces and stiffens when moving from a sitting to a standing position, the nurse should try to clarify the discrepancy through further questioning. Inconsistencies and vagueness in responding to questions may indicate that the client is masking information (see chap. 3). In this situation, the nurse should strive to create an atmo-

TABLE 11-15
Haight's Life Review and Experiencing Form

Childhood:

1. What is the very first thing you can remember in your life? Go as far back as you can.
2. What other things can you remember about when you were very young?
3. What was life like for you as a child?
4. What were your parents like? What were their weaknesses, strengths?
5. Did you have any brothers or sisters? Tell me what each was like.
6. Did someone close to you die when you were growing up?
7. Did someone important to you go away?
8. Do you ever remember being very sick?
9. Do you remember having an accident?
10. Do you remember being in a very dangerous situation?
11. Was there anything that was important to you that was lost or destroyed?
12. Was church a large part of your life?
13. Did you enjoy being a boy/girl?

Adolescence:

1. When you think about yourself and your life as a teenager, what is the first thing you can remember about that time?
2. What other things stand out in your memory about being a teenager?
3. Who were the important people for you? Tell me about them. Parents, brothers, sisters, friends, teachers, those you were especially close to, those you admired, those you wanted to be like.
4. Did you attend church and youth groups?
5. Did you go to school? What was the meaning for you?
6. Did you work during these years?
7. Tell me of any hardships you experienced at this time.
8. Do you remember feeling that there wasn't enough food or necessities of life as a child or adolescent?
9. Do you remember feeling left alone, abandoned, not having enough love or care as a child or adolescent?
10. What were the pleasant things about your adolescence?
11. What was the most unpleasant thing about your adolescence?
12. All things considered, would you say you were happy or unhappy as a teenager?
13. Do you remember your first attraction to another person?
14. How did you feel about sexual activities and your own sexual identity?

Family and Home:

1. How did your parents get along?
2. How did other people in your home get along?
3. What was the atmosphere in your home?
4. Where you punished as a child? For what? Who did the punishing? Who was "boss"?
5. When you wanted something from your parents, how did you go about getting it?
6. What kind of person did your parents like the most? The least?
7. Who were you closest to in your family?
8. Who in your family were you most like? In what way?

Adulthood:

1. What place did religion play in your life?
2. Now I'd like to talk to you about your life as an adult, starting when you were in your twenties up to today. Tell me of the most important events that happened in your adulthood.
3. What was life like for you in your twenties and thirties?
4. What kind of person were you? What did you enjoy?
5. Tell me about your work. Did you enjoy your work? Did you earn an adequate living? Did you work hard during those years? Were you appreciated?
6. Did you form significant relationships with other people?
7. Did you marry?
    (yes) What kind of person was your spouse?
    (no) Why not?
8. Do you think marriages get better or worse over time? Were you married more than once?
9. On the whole, would you say you had a happy or unhappy marriage?

10. Was sexual intimacy important to you?
11. What were some of the main difficulties you encountered during your adult years?
    a. Did someone close to you die? Go away?
    b. Were you ever sick? Have an accident?
    c. Did you move often? Change jobs?
    d. Did you ever feel alone? Abandoned?
    e. Did you ever feel need?

Summary:

1. On the whole, what kind of life do you think you've had?
2. If everything were to be the same would you like to live your life over again?
3. If you were going to live your life over again, what would you change? Leave unchanged?
4. We've been talking about your life for quite some time now. Let's discuss your over-all feelings and ideas about your life. What would you say the main satisfactions in your life have been? Try for three. Why were they satisfying?
5. Everyone has had disappointments. What have been the main disappointments in your life?
6. What was the hardest thing you had to face in your life? Please describe it.
7. What was the happiest period of your life? What about it made it the happiest period? Why is your life less happy now?
8. What was the unhappiest period of your life? Why is your life more happy now?
9. What was the proudest moment in your life?
10. If you could stay the same age all your life, what age would you choose? Why?
11. How do you think you've made out in life? Better or worse than what you hoped for?
12. Let's talk a little about you as you are now. What are the best things about the age you are now?
13. What are the worse things about being the age you are now?
14. What are the most important things to you in your life today?
15. What do you hope will happen to you as you grow older?
16. What do you fear will happen to you as you grow older?
17. Have you enjoyed participating in this review of your life?

Note. Derived from new questions and two unpublished dissertations:
Gorney, J. (1968). *Experiencing and Age: Patterns of Reminiscence Among the Elderly.* (Unpublished Doctoral Dissertation, University of Chicago).
Falk, J. (1969). *The Organization of Remembered Life Experience of Older People: Its Relation to Anticipated Stress, to Subsequent Adaptation and to Age.* (Unpublished Doctoral Dissertation, University of Chicago).
© 1982 Barbara K. Haight, RNC, Dr.P.H. Professor of Nursing, College of Nursing, Medical University of South Carolina, Charleston, SC 29425-2404.

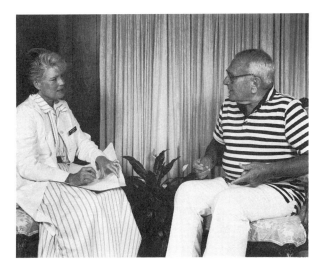

FIGURE 11-4. While listening to the life story, the nurse also can assess coping abilities, outlook in life and personality patterns.

sphere of trust and mutual respect wherein the client feels safe and comfortable sharing information. It is within the context of a trusting relationship that the nurse continues to question the client to clarify discrepancies.

Table 11-1, which outlines adult developmental characteristics, can be used as a guide for identifying what age-appropriate behaviors and changes the nurse should look for at various stages of adulthood. Observation provides a great deal of information about a client's overall state of health. The general appraisal, for example, provides information about the client's state of awareness and level of consciousness, posture and motor activity, grooming and personal hygiene, skin color, sexual development, apparent state of health, and signs of distress. Observations made on general appraisal are then validated on physical examination.

As the nurse examines the client in a systematic manner, the nurse differentiates what are normal age-related findings from those that may be abnormal. For example, loss of hearing, especially of high tones, and a decrease in the ability to taste and smell are physical changes commonly observed in late middle age. However, a young adult presenting with these findings should be referred for further evaluation.

Changes in sensory-cognitive functioning normally occur with aging. As the nurse evaluates cognitive ability and sensory status in an older client, the nurse should be attentive to the subtle differences that may separate normal age-related changes from those related to disease or some underlying problem. For example, increasing forgetfulness, confusion, and difficulty maintaining balance are not normal age-related changes. A client exhibiting these symptoms requires further evaluation.

Psychosocial expectations assist the nurse in evaluating behavior at the various adult developmental stages. In obtaining any developmental assessment, it is essential for the nurse to obtain baseline information about the client's usual behavior and activity. This provides a frame of reference against which to evaluate change in the client.

ADULTS' HEALTH KNOWLEDGE AND PRACTICES

An area of assessment that is important throughout the adult life cycle is knowledge of health, and healthy behaviors. As part of a developmental assessment, the nurse should ask adult clients about their health practices and any changes in health habits over time, including reasons for the change (Walker, Volker, Sechrist, & Pender, 1988).

Healthy behaviors are easily influenced by prevailing social expectations. Healthy behaviors require the ability and motivation to plan for the future (Redeker, 1988). Self-concern and persistence are required to resist such addictive behaviors as smoking, social drinking, or working long hours. Practice of good health habits may change during the life cycle, and certain life stages may precipitate change (Pender, 1987). For example, when physiological changes become noticeable at middle age, adults become more interested in protecting their health and fitness. However, they also may give up good health habits as their bodies become less agile. Table 11-16 lists specific health concerns at three stages of adulthood.

Young adults usually feel quite fit, confirming their notion that they are invulnerable to illness and that healthy behaviors therefore are unimportant. Conscious self-control is necessary to resist peer pressures to drink, use drugs, drive reck-

lessly, and eat and rest erratically. The young adult may relinquish leisure time and hobbies to concentrate on work. Yet young adulthood is the best time for establishing a healthy adult lifestyle.

During middle adulthood, people are models for the younger generation. Their concern for setting an example, combined with noticeable body changes, often increases their interest in health. At this stage people begin to value their health and may be more willing to change lifestyle habits to improve their health and increase their potential life expectancy. The nurse can encourage self-monitoring and self-responsibility for health.

Older people (60–80) today have not adopted as many healthy practices as the 20–40 age group. The reason for this is primarily because social awareness of the importance of fitness had not yet emerged when they were stronger and could take advantage of it. The 60–80 age group is more concerned with managing illnesses than with attaining health. Expectations for good health in this age group are low, and many illness signs are ignored because older people think they are supposed to feel bad.

In older people there is a complex relationship among the perception of health, the reporting of symptoms, and the use of medical services (Levkoff, Cleary, Wetle, & Besdine, 1988). Studies demonstrate the optimism of elderly people in their evaluation of health. They report good health when in fact they may have several chronic illnesses that affect their health negatively (Stoller, 1984). Thus, it seems the older one gets, the fewer aspirations one has for good health. Thirty-nine to 50% of the elderly do not report illness to their physicians simply because they attribute their conditions to aging rather than disease (Levkoff et al. 1988). This is particularly true of those with chronic illness. They tend to cope with symptoms of chronic illness as long as possible before seeking health care. However, there are exceptions to this rule, and a few hypochondriacal elderly overreport symptoms and continually seek medical advice.

The very frail elderly concentrate on conserving energy and often do so by decreasing nonessential activities, planning schedules carefully, and increasing dependence on others (Rhodes, Watson, & Hanson, 1988). Self-care behaviors in this age group are more crisis-oriented than preventive, and often the energy is not available to care for oneself. This group's health behaviors are those of lifetime habit or those that have been newly recommended by a physician. The capacity for self-care in older people is best assessed through the func-

TABLE 11-16
Health Concerns Related to Various Stages of Adulthood

Young Adulthood	Middle Adulthood	Older Adulthood
Understanding of body mechanisms and their maintenance	Menopause and male climacteric	Nutritional intake and patterns
Sexuality	Vision and hearing deficiencies	Dental problems
Pregnancy planning; prevention of sexually transmitted diseases	Decreases in muscular strength and endurance that have implications for safety	Adaptation to sensory and other physical changes affecting safety, especially related to falls and driving
Prenatal care	Decrease in metabolic rate so that weight maintenance requires decreased food intake or increased exercise	Capacity for performing activities of daily living (ADLs)
Nutritional intake		Monitoring for symptoms of disease and for the effects of drugs taken as treatment for symptoms
Eating habits and prevention of obesity	Changes in sleep patterns (less deep sleep and easier arousal) that are influenced by physical, mental, and social activity	Retirement
Dental care		Adjustment to losses of significant others
Rest, relaxation, and sleep	Dental care	Fear of confusion and disability
Exercise and development of leisure activities	Smoking	Alcohol abuse
Moral-religious-ethical development (values provide a sense of purpose and direction in life and as such are health promoting)	Alcohol and drug abuse	
	Response to stress	
Body image and self-concept	Early detection and treatment of symptoms of disease	
Lifestyle options	Cardiovascular disease	
Stress	Cancer symptom detection	
Occupational hazards	Monitoring blood pressure	
Smoking		
Alcohol and drug abuse		
Safety, especially related to motor vehicles		
Breast and testicular examination		
Pap smears		

tional assessment described in Chapter 24. Healthcare providers and investigators have been unable to achieve a composite measure of health based on medical diagnosis and instead have developed measures of function based on the performance of common activities (Ford, Folmar, Salmine, Medalie, Roy, & Galazka, 1988).

Older adults can actively practice healthful habits and monitor their body responses. Some changes in health habits may be necessary. It is never too late to begin practicing the rules for healthful living. Exercise should be initiated gradually. Rhythmic exercise that causes the cardiovascular system to respond (aerobic exercise such as walking, jogging, dancing, swimming, and bicycling—perhaps a three-wheeler) produce more positive physiologic effects and are safer than activities involving quick, jarring movements. The nurse should focus on strengths and how to use them to promote health.

Several indexes or tools are available for assisting adult clients to increase their awareness of various health risks. Table 11-17 lists the seven warning signs of cancer. As people age they become more susceptible to cancer. Knowledge of the warning signs will help them monitor their own risks and practice effective health habits.

The incidence of heart disease also rises with age. Therefore, knowledge of the risk factors for heart disease is essential. Paffenbarger (1978) found, in a study relating exercise to risk of cardiovascular disease, that an individual may reduce the risk of coronary artery disease by 37% through physical activity, 62% by lowering blood pressure, 21% by losing excess weight, and 30% by ceasing smoking. Table 11-18 lists risk factors for heart disease.

Certain personality types also are said to be more at risk for heart disease. Friedman and Rosenman (1974), two cardiologists noticed that their clients were very restless and wore out the edges of the upholstery on the chairs in their office. From

TABLE 11-17
Seven Warning Signs of Cancer

Unusual bleeding or discharge.
Lump or thickening in breast or elsewhere.
A sore that does not heal.
A change in bowel or bladder habits.
Indigestion or difficulty swallowing.
Hoarseness or cough.
A change in a wart or mole.

TABLE 11-18
Risk Factors for Heart Disease

Elevated blood pressure.
Smoking.
Diet high in saturated fats and cholesterol.
Overweight.
Diabetes.
Lack of exercise.
Family history of heart disease.
Psychological and social stress.
Type A behavior pattern.

this observation, they concluded that cardiac types appeared to be more stressed and active. They identified those who were more stressed and at risk as "Type A" personalities and those who were more calm, as "Type B" personalities. Table 11-19 contains a self-test for determining whether a person is a Type A, hard-driving, impatient, and at risk for cardiovascular disease, while Figure 11-5 provides a self-scoring tool for assessing stress and tension levels.

Becoming aware of personality traits that contribute to stress, as well as ways to monitor stress and tension levels, is an important first step in moving to a healthier life style. The nurse can assist clients in this effort by providing the necessary knowledge, skills, and encouragement.

Older adults may find some changes in health habits necessary regardless of their choices. It is never too late to begin practicing the rules of healthy living (Chang, Uman, Linn, Ware, & Kane, 1985). If one has not exercised for some time, exercise should be initiated gradually. Aerobic exercises are especially beneficial if approached in a sensible and careful manner. All people should undergo a physical exam before beginning a new exercise program. Aerobic exercises such as walking, jogging, dancing, swimming, and bicycling are recommended, with a gradual buildup.

NURSING DIAGNOSES RELATED TO ADULT DEVELOPMENT

Adults change in patterned ways throughout the life span. Developmental information helps the nurse formulate individualized nursing diagnoses in several ways, particularly through a better understanding of the client's current situation, special competencies, and deficiencies (Nesbitt, 1988).

An example of such a nursing diagnosis and its use in elderly clients is "feeding-bathing/hygiene-dress/grooming-toileting self-care deficit." As people grow older and more frail, they often lose their abilities to care for themselves and the ability

TABLE 11-19
Are You a Type A?

1. Do you become impatient when asked to perform repetitive tasks?
2. Do people who know you well say that you enjoy a contest and usually try hard to win at whatever you do?
3. Do you read or watch TV while eating alone?
4. Do you get impatient when things don't go as quickly as they could?
5. Do you keep track of what you have accomplished in terms of numbers (of miles, of letters, of parts)?
6. When people talk slowly, do you feel like hurrying them along?
7. Do you know how people are going to finish their sentences and sometimes do it for them?
8. Do you clench your teeth or form your hands into fists without noticing it?
9. Do you walk and eat more rapidly than others?
10. Do you talk explosively, emphasizing words with body gestures and speeding up at the end of sentences?
11. Do you go to your place of work outside normal working hours?
12. Do you bring work home with you or spend leisure time thinking about your job?
13. Do you become irritated when kept waiting for an appointment?
14. Do you try to do two or more things at once?
15. Would you say that your success is due to the fact that you do things faster than other people?
16. When talking to people do you find your mind wandering to things that need to be done?
17. When faced with a deadline, do you make every effort to meet it?
18. Do you get angry when forced to delay work or waste time because someone else is not prompt?
19. Do you find yourself looking for faster ways to do things?
20. Are you uncomfortable when you do nothing for several hours or days?

Note. From *Type A Behavior and Your Heart* by M. Friedman & R.N. Rosenman. Copyright © 1974 by Meyer Friedman. Reprinted by permission of Alfred A. Knopf, Inc.

Behavior	Often	A Few Times a Week	Rarely
1. I feel tense, anxious, or have nervous indigestion.	2	1	0
2. People at work/home make me feel tense.	2	1	0
3. I eat/drink/smoke in response to tension.	2	1	0
4. I have tension or migraine headaches, or pain in the neck or shoulders, or insomnia.	2	1	0
5. I can't turn off my thoughts at night or on weekends long enough to feel relaxed and refreshed the next day.	2	1	0
6. I find it difficult to concentrate on what I'm doing because of worrying about other things.	2	1	0
7. I take tranquilizers (or other drugs) to relax.	2	1	0
8. I have difficulty finding enough time to relax.	2	1	0
9. Once I find the time, it is hard for me to relax.	2	1	0
10. My workday is made up of many deadlines.	2	1	0

Maximum total score = 18. My total score _____

Zone	Score	Tension Level
A	14–18	Considerably above average.
B	10–13	Above average.
C	6–9	Average.
D	3–5	Below average.
E	0–2	Considerably below average.

FIGURE 11-5. Simple Self-Scoring Test for Gauging Stress and Tension Levels (*Note.* Simplified self-scoring test for gauging stress and tension levels. Reprinted from *The American Way of Life Need not be Hazardous to Your Health,* by John W. Farquhar, by permission of W.W. Norton & Company, Inc. Copyright © 1978 by John W. Farquhar. First published in The Portable Stanford, by the Stanford Alumni Association of Stanford, California.)

for self-care is a better measure of how well they function than the presence of disease.

"Self-care deficit" is categorized under the pattern of moving in NANDA (1990) Taxonomy I. Activity is required for an individual to conduct self-care. The goal for the patient with a self-care deficit is to attain the highest level of functioning appropriate for the individual to compensate for lost ability and prevent further disability.

To assess for a self-care deficit one must look in four areas: feeding, bathing, dress, and bathroom habits. A feeding deficit is characterized by the inability to bring food from a receptacle to the mouth. Defining characteristics for a self-bathing/ hygiene deficit include the inability to wash the body or body parts, inability to get to a water source, or inability to regulate water temperature or flow. When one is assessing for a self-dressing/ grooming deficit one must assess ability to put on or take off clothing, ability to replace articles of clothing, ability to fasten clothing and ability to maintain appearance at a satisfactory level. Finally, one should assess bathroom habits by examining

the ability to get to the commode and the ability to sit down or rise up. (Yurick et al., 1984).

The nursing diagnosis of "diversional activity deficit" related to, for example, loss of vision is a frequent diagnosis for elderly clients. This diagnosis describes the situation in which an individual is reluctant or unable to participate in activities that pass the time, provide distraction, or bring pleasure. The sensory and perceptual changes associated with aging can influence an individual's ability and desire to be active. Decreased visual acuity and difficulty hearing can lead the older individual to self-imposed restrictions on activity due to, for example, fear of falling. As a result, the individual may withdraw and avoid opportunities to engage in diversions. Other cues to this diagnosis would be preoccupation with self, napping during the day (more so than usual), apathy or hostility, crying, complaints of boredom, restlessness, and verbalizations of desire for activity.

Another diagnosis categorized under the pattern of moving is "altered growth and development." This diagnosis reflects the state in which an individual demonstrates deviations from his or her age group. Chronic illness, for example, may alter or compromise an individual's development of communication or social skills, thereby delaying the achievement of certain developmental tasks.

When an older client exhibits preoccupation with self, social withdrawal, irritability toward others, disinterest in carrying out activities of daily living, expression of distress at the thought of retirement, and feelings of loss and loneliness related to an impending change in life style, a nursing diagnosis of "anticipatory grieving" related to retirement may be made. This diagnosis, which is categorized under the pattern of feeling, describes the situation in which an individual grieves before an actual loss occurs.

A diagnosis of "fear" is also categorized under the pattern of feeling and describes the feeling of dread related to an identifiable source that the person validates. Fear related to aging, for example, may be used to describe the situation in which a client exhibits increased tension, decreased self-assurance, apprehension, and concentration on or preoccupation with growing older. Once the assessment is made, interventions to manage client problems can be planned. Table 11-20 presents other selected nursing diagnoses that relate to adult development.

TABLE 11-20
Nursing Diagnoses Related to Adult Development

Altered growth and development related to failure to achieve age-appropriate developmental tasks, chronic illness, or depression.

Health-seeking behaviors related to health education or motivation/desire to improve health and fitness.

Altered health maintenance related to knowledge deficit, lack of motivation, cultural values, self-esteem disturbance.

Impaired social interaction related to failure to achieve age-appropriate developmental tasks, depression, self-concept disturbance.

Diversional activity deficit related to sensory-perceptual alteration, impaired mobility.

Feeding-bathing/hygiene-dressing/grooming-toileting self-care deficit related to decreased strength or endurance, pain, sensory or cognitive impairment, depression, impaired mobility.

Anticipatory grieving related to anticipated retirement, loss of home, death of self or loved one.

Dysfunctional grieving related to retirement, loss of job, loss of home, widowhood, chronic illness.

Fear related to aging.

Chapter Highlights

▪ Developmental assessment of an adult is less predictable than that of a child and less dependent on physical change.

▪ Aging is a normal phase of development and is influenced by how an individual lived as a young and middle-aged person.

▪ Knowledge of life span development and transition theories, when used with theories that explain patterns of aging, provide the nurse with a useful framework for assessing adult development.

▪ Mental aging changes occur in both the affective and the cognitive domains. Changes in the cognitive domain, specifically intelligence, memory, and decision-making, are among the most studied.

▪ For many older people the loss of a loved one has a greater psychological effect than the thought of their own impending death.

▪ Grief in the older adult often is misunderstood by health-care providers as depression or confusion.

▪ The life review is a helpful and therapeutic tool for assessing the older adult and may serve as a useful developmental assessment tool, especially during times of change, death, grief, and crises.

Practice Activities

1. Interview two people aged 20 to 80 in different decades and determine how they are accomplishing Erikson's, Havighurst's, and Stevenson's tasks. Discuss differences in each decade.

2. List the developmental (maturational) and situational events you are experiencing. Compare your list with that of a friend close to your own age. What similarities do you see? What differences? What reasons can you determine for those similarities and differences?

3. Visit a senior citizen social center and a nursing home. Conduct a developmental assessment on a person in each setting. Document and record your findings. Formulate appropriate nursing diagnoses. What differences and similarities do you see in the development of these elderly people? Speculate on the reasons for these similarities and differences. What are the implications for nursing care? Share your findings with classmates.

4. Conduct a life review of two individuals aged 20 to 80 in different decades of life. What similarities and differences do you see? Discuss your findings with a colleague and identify their implications for nursing care of the individuals interviewed.

Recommended Readings

Bushy, A. (1990). Rural U.S. women: Traditions and transitions affecting health care. *Health Care of Women International, 11*(4), 503–513.

Brock, A.M., & O'Sullivan, P. (1985). From wife to widow: Role transition in the elderly. *Journal of Psychosocial Nursing, 23*(12), 6–12.

Dimond, M., Lund, D.A., & Caserta, M.S. (1987). The role of social support in the first two years of bereavement in an elderly sample. *The Gerontologist, 27*(5), 599–604.

Farberow, N.L., Gallagher, D.E., & Gilewski, M.J. (1987). An examination of the early impact of bereavement on psychological distress in survivors of suicide. *The Gerontologist, 27*(5), 592–598.

Huss, M.J., Buckwalter, K.C., & Stolley, J. (1988). Nursing's impact on life satisfaction. *Journal of Gerontological Nursing, 14*(5), 31–36.

LaRosa, J.H. (1990). Executive women and health: Perceptions and practices. *American Journal of Public Health, 80*(12), 1450–1454.

Maddox, M.A., & Tillery, B.J. (1988). Elderly image: Seen by health-care professionals. *Journal of Gerontological Nursing, 14*(11), 21–25.

Makuc, D.M., Fried, V.M. & Kleinman, J.C. (1989). National trends in the use of preventive health care by women. *American Journal of Public Health, 79*(1), 21–26.

Penn, C. (1988). Promoting independence: The nurse can communicate an understanding of the self-care deficit, and elicit the client's perspective of the deficit and its meaning to daily living. *Journal of Gerontological Nursing, 14*(3), 14–19.

Rosenkoetter, M.M. (1988, July). Is retirement making your patient sick? *RN*, pp. 17–19.

References

American Association of Retired Persons. (1988). *A profile of older Americans.* Washington, DC: Program Resources Department, American Association of Retired Persons (AARP), and the Administration on Aging (AOA), U.S. Department of Health and Human Services.

Belloc, N., & Breslow, L. (1972). Relationship of physical health status and health practices. *Preventive Medicine, 1*, 409–421.

Botwinick, J. (1985). *Aging and behavior.* New York: Springer-Verlag.

Brooke, V. (1989). How elders adjust: Through what phases do newly admitted residents pass? *Geriatric Nursing, 10*(2), 66–68.

Butler, R.N. (1963). The life review: An interpretation of reminiscence in the aged. *Psychiatry, 26*, 65–76.

Chang, B.L., Ulman, G.C., Linn, L.S., Ware, J.E., & Kane, R.L. (1985). Adherence to health care regimens among elderly women. *Nursing Research, 34*(1), 27–31.

Cumming, E., & Henry, W. (1961). *Growing old: The process of disengagement.* New York: Basic Books.

Daley, E.A., & Futrell, M. (1989). Retirement attitudes and health status: Of preretired and retired men and women. *Journal of Gerontological Nursing, 15*(1), 29–32.

Dessonville-Hill, C., Thompson, L.W., & Gallagher, D. (1988). The role of anticipatory bereavement in older women's adjustment to widowhood. *The Gerontologist, 28*(6), 792–796.

Dimond, M. (1981). Bereavement and the elderly: A critical review with implications for nursing. *Journal of Advanced Nursing, 6*, 461–470.

Ebersole, P., & Hess, P. (1985). *Toward healthy aging: Human needs and nursing response.* Princeton, NJ: Mosby.

Erikson, E.H. (1963). *Childhood and society* (2nd Ed.). New York: Norton.

Ford, A.B., Folmar, S.J., Salmon, R.B., Medalie, J.H., Roy, A.W., & Galazka, S.S. (1988). Health and function in the old and very old. *Journal of the American Geriatrics Society, 36*(3), 187–197.

Friedman, M. & Rosenman, R. (1974). *Type 'A' behavior and your heart.* New York: Knopf.

Fuller, S.S., & Larson, S.B. (1980). Life events, emotional support and health of older people. *Research in Nursing and Health, 3*, 81–89.

Gilligan, C. (1982). *In a different voice: Psychological theory and women's development.* Cambridge, MA: Harvard University Press.

Gioella, E.C., & Bevil, C.W. (1985). *Nursing care of the aging client: Promoting healthy adaptation.* Norwalk, CT: Appleton-Century-Crofts.

Gould, R.L. (1972). The phases of adult life: A study in developmental psychology. *American Journal of Psychiatry, 129*(11), 521–532.

Greenberg, J. (1983). *Comprehensive stress management.* Dubuque, IA: Wm. C. Brown.

Haight, B.K. (1988). The therapeutic role of the life review in homebound elderly subjects. *Journal of Gerontology, 43*(2), 40–44.

Haight, B.K. (1989). Life review: A method for pastoral counseling: Part I. *Journal of Religion & Aging, 5*(3), 17–29.

Havighurst, R.J. (1972). *Developmental tasks and education* (3rd ed.). New York: Longman.

Holmes, T.H. & Rahe, R.H. (1967). The social readjustment rating scale. *Journal of Psychosomatic Research, 11*, 213–218.

Karp, D.A. (1988). A decade of reminders: Changing age consciousness between fifty and sixty years old. *The Gerontologist, 28*(6), 727–738.

Kübler-Ross, E. (1975). *Death: The final stage of growth*. Englewood Cliffs, NJ: Prentice-Hall.

Levinson, D.J. (1978). *The seasons of a man's life*. New York: Knopf.

Levinson, D.J. (1980). Toward a conception of the adult life course. In N.J. Smelser & E.H. Erikson (Eds.). *Themes of work and love in adulthood* (pp. 265–290). Cambridge, MA: Harvard University Press.

Levkoff, S.E., Cleary, P.D., Wetle, T., & Besdine, R.W. (1988). Illness behavior in the aged: Implications for clinicians. *Journal of the American Geriatrics Society, 36*(7), 622–629.

Lindemann, E. (1944). Symptomatology and management of adult grief. *American Journal of Psychiatry, 101*, 141–148.

Lum, T.L. (1988). An integrated approach to aging and depression. *Archives of Psychiatric Nursing, 2*(4), 211–217.

Matteson, M.A. & McConnell, E.S. (1988). *Gerontological nursing: Concepts and practice*. Philadelphia: Saunders.

McCracken, A. (1987). Emotional impact of possession loss. *Journal of Gerontological Nursing, 13*(12), 14–19.

McWeeny, M. (1988). Life span growth and development: A review and application to nursing diagnosis. *Journal of Enterostomal Therapy, 15*(2), 81–86.

Nesbitt, B. (1988). Nursing diagnosis in age-related changes. *Journal of Gerontological Nursing, 14*(7), 6–12.

Neugarten, B.L. (1976). Adaptation and the life cycle. *Counseling Psychologist, 6*, 16–20.

Neugarten, B.L., Havighurst, R., & Tobin, S. (1968). *Personality and patterns of aging*. In B.L. Neugarten (Ed.). *Middle Age and aging* (pp. 22–28.). Chicago: University of Chicago Press.

Pender, N. (1987). *Health promotion in nursing practice* (2nd ed.). Norwalk, CT: Appleton & Lange.

Paffenbarger, R.S., Wing, A.S., & Hyde, R.T. (1978). Physical activity as an index of heart attack risk in college alumni. *American Journal of Epidemiology, 108*(3), 61–75.

Redeker, N.S. (1988). Health beliefs and adherence in chronic illness. *Image: Journal of Nursing Scholarship, 20*(1), 31–35.

Rhodes, V.A., Watson, P.M., & Hanson, B.M. (1988). Patients' descriptions of the influence of tiredness and weakness on self-care abilities. *Cancer Nursing, 11*(3), 186–194.

Sheehy, G. (1976). *Passages: Predictable crises of adult life*. New York: Bantam.

Sheehy, G. (1981). *Pathfinders*. New York: Bantam.

Stevenson, J.S. (1977). *Issues and crises during middlescence*. New York: Appleton-Century-Crofts.

Stoller, E.P. (1984). Self-assessments of health by the elderly: The impact of informal assistance. *Journal of Health and Social Behavior, 25*(3), 260–270.

Walford, R.L. (1983). *Maximum life span*. New York: Norton.

Walker, S.N., Volkan, K., Sechrist, K.R., & Pender, N.J. (1988). Health-promoting life styles of older adults: Comparisons with young and middle-aged adults, correlates and patterns. *Advances in Nursing Science, 11*(1), 76–90.

Yurick, A., Spier, B., Robb, S., & Ebert, N. (1984). *The aged person and the nursing process*. Norwalk, CT: Appleton-Century-Crofts.

PART IV

Psychosocial Assessment

12

Intrapersonal and Interpersonal Assessment

CHAPTER OUTLINE

■ Knowledge Needed to Assess Intrapersonal Functioning
    Perception   Self-Concept   Motivation
    Cognitive Processes   Affect and Mood
    Temperament

■ Knowledge Needed to Assess Interpersonal Functioning
    Social Roles   Stressors and Stress Responses
    Coping Responses

■ The Nursing History and Clinical Appraisal
    Perception/Self-Concept   Motivation
    Cognitive Processes   Affect and Mood
    Temperament   Social Roles   Stressors
    and Stress Responses   Coping Strategies

■ Nursing Diagnoses Related to Intrapersonal and Interpersonal Functioning

OBJECTIVES

Upon completion of this chapter, you should be able to:

■ Contrast the intrapersonal and interpersonal dimensions of a psychosocial assessment.

■ Delineate influences of intrapersonal and interpersonal functioning on health.

■ Analyze theoretical concepts for conducting the intrapersonal and interpersonal assessment.

■ Describe approaches that are useful in performing a psychosocial history and clinical appraisal.

■ Collect information related to intrapersonal and interpersonal functioning.

■ Use selected tools to elicit intrapersonal and interpersonal assessment information.

■ Modify the intrapersonal and interpersonal assessment according to the client's age, cultural background, and health.

■ Formulate valid and appropriate nursing diagnoses for clients with actual or potential alterations in intrapersonal or interpersonal functioning.

Nurses long have been concerned with the psychosocial responses of clients to health and health alterations. The interrelationship of physiological and psychological health requires careful attention to both dimensions within the client's family, cultural, and environmental context, and with consideration of the client's developmental level.

Psychosocial functioning has two components: *intrapersonal* and *interpersonal*. Intrapersonal functioning refers to that which goes on within the individual, whereas interpersonal functioning involves a person's interactions or relationships with others. Intrapersonal and interpersonal behaviors often intertwine. They also influence and are influenced by other dimensions of human behavior such as physiological, developmental, family–cultural, and environmental. For example, fear may elicit a physiological response (e.g., increased heart rate, rapid breathing, release of cortisol). Conversely, a physiological change such as diabetes mellitus or a spinal cord injury precipitates psychosocial responses. Hence, assessment of intrapersonal and interpersonal functioning is often complex and challenging.

Intrapersonal and interpersonal assessmen are sometimes referred to as psychosocial asses ment. The major purpose of such an assessment to evaluate how a client functions individually and in relation to the environment and others. How people interact with and respond to internal and external forces may well determine their responses to altered health, their receptivity to nursing and health care, and ultimately to the nurse's ability to assist them.

Psychosocial assessment skills are defined less clearly and therefore are not learned as easily as assessment techniques that primarily involve technical skills (e.g., blood pressure measurement). Also, the nurse's own attitudes, prejudices, values, and general ease with self and others may play a significant role and thus influence the outcomes of the psychosocial assessment.

Psychosocial assessment information relies heavily on the nurse's own interpretations and cannot be compared easily with a chart of normal findings as can, for example, daily caloric intake or heart rate. Thus, nurses must be cognizant of the role their own biases and subjectivity play when obtaining and interpreting psychosocial information. To assess psychosocial status, the nurse relies primarily on observation and interview. After collecting clinical information about psychosocial status, the nurse considers it in light of all that is known about the client and forms inferences based on what the client said and her or his observable behavior. Congruence of what the client says and what the nurse observes, or lack of it, provides important information about the client.

The ability to make inferences about a client's functioning is an important component of the diagnostic reasoning process (Westfall, Tanner, Putzier, & Padrick, 1986) and is especially critical when assessing psychosocial functioning. Inferring and interpreting the meaning of behavior is complex and can be especially challenging for the beginning nurse. The nurse frequently must look beyond the obvious message and seek to understand more subtle cues. For example, when assessing a client's affect (emotions), the nurse may interpret as anxiety the client's behavioral cues of trembling, rapid respiration, and sweating. However, interpreting the meaning of behavior always is subject to human error. These behavioral cues may instead indicate a hypoglycemic response. The chance of error can be minimized by knowing human processes, gathering information carefully, providing a comfortable environment, being aware of one's own biases, and thoroughly validating cues whenever possible.

During the intrapersonal and interpersonal assessment the nurse's attention should focus on the client's current psychosocial status, with enough history to yield an appreciation of the individual's present "self." For a comprehensive approach, the intrapersonal and interpersonal components of the nursing assessment should not be isolated from other parts of the assessment. For example, while assessing a client's physiological status, the client's interaction with and responses to the nurse provide information about cognitive style, affect, and language.

Collecting intrapersonal and interpersonal information also is necessary to help identify interferences in a client's psychosocial functioning that warrant further attention. Nurses should be able to recognize cues that indicate a client's psychosocial needs are not being met in order to plan interventions to promote or restore psychosocial integrity. Often it is helpful for the nurse to take the initiative by sharing with the client a hunch or inference about the client's psychosocial functioning. Many times such openness facilitates a more comprehensive psychosocial assessment and, ultimately, the development of a plan of care that addresses the client's needs. After sufficient information has been gathered to assess the client's present level of functioning, the nurse continues to use it to anticipate potential problems, to build on the client's strengths, to diagnose further problems, and to detect any changes in psychosocial functioning as they occur.

The intrapersonal and interpersonal assessment is conducted according to the same principles that apply to other dimensions of the nursing assessment. A systematic approach is especially important when dealing with a client's psychosocial functioning because of its more nebulous nature. The use of a structured interview or nursing history format makes it easier to collect information about psychosocial functioning.

KNOWLEDGE NEEDED TO ASSESS INTRAPERSONAL FUNCTIONING

Knowledge of nursing, psychology, and sociology provide a basis for assessing intrapersonal and interpersonal functioning. Because psychosocial assessment relies so heavily on establishing an atmosphere of rapport and trust between client and nurse, the nurse's self-awareness and ability to encourage the client's disclosure also influence it profoundly.

The intrapersonal assessment consists of a number of components, including perception, self-concept, motivation, cognition, affect, and temperament. These components are internal dimensions of a person that may or may not be reflected in observable behavior. In general, *perception* refers to how people view themselves and their circumstances. *Self-concept* has four specific components: body schema, body image, self-ideal, and self-esteem. *Motivation* refers to the influence of needs and desires on a client's behavior and includes the dimensions of hope and spirituality. *Cognition* is the client's way of thinking and includes thought processes, reality orientation, judgment, and language. Cognition is influenced greatly by the client's maturational, or developmental level. *Affect* describes a client's emotional tone, which may change in response to situational variables, whereas *temperament* refers to behavioral style, or style of emotional reaction, which tends to be more stable over time and context.

Interpersonal assessment focuses primarily on gathering information about how an individual interacts with others, the individual's social responsiveness. Interpersonal assessment includes the client's various social roles, relationships with others, stress responses, and coping responses.

Perception

Understanding the relevance of perception to the practice of nursing enhances the nurse's ability to deliver individualized care to clients. In fact, clients' perceptions have a greater impact on their health behavior than do the behaviors of others, such as health education and role modeling (Aaronson, 1989). Perception may be viewed as a process in which a person takes in, interprets, and assimilates stimuli from the internal or external environment (Bunting, 1988). Perception is influenced by several factors, including sensory–neurological functioning, general health, cultural beliefs and values, and situational context. The individual's perceptions of self or circumstances also are shaped by past experiences. For example, a client who was hospitalized previously for skin grafting after a serious burn perceived that nurses and physicians allowed him little participation in his care. His perception of lack of control over his care in previous situations influences the client's perception of his current and future hospital experiences. The client's response is linked directly to stimuli perceived in the environment, in this case the prior behaviors of health-care professionals. Perception may, however, be an individual's intuitive awareness or belief about something not connected to a specific stimuli. For example, a client may believe that nurses are too busy to give individualized care, even though the client has no past or present personal experience on which to base this perception.

Perception is exceedingly important to the practice of nursing. Bunting (1988) suggests that nurses must deal with client's perceptions rather than objective reality. If a client perceives that "the room is spinning," it does not matter that the room is doing nothing of the sort. The nurse must be concerned with the client's perceptions and responses to those perceptions. In essence, what is "real" is the client's personal interpretation of the internal or external world. The client's interpretation may be quite different from the nurse's. The challenge is to strive to understand and respond to what the client perceives. Clients' views or thoughts about questions—such as: "How much control do I have or can I exert over my health . . . my quality of living . . . my quality of dying?" "Can I really change how I feel about myself?" and "Why should anyone be really interested in me and supportive as I experience this illness?"—relate to their perceptions of themselves and may have a significant impact on nursing assessment, diagnosis, and care.

Self-Concept

Self-concept refers to perceptions of self and the relationship of self to others and to life, with values attached to these perceptions. Self-perceptions provide a foundation for a person's interactions with the world. Self-concept is shaped from birth onward through interactions with others and with the environment. Self-concept is influenced greatly by the way significant others respond as the person grows and develops. Impressions of the self that are received from significant others are incorporated into one's self-perceptions.

Variables that influence self-concept include developmental level, sociocultural experiences, interpersonal relationships and roles, and general health. Developmental maturation plays an especially important role in the formation of one's self-concept. A newborn infant has no concept of self as a separate entity. As children grow and develop, they become aware of themselves as distinct beings with clearly defined body and personal space boundaries. As the range of life experiences broadens, self-concept is further developed and refined. Also, cognitive maturation influences the ability to conceptualize one's self as a person. Thus, a young child has a less well-developed self-concept than an adult.

Sociocultural factors also influence the development of self-concept because culture determines many of the experiences to which an individual is exposed during the course of a lifetime. Culture also defines acceptable norms that people use to compare themselves. For example, the predominant American value system promotes a positive concept of rich, thin, beautifully, physically fit people, and a negative concept of poor, fat, out-of-shape, or physically disabled people. In addition, the self-concept of members of certain groups in society, such as women or members of ethnic minority groups, may be influenced by the way the larger society perceives and responds to the group.

Interpersonal relationships and roles also influence self-concept formation. Sullivan (1953), a well-respected interpersonal theorist, suggests that self-concept is the result of an individual's interactions with others, especially significant others, and their responses to the individual. How a person is judged or treated by others influences one's self-perception ("looking glass self"). For example, a child who is reminded repeatedly of her faults rather than praised for her successes is likely to develop a negative self-concept.

Roles are important determinants of self-concept because certain roles are accorded more status than others in society and thus influence how people perceive those who occupy specific roles. For example, one's role as a nurse, parent, teacher, welfare recipient, college student, soldier, company vice president, professional athlete, or homeless person influences perceptions of self as well as perceptions others hold about those who occupy such roles. Social attributions of characteristics to people who occupy particular roles can have a profound impact on self-concept. Stereotyping homeless people as lazy, unwilling to work, or worthless reinforces negative self-perceptions and may influence their ability to change their situation (Bassuk, 1984).

Finally, health affects self-concept in important ways. The presence of mental or physical illness plays a role in how people perceive themselves and how others perceive them. For example, a teenage boy with extensive facial scarring from a childhood burn may have a negative view of himself. People with chronic mental illness or mental retardation may be ignored or avoided by others, leading them to feel alienated, isolated, and unimportant. Society often accords negative attributes to people with mental or physical illness or disability—"crazy," "loony," "stupid," "crippled"—which can affect their self-perceptions.

Body Schema

Body schema, the inner mental picture one has of one's body, is attained from all the senses and is an important component of self-concept. Cues from receptors in the limbs, visceral sensations, and sensory feedback from body position, tone, and movement are used in forming a concept or *schema* of the body as a person grows and develops. Newborn infants experience their bodies through visceral, tactile, and postural sensations. As the sensory–perceptual system develops, the ability to localize sensations emerges. By 7 to 10 months of age, infants are able to perceive themselves as distinct from their environment.

By exploring themselves and the immediate environment, toddlers refine and integrate their sensory and motor experiences. They are able to identify their external body parts and differentiate their own body from others'. Body schema development continues through childhood into adulthood as individuals achieve a conscious awareness of their bodies, their body parts, and their bodily functions. The adult's body schema includes an awareness of the relationship of the body parts to one another and the body's relationship in space (kinesthesia). Knowledge of body schema development is important in working with clients who have disturbances in body schema—a client whose limb has been amputated or one who has suffered a stroke. The pregnant client must incorporate the growing fetus into her body schema.

Body Image

Body image is also a major component of self-concept. It can be defined as the mental picture a person has of the physical self, including its appearance and capabilities. Body image has both objective and subjective components. Objectively, body image is what the individual sees in a mirror or photograph. Subjectively, though, body image is how people feel about what they see, feel about what they can't see (e.g., internal body organs), and how they interpret others' images of them.

Body image is shaped by an individual's past and present experiences and develops in response to other's reactions and feedback, particularly feedback from significant others. If feedback about one's body in early life is positive and pleasurable, a person is likely to feel good about her or his body. If, on the other hand, displeasure or disgust is associated with one's body or bodily functions, then body image is likely to be negative.

Like body schema, body image changes as the person grows and develops. Physical changes associated with growth, such as the development of secondary sexual characteristics during puberty, or with aging, such as skin changes and hair loss, play an important role in people's perceptions of their bodies. Body image also is influenced by alterations in health, such as pregnancy, illness (mental or physical), surgery, or trauma. People with a medical diagnosis of mitral valve prolapse have been shown to experience a change in their body image as a result of the diagnosis (Utz, Hammer, Whitmire, & Grass, 1990). Alterations or disturbances in body image may require the individual to adjust or adapt to a new body image temporarily or permanently. Examples of temporary body image changes include pregnancy, wearing a cast, orthodontic braces, or acne. Permanent changes include disfigurement from burn injuries or trauma, amputation of a body part, spinal cord injury, or cosmetic surgery.

An individual's adaptation to an alteration in body image depends upon such factors as the nature and duration of the change, the meaning of the change to the person, the person's coping abilities, responses of significant others, and level of social support. Clients who may be at risk for body image disturbances are identified in Table 12-1.

In a society that values youth, slenderness, and physical attractiveness, people whose bodies do not compare favorably with the social ideal may develop less positive body images. This depends, however, on the individual's own values and perceptions of what constitutes an acceptable and pleasing physical self. Every person has a unique body image because no two people have exactly the same repertoire of sensory–perceptual experiences or receive the same feedback from the environment. Also, different family and cultural groups value different aspects of the physical self and convey these values to their members. What is "beautiful" to one group may not be so to another. Women in some African cultures are not considered beautiful unless their faces have been decoratively scarred.

Self-Ideal

Self-ideal, a third component of self-concept, refers to a person's comparison of the self with an ideal image or goal. Self-ideal actually serves as the standard against which a person evaluates the real self. The ideal self may be clear, realistic, and attainable

TABLE 12-1
Health Alterations That May Lead to Self-Concept Disturbances

Loss of body part from disease or trauma (limb amputation, mastectomy, colostomy, hysterectomy, nephrectomy, laryngectomy)

Loss or impairment of body function (paraplegia, quadriplegia, cerebral vascular accidents, coronary artery disease, cancer, diabetes, aphasia, incontinence, chronic renal disease)

Disfigurement resulting from disease or trauma (burns, cleft lip, hirsutism, eczema, psoriasis, arthritis, alopecia)

Sensory-perceptual and communication deficits or disabilities (visual and hearing impairments, sensory deprivation or overload, learning disabilities such as dyslexia, autism, speech impairments)

Mental health and illness problems (alcoholism, drug dependency or addiction, child abuse, spouse abuse, schizophrenia, depression, anorexia nervosa)

Neuromuscular disabilities (cerebral palsy, scoliosis, multiple sclerosis, Parkinson's disease)

Obesity

Sexuality changes or problems (AIDS, sexually transmitted diseases, sterilization, infertility, impotence, frigidity, menopause, mastectomy, hysterectomy, mammoplasty, sexual assault, homosexuality or lesbianism, transsexualism)

Maturational and situational crises (puberty, pregnancy, abortion, miscarriage, aging, menopause; role changes—e.g., new parenthood, marriage, divorce, loss of employment, retirement; addition or loss of a family member, natural or man-made disasters—e.g., fires, floods, environmental contamination) or it may be ambiguous, unrealistic, and inappropriate. The ideal self-image includes not only physical attributes the individual would like to achieve but personal and social attributes as well. Self-ideal is to a great extent determined by social and cultural norms, by what society dictates is most desirable.

Self-Esteem

Self-esteem is closely related to self-ideal because self-esteem is determined by the conscious and unconscious comparison of one's self-image with one's self-ideal. Other terms used interchangeably with self-esteem include self-regard, self-acceptance, and self-worth. Self-esteem is determined by the congruency or fit between the self-image and the self-ideal. In other words, does the individual measure up to his or her own expectations? Self-esteem is enhanced when self-image and self-ideal are relatively congruent. If a significant discrepancy exists, self-esteem may be lowered. The development of self-esteem is essentially a lifelong process and is shaped and reshaped by life experiences.

Of all the components of self-concept, self-esteem has been studied most extensively. Positive self-esteem has been linked to good health practices (Muhlenkamp & Sayles, 1986). People who feel positively about themselves are more likely to engage in good health practices. People with greater self-esteem also are likely to cope more effectively with life stressors, such as divorce (Barron, 1987).

Motivation

One of the most prominent contributors to the field of human motivation is Abraham Maslow (1970). Maslow asserts that much of human behavior is motivated by human needs. The needs identified by Maslow are progressive in the sense that "lower order" needs must be met before behavior is directed toward "higher order" needs. Maslow's hierarchy (1970), from lowest to highest need, includes: (1) physiological needs (e.g., food, water, air); (2) safety needs (e.g., security, protection, order); (3) love and belonging needs (e.g., a sense of genuine human connection to others, friendship); (4) esteem needs (e.g., self-respect, recognition, appreciation); and (5) self-actualization needs (e.g., self-fulfillment as one strives to reach one's maximum potential). Kalish (1966) adapted Maslow's hierarchy to distinguish between physiological needs that are essential for human survival and those needed for matura-

tion and growth. Figure 12-1 illustrates the hierarchy of human needs that motivate human behavior.

The hierarchy of human needs provides a useful framework for conceptualizing and ranking a client's needs. For example, people will have difficulty engaging in activities that enhance their affiliations with others (love and belonging needs) if they are concerned about paying monthly bills or keeping their jobs (safety needs). People will have difficulty achieving self-fulfillment and being creative at work (self-actualization needs) if they are experiencing family conflicts (security needs).

Hope and Despair

An important facet of motivation is the level of hope or optimism a person has about fulfilling a need or accomplishing a goal. Hope has been described as an essential life force (Fromm, 1968). In many instances, it is hope that helps the individual tolerate and look beyond the immediacy of a stressful or painful experience and imagine a future that is brighter and more meaningful. In this sense, hope is related intimately to an individual's perception of the probability that what is desired is attainable (Stotland, 1969; Travelbee, 1971). Additionally, hope mobilizes or energizes an individual to take actions to overcome obstacles or cope with life's realities (McGee, 1984; Travelbee, 1971). Hope fortifies a person to cope with the stress and suffering that accompany illness, failure, tragedy, and loneliness (Travelbee, 1971). Baldree, Murphy, and Powers (1982) found that hope was the most frequently cited coping mechanism in a study of dialysis patients.

When an individual is faced with an experience that causes physical or emotional disequilibrium, the presence of hope not only induces the person to cope but also wards off despair. When despair is experienced, a person becomes engulfed by feelings of helplessness, hopelessness, doubt, overwhelming sadness, and grief. Such feelings may immobilize the individual to such a degree that "giving-up behaviors" take over. The individual may become depressed, disorganized, apathetic, and in extreme cases may lose the will to live (Lange, 1978).

Hope and despair may be conceptualized on a continuum. Individuals with hope generally have a solid sense of trust in themselves, in others, and in their futures. Their basic trust plays a significant role in their ability to relate to the world in a way that reflects their belief in themselves and in others (Lange, 1978). Table 12-2 illustrates differences in behaviors that indicate hope and those that indicate despair.

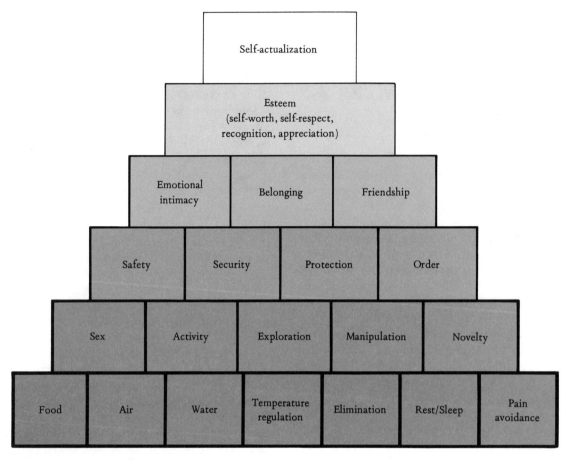

FIGURE 12-1. The Hierarchy of Human Needs.

Hope may be a motivating force that influences how clients respond to actual or potential health problems. Stoner and Keampfer (1985) suggest that hope in people with cancer is related to perceived life expectancy—specific knowledge of predicted life expectancy was found to lessen feelings of hope.

Spirituality

Spirituality, another important component of intrapersonal functioning, has been described as the essence of the self, an intangible core that enables a person to derive meaning and purpose from life (Stoll, 1989). Spirituality involves a sense of who one is and who one is becoming, particularly in relationship with one's self, others, and usually a supreme being, although not necessarily within a particular religious framework. It is important to recognize that religion and spirituality are not interchangeable, although for most people spirituality involves a relationship with a transcendent or personal being. However, a person may be an atheist or nonparticipant in any type of organized religion and still have a very deep spiritual life.

Spirituality is a quality of universal significance that motivates people toward their life goals and aspirations, or self-actualization. Maslow (1970) defines spirituality as "a framework of values, a philosophy of life, a religion or religion-surrogate to live by" (p. 206). A person's spirituality, in effect, transcends the physical and biological self, a "life principle that pervades a person's entire being" (Kim, McFarland, & McLane, 1987).

Highfield and Cason (1983) identify four spiritual needs that reflect spiritual health or distress:

- Need for meaning and purpose of life
- Need to receive love
- Need to give love
- Need for hope and creativity

Examples of healthy behaviors that indicate that each of these needs is being met are outlined in Table 12-3.

Although spirituality transcends the biological and physical self, it is not separate from the other dimensions that make up the whole person. The spiritual self interacts with the physical, biological,

TABLE 12-2
Comparison of Hope and Despair Behaviors

Hope	Despair
Activation	**Hypoactivation**
Feeling vitality, vibrancy	Feeling all excitement, vitality gone
Having energy and drive	Feeling empty, drained, heavy
Feeling inner buoyancy	Being understimulated
Seeming to be more alert and wide awake	Feelings seeming to be dulled
Experiencing everything fully	Feeling tired, sleepy
Feeling interest and involvement	Feeling dead inside
Feeling like singing	Feeling mentally dull
Comfort	**Discomfort**
Having a sense of well-being	Having a lump in one's throat
Feeling harmony and peace within	Sensing loss, deprivation
Feeling free of conflict	Heart seeming to ache
Feeling loose, relaxed	Not being able to smile or laugh
Feeling general release, lessening of tension	Having whole body tense, wound up inside
Feeling safe and secure	Having feeling of being trapped, boxed in
Feeling life is worth living	Being easily irritated, hypersensitive
Feeling optimistic about the future	Feeling under a heavy burden
Moving Toward People	**Moving Away from People**
Having an intense positive relationship with another	Having a sense of unrelatedness
Reaching out	Wanting to withdraw, be alone
Having a sense of being wanted and needed	Lacking involvement
Feeling much respect and interdependence	Not caring about anyone
Wanting to touch, hold, be close	Feeling a certain distance
Sensing empathetic harmony with another	Wanting to crawl into oneself
Competence	**Incompetence**
Feeling strong inside	Feeling that nothing one does is right
Having a sense of sureness	Sensing regret
Feeling taller, stronger, bigger	Feeling vulnerable and totally helpless
Being more confident in oneself	Feeling caught up and overwhelmed
Having a sense of accomplishment, fulfillment	Having no sense of control over situation
Really functioning as a unit	Longing to have things as they were
Being motivated	Feeling unmotivated and afraid to try

Note. From Lange, S.P. (1978). Hope. In C.E. Carlson & B. Blackwell (Eds.)., *Behavioral concepts and nursing intervention* (2nd ed.). Philadelphia: Lippincott, 175.

and cognitive selves in a dynamic, reciprocal process. Spiritual distress may contribute to physical or mental distress, while physical or mental illness may influence spiritual health. Spiritual needs have been shown to be important to people hospitalized for physiological problems (Peterson, 1985). Prayer and trust in God have been identified as important coping strategies among people with chronic health problems (Baldree et al., 1982).

Cognitive Processes

The capacity to think, reason, and communicate with language is a distinguishing hallmark of the human being. Cognitive functioning is highly valued by society, as evidenced by the derogatory terms that are used to label people with cognitive impairment—"stupid," "senile," "idiot," or "im-

becile." Intact cognitive processes are essential to a meaningful and productive life. The ability to orient one's self to the world, to attend to stimuli in the environment, to recall past events, to comprehend and interpret reality, to think logically and rationally, to make competent judgments and decisions, and to use language to communicate with others depends on intact cognitive processes. These processes can be conceptualized on a continuum from logical, coherent thought and rational decision-making to incoherence, disorientation, and memory loss (see Figure 12-2).

Cognition encompasses the mental activities involved in the processes of thinking and reasoning and in the way that thoughts are connected or associated when communicated. Cognition is an intellectual process of knowing and being aware. Cognition is closely connected to and depends on

TABLE 12-3
Spiritual Needs and Healthy Behaviors

Need for Meaning and Purpose in Life	Lives in accordance with own value system.
	Expresses desire to participate in religious or spiritual rituals.
Need to Receive Love	Expresses feelings of being loved by others or God.
	Expresses feelings of forgiveness.
Need to Give Love	Expresses love for others through words and actions.
	Seeks the good and well-being of others.
Need for Hope and Creativity	Sets realistic personal goals.
	Values the inner self more than the physical or biological self.

Note. Adapted from Highfield, M.F., & Cason, C. (1983). Spiritual needs of patients: Are they recognized? *Cancer Nursing, 6,* 188.

perception. The ability to receive, perceive, and interpret sensory information is essential to the other dimensions of cognitive functioning. Cognitive functioning provides the nurse with valuable information relative to a client's overall mental status.

Cognition influences a person's ability to perceive and understand phenomena and events in the environment. How one interprets and copes with life events and interacts with others is influenced to a significant degree by cognitive ability and, therefore, changes over time. Very young children have limited capacity for comprehending, for example, disease or injury in terms of the impact on their daily functioning or future. However, adults who have achieved more complex cognitive ability are able to consider the full range of meaning that an illness, injury, or disability has for them, both now and in the future.

Piaget's theory of cognitive development, discussed in Chapter 10, provides useful knowledge about the development of cognitive abilities throughout life. Table 10-7 outlines cognitive changes that occur as children develop. Table 11-1 delineates cognitive abilities and changes which characterize adult thinking at various life stages.

Thought Processes

Thinking may be stimulated by the need to solve a problem, to analyze a situation, or to perform a task. Regardless of what stimulates it, thinking is a continuous and logical process for most people. Thought processes refer to continuity of thoughts

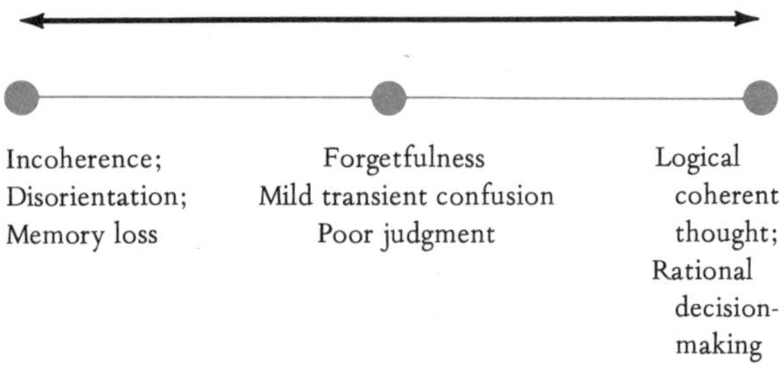

FIGURE 12-2. Continuum of Cognitive Processes. (*Note.* Adapted from Stuart, G.W., & Sundeen, S.J. [1991]. *Principles and Practices of Psychiatric Nursing* [4th ed.]. St. Louis: The C.V. Mosby Co., 571.)

and how they are related to one another. Thought processes include comprehension, memory, attention, reality orientation, and judgment. Disturbances in thought process or content occur when a client's thoughts lose their continuity or logical flow, when thoughts are not tied together in a meaningful way and can be comprehended by others.

Comprehension refers to the capacity for understanding, the ability to grasp information and derive meaning from it. When comprehension is impaired, a client may respond inappropriately or give other cues that understanding is lacking. Variables that may affect comprehension include age, general intelligence, level of education, life experiences, and health.

Attention involves the ability to consciously direct mental energy to a task or activity. Clients with diminished or impaired attention often are distracted easily or exhibit behaviors that suggest disinterest or uninvolvement in a task or conversation.

Memory, another component of cognition, may be short-term or long-term. Short-term or recent memory is the ability to recall information from the immediate past and up to 3 weeks previously. Long-term memory refers to the ability to recall events, places, persons, or things from the distant or remote past. If impairment of memory occurs, recent memory is the first to be influenced. Generally, clients with short-term memory deficits are able to recall only remote meaningful happenings in their lives.

A specific reason for memory failure is damage to the brain. An organic brain insult may be temporary, as in the case of toxic brain syndromes caused by some drugs, or permanent as in the case of irreversible brain damage linked to Alzheimer's disease. A less frequent reason for memory loss is severe depression. In case of severe depression, the client usually experiences temporary or reversible memory impairment.

Reality orientation, another measure of cognitive functioning, refers to one's awareness of and connection to the world. People who are oriented know who they are and are aware of their placement in time and space. Orientation to reality is intimately connected to memory and an ability to project the future. Reality orientation, as well as other aspects of cognitive functioning, varies with the client's maturation, educational level, and life experiences. In general, orientation increases from birth to adulthood, then declines during old age (see chap. 24).

Disorientation results when a person cannot preserve a sense of self in relation to time and the environment. Disorientation may occur in response to a variety of factors, including mind-altering substances (alcohol, certain medications, illicit drugs), social isolation, or neurological disease or trauma (Alzheimer's disease, head injury).

Judgment is a cognitive process of comparing and evaluating facts or cues and their relationships to one another in order to draw appropriate conclusions. The ability to judge, or interpret, sensory information is the basis of all human decision-making and relies on other cognitive processes, such as orientation, attention, and memory. In order to make judgments, or select from alternatives, a person must be oriented to the situation, able to selectively attend to important and valid cues, and refer to stored information (memory) in order to consider all possibilities and their potential consequences.

Language and Literacy

Command of language affects an individual's ability to transmit and receive verbal information. Language requires use of knowledge and the ability to process information in order to communicate with others.

Language serves several purposes. It influences the way events are perceived and enhances memory. Numerous studies have demonstrated that memory for events is increased when language is associated with them. Language also facilitates problem-solving by allowing an individual to represent ideas and alternatives with words, either oral or written. Language is the major tool for human communication.

Language consists of words, which are tools or symbols that represent ideas and feelings or indicate objects. Language development follows a predetermined maturational sequence. However, adequate stimulation from the environment, including appropriate role models, is essential for learning appropriate language skills. In fact, there

is evidence of a critical period (see chap. 10), for acquiring language after which it becomes much more difficult to acquire and use the tools of language.

Language has two major components: receptive and expressive. Receptive language refers to the ability to understand or comprehend spoken words and sentences. Expressive language is the ability to convey thoughts, ideas, and feelings—orally, in writing, or through gestures such as sign language. Receptive language is learned before expressive language. Thus, infants and toddlers are able to comprehend what is being said to them before they can communicate their thoughts to others. Also, people who are learning a foreign language are able to understand the spoken or written word before they can express it themselves. Language barriers between nurse and client may have an adverse effect on nursing assessment and diagnosis, especially the collection and validation of information. An interpreter or at least some assistance in communicating with anyone who speaks a foreign language may be necessary. This is also true for clients who are hearing impaired or who have a neurological deficit that impedes clarity of communication.

A nurse cares for clients from multiple and diverse cultures and social backgrounds. Family and cultural influences on language are many. Clients from lower socioeconomic backgrounds may use simpler grammatical structure. Rate, tone, and dialect of speech vary among geographical locations. Different cultural groups may attribute different meanings to the same words or expressions.

Growing up in a poor learning environment and lacking role models who use language for purposes other than mundane oral communication can have a profound impact on literacy. Only two-thirds of the people in the U.S. are literate (Hirsch, 1987). This means that at least one-third of the population is either unable to read and write or does not have the skills to understand and use printed materials encountered in daily life, such as traffic signs, the newspaper, a job application, or the utility bill. These problems are particularly acute among lower socioeconomic levels and among certain minority groups (Stedman & Kaestle, 1987). For example, 47% of all black 17-year-olds and over one-third of mothers on welfare are functionally illiterate (Kozol, 1985).

The widespread problems of illiteracy have particular implications for the delivery of nursing care. Nurses frequently function as educators, making use of instructional materials in the process. Yet, approximately 50% of clients have serious difficulty with reading or are unable to read instructional materials written at a fifth grade level. (Doak, Doak, & Root, 1985). Many educational materials for clients are written at an inappropriately high level and often contain a significant number of medical terms unfamiliar to clients.

Affect and Mood

Affect is a person's emotional tone. It is subjective and may be communicated behaviorally. Affect is a basic component of human behavior and plays a major part in motivating an individual's interactions with the environment and others. Affect is one aspect of the uniqueness of every individual. It is, for the most part, a stable emotional tone that a person exhibits over time. For example, an individual's affect may be described as "easy-going," "nervous," "flat," or "highly changeable." Mood, on the other hand, is a temporary emotion that usually occurs in response to situational variables. For example, an individual's mood may be exuberant or joyful when a healthy baby is born or despondent over the loss of a job.

Affect and mood are a significant part of the human condition and hence influence clients' psychosocial and physiological functioning. Three common emotions that may influence affect and mood are anxiety, anger, and depression.

Anxiety

Anxiety is a universal human experience that occurs in response to a real or perceived threat. Anxiety is an internal response that cannot be observed directly, but is manifested in a feeling of vague unease. People experiencing anxiety may describe their experience as discomfort, restlessness, uncertainty, or uneasiness. Anxiety leads a person to feel a vague sense of apprehension and dread.

Anxiety is different from fear. Anxiety occurs in response to an ill-defined, intangible threat or conflict. Often the individual is not even aware of exactly what has triggered the response. In contrast, fear is a human response to a known specific threat that lies outside of the person. Anxiety is a much more diffuse response than fear and tends to persist for a much longer period of time. By definition, anxiety and fear are different emotions, although they may occur simultaneously.

Easily recognizable cues of anxiety include tense facial expression, tremors of the extremities, rapid speech, restlessness, palpitations, excessive perspiration, poor concentration, and difficulty solving problems. The physiological and cognitive dimensions of varying degrees of anxiety are presented in Table 12-4.

The ability to focus on what is happening in an anxiety-producing situation is inversely proportionate to the severity of the anxiety: the greater the anxiety, the less the ability to focus. Mild anxiety can be an effective coping mechanism because alertness is increased, whereas a severe or panic level of anxiety inhibits the individual's awareness of what is going on in the immediate surroundings.

As mentioned earlier, anxiety is a subjective response to a real or perceived threat. Since nurses interact with clients who frequently are confronted with health problems that may be perceived as threatening, the presence or absence of anxiety as a human response is of significance.

Anger

Anger is a feeling of intense displeasure directed towards someone or something. Anger results when a person's sense of self-worth is threatened, usually because the person has not been able to reach a goal or has an unmet need. Figure 12-3 illustrates how anger is developed and released.

Anger may be expressed directly or indirectly. Direct and functional expression of anger is difficult for many people because they fear rejection. Fear of expressing anger may be traced to parental disapproval of overt expression of anger during childhood. Some people learn at an early age to "turn the other cheek" or to suppress their anger. However, relief from the buildup of tension from suppressed anger eventually must occur in some manner. For example, an individual may develop a physical illness, such as ulcerative colitis or migraine headaches, or may become depressed or overtly violent. Anger also may be expressed in indirect or passive ways such as humor, sarcasm, gossip, or avoiding the person or stimulus that evokes the anger.

Depression

As a mood state, some degree of depression is experienced by everyone at some time. Some depressions are self-limiting and occur in response to an identifiable life change or crisis, such as failing a test, relocation to a new city, or the death of a loved one. Depression also may be prolonged and not generally associated with a particular life event. It may result from suppression of anger. Typical symptoms of prolonged depression include sleep disorders, self-recriminations, sadness, apathy, decreased activity, and diminished sexual desire.

Depression may manifest itself in one or more of the following areas: affective, cognitive, behavioral, or physical. Affective or emotional responses include feelings of sadness and deriving less plea-

TABLE 12-4
Physical and Psychological Manifestations of Anxiety

	Physical	Psychological
Mild	Increased heart rate Increased respirations Loss of appetite Dilation of pupils Urinary urgency Dryness of mouth Improved visual discrimination Improved auditory discrimination	Increased alertness Restlessness Irritability
Moderate	Increased muscular tension Pounding heart Perspiration Gastric discomfort	Reduced ability to perceive Can attend if directed to do so Selective inattention Talking may not be heard
Severe	Increased symptoms Perceptual field greatly reduced Focus on detail or many scattered details	Unable to observe what is going on even with assistance
Panic	May freeze, unable to function May withdraw physically May paralyze or overwork capabilities	Exclusive focus on event Cannot notice what goes on Behavior of person oriented toward getting immediate relief Automatic behavior not requiring thought used to relieve anxiety.

Note. Adapted from Hays, D.R. Teaching a Concept of Anxiety to Patients, *Nursing Research, 10,* 108 (Spring 1961). Reprinted with permission from American Journal of Nursing Company.

Perceived threat (frustration, unmet expectation, loss of
    self-esteem)

▽

Anxiety is felt

▽

Anxiety is transformed to anger (anger gives a sense of power,
    which results in increased self-esteem, which is a
    stimulus for action)

▽

Anger is expressed

▽

Feel relief (however, if the expression of anger has been
    forbidden, ignored, or ineffective in the past, the
    individual likely will experience guilt or lowered
    self-esteem)

FIGURE 12-3. A Model of Anger. (*Note.* Adapted from McElvain, M.S. [1989]. Suspicious, hostile, and aggressive behavior: The delusional and acting-out behaviors. In B.S. Johnson (Ed.), *Adaptation and growth: Psychiatric mental-health nursing.* Philadelphia: J.B. Lippincott, p. 446.)

sure from life. Crying spells occur frequently. Cognitive manifestations include difficulty with concentration and decision-making and slowing of thought processes. Thoughts of suicide may occur. Behavioral manifestations such as diminished social involvement, excessive dependence, and insomnia may be present. Physical complaints such as amenorrhea, fatigue, loss of appetite, constipation, and various types of somatic complaints, such as headaches or backaches, may occur.

In an attempt to dull or "medicate" the psychic pain caused by depression, some individuals resort to the abuse of alcohol or drugs. Other types of maladaptive responses to the experience of depression include excessive gambling, truancy, promiscuity, and illegitimate pregnancy. These "acting out" behaviors, while self-defeating, often indicate that the individual is struggling against an underlying depression.

Temperament

While affect primarily describes an individual's emotional tone at a particular time or in a particular situation, temperament describes an individual's behavioral style of reacting over time and across situations (Chess & Thomas, 1986). Temperament is primarily an innate attribute, although it may be affected to some extent by interaction with significant others and the social environment.

Buss and Plemin (1975) suggest that temperament has four components:

1. *Level of activity*, or the individual's energy level

2. *Emotionality*, or intensity of the person's reaction

3. *Sociability*, or how the person relates to others

4. *Impulsivity*, the time taken by the person to respond.

For each component of temperament, there is a range of reactions (see Table 12-5). For example, level of activity may range from very active to lethargic. An individual's sociability may be gregarious and outgoing or, at the other extreme, detached and isolated.

Chess and Thomas (1986) pioneered work on temperament in children. They believe that temperament results from an interaction of genetic and environmental factors. Their inductive analysis of data obtained from parent interviews in the New York Longitudinal Study of middle and upper middle class children led to the identification of various temperament styles. These styles are exhibited by infants and children as young as a few weeks. Each style is based upon the infant's or child's behavioral responses in nine categories: activity level, rhythmicity (regularity), adaptability, response to new situations, sensory threshold, intensity of response, quality of mood, distractibility, and persistence and attention span. Each dimension of temperament is described in Table 12-6.

Chess and Thomas (1986) have identified three common patterns of child temperament: "easy child," "difficult child," and "slow-to-warm-up child." Approximately 40% of children are categorized as easy, 10% as difficult, and 15% as slow to

TABLE 12-5
Four Dimensions of Temperament

Dimension	Extremes of the Dimension	Aspect of Behavior
Activity	Active–lethargic	How much
Emotionality	Emotional–impassive	Intensity
Sociability	Gregarious–detached	How close to others (Proximity seeking)
Impulsivity	Impulsive–deliberate	Quickness vs. inhibition of response

Note. From *A Temperament Theory of Personality Development*, by A.H. Buss and R. Plemin. Copyright © 1975 by John Wiley & Sons, Inc., pp. 241–242. Reprinted with permission.

warm up. The temperament variables that characterize each of these styles are shown in Table 12-7. However, it is important to remember that approximately 35% of all children do not exhibit one of these patterns, but instead show varying combinations of the nine temperament variables.

Temperament is a particularly important part of intrapersonal functioning for children, as it shapes the child's responses to the environment and thus may have a profound impact on the child's developmental experiences. The child's receptivity to new experiences, ability to attend to stimuli in the environment, and initiation or avoidance of new experiences are examples of how temperament may affect development.

One of the critical aspects of temperament is the "goodness of fit" between an individual's temperament and the expectations and demands of the environment (Carey, 1990). When a child's behavioral style, capacities, and motivations are consistent with the expectations and demands of the environmental context, such as the parents' own temperament styles and expectations or demands imposed by the school or day care environment, then a good fit exists between the child and the environment. In such instances, developmental and health outcomes are likely to be positive (Carey, 1990). Conversely, a poor fit between the child and the environmental demands and expectations may compromise the child's development and well-being (Carey, 1990).

Carey (1986) describes "temperament assets" as those characteristics that promote a positive fit between the child and the environment, whereas "temperament risk factors" are those that predispose a child to a "poor fit," and consequently to stress, conflict, and developmental problems. For example, a child with a high activity level and high distractibility may fit poorly in a school that requires children to sit still at their desks engaged in quiet learning activities for long periods of time.

KNOWLEDGE NEEDED TO ASSESS INTERPERSONAL FUNCTIONING

A major part of any individual's life relates to interactions with and reactions to other people. Consequently, nurses should be knowledgeable of certain concepts that relate to interpersonal functioning. These concepts include social roles, stress, and coping.

Social Roles

A social role is a set of behaviors expected of a person in a given position or social situation in life. Roles usually involve expectations held by others

TABLE 12-6
Childhood Temperament Variables

I. *Activity level*—the amount of physical activity during sleep, feeding, play, dressing, etc.
(1) high   (2) medium   (3) low

II. *Regularity*—of bodily functioning in sleep, hunger, bowel movements, etc.
(1) fairly regular   (2) variable
(3) fairly irregular

III. *Adaptability to change in routine*—the ease or difficulty with which initial response can be modified in socially desirable way.
(1) generally   (2) variable
adaptable   (3) generally slow at adaptation

IV. *Response to new situations*—initial reaction to new stimuli, to food, people, places, toys, or procedures:
(1) approach   (2) variable
(3) withdrawal

V. *Level of sensory threshold*—the amount of external stimulation, such as sounds or changes in food or people, necessary to produce a response.
(1) high threshold (much stimulation needed)

(2) medium
(3) low threshold (little stimulation)

VI. *Intensity of response*—the energy content of responses regardless of their quality.
(1) generally intense   (2) variable
(3) generally mild

VII. *Positive or negative mood*—amount of pleasant or unpleasant behavior throughout day.
(1) generally positive   (2) variable
(3) generally negative

VIII. *Distractibility*—the effectiveness of external stimuli (sounds, toys, people, etc.) in interfering with ongoing behavior.
(1) easily distractible   (2) variable
(3) non-distractible

IX. *Persistence and attention span*—duration of maintaining specific activities with or without external obstacles.
(1) persistent   (2) variable
(3) not persistent

Note. Adapted from "Revision of the Infant Temperament Questionnaire," by W.B. Carey and S.C. McDevitt, *Pediatrics*, 1978, 61:735–739. Copyright American Academy of Pediatrics 1978.

about what behaviors are appropriate for a given situation and those that are not. Everyone occupies numerous roles in life (e.g., adult, spouse, parent, professional nurse, church member, soccer coach, friend). The various roles that a person assumes influence behavior and shape much of human interaction.

Individuals may have ascribed (assigned) or achieved (acquired) roles. Ascribed roles are roles assigned by virtue of a position associated with birth, marriage, gender, family structure, religious affiliation, or cultural group. Ascribed roles include daughter, sister, wife, parent, Catholic, Mexican-American, or head of the household. Sex roles (boy, girl, man, woman) are assigned roles and reflect those expectations society holds for its male and female members (see chap. 13). Age also determines certain assigned roles. Examples of age-determined roles are parent, child, teenager, and senior citizen. With aging there may be involuntary constriction of social roles owing to retirement (see chap. 11). Groups to which an individual belongs also contribute to how that individual is expected to act in a particular role. For example, certain behavioral expectations exist for people who are "poor," "middle class," "yuppies," "migrants," or "southern Baptists." Marital status (single, married, divorced, widowed) also is considered an assigned role.

Achieved roles refer to roles acquired through education, acquisition of resources, appointment, election, or promotion and include such occupa-

TABLE 12-7
Three Common Temperament Styles

Patterns (% of Children)	Temperament Variables				
	Rhythmicity	Approach/Withdrawal	Adaptability	Intensity	Mood
Easy (40%)	High	Approach	High	Low	Positive
Difficult (10%)	Low	Withdrawal	Low	High	Negative
Slow to warm up (15%)	Moderate	Withdrawal	Low	Low	Negative

Note. From Chess, S., & Thomas, A. (1986). *Temperament in clinical practice.* New York: Guilford Press.

tional and social status roles as teacher, fourth grade student, attorney, laborer, community leader, senator, or country club member. Society has certain expectations of individuals who occupy each of these roles. Generally, the more status afforded the role, the greater the expectations are.

While the expected behaviors of a particular role are defined or enforced by society, an individual may modify them according to what he or she has learned from role models and the person's basic personality. Role modification and refinement lead to the actual performance of a given role. There may be great variability within particular roles. For example, the role of college student includes certain expectations—preparation for and attendance at class, participation in class discussions, satisfactory performance on examinations or written projects, and involvement in extracurricular activities. The range of behaviors exhibited in this role, however, varies widely.

Unfortunately, role-typing may lead to stereotyping. A nurse may hold stereotypical beliefs about particular roles and expect the client to conform. Stereotyping can color the nurse's perceptions of the client and interpretation of the client's behaviors and thus interfere with an accurate nursing assessment.

Individuals often meet the expectations of many roles simultaneously. This can be manageable and quite rewarding when things are running smoothly. However, there are times when role problems occur. Three types of role-related problems are role conflict, role ambiguity, and role strain.

Role conflict usually occurs when a person perceives that the expectations for one role are incompatible with the expectations for another role or when the person's values or beliefs are at odds with role expectations. For example, a teenage father may reject his parental role in favor of spending time with the guys. Another type of role conflict may occur when two or more expectations within a single role are incongruent. For example, a school principal may be faced with the superintendent's expectation that the school operate on a very limited budget and that class sizes increase, while he and the school's teachers, or parents, may believe that class sizes should be reduced. The varying expectations that others have about a particular role can lead to role conflict. Regardless of the type of role conflict, the central concern is role performance expectations that are incompatible and that conflict with each other.

A second type of role problem is role ambiguity. *Role ambiguity* refers to unclear role expectations

and therefore uncertainty in knowing whether one is meeting role expectations. Role ambiguity contributes to feelings of insecurity and at times confusion. An example of role ambiguity is the expectation that professional nurses be assertive, efficient, and independent, and yet acquiesce to the rules and constraints on role performance imposed by hospital bureaucracies.

Role strain indicates that a person may be experiencing role conflict and role ambiguity. Role strain may be expressed as anxiety, worry, frustration, or guilt over a perceived inability to meet role demands or expectations. Also, people experience role changes, whether they assume a new role, shift from one role to another, or experience role loss. Role strain may occur as they try to adapt to role changes. Examples of role changes include adolescence, marriage, parenthood, retirement, job promotion, loss of employment, and change in family roles, such as the birth of a third baby changing the status of the "youngest" to "middle" child.

Stressors and Stress Responses

Stress may be defined as general wear and tear on the body. Stress is an intangible that may be identified indirectly by observing or measuring certain behaviors. Stress is normally present in all individuals and is essential for life and growth. When energy expenditure and energy consumption are balanced, stress is barely perceptible; the individual is unaware of it. This is known as the steady state, or *homeostasis*. Stress is a neutral term, whereas distress indicates a disturbance in the steady state. A stressor is a factor or agent that causes intensification of the stress state.

Stressors may emanate from three sources: internal processes, the physical environment, and the psychosocial milieu. Internal stressors are those related to physiological functioning of the body, such as increased intracranial pressure or hunger. Factors such as the weather and environmental conditions are stressors in the physical environment: extremes of temperature, noise, and air pollution. Of course, internal stressors may be influenced by external factors and vice versa. Genetic, maturational, and perceptual factors also influence the effects of stressors on individuals.

Psychosocial factors that may cause stress include social position, change, conflict, and occupational roles and responsibilities. In a study that examined the influence of stress and social support on expectant mothers' and fathers' health, Brown (1986) concluded that nursing interventions to reduce stress and improve expectant parents' satisfaction with support received from the partner may enhance health.

Psychosocial stressors also elicit physiological responses, and both psychosocial and physiological responses are influenced by a person's perception of the event. In other words, some people may perceive a change in job status or residence as immensely stressful, whereas others may not. Thus, it is the perception or interpretation of a stressor that determines a person's response to it, rather than the stressor itself.

The stress response, as described by Selye (1956), occurs in three stages. The first stage is the alarm reaction. This is a general alert to the body's defenses and prepares the individual for "fight or flight." During the second phase, resistance, the response attempts to limit the effects of stressors. Adaptation may or may not occur in this stage. Attempts to cope with stressors include altering individual behavioral patterns or modifying the environment. During the third phase, exhaustion, adaptation is no longer occurring. The individual has been unable to deal with the stressors imposed. Also, the internal and external resources usually needed to restore adaptive capacity are no longer operating. Without assistance from others or technology (e.g., surgery, medications), death can result.

Physiological alterations that occur with stress may provide the nurse with information about the stress response of clients. These physiological changes are governed by the autonomic nervous system. Table 12-8 presents examples of physiological responses to stress.

Adaptation to stress involves physiological, psychological, sociocultural, spiritual, and developmental factors. All adaptive responses to stress are attempts to maintain homeostasis. However, adaptive mechanisms have limitations and operate within the genetic potential of the individual. Adaptability also varies from individual to individual.

To anticipate or predict behaviors that may occur in response to a stressor, the nurse must consider the client's adaptive capacity (response to stressors). Variables that influence an individual's ability to adapt to stress include: (1) the nature of the stressor itself, (2) the number of stressors an individual must cope with simultaneously, (3) how long the stressor lasts, and (4) the person's previous experiences with similar stressors. A highly stressful event that is short-lived often is better tolerated than a long-term stressful event that requires continuous adaptive behaviors.

TABLE 12-8
Behavioral Manifestations of Stress

Dilated pupils
Skin pallor, clammy palms
Dry mouth
Rapid pulse
Elevated blood pressure
Increased rate and depth of respirations (use of abdominal muscles)
Anorexia
Inability to void or defecate
Muscle tension
Increased observational powers

Note. The above manifestations are the result of stimulation of the sympathetic division of the autonomic nervous system. Because of the proximity of sympathetic and parasympathetic nerve fibers, however, parts of the parasympathetic division are sometimes stimulated in response to perceived threats. When this happens, some manifestations that are the opposite of those listed above may occur (e.g., incontinence, pupil constriction, flushing, increased salivation, nausea and vomiting, bradycardia, dizziness, intellectual disorientation).

Other variables that influence a client's ability to adapt to stress include the client's developmental level, cultural beliefs and values, spirituality, and health. For example, a person who is healthy generally adapts more easily to a stressful situation than one whose adaptive capacity is low because of illness.

Coping Responses

A person's responses to a particular situation or stressor are determined by the situation or stressor itself as well as the social context in which it occurs. When confronted with stressors, people exhibit a variety of coping strategies. Efforts to cope may be cognitive, emotional, or physical. An example of a cognitive response is to think about the situation and consider alternative explanations and ways of resolving the stressor. Yelling, crying, drinking alcohol, or resigning one's self to the situation are examples of emotional responses. Physical coping responses include exercise or sleeping.

Regardless of whether the person's coping responses are cognitive, emotional, or physical, their responses may be constructive or destructive (Stuart & Sundeen, 1987). Constructive coping mechanisms are those that permit the person to recognize the response to a stressor as a warning that something is wrong. The person welcomes the warning as a challenge and an opportunity to clarify and resolve the underlying problem or conflict. Destructive coping mechanisms, on the other hand, protect the person from acknowledging the underlying problem or conflict and thus do not lead to resolution. In fact, destructive coping mechanisms may themselves become a source of stress because they command a high level of emotional energy to maintain.

Jaloweic and Powers (1981) categorize coping mechanisms as "problem-oriented" and "affective-oriented." Problem-oriented strategies are ways of coping with stressors that deal with the stressor or situation itself, whereas affective-oriented strategies focus on dealing with the emotions evoked by the stressor or situation (see Table 12-9 for examples). Jaloweic and Powers (1981) propose that a balance between problem-solving and affective strategies probably is most effective in promoting constructive coping.

Walker (1988) proposes a beginning taxonomy of coping based on her work with siblings of child-hood cancer patients (see Table 12-10). However, she cautions that it can be difficult to classify a particular coping strategy because coping responses are contextually bound and vary from situation to situation.

While it may appear that coping responses are readily observable and the person is aware of using various coping strategies, people often employ unconscious defense mechanisms to cope with their emotional responses to stressors.

Defense mechanisms are mental mechanisms that help people deal with stress and anxiety. Defense mechanisms protect people from perceived threats and thus help them feel more secure. Defenses act to block out or divert people from the unpleasant or anxiety-invoking elements of a situation.

Defense mechanisms may be appropriately or

TABLE 12-9
Coping Strategies

Affective-Oriented Coping Strategies	Problem-Oriented Coping Strategies
Hope that things will get better	Try to maintain some control over the situation
Eat; smoke; chew gum	Find out more about the situation
Pray; trust in God	Think through different ways to handle the situation
Get nervous	Look at the problem objectively
Worry	Try out different ways of solving the problem to see which works best
Seek comfort or help from friends or family	Draw on past experience to help you handle the situation
Want to be alone	Try to find meaning in the situation
Laugh it off, figuring that things could be worse	Break the problem down into "smaller pieces"
Try to put the problem out of your mind	Set specific goals to help solve the problem
Daydream, fantasize	Accept the situation as it is
Get prepared to expect the worst	Talk the problem over with someone who has been in the same type of situation
Get mad; curse; swear	Actively try to change the situation
Go to sleep, figuring things will look better in the morning	Settle for the next best thing
Don't worry about it, everything will probably work out fine	Do anything just to do something
Withdraw from the situation	Let someone else solve the problem
Work off tension with physical activity	
Take out your tensions on someone or something else	
Drink alcoholic beverages	
Resign yourself to the situation because things look hopeless	
Do nothing in the hope that the problem will take care of itself	
Resign yourself to the situation because it's your fate	
Blame someone else for your problems	
Meditation, yoga, biofeedback	
Take drugs	

Note. From Jalowiec, A., and Powers, M.J. Stress and Coping in Hypertensive and Emergency Room Patients. *Nursing Research, 30*: 13. (January–February 1981). Reprinted with permission, American Journal of Nursing Company.

TABLE 12-10
Beginning Taxonomy of Coping

Domain	Theme	Category
Cognitive		
1. Intrapsychic	A. Deliberate	1. Thought stopping
		2. Emotional expression
		3. Convince self
		4. Empathy
		5. Hope enhancement
		6. Wishful thinking
		7. Submit/endure
	B. Subconscious	1. Avoidance/denial
		2. Regression
2. Interpersonal	A. Support	1. Talking to others (family, peers, other cancer siblings, professionals)
		2. Being with others
	B. Substitute	1. Lost relationship
3. Intellectual	A. Seek information	1. Hospital program
		2. Media (books, films)
		3. School project
		4. Parents' teachings
	B. Process information	1. Analyze/learn
		2. Remedy
Behavioral		
1. Self-focusing	A. Attention seeking	1. Somatization
		2. Being nice
		3. Joining in
		4. Acting out
		5. Accidents
	B. Self-soothing activities	1. Repetitive actions
		2. Eating
2. Distraction	A. Solitary	1. Play alone
		2. Music
	B. Group activities	1. Quiet activities
		2. Strenuous activities
3. Exclusion	A. Time out	1. Special place
	B. Escape	1. From family contact
		2. From social contact
		3. Temporary escape

Note. From Walker, C.L. Stress and coping in siblings of childhood cancer patients. Copyright 1988 American Journal of Nursing Company. Reprinted from *Nursing Research*, 1988, 37(4), 208–212. Used with permission. All rights reserved.

inappropriately used, and if overused may prevent the individual from resolving intrapersonal or interpersonal conflicts. Individuals can use adaptive defense mechanisms in healthy, positive ways to increase their abilities to cope with life. If, however, defense mechanisms become a patterned way of eluding problems and conflicts, persons eventually will be overwhelmed by unresolved anxieties and compromise their intrapersonal resources for dealing with their problems.

Adaptive or constructive uses of defense mechanisms include the temporary avoidance of solving emotional conflicts and channeling unresolved, so-cially inappropriate behavior into socially acceptable behavior. Other mature defense mechanisms include humor, altruism, and sublimination. Maladaptive or destructive defense mechanisms include extreme or prolonged denial, repression, aggression, and passive-aggressive behavior, all of which permit the person to avoid confronting uncomfortable or painful situations.

Defense mechanisms serve five major functions. They help an individual:

1. Postpone dealing with the root of a conflict,
2. Hide true feelings, fears, and conflicts,

3. Reduce anxious feelings,

4. Release strong emotions in a socially acceptable manner,

5. Change unacceptable behavior into an acceptable form.

Defense mechanisms relieve conflict and become more sophisticated with experience. As defense mechanisms are learned, they become ingrained and soon operate without conscious awareness. A pattern is established by repeated actions or responses and when used with regularity, strongly influences the person's entire personality.

People use many defense mechanisms in their daily lives. The most common are described in Table 12-11.

THE NURSING HISTORY AND CLINICAL APPRAISAL

Because of the nature of intrapersonal and interpersonal functioning, most of the information needed to assess this dimension of human behavior is obtained from interview and observation. The clinical appraisal of a client's current psychosocial status typically occurs during the nursing history interview. As the nurse gathers information, the client's verbal and behavioral responses are assessed concurrently. The nurse may, when indicated, also choose to use certain tools to supplement or validate information obtained from the nursing history interview and clinical appraisal.

The scope of the intrapersonal and interpersonal assessment varies with each client and depends on the nature of the nurse–client relationship, the purpose of the contact, the interview environment (whether it affords sufficient privacy), and the client's age, cultural background, health, behavioral style, and willingness to disclose certain information.

When assessing intrapersonal and interpersonal functioning, the history and clinical appraisal often overlap. In fact, clinical appraisal of the client's psychosocial status occurs throughout the nursing history interview and during the clinical

TABLE 12-11
Defense Mechanisms

Defense Mechanism	Purpose	Example
Denial	Helps keep intolerable thoughts, feelings, wishes, needs, and experiences in unconscious mind.	A postcoronary bypass client ignores prescribed treatment regimen and continues with presurgical lifestyle activities.
Projection	Helps avoid unpleasant emotions by attributing them to others.	A student fails a course and blames the instructor.
Repression	Helps provide a forgetting type of process whereby unpleasant thoughts, feelings, urges, and memories are kept in the unconscious mind.	A soldier, seeing his best friend killed in combat, becomes amnesic about the details of the experience.
Regression	Allows for a return to a time earlier in development when dependence and nurturance provided comfort.	A teenager ends a relationship with her boyfriend and stays home from school to be cared for by her mother.
Displacement	Helps the person release feelings evoked by one object or person by expressing them to a less threatening object or person.	A man is angry at his boss and goes home and yells at his family.
Rationalization	Helps justify behavior in a plausible yet invalid way.	A mother punishes her child severely and unjustly and justifies her feelings of guilt by saying that he deserves it for all the other times that he was naughty.
Undoing	Allows for the relief of feelings of guilt.	A woman yells at and talks to her neighbor very disrespectfully and two days later sends her a bouquet of roses.
Sublimation	Helps channel instinctive or unacceptable psychic energy into socially acceptable activities.	A high school teacher is sexually attracted to several of his female students and writes poems about the vibrancy, innocence, and naivete of female youth.
Identification	Helps diminish focus on personal inadequacies by imitating the behavior of another person.	A student nurse imitates the empathic behaviors of one of her instructors.

appraisal of physiological functioning and thus is not conducted separately from other portions of the nursing assessment.

Conversing with and observing a client during the nursing history and clinical appraisal provides a wealth of information related to the client's behavioral style, thought processes, self-concept, language ability, and interpersonal skills. Such information helps the nurse make clinical judgments about the extent to which additional psychosocial information is needed.

The psychosocial assessment covers many areas that people usually consider private and personal. Communicating a genuine sense of interest and concern as well as respect for the client is critical for facilitating the client's disclosure of what is often sensitive or very personal information. Clients who perceive that the nurse accepts them and is not making value judgments about the information they choose to share are much more likely to feel safe in the relationship and disclose information. Unnecessary probing, treating clients' concerns lightly, or responding in a judgmental way can inhibit open communication and trust between client and nurse and thereby compromise the validity, reliability, and completeness of psychosocial assessment information.

Table 12-12 outlines the parameters of the intrapersonal and interpersonal nursing history. The nurse should incorporate all these parameters to some extent, although the depth of information obtained will vary, depending on each client's situation.

The major goal of the intrapersonal and interpersonal portion of the nursing history is to reveal a historical and current perspective of the client's psychosocial functioning. Historical information is a background against which current functioning may be compared and future functioning anticipated or predicted. For example, if a client's marital status is divorced or widowed, the nurse should ascertain when the client became divorced or widowed and how this role change affected the client's life. The client's response provides important clues about the meaning of this event, how the client coped with the loss, and how the client might be expected to cope with future role changes.

It is very important to observe the client's response and behaviors as intrapersonal and interpersonal assessment information is revealed. How does the client describe significant events (language, affect, mood)? Is there congruence between the client's affect and thoughts? Are the client's thoughts expressed clearly and logically? Does the client seem capable of emotional intimacy with significant others? Does the client exhibit positive self-

TABLE 12-12
The Intrapersonal/Interpersonal Nursing History

Intrapersonal
Perceptions of current life situation and personal health
Self-concept: body image development and concerns; changes in body image; self-ideal; self-esteem (perception of self-worth)
Motivation: ability to meet basic needs; future goals and aspirations; spirituality—what gives meaning and hope to client's life
Cognitive processes: educational level; level of cognitive development; thought processes (comprehension, coherence, attention, memory, reality orientation, judgment)
Language: ability to understand and express thoughts, ideas, and feelings; primary language, other languages (foreign, signing); special dialects or accents that interfere with clarity of communication; ability to read and write (what grade level)
Affect and mood: usual feeling; occurrences of anxiety, anger, depression (in response to what? how managed?)
Temperament: intensity of responses, energy level, sociability, impulsivity

Interpersonal
Social roles: ascribed roles, achieved roles; role conflict, role strain, role ambiguity
Interpersonal relationships (family, friends, colleagues/peers); ability to get along with others; social activities (type, frequency)
Recent stressors (life changes, illness, etc.)
Coping responses (cognitive, emotional, physical); defense mechanisms

esteem? What coping patterns are evident (support from family and friends? religious or spiritual affiliation? use of alcohol, tobacco, or drugs?)

A client's behaviors and characteristics, such as body language, eye contact, dress, grooming, responsiveness, sociability, affect, and temperament, should be observed carefully throughout the nursing assessment. When recording the intrapersonal and interpersonal assessment, the nurse should describe objectively observations of the client's intrapersonal and interpersonal behavior. For example:

> Dressed in clean, casual clothes; well-groomed; responds to questions in a quiet monotone with eyes cast downward; sits with shoulders slumped; moves slowly and deliberately; flat affect.

Generally, the nursing history and observation of the client's behavioral responses throughout the nursing assessment provide sufficient information for evaluating intrapersonal and interpersonal functioning. However, when the nursing history or clinical observations suggest a potential or obvious problem, the nurse may wish to supplement the information by administering a more in-depth questionnaire or other tool.

Perception/Self-Concept

During the nursing history, the nurse should attempt to ascertain clients' perceptions of self, how they get along in life, and their relationships with others. Using therapeutic techniques, the nurse will be able to ascertain perceptions that relate to the client's sense of well-being and health. Actively listening to the client's verbal and nonverbal messages gives cues about which of the client's perceptions need to be explored in greater depth. The nurse can use those messages to explore further the client's perceptions of particular events. "Earlier in our conversation, I noticed that you looked away when you mentioned your last experience with labor and delivery," the nurse might say. "Tell me some more about what that experience was like for you." Or "As I listen to you, I get the impression that you're feeling pressure to make a decision . . . where's that coming from?" or "What about your past do you view as being to blame for your present situation?"

The above examples illustrate that areas to be assessed about a client's perception are unique to each client. Assessment of perception is highlighted here to emphasize that the nurse must respond to each client's personality and situation. In actual practice, assessment of perception usually occurs in tandem with assessment of other psychosocial dimensions, particularly self-concept.

Interview questions that help assess a client's

self-esteem and self-concept are presented in Table 12-13. Included are questions the nurse can ask parents in order to gather subjective information about a child's self-esteem and self-concept. A child's teacher also may be an important source of information for school-age children, particularly if there is concern about the child getting along in school or if the child is exhibiting withdrawn or depressed behaviors.

The client's interactions with others, nonverbal behaviors, and general appearance give the nurse information for formulating impressions about the client's self-concept. For instance:

Is the client's physical appearance neat or disheveled?

Does the client establish eye contact readily or avert eyes downward when answering questions? (See chapters 2 and 8 for cultural considerations.)

Does the client initiate or seek interactions with others or avoid social contact?

If the client is a child, does he or she eagerly share activities and information about himself or herself?

These behaviors may provide clues to the client's self-concept, although the nurse's impressions should be validated directly with the client.

Questions related to the client's body image and understanding of body parts and functions may be incorporated in the nursing interview. Table 12-13 (questions 4 and 6) offers sample items that may be asked to assess a client's body image and

---

TABLE 12-13
Interview Questions to Assess Self-Concept

1. Describe yourself, using "I" statements. What do you like most about yourself? What would you like to change about yourself? What do others like most about you? What would others like to change about you?

2. Who are the most important people in your life? With whom do you share your feelings, hopes, disappointments? Are these people available to you now?

3. What personal achievements have given you the most satisfaction? What plans and hopes do you have for the future?

4. What do you like most about your body? What would you like to change? What parts of your body are most important to you? Why?

5. What situations make you feel calm and secure? What situations made you feel uncomfortable and anxious?

6. (For a client with an alteration in health or lifestyle). How has (illness, surgery, injury, pregnancy) changed the way you feel about yourself? How has it changed the way others feel about you (respond to you)?

Children (interview questions for parents)

1. What words describe your child? What do you like most about your child? What do you wish were different about your child?

2. How does your child get along with other children? With adults?

Note. Adapted from Bellack, J.P. (1981). Self-concept. *Clinical nursing concepts series* (videotape), Lexington: University of Kentucky College of Nursing.

body schema. Also, for the client undergoing diagnostic testing or surgery, or for the client who has experienced an alteration in body appearance or function, it is important to ascertain the client's understanding of changes in body parts or function and the effects on the client's self-concept and lifestyle.

Because children often do not respond well to direct questioning, projective techniques such as drawings generally are more useful for assessing their understanding of body image and potential body image disturbances. For example, children can be given an outline of a child's body and asked to draw and identify body parts (see Figure 12-4). This technique works well with most children over the age of 4 or 5. This type of drawing allows the nurse to identify any misconceptions children may have about their bodies or to note distortions.

A child also can be given paper, pencil, and crayons and asked to draw a self-portrait. Figure 12-5 shows self-portraits of children of different ages. Missing parts or severely distorted drawings may indicate a disturbance in body image.

A number of scales have been developed for assessing self-concept. These tools include some items that reflect self-esteem. The Tennessee Self-Concept Scale (Fitts, 1965) is designed for individuals who have at least a sixth grade reading level. The Piers-Harris Children's Self-Concept Scale (*The Way I Feel About Myself*, Piers & Harris, 1969) is designed for school-age children and is administered and scored easily. Sample items from the Piers-Harris scale are shown in Table 12-14.

Motivation

A client's motivation can be assessed throughout the nursing history interview using the hierarchy of human needs (Figure 12-1) as a guide. For example, the degree to which a client's basic physiological needs are met will be determined during the physiological and sexuality assessments, as well as during assessment of the client's environment. Ascertaining the client's family relationships, roles, friendships, and social activities allows the nurse to assess the client's motivation for meeting love and belonging needs. The client's values, beliefs, and life goals provide clues to self-actualization needs and the client's attempts to meet them.

Hope may be inferred from the client's expression of thoughts and feelings. Do the client's thoughts and feelings reveal a positive, hopeful outlook on life or one of despair? Assessment of hope includes determining the client's orientation toward the future: Does the client have future goals

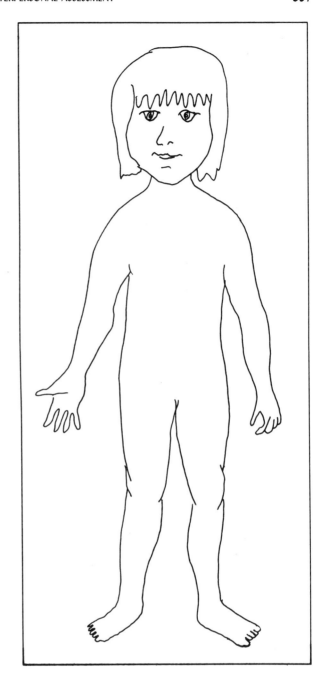

FIGURE 12-4. Body Outline for Drawing Internal Body Parts.

or aspirations? Regardless of the client's level of certainty about health prognosis, does the client anticipate an improved state or relief from the current stress? Anticipation of an improved state or relief from the current stress may indicate a future orientation that relates to life or death.

Another way the nurse can assess hope is by asking the client to fill out a questionnaire. The Miller Hope Scale (Miller & Powers, 1988) is a 40-item Likert scale from "strongly agree" to

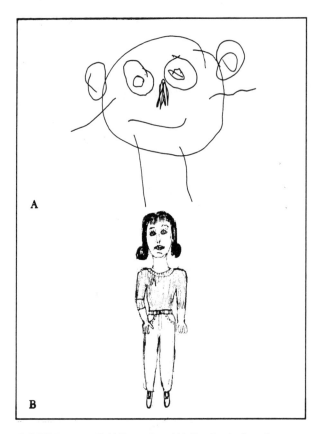

FIGURE 12-5. Self-Portraits. (A) Braden's drawing, age 3. (B) Kristen's drawing, age 10.

delineates observations to be made when assessing spirituality.

Cognitive Processes

Listening to and observing the client's responses during the entire assessment process provide many clues about the client's cognitive functioning. In some instances, the nurse may determine that detailed focus on the specific parameters of cognitive assessment is not necessary. For instance, as the client shares information during the nursing history interview, the nurse may note that the client exhibits logical thinking, sound judgment, and no impairment in memory or orientation. However, there may be times when a more thorough approach to assessing cognition is warranted.

A client's thought processes can be assessed during any verbal exchange with a client. Are the client's thoughts (statements) logical, coherent, and easily understood? Or are they disjointed and difficult to derive meaning from? To assess thought content, the nurse listens to the major topics the client discusses while also attending to major themes in the latent messages communicated by the client. The nurse may also ask, for example, "What kinds of things do you usually think about in a typical day?" The client's response to such a question should indicate whether the client is preoccupied with any particular thought.

Information relative to the client's memory also may be obtained by direct questioning. For example, if the nurse knows the answer to such a question, the client could be asked to recall the menu selections at the most recent meal. Or, the nurse may ask the client to repeat a series of 5 to 7 single numbers. The nurse should say the numbers aloud—"Nine, four, seven, one, five, three, two"—and ask the client to repeat them. Long-term memory may be assessed by asking the client to identify the names of schools attended or to sequentially name the U.S. presidents since World War II.

To assess comprehension, the nurse can ask the client to follow such simple commands as,

"strongly disagree." Examples of statements on the scale are: "I look forward to an enjoyable future" and "I feel trapped, pinned down." The Herth Hope Scale (Herth, 1990) is a 30-item scale that has been used with diverse populations.

Assessment of spirituality far exceeds asking the client to identify a specific religious preference or degree of involvement in religious practices, customs, and rituals. Table 12-15 outlines areas, with sample questions, to be covered in a spirituality interview. Observations of the client's verbal and nonverbal behavior, interactions with others, and the client's personal environment can yield helpful clues to the client's spiritual life. Table 12-16

TABLE 12-14
The Piers-Harris Children's Self-Concept Scale—Sample Items

I am a happy person.	Yes	No	I am often sad.	Yes	No
I am smart.	Yes	No	It's hard for me to make friends.	Yes	No
My looks bother me.	Yes	No	I worry a lot.	Yes	No
I am well-behaved in school.	Yes	No	I do many bad things.	Yes	No
I have good ideas.	Yes	No	I am an important member of my family.	Yes	No
I am shy.	Yes	No	I give up easily.	Yes	No

Note. From Piers, E.V., & Harris, D.B. *The Piers-Harris Children's Self Concept Scale.* Nashville: Counselor Recording and Tests, 1969. Reprinted by permission of Western Psychological Services, 12031 Wilshire Blvd., Los Angeles, CA 90025.

TABLE 12-15
Areas to Be Covered in a Spirituality Interview

Concept of God	1. Is religion or God important to you? If so, can you describe how?
	2. Do you use prayer in your life? If so, does prayer benefit you in any way?
	3. Do you believe God or a deity is involved in your personal life? If so, how?
	4. What is your God or deity like?
Sources of Strength and Hope	1. Who are your support people?
	2. Who is the most important person in your life?
	3. Are people available to you when you are in need?
	4. Who or what provides you with strength and hope?
Religious Practices	1. Is your religious faith helpful to you?
	2. Are there any religious practices that are meaningful to you?
	3. Has your illness affected your religious practices?
	4. Are there any religious books or symbols that are helpful to you?

Note. Adapted from Stoll R., (1979). Guidelines for a spiritual assessment. *American Journal of Nursing, 79,* 1574–1577.

"Close the door," "Sit in this chair," or "Pick up the pencil." Comprehension also can be assessed during clinical appraisal of the sensory–perceptual system (see chap. 15). The client's response or need for additional direction or clarification should be noted. When assessing the client's concentration, the nurse should note the client's intensity in dealing with a task. Is the client able to concentrate or easily distracted? Does the client seem so absorbed in a task that all else is blocked out, or is the client's attention diverted easily to other stimuli?

When assessing reality orientation, the nurse should listen to the client's expressed thoughts and behavior for consistency with reality. Do the client's actions and words reflect an awareness of the present situation? The nurse also should assess the client's orientation to time ("What is today's date?" "What year is this?"), place ("Where are we right now?" "Where do you live?"), and people ("What is your name?" "Who am I?"). Assessment of orientation and level of consciousness is detailed in Chapter 15.

Two useful guides for assessing the cognition of adults and children are presented here. Figure 12-6 presents a diagnostic interview schedule developed by Savitz and Friedman (1981). This

TABLE 12-16
Observations to Be Made in a Spirituality Assessment

Nonverbal behavior	1. Observe affect. Does the client's affect or attitude convey loneliness, depression, anger, agitation, or anxiety?
	2. Observe behavior. Does the client pray during the day? Does the client rely on religious reading material or other literature for solace?
Verbal behavior	1. Does the client seem to complain out of proportion to [the] illness?
	2. Does the client complain of sleeping difficulties?
	3. Does the client ask for unusually high doses of sedation or pain medication?
	4. Does the client refer to God in any way?
	5. Does the client talk about prayer, faith, hope, or anything of a religious nature?
	6. Does the client talk about church functions that are a part of his [or her] life?
	7. Does the client express concern over the meaning and direction of life? Does the client express concern over the impact of the illness on the meaning of life?
Interpersonal relationships	1. Does the client have visitors or does he [or she] spend visiting hours alone?
	2. Are the visitors supportive or do they seem to leave the client feeling upset?
	3. Does the client have visitors from his [or her] church?
	4. Does the client interact with the staff and other clients?
Environment	1. Does the client have a Bible or other religious reading material with him [or her]?
	2. Does the client wear religious medals or pins?
	3. Does the client use religious articles such as statues in observing religious practices?
	4. Has the client received religious get-well cards?
	5. Does the client use personal pictures, artwork, or music to keep his [or her] spirits up?

Note. From Carson, V.B. (1989). *Spiritual dimensions of nursing practice.* Philadelphia: W.B. Saunders, 158.

QUESTION 1 WHY ARE YOU HERE?

1. Adaptive Responses

The persons admit they came because they have a problem. They are able to identify the situation that troubles them and the aspects of the situation that are causing them a problem. In describing the problem, the individuals are able to describe their feeling toward the various people in the situation as well as the behaviors that need to be changed to alleviate the problem. For example, a person might say, "We have a new baby, my husband is gone all day, and I stay in every minute. I love my baby, but I need to make arrangements to get out of the house a couple of times a week."

2. Maladaptive Responses

A. Responses of bored individuals

Bored individuals indicate that they came for help on their own initiative. They display a keen awareness that they have a problem. They indicate that they are emotionally upset and express a desire for relief. For instance, a person might say, "I am frustrated and don't know what to do about it. I'm in a rut — do the same things every day."

B. Responses of confused individuals

Confused individuals indicate they came for help because others prompted them to. Although they can identify their problem situation, they indicate that others are more aware of their problem than they are. For example, a confused person might say, "People say I'm just spinning my wheels and need help. I can't seem to get anything accomplished at work, but I don't know why."

QUESTION 2 WHAT HAS BEEN HAPPENING TO YOU?

1. Adaptive Responses

Individuals describe their activities and their feelings about themselves in relating to their problems. They describe their own contributions to the problems and their responsibility for contributing to the solution. For instance, a person might say, "My difficulty is mainly housework and raising kids. I get angry with my husband because he spoils the kids. I need to control my temper and work out a plan with him.

2. Maladaptive Responses

A. Responses of bored individuals

Bored individuals express a general lack of interest in their activities and a lack of energy to carry them out. They complain that they are not motivated to do anything. For example, a person might say, "I used to do a variety of things, but now I do the same things over and over. I'm tired most of the time."

When they discuss their problem situation, they describe the routine, repetitive tasks they perform without understanding specifically that they suffer from boredom. For example, one might say, "I get up at 6:15. I bathe, I cook breakfast, I clean up, and so on through the whole day."

B. Responses of confused individuals

They describe how others view the events in the problem situation, and how others interpret the factors creating the problem. For example, a person might say, "My friends tell me I'm handling my boss all wrong. They think I should assert myself more. I wish I knew what to do."

In addition, confused people describe the many different things that are overwhelming them without understanding specifically that they are confused by it all. Their description of events seems detached from their feelings. For instance, one might say, "There's too much to do at the office, I never seem to get caught up, I do the work of two people, but I can't get the help I need."

QUESTION 3 WHAT DOES THE FUTURE HOLD FOR YOU?

1. Adaptive Responses

Individuals have no difficulty discussing the future. They convey what they expect to happen and/or what they hope will happen. They describe their short- and long-term goals and tell how they are in the process of pursuing them. For example, one might say, "I am working now and taking courses at night to qualify as a supervisor next year."

2. Maladaptive Responses

A. Responses of bored individuals

Bored people indicate that they expect the future to be the same as the present. They also express little interest in future events, and complain that they do not have the energy to prepare for the future or to influence the future. For example, a person might say, "I expect things to stay the same as now—I eat, take care of the house, cook, go to bed. I can't get with it."

B. Responses of confused individuals

Confused people indicate how others perceive their future. They describe future events as if they were detached and remote from them. For instance, a person might say, "I might want to be a doctor, or a lawyer or an accountant. They make good money. People tell me I would make a good lawyer."

QUESTION 4 CAN YOU PREDICT WHAT TOMORROW WILL BE LIKE FOR YOU?

1. Adaptive Responses

Individuals describe, in general, what they expect to happen to them and comment on the things they are uncertain of, without being troubled by the uncertainty. They communicate a pattern and predictability in their life. However, they describe new and challenging undertakings, the outcomes of which are presently unpredictable. For example, a person might say: "Tomorrow I will get up, and so on, but what surprises the day will bring—I'm not sure. It's interesting."

2. Maladaptive Responses

A. Responses of bored individuals

Bored people provide a detailed description of their daily routine. They show anger and frustration when they comment on their routine. For instance, "I'll get up, wake the children, shower, feed the family toast and bananas, get the children off to school, clean the house, fix dinner, and so on. It's got me down."

B. Responses of confused individuals

Their descriptions are vague and speculative. They have difficulty conveying details or pattern. One might say, "God only knows, my parents want me to go to school, but I don't feel like it. Maybe I'll join the Navy or get a job."

QUESTION 5 WHAT DO YOU ENJOY DOING?

1. Adaptive Responses

Individuals enumerate a number of things they enjoy doing, and partake of at least one enjoyable activity weekly. They communicate that they know what they enjoy. They select enjoyable activities and participate in them. For example, "I enjoy skiing, playing golf, sewing, reading—some I do more often than others. I golf once a week when the weather's right."

2. Maladaptive Responses

A. Responses of bored individuals

They refer to things they might like to do, but they do not see the likelihood of doing them. They do refer to specific situations in the recent past that brought them enjoyment. For instance, "I used to sing, play golf, and so on—now I just do my daily chores. I don't have the time or energy for other things."

B. Responses of confused individuals

Responses indicate that they do not know for sure what brings them enjoyment in the present. The best they can do is refer to a remote situation. For example, "One thing's as good as another. I used to like to play baseball when I was a kid. Someday I hope to travel."

QUESTION 6 WHAT ARE YOUR GOALS?

1. Adaptive Responses

Individuals refer to specific goals they have set, a time frame and plan for achieving them, and are involved in pursuing them. They refer also to what the achievement of the goals will mean to them. For example, "I'm going to night school. In two years I'll get my master's degree. Then I'll get a promotion and raise in salary."

2. Maladaptive Responses

A. Responses of bored individuals

They refer to goals they might like to pursue, but make excuses for not pursuing them. They describe little if any movement toward the goals, and do not regard the goals as attainable under prevailing conditions. For instance, "I wish I could go play tennis, but I don't have the time."

B. Responses of confused individuals

They refer to unrealistic, remote goals or do not define specific goals. If they do state a goal, they do not prescribe a way of achieving it. For example, "One day I will run for political office. I'm not sure which one."

FIGURE 12-6. The Diagnostic Interview for Assessing Cognition. (*Note.* From Savitz, J. and Friedman, M. T., "Diagnosing Boredom and Confusion," *Nursing Research, 30,* 18, January–February, 1981. Reprinted with permission of American Journal of Nursing Company.)

schedule may be used to assess whether an adult client exhibits bored, confused, or adaptive cognitive responses. Using this guide, clients are asked six questions, and their responses are compared with the criteria presented.

The second method is helpful in assessing cognitive functioning of children, but also may be used with adults. Table 12-17 suggests tasks that the nurse can ask the client to complete to determine whether the client's cognitive development is age-appropriate.

Assessment of the client's ability to make sound judgments or solve problems is another important aspect of assessing intrapersonal functioning. To assess judgment, the nurse should ask the client questions that require responses that indicate problem-solving ability. For example, the nurse may ask, "What will you do if your medication runs out before your next clinic appointment?" The nurse can assess judgment by evaluating how realistic the client's plans are.

Assessing a client's ability to comprehend and use language, as well as the client's reading ability, is a critical part of nursing assessment. A person's ability to relay information about his or her health, to receive health information, and to read health education materials and treatment instructions is essential to optimal health and well-being. During the nursing history interview, the nurse should note the client's level of vocabulary, accurate use of grammar and sentence structure, and general clarity of communication. The nurse should clarify meanings of statements and expressions with the client because there can be many variations among cultural groups for meanings of words or expressions.

While expressive language and the client's reported educational level may provide clues to the client's ability to understand oral or written communication, it usually is necessary for the nurse to validate the client's reading and writing abilities. Seeking validation, especially if the nurse suspects

TABLE 12-17
Assessment of Cognitive Development

Age/Stage (Piaget)	Characteristic Cognitive Development	Selected Tasks
Sensorimotor Birth to age 2	Knowledge consists of manipulation of objects in the environment. Shows interest in bright objects and responds to lights and sounds. By age 2, seeks objects placed out of sight (object permanence).	Place infant's play object out of sight and see if infant searches for hidden object. Give bright-colored toy. Observe how infant responds to sound and light. (By 2 years, child should search for hidden object and handle toys, as well as turn head toward stimuli.)
Preoperational age 2–4 years	Develops concepts through use of language. Responds better to visual cues than spoken cues. Egocentric (sees things only from own point of view.) Able to group items according to criteria.	Ask child to place all red blocks together from a group of colored blocks. (By age 4, child should be able to group same color blocks together.)
Intuitive thought age 4–7 years	Major cognitive skill is conservation—ability to understand that the amount of something stays the same regardless of shape or pieces. Also able to form classes of objects and understand numbers.	Given two balls of clay of exact same size, manipulate one ball into a different shape and ask child which one has more clay. (By age 7, child should be able to state that both have same amount.)
Concrete operations age 7–11	Can handle classification problems and is capable of logical operations with concrete things.	Ask the child, "If 'A' is greater than 'B' and 'B' is greater than 'C,' is 'A' greater than 'C'?" The child should be able to answer correctly and offer a logical explanation for why the answer is correct.
Formal operations age 11 and over	Capable of logical thinking with abstractions; can draw conclusions, make interpretations.	Ask the client to define several concrete words (e.g., "apple," "house") and abstract words (e.g., "love," "freedom"). Concrete words should be defined in terms of their categories or classifications (e.g., "fruit," "a place to live"); abstract words should be defined in terms of their qualities (e.g., "affection or deep concern for someone close," "liberty, independence, political and personal rights")

that the client may have a literacy problem, must be done with the utmost sensitivity for the client. When assessing comprehension of verbal or written information, the nurse can ask clients to describe their understanding of what was discussed.

An objective method that is useful for assessing language ability is the Wide Range Achievement Test (WRAT, Jastak & Jastak, 1978). The WRAT offers a quick approximation of a client's functional reading level or approximate grade level for word recognition. The test is designed to measure word recognition, which correlates positively with reading ability (Jastak & Jastak, 1978). The WRAT test usually is perceived as a nonthreatening approach to assessing a client's literacy (Doak, Doak, & Root, 1985). Words included in the WRAT are organized into two levels. Level I words are intended for individuals between the ages of 5 and 11. Examples are "book," "weather," and "quality." Level II words are intended for those older than 11, and include such words as "residence," "luxurious," and "itinerary." The test usually can be administered in less than 10 minutes.

The appropriate word list is presented to the client, who is instructed to read the words out loud. The number of words the client reads correctly are totaled to determined an equivalent grade level.

Assessment of language ability is important for determining appropriate health education methods to use with clients. Jastak and Jastak (1978) recommend teaching methods suitable for use with clients whose word recognition ability is at various grade levels. For example, clients who read below a fifth grade level benefit from demonstrations and visual or audio teaching methods (audiotapes, radio or television announcements). People who read at or above a ninth grade level can be given written materials (up to tenth grade reading level), such as health instruction sheets and booklets.

Affect and Mood

To assess general affect, the nurse should note the client's verbal and nonverbal expressions of emotion. The nurse can ask, "How would you describe your usual mood or emotional state?" Variability in the client's moods and emotional reactions should be noted, including what tends to precipitate changes if that is known. The nurse might ask, "What things make you feel especially happy [or upset]?" The nurse may need to verify response patterns with people who know the client well, such as a parent or spouse. If the client's nonverbal behavior conveys excitement or irritability, the nurse should compare the client's emotional state with prevalent feelings over time. The nurse also may ask how long the client has experienced a particular emotional reaction or mood, especially when it differs from usual.

Older children can be asked, "Tell me how you feel right now" or "Tell me how you feel when . . ." If the child is unable or unwilling to answer, the child can be shown photos or pictures of a child in various situations (home, hospital, school) and asked to describe how the child in the picture is feeling. Younger children respond especially well to this indirect method of assessing their feelings (Lynn, 1987). Children's emotional responses in various situations, such as play or when separating from or reuniting with parents, can be assessed for quality and intensity of feeling.

A tool for assessing the adult client's feelings in a more objective way is the Semantic Differential Scale for Assessing Feelings, developed by Avillo (1978) and depicted in Table 12-18. The client is asked to check the adjective that most closely describes how the client feels. Although this tool was developed for use with hospitalized clients, it may be adapted for use with adults in any setting. It is easy to administer and score and requires a minimal amount of time. Points are totaled, and the score can be used for ongoing assessment and comparison. The high score of 84 indicates positive feelings. This tool may be especially helpful when clients have difficulty identifying positive or negative feelings. Some clients cannot describe their feelings, yet are capable of completing a list of adjectives.

In older individuals, it is important to assess affective changes that accompany aging. These may be assessed by inquiring into the person's responses to growing older. For instance, how satisfied is the client with life, compared to earlier years? What evokes feelings of happiness [sadness] in him or her at this time in life? Chapter 11 discusses in greater depth the process of life review for assessing people's responses to life changes.

Anxiety

Assessment of anxiety, like assessment of other psychosocial parameters, begins with the nurse's awareness of self. Since anxiety is a highly contagious human emotion, nurses must monitor carefully their own behavior and maintain a presence that communicates calmness. If the nurse is highly anxious, the client is apt to become anxious. While preparing a 55-year-old woman for a breast biopsy and possibly a mastectomy, the nurse avoids eye

TABLE 12-18
Semantic Differential Scale for Assessing Feelings

DIRECTIONS: To help give you better care, we'd like to know how you feel about yourself at this time. One way to do this is to measure what certain words mean to you.

On this questionnaire, 12 pairs of adjectives are separated by lines composed of 7 boxes. On each line, place a check in the box that most closely describes your feelings about yourself. For example, which box below best describes you at this time?

	Short						Tall
	1	2	3	4	5	6	7

Score values:	1 Very short	5 Slightly tall
	2 Short	6 Tall
	3 Slightly short	7 Very Tall
	4 Neutral	

If you think you are very tall, place a check in box #7. If you are just tall, place a check in box #6.
The answers you give should apply only to how you feel right now. You may feel differently tomorrow. There are no wrong answers.

	1	2	3	4	5	6	7	
Changeable	☐	☐	☐	☐	☐	☐	☐	Stable
Uncertain	☐	☐	☐	☐	☐	☐	☐	Confident
Dejected	☐	☐	☐	☐	☐	☐	☐	Happy
Detached	☐	☐	☐	☐	☐	☐	☐	Involved
Confused	☐	☐	☐	☐	☐	☐	☐	Organized
Inattentive	☐	☐	☐	☐	☐	☐	☐	Concerned
Indifferent	☐	☐	☐	☐	☐	☐	☐	Enthusiastic
Passive	☐	☐	☐	☐	☐	☐	☐	Active
Uninterested	☐	☐	☐	☐	☐	☐	☐	Interested
Lonely	☐	☐	☐	☐	☐	☐	☐	Friendly
Uncomfortable	☐	☐	☐	☐	☐	☐	☐	Comfortable
Nervous	☐	☐	☐	☐	☐	☐	☐	Calm

Note. From Avillo, L. (1978). Semantic Differential Scale for Assessing Patients' Feelings. In *Instruments for measuring nursing practice and other health care variables* (Vol. 1, pp. 209–211). Health Manpower References, U.S. DHEW Publication No. HRA78-53. Washington, DC: U.S. Government Printing Office. Reprinted with permission.

contact with the client and becomes immersed in tidying the bedside table. The client, feeling the nurse's evasiveness, becomes even more anxious than before.

Conversely, the nurse must avoid allowing the client's anxiety to interfere with the nurse's ability to assess the situation accurately. For example, the nurse may become so uncomfortable when a client is highly anxious that the nurse changes the subject to avoid pursuing it in some depth or even terminates the assessment quickly.

The nurse should observe the client for overt as well as covert cues of anxiety (see Table 12-4). Also, the absence of congruence in the client's verbal and nonverbal behaviors may indicate the presence of anxiety and the client's effort to defend against it. A client's facial expression may be tense or pensive, yet the client says, "I'm not worried about my test results; in fact, I'm not even thinking about them."

Zung (1971) has developed an Anxiety Status Inventory and a Self-Rating Anxiety Scale. The former, which is shown in Table 12-19, can be administered easily in a short time. This tool may be especially useful with clients who are reluctant to disclose their feelings verbally or who evade acknowledging their feelings.

Anger

Assessment of anger requires that the nurse listen, observe, and validate cues that suggest a client is angry. Listening to the content of a client's speech in conjunction with observing such nonverbal behaviors as eye contact, posture, and hand gestures may assist the nurse in recognizing that the client is angry. If anger is the client's response to a threat, its expression may be indirect (passive) or direct (assertive or aggressive). Table 12-20 provides guidelines for assessing the expression of anger.

Depression

Observation of the client's nonverbal and verbal behaviors as well as interactions with others provides clues about the presence or absence of de-

TABLE 12-19
The Anxiety Status Inventory (ASI)

Affective and Somatic Symptoms of Anxiety	Interview Guide for Anxiety Status inventory (ASI)	Severity of Observed or Reported Responses			
		None	Mild	Mod.	Sev.
1. Anxiousness	Do you ever feel nervous and anxious?	1	2	3	4
2. Fear	Have you ever felt afraid?	1	2	3	4
3. Panic	How easily do you get upset? Ever have panic spells or feel like it?	1	2	3	4
4. Mental disintegration	Do you ever feel like you're falling apart? Going to pieces?	1	2	3	4
5. Apprehension	Have you ever felt uneasy? or that something terrible was going to happen?	1	2	3	4
6. Tremors	Have you ever had times when you felt yourself trembling? shaking?	1	2	3	4
7. Body aches and pains	Do you have headaches? neck or back pains?	1	2	3	4
8. Easy fatigability, weakness	How easily do you get tired? Ever have spells of weakness?	1	2	3	4
9. Restlessness	Do you find yourself restless and can't sit still?	1	2	3	4
10. Palpitation	Have you ever felt that your heart was running away?	1	2	3	4
11. Dizziness	Do you have dizzy spells?	1	2	3	4
12. Faintness	Do you have fainting spells? or feel like it?	1	2	3	4
13. Dyspnea	Ever have trouble with your breathing?	1	2	3	4
14. Paresthesias	Ever have feelings of numbness and tingling in your fingertips? or around your mouth?	1	2	3	4
15. Nausea and vomiting	Do you ever feel sick to your stomach or feel like vomiting?	1	2	3	4
16. Urinary frequency	How often do you need to empty your bladder?	1	2	3	4
17. Sweating	Do you ever get wet, clammy hands?	1	2	3	4
18. Face flushing	Do you ever feel your face getting hot and blushing?	1	2	3	4
19. Insomnia	How have you been sleeping?	1	2	3	4
20. Nightmares	Do you have dreams that scare you?	1	2	3	4

pression. Also, certain physiological responses may indicate depression. Table 12-21 provides a guide for assessing affective, physiological, cognitive, and behavioral indicators of depression. As indicated in Table 12-21, there is a wide spectrum of responses to an underlying depression.

Since depression is classified primarily as a disturbance in affect, the client who is depressed often communicates it. The nurse must listen to both manifest and latent messages when assessing a client's feelings. A client may talk about feeling unhappy, despondent, listless, or dissatisfied with life. On the other hand, some clients may communicate their depressed states indirectly by indicating intense worry and agitation. One assessment tool that can be used when a client communicates difficulties with depression is the Algorithm for Depression questionnaire (Orsolotis & Morphy, 1982). The tool, presented in Table 12-22, focuses on such dimensions as social supports, recent losses, suicidal thoughts, various behavioral states, and judgment of the clinician. Zung's (1965) Depression Status Inventory is a brief, easy to administer scale for determining the depth or intensity of depression (see Table 12-23).

Temperament

Since temperament relates to how a client behaves and reacts emotionally over time and across situations, the nurse will need ongoing observations of the client. For example, a newly admitted client may be accompanied to the hospital by several family members and may interact with them in a pleasant manner. The nurse cannot conclude, however, that the client's temperament reflects a functional level of emotionality and sociability. Instead, the nurse must observe ongoing contacts between the client and family.

The nurse may use Buss and Plemin's EASI–III Temperament Survey (see Table 12-24) as a guide for assessing temperament. This tool allows the nurse to assess a client's temperament by comparing the client's general tendencies in the areas of emotionality, activity, sociability, and impulsivity. Much information can be obtained by listening to

TABLE 12-20
Comparison of Passive, Assertive, and Aggressive Behaviors

	Passive	Assertive	Aggressive
Content of speech	Negative Self-derogatory "Can't I" "Will you?"	Positive Self-enhancing "I can't" "I will"	Exaggerated Other derogatory "You always" "You never"
Tone of voice	Quiet, weak, whining	Modulated	Loud, demanding
Posture	Drooping, bowed head	Erect, relaxed	Tense, leaning forward
Personal space	Allows invasion of space by others	Maintains a comfortable distance; claims right to own space	Invades space of others
Gestures	Minimal, weak gesturing, fidgeting	Demonstrative gestures	Threatening, expansive gestures
Eye contact	Little or none	Intermittent, appropriate to relationship	Constant stare

Note. From Stuart, G., & Sundeen, S. (1991). *Principles and practice of psychiatric nursing* (4th ed.). St. Louis: C.V. Mosby, 549.

the client's responses to questions or statements in major categories. Examples of questions or statements include: "What are some things that tend to make you upset [fearful] [angry]?" "How do other people know when you're upset [fearful] [angry]?" "Describe a typical day's activity for you." "What kinds of social activities or experiences do you tend to like [dislike]?" "Talk about some major decisions you have had to make in your life."

Assessment of temperament in infancy and childhood can provide valuable information for helping parents understand their child's responses and for providing guidance in childrearing practices (Carey, 1990). Routine screening of temperament, however, is not usually necessary, but should be done when concern is expressed by parents or when the nurse notes a problem in "fit" between parent and child. For example, parents who are gregarious and outgoing may be frustrated with a child who is shy and withdraws from new situations; parents who are quiet and shy may feel overwhelmed by a child who is boisterous and out-

TABLE 12-21
Behaviors Associated with Depression

Affective	Physiological	Cognitive	Behavioral
Anger	Abdominal pain	Ambivalence	Aggressiveness
Anxiety	Anorexia	Confusion	Agitation
Apathy	Backache	Inability to concentrate	Alcoholism
Bitterness	Chest pain	Indecisiveness	Altered activity level
Dejection	Constipation	Loss of interest and motivation	Drug addiction
Denial of feelings	Dizziness	Self-blame	Intolerance
Despondency	Fatigue	Self-depreciation	Irritability
Guilt	Headache	Self-destructive thoughts	Lack of spontaneity
Helplessness	Impotence	Pessimism	Overdependency
Hopelessness	Indigestion	Uncertainty	Poor personal hygiene
Loneliness	Insomnia		Psychomotor retardation
Low self-esteem	Lassitude		Social isolation
Sadness	Menstrual changes		Tearfulness
Sense of personal	Nausea		Underachievement
worthlessness	Overeating		Withdrawal
	Sexual nonresponsiveness		
	Sleep disturbances		
	Vomiting		
	Weight change		

Note. From Stuart, G., & Sundeen, S. (1991). *Principles and practice of psychiatric nursing* (4th ed.). St. Louis: C.V. Mosby, 432.

TABLE 12-22
Algorithm for Depression

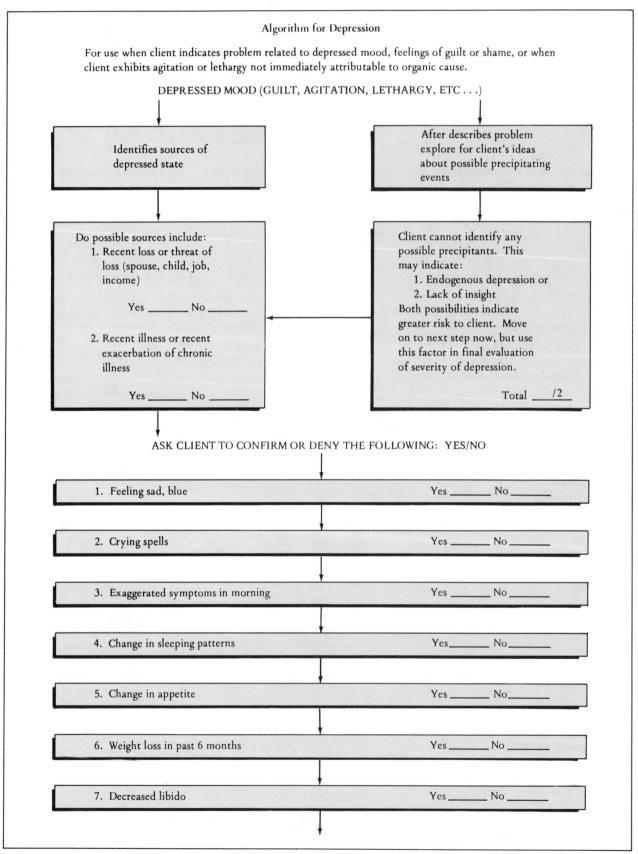

Algorithm for Depression

For use when client indicates problem related to depressed mood, feelings of guilt or shame, or when client exhibits agitation or lethargy not immediately attributable to organic cause.

DEPRESSED MOOD (GUILT, AGITATION, LETHARGY, ETC . . .)

Identifies sources of depressed state

After describes problem explore for client's ideas about possible precipitating events

Do possible sources include:
1. Recent loss or threat of loss (spouse, child, job, income)

    Yes _____ No _____

2. Recent illness or recent exacerbation of chronic illness

    Yes _____ No _____

Client cannot identify any possible precipitants. This may indicate:
    1. Endogenous depression or
    2. Lack of insight
Both possibilities indicate greater risk to client. Move on to next step now, but use this factor in final evaluation of severity of depression.

    Total ____ /2

ASK CLIENT TO CONFIRM OR DENY THE FOLLOWING: YES/NO

1. Feeling sad, blue   Yes _____ No _____

2. Crying spells   Yes _____ No _____

3. Exaggerated symptoms in morning   Yes _____ No _____

4. Change in sleeping patterns   Yes _____ No _____

5. Change in appetite   Yes _____ No _____

6. Weight loss in past 6 months   Yes _____ No _____

7. Decreased libido   Yes _____ No _____

continued

TABLE 12-22 (Continued)

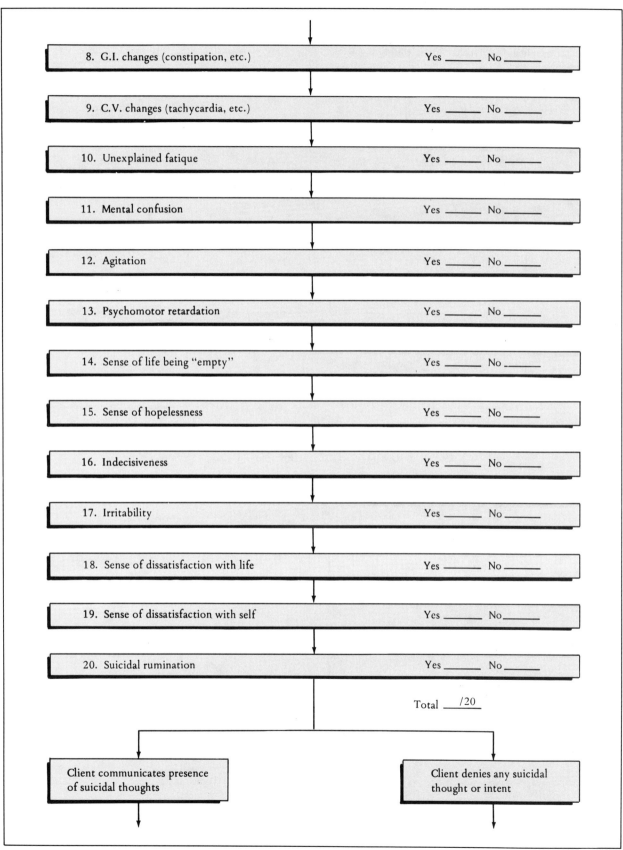

8. G.I. changes (constipation, etc.)   Yes _____ No _____

9. C.V. changes (tachycardia, etc.)   Yes _____ No _____

10. Unexplained fatique   Yes _____ No _____

11. Mental confusion   Yes _____ No _____

12. Agitation   Yes _____ No _____

13. Psychomotor retardation   Yes _____ No _____

14. Sense of life being "empty"   Yes _____ No _____

15. Sense of hopelessness   Yes _____ No _____

16. Indecisiveness   Yes _____ No _____

17. Irritability   Yes _____ No _____

18. Sense of dissatisfaction with life   Yes _____ No _____

19. Sense of dissatisfaction with self   Yes _____ No _____

20. Suicidal rumination   Yes _____ No _____

Total ____/20

Client communicates presence of suicidal thoughts   Client denies any suicidal thought or intent

continued

TABLE 12-22 (Continued)

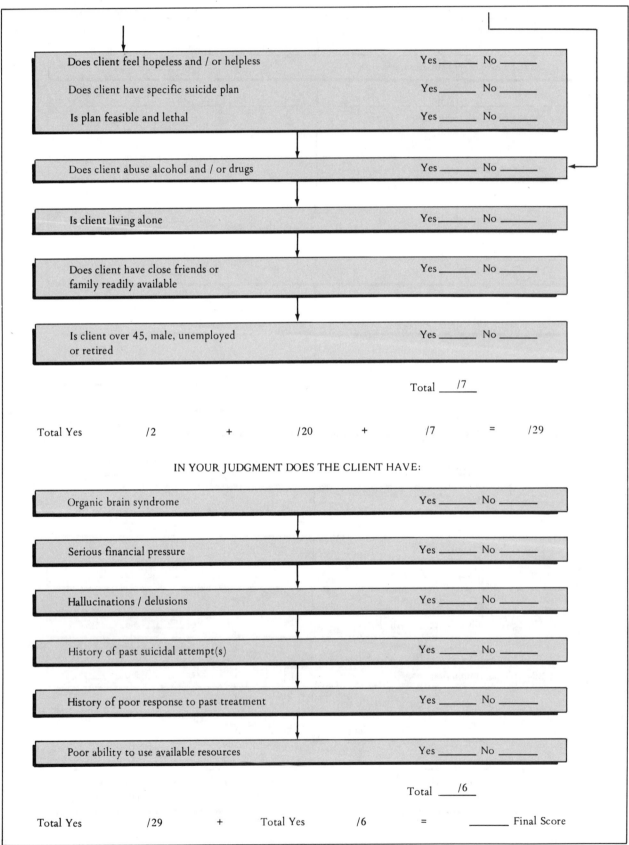

Does client feel hopeless and / or helpless   Yes _____ No _____

Does client have specific suicide plan   Yes _____ No _____

Is plan feasible and lethal   Yes _____ No _____

Does client abuse alcohol and / or drugs   Yes _____ No _____

Is client living alone   Yes _____ No _____

Does client have close friends or
family readily available   Yes _____ No _____

Is client over 45, male, unemployed
or retired   Yes _____ No _____

Total ___/7___

Total Yes   /2   +   /20   +   /7   =   /29

IN YOUR JUDGMENT DOES THE CLIENT HAVE:

Organic brain syndrome   Yes _____ No _____

Serious financial pressure   Yes _____ No _____

Hallucinations / delusions   Yes _____ No _____

History of past suicidal attempt(s)   Yes _____ No _____

History of poor response to past treatment   Yes _____ No _____

Poor ability to use available resources   Yes _____ No _____

Total ___/6___

Total Yes   /29   +   Total Yes   /6   =   _____ Final Score

continued

TABLE 12-22 (Continued)

Admit to psychiatric unit	5. _____
Refer to:	
Day hospital	4. _____
Crisis intervention	3. _____
Outpatient clinic	2. _____
Home (no treatment)	1. _____

To M.D. (Level II or III)	
Confirmation	1. _____
Medical evaluation	2. _____

ALGORITHM SCORING

Add the number of "Yes" responses in each subsection to provide a final score. Scoring has been included in the algorithm's construction from the outset in order to facilitate future analysis of data. Correlations of disposition decisions, and possibly other outcome measures, with these subtotal and total scores can be completed.

Note. Reprinted with permission from *Journal of Psychiatric Treatment and Evaluation*, 4, M. Orsolotis and M. Morphy, "A Depression Algorithm for Psychiatric Emergencies," Copyright 1982, Pergamon Press plc.

going. In such instances, screening with a temperament questionnaire may be indicated.

Carey and McDevitt developed the first temperament questionnaire (Infant Temperament Questionnaire, 1978) based on the temperament styles and accompanying behavioral responses identified by Chess and Thomas (1977). The questionnaire consists of 95 items that assess an infant's responses to such situations as feeding, sleeping, bathing, and diapering. A portion of the Revised Infant Temperament Questionnaire (for 4–8 month-old infants) is presented in Table 12-25.

Since the original Infant Temperament Questionnaire, four additional questionnaires have been developed: the Early Infancy Temperament Questionnaire (1–4 months), the Toddler Temperament Scale (1–3 years), the Behavioral Style Questionnaire (3–7 years), and the Middle Childhood Temperament Questionnaire (8–12 years). The boxed insert gives information for obtaining the complete questionnaires.

Social Roles

To assess a client's social roles and relationships, the nurse can ask the client, "Describe yourself in terms of the roles [responsibilities] you fulfill, such as parent, your work roles, and so forth. Which are most important to you? Which are difficult or create problems for you?" Responses identify the various roles held by the client.

Clients should be asked to describe their perceptions of the expectations they have for themselves and that others have of them in each role. Assessment should include identification of role conflict, role ambiguity, or role strain that the client is experiencing or has experienced:

Do you seek help from others when you feel burdened or overloaded?

Do you feel at odds with yourself or with others and thus dissatisfied with fulfilling expectations in one or more roles?

Do you feel unsure about what to do or how to act in various roles?

The nurse also should note any role changes the client has experienced recently, such as assumption of a new role, shift from one role to another, or loss of a role, and how the changes have affected the client's lifestyle, patterns, and relationships. Examples of role changes include adolescence, marriage, divorce, new parenthood, retirement, widowhood, job promotion, and loss of employment.

TABLE 12-23
The Depression Status Inventory (DSI)

Signs & Symptoms of Depression	Interview Guide for Depression Status Inventory (DSI)	Severity of Observed or Reported Responses:			
		None	Mild	Mod.	Sev.
1. Depressed mood	Do you ever feel sad or depressed?	1	2	3	4
2. Crying spells	Do you have crying spells or feel like it?	1	2	3	4
3. Diurnal variation: symptoms worst in a.m.	Is there any part of the day when you feel worst? Best?	1	2	3	4
4. Sleep disturbance	How have you been sleeping?	1	2	3	4
5. Decreased appetite	How is your appetite?	1	2	3	4
6. Weight loss	Have you lost any weight?	1	2	3	4
7. Decreased libido	How about your interest in the opposite sex?	1	2	3	4
8. Constipation	Do you have trouble with constipation?	1	2	3	4
9. Tachycardia	Have you had times when your heart was beating faster than usual?	1	2	3	4
10. Fatigue	How easily do you get tired?	1	2	3	4
11. Psychomotor agitation	Do you find yourself restless and can't sit still?	1	2	3	4
12. Psychomotor retardation	Do you feel slowed down in doing the things you usually do?	1	2	3	4
13. Confusion	Do you ever feel confused and have trouble thinking?	1	2	3	4
14. Emptiness	Do you feel life is empty for you?	1	2	3	4
15. Hopelessness	How hopeful do you feel about the future?	1	2	3	4
16. Indecisiveness	How are you at making decisions?	1	2	3	4
17. Irritability	How easily do you get irritated?	1	2	3	4
18. Dissatisfaction	Do you still enjoy the things you used to?	1	2	3	4
19. Personal devaluation	Do you ever feel useless and not wanted?	1	2	3	4
20. Suicidal	Have you had thoughts about doing away with yourself?	1	2	3	4

Stressors and Stress Responses

An appraisal of stressors and stress responses in the client's life is another important part of the intrapersonal and interpersonal assessment. The nurse should determine what stressors the client is experiencing as well as the source of the stressor (i.e. internal processes, physical environment, or psychosocial milieu). The timing of the stressor is another important dimension of assessment. When did the stressor occur? What else might have been going on in the client's life at that time? How long has the client been exposed to the stressor? How frequently does the client interact with or experience the stressor? Also, how many stressors has the client experienced within a given time frame? The latter consideration is important because the client may be experiencing a cumulative response to stress.

An individual's ability to adapt to stressors is related to the number of life events and changes. Holmes and Rahe (1967) developed the Social Re-adjustment Rating Scale to assess the potential for stress. Rahe and Arthur (1978) report an association between an increased number of stressful life events and the incidence of chronic illness. In other words, clients with chronic illness are more likely to have experienced a number of life changes.

The Social Readjustment Rating Scale explores life changes in several categories: health, work, home, and family (see Table 12-26). The nurse should ask the client to check or circle events that have occurred during the previous year that involved an adjustment of the client's usual routine. The seriousness of life events is ranked on the questionnaire. The total value of events indicated by the client is scored. Clients with more than 300 "Life Change Units" in the past year have close to an 80% chance of becoming ill (Rahe and Arthur, 1978). Those with 150 to 299 points have approximately a 50% chance of illness in the near future, whereas only 30% of people with fewer than 150 Life Change Units are likely to become ill in the near future.

TABLE 12-24
EASI-III Temperament Survey

Emotionality

General
  I frequently get upset
  I am almost always calm—nothing ever bothers me
  I get excited easily
  I am somewhat emotional
  I often feel like crying

Fear
  I am easily frightened
  I often feel insecure
  I tend to be nervous in new situations
  I have fewer fears than most people my age
  When I get scared, I panic

Anger
  When displeased, I let people know it right away
  It takes a lot to get me mad
  I am known as hot-blooded and quick-tempered
  I yell and scream more than most people my age
  There are more things that annoy me

Activity

Tempo
  I usually seem to be in a hurry
  For relaxation I like to slow down and take things easy
  I like to be off and running as soon as I wake up in the morning.
  I like to keep busy all the time
  My life is fast paced

Vigor
  I like to wear myself out with exertion
  I often feel sluggish
  I often feel as if I'm bursting with energy
  When I do things, I do them vigorously
  My movements are forceful and emphatic

Sociability
  I make friends very quickly
  I am very sociable
  I tend to be shy
  I usually prefer to do things alone
  I have many friends

Impulsivity

Inhibitory Control
  I have trouble controlling my impulses
  Usually I can't stand waiting
  I can tolerate frustration better than most
  I have trouble resisting my cravings (for food, cigarettes, etc.)
  I like to spend my money right away rather than save it for long-range goals

Decision Time
  I often say the first thing that comes into my head
  I often have trouble making up my mind
  I like to plan things way ahead of time
  I often act on the spur of the moment
  I like to make detailed plans before I do something

Sensation Seeking
  I generally seek new and exciting experiences and sensations
  I'll try anything once
  I sometimes do "crazy" things just to be different
  I'm happiest in familiar surroundings
  I get bored easily

Persistence
  I generally like to see things through to the end
  I tend to hop from interest to interest quickly
  I tend to give up easily
  Unfinished tasks really bother me
  Once I get going on something I hate to stop

Note. From *A Temperament Theory of Personality Development*, by A.H. Bussand R. Plemin. Copyright © 1975 by John Wiley & Sons, Inc., pp. 241–242. Reprinted with permission.

Volicer and Bohannon (1975) developed a 49-item scale to identify stressful situations experienced by hospitalized adult clients. Situations that are stressful for an individual client can be identified so that nurses can focus on reducing those stressors. The scale is easy to administer, using a checklist of events (see Table 12-27). The client is asked to check stressors experienced while in the hospital, and the total "stress value" is scored. This stress value may help validate the client's stress level and susceptibility to further alterations in health.

Coping Strategies

During the nursing history interview, the nurse usually is able to determine what modes of coping the client is consciously aware of using when confronted with stressors. In other words, assessment of task-oriented coping strategies usually can be made by conversing with the client. Since many defense mechanisms are outside of conscious awareness, they are much more difficult to assess and may prove impossible to determine. However, as the relationship between the client and nurse evolves and the nurse gets to know and observe the client over time, cues for the client's use of defense mechanisms will become evident.

Questions to ask the client about coping include:

When you feel stressed in your day-to-day life, what do you tend to do?

Tell me about the last time in your life that you

TABLE 12-25
The Revised Infant Temperament Questionnaire—Sample Items (4–8 months)

The mother rates each of the following items as follows:

Almost Never					Almost Always
1	2	3	4	5	6

Category	Description
1. Activity	The infant moves about much (kicks, grabs, squirms) during diapering and dressing. The infant plays actively with parents—much movement of arms, legs, body.
2. Rhythmicity	The infant wants and takes milk feedings at about the same times (within one hour) from day to day. The infant's bowel movements come at different times day to day (over one hour's difference).
3. Approach	The infant accepts right away any change in place or position of feeding or person giving it. For the first few minutes in a new place or situation (new store or home), the infant is fretful.
4. Adaptability	The infant objects to being bathed in a different place or by a different person, even after two or three tries. The infant accepts regular procedures (hair brushing, face washing, etc.) any time without protest.
5. Intensity	The infant reacts strongly to foods, whether positively (smacks lips, laughs, squeals) or negatively (cries). The infant reacts mildly to meeting familiar people (quiet smiles or no response).
6. Mood	The infant is pleasant (smiles, laughs) when first arriving in unfamiliar places (friend's house, store). The infant cries when left to play alone.
7. Persistence	The infant amuses self for half an hour or more in crib or playpen (looking at mobile, playing with toy). The infant watches other children playing for under a minute and then looks elsewhere.
8. Distractibility	The infant stops play and watches when someone walks by. The infant continues to cry in spite of several minutes of soothing.
9. Threshold	The infant reacts even to a gentle touch (startle, wriggle, laugh, cry). The infant reacts to a disliked food even if it is mixed with a preferred one.

Note. From "Revision of the Infant Temperament Questionnaire," by W.B. Carey and S.C. McDevitt, *Pediatrics*, 1978, 61:735–739. Copyright American Academy of Pediatrics 1978.

felt very overwhelmed. What helped decrease those feelings for you?

About how long did it take for you to feel better?

How do you typically handle difficult times in your life?

Many clients are able to respond readily to such questions. However, in some instances, the nurse may have to assist the client in identifying specific coping strategies. This can be done by describing examples of coping efforts. For instance, the nurse could select some of the coping strategies identified in Table 12-9 or Table 12-10, share these with the client, and help the client's focus on coping efforts that have been helpful in the past.

Assessment of coping in young children can be facilitated by various projective techniques, including puppets. The nurse could indicate that the puppet is sick. The child can be asked what the puppet is feeling and what the puppet can do

about these feelings. Lynn (1987) notes that storytelling is useful. By presenting story pictures and asking the child to tell a story about what is happening in the picture, the child's perceptions and interpretations of the events, including the coping strategies used by people in the story, can be ascertained.

NURSING DIAGNOSES RELATED TO INTRAPERSONAL/INTERPERSONAL FUNCTIONING

Generally, much information about intrapersonal and interpersonal functioning has been gathered by the conclusion of the nursing assessment. In the psychosocial area, there are many nursing diagnoses that may emerge from thorough analysis and clustering of the information.

Nursing diagnoses associated with psychosocial functioning are categorized, for the most part,

Where to Obtain Infant and Child Temperament Questionnaires

Early Infancy Temperament Questionnaire
(1–4 months)
Developed by B. Medoff-Cooper, W.B. Carey, &
S.C. McDevitt, 1985–1990

> Barbara Medoff-Cooper, Ph.D., F.A.A.N.
> School of Nursing, University of Pennsylvania
> Philadelphia, PA 19104–6096
> (215) 898-3399

Infant Temperament Questionnaire (4–8 months)
Developed by W.B. Carey & S.C. McDevitt,
revised 1977

> William B. Carey, M.D.
> Division of General Pediatrics
> Children's Hospital
> Philadelphia, PA 19104
> (215) 590-2168

Toddler Temperament Scale (1–3 years)
Developed by W. Fullard, S.C. McDevitt, & W.B. Carey,
1978

William Fullard, Ph.D.
Department of Educational Psychology
Temple University
Philadelphia, PA 19122
(215) 787-6022

Behavioral Style Questionnaire (3–7 years)
Developed by S.C. McDevitt & W.B. Carey, 1975

> Sean C. McDevitt, Ph.D.
> Western Behavioral Associates
> 4626 East Shea Blvd.
> Phoenix, AZ 85028
> (602) 494-0224

Middle Childhood Temperament Questionnaire
(8–12 years)
Developed by R.L. Hegvik, S.C. McDevitt &
W.B. Carey, 1979–80

> Robin L. Hegvik, Ph.D.
> 243 Cohasset Lane
> West Chester, PA 19380
> (215) 296-5602

All of the above listed scales assess the NYLS temperament characteristics by eliciting parent responses to about 97 specific behavioral descriptions. Since the following instruments were developed with minimal financial support, please send a prepaid contribution of $10 for each scale. The forms may be reproduced as often as wished from the one received.

under the response patterns of "relating," "valuing," "choosing," "perceiving," and "feeling." Hence, individuals who have actual or potential psychosocial health problems may have difficulties in such areas as relating to others ("altered role performance," "social isolation"), finding meaning and purpose in life ("spiritual distress"), using coping strategies that encourage a functional response to stress ("decisional conflict," "impaired adjustment," "ineffective denial"), viewing self in ways that do not promote health ("self-esteem disturbance," "body image disturbance," "hopelessness," "powerlessness," "personal identity disturbance"), and feeling anxious or frightened ("anxiety," "fear").

"Ineffective individual coping," a nursing diagnosis categorized under choosing, infers that the individual is impaired in adapting to life's problems, demands, or roles. Validation of this diagnosis stems from nursing history and clinical appraisal that indicate a client is pessimistic, unhappy, hopeless, self-absorbed, and lacks a future orientation. The client also may be detached from social supports and refuse help if it is offered. Factors that may contribute to this nursing diagnosis

include inaccurate appraisal of an event or illness; impairment in responding in a functional way to stressors (for example, difficulty in expressing feelings or behaving in a destructive way towards self or others); inability to develop realistic goals and plans; and a self-perception of being powerless and not in control.

The nursing diagnosis "anxiety," is among those associated with feeling. Anxiety as a diagnosis may be characterized by the client's overt or covert expressions (for instance, reporting worry or apprehensiveness; responses (anger, guilt, and regression) that are inappropriate to the situation; physiological arousal, such as increased heart rate and blood pressure; and difficulty attending to details or concentrating. As with most nursing diagnoses, there are usually many factors that contribute to a diagnosis of anxiety. Loss of a significant other, guilt about past behavior, illness of any nature, and developmental crises are among the possibilities.

Table 12-28 suggests nursing diagnoses that may result from the analysis and interpretation of information about intrapersonal and interpersonal functioning.

TABLE 12-26
The Social Readjustment Rating Scale

Life Event	Mean Value
1. Death of spouse	100
2. Divorce	73
3. Marital separation from mate	65
4. Detention in jail or other institution	63
5. Death of a close family member	63
6. Major personal injury or illness	53
7. Marriage	50
8. Being fired at work	47
9. Marital reconciliation with mate	45
10. Retirement from work	45
11. Major change in the health or behavior of a family member	44
12. Pregnancy	40
13. Sexual difficulties	39
14. Gaining a new family member (e.g., through birth, adoption, oldster moving in, etc.)	39
15. Major business readjustment (e.g., merger, reorganization, bankruptcy, etc.)	39
16. Major change in financial state (e.g., a lot worse off or a lot better off than usual)	38
17. Death of a close friend	37
18. Changing to a different line of work	36
19. Major change in the number of arguments with spouse (e.g., either a lot more or a lot less than usual regarding child rearing, personal habits, etc.)	35
20. Taking out a mortgage or loan for a major purchase (e.g., for a home, business, etc.)	31
21. Foreclosure on a mortgage or loan	30
22. Major change in responsibilities at work (e.g., promotion, demotion, lateral transfer)	29
23. Son or daughter leaving home (e.g., marriage, attending college, etc.)	29
24. [Spouse] beginning or ceasing work outside the home	26
25. Beginning or ceasing formal schooling	26
26. Major change in living conditions (e.g., building a new home, remodeling, deterioration of home or neighborhood)	25
27. Revision of personal habits (dress, manners, association, etc.)	24
28. Troubles with the boss	23
29. Major change in working hours or conditions	20
30. Change in residence	20
31. Changing to a new school	20
32. Major change in usual type and/or amount of recreation	19
33. Major change in church activities (e.g., a lot more or a lot less than usual)	19
34. Major change in social activities (e.g., clubs, dancing, movies, visiting, etc.)	18
35. Taking out a mortgage or loan for a lesser purchase (e.g., for a car, TV, freezer, etc.)	17
36. Major change in sleeping habits (a lot more or a lot less sleep, or change in part of day when asleep)	16
37. Major change in number of family get-togethers (e.g., a lot more or a lot less than usual)	15
38. Major change in eating habits (a lot more or a lot less food intake, or very different meal hours or surroundings)	15
39. Vacation	13
40. Christmas	12
41. Minor violations of the law (e.g., traffic tickets, jaywalking, disturbing the peace, etc.)	11

Note. Reprinted with permission from *Journal of Psychosomatic Research,* 11. T.H. Holmes and R.H. Rahe, "The Social Adjustment Rating Scale," Copyright 1967, Pergamon Press.

TABLE 12-27
The Hospital Stress Rating Scale

Assigned Rank	Stress Value	Event	
1	13.9	Having strangers sleep in the same room with you	____
2	15.4	Having to eat at different times than you usually do	____
3	15.9	Having to sleep in a strange bed	____
4	16.0	Having to wear a hospital gown	____
5	16.8	Having strange machines around	____
6	16.9	Being awakened in the night by the nurse	____
7	17.0	Having to be assisted with bathing	____
8	17.7	Not being able to get newspapers, radio, or TV when you want them	____
9	18.1	Having a roommate who has too many visitors	____
10	19.1	Having to stay in bed or the same room all day	____
11	19.4	Being aware of unusual smells around you	____
12	21.2	Having a roommate who is seriously ill or cannot talk with you	____
13	21.5	Having to be assisted with a bedpan	____
14	21.6	Having a roommate who is unfriendly	____
15	21.7	Not having friends visit you	____
16	21.7	Being in a room that is too cold or too hot	____
17	21.1	Thinking your appearance might be changed after your hospitalization	____
18	22.3	Being in the hospital during holidays or special family occasions	____
19	22.4	Thinking you might have pain because of surgery or test procedures	____
20	22.7	Worrying about your spouse being away from you	____
21	23.2	Having to eat cold or tasteless food	____
22	23.3	Not being able to call family or friends on the phone	____
23	23.4	Being cared for by an unfamiliar doctor	____
24	23.6	Being put in the hospital because of an accident	____
25	24.2	Not knowing when to expect things will be done for you	____
26	24.5	Having the staff be in too much of a hurry	____
27	25.9	Thinking about losing income because of your illness	____
28	26.0	Having medications cause you discomfort	____
29	26.4	Having nurses or doctors talk too fast or use words you can't understand	____
30	26.4	Feeling you are getting dependent on medications	____
31	26.5	Not having family visit you	____
32	26.9	Knowing you have to have an operation	____
33	27.1	Being hospitalized far away from home	____
34	27.2	Having a sudden hospitalization you weren't planning to have	____
35	27.3	Not having your call light answered	____
36	27.4	Not having enough insurance to pay for your hospitalization	____
37	27.6	Not having your questions answered by the staff	____
38	28.4	Missing your spouse	____
39	29.2	Being fed through tubes	____
40	31.2	Not getting relief from pain medications	____
41	31.9	Not knowing the results or reasons for your treatments	____
42	32.4	Not getting pain medication when you need it	____
43	34.0	Not knowing for sure what illness you have	____
44	34.1	Not being told what your diagnosis is	____
45	34.5	Thinking you might lose your hearing	____
46	34.6	Knowing you have a serious illness	____
47	35.6	Thinking you might lose a kidney or some other organ	____
48	39.2	Thinking you might have cancer	____
49	40.6	Thinking you might lose your sight	____
TOTAL			____

Note. From B.J. Volicer, and M.W. Bohannon. A Hospital Stress Rating Scale. Copyright © 1975, American Journal of Nursing Company. Reproduced, with permission, from *Nursing Research*, September–October, Vol. 24, No. 5.

TABLE 12-28
Sample Nursing Diagnoses Related to Intrapersonal or Interpersonal Functioning

Impaired adjustment related to inadequate support systems, effects of chronic illness or disability, or major life change (divorce, adolescence, menopause, widowhood)

Anxiety related to perceived threat to health, situational or maturational crises, values conflict, or loss of control

Body image disturbance related to loss of body part or function, pregnancy, trauma, or aging

Decisional conflict related to multiple sources of information, lack of relevant information, or unclear values/beliefs

Ineffective individual coping related to change in life situation, chronic illness or disability, lack of social support systems, or loss of significant other

Ineffective denial related to perceived threat to health or actual loss (e.g., death of loved one, loss of body part or function)

Fear related to loss of body part or function, language barrier, threat of death, or lack of knowledge

Hopelessness related to depression, social isolation, abandonment, personal failures (e.g., loss of job), or chronic or life-threatening illness

Personal identity disturbance related to role change or developmental crises (e.g., adolescence, divorce, menopause)

Powerlessness related to low self-esteem, cultural roles, role change, poverty, or health-care environment

Altered role performance related to change in employment, family structure, financial status, or health status; developmental crisis,; or ineffective coping

Self-esteem disturbance related to negative childrearing experiences, chronic illness, or personal failure (e.g., school performance, loss of employment, failure to achieve goals)

Impaired social interaction related to low self-esteem, social skills deficit, or communication barriers

Social isolation related to living alone, stressors, inappropriate social behaviors, or inadequate social support systems

Spiritual distress related to values conflict, disruption in usual religious practices, effects of personal or family disasters, or loss of significant others

Altered thought processes related to depression; anxiety; stress; social isolation; memory loss; or effects of illness, medications, or substance abuse

Chapter Highlights

▪ Psychosocial assessment focuses on the intrapersonal and interpersonal functioning of the client.

▪ Psychosocial assessment is guided primarily by knowledge of the behavioral sciences and nursing.

▪ The intrapersonal assessment consists of a number of components—perception/self-concept, motivation, cognition, affect/mood, and temperament.

▪ The interpersonal assessment addresses the client's social responsiveness and includes information related to social roles, stressors, responses to stress, and coping strategies.

▪ The major approaches for conducting the intrapersonal/interpersonal assessment are interview and observation.

▪ When indicated, information from the nursing history and clinical appraisal may be supplemented by use of a test or scale to measure specific parameters of intrapersonal or interpersonal functioning.

▪ Data from the intrapersonal and interpersonal assessment should be analyzed and validated to formulate appropriate nursing diagnoses.

Practice Activities

1. Assess the self-concept of at least one child and one adult using interview questions (Table 12-13), drawings (for the child), and behavioral observations. What inferences can you draw on the basis of the information gathered?

2. Assess the spirituality of at least one adolescent, one middle-aged adult, and one older adult (see Table 12-15). Compare and contrast the information gathered. What inferences can you make?

3. Assess cognitive functioning of at least one child (see Table 12-17) and one adult (see Figure 12-6). Ask the same child and adult to explain the meaning of a metaphor ("Every cloud has a silver lining") and compare their responses.

4. Administer the Semantic Differential Scale for Assessing Feelings to a hospitalized adult client (Table 12-18). What conclusions can you draw on the basis of the client's responses?

5. Obtain a copy of one of the infant or child temperament questionnaires (see boxed insert, p. 373), and assess an infant's or child's temperament. What conclusions can you draw? What temperament assets and temperament risks did you identify?

6. Assess the roles held by at least one adult. Identify any role conflict, role ambiguity, or role strain experienced by the individual. What nursing diagnoses are indicated?

7. Conduct a self-assessment of recent changes in your life using the Social Readjustment Rating Scale (Table 12-26). How do you score? What are the implications for your future health?

8. Administer the Hospital Stress Rating Scale (Table 12-27) to a hospitalized adult. What stressors are identified? What strategies is the client using to cope with the stressors?

9. Ask a client to describe the last significant event in his or her life when coping with stress was an issue. What coping strategies did the client use? Differentiate between affective and problem-solving strategies (see Table 12-9). What inferences can you draw?

10. Conduct a complete intrapersonal/interpersonal assessment of at least one child and one adult. Record your findings. What nursing diagnoses (Table 12-28) are supported by the information?

Recommended Readings

Bruss, C.R. (1988). Nursing diagnosis of hopelessness. *Journal of Nursing and Mental Health Services, 26*(3), 28–31, 38–39.

Bunting, S.M. (1988). The concept of perception in selected nursing theories. *Nursing Science Quarterly, 1*(4), 168–174.

Chess, S., & Thomas, A. (1985). Temperamental differences: A critical concept in child health care. *Pediatric Nursing, 11*(3), 167–171.

Davis, T., & Jenson, L. (1988). Identifying depression in medical patients. *Image: Journal of Nursing Scholarship, 20*(4), 191–195.

Fagin, C.M. (1987). Stress: Implications for nursing research. *Image: Journal of Nursing Scholarship, 19*(1), 38–41.

Geach, B. (1987). Pain and coping. *Image: Journal of Nursing Scholarship, 19*(1), 12–15.

Gobel, B.H., & Donovan, M.I. (1987). Depression and anxiety. *Seminars in Oncology Nursing, 3*(4), 267–276.

Herth, K. (1990). Relationship of hope, coping styles, concurrent losses, and setting to grief resolution in the elderly widow(er). *Research in Nursing & Health, 13*, 109–117.

Hinds, P.S. (1984). Introducing a definition of "hope" through the use of grounded theory methodology. *Journal of Advanced Nursing, 9*, 357–362.

Manderino, M.A., & Bzdek, V.M. (1986). Mobilizing depressed clients: Cognitive nursing approaches. *Journal of Psychosocial Nursing, 24*(5), 23–28.

Panzarine, S. (1985). Coping: Conceptual and methodological issues. *Advances in Nursing Science, 7*(4), 49–57.

Stokes, S.A., & Gordon, S.E. (1988). Development of an instrument to measure stress in the older adult. *Nursing Research, 37*(1), 16–19.

References

Aaronson, L.S. (1989). Perceived and received support: Effects on health behavior during pregnancy. *Nursing Research, 38*, 4–9.

Avillo, L.J. (1978). Semantic differential scale for assessing patients' feelings. In *Instruments for measuring nursing practice and other health care variables* (Vol. 1, Health Manpower References, DHEW Publication No. HRA 78–83). Washington, DC: U.S. Government Printing Office.

Baldree, K.S., Murphy, S.P., & Powers, M.J. (1982). Stress identification and coping patterns in patients on hemodialysis. *Nursing Research, 31*, 109–111.

Barron, C.R. (1987). Women's causal explanations of divorce: Relationships to self-esteem and emotional distress. *Research in Nursing & Health, 10*, 345–353.

Bassuk, E.L. (1984). The homeless problem. *Scientific American, 251*(1), 40–45.

Brown, M.A. (1986). Social support, stress and health: A comparison of expectant mothers and fathers. *Nursing Research, 35*(2), 72–76.

Bunting, S.M. (1988). The concept of perception in selected nursing theories. *Nursing Science Quarterly, 1*, 168–174.

Buss, A.H., & Plemin, R.A. (1975). *A temperament theory of personality development.* New York: Wiley.

Carey, W.B. (1986). The difficult child. *Pediatrics in Review, 8*, 39–45.

Carey, W.B. (1990). Temperament differences in children. *Early Childhood Update, 6*(1), 1–3.

Carey, W.B., & McDevitt, S.C. (1978). Revision of the infant temperament questionnaire. *Pediatrics, 6*, 735–737.

Carson, V.B. (Ed.) (1989). *Spiritual dimensions of nursing practice.* Philadelphia: Saunders.

Chess, S., & Thomas, A. (1986). *Temperament in clinical practice.* New York: Guilford.

Doak, C.C., Doak, L.G., & Root, J.H. (1985). *Teaching patients with low literacy skills.* Philadelphia: Lippincott.

Fitts, W.H. (1965). *Tennessee Self-Concept Scale.* Nashville: Counselor Recording and Tests.

Fromm, E. (1968). *The revolution of hope.* New York: Bantam.

Herth, K. (1990). Relationship of hope, coping styles, concurrent losses, and setting to grief resolution in the elderly widow(er). *Research in Nursing & Health, 13*, 109–117.

Highfield, M.F., & Cason, C. (1983). Spiritual needs of patients: Are they recognized? *Cancer Nursing, 6*, 187–192.

Hirsch, E.D. (1987). *Cultural literacy.* Boston: Houghton Mifflin.

Holmes, T.H., & Rahe, R.H. (1967). The social readjustment rating scale. *Journal of Psychosomatic Research, 11*, 213–218.

Jalowiec, A., & Powers, M.J. (1981). Stress and coping in

hypertensive and emergency room patients. *Nursing Research, 30,* 10–15.

Jastak, J.F., & Jastak, S. (1978). *The Wide Range Achievement Test manual of instructions.* Wilmington, DE: Jastak.

Kalish, R.A. (1966). *The psychology of human behavior.* Belmont, CA: Wadsworth.

Kim, M.J., McFarland, G.K., & McLane, A.M. (1987). *Pocket guide to nursing diagnoses* (2nd ed.). St. Louis: Mosby.

Kozol, J. (1985). *Illiterate America.* New York: New American Library.

Lange, S.P. (1978). Hope. In C.E. Carlson & B. Blackwell (Eds.), *Behavioral concepts and nursing intervention* (pp. 171–190). Philadelphia, Lippincott.

Lynn, M.R. (1987). Projective techniques in research and practice. *Journal of Pediatric Nursing, 2*(2), 129–131.

Maslow, A.H. (1970). *Motivation and personality* (2nd ed.). New York: Harper & Row.

McGee, R.F. (1984). Hope: A factor influencing crisis resolution. *Advances in Nursing Science, 6,* 34–44.

Miller, J.F., & Powers, M.J. (1988). Development of an instrument to measure hope. *Nursing Research, 37,* 6–10.

Muhlenkamp, A.F., & Sayles, J.A. (1986). Self-esteem, social support, and positive health practices. *Nursing Research, 35,* 334–338.

Orsolotis, M., & Morphy, M. (1982). A depression algorithm for psychiatric emergencies. *Journal of Psychiatric Treatment and Evaluation, 4,* 135–137.

Peterson, E.A. (1985). The physical, the spiritual. Can you meet all of your patients needs? *Journal of Gerontological Nursing, 11,* 23–27.

Piers, E.V., & Harris, D.B. (1969). *Piers-Harris children's self-concept scale (The way I feel about myself).* Nashville: Counselor Recording and Tests.

Rahe, R.H., & Arthur, R.J. (1978). Life change and illness studies: Past history and future directions. *Journal of Human Stress, 4,* 3–15.

Savitz, J., & Friedman, M.T. (1981). Diagnosing boredom and confusion. *Nursing Research, 30,* 18.

Selye, H. (1956). *The stress of life.* New York: McGraw-Hill.

Stedman, L., & Kaestle, C. (1987). Literacy and reading performance in the United States, from 1880 to the present. *Reading Research Quarterly, 22*(1), 48–52.

Stoll, R.I. (1989). The essence of spirituality. In V.B. Carson, (Ed.), *Spiritual dimensions of nursing practice* (pp. 4–23). Philadelphia: Saunders.

Stoner, M.H., & Keampfer, S.H. (1985). Recalled life expectancy information, phase of illness and hope in cancer patients. *Research in Nursing & Health, 8,* 269–274.

Stotland, E. (1969). *The psychology of hope.* San Francisco: Jossey-Bass.

Stuart, G., & Sundeen, S. (1991). *Principles and practice of psychiatric nursing* (4th ed.). St. Louis: Mosby.

Sullivan, H.S. (1953). *The interpersonal theory of psychiatry.* New York: Norton.

Thomas, A. & Chess, S. (1977). *Temperament and development.* New York: Brunner/Mazel.

Travelbee, J. (1971). *Interpersonal aspects of nursing* (2nd ed.). Philadelphia: Davis.

Utz, G.W., Hammer, J., Whitmire, V.M., & Grass, S. (1990). Perceptions of body image and health status in persons with mitral valve prolapse. *Image: Journal of Nursing Scholarship, 22*(1), 18–22.

Volicer, B.J., & Bohannon, M.W. (1975). A hospital stress rating scale. *Nursing Research, 24,* 352–359.

Walker, C.L. (1988). Stress and coping in siblings of childhood cancer patients. *Nursing Research, 37*(4), 208–212.

Westfall, U.E., Tanner, C.A., Putzier, D., & Padrick, K.P. (1986). Activating clinical inferences: A component of diagnostic reasoning in nursing. *Research in Nursing & Health, 9*(4), 269–277.

Zung, W.W.K. (1971). A rating instrument for anxiety disorders. *Psychosomatics, 12,* 371–379.

13

Sexuality Assessment

OBJECTIVES

Upon completion of this chapter, you should be
able to:

◼ Recognize your own level of comfort or discomfort with sexuality assessment, and explore
ways to resolve any discomfort.

◼ Describe human sexuality as a complex phenomenon with multiple dimensions.

◼ Delineate reasons the nurse should assess
sexuality as a routine part of a comprehensive
nursing assessment.

◼ Demonstrate a thorough understanding of the
knowledge needed to assess sexuality, including
sexual development across the life span, human
sexual response, cultural variables related to
sexuality, and the effect of changed health on
sexuality.

◼ Compare and contrast selected approaches to
obtaining the sexuality history.

◼ Obtain an appropriate sexuality history considering age, cultural background, and health of
clients.

◼ Examine the breasts of female and male
clients using correct inspection and palpation
techniques.

◼ Examine the external genitalia of male and
female clients, using the correct techniques for
inspection and palpation.

◼ Assess clients for their ability to examine their
own breasts or testes correctly.

◼ Formulate valid and appropriate nursing
diagnoses related to sexuality.

Human sexuality is complex and multidimensional. The World Health Organization (1975) defines healthy sexuality as the "integration of the somatic, emotional, intellectual, and social aspects of sexual being in ways that are positively enriching and that enhance personality, communication, and love" (p. 6). Thus, sexuality is an integral and essential part of life. It involves much more than the biological ability to have sexual intercourse or to reproduce. Sexuality influences our sense of self, our roles and relationships with others, our dress and manner, often our career choices, and our social behavior.

Sexual health is determined by numerous physiological, psychosocial, developmental, and cultural factors. Human sexuality encompasses sexual function, sexual self-concept, sexual adjustment, and sexual roles and relationships (Chapman & Sughrue, 1987; Woods, 1987).

Because sexuality is so important to physiological, mental, and social well-being, it is essential that sexuality be assessed as a routine part of a comprehensive nursing assessment, regardless of the client's age or health. There are several reasons the nurse should assess a client's sexual functioning and health.

Assessment of sexuality provides an opportunity to openly acknowledge the importance of sexuality to the client's general health and well-being. Such recognition reinforces for the client that sexuality is as important as other areas of health. This can encourage clients to gain self-awareness of sexual functioning, relationships, or self-concept and how they contribute to or interfere with general health and well-being.

Sexuality assessment also gives clients an opening to ask questions or share concerns and fears related to sexuality. Clients often are reluctant to raise concerns about sexuality because of embarrassment and social taboos. Incorporating sexuality assessment as a routine part of the nursing assessment gives clients "permission" to disclose their sexual concerns or fears and to ask questions about sexual functioning and health.

Another reason for assessing sexuality is to provide education appropriate to the client's specific needs. During the assessment, the nurse can capitalize on the opportunity by initiating discussion with the client about sexual anatomy and physiology, sexual function, normality of sexual practices, "safe sex" practices, and breast or testicular self-examination. For instance, during sexuality assessment of a teenager, the nurse may have an opportunity to explain the normality of mastur-

bation—that it causes neither mental nor physical disorders, but allows for safe release of sexual tensions.

Finally, sexuality assessment aids in detecting actual or potential problems in sexual functioning, sexual relationships, or sexual self-concept. Early identification of such problems enables appropriate planning and intervention to restore sexual health and well-being. Because problems in sexuality can influence a client's general health and well-being, and problems in other areas of health can affect sexual health, it is essential that sexuality not be overlooked or dismissed as unimportant.

The nursing history and the clinical appraisal should include attention to the areas of human sexual development and response, sexual roles and relationships, cultural variables related to sexuality, and the impact of altered health on sexual well-being. The degree to which each is assessed with a particular client will depend on the reason for the nurse's contact with the client; the client's age, culture, health, and particular concerns; and the rapport between nurse and client.

KNOWLEDGE NEEDED TO ASSESS SEXUALITY

In order to assess sexuality, the nurse must have an adequate understanding of human sexual development throughout life, human sexual response, cultural variables that affect sexuality, and the impact of alterations in health on sexual development and expression. These dimensions of human sexuality are intimately connected to and influence each other. For example, sex role socialization is influenced strongly by cultural variables that, in turn, influence human sexual response and responsiveness. Physical disability, such as severe cerebral palsy or spinal cord injury, may interfere with the expression of the physiological aspects of sexuality in the affected individual. Alcohol, drugs, and certain medications can interfere with human sexual response, as can chronic illness, such as diabetes mellitus and renal dialysis.

Human Sexual Development Across the Life Span

Human sexual development is a complex process that begins at the moment of conception when chromosomal pairing for a male or female is established. Sexuality continues to develop and change throughout life in response to a host of physiological, psychosocial, and cultural factors. Table 13-1 provides a summary of the development of sexual

TABLE 13-1
Sexual Function, Sexual Self-Concept, and Sexual Relationships Across the Life Span

	Sexual Function	Sexual Self-Concept	Sexual Role/Relationship
Infancy	Orgasmic potential present Erectile function present	Gender identity reinforced Association of sexuality and good/bad Distinction between self and others	
Childhood	Genital pleasuring and exploration Sensual activity (e.g., hugging)	Core gender identity solidified (by age 3)	Sex role differences learned Discrimination between male and female role models Sexual vocabulary learned
Preschool	Sex play—exploration of own body and those of playmates Self-pleasuring (masturbation)		Sex roles learned Parental attachment and identification
School-age		Curiosity about sex Sexual fears and fantasies Interest in aspects of sexual development Self awareness as sexual being	Same sex friends
Adolescent, pre-pubertal	Menarche Seminal emissions	Concerns about body image	Same sex friends Sexual experiences as part of friendship
Early adolescence	Awkwardness in first sexual encounter (50% not sexually active) Masturbation, petting	Sexual thoughts, fantasies Anxiety over inadequacy, lack of partner, virginity	Appropriate sex friendships Dating
Late adolescence	May or may not be sexually active	Responsibility for sexual activity	Intimacy in relationships learned Sex role behaviors, life styles explored
Young adult	Experimentation with sexual positions, expression Exploration of techniques	Responsibility for sexual health, e.g., contraception, sexually transmitted disease prevention Development of adult sexual value system, tolerance for others	Giving and receiving pleasure learned Long-term commitment to relationship developed
Middle adult	Adaptation to altered sexual function, e.g., vaginal dryness of menopause, slower erections	Accept body image changes related to aging	Adjustment of relationship as roles change
Late adults	More gradual sexual function	Accept slowed sexual response cycle without ending sexual aspects of relationship	New ways of sharing sexual pleasure and intimacy developed Adaptation to loss or illness of partner

Note. From Woods, N.F. (1987). Toward a holistic perspective of human sexuality: Alterations in sexual health and nursing diagnoses. Reprinted from *Holistic Nursing Practice*, Vol. 1, No. 4, p. 4, with permission of Aspen Publishers, Inc., © 1987.

function, sexual self-concept, and sexual roles and relationships across the life span.

Infancy and Childhood

Numerous events in infancy influence the development of sexuality, such as choice of name, room decor, toy and clothing selections, and parental interactions with their new infant. Lamb (1986) notes that parents interact very differently with girls than with boys. For instance, girls are spoken to more softly, held more gently, and touched more frequently than boys. There are differences between parental responses to infants as well. Mothers are usually more directly involved in caretaking (changing, feeding, dressing), while fathers play more with their infants (Lamb, 1986).

The quality and quantity of sensory stimulation, especially touching through hugging, kissing, stroking, and cuddling, play a major role in the development of sensuality in the infant and toddler, which relates directly to the capacity for sexual expression in later years. Infants and early toddlers typically fondle their genitals and other parts of their bodies. Toddlers become more knowledgeable about and aware of their bodies as they learn to point to and name body parts. They also begin to learn what is acceptable and unacceptable social behavior related to sexuality. For instance, young children typically are taught to keep their clothes on and not to play with their genitals in public.

During the preschool years, the first cognitive understanding of gender differences emerges. This understanding is based on the child's observation of anatomical differences, which marks the beginning of personal sexual identity. At this age, however, maleness/femaleness is perceptual: If a person has male characteristics (dress, voice tone, hair length), the person is perceived as a boy regardless of biological gender.

As children grow, they develop and refine their understanding of sex role distinctions through play, adult modeling, and explicit socialization by the particular cultural group or subgroup (for example, "Big boys don't cry" or "Little ladies shouldn't behave that way"). Rigid gender distinctions are disappearing in Western cultures as particular role behaviors, styles of dress, and occupational choices have become androgynous (not distinctly masculine or feminine) (Woods, 1987). However, many forces continue to reinforce sex role stereotyping, not the least of which are media depictions of traditional male and female roles, and practices in the work environment that continue to relegate women to positions of low status, power, and pay. Bem (1985) suggests that while androgyny appears to be a de-

sirable quality and one that is usually associated with a mentally healthy person, the idea of sexual differences can be very helpful to young children in organizing their social world and minimizing confusion about sex roles.

The development of gender identity, an awareness that one is female, male, or ambivalent, parallels the cognitive development of a sense of self as a distinct human being. Gender identity is a significant part of a child's self-esteem (Coopersmith, 1967) and is well established by age six. The child's anatomy, social experiences, and cues from parents and significant others contribute to the child's sense of self as a boy or girl.

In middle to later childhood there is clear-cut, almost stereotypical male–female role distinction. Boys and girls at this age tend to separate for social activities, such as parties or school recess. Other influences on sexual development in middle childhood include interactions with teachers, the media (television, movies, music), and sex education. For example, most elementary school teachers are women and most principals are men, which transmits certain expectations about appropriate male–female roles. Additionally, teachers have been noted to act differently with boys and girls; boys are disciplined more frequently than girls, even for similar behaviors (Sadker & Sadker, 1985). The mass media play a major role in transmitting information and values about sexuality, including sexual activity, physical appearance, sexual orientation and lifestyles, role distinctions, reproduction, and sexual morality (Meyrowitz, 1985). Sex education classes in school and parent and peer views of sex and sexuality also are instrumental in shaping the school-age child's sexual knowledge and values.

Adolescence

The development of a sense of identity, so important to the adolescent, cannot be separated from sexuality. Puberty brings about dramatic changes in anatomical and physiological functioning that are intimately related to the developing sexual self. The adolescent's body begins this metamorphosis between the ages of 9 and 11 for girls, and between 12 and 14 for boys (see chap. 23).

It is important to note that there is a wide range in the rate of pubertal development. Livson and Peskin (1980) have studied the particular problems faced by early and late maturing adolescents. Early maturing girls and late maturing boys are especially vulnerable, although early maturation in girls has fewer permanent effects than late maturation in boys. Late maturing boys tend to have a lower self-concept and more anxiety than their peers and as adults are less likely to have leadership positions and more likely to express feelings of rejection and inferiority.

The adolescent's choice of friends exerts a profound influence on sexual identity. Adolescents constantly compare their bodies and physical attractiveness with their peers. Adolescents tend to feel anxious about their sexual attractiveness and adequacy (knowing what to do and how to do it) and typically are awkward in their early sexual encounters. Teenagers are subjected to constant peer pressure, whether explicit or subtle, and often make sexual choices in response (Leppink, 1979). Friends are seen as credible sources of sexual information. Adolescents continually are confronted with the conflict between sexual impulses and sexual responsibility, yet they have an unrealistic notion of the consequences of risk-taking behaviors, which may lead to sexual activity without contraception (Sachs, 1986).

Yoos (1987) points out that the characteristics of adolescents' cognitive thought processes interfere with the ability to make rational decisions about sexual practices, including whether to become sexually active and to use birth control or disease prevention methods. Yoos's review of the literature reveals the following characteristics: lack of knowledge or inaccurate knowledge about sexual physiology and reproduction, misperceptions about their vulnerability to pregnancy or disease, inability to anticipate consequences or think about alternatives, feelings of omnipotence (i.e., "It can't happen to me"), and inability to understand probability. Conflicting messages about sexuality presented by the media, parents, and professionals add to these problems.

The first sexual experiences with a partner typically occur in early adolescence and may or may not progress to sexual intercourse. The American Public Health Association (1985) estimates that two-thirds of adolescents will have engaged in sexual intercourse by age 20. Moore and Erickson (1985) studied sexual knowledge, attitudes, and behaviors among adolescents and young adults from four ethnic groups: whites, blacks, Hispanics, and Asians. They found that 59% of the subjects age 16 to 19 had had sexual intercourse, with males in all groups initiating sex at a younger age than females. Blacks and Hispanics became sexually active at a younger age than whites or Asians, while blacks (81%) and whites (79%) had a higher percentage overall of sexually active subjects than Hispanics (61%) or Asians (36%). Hispanics and blacks were at greater risk of teenage pregnancy be-

cause of infrequent contraceptive use and the young age at which they became sexually active.

The numerous converging components of socialization have a dramatic effect on adolescent sexuality. How an adolescent responds to the many forces shaping sexual self-concept and behavior depends on relationships with parents, peers, and other significant people. As adolescence nears an end, the emerging young adult has a complex perception of human sexuality, and the potential for greater understanding, less fear, and more responsible sexual decision-making and behavior.

Adulthood

Adult sexuality has been the topic of much study, from the early research of Kinsey and colleagues (1948; 1953) and Masters and Johnson (1966) to the more recent work of sociologists, psychologists, and nurses (Bernhard & Dan, 1986; Huston, 1985; Weg, 1983; Woods, 1987). It is beyond the scope of this chapter to focus on the wide variety of issues related to adult sexuality. Instead, the continuing evolution of sexual identity and sex role behavior is emphasized, as well as the impact of aging.

Given their early social experiences, men typically emerge from adolescence with more confidence and independence in sexuality than women. This behavior occurs in response to social expectations that men must be strong and protective and demonstrate mastery in their lives (Livson, 1983). Women, on the other hand, are socialized to be more communal, in preparation for motherhood and the traditional duties of home management. While economic and social changes have forced a reexamination of masculine and feminine sex role behaviors, recent studies indicate that many traditional male–female roles still prevail (Barnett & Baruch, 1987; Huston, 1985). Livson (1983) suggests that traditional gender roles may delay the development of a sense of identity for women well into the adult years, and that it isn't until midlife, when parenting is no longer a significant factor, that women fully realize their worth and autonomy. By contrast, men are socialized to understand their worth and "selfhood" much earlier in life. These differences can have profound effects on adult sex role development and behavior.

As men and women move through midlife, however, there is a convergence of sexual identity (Gutman, 1985). There tends to be greater flexibility in sex roles and behaviors, as well as changes in perception of sexuality. With changing physical ability, men become less rigid in their sex roles and more affiliative, while women exhibit greater independence and self-assurance. The all-encompass-ing duties of parenthood may reduce sexual activity and have an impact on merging sex roles (Gutman, 1985).

Despite increased experience and experimentation with sex, many adults lack adequate or accurate knowledge of male and female sexual anatomy, human sexual response, reproduction, contraception, and sexually transmitted diseases (Masters, 1986). Misinformation and misunderstanding can influence sexual behavior and ultimately affect sexual health, whether physiologically, psychosocially, or both. For instance, the myth that withdrawal during intercourse is an effective method of contraception can lead to unwanted pregnancy. Lack of knowledge about the female sexual response can result in frustration during sex for both partners (Masters, 1986).

Older Adulthood

As adults age, they reevaluate their sexual identity and reexamine their sexual roles. In our youth-oriented society, many older adults become concerned about the physical changes associated with aging (see chap. 11) and about their sexual adequacy. Women tend to be more concerned with their physical appearance as they age, whereas men worry about sexual adequacy (Robinson, 1983). Most older adults are comfortable with their sex roles and activity. While there may be a decrease in frequency of sexual interest and activity with aging, there are wide variations among individuals, which should be considered when assessing sexuality in older adults.

Sexual activity among older adults generally is viewed more positively than in the past (Dressel & Avant, 1983). Dressel and Avant (1983) identify several themes that apply to sexuality in the later years:

1. With reasonable health and a partner, sexual relations are possible into the seventh, eighth, and ninth decades of life.

2. Sexual drive varies greatly from person to person and in one person from time to time.

3. Overall there is a pattern of decline in sexual interest with increasing age but sexuality holds a place of importance for most older people.

4. Sexual patterns tend to persist throughout a lifetime, with those who were most active in their younger years being most active in later years.

5. Maintenance of [sexual] capacity and activity are dependent upon opportunity for expression. (pp. 199–200)

Retirement and relief from financial and parenting burdens may bring renewed interest in sex.

In some cases, physiological changes actually enhance sexual enjoyment. For example, the older man needs a longer time to achieve an orgasm, thus creating more time for foreplay (Robinson, 1983).

The physiological changes that affect sexuality as people age alter sexual response for both men and women. The most notable physiological change associated with aging is menopause in women. The cessation of menses signals the end of the childbearing years, although the vast majority of women choose to relinquish their childbearing role at an earlier age with the assistance of effective contraceptives. Although no single event characterizes changing sexuality in men, men do experience significant physiological changes that may affect their sexual functioning, as well as their sexual self-concept and relationships.

Among women, the mean age for menopause is 50. Menopause is considered definitive after one year of amenorrhea. Changes that occur during the perimenopausal period include decreased frequency of menstrual periods, increased variability in the menstrual cycle, and a gradual decline in the duration and intensity of sexual response. Less estrogen is produced by the ovaries, which results in atrophic changes in the internal and external genitalia, lessened elasticity of pelvic and vaginal tissues, vaginal dryness, and the "hot flashes" experienced by nearly three-fourths of all perimenopausal women.

As they age, men also experience atrophic changes in the genitalia, including reduced testicular volume, decreased spermatogenesis, and delay in achieving erection and ejaculation. These changes sometimes are referred to as "male menopause." Impotence in men is more likely to result from psychosocial stressors, chronic illness, or drug therapy than from the physiological changes of aging. These changes also may affect the desire for sexual activity. Table 13-2 summarizes the normal sexual changes associated with aging.

In addition to physiological changes that affect sexuality in the later years, a number of other factors can influence sexual health and well-being. The loss of a sexual partner through death or debilitating illness can mean lost opportunity for sexual expression with another. Role changes resulting from retirement or illness can affect self-esteem and, therefore, sexual desire and responsiveness. Changes in living arrangements may inhibit opportunities for sexual expression. The move to a retirement home or convalescent facility without a private bedroom and with unpredictable interruptions by staff prohibits the privacy that Western culture deems essential for sex.

TABLE 13-2
Sexual Changes Associated with Aging

Male	Female
Desire—average frequency of sexual activity decreases with advancing age	*Desire*—varies, but may increase owing to relative stability of androgens while estrogens decrease
Serum testosterone gradually decreases	
Excitement phase—	*Excitement phase*— decreased estrogen
Increase in time to attain full penile erection	Decreased vaginal lubrication
Decrease in vasocongestion of scrotum	Atrophy and friability of vagina
	Decreased acidity of vaginal secretions; increased vaginal infections
	Decreased vaginal elasticity
Plateau phase—	*Plateau phase*—decreased general muscle tension with arousal
Increased ejaculatory control	Decreased uterine elevation
Decreased firmness or fullness of erection	Decreased labial elevation
Decreased seminal fluid volume	Decreased clitoral size
Decreased warning of inevitability of ejaculation	
Orgasmic phase—	*Orgasmic phase*—
Ejaculation less powerful	Decreased duration of orgasm, though still capable of multiple orgasm
Resolution phase—	*Resolution phase*—
Occurs more quickly	Occurs more quickly
Refractory period is prolonged	

Note. Adapted from *Topics in Clinical Nursing*, Vol. 3, No. 1, pp. 59–70, with permission of Aspen Publishers, Inc., © 1981.

The older adult's adjustment to physiological and psychosocial changes that affect sexual self-concept and sexual activity depends on a variety of factors, such as a supportive partner, opportunities for privacy, and willingness to experiment with ways other than intercourse to express sexuality and experience sensual pleasure. Assessment of sexuality in the older adult should include attention to the many factors that influence sexual self-concept, roles and relationships, and sexual function and activity.

Human Sexual Response

Masters and Johnson (1966) were the first researchers to study definitively the physiology of human sexual response. Their work provided the first scientific explanations of sexual physiology in both men and women during sex. Specifically, Masters and Johnson defined the human sexual response cycle as consisting of four phases: *excitement, plateau, orgasm,* and *resolution.*

The excitement phase occurs in response to sexual arousal and is manifested by vasocongestion and muscle tension throughout the body. This phase may last a few minutes to several hours. If sexual stimulation continues, the plateau phase ensues. The result is engorgement of genital blood vessels and increased muscle tension, with this phase lasting 30 seconds to 3 minutes. The orgas-

mic phase follows, characterized by an involuntary release of muscle tension through a sequence of contractions that last 3 to 15 seconds. The last phase, the resolution phase, is manifested by gradual dissipation of remaining vasocongestion and muscle tension. The length of the resolution phase depends on whether orgasm occurred, lasting much longer if it did not. During the resolution phase, women are capable of being restimulated to orgasm, whereas most men need a refractory period before they can be stimulated to orgasm again.

Masters and Johnson (1966) and Kaplan (1979) identify several common sexual dysfunctions and difficulties. These range from difficulty with achieving or maintaining an erection to inability to reach orgasm in females to sexual disinterest. Common sexual problems during the various phases of the human sexual response cycle are summarized in Table 13-3.

Cultural Variables Related to Sexuality

Human sexual development, while directed by maturational forces, is also a social and cultural process. Sexual behavior and sex role differentiation are affected continually by cultural and subcultural cues and conditioning. Acceptable sexual behavior varies from culture to culture and from generation to generation. What may be acceptable

TABLE 13-3
Common Sexual Dysfunctions and Difficulties

Dysfunctions	Difficulties
Women:	*Men and Women:*
Difficulty with sexual arousal	Partner chooses inconvenient time
Difficulty maintaining sexual excitement	Dissatisfaction with frequency (too much or too little)
Difficulty in reaching orgasm	Inability to relax
Inability to reach an orgasm	Attraction to person other than mate
Dyspareunia (difficult or painful vaginal intercourse)	Disinterest
Vaginismus (vaginal wall muscle spasms making penetration difficult or impossible)	Attraction to person of same sex
Inadequate vaginal lubrication	Different sexual practices or habits
	Value conflicts related to different sexual practices or habits
Men:	Too little foreplay before intercourse
Difficulty getting an erection	Too little "tenderness" after intercourse
Difficulty maintaining an erection	
Ejaculating too quickly	
Difficulty in ejaculating	
Inability to ejaculate	

Note. Adapted from Chapman, J., & Sughrue, J. (1987). A model of sexual assessment and intervention. *Health Care for Women International, 8,* 89.

within a particular generation may conflict with cultural mores. For example, unmarried teenagers who are sexually active risk disapproval of the larger cultural group.

Caplan (1987) identifies commonly held values related to sexuality in Western cultures:

1) sexual desire is a basic urge, drive, or instinct that "demands" release,

2) there are clear male–female differences in the expression and satisfaction of the sex drive,

3) "sex" is equated with intercourse,

4) "normal" sexual expression is heterosexual,

5) pleasurable sex is just as acceptable as reproductive sex,

6) legitimate outlets for sex are necessary for optimal mental health, and

7) sexual mastery is a part of the developmental process.

These values reflect middle, upper middle, and upper socioeconomic norms that are well established in Western educational and political institutions. However, while there is general agreement within Western culture about acceptable and unacceptable sexual roles, behaviors and practices, there is wide variability among specific cultural and subcultural groups (Caplan, 1987). For instance, there is greater acceptance of early adolescent sexual activity among lower socioeconomic groups than upper middle income groups. Religious and moral values play a major role in shaping sex role behavior. There tends to be greater

male–female sex role differentiation within groups that hold strong, traditional religious values, such as Hispanic Catholics, Southern Baptists, or Islamic Arabs. Thus, assessment of culture and, in particular, cultural values and norms related to sexual roles and practices, should be an essential part of a comprehensive nursing assessment.

Sexuality and Health

As noted earlier, sexuality and health are reciprocal. Alterations in sexuality, such as a poor sexual self-concept, conflicts in sexual relationships, or sexual dysfunctions can affect adversely a person's health and well-being, leading to such mental health disturbances as depression, anxiety, and alcoholism. Conversely, alterations in general health, such as alcoholism, depression, situational stressors, chronic illness, loss of a body part (e.g., mastectomy or limb amputation) or medications, can affect the expression of sexuality.

One of the challenges of sexuality assessment is to determine whether a complaint is a sexual problem or symptom of some other problem (Woods, 1984). Is a client depressed because sexual desire is decreased, or is the decrease in desire the result of depression?

Alterations in sexuality include problems of sexual self-concept, sexual relationships, and sexual dysfunction. These problems may be primary or may be the result of underlying health problems. Health problems that interfere with sexuality may involve anatomical disruptions or physiological alterations. Such alterations may or may not be reversible, and the associated sexual dysfunctions may be temporary or permanent. Although health changes need not produce sexual dysfunction, they may if the sexual concern or problem is not identified and treated. For example, men who have suffered a myocardial infarction are often fearful about resuming sexual intercourse. Failure to identify such a concern may lead to problems in sexual function and self-concept, as well as sexual roles and relationships.

Nearly any type of health problem has the potential to interfere with sexuality. Some problems result in primary sexual dysfunction, whereas others interfere with sexual self-concept and sexual relationships, leading to secondary sexual dysfunction. Examples of common health problems or developmental experiences that can interfere with sexual response, sexual self-concept, or sexual roles and relationships are summarized in Table 13-4.

Pharmacological agents—prescribed, over-the-counter, or recreational—also can affect sexuality, either positively or adversely. Antihypertensives interfere with innervation of the genitals and thus may inhibit sexual desire and responsiveness. Nic-

otine, which causes vasoconstriction, may reduce blood flow to the sex organs and interfere with erections. Codeine and other opiates depress the central nervous system and, while they may reduce sexual inhibitions, they also decrease sexual desire and may cause impotence. Small amounts of alcohol temporarily enhance sexual arousal, but large amounts can lead to impotence or premature ejaculation. Some drugs may cause permanent interferences with the human sexual response cycle: cocaine, high doses of sedatives or hypnotics, corticosteriods, and antiandrogenic hormone preparations.

Sexually transmitted diseases (STDs) can disrupt sexual functioning and affect sexual self-concept and relationships. STDs such as herpes or vaginal infections can cause pain with intercourse. The stigma and embarrassment associated with having a sexually transmitted disease can have an adverse effect on a person's self-concept and cause reluctance or fear of engaging in sexual relationships. Fear of acquired immune deficiency syndrome (AIDS) and its increasing incidence in the population also may have an adverse effect on a client's sexual relationships: the selection and frequency of sexual partners, willingness to trust the

---

TABLE 13-4
Examples of Health Problems That Can Interfere with Sexuality

Congenital Anomalies of the Genitalia
  Adrenogenital syndrome
  Hypospadius, epispadius
  Congenital absence of the vagina or penis

Developmental Disabilities
  Mental retardation
  Cerebral palsy
  Spina bifida

Musculoskeletal and Degenerative Disorders
  Herniated disc
  Arthritis
  Multiple sclerosis
  Muscular dystrophy
  Myasthenia gravis

Metabolic and Cardiovascular Disorders
  Diabetes mellitus
  Addison's disease
  Cushing's disease
  Cerebral vascular accident (stroke)
  Myocardial infarction
  Cardiac surgery

Infectious Disease
  Sexually transmitted infections of the female and
    male genitourinary tracts
  Acquired immune deficiency syndrome (AIDS)

Trauma (physical, psychological, sexual)
  Spinal cord injury
  Disfigurement (burns, scarring)
  Obstetric trauma; poor episiotomy
  Rape, sexual assault
  Child sexual abuse, incest
  Battering, spouse abuse

Body Image or Sexual Self-Concept Alterations
  Obesity
  Anorexia nervosa
  Breast size (too small, too large, inverted nipples)
  Mastectomy
  Limb amputation
  Ostomies (ileostomy, colostomy)
  Hysterectomy
  Total pelvic exoneration
  Orchiectomy
  Transsexualism

Cancer and Cancer Therapies (radiation, chemotherapy)

partner, and specific sexual practices (e.g., use of condoms, avoiding anal intercourse, or abstinence).

It is important to recognize that different people respond differently to problems related to their sexuality. Their responses depend on the nature of the problem, their usual pattern of coping, the extent of the change (in health or sexuality or both), and the value they attach to the change. Interferences with sexuality may be particularly difficult during vulnerable developmental phases, such as adolescence or retirement, or during situational crises, such as death of a partner or loss of a body part due to surgery or trauma. Other factors that affect an individual's response to alterations in sexuality are the abruptness of the change and whether it is reversible.

In the following two situations, consider the variables that are likely to affect the person's sexuality:

Client A is a 19-year-old male college sophomore. Three weeks ago, he suffered a severe spinal cord injury that resulted in permanent paralysis. The nursing history reveals the client has been sexually active ("I've made it with a lot of chicks") since age 15; he has been withdrawn and depressed the past 4 days.

Client B is a 53-year-old woman hospitalized for an elective hysterectomy for extensive uterine fibroids. She tells the nurse, "I'm glad to be getting rid of this problem once and for all."

In the first situation, the client has suffered a major change in health. The injury was sudden and is irreversible. The value the client places on his sexual ability is likely to be high, and the injury has resulted in a permanent physiological sexual dysfunction with profound psychological and social consequences. In addition, he is making a transition from adolescence to young adulthood, a time when sexuality assumes major importance. On the other hand, Client B has had time to prepare herself psychologically for loss of her reproductive organs. She is past her childbearing years and has expressed a desire to have the operation. Also, she will have no lasting health impairment that will interfere with her ability to resume an active sex life. The nurse should keep in mind that reintegration following a sexual disruption will be gradual, and the client first must mourn the loss.

Nursing assessment of sexuality should incorporate all the dimensions discussed above—human sexual development, sexual function, sexual self-concept, and sexual roles and relationships. These dimensions should be considered in the context of the client's cultural background, values, and life experiences and also should take into account actual or potential health alterations that may interfere with sexuality. Because human sexuality is a sensitive area, specific approaches to assessing sexuality can be helpful in reducing discomfort and embarrassment for both client and nurse.

APPROACHES TO SEXUALITY ASSESSMENT

Unfortunately, age-old taboos surrounding sexual matters may cause anxiety on the part of either the nurse or the client and may interfere with assessing sexuality. In particular, the client may be vague in asking questions or voicing concerns, and the nurse may be equally vague in phrasing questions related to sexuality and in providing sexual information. The level of anxiety will, of course, depend on a number of factors, such as the nurse's and client's ages, their own life and sexual experiences, cultural backgrounds, religious beliefs, and so forth. Additionally, mutual retreat may occur in the nurse–client relationship because either nurse or client feels uncomfortable. To minimize nurse–client anxiety and to promote an environment conducive to discussing sexuality, several principles should be considered.

The nurse's comfort with sexuality assessment is of primary importance. "Comfort" presumes that nurses are aware of their feelings regarding their own sexuality, sexual identity, and sex role behavior *and* find them acceptable. Nurses who feel uncomfortable asking clients about sexuality or handling clients' questions about or expressions of sexuality should work to overcome their inhibitions. A college course in human sexuality, reading, discussion groups, and individual counseling are some ways to help lessen discomfort with this important human dimension.

Nurses should examine their own beliefs and value systems in order to accept those who differ. It is essential that the nurse maintain a neutral attitude toward the client's expressions of sexuality. One way to avoid being judgmental is by using appropriate words. For example, the nurse should couch questions or comments in terms of sexual relationships, partners, or experiences without using such words as "promiscuous" or "unfaithful."

While a nonjudgmental attitude is important, so is responding genuinely. The nurse whose beliefs conflict with the client's behaviors or beliefs can use the reaction constructively instead of responding in a value-laden way. For example, if the nurse disapproves of a client's negative feelings about touching herself while inserting a diaphragm, chastising the client or minimizing her feelings will be less effective than exploring and discussing them to help the client arrive at a decision about birth control. In addition, avoiding either over- or underreactions is important. Underreactions tend to convey lack of concern; overreactions reflect intolerance of others. Combining a neutral attitude with genuine responses conveys trust, acceptance, and respect for the client.

Yet another factor in minimizing nurse–client anxiety is the nurse's own education. Current information about human sexuality and sexual functioning is vital. Nursing education programs often provide only basic information, and the nurse may need to seek out formal academic courses, workshops, readings, or other resources to achieve adequate grounding in human sexuality. Nurses must be aware of their limitations and should seek not only to improve their skills but know when to refer the client to other professionals. Typically, the professional nurse may not possess adequate knowledge or experience to address the client's sexuality needs, particularly if the client is experiencing problems related to sexual function or sexual relationships. The assessment roles that the nurse may assume and the professional competence required are summarized in Table 13-5.

Establishing a conducive environment includes providing privacy and assuring confidentiality. Moreover, providing a casual setting, one with equal status seating, may help overcome social inhibitions for a discussion of sexuality.

A number of communication skills also may encourage nurse–client rapport (see chap. 2). The following guidelines are especially important to consider when conducting the sexuality assessment:

Bring the subject up as part of the overall health assessment so that the client realizes sexuality is a legitimate health issue. Do not wait until the physical assessment, when the client is undressed and vulnerable.

Be sensitive to nonverbal behavior. For example, an individual may deny sexual concerns yet display contradictory body language. Signs of discomfort may include a defensive posture with arms and legs crossed, eyes averted, and fidgety hands.

If clients seem uncomfortable with questions, the nurse may *acknowledge their apparent discomfort* and suggest discussion at a later time.

Organize questions and the examination pertaining to sexuality as a sequential part of the total assessment: They should follow logically from the obstetric-gynecological–menstrual history and examination in women and the genitourinary system history and examination in men.

Use "bilateral" language. A nurse should not presuppose meanings and should clarify and summarize the client's terminology. Paraphrasing and summarizing offer the nurse an opportunity to teach an appropriate vocabulary that may help nurse and client discuss their concerns more comfortably. The nurse, of course, must know sexual terminology, from the vernacular to the scientific, and may need to practice using the terms to be comfortable during the nurse–client interview. For example, a woman may complain of a discharge from her "bottom." The nurse should clarify whether this refers to urethral, vaginal, or rectal discharge. Table 13-6 compares formal and slang expressions for some sexual terms. In addition, maintaining a sense of humor about sexual words may help decrease tension. In response to a new word or phrase, the nurse might say, "I haven't

TABLE 13-5
A Model for Assessing Sexuality

	Professional Competence Required	Levels of Assessment
Level 1	Professional nurse	Health history: screen for sexual concerns, functions, and dysfunctions
Level 2	Experienced professional nurse or one postgraduate course in human sexuality	Complete sexuality history
Level 3	Professional nurse, physician, psychologist, social worker—certified as sex therapists	Sexual problem history
Level 4	Masters or doctorally prepared psychiatric nurse clinician, physician, psychologist, social worker—with intensive specialization in sex therapy	Detailed psychiatric and psychosexual history

There is a linear relationship between the depth of a client's sexual problem and the kind of professional competence that is needed to assess and treat it.

Note. Adapted from Watts, R.J. (1979). Dimensions of sexual health. *American Journal of Nursing, 79,* 1570.

heard that phrase (word) before! Could you explain what you mean?"

Progress from less sensitive topics to more sensitive areas. This technique also is helpful in reducing anxiety. For example, one might discuss nocturnal emissions with men and menstruation with women before proceeding to a discussion of masturbation or intercourse.

Use the techniques of universality, ubiquity, and unloading. These terms refer to the following approaches:

Universality—"Many people experience. . . ."
Ubiquity—"How or when did you begin. . . ."
Unloading—"Some people have this experience, others not at all, and others rarely. . . ."

Additional measures may include the following:

Use of silence. A nurse who is uncomfortable with the topic may find this technique difficult. Sometimes one must deliberately pause and await the client's response to allow adequate time for thinking through feelings and thoughts. Using silence becomes easier with practice.

Use of open-ended questions and a matter-of-fact approach, with emphasis on acceptable behavior. For example, while interviewing a pregnant woman, the nurse might say, "Many women find that their sexual drives and those of their partners change during pregnancy. What has your experience been?"

Ascertaining the client's "ideal" rather than real experiences. If the nurse asks, "What kind of mother would you like to be?" the client can describe first the ideal, then the real. The nurse then can ascertain discrepancies in role expectations.

"Reviewing" information with the client as a colleague. The nurse may avoid a patronizing attitude by using the approach, "You may remember . . ." rather than, "This is how it is. . . ."

TABLE 13-6
Slang Expressions for Sexual Terms

Formal Term	Slang Expressions
Breasts	Tits, sacks, front, headlights, knockers, boobs, bonkers, bust, jugs, buds, hooters, bodacious ta-tas
Climax	Come, go off, shoot, cream, blast off; the clouds and the rain (Asian)
Clitoris	Bad fellow, little gem, gaiety, narrow strip
Cunnilingus	Eating it, going down, eating pussy
Erection	Hard on, stiff, bone, boner, hot rocks, lover's nuts
Fellatio	Going down, sucking, blowing, getting a blow job, giving head, cocksucking
Homosexual	Fairy, fag, faggot, gay, queen, nellie, homo, swish, pervert, pansy, lez, sister, lesbo, dyke, bull dyke
Hymen	Cherry, membrane, maidenhead
Impotence	Couldn't get it up, couldn't get a hard on
Intercourse (Coitus)	Make love, screw, fuck, get down, ball, make it, get laid, boff, mess around, score, bang, jive, grig, get a piece, sleep with, get some tail; schtup (Yiddish)
Masturbation	Jack off, jerk off, pocket pod, hand fuck, circle jerk, beat the meat, hand job
Mutual Oral-Genital Stimulation	Sixty-nine, give head, go down on
Orgasm	Come, climax, get it, get a nut
Penis	Joystick, worm, dick, prick, stick, peter, rod, john, third leg, middle leg, joint, glans, cock, organ, thing; schmuck, putz (Yiddish); yang, steaming stalk (Asian)
Pubic Hair	Beaver, bush, pubes
Semen	Come, juice, egg white, cream
Sexual Choice	Straight (heterosexual), gay, lesbian (female homosexual), AC-DC (bisexual)
Testes	Balls, nuts, cojones
Vagina	Pussy, hole, cunt, cat, pocketbook, treasure, twat, furburger, box, beaver, snatch, tunnel; yin, jade gate, golden gulley (Asian)

Note. Adapted from *Human Sexuality: A Nursing Perspective*, by R. Hogan (Ed.). Copyright © 1980 by Appleton-Century-Crofts. Reprinted by permission.

Recording information during the sexuality assessment may be inhibiting, since the information often is of a sensitive nature. The nurse may have to learn to condense information and use abbreviations. Furthermore, it may be helpful to share with the client what is being written. Tape recordings may be used, with the client's consent, of course.

The nurse must be knowledgeable, approachable, and comfortable with sexuality in order to provide an atmosphere conducive to assessing sexuality. The sexuality assessment should include a sexuality history, clinical appraisal, and screening for particular problems, specifically breast and testicular masses.

THE SEXUALITY HISTORY

A sexuality history should be obtained routinely as part of the nursing history, not simply when a problem is suspected. Using a standard approach and practicing repeatedly will make the nurse more comfortable with the topic. The extent to which sexuality is assessed depends on the purpose of the health contact, the client's age and health, and the setting. For instance, a sexuality history is not an immediate priority for a client newly hospitalized with a myocardial infarction. But at some point during recovery and prior to discharge from the hospital, the nurse should obtain a sexuality history to help the client plan for resumption of sexual activities. For hospitalized patients who are less acutely ill, the sexuality history may follow logically from the admission interview when daily activities are being discussed. In the primary care setting, the usual approach is to include the sexuality history with the reproductive history for women and the elimination history for men. Asking questions chronologically often reduces anxiety. For example, it is usually less stressful to inquire about sex education, menarche, and first experiences with sex before moving to more sensitive areas.

The sexuality history should incorporate questions related to several areas: sexual physiology and development, sexual self-concept, including gender identity, sexual relationships, and sexual functioning and problems. The nurse should inquire about the client's practice of breast or testicular self-examination and, when appropriate, ascertain the client's menstrual, reproductive, and contraceptive history. The client also should be asked about the occurrence of sexually transmitted disease.

Modifications in the sexuality history will depend upon the client's age, cultural background, and health. For instance, the parent may have to provide information for a young child. A client whose cultural beliefs prohibit open discussion of sexuality may require greater time and sensitivity on the nurse's part. Or, the nurse may need to spend more time with a chronically ill client exploring how illness has influenced the client's sexuality.

Sexual Physiology and Development

It usually is easier and less embarrassing for the client to focus on sexual development and issues related to reproduction and contraception as a lead-in to the remainder of the sexuality history. Clients expect to be asked such questions because physical development, reproduction, and contraception are areas typically associated with health. The following information should be gathered:

- sexual development—age of onset of secondary sex characteristics; problems

- menstrual history—age of onset, frequency, duration; characteristics, such as flow, presence and severity of cramps, perimenstrual stress or tension; problems

- obstetric history—gravida, para; abortions or miscarriages, fertility problems, obstetric complications

- contraceptive history—type, duration of use, side effects; accuracy of knowledge about types and use

- history of vaginal or genitourinary infections; specific symptoms, how treated

- sexually transmitted diseases—type, when diagnosed, how treated, response to treatment; accuracy of knowledge, practices to prevent recurrence

- practice of breast or testicular self-examination—knowledge of correct technique; frequency, regularity of timing (same day each month or immediately following menstrual period); problems noted; history of breast cancer in family

- presence of symptoms associated with menopause, and client's responses to these changes.

These questions help set the stage for further inquiry related to sexuality and generally enhance the level of comfort for the nurse and the client in discussing more sensitive areas, including sexual self-concept, sexual relationships, and sexual functioning.

Sexual Self-Concept

Questions related to the client's knowledge of sex and sexuality, feelings of masculinity or femininity, and sex roles are important to include in the sexuality history. Lack of accurate or adequate knowledge about sex can place the client at risk for a number of problems, such as unwanted pregnancy, sexually transmitted disease, concerns about normality of sexual practices, or feelings of sexual inadequacy.

It is important to determine the client's perceptions of appropriate sex roles and sex role behaviors including feelings of satisfaction or dissatisfaction in achieving role expectations (whether his or her own or those of significant others, such as parents, spouse/partner, or peers). The nurse should, therefore, inquire about

- the client's sources of information about reproduction, contraception, STDs, and sexual practices

- adequacy and accuracy of client's knowledge (appropriate to client's age and context)

- client's satisfaction with self as a man or a woman

- client's perception of sex roles and level of comfort or satisfaction in fulfilling sex role expectations (those of self and others)

- past or current problems, such as illness, disability, or loss, that have influenced client's view of self as a sexual person.

Sexual Relationships

The client's sexual relationships are connected intimately to sexual self-concept. People who are comfortable with their sexual identity, knowledgeable about sexual functioning and practices, and satisfied with their sex roles typically enjoy satisfying sexual relationships. Problems in sexual relationships, however, may occur if there are problems in sexual self-concept or in other areas of relationships with sex partners. For example, clients who are experiencing discord related to life stresses, such as illness, financial problems, loss of employment, or parenting demands, also may experience problems in their sexual relationships. Thus, it is important to determine whether the client is experiencing problems in sexual relationships with others and, if so, what factors are contributing to these problems. This can help pinpoint whether the problem can be attributed primarily to the sexual relationship itself or whether problems in the sexual relationship are secondary to other stressors.

Sexual Functioning and Sexual Problems

Facilitating a client's disclosure about sexual functioning or sexual problems requires sensitivity and expertise and may not be an appropriate area for a routine sexuality history or one being obtained by a novice. Generally, an indirect approach is best because it places responsibility on the client to initiate the discussion. The following areas should be included when assessing or trying to identify problems in sexual functioning:

- client's satisfaction with or concerns about quality and frequency of past and current sexual functioning, including sexual response and normality of practices

- recent changes in interest or desire for sexual activity

- illness (acute or chronic), disfigurement, or disability that may affect the client's desire or ability for sexual expression

- use of medications, alcohol, or recreational drugs—effects on sexual desire and functioning

- past history of problems that may affect sexual functioning, such as sexual abuse as a child or sexual assault (rape)

- specific problems the client is experiencing in sexual functioning, such as difficulty maintaining an erection, difficulty achieving orgasm, lack of desire, or pain.

It is especially important to conclude the sexuality history, however brief it may be, with an open-ended question, such as "What other concerns or questions about sexuality do you have?" If a specific problem is identified by the client, the nurse should ask the client to describe the problem, including onset, duration, the client's perception of the cause, interventions (self-help or other), and outcomes, as well as the client's expectations for intervention. Some situations, such as sexual abuse of a child or rape, require immediate referral to an appropriate resource.

Table 13-7 summarizes the sexuality history and identifies key information that should be obtained.

Modifying the Sexuality History

The sexuality history should be modified or adapted so it is appropriate to the client's age. This is especially important for children, adolescents, and older adults, each of whom have unique needs related to sexuality.

Infancy and Childhood

Obviously, the newborn and very young child cannot answer questions; therefore, the parents usually are interviewed. Assessment at these ages usually is performed to determine whether the

TABLE 13-7
The Sexuality History

Sexual Physiology and Development (modify as appropriate for age, sex, and health)

Sexual development—age of onset of secondary sex characteristics; problems in sexual development

Menstrual history—age of onset, frequency, duration; characteristics, such as flow, presence and severity of cramps, perimenstrual stress or tension; problems

Obstetric history—gravida, para; abortions or miscarriages, fertility problems, obstetric complications

Contraceptive history—type, duration of use, side effects; accuracy of knowledge about types and use

Vaginal or genitourinary infections—specific symptoms, how treated

Sexually transmitted diseases—type, when diagnosed, treatment, response to treatment; accuracy of knowledge about the disease, practices to prevent recurrence

Practice of breast or testicular self-examination—knowledge of correct technique; frequency, regularity of timing, problems noted; history of breast cancer in family

Menopause—symptoms; responses to changes in sexuality associated with aging

Sexual Self-Concept

Source(s) of information about reproduction, contraception, sexual practices, risks (e.g., STDs, pregnancy)

Knowledge about sex (appropriate to client's age and context)

Satisfaction with gender

Values and beliefs about sexuality; expressions of fear, confusion, or guilt about sexuality

Perceptions of sex roles; level of satisfaction with current sex roles (expectations of self and others)

Past or current problems, such as illness, disability, or loss, that influence client's sexual self-concept

Sexual Relationships

Sexual orientation (heterosexual, homosexual, bisexual)

Satisfaction with sexual orientation and sexual relationships

Current stressors or problems affecting sexual relationships

Sexual Functioning

Satisfaction with or concerns about quality and frequency of sexual functioning, including sexual response and normality of practices

Recent changes in interest or desire for sexual activity

Illness, disfigurement, or disability that may be affecting client's desire or ability for sexual expression

Use of medications, alcohol, or recreational drugs—effects on sexual desire and functioning

Past history of problems that may affect sexual functioning, such as sexual abuse as a child or sexual assault

Specific current problems in sexual functioning (lack of desire, impotence, etc.)—onset, duration, perception of cause, interventions (self-help or other), outcomes

Other Concerns or Questions About Sexuality (not covered above)

---

parents need to learn about infant hygiene, hormonal influence on breasts and genitalia at birth, and sex-typing of infants.

During childhood, parents often are concerned about sex education (reproductive aspects) and sexuality education (fears, feelings, and the responsibilities of sexuality). Some parents may desire information so they can provide sex education for their children, whereas others may delegate this responsibility to the school, the church, the nurse, or others. Therefore, it is pertinent to interview the parents about this need. Aquilino and Ely (1985) interviewed parents of preschoolers about their knowledge of preschool sexuality, how they would respond to common sexual behaviors of preschoolers (such as masturbation or curiosity), and their level of comfort in handling such situations. The researchers found that parents who were more knowledgeable also felt more comfortable with childhood sexuality, yet there was no significant re-

lationship between their knowledge and their response or between their response and their level of comfort. The authors conclude that parents need more than information about childhood sexuality: they need assistance in responding constructively to their children's expressions of sexuality. Aquilino and Ely (1985) suggest including assessment of parents' concerns about their child's sexuality as a natural part of the nursing history. Assessment often focuses on helping parents assess their children's knowledge of and need for sexuality education. Some areas to assess with parents include:

▪ parents' knowledge of childhood sexual development

▪ how parents respond to the child's questions about sex and reproduction; parents' level of comfort with providing sexual information to the child

▪ parents' observations of child's sexual activity (masturbation, exploration with other children); how parents respond to such activity

- concerns parents have about the child's relationship with friends or family members

- what assistance parents want to help them foster healthy sexuality in their child.

Adolescence

The adolescent sexual history involves more than obtaining a menstrual history and information about onset of secondary sex characteristics. It also should include assessment of sexual knowledge and activity. Peach (1980) suggests that the nurse should consider three points before asking about sexual activity in adolescent clients:

The adolescent's social activity: whether the teenager attends primarily same sex parties or goes to unchaperoned, mixed parties.

Whether the adolescent is homeless.

Whether the adolescent has been seen repeatedly for genitourinary infections.

According to Peach (1980), other issues the nurse must be aware of include knowledge of state laws regarding treatment of minors for sexually transmitted disease and birth control, the importance of genuineness and confidentiality, semantics (i.e., the importance of clarifying meanings with both adolescents and their parents), and awareness of the adolescent's cognitive development (i.e., is the adolescent a present-oriented, concrete thinker or an abstract, future-oriented thinker?).

When interviewing the adolescent or preadolescent, then, the nurse should collect information about sexual knowledge and activity. In addition, the adolescent (or parents, when appropriate) should be interviewed for information regarding menarche, nocturnal emissions, and the development of secondary sex characteristics, such as axillary and pubic hair, and breast development in young women.

Teenagers frequently need education about their body changes, especially menstruation and nocturnal emissions. Green (1979) suggests using the concepts of universality and normality when discussing these topics. For example, when discussing menstruation the nurse might say, "While growing up, we sometimes hear rumors or get no information regarding body changes that usually occur between eleven and fourteen, such as menstrual periods. What do you know about what to expect, what this means?" For adolescent males the nurse might say, "Many guys have dreams with sex in them and awaken to find their pajamas, underwear, or sheets stained or wet. Has this happened to you?"

In addition, adolescents may raise their own questions about sexuality. Referring them to their parents for information should be avoided, since this indicates the nurse is unwilling to discuss sexuality and may make the adolescent feel like a dependent child who requires parental permission to discuss sexual matters. However, it is important to ascertain whether adolescents are able to discuss sex openly and comfortably with their parents.

In general, adolescents are concerned with physiological growth and development as well as physical appearance. This becomes an even greater concern for the adolescent with a condition that affects (or is perceived as affecting) normal growth and development or physical appearance, such as school failure, acne, scoliosis, or cerebral palsy (Frauman & Syphert, 1979). A sensitive nurse will be able to identify such conflicts with a thorough history.

Middle and Older Adulthood

Questions should be directed toward eliciting what middle-aged clients need to know about male and female menopause and sexual changes related to aging. Some clients may be misinformed about these and other matters related to sexuality. In questionnaires used in a study by LaRocca and Polit (1980), women aged 40 to 60 revealed that their primary concern was what to expect during or as a result of menopause.

Elderly clients may be concerned whether sexual activity at their age is "normal." Society tends to sexually disenfranchise older people, even those in later middle age. Adolescents and young adults often are shocked to discover that their parents or grandparents have active sex lives. Nurses, especially, must recognize that growing old does not signify an end to the sexual self. Pfeiffer (1979) interviewed men and women aged 60 to 94 and found the majority had not lost interest in sex. Many reported continued sexual intercourse at regular intervals. A number of factors were related to sexual expression in old age, including previous sexual activity ("Use it or lose it!"), general health, adequacy of income, and general life satisfaction. In addition, Friedeman (1979) reported that age, religious orientation, social norms, previous sexual expressiveness, knowledge of changes in sexual function, extent of privacy, and psychological/emotional health affect sexual expression in later years. Psychological health is especially important, since depression is one of the most common psychological problems of old age, and one of its most frequent manifestations is decreased libido.

Combining the concepts of universality and normality can be helpful in obtaining the sexuality history from an aging client. For example, the nurse might say, "Many older people find that sexual activity remains an important part of their lives, but they may wonder whether this is normal. Do you think about sex differently now than when you were younger? How has your sex life changed? Are you concerned about some aspects of it?"

Growing old may be accompanied by health limitations or loss of a longtime sexual partner. Clients in late adulthood may need information about alternative means for expressing sexual desires and relieving sexual tensions. Nurses can help by supporting clients' efforts to retain their sexual identities in socially acceptable ways. A nurse sometimes can help both client and family by explaining to younger members that sexuality is a natural part of life at any age, and that older family members who continue to express interest in sexual activity are not only acting normally but may well be promoting their continued health and well-being.

CLINICAL APPRAISAL

Clinical appraisal of sexuality may be embarrassing and considered intrusive by the client. Therefore, the nurse should use a sensitive yet matter-of-fact approach and should explain to the client the purpose of each portion of the examination. A thorough clinical appraisal of sexuality includes observation and inspection of visible sexual characteristics, examination of the breasts (women and men), inspection of the external genitalia, and observation of the client's performance of breast or testicular self-examination.

Numerous opportunities for teaching clients about sexuality may arise during the examination. For example, the nurse may teach the client breast or testicular self-examination or may use mirrors to teach anatomy and physiology of the sexual organs.

The initial appraisal of sexuality should include noting outward signs of male or female sexual identity, including clothing, hairstyle, use of makeup, visible secondary sex characteristics (voice pitch, facial hair, breast development), and mannerisms. Many of these manifestations are culturally dictated, which will influence the interpretations the nurse makes. For example, acceptable hair length and clothing vary with current styles, cultural context, or geographic region. Men who use makeup or who have effeminate mannerisms

may be experiencing problems with sexual identity, necessitating further assessment.

The remainder of the physical appraisal of sexuality should include an examination of the breasts and the external genitalia.

Assessment of the Breasts*

There is a high incidence of disease of the breast; therefore, it is a very important part of the routine assessment of sexuality. The breast is the second most common site of cancer in women. Men also can develop breast carcinoma, although the incidence is low (1–5% of cases). The nurse plays a vital role in screening for early detection of breast cancer and in health education. The American Cancer Society (1988) recommends that women aged 20 to 40 should have their breasts examined by a health professional every three years (in addition to practicing monthly breast self-examinations). Women over 40 are advised to have a professional examination of their breasts annually (American Cancer Society, 1988). Clients need to know the why, when, and how of breast self-examination and the importance of follow-up if any abnormalities are detected.

Structure and Function of the Breasts

During the prenatal period, estrogen from the mother crosses the placenta. The estrogen may produce hypertrophy of the breasts of the newborn, a not uncommon condition. The hypertrophy may be either unilateral or bilateral and may be present for as long as 1 to 2 months. In addition, there may be milky secretions, but they are of no significance unless accompanied by signs of inflammation.

Figure 13-1 shows how the breast is anatomically divided into four quadrants (upper and lower medial quadrants and upper and lower lateral quadrants). The areolae of the female breasts contain Montgomery's glands (sebaceous glands). With lactation, they secrete a lipoid substance to protect the nipple during breastfeeding. Prominence of Montgomery's glands may occur from edema of the breast.

Changes in the breast occur with aging. Weakening ligaments and a decrease in subcutaneous tissue caused by reduced estrogen levels result in the characteristically flaccid, droopy appearance of the breasts in elderly women. Nipple size and the

---

*This section is adapted from Grimes, J. & Burns, E. (1987). *Health assessment in nursing practice* (2nd ed.). Boston: Jones and Bartlett Publishers, 279–289.

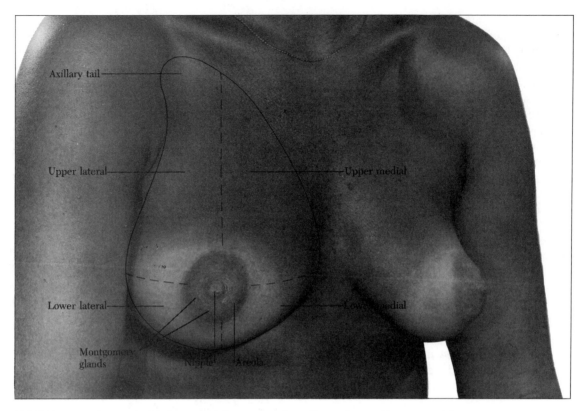

FIGURE 13-1. Anatomical Divisions of the Breast. (*Note.* From Grimes/Burns: *Health Assessment in Nursing Practice,* Second Edition, © 1987. Boston: Jones and Bartlett Publishers, p. 280.)

ability of the nipple to become erect also diminish. Ludwick (1988) notes that detection of a breast mass usually is easier in older women because of the decrease in fatty tissue.

Elderly women may be at greater risk of delayed detection of breast cancer than younger women. Because older women's visits to health professionals occur for specific health problems usually unrelated to the breasts, they are less likely to receive routine breast screening examinations or to request them (Rudolph & McDermott, 1987). The elderly client also is more likely to be modest about exposing her breasts for examination. Her self-consciousness can be reduced by careful draping or use of a special gown that fastens in the front (Ludwick, 1988).

Elderly men may exhibit hypertrophy or gynecomastia of the breasts, with onset occurring between 50 and 70 years of age. These conditions are typically bilateral and may be accompanied by breast tenderness, which aids in differentiating the normal changes of aging from a breast mass (Ludwick, 1988). Although breast cancer in men is rare, its highest incidence occurs in those over 65 years of age.

The breast is affected by many diseases, but probably the most dreaded is cancer. The most common site of breast cancer in the female is the upper lateral quadrant; in the male it is directly under the areola. Early detection is of prime importance for successful treatment. In assessing the breasts, the same sequence of steps should be followed for both male and female clients.

Inspection

Inspection of the client's breasts (see boxed insert, p. 398) should be performed with the client in both the sitting and supine positions. The nurse should examine the skin of the breasts for any lesions, increased vascular patterns, color changes, edema, or irregularities of the surface, such as dimpling or retraction. Retraction can be the result of scarring following inflammation or trauma, but most often it is an indication of malignancy.

As in Figure 13-2, the breasts should be inspected closely as the client forcibly presses hands on hips (A), as the arms are raised overhead (B), and while the hands are pushed together in front (C). Women, in particular, should become familiar with the shape and feel of their own breasts. The nurse also should inspect the axillary and clavicular areas for any erythema or bulging, as they are the chief regions of lymphatic drainage of the breasts.

The areolae are a darker color in dark-haired

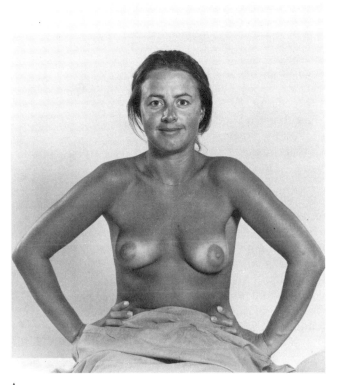

A

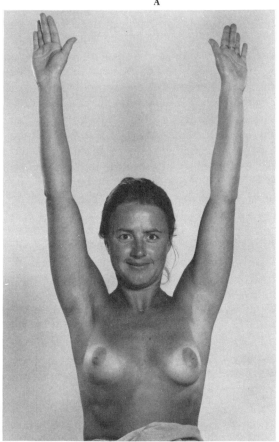

B

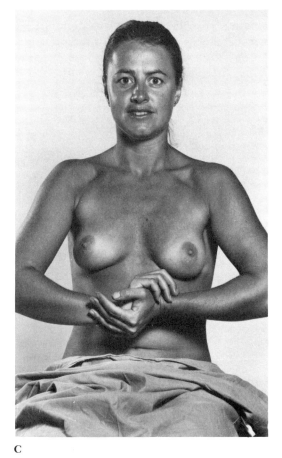

C

FIGURE 13-2. Method of Breast Inspection. (A) While client presses hands on hips. (B) With client's arms raised overhead. (C) With client's hands pushed together in front. (*Note.* From Grimes/Burns: *Health Assessment in Nursing Practice,* Second Edition, © 1987. Boston: Jones and Bartlett Publishers, p. 282.)

people and a light pinkish hue in blondes. Clients who are pregnant, those taking oral contraceptives, and dark-skinned clients will have darker areolae.

Clients should be made aware of the fact that there is a slight asymmetry of the breasts. This is most noticeable in the sitting position. Although the left breast generally is larger than the right, the nipples should be symmetrical on the breasts. Underlying skin retraction often will cause the nipple to turn toward an involved area, so that the nipple points to a lesion.

The nurse should note whether the nipples are inverted or erect. Inverted nipples may be congenital, but any recent inversion of the nipple is significant and could be the result of inflammation or abscess, as well as malignancy. The nipples also should be inspected for any scaling, crusting, or fissures (cracks). Bilateral involvement usually is observed in dermatological conditions. Paget's disease, a slow intraductal carcinoma, is usually unilateral and begins as scaling and erythema, which eventually progresses into ulceration.

Palpation

Palpation of the female breasts should be performed both in the sitting position, as shown in Figure 13-3, and in the supine position, as shown

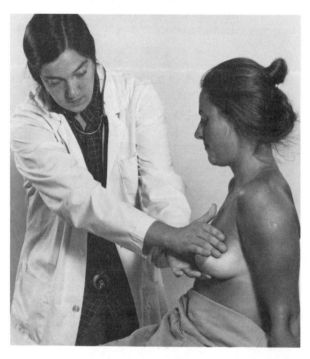

FIGURE 13-3. Bimanual Palpation of the Breast with Client in Sitting Position. (*Note.* From Grimes/Burns: *Health Assessment in Nursing Practice,* Second Edition, © 1987. Boston: Jones and Bartlett Publishers, p. 284.)

Technique for Inspection of the Breast

1. Provide adequate lighting, warm room, and privacy.
2. Client is exposed to the waist.
3. Client is sitting, preferably before a mirror.
4. Explain each step (health teaching).
5. Note characteristics: contour and size, skin, nipples, areolae, axillary and clavicular lymph node areas, abnormalities (lesions, color changes, increased vascular patterns, edema, dimpling, retraction).
6. Ask client to raise arms overhead: inspect.
7. Ask client to press hands on hips: inspect.
8. Ask client to push palms of hands together: inspect.
9. Ask client with large or pendulous breasts to stand and lean forward as you hold her hands in yours: Inspect the breasts while suspended.

Note. From Grimes/Burns: *Health Assessment in Nursing Practice,* Second Edition, © 1987. Boston: Jones and Bartlett Publishers.

---

in Figure 13-4. The supine position provides the most accurate findings. In the sitting position, palpation of the breasts, the axillary region, and the clavicular region should be performed first with the client's arms down at her sides and then with her arms raised overhead. The axillary and clavicular regions contain the lymph nodes responsible for draining the breast area. It is important to palpate all these lymph node groups. Figure 13-5 illustrates their anatomical location. A bimanual technique, particularly with large breasts, may prove beneficial in detecting small, deep-seated masses. In the supine position a small pillow or folded towel placed under the shoulder of the side being palpated helps to spread the breast tissue more symmetrically over the chest wall. The arm on the side being palpated should be extended over the head. As with the sitting position, the axillary and clavicular nodes also should be examined, first with the arms raised and then with the arms at the client's sides.

Palpation (see boxed insert, p. 404) should begin in the upper lateral quadrant. Using a gentle "to and fro" rotary motion with the palmar aspects of the fingers, the examiner's hands should move from the periphery to the areola. Figure 13-6 shows how palpation should move clockwise about the periphery of the breast, each time proceeding from the areola. A tracing of the sequence would look like a wheel with spokes. After light palpation, the breast should be examined with deep palpation. The nurse should begin at the top of the upper lateral quadrant and feel in a clockwise motion full circle, then move on inch toward the nipple and

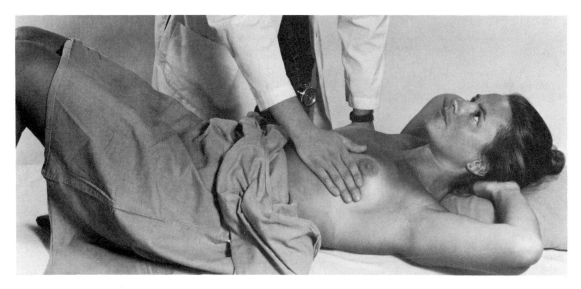

FIGURE 13-4. The Supine Position for Breast Palpation. (*Note.* From Grimes/Burns: *Health Assessment in Nursing Practice,* Second Edition, © 1987. Boston: Jones and Bartlett Publishers, p. 284.)

repeat. This procedure should be repeated at least twice more, followed by palpation of the nipple area last. This is called the spiral technique and is recommended by the American Cancer Society (Figure 13-7). Careful palpation of the areolar area, the axillary region, and the clavicular region is es-

pecially important in the male, as there is early metastasis of breast carcinoma to the lymphatics because of the paucity of breast tissue in males.

Should a mass be detected, the following characteristics should be described in recording the findings:

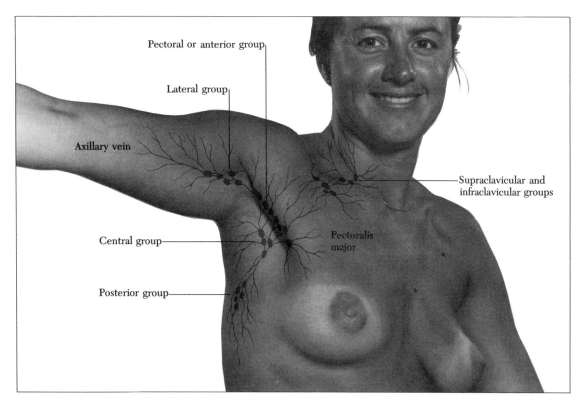

FIGURE 13-5. Location of the Lymph Nodes. (*Note.* From Grimes/Burns: *Health Assessment in Nursing Practice,* Second Edition, © 1987. Boston: Jones and Bartlett Publishers, p. 285.)

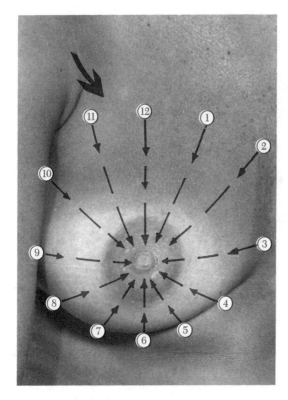

FIGURE 13-6. Sequence of Palpation of the Breast. Palpation begins on the upper lateral quadrant (arrow) and proceeds in a clockwise direction around the periphery of the breast and moves inward toward the areola. Locations of masses are documented in the o'clock axes (circles). (*Note.* From Grimes/Burns: *Health Assessment in Nursing Practice,* Second Edition, © 1987. Boston: Jones and Bartlett Publishers, p. 285.)

1. *Location*—Cite distance from the nipple, in the schema of a clock, and indicate whether the client's arms were at the sides or extended overhead, as these positions may change the location. For example: "Located at 3:00 axis of left breast 1 cm from the areolar border with arms extended overhead." (See Figure 13-8).

2. *Size*—State three dimensions, if possible (length, width, and thickness). If unable to determine discrete margins, record this also.

3. *Surface*—Indicate whether smooth and regular or irregular contour.

4. *Discreteness*—Note whether margins are difficult to determine or easily detected (a discrete mass).

5. *Consistency*—Indicate whether soft, firm, or stony hard.

6. *Mobility*—Note whether mass is movable or firmly or moderately fixed.

7. *Tenderness*—Note whether mass is painful or not.

The presence of any mass or other serious abnormalities in one or both breasts warrants immediate referral. Table 13-8 delineates the common characteristics of benign and malignant breast lesions.

Assessment of the External Genitalia*

Deferral of this portion of the sexuality assessment may be appropriate in some circumstances, such as embarrassment in a school-age child (assuming the sexuality history reveals no problems), but usually is attributable to discomfort on the part of the examiner. Because problems that affect the external genitalia can have an impact on the client's health, it is important to include examination of the external genitalia whenever a thorough appraisal of the client is being conducted. This particular portion of the physical assessment may be embarrassing and uncomfortable, so proper preparation of the client and support during the assessment are essential. The environment should be arranged to provide comfort and privacy. Each step should be explained to the client prior to performing it.

Males

On inspection of the male genitals, pubic hair distribution should be noted. This may vary somewhat from person to person; only the absence or extreme sparseness of pubic hair in the adult male need be reported. Usually a diamond or triangular pattern is observed (see Figure 13-9).

Figure 13-9 shows the normal male penis. Inspection will reveal the size of the penis, which also varies from person to person. Usually the left testis will be lower than the right. The skin of the penis should be inspected to detect the presence of any abnormalities. Inspection of the skin for lesions or scars can be accomplished simultaneously with palpation (see boxed insert, p. 406).

Whether the client is circumcised or uncircumcised should be noted. In uncircumcised men, a small amount of thick white secretion may be observed between the foreskin and the glans; this a normal secretion called smegma. The penile shaft may be palpated for any signs of tenderness or induration (hardening). Normally the urethral meatus is present at the distal end of the penis. To inspect the urethra, the thumbs should be used to separate the meatus, as shown in Figure 13-10. A culture should be taken if a thick, purulent discharge is noted, as it suggests gonorrhea. Gonor-

---

*This section is adapted from Grimes, J. & Burns, E. (1987). *Health assessment in nursing practice* (2nd ed.). Boston: Jones and Bartlett Publishers, 371–381.

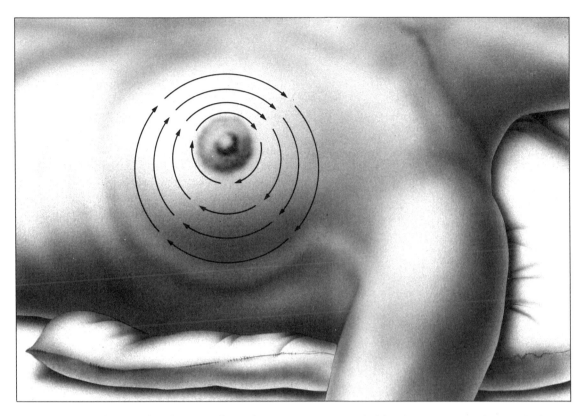

FIGURE 13-7. The Spiral Technique. This technique is recommended for clients' use in palpating the breast and should be performed in both sitting and supine positions. (*Note.* From Grimes/Burns: *Health Assessment in Nursing Practice,* Second Edition, © 1987. Boston: Jones and Bartlett Publishers, p. 286.)

rhea also is associated with urinary symptoms. A thin, mucoid discharge may indicate urethritis.

If during the elimination history the client has complained of dysuria or a change in urination stream, the nurse should try to observe the client voiding, if possible. A deviated or poor stream may suggest urethral stricture or obstruction.

The scrotum should be observed for any redness, swelling, lesions, or scaly patches ("jock itch"). Gentle palpation of the testes may be performed. Normally the testes are tender. The testes are 2 × 4 cm in size and are rubbery (neither hard nor soft) in consistency. They become softer and decrease in size during middle age. The nurse's thumb should be placed on the anterior surface of the scrotum and the index finger behind the scrotum. This same technique of using the thumbs on the anterior surface is explained to men when teaching them how to perform the testicular self-examination (TSE). Any nodule found within the testes warrants medical referral.

Women

The female client should be supine with her knees flexed and feet flat on the surface. The client should be draped for privacy. Adequate lighting is

essential. The client should be instructed to relax and allow her knees to fall apart. Inspection of the external genitalia (mons pubis and vulva) should include observation of hair growth, pigmentation and distribution; inflammation (redness or swelling); and the presence of lesions or discharge. If indicated, the nurse may separate the labia after preparing the client for what to expect. The interior aspects of the outer labia and the characteristics of the inner labia should be examined, as should the clitoris, vestibule, urethral meatus, vaginal introitus, and perineum (see Figure 13-11). The nurse should note the presence and location of any erythema, edema, nodules, lesions, or other abnormality. If abnormalities are noted, the client should be referred for a complete pelvic examination.

Breast and Testicular Self-Examination

Breast self-examination (BSE) should be practiced routinely and systematically by all postpubescent females. The American Cancer Society has concluded that breast self-examination need not be performed by men unless they exhibit gynecomastia.

Massey (1986) investigated the relationship be-

Technique for Palpation of the Breast

1. Client in sitting position.
2. Use palmar aspects of your fingers to knead breast tissue.
3. Palpate axillary and clavicular lymph nodes with a cupped hand, first with client's arm raised and supported at the wrist with your hand and then with client's arm at the side.
4. Begin palpation of breast with the axillary tail and upper lateral quadrant.
5. Lightly palpate from periphery to nipple, like spokes of a wheel.
6. Repeat palpation of breast using deep palpation performed in a spiral technique. Palpate the nipples last.
7. Compress nipple between thumb and forefinger. Note any discharge.
8. Perform bimanual palpation of each breast particularly when client's breasts are large.
9. Place client in lying position.
10. Place small pillow or folded towel under shoulder of side to be inspected and palpated.
11. Ask client to extend arm overhead on side being examined.
12. Repeat inspection of each breast.
13. Repeat above palpation steps (2–7) for each breast.
14. Transfer small pillow or towel to the opposite side when inspecting and palpating the remaining breast.

Note. From Grimes/Burns: *Health Assessment in Nursing Practice*, Second edition, © 1987. Boston: Jones and Bartlett Publishers.

tween perceived susceptibility to breast cancer and the practice of BSE. She found that women who perceive themselves as susceptible reported more frequent practice of BSE. Younger women were more likely to practice BSE than women over 50 because they perceived themselves as more susceptible to breast cancer, even though in fact the older population is more susceptible. Rutledge (1987) found that high benefits and low barriers perceived for BSE related directly to the frequency with which BSE was practiced by a group of upper middle class subjects. Both studies have implications for nursing assessment. Women should be asked about their knowledge and practice of BSE, whether they perceive themselves as susceptible to breast cancer, and what barriers interfere with their regular performance of BSE. The nurse also should assess the client's self-concept, since women who have a positive self-concept are more likely to practice BSE (Rutledge, 1987).

Women of childbearing age should be advised to perform BSE immediately after each menstrual period. Postmenopausal women should perform BSE on a designated day each month, such as the first or last day of the month, so they do not forget.

Ludwick (1988) notes that many of the changes associated with the aging process may interfere with the elderly client's ability to practice BSE. Specifically, she cites decreased range of motion, diminished sensation in the fingertips, vision impairments, and decreased agility as factors that may compromise the thoroughness and accuracy of BSE in elderly clients. The process of BSE in the elderly often will require more time and may require the use of special devices, such as a magnifying glass, large mirror, and talc to increase finger sensitivity (Ludwick, 1988).

The correct technique for self-examination of the breasts has been recommended by the American Cancer Society (1990) and is illustrated in Figure 13-12. The nurse should observe the client perform breast self-examination to verify that the client is using this technique. Clients who are embarrassed about examining their own breasts while the nurse watches may demonstrate the technique on a breast model.

Testicular cancer is one of the most common cancers in men aged 15 to 40. Testicular self-examination, like BSE, is essential for early detection and cure. The client's knowledge of testicular self-examination (TSE), his perceived susceptibility to testicular cancer, and the frequency of practice of TSE should be assessed during the sexuality history.

Reno (1988) studied men's knowledge and health beliefs about testicular cancer and TSE and found a highly significant relationships between perceived susceptibility to testicular cancer and beliefs about the importance of TSE. Men who were aware of the risk of testicular cancer were more likely to believe in the regular practice of TSE. The client should be asked to demonstrate testicular self-examination, or if he does not know the correct technique, the nurse should demonstrate on the client or by using a model.

The best time for performing TSE is after a warm bath or shower when the scrotal skin is more relaxed. The examination takes approximately 3 minutes and should be performed monthly. The client should roll each testicle gently between the thumb and fingers of both hands as illustrated in Figure 13-13. If any hard lumps or nodules are found, a physician should be consulted promptly.

NURSING DIAGNOSES RELATED TO SEXUALITY

The information obtained from the sexuality assessment should be analyzed to determine whether it suggests potential or actual alterations

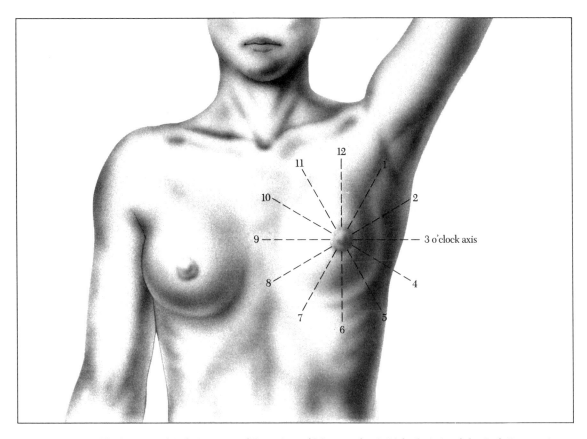

FIGURE 13-8. Clock Axes of Left Breast and Location of Mass at the 3 O'clock Axis of the Left Breast, 1 cm from the Areolar Border with Arm Extended Overhead. (*Note.* From Grimes/Burns: *Health Assessment in Nursing Practice*, Second Edition, © 1987. Boston: Jones and Bartlett Publishers, p. 287.)

TABLE 13-8
General Characteristics of Benign and Malignant Lesions*

Characteristics	Benign	Malignant
Surface	Smooth and regular	Uneven
Discreteness	Well-defined margins	Discrete in early stage, irregular borders
Consistency	Soft	Generally firm to hard
Mobility	Easily movable	Fixed as progresses to invasion of underlying tissues
Tenderness	Usually tender	Generally nontender
Transillumination	May or may not; if cyst, usually will	No
Retraction	Rarely	Often present
Incidence	Young women, men over 50 years old	1 out of 10–15 women; most common in middle-aged and elderly; 1–5% of cases of breast carcinoma in men
Lymph node involvement	Rarely	Most common site (females): upper outer quadrant; variable involvement Most common site (males): under areola with early metastasis to axillary lymph nodes

*Note that these are general characteristics and are not diagnostic of either benign or malignant lesions. Carcinoma of the breast is diagnosed only by biopsy.
Note. From Grimes/Burns: *Health Assessment in Nursing Practice*, Second Edition, © 1987. Boston: Jones and Bartlett Publishers.

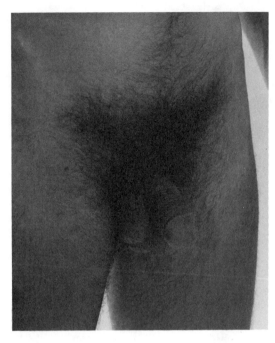

FIGURE 13-9. Normal Male Genitals. (*Note.* From Grimes/Burns: *Health Assessment in Nursing Practice*, Second Edition, © 1987. Boston: Jones and Bartlett Publishers, p. 373.)

Techniques for Inspection and Palpation of Penis and Scrotum

1. Arrange for client's comfort and privacy.
2. Have adequate lighting.
3. Sit on chair facing client.
4. Put on gloves.
5. Explain each step prior to doing it.
6. Characteristics of inspection:
   Hair distribution
   Size and contour
   Skin surfaces
   Position of urethral meatus
   Abnormalities
7. Palpate penile shaft between thumb and first two fingers.
8. Retract foreskin.
9. Separate meatus with thumbs.
10. If client complains of dysuria or change in urination stream, observe client voiding.
11. If thick, purulent urethral discharge, take culture of discharge.

Note. From Grimes/Burns: *Health Assessment in Nursing Practice*, Second Edition, © 1987. Boston: Jones and Bartlett Publishers.

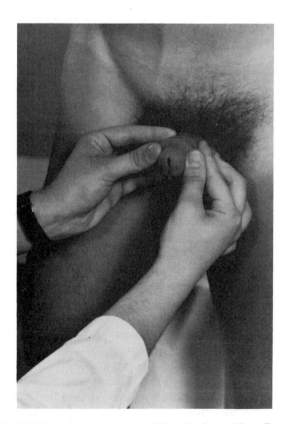

FIGURE 13-10. Inspection of the Urethra. (*Note.* From Grimes/Burns: *Health Assessment in Nursing Practice*, Second Edition, © 1987. Boston: Jones and Bartlett Publishers, p. 373.)

in the client's sexuality patterns or the presence of sexual dysfunction. The nursing diagnosis, "altered sexuality patterns," is categorized in the North American Nursing Diagnosis Association (NANDA) Taxonomy I (1990) under the human response pattern of relating, implying a problem with interpersonal bonds or relationships. To support this diagnosis, information from the nursing history or clinical appraisal should reflect physiological or psychological difficulties, limitations, or changes that have altered the client's usual patterns of sexuality or sexual responses. Factors that may contribute to alterations in sexuality patterns include illness, loss, intrapersonal conflict about sexual orientation, absence of a partner, pain, body image disturbances, or fatigue. The client who is experiencing a life change or transition, such as pregnancy, childbirth, trauma, menopause, or surgery, may lack adequate knowledge about alternatives to ensure continued healthy sexual self-concept, sexual expression, or sexual functioning.

The accepted nursing diagnosis, "sexual dysfunction," also is categorized under the human response pattern of relating. Within the NANDA Taxonomy I Revised, however, it is identified as a specific problem of "altered role performance." Sexual dysfunction is characterized by unrewarding or inadequate sexual health or functioning: impotence, delayed development of secondary sex characteristics, sex role conflicts, sexual dissatisfac-

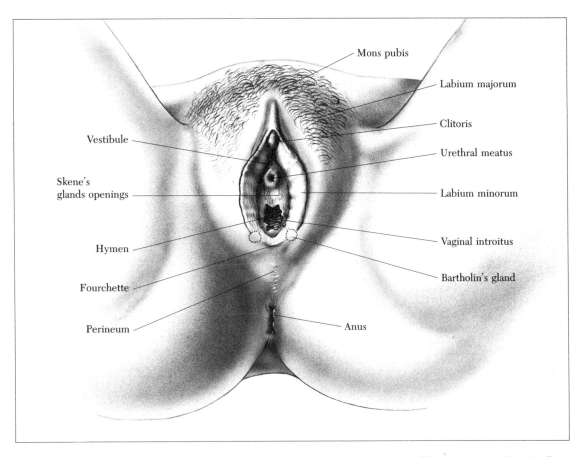

FIGURE 13-11. The Female External Genitals. (*Note.* From Grimes/Burns: *Health Assessment in Nursing Practice,* Second Edition, © 1987. Boston: Jones and Bartlett Publishers, p. 377.)

tion, or variant sexual expression, such as transvestism, voyeurism, or exhibitionism. The latter problems usually are diagnosed by a practitioner with advanced education in mental health or sex therapy.

Other NANDA-approved diagnoses related to sexual self-concept or functioning are categorized under the human response pattern of feeling and include "rape-trauma response" with the more specific diagnoses of "rape-trauma syndrome: compound reaction" and "rape-trauma syndrome: silent reaction," all of which are related to trauma resulting from sexual assault. Rape-trauma syndrome is characterized by an acute phase of disorganization followed by a long-term phase of reorganization and reintegration. Nursing diagnosis of rape-trauma syndrome in the immediate posttrauma phase is determined by the client's description of events and, when possible, confirming evidence from the clinical appraisal. Confirming physical data include evidence of trauma, such as the client's general appearance and emotional state, bruises, as well as findings of a vaginal, rectal, or oral examination. Nursing diagnosis of rape-trauma syndrome may be made retrospectively in

clients who did not seek assistance immediately after the assault, but later seek help for other problems arising from the experience. Such problems may include sexually transmitted disease, pregnancy, physical symptoms (pain, muscle tension, sleep problems, or gastrointestinal upset), depression, anxiety, self-blame, fear of being alone, or inability to establish (or reestablish) intimate relationships. In any event, the nurse should be sensitive to and supportive of any client whose history or behavior indicates the possibility of rape-trauma response.

Woods (1987) offers a holistic perspective of nursing diagnoses related to sexuality. She points out that sex therapists typically classify sexuality problems in terms of sexual dysfunction and thus do not address the dimensions of sexual self-concept or sexual relationships, which can have profound influences on sexual health. Woods proposes a diagnostic taxonomy that includes alterations in sexual function, sexual self-concept, and sexual relationships. Alterations in sexual function include 1) alterations in sexual desire, 2) alterations in sexual arousal, and 3) alterations in orgasm. Specific examples of diagnoses related to

■ WHY DO THE BREAST SELF-EXAM?

There are many good reasons for doing a breast self-exam each month. One reason is that breast cancer is most easily treated and cured when it is found early. Another is that the more you do it, the better you will get at it. When you get to know how your breasts normally feel, you will quickly be able to feel any change. Another reason, it is easy to do.

■ WHEN TO DO BREAST SELF-EXAM

The best time to do breast self-exam is after your period, when breasts are not tender or swollen. If you do not have regular periods or sometimes skip a month, do it on the same day every month.

Remember: A breast self-exam could save your breast—and save your life. Most breast lumps are found by women themselves, but, in fact, most lumps in the breast are not cancer. Be safe, be sure.

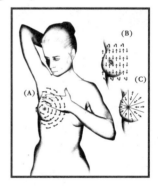

■ NOW, HOW TO DO BREAST SELF-EXAM

1. Lie down and put a pillow under your right shoulder. Place your right arm behind your head.

2. Use the finger pads of your three middle fingers on your left hand to feel for lumps or thickening. Your finger pads are the top third of each finger.

3. Press firmly enough to know how your breast feels. If you're not sure how hard to press, ask your health care provider. Or try to copy the way your health care provider uses the finger pads during a breast exam. Learn what your breast feels like most of the time. A firm ridge in the lower curve of each breast is normal.

4. Move around the breast in a set way. You can choose either the circle (A), the up and down line (B), or the wedge (C). Do it the same way every time. It will help you to make sure that you've gone over the entire breast area, and to remember how your breast feels.

each month.

5. Now examine your left breast using right hand finger pads.

6. If you find any changes, see your doctor right away.

■ FOR ADDED SAFETY:

You might want to check your breasts while standing in front of a mirror right after you do your breast self-exam each month. See if there are any changes in the way your breasts look: dimpling of the skin, changes in the nipple, or redness or swelling.

You might also want to do an extra breast self-exam while you're in the shower. Your soapy hands will glide over the wet skin making it easy to check how your breasts feel.

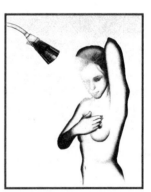

FIGURE 13-12. Breast Self-Examination Techniques. (*Note.* Reprinted with permission, American Cancer Society, 1990.)

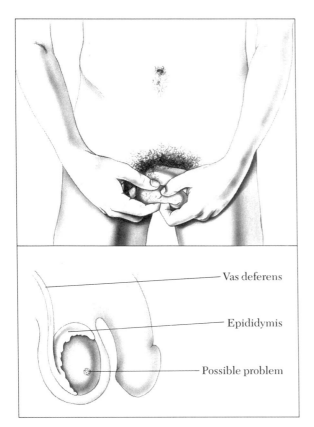

Vas deferens

Epididymis

Possible problem

FIGURE 13-13. Testicular Self-Examination. This is a 3-minute monthly examination that should be performed by all postpubertal males. Preferably, the exam should be done after a warm bath or shower when the scrotal skin is more relaxed. Each testicle should be rolled between the thumb and first two fingers of both hands. If any hard lumps or nodules are detected, the client should seek immediate medical attention.

these respective alterations are "low sexual desire related to chronic pain," "decreased vaginal lubrication related to aging," and "premature ejaculation related to performance anxiety" (Woods, 1987). Examples of alterations in sexual self-concept include "anxiety about sexual encounters related to body image changes" and "altered sexual self-concept related to illness" (Woods, 1987). Examples of alterations in sexual relationships include "dissatisfaction with sexual frequency (or type and amount of sexual stimulation)" and "value conflicts related to alternative forms of sexual expression" (Woods, 1987).

When the nursing history and clinical appraisal reveal no immediate or past problems related to sexuality, the client is judged to be sexually healthy. It is important, however, that the nurse identify potential concerns or problems in the area of sexuality. For instance, a prepubescent child may lack knowledge about the physical and emotional

TABLE 13-9
Sample Nursing Diagnoses Related to Sexuality

Altered sexuality patterns related to chronic illness, fear of acquiring a sexually transmitted disease, separation from partner, or extreme fatigue

[Sexual] self-esteem disturbance related to values conflict, performance failure, or body image changes (e.g., mastectomy, pregnancy, aging, or burn injury)

Sexual dysfunction related to depression, body image disturbance, effects of disease or therapy (e.g., hemodialysis, chemotherapy, or radiation), substance abuse, or dysfunctional interpersonal relationships

Rape-trauma response related to sexual assault
Rape-trauma syndrome: compound reaction
Rape-trauma syndrome: silent reaction

changes that accompany the onset of puberty and therefore may be at risk for an alteration in sexuality if appropriate guidance and education are not provided. The nurse should expect that a sexually active and sexually healthy adult who undergoes surgery or who is diagnosed with a chronic illness may experience altered sexuality patterns, especially if appropriate education and support in this area are not provided.

Table 13-9 lists the NANDA Taxonomy I Revised (1990) diagnoses related to sexuality. Defining characteristics and additional related factors may be found in Chapter 6 (color-highlighted pages).

Chapter Highlights

■ Human sexuality is a complex phenomenon influenced by physiological, developmental, psychosocial, and cultural factors.

■ Assessment of sexuality is an essential aspect of a comprehensive nursing assessment, regardless of the client's age or health.

■ The nurse's own self-awareness, attitudes toward and knowledge of sexuality will influence the quality and completeness of the sexuality assessment.

■ To assess sexuality, the nurse must have an adequate understanding of human sexual development across the life span, human sexual response, cultural variables that influence sexuality, and the impact of changed health on sexual development and expression.

■ Several approaches to obtaining sexuality information, including universality ("Many people experience . . ."), sensitivity, confidentiality, and appropriate use of humor, can assist in lessening discomfort for the nurse and the client, thereby enhancing the completeness and validity of the information collected.

■ The sexuality history should incorporate questions related to sexual physiology and development, sexual self-concept, sexual relationships, and sexual functioning.

■ Modifications in the sexuality history will depend upon the client's age, cultural background, and health.

■ The aging process results in changes in sexual physiology and functioning. The older adult's adjustment to these changes depends primarily on psychosocial and cultural factors.

■ Clinical appraisal of sexuality should include observation and inspection of visible sexual characteristics, examination of the breasts (women and men), inspection of the external genitalia, and assessment of the client's practice of breast self-examination or testicular self-examination.

■ Data obtained from the sexuality history and clinical appraisal should be analyzed carefully and appropriate nursing diagnoses should be formulated.

■ Nursing diagnoses should delineate problems related to the various dimensions of sexuality, leading to an appropriate plan for nursing care.

Suggested Practice Activities

1. Respond in writing to the following questions and include your feelings. Discuss your responses with classmates.
   a. If the topic of sex were unexpectedly introduced while you were with others, would you feel your privacy had been invaded? Would you worry about the feelings of other people in the group?
   b. Would you talk about sex differently if you were talking to a man than if you were talking to a woman? A boy? A girl?
   c. Would you ask different questions about sex if you were asking a man than if you were asking a woman? A boy? A girl?
   d. Some people enjoy sexual humor. Do you? Do you feel it is appropriate to express sexual humor in mixed company? Do you have a favorite "dirty" joke?
   e. There is street language for terms related to sex and sexuality. Refer to Table 13-6. Are you familiar with street language other than in the table? Do you remember when you first became aware of these words? Are some words more difficult to say than others? Which ones? Are there circumstances in which it is appropriate to use street language? If so, what might they be? How would you feel if a client used street language during the sexuality history? How would you respond?
   f. Think about a recent interaction you had with a client. Was touch part of the interaction? What are some of the nonverbal techniques you use to show comfort with and acceptance of the client as a person?
   g. In a client interaction, would you feel more comfortable touching a man or a woman? A boy or a girl? Where would you feel comfortable touching a man? A woman? A boy? A girl? How do you think you learned your touching behavior?
   h. Imagine examining your own genitalia with a hand mirror. What kinds of feelings might you have? Anxious? Embarrassed? Ashamed? Childlike? Happy? Pleased? Interested? Disgusted? Turned on? Turned off?

2. Review nursing or health history forms from at least two health agencies, and
   a. critique for inclusion of sexuality assessment.
   b. suggest ways of incorporating areas not included.
   c. suggest ways to modify forms according to age, culture, and health.

3. Using the sexuality history in Table 13-7, role-play obtaining a sexuality history. What areas or questions did you have difficulty with? What factors contributed to your discomfort?

4. Assess the sexuality of at least one healthy child and one healthy adult, including history and clinical appraisal, and formulate appropriate nursing diagnoses.

5. Assess sexuality of at least one client with one of the following alterations in health:
   a. Pregnancy or postpartum
   b. Developmental disability
   c. Postsurgery (e.g., mastectomy, amputation, ostomy)
   d. Post-myocardial infarction
   e. Chronic illness (e.g., diabetes mellitus, chronic renal failure)

6. Perform a breast or testicular examination on yourself using the guidelines provided in this chapter. Record your findings.

Recommended Readings

Allen, M.E. (1987). A holistic view of sexuality and the aged. *Holistic Nursing Practice, 1*(4), 76–83.

Andrist, L.C. (1988). Taking a sexual history and educating clients about safe sex. *Nursing Clinics of North America, 23*, 959–973.

Aquilino, M.L., & Ely, J. (1985). Parents and the sexuality of preschool children. *Pediatric Nursing, 11*(1), 41–46, 73.

Brink, P.J. (1987). Cultural aspects of sexuality. *Holistic Nursing Practice, 1*(4), 12–20.

Friend, R.A. (1987). Sexual identity and human diversity: Implications for nursing practice. *Holistic Nursing Practice, 1*(4), 21–41.

Ludwick, R. (1988). Breast examination in the older adult. *Cancer Nursing, 11*(2), 99–102.

Moore, D.S., & Erickson, P.I. (1985). Age, gender, and ethnic differences in sexual and contraceptive knowledge, attitudes, and behaviors. *Family and Community Health, 8*(3), 38–51.

Muscari, M.E. (1987). Obtaining the adolescent sexual history. *Pediatric Nursing, 13*, 307–310.

Reno, D.R. (1988). Men's knowledge and health beliefs about testicular cancer and testicular self-examination. *Cancer Nursing, 11*(2), 112–117.

Rutledge, D.N. (1987). Factors related to women's practice of breast self-examination. *Nursing Research, 36*, 117–121.

Steinke, E.E. (1988). Older adults' knowledge and attitudes about sexuality and aging. *Image: Journal of Nursing Scholarship, 20*, 93–95.

Woods, N.F., Most, A., & Longenecker, G.D. (1985). Major life events, daily stressors, and perimenstrual symptoms. *Nursing Research, 34*, 263–267.

References

American Cancer Society. (1990). *Breast self-examination techniques*. New York: Author.

American Cancer Society. (1988). *Cancer facts and figures*. New York: Author.

American Public Health Association. (1985). Major study shows change in contraception, fertility. *The Nation's Health, 1*, 3.

Aquilino, M.L., & Ely, J. (1985). Parents and the sexuality of preschool children. *Pediatric Nursing, 11*(1), 41–46, 73.

Barnett, R.C., & Baruch, G.K. (1987). Determinants of fathers' participation in family work. *Journal of Marriage and the Family, 49*, 29–40.

Bem, S. (1985). Androgyny and gender schema theory: A conceptual and empirical integration. In T.B. Sondegegger (Ed.), *Nebraska symposium and motivation: Psychology and gender*. Lincoln: University of Nebraska Press.

Bernhard, L.A., & Dan, A.J. (1986). Redefining sexuality from women's own experiences. *Nursing Clinics in North America, 21*, 125–136.

Caplan, P.C. (Ed.) (1987). *The cultural construction of sexuality*. London: Tavistock.

Chapman, J., & Sughrue, Jr., J. (1987). A model for sexual assessment and intervention. *Health Care for Women International, 8*, 87–99.

Coopersmith, S. (1967). *The antecedents of self-esteem*. San Francisco: Freeman.

Dressel, P., & Avant, W. (1983). Range of alternatives. In R. Weg (Ed.), *Sexuality in later years: Roles and behavior* (pp. 185–207). New York: Academic.

Frauman, A.C., & Syphert, N.S. (1979). Sexuality in adolescents with chronic illness. *MCN: The American Journal of Maternal–Child Nursing, 4*, 371–375.

Friedeman, J.S. (1979). Sexuality in older persons: Implications for nursing practice. *Nursing Forum, 18*, 92–101.

Green, R. (Ed.). (1979). *Human Sexuality: A health practitioner's text* (2nd ed.). Baltimore: Williams & Wilkens.

Grimes, J., & Burns, E. (1987). *Health assessment in nursing practice* (2nd ed.). Boston: Jones & Bartlett.

Gutman, D. (1985). The parental imperative revisited: Toward a developmental psychology of later life. *Contributions to Human Development, 4*, 31–60.

Huston, A.C. (1985). The development of sex typing: Themes from recent research. *Developmental Review, 5*, 1–17.

Kaplan, H. (1979). *Disorders of sexual desire and other concepts and techniques in sex therapy*. New York: Brunner/Mazel.

Kinsey, A.C., Pomeroy, W.B., & Martin, C.E. (1948). *Sexual behavior in the human male*. Philadelphia: Saunders.

Kinsey, A.C., Pomeroy, W.B., Martin, C.E., & Gebhard, P.H. (1953). *Sexual behavior in the human female*. Philadelphia: Saunders; New York: Pocket Books.

Lamb, M.E. (1986). The emergent American father. In M. Lamb (Ed.), *The father's role: Applied perspectives*. New York: Wiley.

LaRocca, S.A., & Polit, D.F. (1980). Women's knowledge about the menopause. *Nursing Research, 29*, 10–13.

Leppink, M.A. (1979). Adolescent sexuality. *Maternal Child Nursing Journal, 8*, 153–161.

Livson, F.B. (1983). Gender identity. In R.B. Weg (Ed.), *Sexuality in the later years: Roles and behavior*. New York: Academic.

Livson, N., & Peskin, H. (1980). Perspectives on adolescence from longitudinal research. In J. Adelson (Ed.), *Handbook on adolescent psychology*. New York: Wiley.

Ludwick, R. (1988). Breast examination in the older adult. *Cancer Nursing, 11*(2), 99–102.

Massey, V. (1986). Perceived susceptibility to breast cancer and practice of breast self-examination. *Nursing Research, 35*, 183–185.

Masters, W.H. (1986). Sex and aging: Expectations and reality. *Hospital Practice, 21*, 175–198.

Masters, W.H., & Johnson, V.E. (1966). *Human sexual response*. Boston: Little, Brown.

Meyrowitz, J. (1985). *No sense of place*. New York: Oxford.

Moore, D.S., & Erickson, P.I. (1985). Age, gender, and ethnic differences in sexual and contraceptive knowledge, attitudes, and behaviors. *Family and Community Health, 8*(3), 38–51.

Peach, E.H. (1980). Counseling sexually active very young adolescent girls. *MCN: The American Journal of Maternal-Child Nursing, 5*, 191–195.

Pfeiffer, E. (1979). Sexuality and the aging patient. In R. Green (Ed.), *Human sexuality: A health practitioner's text* (2nd ed., pp. 124–135). Baltimore: Williams & Wilkins.

Reno, D.R. (1988). Men's knowledge and health beliefs about testicular cancer and testicular self-examination. *Cancer Nursing, 11*(2), 112–117.

Robinson, P.K. (1983). The sociological perspective. In R.B. Weg (Ed.), *Sexuality in later years: Roles and perspectives*. New York: Academic.

Rudolph, A., & McDermott, R.J. (1987). The breast physical examination: Its value in early cancer detection. *Cancer Nursing, 10*(2), 100–106.

Rutledge, Dana N. (1987). Factors related to women's practice of breast self-examination. *Nursing Research, 36*(2), 117–121.

Sachs, B. (1986). Reproductive decisions in adolescence. *Image: Journal of Nursing Scholarship, 18*(2), 69–72.

Sadker, M., & Sadker, D. (1985). Sexism in the schoolroom of the 1980s. *Psychology Today, 19*(3), 54–57.

Tanner, J.M. (1962). *Growth at adolescence* (2nd ed.). Oxford: Blackwell Scientific.

Watts, R.J. (1979). Dimensions of sexual health. *American Journal of Nursing, 79*, 1568–1572.

Weg, R.B. (1983). *Sexuality in the later years: Roles and behavior*. New York: Academic.

Woods, N.F. (1984). *Human sexuality in health and illness* (3rd ed.). St. Louis: Mosby.

Woods, N.F. (1987). Toward a holistic perspective of human sexuality: Alterations in sexual health and nursing diagnoses. *Holistic Nursing Practice, 1*(4), 1–11.

World Health Organization. (1975). *Education and treatment in human sexuality: The training of health professionals*. Report of a WHO Meeting. Technical Report Series No. 372. Geneva: WHO.

Yoos, L. (1987). Adolescent cognitive and contraceptive behaviors. *Pediatric Nursing, 13*(4), 247–250.

Yoselle, H. (1981). Sexuality in the later years. *Topics in Clinical Nursing, 3*, 59–70.

PART
V

Physiological Assessment

14

Physical Integrity Assessment

CHAPTER OUTLINE

■ Knowledge Needed to Assess Physical Integrity
General Appraisal   Physical Growth   Vital Signs   Skin Integrity   Immune Response   Approach to Physical Integrity   Variables That Influence Physical Integrity

■ The Physical Integrity History

■ Clinical Appraisal and Screening
General Appraisal   Measurement and Interpretation of Physical Growth   Vital Signs   Integumentary Assessment   Assessment of the Lymphatic System

■ Nursing Diagnoses Related to Physical Integrity

OBJECTIVES

Upon completion of this chapter, you should be able to:

■ Explain the importance of general appraisal, integumentary and lymph node assessments, and accurate measurement of vital signs and growth in evaluating a client's health.

■ List the major components of the physical integrity assessment of a client.

■ Describe the correct methods of assessing a client's physical growth and vital signs.

■ Describe the components of the integumentary and lymph node assessments of a client.

■ Conduct an assessment of a client's physical growth, vital signs, lymph nodes, skin, hair, and nails.

■ Explain how the physical integrity assessment should be modified according to the client's age, race, cultural background, and health.

■ Use information obtained from the physical integrity assessment to formulate valid and appropriate nursing diagnoses.

Physiological assessment begins with an appraisal of the client's general appearance and skin integrity, including hair and nails. These checks, in combination with measurements of vital signs and physical growth, are referred to as *physical integrity* because they are valuable indicators of the client's general state of health. They can help identify problem areas that should be evaluated more thoroughly in subsequent parts of the assessment.

More important, the nurse should begin the assessment with the client's general appearance and skin because this appraisal is not invasive and thus is less threatening initially to the individual, whether adult or child. Since the client's general appearance, hair, and skin of at least face and hands are readily visible, the nurse can conduct a general appraisal while establishing rapport with the client. The initial part of any meeting can be used to begin the physiological assessment, but the time devoted to assessing physical integrity is especially useful for helping the client feel at ease. This interlude sets the stage for the remainder of the assessment. It is impossible to overstress the importance of being attentive to the client's comfort, talking with the client, and maintaining the client's privacy to promote the client's sense of well-being, to foster the client's positive feelings about health care, and to obtain an accurate assessment of the client's physiological state.

KNOWLEDGE NEEDED TO ASSESS PHYSICAL INTEGRITY

The importance of measuring vital signs and physical growth cannot be underestimated in evaluating a client's health. Changes in temperature, pulse, respiration, and blood pressure occur with changes in body functions, disease, and emotional states. Often a change in vital signs is one of the first indications of a change in the individual's health. Height and weight are particularly important factors to consider, especially in children. In an adult, a change in weight may indicate a disease, but weight also may predispose an individual to certain diseases such as obesity, which has been related to cardiovascular disease.

Systemic diseases often manifest themselves in changes in the integumentary system, such as the pallor of anemia or jaundice of liver disease. In addition to reflecting problems in other systems, the skin itself performs functions that are vital to the well-being of the human organism. The immune system also performs functions that are critical. Through a complex, but integrated number of components, the immune system maintains homeostasis through protective mechanisms. Knowledge of the signs that reflect physical integrity and immune response (specifically, the lymphatic system and lymph node assessment) is necessary for accurate assessment.

General Appraisal

The general appraisal or general survey is a broad assessment of the individual's overall state of health. The general appraisal includes an evaluation of overall appearance, physical growth, and vital signs. These are important general indicators of health and are assessed at the beginning.

Aspects to consider in a general appraisal include the client's sex, race, gait, posture, body build, grooming and hygiene, level of consciousness, mood, affect, and cognitive abilities. Any signs of discomfort or ill health also should be noted. Information about these dimensions provides clues to health status. For example, how people feel about themselves often is reflected in how they dress and carry themselves. The content and patterns of an individual's speech and the appropriateness of the responses reflect the cognitive abilities of the client. Posture, affect, facial expressions, gait and body movements may indicate anger, depression, pain, or fear or they may be the outward signs of a specific underlying disease, such as the blank stare and shuffling gait associated with Parkinson's disease. As the nurse engages the client in conversation during the initial moments of the clinical appraisal, the nurse begins, through careful observation, to form a general appraisal of the client. This initial appraisal then is validated further during the course of the entire assessment.

Physical Growth

The concepts of human growth and development are important for understanding of changes during the life cycle. Growth refers to an increase in the number and size of the cells while development refers to the increasing functional ability of cells (Williams & Worthington, 1988). At different periods in the life cycle, the rate or movement of the growth along a specific course will vary. At certain points growth will accelerate: in the early years of development and then at puberty, after which the growth rate "decelerates and maintains a slower and gradually declining velocity through adulthood" (Williams & Worthington, 1988, p. 26).

Gross body composition for an adult remains relatively stable from young adulthood through old age. There are, however, individual differences due to genetic makeup and lifestyle. There are also differences between men and women (Table 14-1). *Reference standard* does not mean that all men and women must achieve the specific body composition listed, "nor that the reference man and woman are in fact average" (Shangold & Mirkin, 1988, p. 31). The model presents only a useful frame of reference for comparisons.

In the young adult years (18–40), women have larger fat cells and larger body fat mass. Women also are smaller in size, height, and weight. Men, on the other hand, evidence a larger skeletal muscle mass, body size, height, and weight. There are a gradual decline in lean body mass and an increase in body weight as one moves into the middle years (40–60). As an individual approaches the later years, marked changes in body composition occur and overall height decreases. Subcutaneous fat is lost and bony prominences are evident. The use of skinfold measurements to assess body fat in older adults is less accurate than in earlier years due to changes in skin compressibility and the presence of pendulous and redundant fat folds (Williams & Worthington, 1988).

Vital Signs

Temperature, pulse, respiration, and blood pressure reflect a client's health. Because of their importance as indicators of psychological functioning, they are referred to as *vital signs*. The physiological mechanisms controlling the vital signs are extremely sensitive and maintain these indicators within very narrow limits. Along with other physiological factors, the vital signs form the basis of clinical problem-solving. The nurse's ability to ac-

curately measure these factors is important for identifying the presence of problems.

Body Temperature

Body temperatures change throughout the day with the lowest temperature 36.5°C occurring between 1:00 A.M. and 4:00 A.M. and peaking between 4:00 P.M. and 6:00 P.M. The normal range of body temperature is 36.1°C (97°F) to 37.6°C (99.6°F). Table 14-2 provides the equivalents of centigrade and Fahrenheit for body temperature. Relative stability of the temperature with these limits usually is maintained by the temperature-regulating mechanism of the hypothalamus. The hypothalamus serves as the central thermostat. Two centers within the hypothalamus control the conservation or dissipation of heat. The anterior hypothalamus regulates heat dissipation and the posterior hypothalamus regulates heat conservation. If the thermoreceptors of the anterior hypothalamus sense that the blood is too warm, heat-dissipating mechanisms are activated. Sweating is stimulated, and there is an increase in blood flow to superficial capillaries of the skin through vasodilation. If the thermoreceptors of the posterior hypothalamus sense that the blood is too cold, peripheral vasoconstriction occurs to prevent loss of heat, and metabolic activity is increased to increase heat production. Shivering is a physiological response that produces heat by means of muscular activity.

The heat produced by the body must equal the amount of heat lost in order for the body's temperature to remain constant. Heat is produced in the body as a by-product of the metabolism of food.

TABLE 14-1
Gross Body Composition of a Reference Man and Woman for Muscle, Fat, and Bone

Reference Man	Variable	Reference Woman
20–24	Age, yr	20–24
68.5	Height, in	64.5
154	Weight, lb	125
69 (44.8%)	Muscle, lb	45 (36.0%)
23.1 (15.0%)	Total fat, lb	33.8 (27.0%)
4.6 (3.0%)	Essential fat, lb	15.0 (12.0%)
18.5 (12.0%)	Storage fat, lb	18.8 (15.0%)
23.0 (14.9%)	Bone, lb	15.0 (12.0%)
136	Lean body weight, lb	—
—	Minimal weight, lb	107

Note. From Shangold, M., & Murkin, G. (1988). *Women and Exercise: Physiology and Sports Medicine.* Philadelphia: Davis, p. 31.

Adapted from McArdle WD, Katch Fl, and Katch VL. *Exercise Physiology,* ed. 2. Lea and Febiger, Philadelphia, 1986.

TABLE 14-2
Centigrade–Fahrenheit Equivalents

Centigrade	Fahrenheit
35.0	95.0
35.5	95.9
36.0	96.8
36.5	97.7
37.0	98.6
37.5	99.5
38.0	100.4
38.5	101.3
39.0	102.2
39.5	103.1
40.0	104.0
40.5	104.9
41.0	105.8
41.5	106.7

The index for measuring the rate of energy (heat) the body uses during rest is the basal metabolic rate. Heat is lost from the body through four basic mechanisms: radiation (approximately 60%), evaporation (approximately 25%), convection (approximately 12%), and conduction (approximately 3%). An alteration of these mechanisms will result in an increase in body temperature.

Pulse

The heart rate is regulated by the autonomic nervous system and normally is set by the sinoatrial node, or pacemaker, situated in the right atrium. Parasympathetic stimulation leads to slowing of the heart rate, whereas sympathetic stimulation increases the rate. The arterial pulse is produced by the ejection of blood into the aorta following ventricular systole. This action produces a pressure wave throughout the arterial system. The palpation of this pulse wave in a peripheral artery is referred to as an arterial pulse. The pulse rate is defined as normal, tachycardic, or bradycardic. In an adult, the average pulse ranges from 60 to 100 beats per minute. Tachycardia refers to a rate over 100, and bradycardia is a rate under 50 beats per minute.

Pulse rates vary greatly with age. Normal pulse rates also vary according to sex, usual activity level, and time of day. Starting at approximately age 12, females have pulse rates 5 to 10 beats per minute higher than males. Athletes have lower average pulse rates than others, often as low as 40 to 50 beats per minute.

A medication, such as digitalis, will decrease the pulse rate because it stimulates the vagus nerve, which decreases cardiac contractions. Factors such as pain, exercise, strong emotions, prolonged application of heat, elevated temperature, and a decrease in blood pressure (due to blood loss) will result in an increase in the pulse rate. As with temperature, pulse rates follow a circadian rhythm and generally are lowest in the early morning and highest in the late afternoon.

Respiration

Respiration is controlled by the respiratory center in the medulla oblongata. As with the pulse, respiration is dependent not only on neurological stimulation, but also on the condition of the pulmonary system, including pulmonary circulation, the respiratory tract, and pulmonary musculature. Abnormalities in any of these areas will affect respiration. Other factors such as age, emotional states, exercise, acid-base balance, oxygen and carbon dioxide levels also will affect respiration. For the adult, the range of normal respirations is 12–20 respirations per minute.

Blood Pressure

Blood pressure is determined by the total peripheral resistance and cardiac output (amount of blood pumped with each ventricular contraction) multiplied by the heart rate. Blood pressure is regulated by a complex combination of nervous, hormonal, and renal factors. Blood pressure, like pulse and respiration, varies with age. For the adult, normal blood pressure values range from 95–140 mm Hg systolic over 60–90 mm Hg diastolic. Alterations in blood pressure may be related to changes in the blood vessels, blood volume, or the heart's pumping ability, as well as to nervous, endocrine, or renal disorders. It is important to consider what is normal for an individual as well as what is normal for the population in assessing blood pressure.

Vital signs can provide valuable clues to many underlying problems, but numerous factors can cause similar changes in any one or all of the vital signs. In interpreting findings, therefore, the nurse also must evaluate data from other parts of the client's assessment before drawing conclusions about what may be causing any change or abnormality in the vital signs.

Skin Integrity

The skin is made up of three layers (Figure 14-1). The outermost layer is the epidermis. This thin, avascular layer is itself composed of two parts: a horny layer of dead cells that are sloughed and replaced, and a basal cell layer consisting of living cells that contain melanin. The amount of melanin, and thus the color of an individual's skin, is determined by heredity, hormones, sun exposure, and irritants. The middle skin layer is the dermis. It is made up of connective tissue, has a good blood supply, and contains nerve endings. The dermis tends to be thicker on the palms, soles, and dorsal and lateral surfaces; it is thinner on the eyelids, penis, scrotum, and ventral and medial surfaces. The innermost layer consists of subcutaneous tissue, which stores fat and thus acts as an insulator.

In addition to these three layers are the hair follicles, sebaceous glands, eccrine glands, and apocrine glands, which extend down from the surface into the dermis and subcutaneous tissue. The sebaceous glands secrete sebum, which lubricates the skin. The eccrine glands are widely scattered over the body and secrete salt and water in response to elevated temperatures and sympathetic nervous

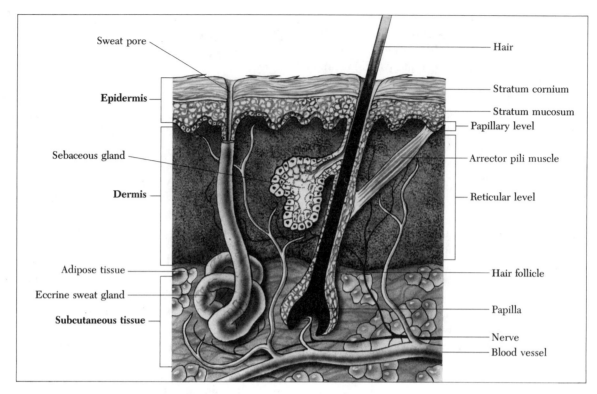

FIGURE 14-1. Anatomy of the skin.

stimulation. In contrast to these odorless secretions, the apocrine glands found in the axillary and genital areas produce secretions that decompose in the presence of bacteria, leading to the characteristic body odor.

The skin itself performs vital functions. The integument helps prevent fluid and electrolyte loss and allows for the elimination of certain waste products, such as urea and bilirubin. The skin aids in maintaining normal body temperature; sweat glands permit heat loss, whereas subcutaneous tissue acts as insulation to conserve heat. The skin is a sense organ for pain, temperature, and touch, warning the body of harmful or noxious stimuli. Last but not least, the skin acts as the body's first line of defense, protecting deeper tissue from invasion by foreign material and organisms.

The hair covering the body is of two types: vellus (tiny, small hairs covering the entire body with the exception of the soles and palms) and terminal (coarse, long, thick and easily visible on the scalp, axillary, and pubic areas). The oil from the sebaceous glands within the hair follicle lubricates the hair. The nails are keratinized appendages of the epidermis. The nails should be smooth, convex, transparent, not tender, and firm. The nail beds should be pink.

The condition of the skin, hair, and nails can provide important clues to the individual's overall health. Their condition is influenced by such factors as age, race, health, environmental elements, and medications, which will be addressed in a later section of this chapter.

Immune Response*

Through a complex and integrated number of components, the immune system maintains homeostasis by protecting the body from invasion by foreign agents and preventing their growth. These protective mechanisms or body defenses are classified as nonspecific and specific.

The nonspecific body defenses are the primary defenses. These include the physical and chemical barriers located throughout the body (skin, bacterial flora, tears, sneezing, and coughing, blinking, cilia, saliva, nasal secretions, urine, and vaginal secretions), the phagocytic action of white blood cells, the cellular production of the protein interferon, and the inflammatory process. The nonspecific body defenses provide immunity by preserving the internal environment of the body.

The specific body defenses are referred to as

---

*Adapted from Servonsky, J., & Opas, S.R. (1987). *Nursing Management of Children.* Boston: Jones and Bartlett Publishers.

the secondary defenses and include humoral (antibody-mediated) immunity, cellular (cell-mediated) immunity, complements (serum proteins, which enhance antigen–antibody reaction), and phagocytosis. These body defenses provide immunity by stimulating the immune response.

If an organism or foreign agent passes through the nonspecific body defenses and survives, the agent or organism must overcome the specific defenses of the body. The primary defenses of the body provide resistance to all microorganisms, while the secondary defenses resist only those organisms to which they are exposed.

The lymphatic system plays a key role in the immune response. One of its functions is to develop, maintain, and repair the immune system. Microorganisms in interstitial spaces are collected by the lymphatics and taken to the lymph nodes. There the lymphocytes and macrophages encircle the microorganisms.

In addition to its protective mechanism, the lymphatics also collect proteins and fluid from the interstitial spaces. These are then transported to the venous system thus helping to prevent edema. There are more than 500 lymph nodes in the body. They may be found in clusters or chains and may be deep or superficial. With age, the size and number of lymph nodes decrease (McConnell, 1988).

Approach to Physical Integrity

Specific approaches for each component of the physical integrity assessment will be discussed later. However, some general principles are applicable to all aspects of the physiological portion of the nursing assessment.

Head-to-Toe

As with any assessment, it is important to be systematic. Generally speaking, a cephalocaudal (head-to-toe) approach works best. The nurse begins the appraisal with the head and progresses down the body to the upper extremities, trunk, and lower extremities, carefully inspecting each part, front and back. If a systematic approach is not used, the nurse may overlook portions of the assessment.

General-to-Specific

Having made a thorough general observation, the nurse should proceed to closer examination of any abnormalities noted. For example, if there is a rash on the client's arm, its extent and specific characteristics should be determined. There is good reason for completing the general observations first,

then going back to make a more specific assessment. It is easy to become distracted by an abnormality, getting involved in describing it in exact detail, to the extent that one can neglect entirely the remainder of the general appraisal.

Although the components of the assessment will be essentially the same regardless of age, culture, or health, the approach may need to be altered to accommodate these factors. For example, with an adult the nurse can, after a brief statement of what is to be done, simply begin the physical examination either by taking the client's vital signs or inspecting and palpating the head. This is not likely to be successful with a young child, however. Whether young or old, if the individual is not feeling well, adjustments in approach may be necessary. If the client is confined to bed and has difficulty moving, it may be necessary to first examine the front of the body and then the back, rather than assessing the front and back of each body part before proceeding to the next part. For the older client, the nurse may need to minimize the number of position changes during the examination in order to avoid fatiguing the client.

It is not possible to describe here each modification that may be necessary as a result of a client's health. The important part is that the nurse should be alert to the need for varying the approach. Thus, the manner of approach and the specific order of the examination should be adjusted to the individual client, rather than conforming to a set outline. The only standard guideline is that the assessment should be systematic and, therefore, as complete as possible.

Variables That Influence Physical Integrity

Variations related to the age, racial background, and health of the client must be taken into account when performing a nursing assessment of physical integrity.

Age

Findings in several areas of the general appraisal will vary with the age of the client. The first of these is mental status.

The elderly client, for example, may be slow in responding or may not respond at all to questions or commands. This slowness, which can appear to be an intellectual deficit, may instead be due to age-related hearing and vision loss. The client should be observed for signs of confusion, including limited attention span, loss of recent memory, and poor judgment. Such confusion may be associated with a variety of physical disorders, including oxygen deficiency, metabolic disturbances, and neurological disease, but it may also be the result of being placed in an unfamiliar environment. This is seen frequently at night in the hospital when clients awaken and temporarily cannot remember where they are.

The examples noted above show how one should consider first simple explanations for variations from normal rather than assuming that abnormal findings must be due to disease.

The other aspects of general appraisal to consider are body proportions and movements. In the infant, the head appears large in relation to the rest of the body. Also, when first learning to walk, children have a poorly balanced, wide-based gait; their walk does not become steady until the latter half of the second year of life. In the elderly, gait will change, once again becoming less stable and also slower.

With aging, changes can be expected in the skin, hair, and nails. As in the case of the very young, the skin of the older adult becomes thinner. With loss of sebaceous glands, the skin is drier, less elastic, and prone to wrinkling. As a result of these changes, the skin is again more sensitive to trauma. Also, since regenerative capacity is decreased, healing takes longer in older clients. Areas of hyperpigmentation and hypopigmentation are common.

Several skin lesions occur normally in older individuals (Miller, 1990). Seborrheic keratoses are light tan to black, raised lesions up to 3 cm in diameter with rough surfaces. Skin tags are small (up to 1 cm), tan lesions that appear to hang from the neck, face, or axillae, while senile angiomas are small (up to 5 mm), red or purple dome-shaped lesions occurring on the trunk and extremities.

Nails tend to become thicker and more brittle with age, and hair begins to turn gray; the age at which this graying starts is highly variable and individual. Recession of hair on the scalp begins fairly early in life, by age 20 in men and by age 40 in women; in women this recession is bitemporal. In addition to recession of hair, there is a general thinning of scalp, leg, axillary, and pubic hair with age. Conversely, many women develop increased facial hair, and the eyebrows and nasal hair of men tend to lengthen.

The young as well as the old experience differences in temperature regulation. While infants and children demonstrate less well-regulated temperature, the older adult has a decreased ability to respond to changes in environmental temperature because sweat glands atrophy with age and the ability of the blood vessels to dilate or constrict de-

clines (Miller, 1990). In addition, there is a general decrease in body temperature with age that is secondary to lowered metabolic rate and activity as well as poor circulation (Burnside, 1988). Therefore, as with infants, hypothermia and hyperthermia are major concerns.

Blood pressure, like pulse and respiration, varies with age. In general, there is a gradual increase in blood pressure after age 20. Blood pressure is normally lower in women than men. It is also lower in the early morning and highest in the late afternoon. Exercise, emotional upset, and pain will increase blood pressure.

In most healthy individuals, with the exception of newborns and the elderly, the rhythm of respiration is fairly regular. In the very young, the respiratory rate is normally irregular—rapid breaths alternate with short periods of apnea. During sleep, elderly individuals may have periods of deep respiration alternating with periods of cessation of breathing (apnea). Respiration is cyclical: It becomes increasingly shallow, progresses to apnea, and then becomes increasingly deeper. This periodic breathing, or Cheyne-Stokes respiration, also is seen in severely ill individuals such as those with brain damage, heart failure, or renal failure.

Health

Both the approach to and the findings in the general appraisal will vary with the health of the client. Certain areas may need to be omitted. For example, if an individual is confined to a bed or a wheelchair, either at home or in the hospital, it will not be possible to assess gait or to assess posture in all three positions—lying, sitting, and standing. Also, if a hospitalized client must push an IV pole or carry some other equipment while walking, an abnormality of gait is more likely to reflect this encumbrance rather than an underlying neurological or muscular disorder.

Another aspect of the general appraisal that may vary with the health of an individual is mental status. Disorientation and lethargy may indicate a neurological deficit related to trauma or an underlying disease. Alternatively, these signs may be the result of a number of other factors, such as medications the client is receiving, oxygen deficiency, or acidosis. As noted earlier, with the hospitalized client confusion also may be the result of being placed in an unfamiliar environment.

The last aspect of general appraisal to be considered here is hygiene, dress, and grooming. Bedridden or handicapped clients may be dependent on assistance from others in these areas. Thus, their hygiene, dress, and grooming may reflect the availability of such assistance rather than their self-concept or sociocultural values. Information about the client's usual hygiene practices and patterns should be obtained on admission. It is important to assess the client's reaction to his or her state of hygiene while hospitalized. Lack of concern for hygiene may indicate depression, excessive fatigue, or pain with movement. On the other hand, lack of hygiene care can be distressing to clients and may add to their discomfort.

Careful temperature recording for febrile patients is important, since the pattern of a fever may provide clues to its origin. A continuous or sustained fever in which there is a consistently elevated temperature without diurnal variation is seen in typhoid and scarlet fever. An intermittent fever, characterized by wide daily variations and a normal morning temperature, is seen with abscesses. A remittent fever with wide daily fluctuations but without a return to a normal temperature is found in septicemia. A relapsing fever, as in malaria, or Hodgkin's disease, is one in which periods of elevated temperature alternate with periods of normal temperature.

In evaluating fevers, it is helpful to remember that infants and elderly clients may not show the same responses to illness as others do because of their poor thermoregulatory capabilities. At both ends of the age span, there may be a slow or limited rise in temperature in response to infection. The nurse must therefore be alert to smaller variations in temperature in these clients.

In addition to the foregoing causes, elevated temperatures may be caused by hormones (such as thyroid hormone and progesterone), drugs that reduce sweating (such as atropine), hypermetabolic conditions (such as hyperthyroidism), and disorders of the central nervous system that interfere with the temperature-regulating center. With central nervous system diseases or damage, hyperpyrexia, a temperature over 41.1°C [106°], can occur.

Disease does not always result in a temperature elevation. Hypothermia can occur with severe infections in newborns and the elderly. Central nervous system depression also may cause a decrease in body temperature.

Alterations in blood pressure may be related to changes in the blood vessels, blood volume, or the heart's pumping ability, as well as to nervous, endocrine, or renal disorders.

In approximately 90% of adults and 20 to 30% of children with high blood pressure, the cause is unknown, and the condition is called essential or primary hypertension. Secondary hypertension is high blood pressure related to some identifiable underlying disease. The specific disease processes that can cause hypertension are too numerous to mention, but as noted previously, neural, endocrine, renal, and cardiovascular problems all are potential causes of hypertension. Hypotension, on the other hand, may occur with hypovolemia due to hemorrhage or dehydration, heart failure, medication, or sepsis.

Assessment of the skin has special implications for individuals who are ill, immobilized, or hospitalized. These individuals are more prone to skin problems, particularly skin breakdown, than others. Skin integrity depends on an adequate supply of nutrients and the removal of waste products. Anything that interferes with either of these, such as poor circulation or malnutrition, predisposes the individual to skin breakdown. Limited circulation can result from pressure (especially over bony prominences) or disease (such as arteriosclerosis or diabetes). Other factors that contribute to skin breakdown include friction, moisture, and irritating substances.

Individuals who must remain in bed or in a chair are prone to the development of pressure sores (decubitus ulcers). If they lie or sit in any one position for a period of time, points of contact between their bodies and the chair or bed suffer from diminished blood flow secondary to pressure, which may in turn lead to skin breakdown. This is true even for a basically healthy individual.

Individuals with underlying health problems are especially susceptible to skin breakdown. For example, the chronically ill or debilitated client may be underweight, having less subcutaneous tissue to act as a cushion or protection against pressure. In those who are anemic, arteriosclerotic, vitamin deficient, or hypoproteinemic, the skin is not receiving sufficient nutrients for cell maintenance. Perspiration, urine, and feces are irritating to the skin, thus increasing the chance of skin breakdown in the febrile or incontinent client. Any of the foregoing factors only add to the problems created by pressure from lying in bed or sitting in a chair for prolonged periods.

One other group of individuals deserves particular mention—those who are immobilized. Normally, individuals move frequently to relieve and redistribute pressure. Individuals with spinal cord injuries and neurological disorders, such as strokes, cannot readily move and often spend many hours in one position; in addition, they may not be able to sense ischemia through tingling and numbness, so they do not receive this normal stimulus to relieve pressure by moving. Others who cannot move include those who are unconscious, paralyzed, sedated, or restrained. Casts, braces, and splints also may cause skin breakdown through pressure and friction.

Clients with ostomies also deserve specific consideration relative to skin integrity. Because of the irritating nature of excretions through ostomies and sometimes of the appliances used to collect excretions, the nurse (or client) must carefully and regularly examine the surrounding skin for redness and excoriation. Assessment and avoidance of skin breakdown is a clearly significant concern for the nurse.

Race

Modifications of the physical integrity assessment related to racial characteristics primarily have to do with the integument (see Table 14-3). The components of the exam are the same, but the approach requires some modifications for dark-skinned clients. The nurse must listen carefully to the client's or family's assessment of changes in the integument, particularly in an initial assessment and if the changes are subtle.

As with any client, color changes are observed most easily in the least pigmented areas: sclerae, conjunctivae, nail beds, lips, and mucous membranes. The palms of the hands and the soles of the feet, which also generally contain less pigment, are not as useful in evaluating changes in skin color; when calloused, these areas take on an opaque, yellowish color that obscures other changes in skin color. The sclerae are normally white and the conjunctivae pink; however, in many individuals with dark skin there are subconjunctival fat deposits that give a yellowish hue to the conjunctivae and adjacent sclerae. This normal variation may be misinterpreted as the beginning of jaundice. The nail beds, lips, and mucous membranes are usually pink, yet bluish lips are normal in some dark-skinned clients, especially those from the Mediterranean. Also, some blacks normally have slightly bluish gums. These findings may be mistaken for cyanosis. Awareness of such differences can prevent errors in assessment..

Pallor was described earlier as a decrease in the normal underlying red tones related to a decrease in oxygenated hemoglobin. In the black client, this decrease results in an ashen-gray appearance, and in the brown-skinned client a yellowish-brown color is evident.

The redness associated with flushing is less easily seen in those with dark skin. However, since flushing generally is associated with an increased blood flow to an area, the temperature of the skin is likely to be warmer. Thus, it may be possible to "feel" redness or flushing more easily than to see it.

Cyanosis can be difficult to detect in dark-skinned clients, especially since the lips and gums may have a normally bluish tinge, but careful inspection will enable the nurse to identify cyanosis. The area around the mouth will appear grayish, while the nail beds, tongue, and buccal mucosa will appear bluish.

With jaundice, the sclerae of dark-skinned clients will become yellow. In order not to be confused by the yellow tinge from subconjunctival fat deposits, the nurse should inspect the sclerae nearest to the center of the eye. The other area that will aid in detecting jaundice, and thus should be inspected, is the mouth. The oral mucosa, particularly in the area of the palate, will become a muddy yellow if the client is jaundiced.

As with all clients, areas of hyperpigmentation and hypopigmentation should be noted in dark-skinned persons. Areas of hypopigmentation, such as vitiligo, are particularly distressing to dark-skinned clients since they are much more noticeable than similar areas would be on light-skinned individuals. Another common type of hypopigmentation is that associated with healing of injuries and inflammation of the skin. Hyperpigmentation also may follow injury or inflammation; the exact cause of these changes in pigment is not known, but the changes usually resolve with time.

Skin lesions, such as rashes, can be particularly difficult to see on a dark-skinned client. For this reason, careful palpation is generally more helpful than inspection in detecting lesions. Blacks are prone to the same type of skin lesions as others, but some lesions, such as keloids, occur more frequently in blacks than in other racial groups.

Finally, there are a few points relative to hair that are worthy of note (see Table 14-3). In general, Asians and native Americans tend to have less body hair than those from other racial backgrounds. Most blacks have curly hair; in men, this frequently leads to a problem known as pseudofolliculitis. When the hair is shaved it curls back on itself and the cut end penetrates the skin, creating an inflammatory reaction. A second hair problem common to blacks is alopecia secondary to use of a hair pick or tight braiding of the hair. Picking tends to break hair shafts, while tight braids create a constant pull on the hair roots.

TABLE 14-3
Racial or Ethnic Variations of the Integumentary System

Racial or Ethnic Group	Predominant Skin Color	Predominant Hair Color and Texture
Black	Light brown to deep brown tones	Black; curly and wooly
Raza and Latino (Mexican or Chicano, Puerto Rican, Cuban, Spanish, Central and South American)	Tan, olive, to dark brown tones	Black or dark brown; wavy, curly or straight
Filipino	Brown tones	Black; coarse, straight or wavy
Chinese	Yellow tones	Black; coarse, straight or wavy
Japanese	Yellow tones	Black or brown-black; coarse, straight or wavy
Vietnamese	Brown tones	Black; coarse, straight or wavy
Eskimo and Aleut	Yellow tones	Black; straight
American Indian	Brown-red tones	Black; straight
Caucasian	Pale pink, tan, olive tones	Black, brown, red, or blond; straight to curly, coarse to very fine

Note. From Servonsky/Opas: *Nursing Management of Children*, © 1987. Boston: Jones and Bartlett Publishers.
Compiled from *Ethnic nursing care: a multicultural approach*, by M. Orque, B. Bloch, and L. Monrroy (St. Louis: The C.V. Mosby Company, 1983), pp. 102, 139, 169, 197, 263, and 290.

THE PHYSICAL INTEGRITY HISTORY

The physical integrity history provides information on a number of important aspects that reflect the client's overall health. These aspects include general appraisal (appearance, mental status, body characteristics, signs of distress), vital signs, and integumentary status. As the nurse engages the client in conversation, the nurse begins to form a general appraisal of the client. Careful questioning of the client with regard to personal hygiene habits, frequency of bathing and shampooing, preference for dress, and routine care of the skin, hair, and nails provides important nursing history information. With regard to dress, the nurse must consider what is appropriate for the client's age, time of year, as well as what is culturally or socially in vogue at the time. An older client in an uncoordinated outfit should not be described as eccentric or unkempt based on dress. The client may have difficulty perceiving color and not be aware of color differences, a common occurrence with aging.

The presence of body odors should be explored. While they may indicate poor hygiene, they also may reflect health problems, such as the acetone breath associated with diabetes or alcohol abuse.

Indications of the mental status of a client are discerned through conversation with the client. In this manner, the nurse observes the client's orientation, attention span, and thought processes. Speech is noted as the client easily or with difficulty responds to questions. The nurse observes the behavior of the client, noting appropriateness for age and the setting. Congruence of verbal and nonverbal behavior should be noted. The client's descriptions of general mood and handling of stress provide clues to coping ability and personal resourcefulness. The nurse should explore any problems related to loss of consciousness, dizziness, falls, head injuries, or the use of recreational drugs. Past or current use of psychotropic drugs and professional counseling should be noted as well. Any family history of mental illness should also be documented.

Height and weight are measured during the clinical appraisal; it is important for the nurse to determine whether there has been a change in the client's weight or height. For example, sporadic dieting may result in the frequent fluctuation of a client's weight and the inability to maintain a stable weight. Older adults may lose anywhere from 2.5 to 10 cm. in height as they age. Loss of height may be subtle over time and this needs to be explored with the client. A client's comment that clothes are not fitting properly or seem to be getting longer provides important information.

Signs of distress usually are observed early in the client–nurse interaction and need to be explored. The tense and anxious client may be experiencing respiratory difficulty, not simply feeling anxious about seeking medical care.

Vital signs are valuable indicators of health and it is important to determine what is normal for the client. Vital signs are influenced by a variety of factors such as age, stress, exercise, illness, climate, and medications. Obtaining data on these aspects is important. A family history of respiratory or cardiac problems should be documented and alerts the nurse to explore the client's risk factors as well as preventive measures.

Like the vital signs, the skin is an important indicator of overall health. Characteristics of the client's skin should be explored and any changes described. Routine care of the skin (lotions, frequency of bathing) should be noted. Along with the skin, the nurse obtains data about the hair and nails. Determining what is normal for the client and how long this has been the case is important. Thinning hair of long standing may be familial and thus not an indicator of a change in the client's health. In obtaining information about the skin, hair, and nails, the nurse should explore the client's nutrition for indications of deficiencies. This is especially important if problems are evident or suspected. A family history of allergies, skin cancer, psoriasis, or alopecia also should be documented. A careful and thorough history of physical integrity (see Table 14-4) guides the nurse in performing the clinical appraisal.

CLINICAL APPRAISAL AND SCREENING

The clinical appraisal and screening for physical integrity are assessments of the client's general appearance, vital signs, growth, and skin integrity and include assessment of the lymphatic system (see boxed insert, p. 424). Observation, inspection, and palpation are the techniques used.

General Appraisal

The general appraisal is a broad assessment of the individual's overall health. The data for this assessment are gathered from the moment the nurse first meets the client and continues throughout the time they spend together. Information is collected through observation and inspection, involving not only vision, but also hearing and smell.

Appearance

Although seemingly obvious, it is important to note the client's sex and race. These two factors should be kept in mind when obtaining the health history, doing a physical appraisal, and evaluating the information gathered, because some problems are more prevalent in a particular sex or race.

Next to be considered is the client's apparent age in comparison with stated chronological age. Great variations can occur because of heredity, sex, prior illnesses, and life experiences. Despite this normal variation, it is important to consider gross differences between apparent age and chronological age. Adults who appear much older than their stated ages may be suffering from acute or chronic stress, which may be physical or emotional. A child may be developing secondary sex characteristics prematurely, indicative of precocious puberty.

Hygiene, dress, and grooming may reflect an individual's self-concept, access to cleansing agents and makeup, physical disabilities, or socio-cultural values. The client should be asked about usual personal hygiene habits: How often does the client bathe or shower? At what time of day? What soaps, lotions, or oils are used? How often does the client shampoo? Other personal hygiene habits, such as use of deodorants, foot care, nail care, shaving, and use of makeup, should be elicited. If the client is a small child, an elderly person, or a physically disabled individual, the nurse should inquire what assistance the client needs with personal hygiene.

The nurse should appraise the client's hair, skin, and nails for cleanliness, bearing in mind that with some occupations (such as an auto mechanic) and with some pastimes (such as gardening) it is difficult or impossible to maintain clean nails. Moreover, a normally clean client might appear dirty in an emergency situation, owing to activities when an accident or sudden illness (e.g. heart attack) occurred. In such situations, a valuable clue to "normal" status might be whether the hair is cut and trimmed, whether dyed hair has grown out, and similar details.

The fit and cleanliness of clothes should be noted. Poorly fitting clothes can indicate a recent gain or loss of weight or may be a reflection of socioeconomic status. Although the nurse should consider whether or not dress is appropriate, one should remember that this varies greatly with age, culture, climate, economic status, and lifestyle. Not every client will be clothed in a fashion the nurse from a middle class background is accustomed to.

Body odor can result from poor hygiene, strenuous work, or exercise, as well as from disease. Acetone breath is present in diabetes, starvation, or as a result of certain fad diets (e.g., liquid protein). The smell of ammonia is evident in renal failure, and foul-smelling breath may be due to an oral in-

TABLE 14-4
Physical Integrity History

General Appraisal

Appearance
  Sex
  Race
  Apparent age versus chronological age
  Appropriate weight for height
  Usual personal hygiene habits—bath, shower (time of day); use of soaps, lotions, and frequency of shampooing
  Presence of body odor
  Dress—fit, cleanliness, appropriate for age, time of year, and what is culturally/socially acceptable

Mental Status
  Level of consciousness
  Orientation to people, place, and time
  Behavior appropriate to age and setting
  Speech appropriate to age; clarity; presence of speech impediments
  Thought process logical, attention span appropriate for age
  General mood and ability to handle stress
  Problems with loss of consciousness, dizziness, falls, recreational drug use
  Use of prescribed medications and professional counseling
  Personal and family history of mental illness

Body Characteristics
  Size and shape—proportionate and symmetrical
  Posture—erect, stooped, presence of deformity
  Movement—pattern of gait, general gross and fine motor movements appropriate for age, presence of any difficulties with movement

Signs of Distress
  Posture—relaxed or tense
  Facial expression—relaxed or tense, congruent with what is verbally communicated
  Breathing pattern—slow, regular, or increased
  Verbalization of pain explored with respect to location, onset, duration, associated signs/symptoms, relief efforts

Vital Signs

Temperature
  Normal temperature for client
  Patterns of elevation during illness
  Method usually used to take temperature (oral, axillary, rectal)

Pulse
  Normal rate for client
  Regularity of pulse; episodes of increased or decreased pulse rate or irregularities

  Use of medications to regulate pulse rate
  Response to exercise
  Last electrocardiogram (EKG) and findings
  Personal or family history of heart disease

Respiration
  Normal rate for client
  Regularity and ease of respiration
  Response to exercise
  History of respiratory problems (asthma, allergies, chronic obstructive lung disease, frequent colds)
  Presence of dyspnea, cough, sputum
  Smoking history
  Last chest x-ray and findings
  Current medications to improve breathing
  Personal or family history of respiratory problems

Blood Pressure
  Normal reading for client
  Regularity of blood pressure
  History of headaches, light-headedness, falls
  Response to exercise
  Personal or family history of hypertension, cardiovascular disease, or stroke
  Current medications
  Last blood pressure reading and finding

Integumentary Assessment

Skin
  Client's normal skin temperature, sensation, moisture, texture, thickness, and turgor
  Integrity of the skin—presence of infection, lesions or rashes
  Changes in any lesions of the skin over time
  Presence of wounds, ostomies
  Routine care of the skin
  Personal or family history of skin problems (cancer, allergies, psoriasis)
  Signs of nutritional deficiencies

Hair
  Cleanliness, frequency of shampooing
  Quality of the hair—texture, dryness
  Quantity and distribution
  Change in quantity, quality, or distribution
  Condition of scalp; presence of flaking, dandruff, or head lice
  Signs of nutritional deficiencies

Nails
  Normal color and consistency for client
  Contour—evidence of deformities
  Adherence to the nail beds
  Routine care of nails
  Signs of nutritional deficiencies

Sequence of Clinical Appraisal of Physical Integrity

General Appraisal
General Appearance
Mental Status
Body Characteristics
Signs of Distress

Physical Growth
Measurement
  Height
  Weight

Vital Signs
Measurement
  Temperature
  Respirations
  Blood Pressure
  Pulses

Integumentary System
Skin
  Inspection
    Color
    Vascularity
    Lesions
  Palpation
    Moisture
    Temperature
    Sensation

    Texture and thickness
    Turgor
    Lesions
Hair
  Inspection
    Color
    Quantity
    Distribution
  Palpation
    Texture
Nails
  Inspection
    Color
    Shape
    Lesions
  Palpation
    Texture

Lymphatic System
Inspection and Palpation of Lymph Nodes
  Cervical
  Supraclavicular and Infraclavicular
  Axillary
  Epitrochlear
  Superficial Inguinal

fection or to poor oral hygiene. Other odors, such as the smell of alcohol, should be noted.

Mental Status

This part of the evaluation should include the client's level of consciousness, orientation, behavior (and whether this behavior is reasonable for age and the setting), speech, mental capacity, and mood. For the purposes of the general appraisal, these factors need not be examined in detail and can be observed primarily through the client's responses to questions in the health history. In evaluating mood, the nurse also should observe the client's body language (posture and face). Further discussion of the mental status assessment may be found in chapter 15.

Body Characteristics

A third aspect of the general appraisal involves the size, shape, and movement of the body. The body should be proportionate and symmetrical. Arm span should approximately equal the client's height, and the symphysis pubis should be the midpoint between the top of the head and the feet. Atrophy, hypertrophy, or gross deformities of body parts should be noted, as should fat distribution. Atrophy occurs with lack of use, as in musculoske-

letal or neurological disorders. Enlargement of a part can be due to increased use, as in muscles of an athlete, to fat deposition, or to disease such as a neoplasm. Abnormal fat deposits in the face, neck, and trunk occur in Cushing's disease and from taking steroids.

Height and weight will be discussed in detail later. However, in the initial appraisal the nurse can observe for obvious undernutrition or obesity.

Posture should be observed with the client standing, sitting, and lying. Posture can indicate tension, depression, pain, or distress. For example, the client in respiratory distress will not lie flat in bed and often will sit forward in a chair to make breathing easier. The client who is depressed may slouch in a chair.

The client's gait should be inspected, including relative position of arms, trunk, and legs. Body movements should be deliberate, smooth, and coordinated. Abnormalities in gait, tremors, or difficulty with movement of a part occur in a variety of neurological and muscular disorders as well as with the use of drugs and alcohol.

Signs of Distress

The last aspect of general appraisal is looking for any signs of distress. As noted earlier, distress can be seen in the client's posture. Facial expressions, such as wincing or grimacing, and labored breathing also reflect discomfort. Certainly not to be overlooked are the client's reports of pain.

Measurement and Interpretation of Physical Growth

When measuring height (length) and weight it is important to use the same technique as well as the same measurement scale (i.e., centimeters or inches, kilograms or pounds) each time. Without this consistency, changes may be obscured or artificially inflated or deflated. If charts or tables of normal values are used for comparison, any specifications for method of measurement should be noted and either followed or adjusted appropriately. For example, some height charts give height for women in shoes with two-inch heels. If height is measured without shoes, then two inches should be added to the figure obtained from the chart.

Height

Except for young children, height should be measured with the client standing. For adolescents and adults this measurement can be made with the height attachment of a stand-up scale. The client should be asked to stand up straight, and a bar perpendicular to the scale should be placed on top of the client's head for accuracy of measurement. The height can simply be read from the scale.

Weight

For the individual who can stand without difficulty, a standard scale can be used for determining weight. The client who cannot stand or who is unstable in a standing position should be weighed lying on a bed scale. The scale should be balanced at zero before the client is weighed. Ideally, for complete accuracy, weight should be measured without clothing. However, in most instances, especially in the outpatient setting, weight is measured with the client in indoor clothing, but without shoes.

If weights are to be determined on consecutive days or weeks to check for changes, the measurement should be made on the same scale, with the client wearing the same amount of clothing, at the same time each day. Weights on different scales can vary as much as several pounds. Whether the client is weighed before or after eating also can alter the measurement. These factors can make a significant difference, especially if the weights are being used to assess dehydration or fluid retention and

this is serving as a basis for client management. A change in weight of 1 kilogram is equivalent to the gain or loss of 1,000 ml of fluid. This can be critical to an individual who is losing fluid as a result of a burn or to a client retaining fluid secondary to cardiac or renal problems. Observing for changes in weight also is important in assessing nutrition. Situations in which such information is valuable include, among others, the hospitalized or elderly client who is eating poorly and the obese client who is on a weight-loss program.

After height and weight are measured, the findings should be compared with expected norms for the client's age and sex (cross-sectional comparison). It is imperative to compare values with previous measurements of the same client to note any changes (longitudinal comparison).

For the adult who has completed physical growth, measurements of height are used primarily to determine appropriate weight ranges. Often, body build as well as height is considered in determining weight range. Commonly accepted standards of desirable weight for height for adults are given in Table 14-5.

Vital Signs

The client's temperature, pulse, respiration, and blood pressure usually are obtained at the same time. The order in which the vital signs are measured depends on the client. If taking one measurement is likely to upset the client, it should be left until the end. For example, if an adult is embarrassed about having a rectal temperature taken, the other signs should be taken first. Then the more stressful procedure of a rectal temperature can be carried out. It is preferable to determine vital signs when clients are calm and at rest since exercise and emotions can alter the vital signs.

The client's status and hospital or agency policy govern how frequently vital signs are assessed. For example, a client with an elevated temperature usually is assessed every four hours or more frequently depending on the temperature reading. A client returning to the clinical unit following surgery is assessed frequently (as often as every 15 minutes or every 30 minutes depending on the protocol) until vital signs are stable. Whenever possible the nurse should make the initial assessment of a client's vital signs rather than delegating it to auxiliary nursing personnel who may have less knowledge and skill.

Measuring Body Temperature

Body temperature can be measured orally, rectally, or under the armpit (axilla). There are advantages

TABLE 14-5
Metropolitan Life Insurance Company Height.Weight Data, Revised 1983

Height–Weight Tables for Adults (1983)

Women					Men				
Height		Frame*			Height		Frame*		
Ft	In	Small	Medium	Large	Ft	In	Small	Medium	Large
4	10	102–111	109–121	118–131	5	2	128–134	131–141	138–150
4	11	103–113	111–123	120–134	5	3	130–136	133–143	140–153
5	0	104–115	113–126	122–137	5	4	132–138	135–145	142–156
5	1	106–118	115–129	125–140	5	5	134–140	137–148	144–160
5	2	108–121	118–132	128–143	5	6	136–142	139–151	146–164
5	3	111–124	121–135	131–147	5	7	138–145	142–154	149–168
5	4	114–127	124–138	134–151	5	8	140–148	145–157	152–172
5	5	117–130	127–141	137–155	5	9	142–151	148–160	155–176
5	6	120–133	130–144	140–159	5	10	144–154	151–163	158–180
5	7	123–136	133–147	143–163	5	11	146–157	154–166	161–184
5	8	126–139	136–150	146–167	6	0	149–160	157–170	164–188
5	9	129–142	139–153	149–170	6	1	152–164	160–174	168–192
5	10	132–145	142–156	152–173	6	2	155–168	164–178	172–197
5	11	135–148	145–159	155–176	6	3	158–172	167–182	176–202
6	0	138–151	148–162	158–179	6	4	162–176	171–187	181–207

Note. Based on a weight–height mortality study conducted by the Society of Actuaries and the Association of Life Insurance Medical Directors of America, Metropolitan Life Insurance Company, revised 1983.

*Weights at ages 25 to 59 based on lowest mortality. Height includes 1-in heel. Weight for women includes 3 lb. for indoor clothing. Weight for men includes 5 lb. for indoor clothing.

and disadvantages for each. While the rectal temperature has long been considered the most reliable, this belief is being challenged. A study by Guiffre, Heidenreich, Carney-Gersten, Dorsch, and Heidenrich (1990) found that axillary temperature is accurate and adequately reflects the core body temperature.

Differences between oral, axillary, and rectal temperatures have been found to vary according to individual differences, how long the thermometer is left in place, and the type of thermometer used. In general, if care is taken with placement of the thermometer, if it is left in place for a sufficient length of time, and if the same thermometer is used each time, the nurse can obtain an accurate reflection of the client's body temperature and any changes in temperature with any one of the three methods. It is important to use the same thermometer each time, just as it is important to use the same scale for determining weight, since there may be significant differences between instruments.

For oral readings, at least 2 minutes are needed while rectal readings require only 2 to 3 minutes. Axillary readings, on the other hand, require approximately 10 minutes. Timing generally is not a problem with electronic thermometers, which register in a minute or less, regardless of the site used.

The rectal method should be avoided with clients who have rectal diseases, diarrhea, irritation of the rectum, or who have had rectal surgery. The thermometer should always be lubricated prior to insertion and should be inserted about 1 to 1½ inches in adults. If a glass thermometer is used, one with a blunt bulb should be selected to prevent damage to the rectum.

The oral method is contraindicated for clients who are unconscious, irrational, prone to seizures, or receiving oxygen. Oral temperatures also are contraindicated for those with oral diseases and in those under the age of 5 or 6. In addition, an oral temperature should not be taken if the client has just finished smoking or drinking something. Under these circumstances, the nurse should wait 15 minutes before taking the client's temperature. If a glass thermometer is used, either a long or blunt bulb is acceptable. The thermometer should be placed in the posterior sublingual pocket at the base of either side of the tongue, and the client's mouth should remain shut while the thermometer is registering.

The axillary method is used in those instances in which both oral and rectal methods are contraindicated. Also, because of the danger of perforating the gastrointestinal tract if a rectal thermometer is inserted too far into an infant or young child, axillary temperatures are recommended sometimes for this age group. With glass thermometers, a long bulb should be used because it has a greater surface. The thermometer should be placed in the axilla with the client's arm held close to the side.

Assessing Pulse

Pulse rates can be measured radially or apically. In adults the radial site usually is selected. In those clients with irregular or rapid heart rates, measuring the pulse apically is recommended for greatest accuracy. The apical pulse rate is obtained by listening with a stethoscope over the apex of the heart, in the 5th left intercostal space, at approximately the midclavicular line (Figure 14-2). The radial pulse rate is obtained by placing two fingers lightly over the radial artery (Figure 14-3). Use sufficient pressure to feel the pulsation. The radial artery is palpated readily on the lateral, palmar surface of the wrist.

Pulse rate should be counted for 30 seconds (beginning with a count of "0" (0 . . . 1 . . . 2, etc.) and then doubled to obtain the rate per minute, unless the pulse is irregular, in which case the pulse should be counted for a full minute. According to a study by Hollerbach and Sneed (1990), a 30-second counting interval was the most accurate and efficient method of taking the radial pulse. The study also concluded that 15-second counting intervals produce inaccuracies for rates faster than 100 beats per minute. When taking the pulse, the nurse should assess its rate, rhythm, and quality. These characteristics reflect the condition of the heart itself, the condition of the vascular system, and the oxygen and nutrient requirements of the body.

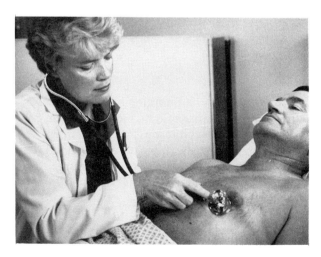

FIGURE 14-2. Site for Auscultating the Apical Pulse.

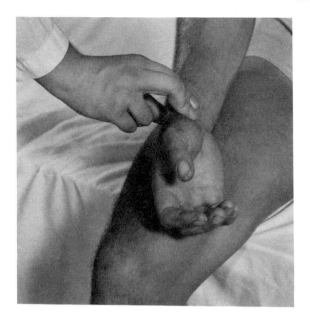

FIGURE 14-3. Palpation of the Radial Artery. (*Note.* From Grimes/Burns: *Health Assessment in Nursing Practice,* Second Edition, © 1987. Boston: Jones and Bartlett Publishers, p. 256.)

The pulse rhythm should be described as regular or irregular. With a regular rhythm, the heart beats at evenly spaced intervals. Disruptions of rhythm are known as *arrhythmias*. The immediate cause of an arrhythmia is an abnormality in the electrical system of the heart, and may be related to any one of numerous underlying problems in the heart. With palpation or auscultation, the nurse can determine only whether the rhythm is regular or irregular. An electrocardiogram (ECG or EKG) is necessary to further define an arrhythmia.

The quality of the pulse is determined by palpation and ranges from absent to bounding. Generally, this is recorded on a scale of 0 to 4 as follows:

0—pulse is absent
1—pulse is thready or weak
2—pulse can be obliterated with pressure
3—pulse is easily felt (normal)
4—pulse is bounding or difficult to depress.

In addition to the radial pulse, a full evaluation of peripheral pulses should include palpation of:

Brachial pulse: In the antecubital fossa medial to the biceps (Figure 14-4)

Femoral pulse: At the midpoint of the inguinal ligament (Figure 14-5)

Popliteal pulse: Behind the knee, most readily felt with the client's knee flexed (Figure 14-6)

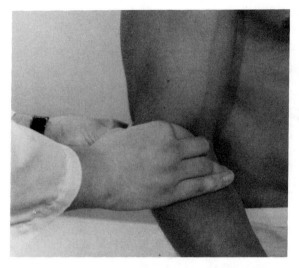

FIGURE 14-4. Palpation of the Brachial Artery. (*Note.* From Grimes/Burns: *Health Assessment in Nursing Practice*, Second Edition, © 1987. Boston: Jones and Bartlett Publishers, p. 257.)

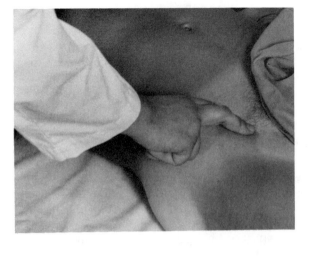

FIGURE 14-5. Palpation of the Femoral Artery. (*Note.* From Grimes/Burns: *Health Assessment in Nursing Practice*, Second Edition, © 1987. Boston: Jones and Bartlett Publishers, p. 257.)

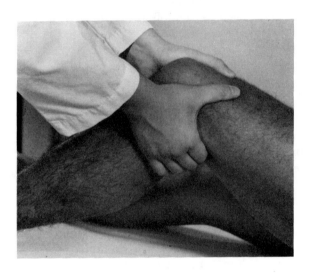

FIGURE 14-6. Palpation of the Popliteal Artery. (*Note.* From Grimes/Burns: *Health Assessment in Nursing Practice*, Second Edition, © 1987. Boston: Jones and Bartlett Publishers, p. 257.)

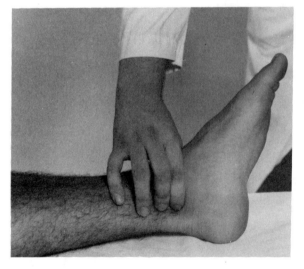

FIGURE 14-7. Palpation of the Posterior Tibial Artery. (*Note.* From Grimes/Burns: *Health Assessment in Nursing Practice*, Second Edition, © 1987. Boston: Jones and Bartlett Publishers, p. 258.)

Posterior tibial pulse: Behind and below the medial malleolus (may be congenitally absent) (Figure 14-7)

Dorsalis pedis pulse: On the dorsum of the foot (may also be congenitally absent) (Figure 14-8)

The carotid arterial pulse can be palpated in the groove between the trachea and the sternocleidomastoid muscle (Figure 14-9). Care should be taken to palpate only one side at a time as massage of the carotid sinus slows the heart rate.

Assessment of the peripheral pulses always is included in the cardiac examination. However, because the pulse is a parameter of physical integrity, a discussion of the techniques for assessing all the pulses is included here. The important point is that assessment of the peripheral pulses must be included and this can be done at several points in the physical examination.

The pulse may be weak or absent if there is obstruction to the blood flow in the area being assessed, such as with arteriosclerosis or coarctation

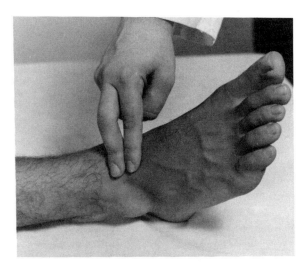

FIGURE 14-8. Palpation of the Dorsal Pedal Artery. (*Note.* From Grimes/Burns: *Health Assessment in Nursing Practice*, Second Edition, © 1987. Boston: Jones and Bartlett Publishers, p. 258.)

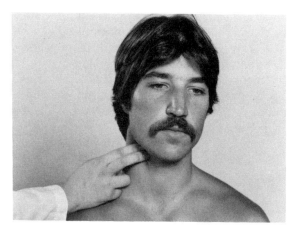

FIGURE 14-9. Palpation of the Carotid Artery. (*Note.* From Grimes/Burns: *Health Assessment in Nursing Practice*, Second Edition, © 1987. Boston: Jones and Bartlett Publishers, p. 256.)

of the aorta. In the latter, the pulses characteristically are strong in the upper extremities and weak in the lower extremities. The pulse may be weak throughout the body in hypovolemia and hypotension, or when the heart muscle cannot contract effectively, as in myocardial damage or heart failure. Strong, bounding pulses usually are noted in hypervolemia, hypertension, and hyperkinetic conditions such as occur with exercise, fever, and anxiety. In some instances, such as severe hypertension, left-sided heart failure, and coronary artery disease, the pulse will alternate between strong and weak, with every other beat being weak. Such a pulse, in which the rhythm is regular but the quality irregular, is known as *pulsus alternans*. If the quality alternates and the rhythm is irregular, a bigeminal pulse, caused by a disruption in the conduction system of the heart, is present.

Changes or abnormalities in a client's heart rate may be due to any number of factors. Some involve an underlying disease state; others do not. Any factor that causes sympathetic stimulation will increase the heart rate, including sympathomimetic drugs and such emotions as anger, anxiety, or fear. The heart rate will increase to meet the additional oxygen demands that accompany increases in the metabolic rate such as occur with fever, hyperthyroidism, and exercise. In some instances, such as anemia, hypovolemia, and hypoxia, the heart rate will increase to meet the normal oxygen demands of the body. Abnormal electrical discharges in the heart are another cause of increased rate and can lead to serious tachycardia.

Blocks in the conduction system of the heart, where the electrical impulses are slow in conducting or do not conduct at all, can cause slowing of the heart rate. Additional causes of bradycardia are parasympathetic (vagal) stimulation, drugs (digoxin, beta blockers), and damage to the heart muscle.

Assessing Respiration

In evaluating respiratory status, the nurse must consider the rate, rhythm, and quality of respiration. Respiratory rates can be counted either by observing chest movements or by listening for breath sounds with a stethoscope. Unless respiration is very shallow or irregular, the rate usually can be counted easily by observing the rise and fall of the chest for 30 seconds and doubling the value obtained. In men and young children, respiration usually is diaphragmatic, so the abdomen should be watched for movement. In women, the thoracic cage will move with respiration. If respiration is shallow or irregular, the rate should be counted for one full minute while listening to the chest with a stethoscope.

Respiratory rates vary with age. Generally speaking, there is an inverse relationship between the client's age and respiratory rate (the older the client, the lower the rate).

Abnormal rates are described with the following terms: tachypnea for rapid rates, bradypnea for slow rates, and apnea for cessation of respiration. A rapid respiratory rate, or tachypnea, is observed with fever, metabolic acidosis, pain, any condition in which carbon dioxide levels are increased or oxygen levels are reduced, exercise, and emotional distress. Rates will decrease in the presence of some drugs, such as central nervous system depressants, metabolic alkalosis, and with increased intracranial pressure.

The nurse should observe the quality of respiration, including depth, any difficulty breathing, or any adventitious sounds such as wheezing. Hyperventilation, or hyperpnea, is an increase in the rate and/or depth of respiration, and may have a neurological, metabolic, pulmonary, pharmacological, or emotional origin. One specific type of hyperventilation that accompanies metabolic acidosis is Kussmaul breathing. The body is attempting to neutralize the effects of excess acids in the body by blowing off carbon dioxide, and so respiration is deep and rapid. Hypoventilation, which is a decrease in the rate and depth of respiration, occurs with central nervous system depression.

With dyspnea, the individual has audible respiration, nasal flaring, mouth breathing, and an anxious expression and may be using accessory muscles, such as the trapezius and sternocleidomastoid muscles. Insufficient oxygenation of the blood for whatever reason will cause dyspnea. Orthopnea, in which the individual must sit upright or stand in order to breathe, is observed in clients with obstructive lung disease, asthma, and severe cardiac disease. Adventitious sounds will be discussed later, in Chapter 17, on oxygenation assessment.

Measuring Blood Pressure

The measurement technique used to assess blood pressure can greatly affect the reading obtained. Therefore, it is important to use the correct technique and to consistently use it in order to assess a client's blood pressure accurately and to evaluate any changes. For example, blood pressure will vary according to where it is taken and the position of the client at the time of measurement. The blood pressure in an individual client may vary as much as 10 to 15 mm Hg between the right and left arm.

Blood pressure will decrease when the client stands up, and the pressure is normally greater when sitting than when lying down. The client's activity level or emotional state prior to taking the measurement will affect the blood pressure, as noted earlier. Ideally the client should be in a calm and restful state. To monitor a client for changes in blood pressure, readings should be taken in the same extremity, with the client in the same position and preferably in a similar state of rest and

comfort. The latter factor is less easy to control than the former two.

Cuff size also should be constant. The width of the cuff bladder should be approximately 1.2 times the diameter of the arm or thigh, which is equivalent to 40 to 50% of the circumference or two-thirds the length of the upper arm or thigh. The bladder should be long enough to completely encircle the extremity used, or approximately 80% of the extremity's circumference (Hill & Grim, 1991). If the cuff bladder is too narrow or too short, the reading will be high; if the bladder is too large, the reading will be lower than the actual blood pressure.

There are several methods of obtaining a blood pressure reading (Table 14-6). The most commonly used is the auscultory method. Before proceeding, the nurse should make sure there are no contraindications to using a blood pressure cuff. For example, a renal dialysis patient who has had a shunt or an arteriovenous fistula implanted should not have blood pressure taken in the affected arm. Doing so could damage the fistula. The client should be positioned with the arm at heart level and the elbow flexed. The cuff should be placed over the bare arm

TABLE 14-6
Blood Pressure Reading Methods

Palpatory Systolic Pressure	Auscultatory Method
1. Place client's arm at heart level.	1. Place client's arm at heart level.
2. Avoid clothing constriction.	2. Avoid clothing constriction.
3. Cuff evenly over brachial artery.	3. Cuff evenly over brachial artery.
4. Palpate radial pulse.	4. Palpate radial pulse.
5. Inflate cuff until radial pulse disappears.	5. Inflate cuff until radial pulse disappears.
6. Inflate cuff 30 mm Hg more.	6. Inflate cuff 30 mm Hg more.
7. Release pressure of cuff slowly.	7. Place stethoscope over brachial artery in anticubital space.
8. Read systolic blood pressure at return point of radial pulse.	8. Release cuff pressure.
	9. The point at which you hear the first sound is systolic pressure. Damping or muffling is diastolic pressure.
	10. Also record the final sound. Example: 116/80/76.

Note. From Grimes/Burns: *Health Assessment in Nursing Practice,* Second Edition, © 1987. Boston: Jones and Bartlett Publishers.

with the center of the bladder over the brachial artery. The cuff should be 2 to 3 cm above the antecubital fossa in an adult. The brachial artery should be palpated and the cuff inflated until the brachial pulse disappears in order to estimate the approximate systolic pressure. The cuff is deflated, and the bell of the stethoscope should be placed over the area of the brachial pulsation. The bell is used because the sounds to be listened for, the Korotkoff sounds, are of relatively low frequency. While the diaphragm works well in most instances, the bell should be selected when the nurse has a choice (Hill & Grim, 1991).

The cuff then is reinflated 20 to 30 mm above the level at which the brachial pulsation was felt to disappear. The cuff should be deflated at 2 to 3 mm Hg per second while the Korotkoff sounds are auscultated. These are the sounds associated with changes in blood flow as the artery goes from a state of occlusion to patency with cuff deflation (Figure 14-10). The first sound is the systolic pressure. This is soft initially but gradually becomes louder. There then may be a gap or silence for up to 40 mm Hg, followed by the second sounds, which are described as swishing. The sounds become louder and clearer in phase 3. The sounds then become muffled (phase 4) and finally disappear (phase 5). In adults the fifth stage is considered to be the diastolic pressure, while in children, especially before puberty, the fourth phase is thought to be a more reliable indicator of diastolic pressure. If the blood pressure is measured in the thigh, the approach is the same except that the popliteal artery is used.

Regardless of the method of measuring blood pressure, care should be taken to have the dial of an aneroid sphygmomanometer in direct view or the mercury manometer at eye level. If this is not done, readings may be inaccurate. Also, if a complete evaluation of blood pressure is being made, readings should be taken in both arms and one leg as well as with the client seated, lying, and standing. A summary of important tips for accurate blood pressure measurement is included here (boxed insert, p. 432). These guidelines will assist the nurse in taking accurate blood pressure readings.

Definitions of the lower limits of hypertension in adults vary from 140/90 to 165/95. Hypotension in an adult is a blood pressure less than 90/50. It is important to consider what is normal for an individual as well as what is normal for the population in assessing blood pressure. A change in systolic and/or diastolic pressure of 20 mm Hg deserves investigation for the cause. The first step with any unexpected reading is to retake the blood pressure,

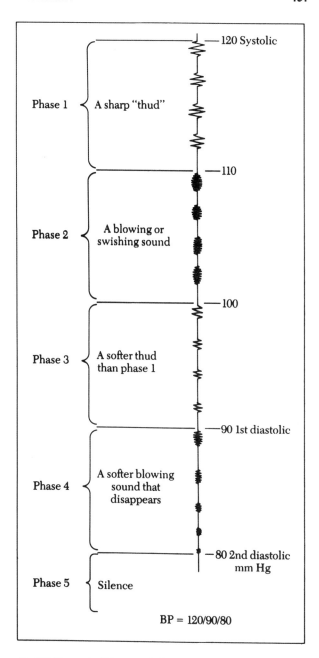

FIGURE 14-10. Phases of the Korotkoff Sounds. (*Note.* From Burch, G.E., and DePasquale, N. P.: *Primer of Clinical Measurement of Blood Pressure.* Copyright © 1962. C.V. Mosby Co. Reprinted by permission of the author.)

waiting 15 to 30 seconds between readings. If the second reading is similar to the first, the cause of the abnormal reading should be investigated.

Integumentary Assessment

Assessment of the skin, hair, and nails involves inspection and palpation. As noted earlier, a systematic approach is necessary to assure a comprehensive evaluation. All skin areas should be

---

Tips for Accurate Blood Pressure Measurement

Select the proper cuff size:
Adult cuff size is 12 to 14 cm wide and 30 cm long.
Pediatric cuff size is 8 to 10 cm wide and 26 cm long.
Larger adult cuff size is 18 to 20 cm wide.

Ensure that equipment is properly assembled and calibrated:

Cuff bladder should be intact inside the cuff.
Sphygmomanometer should be calibrated to 0 mm Hg every few months to ensure reliability.
Cuff must be placed above the area to be auscultated (e.g., if right arm used, the cuff is placed above the brachial artery).

Follow these steps to ensure correct blood pressure measurement and recording:

After the brachial or radial pulse is palpated, the cuff is inflated 30 mm Hg above the level at which those pulses disappear. The cuff is released slowly to palpate the systolic pressure. The cuff is reinflated and systolic and diastolic pressures are auscultated. The auscultated pulses are referred to as Korotkoff's sounds.
Measurements should be recorded on both arms to rule out dissecting aortic aneurysm, coarctation of the aorta, vascular obstruction, and possibly errors in measurement. Subsequent readings should be done on the extremity with the highest pressure.
If arms are inaccessible (after amputation or mastectomy) pressures can be obtained using the client's thigh or calf. The popliteal artery or posterior tibial artery, respectively, is auscultated.
The nurse obtains and records blood pressure with the client in different positions, including supine, sitting, and standing.
The position of the client and the site used to obtain the blood pressure are recorded.

Note. From Ignatavicus, D., & Bayne, M. (1991). *Medical-surgical nursing: A nursing process approach.* Philadelphia: W.B. Saunders Co., p. 2093.

---

examined, with special care taken in the areas of skin folds. Because these areas are warm and moist, they are more prone to breakdown, and they provide an excellent environment for bacterial and fungal growth. While making a thorough assessment, the nurse should be conscientious about maintaining the client's privacy, uncovering only one part at a time. This also helps protect the client from getting cold, which can alter at least one aspect of the examination—skin color—in addition to creating discomfort for the client. One other environmental factor to be considered is the lighting. To see fine changes in skin color or initial stages of rashes and other lesions, good lighting is essential. Some types of lighting, especially fluorescent, can lend a deceptive appearance to skin color.

Skin Color

Skin assessment starts with inspection for color or pigmentation. When assessing the skin, the nurse should consider what is normal for the client's racial background. During initial assessment, color should be noted and carefully documented so that changes may be more readily identified. A general assessment is discussed here; specific modifications according to age and race were presented in an earlier section.

Oxygenated hemoglobin gives skin its normal underlying red tone. Therefore, pallor is seen in anemia and in any condition related to decreased blood flow to an area, as with blood loss or shock. Pallor also is evident in edema since the distance between the surface and the underlying vasculature is increased. Pallor is best seen in the conjunctivae, mucous membranes, nail beds, and palms.

Redness or flushing occurs with an increased blood flow to an area, as in an inflammatory response, blushing, or fever. Flushing may be seen on any portion of the body but generally is most evident in the vascular flush areas: cheeks, bridge of the nose, neck, upper chest, and flexor surfaces of the extremities.

Cyanosis, which is due to an increased amount of deoxygenated hemoglobin, is best seen in the mucous membranes, lips, and nail beds. Central cyanosis, which is a more generalized cyanosis, occurs with some cardiac and respiratory abnormalities. Peripheral cyanosis occurs with slow peripheral capillary circulation. In polycythemia, the skin appears to be reddish blue because of the combined effects of an increase in the overall amount of hemoglobin and an increase in deoxygenated hemoglobin related to the sluggish circulation of polycythemic blood through peripheral capillaries.

Skin Temperature

Skin temperature is evaluated by palpation as an indication of circulatory status and body temperature of the client. The evenness of skin temperature should be considered with particular attention to symmetrical body parts: bilateral coolness of the feet may be normal, whereas unilateral coolness may indicate circulatory impairment. Temperature of the skin is decreased in any situation in which blood flow to the dermis is decreased. If the decrease in blood flow is generalized, as in shock, temperature decrease also is generalized. With localized reductions in flow, as in arteriosclerosis or thrombotic occlusions of vessels, skin temperature decreases locally. Skin temperature also will vary with the temperature of the external environment.

Sensation

The sensitivity of the skin to temperature, pain, touch, and itching should be noted. Of particular concern are areas of decreased sensation. Such areas are prone to damage or breakdown because they lack the normal warnings provided by these sensations. For example, if the lower extremities have decreased temperature sensation, a foot placed near an electric heater or into hot bath water could be seriously burned before the individual has noticed anything is wrong. Sensory assessment is considered in detail in Chapter 15.

Skin Moisture

As used in this discussion, moisture means both wetness and oiliness, which can be assessed through inspection and palpation. Moisture of the skin varies in any one individual: The palms, soles, intertriginous areas, and face tend to be more moist than other areas of the body. Moisture also varies with activity level, temperature, emotional status, and age. Exercise, fever, warm environmental temperatures, and anxiety lead to increased perspiration. Excessive oiliness is seen in individuals with acne and seborrhea. Skin breakdown is a concern in areas of excessive moisture, especially skin folds, so these areas should be observed carefully.

Skin tends to be drier in winter and in dry climates; older individuals also tend to have dry skin. Abnormal dryness is known as xerosis. This occurs in dehydration and is readily checked by examining the buccal mucous membranes. Cracking of the skin is seen often with excessive dryness; a good example is the chapped lips that occur so frequently in winter.

Skin Texture and Thickness

The fineness or coarseness and the thickness of the skin should be evaluated by inspection, especially by palpation. Roughness and thickness occur in areas exposed to pressure, friction, or other irritation. This is to be expected in such areas as the soles of the feet and the palms of the hands but should still be noted, as should unexpected areas of coarseness. Changes in skin texture may be associated with disease: dry, rough skin is seen in hypothyroidism, while soft, smooth skin occurs with hyperthyroidism.

Skin Turgor

As with texture, skin turgor can be assessed through observation but is best assessed through palpation. The amount of fluid in the surrounding tissue and the elasticity of the skin are assessed. With fluid loss or a decrease in subcutaneous fat, as in weight loss and with aging, the skin becomes loose and inelastic. This is evident when pinching a piece of skin. Normally the skin should immediately return to its prior condition. If skin turgor is poor, the skin returns to its original state only slowly or not at all. This "tenting" occurs in dehydration—the skin remains pinched up even after it has been released.

Any edema, or fluid buildup, should be noted and palpated to determine the degree to which it remains indented when pressed. Edematous skin will appear shiny and taut. To determine the presence of edema, the tissue should be firmly pressed for 5 to 10 seconds. If the tissue does not return rapidly to the normal contour, pitting edema is present (Figure 14-11). The classification of edema may vary according to the examiner's preference and the method favored in a particular health-care setting. Several of the scales commonly used to classify degree of edema are:

Time Classification

0	No pitting
1+	Trace
2+	Moderate, disappears in 10–15 seconds
3+	Deep, disappears in 1–2 minutes
4+	Very deep, disappears in 5 minutes

Extent Classification

1+	Shallow pit formed by thumb pressure
2+	Deep pit formed by thumb pressure
3+	Signs of pitting in a dependent part of the body (e.g., limb is 1½ times the normal size)
4+	Generalized deep-pitted edema accompanied by ascites (as in severe congestive heart failure)

Extent Classification

1+	Barely detectable
2+	Indentation of less than 5 mm
3+	Indentation of 5–10 mm
4+	Indentation of more than 1 cm

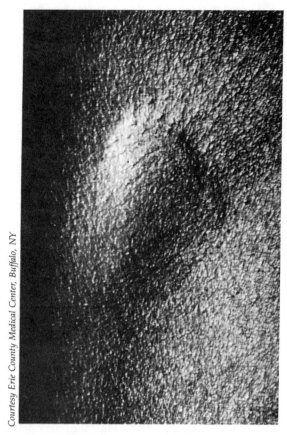

Courtesy Erie County Medical Center, Buffalo, NY

FIGURE 14-11. Indentation of Pitting Edema. (*Note.* From Grimes/Burns: *Health Assessment in Nursing Practice*, Second Edition, © 1987. Boston: Jones and Bartlett Publishers, p. 164.)

Skin Integrity

The last aspect of the skin to be assessed is integrity. Any disruptions of the skin, such as bites, birthmarks, or lesions, must be fully identified through inspection and palpation. The following should be noted: location on the body, color, size, configuration, discharge, morphology, and any changes over time. Lesions should be measured. Configuration is the grouping of lesions; it can provide clues to the underlying etiology of the lesions, since certain diseases are associated with distinctive configuration patterns (Figure 14-12). For example, ringworm is circular, and poison ivy is linear. Other commonly found configurations are clustered, serpiginous (wavy, snakelike lines), iris (concentric circles), and irregular patterns. The nurse should consider whether the configuration of the lesions fits the history of the problem; bruises that cannot be explained may be due to abuse. The color, consistency, amount, and odor of any discharge should be noted.

In terms of morphology, there are three categories of lesions. Primary lesions occur without any prior skin changes. Secondary lesions result from a change in a primary lesion. The third group includes vascular lesions. The various types of lesions are described and depicted in Table 14-7.

There are several types of vascular markings:

Petechiae, which occur in bleeding disorders, are small, red, hemorrhagic spots.

Ecchymoses, commonly known as bruises, are purplish-blue areas of hemorrhage under the skin that fade to greenish-brown or yellow with time.

Telangiectasis is a dilatation of superficial blood vessels in a localized area. Such lesions are seen in liver disease but also in normal individuals.

The foregoing are the more common lesions the nurse may observe, but this is by no means a comprehensive list. Any variation from the normal, clear, intact skin should be carefully inspected and palpated, and the findings clearly described and documented.

Hair

Several aspects of the hair should be evaluated, including cleanliness, quality, quantity, and distribution. As noted earlier, cleanliness may reflect self-concept, the availability of soap and water, and cultural values. In addition to observing the cleanliness of the hair itself, insect infestation in the hair and on the scalp, such as pediculosis (lice), should be looked for.

Two aspects of hair quality should be assessed and noted: texture and dryness. Changes can indicate disease: hair is dry and coarse in hypothyroidism and is fine and silky in hyperthyroidism. Protein-calorie malnutrition results in fine hair that is easily pulled out. Brittleness can occur with frequent use of hair dryers and electric curlers and frequent use of hair dyes and tints.

Normally, pubic hair begins to develop sometime between 8 and 12 years of age (see chap. 23). Axillary hair develops shortly thereafter, followed by facial hair in males.

Changes in quantity and distribution of hair can reflect underlying disease. For example, increased hairiness (hirsutism) occurs in Cushing's disease. A decrease in hair growth is seen in hypopituitarism and hypothyroidism. Infections also can cause decreased hair growth or patchy loss of hair, such as the bald spots seen in ringworm.

Nails and Nail Beds

Nail color, contour, consistency, and adherence to the nail bed all are important factors to evaluate

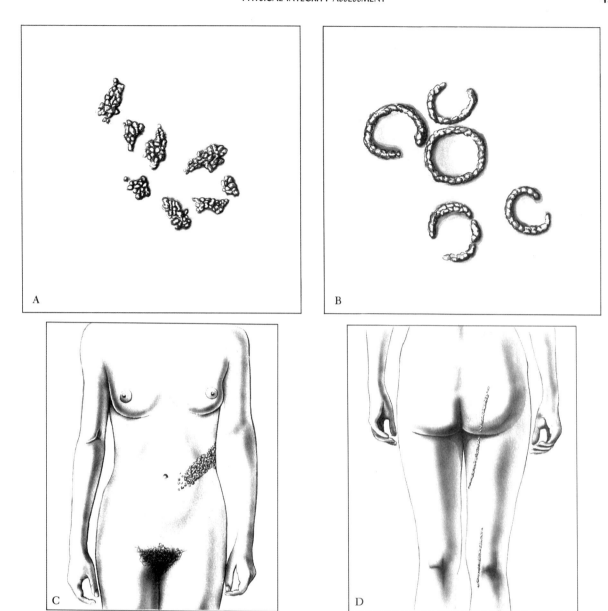

FIGURE 14-12. Lesion Configurations. (A) Clustered. (B) Annular. (C) Zosteriform. (D) Linear.

when assessing the nails. The color of the nail bed was discussed earlier in terms of detecting cyanosis and pallor, both of which are easily seen in this area. The nurse should check blanching of the nail bed to assess circulatory status by pressing down on the nail until the nail bed whitens (blanches), then releasing while observing for the color to return. This determines the time required for the capillaries of the nail bed to refill—normally 1 to 2 seconds. Sluggish capillary refill may indicate some sort of circulatory insufficiency, which may be localized, as in obstruction of a vessel, or generalized, as in hypovolemia. One other aspect of color that should be noted is any redness of the nail or around the nail, generally indicative of infec-

tion. Infection of the nail bed (paronychia) is accompanied by warmth and tenderness of the area.

The general shape or contour of the nails should be examined. The edges of the nail should be smooth, not bitten or ragged. Clubbing of the nails is a sign of oxygen deficiency secondary to respiratory or cardiac disease. Normally, the angle between the nail and the base of the nail is 160°. In the early stages of clubbing, this angle reaches 180° and the nail base is springy or spongy. As the disease progresses, the angle will increase beyond 180° and the nail base becomes obviously swollen (Figure 14-13).

Spooning of the nails, koilonychia, is sometimes seen in iron deficiency anemia; here, the nail

TABLE 14-7
Primary and Secondary Skin Lesions

Primary Lesions

Type	Definition	Examples
Macule	A flat, nonpalpable area of change in skin color less than 1 cm in diameter	Measles, scarlet fever, freckle, flat nevus, drug rash
Papule	A solid elevation of skin less than 1 cm in diameter, caused by thickening of the epidermis; definitely palpable	Wart, raised scaley area of psoriasis, pityriasis rosea
Vesicle	An elevation of the skin less than 1 cm in diameter, caused by clear fluid filling the upper layers of skin; palpable	Fever blister, chickenpox, smallpox, poison ivy, second degree burn, herpes simplex, herpes zoster, eczematous dermatitis
Nodule	A solid mass less than 1 cm in diameter, extending deeper into dermis than a papule; moves with skin when palpated (some may extend into subcutaneous tissue; when palpated at this level skin will slide over nodule)	Area of poorly absorbed injection, dermatofibroma, subcutaneous nodule in rheumatic fever (especially with severe carditis and generally near occipital protuberances or over joints)
Plaque	Like a macule or papule but larger than 1 cm in diameter	Vitiligo, mongolian spot, plantar wart, xanthoma, psoriasis, pityriasis rosea, discoid lupus erythematosus
Bulla	Like a vesicle but larger than 1 cm in diameter; palpable	Pemphigus, some lesions in contact dermatitis, burn, sunburn, poison oak, poison ivy, bullous impetigo; on palms and soles with scarlet fever or congenital syphilis.
Tumor	Like a nodule but larger than 1 cm in diameter; may be firm or soft	Lipoma, fibroma, carcinoma
Pustule	Like a vesicle or bulla but pus-filled	Acne, impetigo, furuncles (arising from hair follicles), carbuncles (arising from sebaceous glands)
Wheal	A circumscribed elevation of the skin caused by escape of serum into the dermis (the larger the amount of the edema, the paler the wheal on a red to pale color continuum)	Urticaria, insect bite, poison sumac, poison ivy
Cyst	An encapsulated, fluid-filled area in the dermis or subcutaneous tissue (generally nontender and may transilluminate light)	Sebaceous cyst, epidermoid cyst

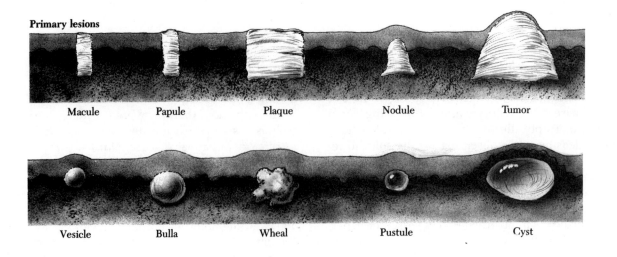

Primary lesions

Macule   Papule   Plaque   Nodule   Tumor

Vesicle   Bulla   Wheal   Pustule   Cyst

TABLE 14-7 (Continued)

Secondary Lesions

Type	Definition	Examples
Scale	A flake of desquamated dead epithelium	Psoriasis, seborrheic dermatitis, pityriasis rosea, exfoliative dermatitis
Excoriation/erosion	An absence of superficial epidermis	Superficial scratch, syphilitic chancre
Crust	A dried serum of blood exudate as found on the surface of an abrasion or excoriation or on the site of ruptured blisters	Fever blister, impetigo
Fissure	A crack in the epidermis	Chapping, cracking of lips as seen in severe dehydration or fever
Ulcer	A necrotic loss of epidermis	An open sore seen sometimes on the leg with sickle-cell anemia or on the leg and pressure areas with vascular insufficiency
Scar (cicatrix)	A connective tissue replacing skin damaged to depth of dermis during healing process	Healing site of trauma, wound, or surgery
Keloid	An overproduction of scar tissue that has a red, raised, smooth appearance, contains blood vessels, is sometimes irritable; has high incidence of occurrence in Blacks	Keloid

Secondary lesions

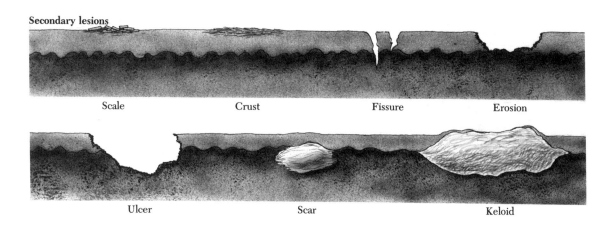

Scale   Crust   Fissure   Erosion

Ulcer   Scar   Keloid

Vascular lesions

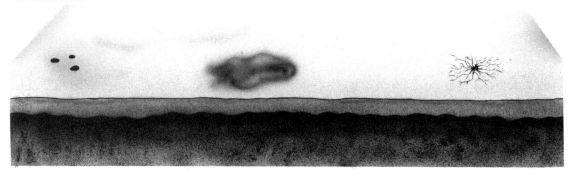

Petechia   Ecchymosis   Telangiectasis

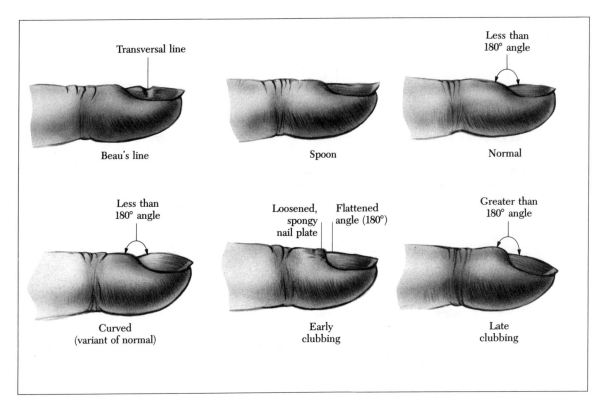

FIGURE 14-13. Normal and Abnormal Nails.

curves upward from the nail bed. Beau's lines are horizontal depressions in the nail that occur with trauma to the nail or in severe illness.

Nails should be of uniform thickness, smooth, and hard. Thickening of the nails occurs with trauma and fungal infections. Excessive brittleness occurs with general malnutrition and specifically with iron and calcium deficiencies.

Finally, the nail should be firmly attached to the surrounding structures. As noted above, a spongy nail base is seen with clubbing. Also, with severe infections or trauma, the nail may begin to separate from the nail bed.

Assessment of the Lymphatic System

Lymph nodes are found in clusters or chains in subcutaneous connective tissue or deep below the muscular fascia and in body cavities. Superficial lymph nodes are palpable, while deep lymph nodes usually are not.

Lymph nodes vary in shape and size. They may be round, oval, flat, or cylindrical. Nodes lying near the periphery are usually larger than those found near the midline of the body. The smallest node may not be palpable, while the largest (the size of an olive) may be readily apparent (McConnell, 1988). The size of lymph nodes de-

creases with age as lymphoid elements are replaced by fatty and fibrous tissue.

The clinical significance of a palpable node depends on a number of factors such as the client's age, location of the node, and the client's health. Usually lymph nodes are not seen or felt. An increase in the size of a node is regarded as pathological and should be evaluated. However, an enlarged node does not always indicate a problem. It is not unusual for a lymph node to remain permanently enlarged (and not tender) following a serious infection (McConnell, 1988).

Inspection and palpation are the techniques used to assess the lymphatic system. Careful inspection of each lymph node group (head and neck, axillary, epitrochlear, inguinal and femoral) precedes palpation. Following inspection, the nurse palpates the lymph nodes using the middle and index fingers in a slow, gentle, circular motion. The nurse should exert some pressure but avoid using too much pressure lest the nodes be lost in the underlying tissue (McConnell, 1988).

As the nurse palpates the lymph nodes, contralateral sides are compared to determine shape and size, location, consistency, symmetry, surface characteristics, mobility, discreteness, and tenderness or pain. In discerning the shape and size of lymph nodes, the nurse determines whether they are oval, round, cylindrical, or flat. The shape may vary. If a node is enlarged, the size should be approximated, noting its thickness and width and length in centimeters. The region and structures drained by the lymph nodes also should be examined. For example, the head and neck nodes drain the throat, mouth, abdomen, breast, thorax, and arms.

The location of lymph nodes should be identified in relation to bony prominences or landmarks. Drawing a picture may be helpful to pinpoint the specific location of an enlarged node. *Consistency* refers to whether a mode is soft, firm, or hard. Nodes also may be described as *spongy, cystic,* or *resilient. Symmetry* implies that the nodes on corresponding sides of the body are similar in their characteristics. The nurse should note whether the nodes are symmetrical or whether there is a difference between the sides.

The way the lymph node feels under the surface of the skin is referred to as *surface characteristics.* In this regard, nodes usually are described as *modular, irregular,* or *smooth. Mobility* denotes whether the lymph node is movable or fixed to adjacent tissues or structures. When palpating a fixed node, it is important to determine whether it is fixed to overlying or underlying tissue and the extent of fixation. Lymph nodes are described as *discrete* if they can be palpated separately. Nodes that are not distinct or separate are referred to as *matted.*

While examining the various lymph node groups, the nurse should observe whether the client experiences pain or tenderness on palpation. If pain or tenderness is observed, the nurse should carefully evaluate surrounding tissues and structures drained by the lymph nodes (McConnell, 1988). The skin surrounding a lymph node group also is evaluated. The nurse should look for signs such as edema, warmth, or erythema. Fixed, matted, enlarged, or tender nodes are indicative of a problem and should be evaluated further (McConnell, 1988).

Examination of the entire lymph system may be done by moving systematically from one lymph node group to the other. This is often done when generalized infection or malignancy are in question. Usually, however, the various lymph node groups are examined as part of other system exams. For example, the head and neck nodes are evaluated during the examination of the structures of the head and neck. The axillary and epitrochlear nodes are evaluated during the breast examination, and the inguinal and femoral nodes maybe included in either the abdominal or peripheral vascular examinations.

Before the nurse begins to palpate the nodes of the head and neck, the client's neck should be slightly flexed. In this relaxed position, the nurse is able to palpate the nodes and underlying areas more readily. It also is important for the nurse to look for symmetry of the nodes by sitting or standing in front of the client before beginning palpation. The lymph nodes on either side of the head and neck may be palpated simultaneously to allow for immediate comparison or one side may be palpated followed by the other side. With either technique, comparing contralateral sides is important. Each of the lymph nodes in the head and neck then is palpated carefully and its characteristics noted (see Figure 14-14).

The axillary nodes are examined following the breast examination (Figure 14-15). These node groups drain the breasts, arms, hands, and chest wall. With the client in a sitting or supine position, the nurse carefully palpates each of the axillary nodes. To assess the central nodes, the nurse must palpate high up in the axilla in the mid-axillary line. The remaining nodes are assessed by pressing the fingertips against the muscles of the axilla and the chest wall (McConnell, 1988). The epitrochlear nodes are located above the medial epicondylus of the humerus and drain the ulnar surface of the forearm and several fingers of the hand. With the arm in a relaxed position, the nurse palpates the area just above the elbow for the presence of nodes.

The last group of lymph nodes to be evaluated is the inguinal and femoral nodes (Figure 14-16), which drain the legs. Only the superficial lymph system is accessible to examination. These nodes are examined with the client supine. Again, the nodes are palpated with the fingertips. These nodes lie close to the inguinal ligament and the upper part of the saphenous vein. In addition to the inguinal and femoral nodes, the popliteal lymph nodes also are examined. However, most of the lymph drainage from the legs is delivered to the inguinal nodes. Any abnormal or unusual findings should be fully described and documented. The lack of palpable nodes on examination always is specified.

NURSING DIAGNOSES RELATED TO PHYSICAL INTEGRITY

A careful and thorough assessment of physical integrity enables the nurse to formulate appropriate nursing diagnoses for actual or potential problems. Once problems are identified, a plan of care can be developed.

A variety of nursing diagnoses related to physical integrity are listed in Table 14-8. These diag-

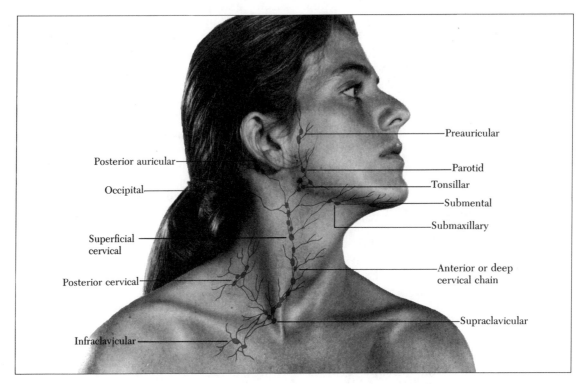

FIGURE 14-14. Location of the Lymph Nodes of the Neck. (*Note.* From Grimes/Burns: *Health Assessment in Nursing Practice,* Second Edition, © 1987. Boston: Jones and Bartlett Publishers, p. 178.)

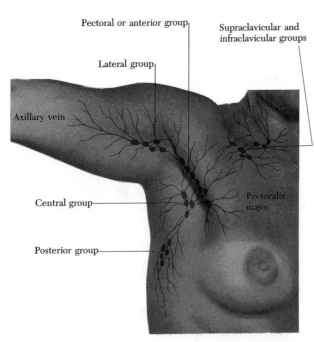

FIGURE 14-15. Location of the Lymph Nodes. (*Note.* Adapted from Grimes/Burns: *Health Assessment in Nursing Practice,* Second Edition, © 1987. Boston: Jones and Bartlett Publishers, p. 285.)

noses are categorized in the North American Nursing Diagnosis Association (NANDA) Taxonomy I under the human response pattern of "exchanging." This pattern implies mutual giving and receiving. A nursing diagnosis of "body temperature, potential altered," reflects a state in which a client's ability to maintain body temperature within normal limits is jeopardized. The physiological activities that regulate heat production and heat loss are influenced by a number of factors such as age, activity and exercise, exposure to extreme temperatures, alcohol and/or drugs, and illness or compromised health.

A diagnosis of "body temperature, potential altered, related to extremes of age," for example, may be appropriate for an older client. With age, sweat glands atrophy and blood vessels lose elasticity and do not readily constrict and dilate. In addition, the metabolic rate generally is lowered (see chap. 24). These factors influence temperature that may be subnormal in the older adult. With the presence of infection, a rise in temperature is not as dramatic in the older adult. Therefore, it is important for the nurse to evaluate even a slight rise in temperature.

For a nursing diagnosis of "hyperthermia," data from the nursing history and clinical appraisal may reflect various findings. The diagnosis of hy-

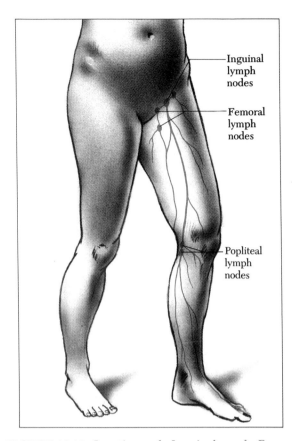

FIGURE 14-16. Location of Inguinal and Femoral Lymph Nodes. (*Note.* From Grimes/Burns: *Health Assessment in Nursing Practice,* Second Edition, © 1987. Boston: Jones and Bartlett Publishers, p. 311.)

perthermia is made when a client's temperature is above normal for the client. An example would be the client who relates prolonged exposure to a hot environment and inadequate replacement of fluids while exposed to the extreme heat. Physical findings may reveal an increase in body temperature, respiratory rate, heart rate, and blood pressure. In addition, the skin may appear flushed and warm. The client also may complain of a headache and generalized aching and may appear confused and restless.

A nursing diagnosis of "skin integrity, impaired" on the other hand, reflects the state in which a client's skin is adversely altered. The client with a diagnosis of "skin integrity, impaired, related to nutrition," for example, may relate a history of strict dieting with limited intake of nutrients for a period of several months. The physical findings demonstrated with this diagnosis can include dull, dry, or sparse hair, decreased subcutaneous fat, loss of skin turgor and elasticity, and dry, pale, rough skin. In addition to impaired skin integrity, nutritionally compromised patients may exhibit

TABLE 14-8
Nursing Diagnoses Related to Physical Integrity

Body temperature, potential altered related to dehydration, sedation, or extremes of age.

Hyperthermia related to exposure to hot environment, inability or decreased ability to perspire, dehydration, or increased metabolic rate.

Hypothermia related to exposure to cool or cold environment, inability or decreased ability to shiver, medications causing vasodilation, or inactivity.

Infection, potential for related to inadequate primary defenses (broken skin, traumatized tissue, stasis of body fluids), inadequate secondary defenses (leukopenia), malnutrition, or effects of chronic disease.

Oral mucous membrane, altered related to effects of chemotherapy, dehydration, immunosuppression, infection, or inadequate oral hygiene.

Skin integrity, impaired related to altered nutritional state, decreased circulation, skeletal prominence, or immobility.

Skin integrity, potential impaired related to infection, edema, allergy (drug, food), or shearing force.

Thermoregulation, ineffective related to effects of trauma or illness, sedation, or medications causing vasoconstriction or vasodilation.

Tissue integrity, impaired related to nutritional deficit, irritants (chemical), altered circulation, or effects of therapeutic radiation.

musculoskeletal, cardiovascular and neurological changes. The extent of these changes depends on such factors as the client's initial weight, amount of weight lost, period of time over which weight loss occurred, and the overall health of the client.

Chapter Highlights

▪ The general appraisal or general survey is a broad assessment of the individual's overall health and includes such aspects as general appearance, physical growth, and vital signs.

▪ The physiological mechanisms controlling the vital signs are extremely sensitive and maintain the indicators within narrow limits.

▪ Because numerous factors can cause changes in any one or all of the vital signs, the nurse also must evaluate data from other parts of the client's assessment before drawing conclusions about what may be causing any change or abnormality in the vital signs.

▪ The skin performs functions vital to the well-being of the human organism, among them prevention of fluid and electrolyte loss, elimination of certain waste products, maintenance of normal body temperature, and protection from invasion by foreign material and organisms.

■ The approach to assessment of physical integrity should be cephalocaudal (head-to-toe) and general-to-specific to ensure that components of the assessment are systematically evaluated and segments not overlooked.

■ When measuring height and weight it is important to use the same technique as well as the same measurement scale lest actual changes be obscured or artificially inflated or deflated.

■ Pulse rate should be counted for 30 seconds beginning with a count of "0" (0 . . . 1 . . . 2, etc.) and then doubled to obtain the rate per minute, unless the pulse is irregular, in which case the pulse should be counted for a full minute.

■ When monitoring a client for changes in blood pressure, readings should be taken in the same extremity, with the client in the same position, and preferably in a similar state of rest and comfort.

■ Integumentary assessment considers the following skin characteristics: color, temperature, sensation, moisture, texture and thickness, turgor, and integrity.

■ In palpating lymph nodes the nurse compares contralateral sides and notes the following characteristics: location, symmetry, size and shape, surface characteristics, mobility, tenderness or pain, and skin color and warmth.

■ Appropriate nursing diagnoses related to physical integrity are based on an analysis and synthesis of the information found from the history and clinical appraisal.

Practice Activities

1. Measure and record vital signs on at least five adults of varying ages:
   a. Describe pulse and respiration for each individual in terms of rate, rhythm, and quality.
   b. Compare blood pressure readings in the sitting, lying, and standing positions.
   c. Compare temperature readings taken orally, rectally, and under the axilla.
   d. Determine whether findings are within normal limits.
   e. List possible causes for any alterations from normal.
   f. Record findings. What conclusions can you draw?
2. Perform a clinical appraisal of integumentary status on three adults of varying ages and from different racial backgrounds.
   a. Describe findings.
   b. Identify possible causes and/or meaning of any variations from normal.
   c. Indicate appropriate nursing diagnoses.
3. Perform an assessment of general appearance and physical growth on at least five adults of varying ages and ethnic backgrounds.
   a. Describe findings.
   b. Identify possible meaning of any variation from expected.
   c. What conclusions can you draw?
4. Assess the lymph system of several adults of varying ages. Contrast and compare your findings. What conclusions can you draw?

Recommended Readings

Baker, N.C., Cerone, S.B., Gaze, N., & Knapp, T.R. (1984). The effect of type of thermometer and length of time inserted on oral temperature measurements of afebrile subjects. *Nursing Research, 33*(2), 109–111.

Bergstrom, N., Braden, B.J., Laguzza, A., & Holman, V. (1987). The Braden scale for predicting pressure sore risk. *Nursing Research, 36*(4), 205–210.

Birdsall, C. (1985a). How do you handle heat loss? *American Journal of Nursing, 85*(4), 367.

Birdsall, C. (1985b). How do you interpret pulses? *American Journal of Nursing, 85*(7), 1414.

Frantz, R., & Kinney, C. (1986). Variables associated with skin dryness in the elderly. *Nursing Research, 35*(2), 98–100.

Gift, A.G., & Soeken, K.L. (1988). Assessment of physiologic measures. *Heart and Lung, 17*, 128–133.

Gurevich, I. (1985). Fever, when to worry about it. *RN, 48*, 14.

Hayter, J. (1980). Hypothermia, hyperthermia in older persons. *Journal of Gerontological Nursing, 6*, 65–68.

Stone, S. (1986). A new concept in routine vital signs measurement. *Nursing Management, 17*(2), 28–29.

References

Burnside, I. (1988). *Nursing and the aged* (2nd ed.). New York: McGraw-Hill.

DeWitt, S. (1990). Nursing assessment of the skin and dermatological lesions. *Nursing Clinics of North America, 25*(1), 235–245.

Folk-Lighty, M. (1984). Solving the puzzles of fluid imbalances. *Nursing, 14*(2), 34–41.

Giuffre, M. Heidenreich, T., Carney-Gersten, P., Dorsch, J., & Heidenreich, E. (1990). The relationship between axillary and core body temperature measurements. *Applied Nursing Research, 3*(2), 52–56.

Guyton, A.C. (1990). *Textbook of medical physiology* (8th ed.). Philadelphia: Saunders.

Hill, M., & Grim, C. (1991). How to take a precise blood pressure. *American Journal of Nursing, 91*(2), 38–42.

Hollerbach, A., & Sneed, N.V. (1990). Accuracy of radial pulse assessment by length of counting interval. *Heart and Lung, 19*(3), 258–264.

Ignatavicius, D., & Bayne, M.W. (1991). *Medical–surgical nursing.* Philadelphia: Saunders.

Lukasiewicz, P. (1986). Rectal temperatures are as accurate as oral temperatures in patients receiving oxygen therapy. *Critical Care Nurse, 6*(1), 72–73.

McConnell, E. (1988). Getting the feel of lymph node assessment. *Nursing, 18*(8), 54–57.

Miller, C. (1990). *Nursing care of older adults.* Glenview, IL: Scott, Foresman.

Samples, J.F., Van Cott, M.L., Long, C., King, I.M., & Kersenbrock, A. (1985). Circadian rhythms: Basis for screening for fever. *Nursing Research, 34*(6), 377–379.

Shangold, M., & Mirkin, G. (1988). *Women and exercise: Physiology and sports medicine.* Philadelphia: Davis.

Tachovsky, B. (1985). Indirect auscultatory blood pressure measurement at two sites in the arm. *Research in Nursing and Health, 8,* 125–129.

Utley, R. (1990). Midarm circumference: Estimating patient's weight. *Dimensions of Critical Care Nursing, 9*(II), 75–81.

Williams, S., & Worthington, B. (1988). *Nutrition throughout the life span.* St. Louis: Times Mirror/ Mosby.

Sensory–Perceptual–Neurological Assessment

OBJECTIVES

Upon completion of this chapter, you should be able to:

■ Explain the purposes and parameters of a sensory–perceptual–neurological assessment.

■ Obtain subjective and objective data related to sensory–perceptual–neurological function.

■ Conduct and document a complete sensory–perceptual–neurological assessment.

■ Identify the components of a neurological check and examples of the types of situations in which a neurological check should be performed.

■ Discuss the phenomenon of pain.

■ Examine several pain assessment methods.

■ Perform a systematic assessment of a client experiencing pain.

■ Modify the sensory–perceptual–neurological assessment according to the client's age, culture, and health.

■ Develop valid and appropriate nursing diagnoses for clients with alterations in sensory–perceptual–neurological status or clients with pain.

Examination of the client's sensory–perceptual–neurological status is a vital component of a comprehensive nursing assessment because the integrated functioning of these systems affects an individual's interaction with the environment. Impairments or deficits involving thought processes, judgment, language, affect or mood, coordination and balance, or sensory perception may, to a lesser or greater degree, interfere with a client's ability to function in society. An understanding of sensory–perceptual–neurological functioning is essential for thorough assessment and the development of nursing interventions for clients who have deficits.

KNOWLEDGE NEEDED TO ASSESS SENSORY–PERCEPTUAL–NEUROLOGICAL FUNCTIONING

The ability to interact with one's environment requires the integrated functioning of the sensory–perceptual–neurological systems. The major areas of the cerebrum, cerebellum, brain stem, and spinal cord are responsible for the functions of conscious thought, memory, personality, interpretation of symbols, perception of sensations, and movement (Figure 15-1).

The major portion of the human brain is the cerebrum. It is responsible for thought, personality, sensations, and voluntary activity. Posterior and inferior to the cerebrum is the cerebellum. This area of the brain controls equilibrium and coordination. The brain stem houses all of the cranial nerves with the exception of the olfactory nerve, which originates in the cerebrum. The brain stem also contains the respiratory and vasomotor centers, which are assessed during the respiratory and cardiac examinations. Impulses are transmitted to and from the brain through the spinal cord. Sensory, motor, and reflex activity are mediated through the spinal cord (Grimes & Burns, 1987).

Sensory–Perceptual Functioning

Sensation is a very personal concept influenced by culture, environment, and psychological factors. One's ability to function and survive is based on the ability to receive, process, and act on different environmental stimuli (Metcalf, 1988). The ability to collect data through the five senses is referred to as *sensory reception*. The ability to organize and translate stimuli into meaningful information is referred to as *sensory perception*.

The senses of sight, hearing, smell, and taste are regulated by cranial nerves, while the sense of touch is controlled by the sensory system. The sensory system is composed of pathways that enable the transmission of various sensory impulses (via the spinal cord) to the thalamus for awareness and then to the cerebrum for location and intensity. Several tracts within this system are particularly important. Sensations of pain, temperature, and crude touch are transmitted via the spinothalamic tract. Sensations of position, vibration, and fine touch are transmitted through the posterior column in the spinal cord. Ascending tracts cross over to the opposite side before reaching the cerebrum. Thus, sensory information from the right side of the body is interpreted in the left cerebral cortex and vice versa (Stevens & Becker, 1988). Sensory function is often broken down into primary and secondary modalities. The primary modalities include pain, temperature, light touch, position, and vibration senses. The secondary modalities involve graphesthesia, stereognosis, and two-point discrimination (see Table 15.4 later in this chapter).

Mental Status

Mental status reflects cerebral function. The frontal lobe regulates thought processes, personality, and behavior. The parietal lobe controls the organization and expression of speech, the ability to interpret symbols, and the ability to engage in hand skills. Sensory and motor areas regulate interpretation and response to a variety of stimuli. For example, a lesion in a specific sensory area may result in a tingling or numbness, while a lesion in a specific motor area may result in paralysis. Mental status is evaluated through appearance, behavior, and conversation.

Special Senses

The special senses of smell (olfaction), taste, vision, hearing, and touch are the core of the sensory–perceptual assessment. The sensory–perceptual system is central to the individual's survival. In the client with normal function, these senses are highly integrated; they permit complex interactions between the internal and external environments. Alteration or absence of any one sense can severely impair the individual's adaptation to changing conditions. For example, an elderly person with an impaired sense of olfaction may not detect the smell of smoke that signals a house fire and thus may be overcome. A diabetic client with peripheral neuropathy affecting the feet may be insensitive to the heat of bath water and thus may be severely burned when stepping into the tub.

To perform an adequate assessment, a nurse

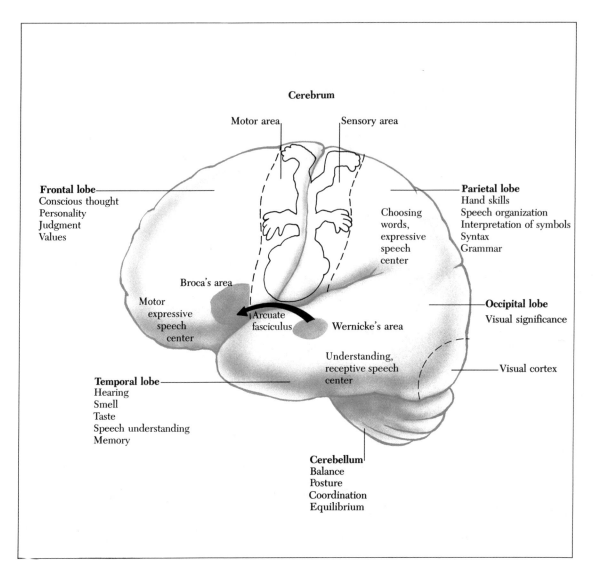

FIGURE 15-1. Functions of the Cerebrum and Cerebellum, Including Three Major Speech Centers in the Frontal, Parietal, and Temporal Lobes. (*Note.* From Grimes/Burns: *Health Assessment in Nursing Practice,* Second Edition, © 1987. Boston: Jones and Bartlett Publishers, p. 340.)

must know about development and deterioration of the special senses, since age-related variations normally exist. Also, the client's health may influence findings or may prevent performance of some or all of the examination.

Smell (Olfaction)

Although present at birth, the sense of smell is not well defined. As this sense becomes more acute, it can influence an individual's willingness to enter into and participate in new situations such as trying unfamiliar foods. The sense of smell originates from a small area of mucous membrane, the olfactory mucosa, deep inside the nose. This small area is made up of millions of tiny endings of the olfac-

tory nerve, Cranial Nerve I (CN I). As one chews food, a small amount of air movement is created by the action of the palate and throat. This air carries odorous material up to the area of the olfactory mucosa where sensitive receptors are stimulated (Geldard, 1972).

The olfactory receptors adapt rapidly, and in approximately one second the awareness of an odor decreases about 50% (Guyton, 1987). Because of this adaptation, strong odors seem to disappear in a few seconds. This phenomenon accounts for the individual's desensitization to certain smells such as cooking odors and adaptation to environmental stimuli such as body odors or noxious smells from factories or sewage treatment plants.

With advancing age, the number of olfactory

nerve fibers decreases and the remaining fibers atrophy to varying degrees. The ensuing decreased acuity in the sense of smell may result in malnutrition of the elderly. Nasal trauma or head injury sustained at any point in the life cycle also may impair olfaction.

Taste

Although present in utero, the sense of taste becomes more acute in the first several months after birth. The sense of taste results from the function of taste buds distributed over the entire surface of the tone. The anterior two-thirds of the tongue contain smaller taste buds, which elicit sweet and salty tastes. Bitter and sour tastes are elicited over the posterior third of the tongue. There are approximately 100,000 taste buds on the surface of the tongue in an adult (Peele, 1977).

Both peripheral and central pathways are involved in the sense of taste (Metcalf, 1988). Input from CN VII (auditory or acoustic), CN IX (glossopharyngeal), and CN X (vagus) makes up the peripheral pathway, which passes eventually into the medulla. The central pathways appear to be secondary solitariothalamic fibers, which ultimately synapse in the thalamus (Peele, 1977).

For taste buds to be stimulated, the tongue must be moist. The sense of taste is diminished greatly when the tongue is dry. The sense of taste also depends on the sense of smell to appreciate fully the vast number of food flavors (Metcalf, 1988).

A generalized deterioration of taste buds begins after age 45, leading to a decreased discrimination in taste. Older people, therefore, often greatly increase their use of seasonings to derive a sense of satisfaction from the taste of foods. They also may eat less because food has less taste.

Taste is a dynamic sense, changing throughout the life span. It is closely linked to cultural/family food practices and influences food preferences. Taste, however, is not the only determinant of food preferences, since sight, smell, and texture are also influential factors.

Vision

Although present at birth, the ability to visualize objects is not totally developed until about 6 years of age. After this time there is minimal further development.

Vision is a complex sense that involves a number of cranial nerves. The optic nerve (CN II) controls the sensory functions involved in both visual acuity and peripheral vision. The ability of the eye to move (ocular muscle movement) is controlled by three cranial nerves. These are the oculomotor (CN III), the trochlear (CN IV), and the abducens (CN VI). In addition to innervating certain extraocular muscles of the eye, the oculomotor nerve elevates the eyelid, contracts the iris muscle, and constricts the pupil.

The ability of the lens to accommodate begins to diminish around age 42, resulting in an inability to focus properly. With further aging, the ability of the eye to adapt to darkness diminishes, so that older people require brighter light to see well. The eyelids also lose elasticity, which may interfere with vision. Further age-related changes include decreased production of tears, decreased peripheral vision, and diminished color and depth perception (see chap. 24). Health problems such as diabetes, hypertension, and, of course, cataracts and glaucoma, also can seriously impair vision.

Hearing

After birth, the ability to finely discriminate among sounds and respond to different sounds increases with maturity. The ability to hear affects language development and the child's learning to speak normally.

Both peripheral and central components contribute to the sensation of hearing. The auditory nerve (CN VIII) along with the outer, middle, and inner ear comprises the peripheral component. The central component includes pathways through the brainstem and thalamus, which eventually terminate in the temporal lobe of the cerebral cortex. It is in this area (auditory cortex) that sound is discriminated and pitch and intensity are determined (Metcalf, 1988).

It is estimated that by age 65, one third of the population loses some auditory acuity. The perception of high frequency sounds associated with speech diminishes first. In addition, the cilia lining the ear canal become stiff and coarse. Their functional ability decreases, so that more cerumen accumulates in the ear and the passage of sound waves diminishes. The aging ear is also prone to otosclerosis, which can cause a significant hearing loss.

Touch

While the ability to respond to tactile stimulation is highly developed at birth, the ability to determine the area of cutaneous stimulation improves as touch receptors mature and multiply. Unlike the other special senses, which result from the function of cranial nerves, the sense of touch occurs as a result of the activity of superficial sensations that flow from the skin receptors, or *dermatomes*, to spinal nerves and onto a specific segment of the spinal cord. Pain and temperature sensations pass without interruption to the thalamus for immediate reaction. Touch, a more complex sensation, follows a route through the thalamus to the cerebral cortex for higher interpretation. This higher level cortical interpretation also enables a person to distinguish or identify familiar objects simply by touching them.

With aging, distal peripheral nerve degeneration may lead to impairment in the sense of touch. Peripheral vascular changes also may contribute to this deterioration. Another significant degenerative change is a decrease in nerve conduction velocity. This results in a prolonged transmission of impulses from the touch receptors in the skin that may be incorrectly interpreted as delayed motor responses.

NEUROLOGICAL FUNCTIONING

The ability to maintain balance, posture, and equilibrium as well as engage in coordinated movement are functions of the cerebellum.

Coordination and Balance

Three motor systems enable voluntary muscle movement and control. These are the corticospinal (pyramidal), extrapyramidal, and the cerebellar systems. The functioning of all three systems is necessary for movement to be willful, smooth, and coordinated.

Voluntary fine motor movement is controlled by the corticospinal or pyramidal system. This system originates in the motor cortex of the cerebrum and travels down the spinal cord crossing over to the opposite side below the medulla. Impulses continue to travel down the cord until they synapse in the anterior horn cell and then travel via efferent nerve fibers to the muscle. The ability to engage in voluntary movement will be affected if an individual sustains injury to this system. Reflex activity, however, will remain intact.

Muscle tone and gross body movement are controlled by the extrapyramidal system. This system lies outside the pyramidal system and comprises motor pathways that connect the cerebrum, brain stem, and spinal cord. These pathways, some of which cross over to the opposite side in the brain stem, travel down the cord to the anterior horn cell and then travel via efferent nerve fibers to the muscle. Injury to this system can result in hyperactive muscle tone, which is evidenced by resting tremors or a shuffling gait.

Equilibrium, balance, and posture are controlled by the cerebellar system. This system is not a distinct system like the systems mentioned above. Its function is to serve as a check-and-balance mechanism, correcting errors in the other two systems when they arise. Injury to this system can result in a loss of equilibrium and a decrease in one's ability to coordinate movement.

Reflexes

A reflex is obtained by applying a "sensory stimulus that initiates the transmission of a muscle-stretch impulse or a cutaneous stimulation through the reflex arc in the spinal cord" (Grimes & Burns, 1987, p. 362). Through this mechanism, sensory nerve pathways (afferent) carry impulses to the posterior horn cell. The impulses then synapse in the anterior horn cell and travel via motor nerve pathways (efferent) back to the muscle. An interruption of any of the fibers in the reflex arc will result in the inability to elicit the reflex (lower motor neuron damage). The upper motor neurons of the cerebral cortex govern the briskness of intact reflexes.

PAIN

Pain is an elusive and complex phenomenon that is both sensory and perceptual in nature (Donovan & Girton, 1984). Pain has been defined in a variety of ways. Sternback (1968) described pain as a "personal, private sensation of hurt, a harmful stimulus which signals current or impending tissue damage and a pattern of response to protect the organism from harm" (p. 12). This definition addresses the psychological, physiological, and sociological nature of pain. Probably one of the most personal and clinically useful definitions of pain is offered by McCaffery (1979), who states that pain "is whatever the experiencing person says it is and exists whenever he says it does" (p. 11). This makes the client the expert on the pain and recognizes the highly personal nature of the experience. All pain is a complex phenomenon composed of physiological and psychological aspects. Even if the primary source of pain is within the mind, physiological changes may occur. Conversely, pain of a purely physiological origin triggers psychological effects.

Theories of pain have undergone evolutionary change. Clinical observations, along with physiological and psychological evidence, have increased our knowledge and understanding of pain (Kim, 1980). The experience of pain involves the processes of *reception, interpretation,* and *response* (Jacox, 1977). Two early theories about reception and interpretation of pain were specificity theory (1800s–1900s) and pattern theory (early 1900s).

According to the specificity theory, specific pain receptors (nerve endings) throughout the body generate pain impulses and are then transmitted through the spinal cord to a pain center in the thalamus. This theory was questioned for many reasons, among them the fact that no one has been able to identify actual "pain receptors" in the body. Pattern theory, on the other hand, states that there are two major pain fibers transmitting impulses, a slow conducting fiber and a rapid conducting fiber. These fibers converge at the spinal cord and transmit information to higher centers in the brain. This convergence of impulses at the spinal cord and their transmission to the brain enabled the interpretation of characteristics such as the intensity, amount, character, and quantity of the pain. Both theories are limited, however, in that they do not address "factors that alter the perception of pain, such as anxiety, depression, and hypnosis or explain the failure of pain to resolve after surgical transection of the pain pathways and spinal cord," note Ignatavicius and Bayne (1991, p. 108).

Currently, the most clinically useful and commonly accepted theory of pain is the gate control theory (Melzack & Wall, 1965), which addresses the multidimensional nature of pain. According to this theory, many neurological processes influence the body's interpretation and response to painful stimuli. These neurological processes occur in the spinal cord, thalamus, and the cerebrum (Eland, 1981).

According to a somewhat oversimplified explanation of the gate control theory, certain neurological processes or mechanisms modify or intensify pain impulse transmission by opening or closing the gate.

Pain perception is diminished by:

Inhibition of small diameter nerve fibers by the activity of large diameter fiber "sensations,"

Inhibition from the brain stem stimulated by imagery and relaxation,

Inhibition from the cerebral cortex and thalamus to diminish anxiety.

Gate-opening mechanisms that increase pain perception include:

Small diameter nerve fiber activity stimulated by pain or tissue damage,

Facilitory impulses from the brain stem initiated by a decrease in stimuli,

Facilitory impulses from the cerebral cortex and thalamus that occur as fear and anxiety are experienced (McCaffery, 1979).

"It is thought that with chronic pain the input from the large-diameter fibers to the substantia gelatinosa is minimized or even eliminated, leaving the gate permanently open" (Eland, 1981, p. 168). Without a "gating" mechanism to modify or inhibit pain transmission, pain messages are readily referred to higher brain centers.

The ability of central control processes (higher brain centers) to exert a modifying effect on pain transmission also is believed to be altered in chronic pain. Years of suffering and memories of failed attempts to manage pain deplete cognitive control and, therefore, maximize the intensity of the pain (Eland, 1981).

Current research into the nature and activity of neurotransmitters—the chemicals that open and close the "gates" to allow transmission of nerve impulses—may provide more information on the complex phenomena involved in pain perception.

Pain may be either short-term (*acute*) or long-term (*chronic*). Acute pain is temporary and reversible. It usually has an identifiable cause and, if caused by injury, diminishes as healing occurs. Acute pain usually is described in terms of sensory qualities, such as sharp, dull, or stabbing. Acute pain has a positive aspect in that it tends to avert further injury to the organism by restricting activity; the rare individual who cannot feel pain will have great difficulty surviving.

Initially, acute pain (predominantly a sympathetic response) causes measurable physiological changes, such as increased or decreased blood pressure, increased pulse and respiration, dilation of the pupils, diaphoresis, and other autonomic responses. Some behaviors may be centered on relief of pain and tension (rubbing, rocking, holding the affected area) or may express discomfort (crying, groaning, wincing). Muscular tension, apprehension, anxiety, restlessness, and impaired thinking also may be present. The client's entire attention often is focused on the pain.

While chronic pain may have an identifiable cause, often the cause is unknown. In addition, chronic pain frequently does not respond to usual therapy. It has an indeterminate duration or may recur over time. It often becomes more debilitating and exhausting than warranted by the apparent physical changes or may take on a meaning of its own. For example, clients with arthritis often focus primarily on the pain rather than the disease or its cause. To maintain function in activities of daily living, the client may choose to perform activities that actually increase the pain. This is a form of adaptation.

The physiological responses seen in acute pain

tend to disappear with chronic pain (predominantly a parasympathetic response). As the client adapts to chronic pain, the autonomic nervous system returns to a near normal state. Psychological responses also assume a totally different pattern. A blank expression, disinterest in talking about the pain, or exhaustion may occur. Depression, not anxiety, usually characterizes the client in chronic pain (Donovan & Girton, 1984; Copp, 1974; McCaffery, 1979). Chronic pain actually may become incorporated in the client's body image. Unlike the pain behaviors seen with acute pain, overt pain behaviors over an extended period of time are not viewed as appropriate or socially acceptable.

Clients who have experienced chronic pain for years may show different responses to an acute pain episode. It is not unusual to have an elderly client refuse pain medication postoperatively, telling the nurse that "compared to the daily pain of arthritis, this pain isn't really so bad." The nurse should not interpret this adaptive response as signifying lack of pain, but rather a change in response to pain. Clients who describe chronic pain often use affective terms such as "awful," "hateful," "sickening," and "wearing."

Once the central nervous system reaches maturity, the threshold for pain is uniform for all healthy individuals; in all individuals an identical amount of painful stimulus is required to produce transmission along the pain fibers. Factors such as changes in concentration or attention, injury to tissues exposing nerve endings, anesthesia or analgesia may alter an individual's pain threshold and therefore the individual's response to a painful stimulus (Eland, 1981). Response is the component of the pain process that shows great individual variation. *It is the response to the painful stimulus that differs among individuals.* It is this component upon which the nursing assessment of pain actually is based. Among the many factors that influence a client's response to pain are age and level of development, gender, culture, values and attitudes, emotional status, will and self-control, personality, body image, previous experiences and coping behaviors, anticipation, the meaning of pain, the environment, and physical condition. These factors must be noted in the pain assessment along with the history and any measurable physiological changes.

Research on pain in the elderly presents some differing conclusions. Miller (1990) notes that while cutaneous nerves responsible for pain sensation are not affected by age-related changes, evidence exists to support the conclusion of a decline in pain sensitivity beginning around age 50 and

progressing with time (Kligman, Grove, & Balin, 1985). This has important implications for clients' safety (increased susceptibility to burns due to diminished tactile sensitivity) and the analgesic management of pain in older adults (undertreatment of pain). The aged, like the child, also may suffer from an inability to express pain.

VARIABLES THAT INFLUENCE SENSORY-PERCEPTUAL-NEUROLOGICAL STATUS

A number of variables influence sensory-perceptual-neurological status. Age and health are among the most significant.

Age

Developmental (age) differences in sensory-perceptual-neurological function must be taken into account during assessment. These are particularly prevalent in the young, in whom they are due to immaturity of the sensory-perceptual system and the elderly in whom deterioration of the sensory-perceptual system is occurring. These developmental differences are detailed in chapters 21, 22, and 24.

Health

Various common health alterations may affect sensory-perceptual-neurological status.

Cerebral Vascular Accident (Stroke)

Cerebral vascular accidents may occur anywhere within the cranial arterial system. Major arterial systems involved include cerebral, vertebral, carotid, and basilar. The extent of damage to the brain is directly related to the arteries involved and degree of disruption of blood flow. The area of brain perfused by the involved arterial system correlates with symptoms produced.

If the lesion involves the dominant side of the brain, higher sensory functions such as speech, memory, and interpretation may be affected to varying degrees. Terminology used to describe some of these effects includes:

Aphasia
expressive (inability to speak)
receptive (inability to understand speech)
visual (inability to recognize figures or words)
Amnesia (impaired memory)
Agnosia (impaired sensory-perceptual ability to recognize objects)

Apraxia (inability to perform purposeful movement or comprehend events)

Motor function defects will not appear so severe, since the contralateral side of the body is involved and the ipsilateral side is not affected. Therefore, a right hemisphere dominant person who experiences a lesion in the dominant hemisphere has impairment of motor abilities on the left side.

If the lesion involves the nondominant hemisphere, higher sensory functions such as speech are not affected but motor abilities may be severely impaired.

Visual impairments resulting from strokes vary greatly, because of the pattern of innervation of the optic nerve tracts. Each optic nerve begins in one hemisphere, with half the fibers crossing at the optic chiasm and terminating in the opposite hemisphere and half remaining in the side where the nerve originates. Thus, a stroke is more likely to affect portions of the visual fields of both eyes rather than one eye only.

A stroke in the basilar arterial system tends to produce symptoms that affect the entire body, since the cerebellum, pons, and brain stem are involved. The severity of strokes in this area is often greater because the vital functions are affected.

Symptoms such as unilateral weakness, headaches, forgetfulness, and visual changes may be early signs of a stroke. The extent of damage cannot be assessed immediately, since further occlusion or bleeding may evolve. The client must be monitored closely throughout the evolution of the stroke until maximum damage has occurred and rehabilitation can begin. The neurologic check for this client consists, therefore, of level of consciousness, pupil response, coordination/muscle tone, reflexes, vital signs, and other assessments directed toward identifying the location and severity of the stroke.

Seizures

Seizures are a significant neurologic problem affecting all age groups. Nursing assessment can be important in monitoring and controlling this condition. Seizure disorders may be idiopathic or acquired; recurrent or nonrecurrent; generalized, partial (focal), or other.

Idiopathic seizures have no known cause. Acquired seizures may result from brain trauma, hypoxia, tumors, infections, toxins, hypoglycemia, and so forth. Generalized seizures involve both hemispheres of the brain symmetrically and usually result in loss of consciousness. An aura of warning may precede the attack. Partial seizures (focal) originate in the specific area of the brain but may spread to other areas of the brain following a consistent pattern. Loss of consciousness may or may not occur. It is important to have the client describe, if possible, the course of the seizure in detail, as this can pinpoint the location of the seizure activity.

Other seizures may not be classified in either of these broad categories, since the precipitating stimulus does not originate in the brain. Some examples include febrile, alcohol or drug withdrawal, and toxic seizures.

In some cases seizures may progress to status epilepticus. This is a serious condition consisting of continuous seizure activity that may lead to cerebral anoxia or death if untreated.

Since loss of consciousness and amnesia are often components of seizure activity, it is important that the nurse either interview someone who has observed the seizure or observe the seizure activity personally. Even if the client is capable of describing it, it is better if the nurse can observe and describe the event. Observations should include:

Onset, including precipitating events and aura

Activity, including where the seizure started and how it progressed

Duration

Associated findings, including loss of consciousness, incontinence, pupil changes, character of respirations

Postictal (postseizure) state

A neurologic check following seizure activity will reveal variable findings depending upon the type of seizure and presence or absence of a postictal state. This check includes level of consciousness, pupil response, and vital signs. The client's tongue and mouth should also be inspected for injury. The client should also be assessed for incontinence during the seizure and for confusion after the seizure.

Increased Intracranial Pressure

Increased intracranial pressure may result from a wide variety of conditions including trauma or tumors. The symptoms of increased intracranial pressure are related to pressure exerted by the fluid or the lesion on the surrounding cranial tissue. Pressure may be so great that portions of the brain are forced through the tentorial notch or foramen magnum. Local symptoms are dependent upon the portion of brain affected by the lesions. General early symptoms of increased intracranial pressure may include any combination of the following:

Headache
Change in level of consciousness
Sensory loss
Hemiplegia
Monoplegia
Papilledema
Widening pulse pressure
Bradycardia
Vomiting
Personality change
Seizures

Later signs may include:

Fixed unilateral or bilateral pupil dilation
Decreased blood pressure
Increased pulse
Respiratory depression

Death may ensue. Thus, the neurologic check for a client with increased intracranial pressure usually includes level of consciousness (orientation and state of awareness), pupil response, equality and strength of motor responses, sensory response, and vital signs.

THE SENSORY-PERCEPTUAL-NEUROLOGICAL HISTORY

To assess the status of the client's sensory–perceptual–neurological functioning adequately, a complete and accurate history is necessary. Interpretation of information gained from the history will help the nurse accurately focus the clinical appraisal on areas of potential problems.

The health history used for an adult is based on the format in Table 15-1, which lists general categories from which the nurse may develop questions to match the client's level of knowledge and understanding. Categories include areas of concern, past or present problems, and medications taken. If the client responds affirmatively to questions about past or present problems, it is important to explore onset, frequency, duration, and similar details. In addition, a complete medication history should be obtained, since use of prescribed or over-the-counter medications may be related to sensory–perceptual–neurological disturbances. Use of certain medications may place the client at great risk. For example, use of atropine in the client

with glaucoma may dangerously increase intraocular pressure.

While taking the history it is important to observe the client's physical appearance, since sensory changes may result in problems about which the client is unaware. Sensory deficits, for example, may result in apparently abnormal findings in other areas. A hearing impaired client may misinterpret and respond to questions inappropriately, giving the inaccurate appearance of confusion. A reliable history cannot be obtained from a confused client. The nurse also should be aware of nonverbal behaviors from which much information can be gained. Data concerning prior vision/hearing exams or their lack can reveal information about health behaviors and may open this area to exploration.

Mental Status History

The nurse begins with the collection of information on mental status. While asking questions, the nurse observes the facial expression of the client, body posture, and motor behavior (appearance of behavior). Is there congruence between verbal and nonverbal behavior? Does the patient's body posture indicate a relaxed, calm state or one of constant motion and fidgeting?

In addition, the nurse observes the dress, grooming, and hygiene of the client. Is the client dressed appropriately for his or her age and for the occasion? Is the dress appropriately applied? Clients with chronic brain syndrome, for example, have difficulty dressing themselves and may apply their outer clothing first and their undergarments on top of the outer clothing. The colors of the client's clothing also should be observed. Older clients may experience difficulty perceiving certain colors. The client exhibiting this normal, age-related change needs to be differentiated from the client with a manic personality who exhibits eccentric combinations in dress. Poverty and homelessness also can affect dress.

Mood is explored by asking the client to describe how she or he generally feels (happy, content, anxious). Does the client experience mood swings? Is the client's affect appropriate to the types of questions asked and the responses given during the nursing history?

The client's thought processes, content of communication, and perceptions also are evaluated carefully. Is the thought process logical? Does the conversation make sense? Is the client able to clearly articulate thoughts and feelings? Is a client's hesitance to answer questions related, for example,

TABLE 15-1
The Sensory–Perceptual–Neurological History

Appearance of Behavior
1. Ability to dress appropriately for occasion and age.
2. Dress appropriately applied.
3. Client's perception of own physical appearance.
4. Ability of the client to be responsible for physical appearance.
5. Change in ability to care for one's physical appearance.
6. Body build, height, and weight.
7. Recent changes in weight.

Mood
1. Client's description of how he/she generally feels (happy, sad, calm, angry).
2. Recent change in client's mood.
3. Ability of the client to relate:
   - ability to cope with stress
   - feelings about self
   - attitudes
   - relationships with family members
   - ability to deal with frustration
   - goals
4. Past or present problems such as:
   - acute infection or trauma
   - chronic illness
5. Use of alcohol or mood-altering drugs

Thought Processes, Content, Perceptions
1. Oriented to time, place, and person.
2. Clarity of communication.
3. Speech—coherence, articulation, appropriateness.
4. Recent changes in orientation or thought processes.
5. Client's perception of the world around him/her.
6. Past or present problems with:
   - seizures
   - loss of consciousness
7. Use of medications: anticonvulsants, antidepressants, tranquilizers.

Cognitive Functions
1. Educational history.
2. Ability to conceptualize and make appropriate judgments.
3. Understanding of present condition.
4. Recent and remote memory functions appear intact.
5. Change in memory function.
6. Ability to make simple calculations.
7. Client's awareness of things considered to be common knowledge.

Smell
1. Ability to discriminate among and distinguish between specific odors.
2. Recent change in sense of smell. (If no, proceed to number 4.)
3. Manner in which sense of smell changed.
4. Past or present problems such as:
   - Difficulty in breathing through the nose, mouth breathing (nasal obstruction).
   - Nasal discharge (rhinorrhea).

- Nosebleeds (epistaxis)
- Hay fever (seasonal rhinitis)
- Allergies
- Frequent colds
- Change in sense of taste (changes in taste are often reported when pathology actually involves sense of smell)
5. Past injury to head or nose.

Taste
1. Ability to differentiate among the four tastes (bitter, salty, sour, sweet).
2. Changes in sense of taste. (If no, proceed to vision.)
3. Effects of changed sense of taste on food preferences or amount of seasoning used.

Vision
1. Date of last vision test. Results; person performing the exam. Tested for glaucoma (over age 40) or cataracts (over age 60).
2. Use of glasses or contact lenses. If yes, when last checked or changed.
3. Type of corrective lenses worn.
4. Change in visual acuity.
5. Reason to believe that vision is not as good as it should be?
6. Past or present problems such as:
   - difficulty seeing
   - blurred vision
   - diplopia (double vision)
   - pain or burning in or around the eyes
   - itching
   - redness or irritation
   - excessive tearing
   - increased sensitivity to bright light (photophobia)
   - night blindness
   - blind spot
   - halo vision
   - tunnel vision
   - swollen eye
   - eye infections
   - frequent headaches
   - trauma to eye
   - eye surgery
   - glaucoma
   - cataracts
   - diabetes
   If the client responds affirmatively to any of the above problems, obtain a complete medication history.
7. Wear a prosthesis.
8. Use of eye medication—prescribed or over-the-counter. Type, frequency, and reason.

Hearing
1. Date of last hearing examination. Results; person performing the exam.
2. Family history of hearing loss. Describe.
3. Live, work in a high noise area.
4. Change in ability to hear.

(continued)

TABLE 15-1 (Continued)

5. Reason to believe hearing is not as good as it should be?
6. Past or present problems such as:
   - Hearing unusual sounds: tinnitus (ringing), buzzing, other noises (describe)
   - Loss of balance, dizziness, vertigo.
   - Hearing better out of one ear? Which ear?
   - Ear pain or itching, earache, infection, discharge.
   - Ear surgery.
   If client responds to any of the above problems, obtain a complete history.
7. Use of corrective devices (hearing aid)? If yes, describe type and effectiveness.

Touch
1. Ability to detect differences in temperature.
2. Difference in sensation on opposite sides of the body?
3. Difficulty discriminating between or identifying familiar objects by touch?
4. Past or present problems such as:
   - Paresthesia (numbness, tingling)
   - Hyperesthesia (increased sensitivity)
   - Hypoesthesia (decreased sensitivity)
   - Anesthesia (total loss of sensation)

- Paralysis
- Asthenia (muscle weakness)
- Tremors
- Diabetes
- Multiple sclerosis or any other nerve disease
- Diminished or absent perspiration
- High arches

Coordination and Balance
1. Ability to maintain balance?
2. Client's use of assistive devices (walker, tripod cane, wheel chair)
3. Smoothness and accuracy of movements
4. Change in ability to coordinate movement?
5. Past or present problems such as:
   - difficulty maintaining balance or grasping objects
   - trauma to head, spinal cord
   - weakness or gait disorders
   - tremors
   - dizziness
   - limited range of motion
   - muscle weakness
6. Medications: anticholingeric antivertigos

---

to a speech impediment such as stuttering or have thought processes been affected by cerebral trauma or disease?

The client's memory, ability to focus (attention), use of language, and the abilities to conceptualize and make appropriate judgments are evaluated as the nurse obtains information about the client's cognitive functions. Has the client experienced loss of memory, or has the ability to remember people, events, or details changed recently?

Culture, age, education, and life experience must be considered when obtaining a mental status history. These factors influence clients' perceptions of health and illness.

Olfactory History

A change in the sense of smell, without any apparent injury or aging, may suggest the existence of significant pathology. If the sense of smell has changed so that formerly pleasant odors become noxious, pathological conditions such as cancer or hepatitis may be present. Cancer patients receiving chemotherapy continue to report significant distortions of smell for a year or more after treatment. Odors as well as sights that caused distress during treatment continue to do so for a time after treatment is completed.

Taste History

The sense of taste is linked closely to the sense of smell. Therefore, the client who reports significant changes in the sense of smell also usually experiences alterations in taste. A sudden change in the client's sense of taste, with formerly pleasant foods becoming aversive, may also indicate the presence of systemic diseases such as hepatitis or cancer. Selected medications also may affect the sense of taste (Table 15-2).

Some objective measure of taste usually can be gained by asking, "How many spoonsful of sugar does it take to make your coffee (cereal, etc.) sweet?" or, "How much salt do you put on your food to make it taste good?" The client then can be asked if this amount recently has increased, a finding often noted in elderly clients as the sense of taste diminishes.

Vision History

While obtaining the history the nurse should observe the client for cues indicating visual impairment such as inability to make or maintain eye contact, squinting, or apparent clumsiness. Problems such as periorbital pain, redness, and itching may be indicative of infection. Headaches, tearing, photophobia, and other associated symptoms may

TABLE 15-2
Selected Medications Affecting the Special Senses

Ototoxic	Oculotoxic	Gustatory effects
salicylates	salicylates	metronidazole (Flagyl)
aminoglycosides (digitalis and derivatives)	anticholinesterase	penicillamine
	antihistamines	chloramphenicol
chloroquine	chloramphenicol	arsenic
erythromycin	chloroquine	phosphorus
gallium nitrates	chlorpromazine	
gentamicin	clonidine	
minocycline (vestibular effects also)	cocaine	
	steroids	
neomycin	ethambutol	
streptomycin	5-fluorouracil	
tobramyclin	neuroleptic agents	
vancomycin	penicillamine	
kanamycin	thrombolytic agents	
capreomycin	local anesthetics	
Butazolidin	isoniazid	
cisplatin		
ethacrynic acid		

be seen in clients who experience migraine headaches. Symptoms such as halo vision and tunnel vision, especially in clients over 40, suggest glaucoma.

If the client reports having diabetes, a detailed visual history and appraisal must be done, since complications of diabetes, along with glaucoma and cataracts, are leading causes of blindness in the United States. It is important to refer these clients to an ophthalmologist. Conditions such as homonymous hemianopsia (loss of vision in the same half of the visual field in each eye) might be suspected when the client appears to see from one side only. Other disorders such as bitemporal hemianopsia (blindness in the temporal portion of each eye) or tunnel vision from glaucoma might be suspected if a client can see an object only when it is directly in the line of vision. Selected medications also may affect vision (Table 15-2).

It is also important to ask about or observe the amount of light the client requires to see well, since diminished ability to accommodate is common in the elderly.

Hearing History

Certain factors may expose the client to a greater than normal risk for developing hearing problems. These factors may range from repeated exposure to loud noise to medications that produce auditory alterations (see Table 15-2).

Listening closely to the speech of clients as they respond to questions is a simple way to recognize speech and/or hearing deficits or other problems. For example, a loud voice, monotonous tone, or distorted speech, which initially may be interpreted as confusion or speech impairment, later may be documented as signs of a hearing deficit. The nurse also must be aware that the client with a significant hearing impairment may consciously or unconsciously lip read and focus on gestures as an adjunct to hearing. Such clients thus may be able to respond quite appropriately despite a hearing deficit. Nonverbal cues, such as turning the head to one side, may indicate a hearing loss in the opposite ear.

The client who acknowledges the presence of tinnitus should be asked about the use of aspirin. Since the elderly often have arthritis, they may be ingesting excessive amounts of aspirin.

Use or nonuse of a prescribed hearing aid should be investigated.

Touch History

While obtaining the history, the nurse should assess for injuries to the hands or feet that may have occurred without the client's knowledge. Such trauma may be related to diminished sensitivity.

The client must understand that questions about temperature discrimination refer not only to overall body temperature but also to specific areas of the body. This may be clarified by such questions as "Do you have trouble regulating the temperature of your bath water?" "Do you find that although the temperature seems correct on your feet, it is too hot when you start to sit down?" If diminished local temperature sensitivity exists, the client should be questioned about diabetes or other diseases causing peripheral nerve alterations. Referral for further testing may be indicated.

If the client appears to exhibit tremors or muscle weakness, questions about conditions such as Parkinson's disease, multiple sclerosis, or any central or peripheral nerve disease are appropriate. If severe peripheral sensory deficits are found, the client reports absence of perspiration, and examination discloses high palatal arches, severe nervous system disease may be present The client should be referred for further testing.

In addition to the special senses, other function are regulated by the cranial nerves and information on these also must be obtained in the nursing history. These functions include swallowing and phonation. Any change in the client's ability to swallow needs to be carefully evaluated in terms of onset, length of time, modifications made (e.g., diet), and other accompanying symptoms (e.g., weight loss, fatigue).

The ability to speak involves a number of functions, among them movement of the tongue, palate, soft pharynx, and larynx. Any problems or changes in these functions also should be explored.

Coordination and Balance History

The nursing history should explore any changes in the client's ability to maintain balance and perform coordinated movement. Bruises on the client's skin can alert the nurse to explore the issue of falls. Of course, bruises also may be the result of abuse, indicate trauma due to decreased tactile sensation (age-related change) or result from hematological disorders. The nurse should question the client about past or current problems, such as weakness, dizziness, and tremors. Obtaining a medication history is also important in order to determine whether medications are taken for problems with coordination or balance or have an untoward effect on these functions.

Pain History

To adequately assess pain, a pain history must be obtained from the client (Table 15-3). Since pain is so subjective, the client should be encouraged to verbalize feelings. Some aspects of the pain history and clinical appraisal are linked closely. For example, a client may be able to express the intensity of

pain more clearly with the use of a pain intensity measurement scale (discussed in the clinical appraisal section) than with a verbal description.

The setting in which a painful experience occurs can influence greatly the amount of pain reported since psychological factors cannot be separated from the experience. If the environment is tense or seen as threatening, the client's anxiety may significantly increase the pain. If the client lacks privacy, an apparent lack of response may simply be due to embarrassment. Some people often are very sensitive to nonverbal signals from the nurse and others that certain responses are not acceptable. This sensitivity may significantly inhibit the client from expressing an accurate and appropriate pain response. Conversely, an open, relaxed, accepting atmosphere provided by the nurse may allow the client the freedom to respond honestly.

Age and sex are related to response in less direct ways. In cultures where sex roles are precisely defined, male and female responses to pain may be quite different. Age also may be an indirect determinant of pain response. The geriatric client may be "expected" either to complain more or to tolerate more; these expectations of others actually may be attributed to age alone.

The influence of nurses' attitudes on pain management in older adults was observed in a study by Faherty and Grier (1984) that examined

TABLE 15-3
Pain History (Current or Significant Past Reports of Pain)

1. Location (have client point to area)
2. Intensity (mild, moderate, severe)
3. Quality (aching, burning, prickling, stabbing, throbbing, sharp, dull, shooting)
4. Chronology (acute, chronic, recurrent, intermittent, constant, onset, duration of episode)
5. Precipitating factors (injury, onset in relation to any event or period in time)
6. Associated symptoms (pain may cause nausea, crying, constipation)
7. Effect upon activities of daily living
8. Factors that aggravate the pain (movement or exercise may increase some types of pain)
9. Measures used to relieve pain (analgesic and nonanalgesic)
10. Analgesic history (medication taken, amount, frequency, effect)
11. Beliefs about pain (cultural, religious influences)
12. Previous experience with pain
13. Mood (how would client describe self)
14. Support systems

the analgesic management of older clients post surgery. The study found that less analgesic medication was prescribed and administered to older clients than younger clients. In addition, nurses gave less than the prescribed dose. Lack of knowledge, misinformation, and unfounded claims contribute to this kind of inconsistent behavior (Ignatavicius & Bayne, 1991).

Culture also affects the client's response to pain (see chap. 8). Moreover, the nurse's own background may influence assessment of the client's pain. For example, a nurse who believes that people should bear pain stoically may think that a postoperative client who is groaning with abdominal pain is overreacting. This perception may lead the nurse to overlook potential complications such as an intestinal obstruction. Nurses must understand that there are ways other than their own of responding to pain. The nurse should explore variations in culture, not to stereotype clients but to understand differences and appreciate diversity. The study of other cultures enables a nurse to learn what are acceptable and appropriate responses to pain and how pain is managed as well as beliefs about pain and its significance (McCaffery, 1979). Awareness of these values and influences reduces the likelihood that they will interfere with the assessment process.

A pain history should include details about the nature of the client's pain. Asking the client to point to the painful area is very helpful and enables the nurse to specifically identify the location. Information also is sought about the intensity and quality of the pain. When clients refer to pain as mild or severe, for example, it is important for the nurse to understand (and not presume) what mild or severe means to the client. Asking a client to rate the pain on a scale of 1 to 10 (1 = no pain; 10 = severe pain) may provide a more accurate reading of the intensity.

Having the client describe the pain (what it feels like) offers further information about the quality of the pain. It is best initially to let the client respond to the question "What does the pain feel like?" rather than cue the client with words, such as "stabbing," "dull," or "aching." If the client has difficulty describing the pain, then cuing the client becomes necessary.

Information about the chronology of the pain along with associated symptoms and precipitating factors is important for diagnosis as well as management. One of the most helpful ways to determine the impact of pain on the client is to ask what effect the pain has had on activities of daily living. A client may state that "my pain is not so bad" and

then relate the inability to go to work or handle all on-the-job responsibilities.

The client's previous experience with pain also provides valuable information. Previous experience can offer insight into coping abilities, personal resourcefulness, measures used to relieve pain (analgesic as well as nonanalgesic), and the client's support system.

Exploring support systems is important to comprehensive pain assessment. Pain, particularly chronic pain, can be a very isolating experience. A support system can buffer the negative effects such as isolation and depression and positively assist clients to cope better.

The importance of a thorough pain history cannot be overemphasized. Pain is a very personal and complex phenomenon. The more the nurse understands the multidimensional nature of pain, the better prepared the nurse will be to develop pain management strategies for each client.

CLINICAL APPRAISAL AND SCREENING

The clinical appraisal of a client's sensory–perceptual–neurological status involves the evaluation of mental status, the special senses, coordination, and balance as well as the reflexes. Cerebral function or mental status is evaluated at the beginning of the examination (see boxed insert, p. 458).

Mental Status

In assessing mental status, the nurse initially focuses on the overall appearance of the client. The nurse notes the patient's general appearance, dress, and personal hygiene. As the nurse engages the client in conversation, the nurse evaluates the client's ability to relate health information. Does the client maintain the train of thought? As the client details information, the nurse also observes the client's language and speech. Does the client talk smoothly? What is the rate and rhythm of the speech?

Throughout the assessment of mental status, the nurse is observant of the client's mood, that is what the client says in regard to how he or she is feeling. This is different from affect. "Affect is the emotional state of the client—the way the client appears to others" (Grimes & Burns 1987, p. 74). Does the client appear happy, sad, anxious, depressed, or unusually alert? How is the client describing his or her mood? Are verbal and nonverbal behaviors congruent?

Assessment of cognitive function begins with a determination of orientation to person, place, and

---

Mental Status

A. Appearance of behavior
   1. Level of consciousness
   2. Posture and motor behavior
   3. Dress, grooming, hygiene
   4. Facial expression
   5. Speech
      a. Quality
      b. Rate and rhythm
      c. Volume
      d. Quantity
B. Mood
C. Cognitive functions
   1. Orientation
   2. Attention
   3. Memory
   4. Language
   5. Higher intellectual functions
      a. Information
      b. Vocabulary
      c. Thought processes
      d. Abstract reasoning—proverbs, metaphors
      e. Judgment
      f. Calculation

---

time. The nurse asks the client his or her name, where he or she is, and the date. If the client is unsure of the date, does the client know the month or the season? The nurse might ask the client which holiday is coming up or has just passed. Orientation can also be assessed by asking the client the names of siblings, a spouse, or doctor.

Attention span can be assessed as the client responds to questions. Does the client respond readily when asked a question or ask to have the question repeated? Does the client look away or fidget during conversation?

Immediate, recent, and remote memory are assessed next. To evaluate immediate memory, the nurse can ask the client to repeat a series of numbers right after the nurse says them. Recent memory also can be determined by asking the client to recall at the end of the examination three words given by the nurse at the beginning of the session. The nurse also could ask the client about a family event that happened during the week. Obviously, this would need to be verified with a family member. The nurse may ask about a local or national event that occurred during the week. This may not be appropriate for the individual who indicates

that he or she does not read the paper or watch television. Remote memory may be determined by asking the client's birth date or the client's ZIP code. Obviously, the nurse would have this information in hand in order to verify its accuracy.

When testing for higher intellectual functions, the nurse must remember that levels of education and interests vary widely. Testing for general information, for example, is not a test of intelligence but a way to assess current general knowledge. Asking the client who is the current vice-president or governor of the state may be difficult for a particular client. However, the same client may be able to name the World Series winner or the Superbowl champion. Obviously, the nurse should not ask a question for which the nurse does not know the answer. As the client responds to questions, the nurse is able to assess whether thought processes are logical and coherent (see chap. 12).

When the nurse is testing for abstract reasoning ability (interpretation of proverbs), the proverb given to the client for interpretation should fit the client situation. An individual who is not fluent in English may never have heard of the expression, "People in glass houses shouldn't throw stones." Also, if the nurse asks the client to interpret the meaning of a particular word or phrase, the client's educational level and life experience must be considered. The purpose of this examination is to determine mental status, not level of intelligence.

To test for judgment, the nurse might ask the client, "What would you do if you saw a stamped letter on a sidewalk near a mailbox?" Asking, "What would you do if your house was on fire?" would be another way to assess judgment. Again, educational level and the client situation should be considered when constructing questions.

The nurse should use caution when assessing the client's ability to calculate. Someone with a minimal level of education may have great difficulty counting backward from 100 by three's. It may be more appropriate to ask the client how much change would be returned from $1.00 for an item costing 85 cents.

Special Senses

Data gathered from the history should be interpreted and used to determine the extent of the sensory clinical appraisal needed. For example, if no abnormal findings in the senses of taste and smell have been reported by the client during the history and if none is suspected by the nurse gathering the information, tests of smell and taste need not be done. However, it is possible to miss a unilateral loss of smell if this sense is not tested, because the client may not report any problems with olfaction. The remainder of the sensory clinical appraisal is done to confirm positive findings from the history and to detect deficits not identified through the history alone.

Clients who are unable to respond or cooperate, such as confused or comatose clients, cannot be tested reliably for all special senses by means of the usual nursing assessment techniques. The comatose client would not be tested for these senses except for responses to pain and selected portions of the vision examination. A neurological check included later in this chapter is likely to be more appropriate for the comatose client.

Appraisal of Smell

The following equipment is needed to perform an adequate appraisal of the sense of smell:

> 2 to 3 clean, stoppered test tubes or vials
>
> substances such as coffee, peanut butter, chocolate, vanilla extract, or tobacco

Small amounts of mildly volatile substances that will not stimulate the gustatory or trigeminal receptors should be used rather than highly volatile substances such as ammonia or alcohol. The nasal passages must be clear for the sense of smell to be accurately assessed. To facilitate this the client should blow the nose. The client then should be instructed to close both eyes so that sight will not influence the sense of smell. One nostril is occluded while the sense is tested by placing the open vial containing the substance under the client's nose and eliciting a response. The procedure is repeated for the other side.

The client with a normal sense of smell (intact cranial nerve I) should be able to discriminate among substances and perhaps identify each. There should be no discernible difference in the acuity of smell between the nostrils if both are patent. It would be inappropriate to test clients who cannot breathe nasally such as a client with a tracheostomy. Care should be used in testing the cancer patient who has received chemotherapy, as formerly pleasant odors often become noxious and trigger nausea and vomiting. This change in smell also may result in an interference with the cancer patient's nutritional intake.

Abnormalities in the sense of smell may be caused by nasal disorders such as obstruction, mucosal damage, or neurological changes following nasal surgery. Unilateral loss of smell may be diagnostic of frontal lesions or injuries.

Appraisal of Taste

The following equipment is needed to perform an adequate appraisal of the sense of taste:

> 4 bottles containing sugar water (sweet), a weak concentration of salt water (salty), lemon juice (sour), and quinine (bitter)
>
> 4 eyedroppers or 8 cotton swabs (1 eyedropper or 2 cotton swabs for each solution)
>
> 1 glass of cool water
>
> 1 emesis basin

The client should open the mouth and extend the tongue. The nurse tests each side and section of the tongue separately, asking the client to rinse the mouth with water between tests. No set order for testing has been developed, but moving from pleasant to less pleasant tastes seems appropriate. An eyedropper or cotton swab is used to place a small amount of sugar water on the right anterior portion of the tongue. The client then is asked to describe the taste sensation. The mouth is rinsed with water, and the left anterior portion of the tongue is tested in the same manner, using the eyedropper or a clean cotton swab. In the order shown on Figure 15-2, salty, sour, and bitter taste bud sensitivity then should be tested. A greater concentration of all substances, especially sweet, may be

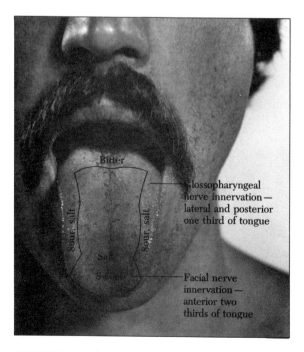

FIGURE 15-2. Locations on the Tongue to Elicit Specific Taste Sensations. (*Note.* From Grimes/Burns: *Health Assessment in Nursing Practice,* Second Edition, © 1987. Boston: Jones and Bartlett Publishers, p. 359.)

required to elicit the normal taste sensation in the elderly.

The client with a normal sense of taste (intact sensory components of cranial nerves VII and IX) should be able to discriminate among the four substances. Taste acuity is highest before meals and diminishes with satiety. The sweet and salty tastes should be elicited from the anterior two thirds of the tongue; bitter and sour from the posterior third. There should be no reported difference between the right and left sides.

Abnormalities in the sense of taste may be unilateral or bilateral. Unilateral loss of taste correlates with cranial nerve lesions or brain damage from cerebral vascular accidents. Bilateral loss of taste can be diagnostic of a lesion in the pons, the pathway for taste transmission. Other abnormalities in taste may result from a variety of problems, including tongue lesions and the loss of the sense of smell. Increased threshold to bitter tastes (and salty and sour to a lesser degree) and decreased threshold to bitter tastes before degenerative changes in the taste buds would normally be expected may be a result of cancer.

Although many individuals report a loss of sense of taste when the sense of smell is diminished, such as with a severe cold, the actual physiological sense of taste is not altered. What often is described as taste is largely the sense of smell.

Cultural food preferences or aversions vary, but no physiological difference in the taste buds has been identified in people from different ethnic groups. Thus, the previously described technique for appraisal of taste is appropriate for all cultural groups.

Appraisal of Vision

To adequately assess vision, the following equipment is needed:

A Snellen E and/or a Snellen alphabet chart (Figures 15-3 and 15-4)

A Jaeger chart or newsprint

The Ishihara plates or other pseudoisochromatic plates

A penlight

A cotton ball

A yardstick

A 3" × 5" card, paper cup, or other covering device

An ophthalmoscope

Testing Distant Visual Acuity. In a well-lighted room, the Snellen chart should be positioned ex-

actly 20 feet from and level with the client's eyes. Selection of the Snellen E chart (see chap. 22) or the Snellen alphabet chart depends upon the literacy and the language of the client.

Eyes are tested separately and then together. The client is instructed to cover one eye using the covering device but to avoid applying pressure to it, as this may later cause blurred vision. The importance of keeping the eye covered completely, but open, is emphasized so that accurate test results can be obtained. If the client wears corrective lenses for distance vision, the test is performed with the lenses in place and then with the lenses removed.

The client should be instructed to read the smallest line possible, identifying either the letters or the direction in which each "E" is pointing. The smallest line that the client can read completely and accurately denotes visual acuity (intact cranial nerve II). Each line on either Snellen chart is marked with the number of feet from which a person with normal vision can read that line. The number by the line that the client reads completely and accurately then is compared to the client's distance from the chart, 20 feet. For example, if the client is able to read only the first line, marked 200, the vision in that eye is expressed 20/200. In this instance, the numerator represents the distance of the client from the chart, and the denominator represents the distance at which a normal eye can read the line. Normal vision is expressed as 20/20. In the adult, abnormal visual acuity is anything less than 20/20 vision. This may indicate myopia and requires referral to an ophthalmologist.

Testing for Near Vision. Near vision may be assessed using the Jaeger Chart or newsprint held 14 inches from the client. A client who wears corrective lenses for reading should wear them during the test. If the client is unable to read the words, the test device is moved to a readable distance either closer or farther away. Near vision is expressed by comparing the distance in inches at which the chart can be read by a person with normal vision—14 inches (intact cranial nerve II).

Loss of near vision, or hyperopia, often is associated with aging. Since hyperopia may be confused with presbyopia (degenerative lens changes with decreased ability to focus), the client should be referred to an ophthalmologist. Hyperopia is treated with corrective lenses, whereas presbyopia is treated with magnifying lenses.

Testing for Color Vision. Testing for color vision is not usually done in a routine physical examination. If the client reports some difficulty with color

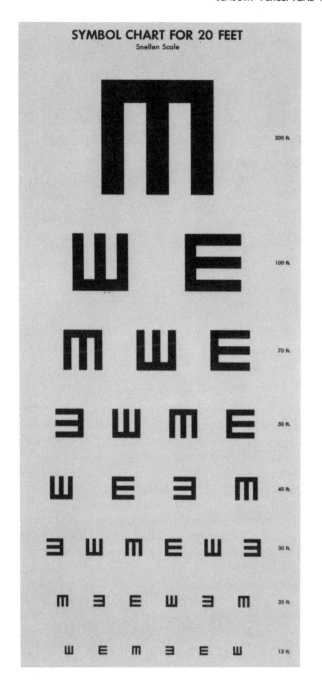

FIGURE 15-3. Snellen "E" Symbol Chart for 20 Feet. (*Note.* Reprinted with permission, National Society to Prevent Blindness, New York City.)

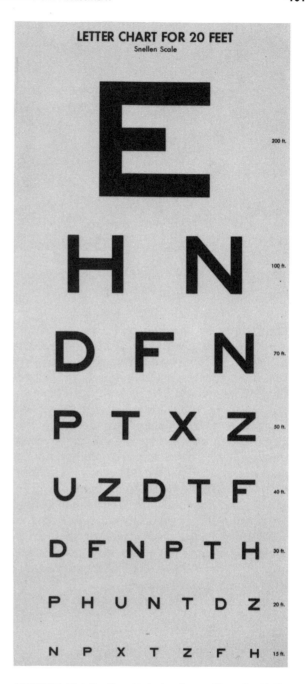

FIGURE 15-4. Snellen Alphabet Letter Chart for 20 Feet. (*Note.* Reprinted with permission, National Society to Prevent Blindness, New York City.)

perception, the nurse can screen for color vision by asking the client to distinguish the primary colors. When there is a need to test for color vision, the *Ishihara Plates* or similar pseudoisochromatic plates can be used (see chap. 22). Color deficits are not correctable, but awareness of the deficiency is important, as it may influence driver education and career choices.

Testing for Peripheral Vision. The test for peripheral vision or visual fields begins with the client and the nurse facing one another, at the same eye level, approximately two feet apart (Figure 15-5). The client covers one eye with the cover card in the same manner described for far vision testing. The opposite eye of the nurse is covered, and each participant focuses directly on the other's open eye.

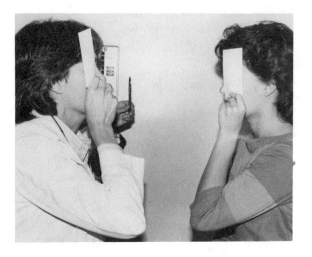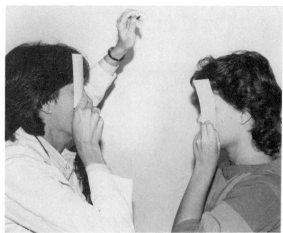

FIGURE 15-5. Assessment of Peripheral Vision.

The four peripheries of each eye—temporal, nasal, upward, and downward—are tested. The nurse tests temporal vision by holding an object (penlight) with arm extended laterally and positioned midway between them. The object is slowly moved inward until the client indicates it is seen. The nurse then records peripheral vision by approximating the angle between the straight line of vision and the point where the object is seen. In a similar manner the nasal, upward, and downward peripheries are checked and recorded for both eyes. The nurse is assumed to have normal peripheral vision, as this confrontation method uses the nurse as the norm. Both client and nurse therefore should see the object at approximately the same point. Normal findings would document that the client's visual fields approximate examiner's. Testing of peripheral vision further tests the function of cranial nerve II.

In an alternative and somewhat more exact method, the nurse records peripheral vision by approximating the angle between the straight line of vision and the point at which a test object (penlight) is seen. Another object is positioned directly in front of the client, who is asked to focus one eye on it while covering the other. The nurse slowly moves the test object into the client's line of peripheral vision. Again, each periphery and each eye is measured separately. The client must continuously focus straight ahead and must not move the uncovered eye toward the test object, thus invalidating the results.

Either test may be used with a cooperative client 3 years of age or older. Normal peripheral vision is:

Temporal—90°
Nasal—60°
Upward—50°
Downward—70°

Decreased perception in all visual fields may be a symptom of glaucoma, and the client should be further tested with tonometry (see below). Lesions of the optic nerve and tract produce variations in visual field loss depending on the position of the lesion. A lesion in the optic chiasm produces bitemporal hemianopsia (loss of temporal vision). A lesion in either optic tract produces homonymous hemianopsia (loss of the corresponding half of the visual field in each eye) (Figure 15-6). A lesion in the right tract produces left homonymous hemianopsia, whereas a lesion in the left tract produces right hemianopsia. Symptoms associated with this loss, such as clumsiness due to inability to see objects in the lost visual field, may be mistaken as signs of other neurological disorders.

Testing of Extraocular Movements. The six cardinal fields of gaze are shown in Figure 15-7. Extraocular movements (evaluation of cranial nerves III, IV, VI) may be tested by having the client follow the nurse's finger, or penlight, through the six fields (Figure 15-8). Both eyes should move through each field smoothly and in unison. Minimal nystagmus may occur if the temporal position is held for too long. Inability to move both eyes simultaneously, in a coordinated and parallel fashion, through any of the six cardinal fields of gaze may indicate paralytic or nonparalytic cranial nerve damage. Sustained nystagmus is abnormal,

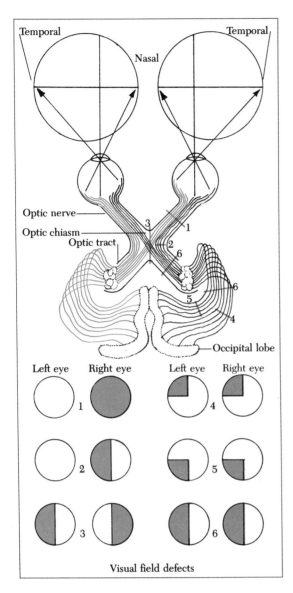

FIGURE 15-6. Lesions of the Optic Tract and Resultant Visual Field Defects. (*Note.* From Grimes/Burns: *Health Assessment in Nursing Practice,* Second Edition, © 1987. Boston: Jones and Bartlett Publishers, p. 356.)

indicating the possibility of neurological damage, and the client must be referred to an ophthalmologist for further testing.

Testing for Strabismus (Cover–Uncover Test). To test for strabismus, the client is asked to stare straight ahead at a near or distant object while the nurse covers one of the client's eyes with a cover card. The uncovered eye must be closely watched for movement. When the cover is removed, the previously covered eye is observed for any movement. This procedure is repeated for the opposite eye. No movement should be noted in either eye.

Testing of Pupil Response. To evaluate direct and consensual pupil response the client is seated in a partially darkened room and instructed to stare straight ahead at a fixed point. While observing the left eye, the nurse brings the lighted penlight from the temporal region inward until it shines directly on the pupil. The illuminated, dilated pupil should constrict in direct response. This procedure is repeated while the right eye is observed. It should constrict in consensual response to illumination of the left eye. The identical procedure is used to test the right eye. Normal pupils are equal in size and ability to constrict in response to light (intact cranial nerve III). Referral is necessary if the pupils are unequal in size and reaction to light, although this may be a normal variant in the absence of any other abnormal neurological signs. Bilateral, fixed, pinpoint pupils in a client not using miotics may indicate presence of central nervous system depressant drugs such as morphine or heroin. In a comatose client, it may indicate hemorrhage in the pons. Small, irregular, fixed pupils may be diagnostic of central nervous system syphilis. Bilateral, fixed, dilated pupils in a client not using mydriatic drugs can be caused by anticholinergics and certain other drugs, including glutethimide poisoning. In a comatose client, this condition is diagnostic of severe brain damage and cerebral anoxia.

Nonresponse to direct light stimulation in an eye that responds normally to consensual stimulus indicates that the eye tested for direct response is blind but oculomotor and optic nerves are intact in both eyes.

Testing the Corneal Reflex. The client should be asked to remove corrective lenses, including contact lenses, before this test begins. The client then is asked to face forward, keep both eyes open, and look upward. The nurse lightly touches the cornea of one eye with a wisp of cotton. Both eyes should blink in response. The opposite eye is tested in an identical manner. Absence of the corneal reflex is diagnostic of damage to cranial nerve V.

Testing the Corneal Light Reflex. The client should stare straight ahead with both eyes open. The penlight is held a short distance from the client's face, at the midline so that the light shines on both corneas (Figure 15-9). The light reflection should appear symmetrical in both eyes. Asymmetry of the corneal light reflex indicates extraocular muscle weakness, and the client should be further evaluated.

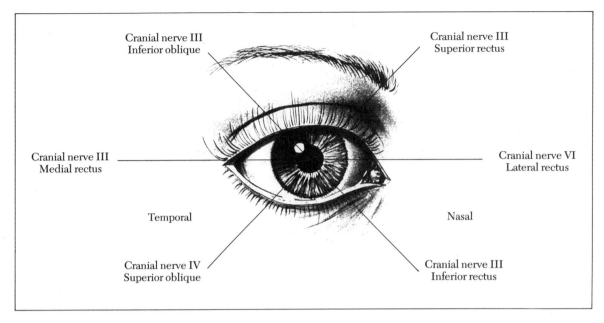

FIGURE 15-7. Six Cardinal Fields of Gaze and Corresponding Cranial Nerves.

Testing for Accommodation. With the client staring straight ahead at a fixed point, an object such as a penlight is held about 4 inches in front of the client's face at the midline. While the nurse closely observes the client's eyes, the client is asked to refocus on the near object. The eyes should converge and the pupils constrict symmetrically as they refocus (intact cranial nerve III).

Inability of the eyes to accommodate is symptomatic of degeneration of the optic lens. As a result the eyes do not converge symmetrically nor do the pupils constrict, and the ability to focus on near objects is lost.

Testing for the Red Reflex. The "red eyes" often noticed in snapshots taken with flashbulbs are caused by the so-called red reflex, which is best elicited in a darkened room. After the client has removed glasses or contact lenses, if any, the ophthalmoscope is set at zero diopters. While looking through the lens of the ophthalmoscope, the nurse directs the light into one of the client's pupils. A flash of red should be visible in the pupil tested. Absence of the red reflex is diagnostic of cataracts, a common occurrence in elderly clients. Another condition in which the red reflex is diminished is pterygium (thickening of the bulbar conjunctiva that may cover the cornea).

Tonometry. Tonometry is a means of measuring intraocular pressure that is used to screen for glaucoma. Although tonometry is not a routine component of the nursing assessment, the nurse should be aware of the importance of tonometry as a routine visual screening measure after age 40. Normal intraocular pressure is 12 to 22 mm Hg. An intraocular pressure greater than 25 to 35 mm Hg may be indicative of glaucoma.

Examination for glaucoma should be included as part of the routine visual clinical appraisal after age 40.

Ophthalmoscopic Examination. Examination of the internal eye structures (CN II) enables the nurse to screen for health problems and refer clients for further evaluation when appropriate.

Using the ophthalmoscope (see chap. 3) the nurse inspects the internal eye, noting:

- red reflex
- color and clarity of the optic disc
- arterioles and veins, particularly arteriovenous crossings
- condition of the retina
- macular area

The usual findings for a healthy adult would include the presence of the red reflex and a well-delineated optic disk, pale yellow in color (Figure 15-10). The arterioles (small and bright red) and the veins (larger and darker red) are distinct with no narrowing or nicking noted. The retina is diffusely red and may appear darkened in a dark skinned individual.

In addition to the internal structures of the eye, the external structures are inspected as well. These

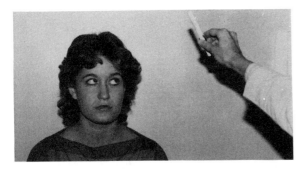

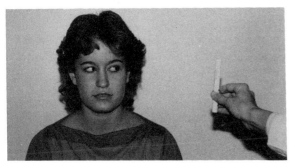

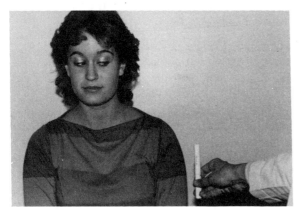

FIGURE 15-8. Assessing Extraocular Muscle Function by Having the Client Follow the Nurse's Finger or Penlight Through the Six Cardinal Fields of Gaze.

structures include the lacrimal apparatus, eyelids, brows and lashes, conjunctiva, sclera, cornea, and iris (see Figures 15-11 and 15-12).

Conducting an ophalmoscopic examination is an advanced skill and requires a great deal of practice. It usually is not part of a routine nursing assessment.

Appraisal of Hearing

There are three major categories of hearing loss: conductive, sensorineural, and central auditory dysfunction. Some individuals may experience loss in more than one category. Conductive losses of sound transmission through bone or air involve defects in the external ear, tympanic membrane, or middle ear. Sensorineural losses involve defects in

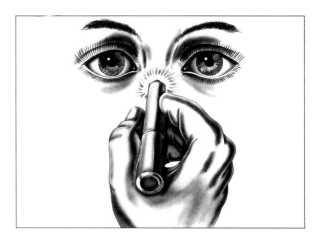

FIGURE 15-9. Corneal Light Reflex Test.

the eighth cranial (acoustic) nerve, inner ear, or central nervous system. Central auditory dysfunctions involve normal hearing ability but a deficit in the ability to process the sounds heard.

The following equipment is needed to grossly assess hearing:

A tuning fork

Two coins

There are some initial gross tests to determine whether an adult has a hearing loss in the speech frequency range. Speaking to the individual in a whisper, a normal tone of voice, and a shout should elicit observable responses at each intensity.

High frequency hearing ability can be tested by several methods, including quickly rubbing the fingers together or clicking two coins near the ear. The individual with normal hearing should be able to correctly acknowledge hearing the sound production equally in both ears. In addition, the nurse should note the distance at which the sound is no longer heard. Sensorineural losses are often in the high frequency range and are the most common hearing loss in the elderly.

Two additional tests use a tuning fork to aid in differentiating between a sensorineural or conductive hearing loss. They do not indicate the severity of the loss, however.

Weber Test. In the Weber test, the stem of a vibrating tuning fork is placed against the skull in the midline or on the center of the forehead (Figure 15-13). If hearing is normal, the sound should be heard equally well in both ears. If the sound is lateralized, or reported "better" in one ear, this may indicate an air conduction loss in that ear. The loss can be detected because the affected ear is not distracted by usual environmental noise. This test

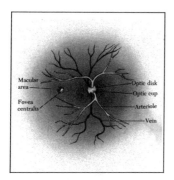

FIGURE 15-10. Retinal Structures.

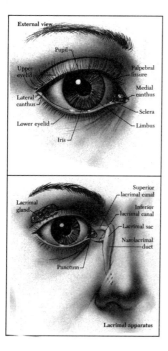

FIGURE 15-11. The External Eye.

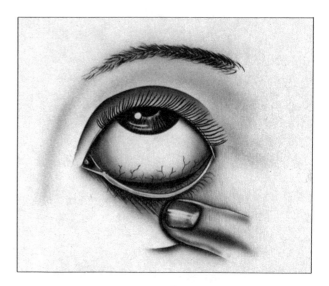

FIGURE 15-12. Inspection of the Sclera and Conjunctiva.

ternal ear, air conduction through the external and middle ear is affected.

Otoscopic Examination. Examination of the auditory canal and tympanic membrane enables the nurse to screen for health problems and refer clients for further evaluation when appropriate.

Using the otoscope (see chap. 3) the nurse examines the auditory canal and the tympanic membrane. The canal is inspected for color, cerumen, discharge, foreign objects, or lesions. The tympanic membrane is evaluated for condition, color, retraction, or bulging. Specific landmarks also are noted. These landmarks are the cone of light, malleus, pars tensa, and pars flaccida (Figure 15-15).

The usual findings for a healthy individual include a clear, smooth canal, pale yellow in color with a small amount of yellow to brown cerumen. The tympanic membrane is intact, semitranslucent and pearly grey in color. No retraction or bulging should be noted. The cone of light and the malleus are distinct.

Performing an otoscopic examination also requires a great deal of practice. Like the ophthalmoscopic examination, it usually is not part of a routine nursing assessment. Whether these examinations are performed by the nurse depends on the client's situation and the knowledge and skill of the nurse in performing these examinations.

In addition to the internal structures of the ear, the external structure, the auricle, is inspected. Examine the auricle for color, shape, lesions, or discharge. Palpate the auricle for tenderness or nodules. Then, palpate the mastoid process for tenderness (Figure 15-16).

may also detect a sensorineural hearing loss, since damage to the inner ear or nerve will result in diminished ability to detect vibrations from the bone. The client would continue to report lateralization of sound to the "better" ear, but in this case, loss is in the opposite ear.

Rinne Test. The Rinne test consists of holding the stem of a vibrating tuning fork against the mastoid process until the client no longer hears the sound (Figure 15-14). The fork then is repositioned near to but not touching the external ear. Since the tuning fork will still be vibrating, the client with normal hearing is expected to report hearing the sound. This procedure is repeated to assess the opposite ear. If the client indicates that the vibrating tuning fork is not heard when placed near the ex-

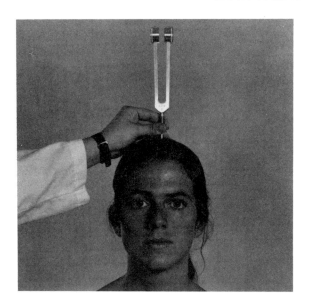

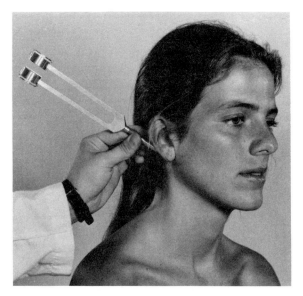

FIGURE 15-13. The Weber Test. (*Note.* From Grimes/ Burns: *Health Assessment in Nursing Practice,* Second Edition, © 1987. Boston: Jones and Bartlett Publishers, p. 215.)

The usual findings for a healthy individual include a smooth auricle varying in color (pink, tan, brown). No deformities, lesions, discharge, or tenderness should be noted.

Appraisal of Touch

The following equipment is needed to assess the sense of touch:

A wisp of cotton

Several sterile hypodermic needles

Two test tubes; the first containing hot water and the second cold water

A tuning fork

A familiar object such as a coin, button, or paper clip

A two-pronged compass

Assessment of sensory function evaluates a number of primary and secondary sensory modalities (see boxed insert, p. 468). Touch may be classified as primary and secondary sensations. *Primary sensations* involve basic identification of the stimulus. *Secondary sensations* coordinate the stimulus reception with cerebral interpretation. Table 15-4 identifies the sensations to be tested, appropriate techniques, and normal and abnormal responses.

This examination is performed to determine the intactness of the sensory nerve fibers, or dermatomes, and the peripheral nervous system. The examination is done bilaterally to compare re-

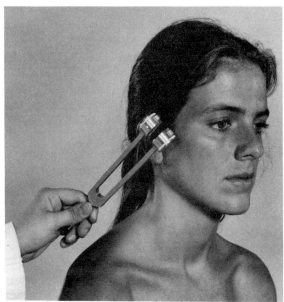

FIGURE 15-14. The Rinne Test. (*Note.* From Grimes/ Burns: *Health Assessment in Nursing Practice,* Second Edition, © 1987. Boston: Jones and Bartlett Publishers, p. 215.)

sponses in contralateral areas. A minimal exam must include one site on each side of the forehead; each cheek; both hands, lower arms, and feet; both legs, and both sides of the abdomen. If light touch and pain are normal, temperature need not be tested. All tests are done with the client's eyes closed. Areas are first tested distally, then proximally (e.g., the foot before the leg), since most abnormalities are first noted in distal areas. However, in testing for proprioception (joint motion sense and position) it is not necessary to test position sense of proximal joints if position sense is intact in

Sensory Function

- Light Touch
  Perception of sensation
- Pain
  Superficial
    Ability to distinguish sharp and dull
  Deep
    Perception of pain
- Temperature
    Ability to differentiate heat and cold
- Position Sense (proprioception)
  Perception of direction of movement
- Vibration
  Ability to identify presence of vibration
- Discriminative Sensations
  Ability to identify objects, numbers and simultaneous stimulation

the distal joints. With organic lesions, position sense is always lacking distally.

Complete dermatome and peripheral nerve (Figures 15-17 and 15-18) testing need not be done unless abnormalities are found on gross screening. Complete dermatome testing is done by performing the complete touch appraisal for each specific dermatome. Peripheral nerves are tested in a like manner.

A clinical appraisal of the special senses evaluates all the cranial nerves with the exception of the motor components of cranial nerves V, VII, X, XI, and XII, and the motor and some sensory compo-

nents of IX (see boxed insert). Assessing these remaining aspects can be done easily following the clinical appraisal of the special senses.

The strength of the temporal and masseter muscles (CN V) can be evaluated by palpating these muscles (the muscles of mastication) as the jaw is clenched. This technique will assist in determining any muscle paresis or paralysis. The nurse also may assess muscle strength by asking the client to open his or her mouth while the nurse exerts resistance (nurse's hand under the lower jaw).

The motor component of CN V can be evaluated by having the client assume a number of facial expressions. Asking the client to smile, frown, raise eyebrows, puff out cheeks, and close eyelids tightly tests the strength of the facial muscles.

The muscles for phonation and swallowing (CN IX) and the movement of the palate, larynx, and pharynx (CN X) are tested together because they are closely related anatomically and functionally. Lightly touching both sides of the pharynx will determine the presence of sensation and the gag reflex. Asking the client to say "ah" should result in the symmetrical rising of the uvula in the midline.

To evaluate the function of the spinal accessory nerve, the nurse asks the client to shrug the shoulders against the nurse's hands (applied resistance). This technique assesses the strength of the trapezius muscle. The nurse also asks the client to turn the head from side to side against applied resistance and to flex the head against the resistance of the nurse's hand on the client's forehead. These maneuvers test the strength of the sternocleido-

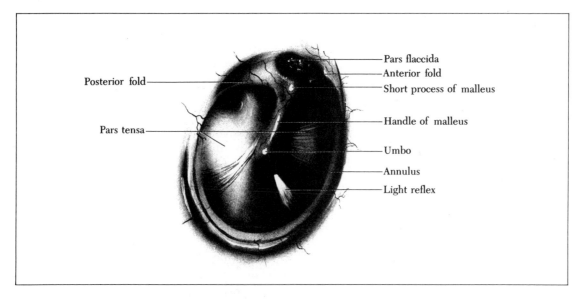

FIGURE 15-15. Diagram of the Right Eardrum.

Cranial Nerves

I — Olfactory: Sensory—smell

II — Optic; Sensory—visual acuity, peripheral vision, funduscopic evaluation

III — Oculomotor: Motor—most extraocular movement, pupillary constriction, accommodation, lid elevation

IV — Trochlear: Motor—inward and downward eye movement

V — Trigeminal: Sensory—facial sensation (pain, light touch); Motor—strength of temporal and masseter muscle corneal reflex

VI — Abducens: Motor—lateral eye movement

VII — Facial: Motor—facial muscle strength (smile, frown, raise eyebrows, puff cheek, lid closure); Sensory—taste on anterior two-thirds of tongue, sensation to pharynx

VIII — Acoustic: Sensory—auditory acuity and position in space (balance)

IX — Glossopharyngeal: Sensory—taste in posterior one-third of tongue, gag reflex, sensation of nasopharynx; Motor—voluntary muscles for phonation and swallowing

X — Vagus: Sensory—larynx and pharynx; Motor—movement of palate, pharynx and larynx

XI — Spinal accessory: Motor—tone and strength of trapezius and sternocleidomastoid muscles

XII — Hypoglossal: Motor—strength and movement of tongue for phonation and swallowing

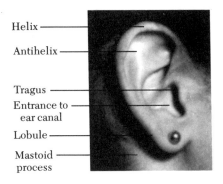

FIGURE 15-16. Inspection of the Auricle and Palpation of the Mastoid Process.

mastoid muscle and complete the evaluation of CN XI.

Movement of the tongue is tested by asking the client to stick the tongue out and then move the tongue from side to side in the mouth. The strength of the tongue is evaluated by having the client push the tongue against the sides of the mouth while the nurse applies resistance on the outside of the cheek with a finger. Both techniques are used to evaluate CN XII.

Coordination and Balance*

Clinical appraisal of coordination and balance evaluates cerebellar function (see boxed insert). As the client performs the various tests, the nurse should closely observe for any abnormalities in smoothness and rhythm.

Coordination is evaluated in both upper and lower extremities, one limb at a time. The *finger-to-nose test* is performed to assess coordination of upper extremities. For this test, the nurse instructs the client to touch his or her nose and then the nurse's finger. The nurse changes finger position and asks the client to follow the same procedure. Holding a fixed finger position, the nurse asks the client to close the eyes and repeat the procedure.

Test the lower extremities by asking the client to perform the *heel-to-shin test*. This test involves placing the heel of one foot on the knee of the opposite leg and moving it down the shin. This test is done with eyes open and closed. It is normally performed without difficulty.

Another test of coordination is the performance of *rapid alternating movements*. For this test, ask the client to rapidly alternate pronation and supination of both hands. To test the lower extremities, ask the client to tap the toes of both feet on the palms of the nurse's hands (clients seated on the examining table) or on the floor (client seated in a chair).

Assessment of balance is evaluated in several ways. Initially, observe the client's gait. Gait is best assessed by having the client walk barefoot across

---

*Adapted from Grimes/Burns: *Health Assessment in Nursing Practice*, Second Edition, © 1987. Boston: Jones and Bartlett Publishers.

Cerebellar Function

Coordination
   Rapid rhythmic alternating movement
   Accuracy of movement

Balance
   Gait
   Equilibrium

TABLE 15-4
Clinical Appraisal: Touch/Proprioception

Sensation	Technique	Normal Adult Response	Abnormal Response
Primary Sensation			
Light touch	A wisp of cotton is touched to each of the designated areas bilaterally to elicit sensation.	Perceives and identifies the area lightly touched.	Anesthesia, hyperesthesia.
Pain/ temperature			
Superficial	Superficial sharp and dull points tested using a hypodermic needle and its hub. Each area is tested bilaterally for sharp and dull.	Easily and bilaterally distinguishes sharp and dull.	Hypoesthesia, hyperesthesia, paresthesia, anesthesia.
Deep	Achilles tendon or biceps squeezed.	States pain is felt.	
Temperature	Hot or cold temperature is tested bilaterally in all designated areas (if pain tests abnormal).	Easily and bilaterally differentiates heat and cold.	
Vibration	Vibrating tuning fork is applied over bony prominences (ankle or wrist) to elicit sensation.	Easily identifies when vibrations felt and when they stop.	Hypoesthesia, anesthesia.
Kinesthesia/ proprioception			
Position sense	With the client's finger or toe in a neutral position, the examiner gently elevates or depresses the digit to elicit position sense.	Easily distinguishes whether digit is elevated or depressed.	Unable to correctly identify position.
Secondary Sensation			
Graphesthesia	A blunt object is used to draw a number or letter on the client's hand, arm, or back.	Easily identifies number or letter bilaterally.	Unable to identify or identifies incorrectly.
Stereognosis	A familiar object is placed in the client's hand, and after feeling it the client is asked to identify the object (paper clip, button, coin).	Easily, correctly, and bilaterally identifies object.	Unable to identify or identifies incorrectly.
Two-point discrimination	Using a compass or two sharp objects, the examiner touches client simultaneously with both points and asks if one or two points are felt.	Two points can be discriminated at the following separations: ■ fingertips 2.8 mm ■ toes 3–8 mm ■ chest and forearm 40 mm ■ back 40–70 mm	Unable to identify or identifies incorrectly.

the room away from the nurse and back. Note the width of the stance, size, and speed of steps, movement of the extremities, and position of the torso.

Next have the client stand up straight, place feet together, and then close the eyes. When asking the client to perform this test of balance, the nurse should stand nearby to stabilize the client if necessary. A small degree of swaying during this test is normal. *Romberg's sign*, the inability to stand with

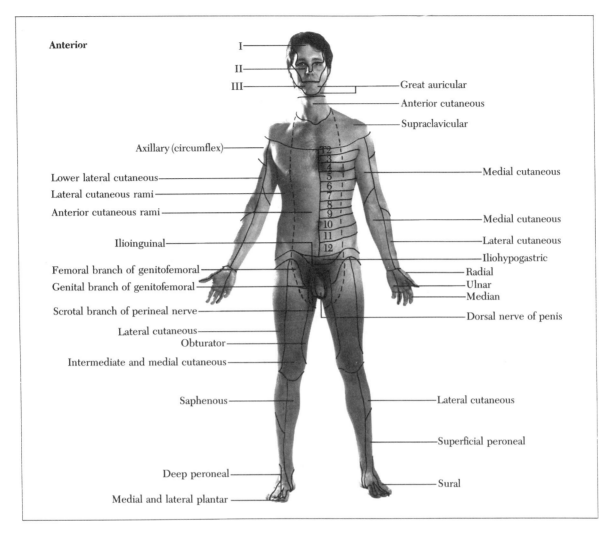

FIGURE 15-17. Dermatomal Areas of the Major Nerves, Anterior View. (*Note.* From Grimes/Burns: *Health Assessment in Nursing Practice,* Second Edition, © 1987. Boston: Jones and Bartlett Publishers, p. 344.)

feet together and eyes closed, may indicate cerebellar disease, among others.

If the client has difficulty with these tests, the nurse can ask the client to perform several additional tests to verify a suspected finding of loss of balance: (1) *tandem walking:* walking in a straight line alternating the placement of the heel of one foot in front of the toe of the opposite foot, (2) *hop on one leg,* then the other, and (3) *deep knee bend,* first on one leg and then the other.

Reflexes*

To elicit and accurately evaluate the neurological reflexes (see boxed insert, p. 472), it is very important for the client's muscles to be relaxed. Stimulus

then is applied evenly to corresponding sides of the client's body and the results compared. Three basic categories of reflexes are considered for assessment purposes: deep tendon reflexes (DTRs), superficial (cutaneous) reflexes, and pathological reflexes. The most common DTRs are presented in Table 15-5. A grading system for tendon reflexes is depicted in Table 15-6. Figure 15-19 provide an example of how the grading system is supplemented for a client with normal tendon reflexes.

The commonly tested superficial reflexes are the abdominal, cremasteric, plantar, and anal (Table 15-7). A pointed object (tongue blade, key, or end of applicator) is used to stroke the skin in order to elicit the abdominal, cremasteric, and plantar reflexes.

Pathological reflexes are documented as being absent or present. They should be absent in healthy adults. The Babinski is normally tested during a routine clinical appraisal because the tech-

---

*Adapted from Grimes/Burns: *Health Assessment in Nursing Practice,* Second Edition, © 1987. Boston: Jones and Bartlett Publishers.

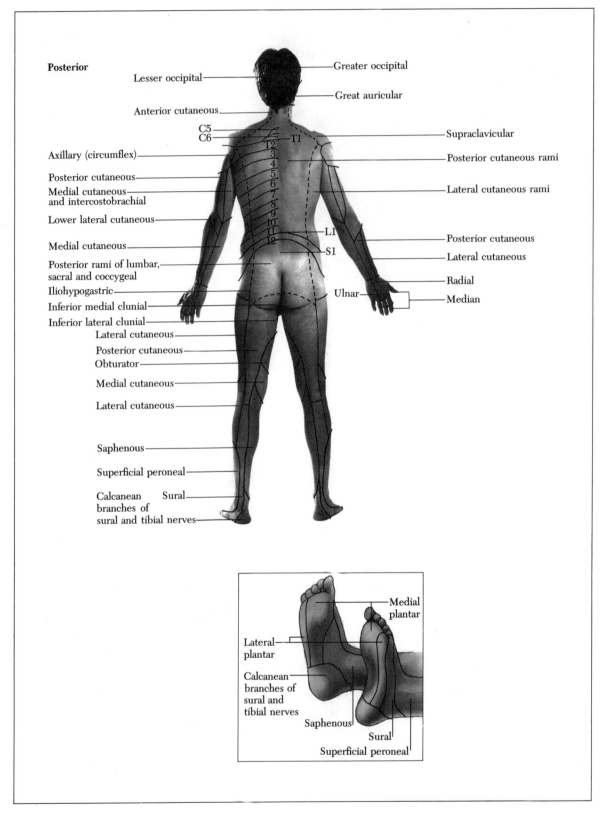

Posterior

Lesser occipital

Anterior cutaneous

C5
C6

Axillary (circumflex)

Posterior cutaneous

Medial cutaneous
and intercostobrachial

Lower lateral cutaneous

Medial cutaneous

Posterior rami of lumbar,
sacral and coccygeal

Iliohypogastric

Inferior medial clunial

Inferior lateral clunial

Lateral cutaneous

Posterior cutaneous

Obturator

Medial cutaneous

Lateral cutaneous

Saphenous

Superficial peroneal

Calcanean   Sural
branches of
sural and tibial nerves

Greater occipital

Great auricular

Supraclavicular

Posterior cutaneous rami

Lateral cutaneous rami

Posterior cutaneous

Lateral cutaneous

Radial

Median

Ulnar

T1
T2
3
4
5
6
7
8
9
10
11
12

L1
S1

Medial
plantar

Lateral
plantar

Calcanean
branches of
sural and
tibial nerves

Saphenous

Sural

Superficial peroneal

FIGURE 15-18. Dermatomal Areas at the Major Nerves, Posterior View. (*Note.* From Grimes/Burns: *Health Assessment in Nursing Practice*, Second Edition, © 1987. Boston: Jones and Bartlett Publishers, p. 345.)

Reflexes and Spinal Segments	
Reflexes	*Spinal segments*
Deep	
Biceps	Cervical 5, 6
Triceps	Cervical 6, 7, 8
Bracioradialis	Cervical 5, 6
Patellar	Lumbar 2, 3, 4
Achilles	Sacral 1, 2
Plantar	Lumbar 4, 5 and Sacral 1, 2
Superficial	
Abdomen	
Upper	Thoracic 7, 8, 9
Lower	Thoracic 10, 11, 12
Cremasteric	Thoracic 12 and Lumbar 1, 2

nique to elicit this reflex or sign is the same as the one used to elicit the plantar reflex. The client with a Babinski reflex would demonstrate extension of the great toe and fanning of the toes. A pathological reflex such as the Babinski is a significant sign of upper motor neuron (cortex) damage. Table 15-8 differentiates between upper and lower motor neuron lesions. The presence of Kernig's sign and Brudzinski's signs (see neurological check) are observed when meningeal irritation is suspected.

The ability to accurately and quickly screen for sensory–perceptual–neurological status is also an important aspect of nursing assessment. A screening exam is useful in a health appraisal of clients of all ages to detect potential problems. The following techniques are included in a screening exam of sensory–perceptual–neurological status (Leslie 1988):

1. Determine mental status (cerebral function)

2. Assess cranial nerves II, III, IV, V, VI and VII (The remaining cranial nerves will be tested during other systems' assessments)

3. Evaluate balance and gait (cerebellar function)

4. Assess wrist, arm and knee extension and flexion (motor function)

5. Assess sensation in both legs and arms (sensory function)

6. Evaluate the following reflexes: biceps, triceps, patellar and Achilles)

Pain

Clients who cannot communicate their pain verbally must be observed for behaviors that may indicate pain. Pain behaviors include crying, restlessness, insomnia, anorexia, rigid body posture or refusal to move, grimacing, and dependent behavior. One method of assessing the specific location of pain in any client is to look for rubbing, splinting, drawing up of the legs to the abdomen, or other gestures that call attention to the painful body part.

In some cases observation may be more reliable than the client's statements about pain, since the client can control the amount of information given to the nurse. Fear of pain from an injection or procedure may be so great that the client refuses to verbally acknowledge any distress. In addition, some clients may expect the nurse to automatically know about the pain they are experiencing. Occasionally, the pain may have lasted so long that the client no longer remembers what it is like to be without pain.

Clients who experience chronic pain develop behavioral adaptations that enable them to continue with daily life. Decreased affect, unwillingness to talk about the pain, and apparent depression are adaptive behaviors and should not be confused with absence of pain.

A number of formal and informal assessment tools may help overcome the reluctance or inability of some clients to accurately relate the pain experience. Two of these tools are Effects of Pain on Daily Life (Table 15-9), and the Pain Ruler (Figure 15-20). These self-rating scales assist in determining the intensity of a client's pain and may also assess the impact of the pain on aspects of daily life. Some scales ask clients to rate their pain on a variety of aspects using the verbal descriptors of "none, mild, moderate" (verbal descriptor scales). Others, like the Pain Ruler, require clients to indicate the intensity of their pain along a line or continuum (visual analogue scale).

The format of the pain assessment tool should be appropriate for the client and the situation. A tool typically used with clients who have chronic pain is the McGill-Melzack Pain Questionnaire (1975). The tool is helpful in assessing the quality and intensity of pain. Administering the tool before and after pain intervention can assist in evaluating the effectiveness of pain relief measures. A client with a low level of literacy may describe the pain more accurately with a visual analogue scale than a verbal description.

Pain itself may indicate an abnormality. The client's description of pain, however, should never be considered abnormal even though the existence of pain may be. Pain assessment is one of the more difficult evaluations, since the client's experience is highly subjective and individualized. At the same time, it is vital that the nurse maintain an objective attitude when performing this assessment.

TABLE 15-5
Deep Tendon Reflexes

Reflex	Percussion Site	Response
Biceps	Biceps tendon	Biceps contraction
		(Place your thumb on tendon cord in midantecubital space with client's elbow flexed. Strike your thumbnail with percussion hammer.)
Triceps	Triceps tendon	Elbow extension; triceps contraction
		(Strike tendon with percussion hammer about 1.5 inches above the olecranon process.)
Brachioradialis	Styloid process of radius	Pronation of forearm and hand
		(Strike tendon about 2 inches above the wrist on the radial [thumb] side of the arm.)
Patellar	Patellar tendon	Knee extension
		(Strike tendon immediately below the patella [knee cap].)
Achilles	Achilles tendon	Plantar flexion of foot
		(Strike heelcord as you gently apply pressure to bottom of foot.)

Note. Adapted from Grimes/Burns: *Health Assessment in Nursing Practice*, Second Edition, © 1987. Boston: Jones and Bartlett Publishers, p. 364.

TABLE 15-6
Grading System for Tendon Reflexes

Grade	Symbols	Interpretation
0	0	Absent (indicate whether reinforcement used)
1	+	Diminished but present
2	+ +	Normal; average
3	+ + +	Normal; brisker than average—may or may not indicate pathology
4	+ + + +	Hyperactive; very brisk—most often pathologic
5	+ + + + +	Hyperactive with clonus

Note. From Grimes/Burns: *Health Assessment in Nursing Practice,* Second Edition, © 1987. Boston: Jones and Bartlett Publishers, p. 365.

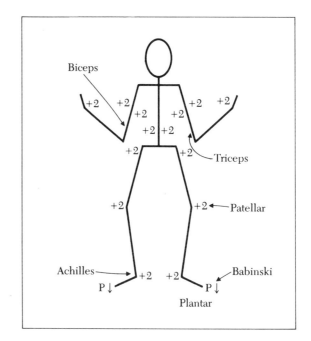

FIGURE 15-19. Normal Reflexes. A similar stick-figure drawing may be used to record findings of assessment of reflexes in the client's health record.

TABLE 15-7
Superficial Reflexes

Reflex	Stimulus site	Response
Abdominal	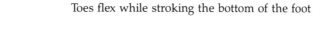	Umbilicus moves toward area briskly stroked
Cremasteric		Scrotum elevates by stroking the inner aspect of each thigh.
Plantar		Toes flex while stroking the bottom of the foot
Anal	Rectal stimulation by gloved finger	Contraction of anal sphincter

Note. Adapted from: Grimes/Burns: *Health Assessment in Nursing Practice,* Second edition, © 1987. Boston: Jones and Bartlett Publishers, p. 366.

TABLE 15-8
Characteristics Associated with Location of Neuron Lesions

Lesion Site	Associated Characteristics
Upper motor neuron	Hyperreflexia
	Contralateral spasticity and atrophy of opposing muscles
	Clonus
	Cogwheel rigidity
	Babinski sign
Lower motor neuron	Hyporeflexia
	Ipsilateral flaccid paralysis and muscle weakness
	Steppage
	Plantar reflex

Note. From Grimes/Burns: *Health Assessment in Nursing Practice,* Second Edition, © 1987. Boston: Jones and Bartlett Publishers.

THE NEUROLOGICAL CHECK

The components of a modified neurological examination, the neurological check, are listed in Table 15-10. This is not a complete neurologic exam, but an abbreviated format that enables the rapid assessment of parameters that provide baseline data on the neurological status of a client. It is used in clinical situations in which the neurological status of a client must be monitored closely. Such situations would include observation of a client with a head injury, loss of consciousness, increased intracranial pressure, central nervous system infection, changes in balance or coordination, spinal trauma, visual disturbances, and personality or mood changes. Subsequent checks provide additional data enabling the nurse to note improvement, deterioration, or stability of the neurological state. The frequency of and specific components included in the check depend upon the nature and severity of the condition and rapidity with which change could occur.

Level of Consciousness

Level of consciousness is assessed several ways. This is done by checking a client's orientation to person, place, and time, state of awareness, and response to painful stimuli.

Orientation to Person, Place, Time

Level of consciousness can be determined by assessing orientation to person, place, and time. When asked, "What is your name?" an adult should be able to state a full name. In response to

TABLE 15-9
Effects of Pain on Daily Life Scale

Sleep
Appetite
Concentration
Work/school
Interpersonal relationships
Marital relations/sex
Home activities
Driving/walking
Leisure activities
Emotional status (mood, irritability, depression, anxiety)

On a scale of 0 (no pain) to 5 (maximum pain) the client should indicate the areas of life currently affected and the severity of the interference. If the client's current level of pain is less than that usually felt, the client should be asked to rate the most pain ever experienced in these areas.

Note. From E. Matassarin-Jacobs, unpublished presentation, "Pain Assessment," Chicago, Illinois, May 1981. Reprinted with permission.

the question, "Where are you?" the client should give an approximate location. An older person may respond "in my bed" or "in my room" as an acceptable answer for orientation to place.

Orientation to time does not require knowledge of the exact time, since clients in health-care settings easily lose track of exact time but still may be oriented. Answers that give the correct year, month, or season are acceptable, as are responses related to daily events, such as meals. Loss usually occurs first in time orientation (e.g., organic brain syndrome, depression, anxiety), then place (e.g., organic brain syndrome, psychiatric disorders), and lastly people (e.g., amnesia, seizures, cerebral trauma). Rather than label a client disoriented, it is more useful to describe the area of loss.

State of Awareness

Assessment of the client's state of awareness is based on observation of behaviors as shown in the definition of terms in Table 15-11. It is more accurate to describe the behavior than to characterize or label it using a single term. What is lethargic to one person may be stuporous to another. Describing the behavior decreases confusion and minimizes error.

The Glasgow Coma Scale was developed to quantify arousability in clients with acute head injuries (Teasdale & Jennett, 1974). The scale is used to evaluate three dimensions of behavioral response: movement, verbalization, and eye open-

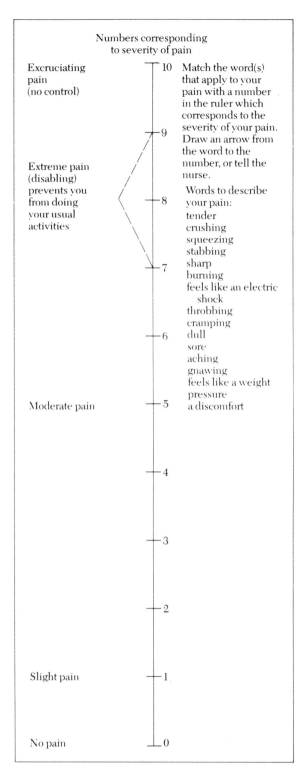

Numbers corresponding
to severity of pain

Excruciating
pain
(no control)

— 10 Match the word(s)
that apply to your
pain with a number
in the ruler which
corresponds to the
severity of your pain.
— 9 Draw an arrow from
the word to the
number, or tell the
nurse.

Extreme pain
(disabling)
prevents you
from doing
your usual
activities

Words to describe
— 8 your pain:
tender
crushing
squeezing
stabbing
— 7 sharp
burning
feels like an electric
shock
throbbing
cramping
— 6 dull
sore
aching
gnawing
feels like a weight
pressure
Moderate pain — 5 a discomfort

— 4

— 3

— 2

Slight pain — 1

No pain — 0

FIGURE 15-20. The Pain Ruler. Clients match the words that describe their pain to a number that corresponds to the intensity of their pain. (*Note.* From Bourbonnais, F. "Pain Assessment: Development of a Tool for the Nurse and the Patient." *Journal of Advanced Nursing,* 6, 280, 1981. Reprinted with permission of Blackwell Scientific Publications Limited.)

TABLE 15-10
The Neurologic Check*

Level of Consciousness
Orientation to person, place, and time
State of awareness
- alert
- lethargic
- stuporous
- unconscious
- comatose
    —decorticate posturing
    —decerebrate posturing
Response to painful stimuli

Eye Movement
Pupil response
- direct
- consensual
Movement/position
- doll's eyes
- sunset eyes
- nystagmus

Coordination/Muscle Tone
Upper extremities
- bilateral hand grasp
Lower extremities
- plantar flexion against resistance

Reflexes
Protective
- corneal
- gag, swallow
Other
- biceps or triceps
- patellar
- Achilles
- plantar

Tests for Meningeal Irritation
Nuchal rigidity
Brudzinski's sign
Kernig's sign

Vital signs

Observations for Associated Symptoms

*Any part(s) may be done at specific frequent intervals based on the client/condition being assessed.

ing. It provides an objective and consistent method for assessing level of consciousness (Table 15-12).

Response to Painful Stimuli

The nurse may note response to painful stimuli according to the terms in Table 15-11 or may simply note its presence or absence. This component of

TABLE 15-11
Descriptive Terms for States of Awareness

Alert: Awake, displays maximum level of consciousness; capable of responding normally.

Lethargic: Diminished level of consciousness, easily awakened, and responsive to minimal stimulation.

Stuporous: Significantly decreased level of consciousness; vigorous stimulation elicits brief, possibly confused response.

Unconscious: Responds only to painful stimuli.

Comatose: Unresponsive, even to painful stimuli.

Decorticate posturing: Usually caused by a lesion in or near cerebral hemisphere. Arms, hands, and fingers adducted and flexed against the palmar surface; legs extended, internally rotated, with plantar flexion of the feet.

Decerebrate posturing: Opisthotonos; extension, adduction, and pronation of arms; flexion of fingers; extension and plantar flexion of the lower extremities, resulting from a severe lesion of pons, midbrain, and diencephalon.

TABLE 15-12
Glasgow Coma Scale Scoring System

Parameter	Observation	Score[a]
Eye opening	Spontaneously	4
	To voice	3
	To pain	2
	None	1
Best verbal response	Oriented	5
	Confused	4
	Inappropriate words	3
	Incomprehensible sounds	2
	None	1
Best motor response	Obeys commands	6
	Localizes	5
	Flexion withdrawal[b]	4
	Abnormal flexion	3
	Abnormal extension	2
	None	1

[a]Maximum score 15 (awake and aware), minimum score 3 (coma).

Note. From Mitchell, P. (1988). Consciousness: An overview. In P. Mitchell, L. Hodges, M. Muwaseves, & C. Wallach (Eds.), *AANN's neuroscience nursing* (p. 64). Norwalk, CT: Appleton-Lange.

the examination is done on unconscious or comatose clients to assess the depth of loss of consciousness. Methods used to induce pain include pinching the Achilles tendon or the biceps muscle. Attempted withdrawal from the painful stimuli, even if unsuccessful, should be considered purposeful.

Eye Movement

The reactivity and size of the pupils, along with the position and movement of the eyes, are carefully evaluated in a neurological check.

Pupil Response

Pupils are checked for size and reactivity to light directly and consensually (see vision exam). Exact measurement of pupil size or reactivity, extreme dilatation or constriction, or inability of pupils to react may be pathological. Metabolic coma does not usually affect pupil size or reactivity.

Movement/Position

The alert client is capable of conscious, deliberate control of eye movement. A phenomenon known as "doll's eyes movement" (oculocephalic reflex) may be seen in a comatose client with an intact brain stem. When the client's head is turned rapidly in one direction, the eyes involuntarily move in the opposite direction, giving the appearance of a fixed gaze in the initial position.

Absence of doll's eyes movement usually is noted in the client with a lesion of the midbrain or pons and indicates damage to the brain stem. In this case, when the client's head is turned, the eyes remain in a fixed position, gazing forward. Nystagmus, or rhythmic involuntary movement of the eyeball, may be observed in the presence of neurological disease.

Coordination/Muscle Tone

The client should be observed for general body position and movement. Abnormal posturing, spasticity, hypotonia, asymmetry of movement, or frequent tremors may be pathological. Coordination and muscle tone may be assessed in several ways. It is important to test bilaterally and simultaneously, if possible, to note any differences in strength or weakness between sides. The adult client who is not comatose should be able to grasp and squeeze the nurse's fingers, lift the legs, or plantar flex the feet against the nurse's hand when asked. Muscle strength and coordination should be equal bilaterally. Plantar flexion of the feet against the nurse's hand should not be included for individuals with increased intracranial pressure. In the unconscious or comatose client, the nurse may assess unilateral paresis or paralysis by simultaneously lifting both arms and releasing them. The arm on the affected side will fall to the bed more rapidly.

Reflexes

The protective corneal and gag reflexes should be checked on unconscious or comatose clients. Absence of these reflexes mandates immediate intervention to prevent corneal drying or occlusion of the airway.

Several reflexes should be tested for both structural intactness and potential upper motor neuron lesions. These reflexes may include triceps or biceps for upper extremities, and patellar, Achilles, and plantar for lower extremities (refer back to Table 15-4).

Absent or diminished reflexes may indicate structural damage within the reflex arc. Hyperreflexia suggests upper motor neuron (corticospinal) lesions, since the inhibitor control from higher centers is interrupted. The Babinski sign or reflex is a significant finding suggesting upper motor neuron lesions. Following a seizure, a client may exhibit a plantar reflex that alternates with a Babinski sign.

Tests for Meningeal Irritation

Signs that may indicate meningeal irritation, such as occur in meningitis, include:

Nuchal rigidity (inability to flex neck, or pain and resistance on passive flexion),

Brudzinski's sign (flexion of hip and/or knees in response to passive neck flexion),

Kernig's sign (pain or resistance upon extension of a flexed knee).

Kernig's sign also occurs with disorders of the spinal cord and spinal nerves.

Vital Signs

Although wide fluctuations in vital signs may occur, certain characteristic patterns are associated with various conditions. It is important to establish a baseline of all vital signs so that changes can be noted and treated as necessary.

Most respiratory abnormalities such as central hyperventilation and apneustic, cluster, and ataxic breathing suggest brain stem involvement. Cheyne-Stokes respirations usually are seen with metabolic, pharmacological, or physiological involvement of the cerebral hemispheres. Fluctuations in body temperature may be observed after injury to the brain, especially that involving the hypothalamus.

NURSING DIAGNOSES RELATED TO SENSORY-PERCEPTUAL-NEUROLOGICAL FUNCTIONING

The information obtained during assessment is extremely important. The nurse analyzes the data to determine whether problems of a sensory-perceptual-neurological nature exist. If problems exist, nursing diagnoses are identified and provide the first step in planning individualized care.

A number of nursing diagnoses related to sensory-perceptual-neurological functioning are listed in Table 15-13. These nursing diagnoses are categorized in the North American Nursing Diagnosis Association's Taxonomy I (NANDA) under several human response patterns. These include *feeling* (pain and chronic pain), *perceiving* (sensory-perceptual alterations), *moving* (impaired swallowing) and *exchanging* (altered tissue perfusion).

The diagnosis of "sensory-perceptual alteration" describes the state in which an individual experiences a change in the patterns or degree of incoming stimuli, accompanied by a diminished, exaggerated, distorted, or impaired response to each stimuli. Alterations in sensory-perceptual status affect an individual's ability to perceive the environment. Alterations of this type commonly occur with aging because the five senses become less efficient with time and interfere with daily activities and overall well-being (Eliopoulos, 1987). Nursing diagnoses that reflect alterations in vision or hearing, taste or touch therefore are frequently identified in an older client population.

TABLE 15-13

Nursing Diagnosis Related to Sensory–Perceptual–Neurological Functioning

Pain related to trauma, chemical irritants, diagnostic tests, or immobility/improper positioning.

Pain, chronic, related to inflammation, pressure points, overactivity, arthritis or stress.

Sensory perceptual alternation: visual, auditory, kinesthetic, gustatory, tactile, olfactory, related to trauma, aging, stress, or environmental factors.

Swallowing, impaired, related to neuromuscular deficit, anesthesia, fatigue, limited awareness, or altered sense of taste.

Tissue perfusion, altered: cerebral, related to trauma, dehydration, sensory-perceptual change associated with aging, medications, or anesthesia.

The history and clinical appraisal of an older adult with sensory–perceptual alterations, in vision, for example, may include the inability to distinguish the fine details of objects within the field of vision, loss of near vision (presbyopia), difficulty driving at night due to problems with glare, difficulty seeing in dimly lit areas and at night (dark and light adaptation), altered color perception, and a decrease in peripheral vision. Older clients can also readily relate the frustrations that accompany changes in vision as well as the concerns for personal safety when vision is impaired. Consequently, self-imposed restrictions on certain activities may become apparent as the older client describes the effect of a sensory–perceptual loss on independence and lifestyle.

A diagnosis of "impaired swallowing," on the other hand, implies a human response pattern involving activity. This diagnosis is used to describe the state in which an individual has difficulty passing fluids and/or solids voluntarily from the mouth to the stomach. The history and clinical appraisal of a client with impaired swallowing could reflect a number of findings. The client may relate either a gradual or fairly sudden decrease in the ability to swallow food or fluids. Dietary modifications, weight loss, and fatigue may also be noted.

Difficulty swallowing may be the result of a neuromuscular impairment such as decreased muscle strength or a mechanical obstruction such as tumor or edema. Fatigue and a general decreased sense of awareness, as observed with Alzheimer's disease, are other factors that can affect a client's ability to swallow.

The diagnoses of "acute pain" and "chronic pain" involve the human response pattern of feeling. Such diagnoses would yield some similar as well as different findings in the nursing history and clinical appraisal. Both types of pain have psychological components, but the anxiety observed with acute pain gives way to the depression characteristically associated with chronic pain. For clients experiencing chronic pain, the pain often becomes a way of life. It is a constant reality that can become part of a client's body image and perception of self.

Pain behaviors are usually more apparent with acute pain than with chronic pain. However, the absence of pain behaviors should in no way minimize the pain experience of the client. The ways in which clients manage pain or other sensory–perceptual–neurological deficits will cue the nurse to such aspects as coping abilities, support systems, and personal resourcefulness. This information is valuable in the development of nursing interventions that capitalize on the client's personal strengths and assets.

Chapter Highlights

■ The integrated functioning of the sensory–perceptual–neurological system makes possible the individual's interaction with the environment. Impairments or deficits in this system may, to a lesser or greater degree, interfere with the client's ability to function in society.

■ Components of a sensory–perceptual–neurological assessment include a nursing history and clinical appraisal of the cranial nerves, mental status, coordination and balance, sensory status, muscle tone and strength, and reflexes.

■ Inspection is the primary assessment technique used in evaluating the sensory–perceptual–neurological system.

■ Pain is a sensory–perceptual experience involving reception, interpretation, and response.

■ Assessment of the client with acute or chronic pain should include the client's subjective description of the pain experience as well as the clinical appraisal of objective behavioral manifestations.

■ Developmental and cultural influences on the perception and expression of pain are critical parameters that should be assessed in clients who state they have pain or whose observable behaviors indicate the presence of pain.

■ Data obtained from an assessment of sensory–perceptual–neurological functioning are analyzed to formulate appropriate nursing diagnoses.

Practice Activities

1. Obtain a sensory–perceptual–neurological history from a friend or classmate. Discuss findings.

2. Practice performing a sensory–perceptual–neurological clinical appraisal with the same friend or classmate. Identify findings.

3. Perform a thorough sensory–perceptual–neurological assessment, including history and clinical appraisal, on at least three healthy adults of differing ages. Describe findings. Formulate appropriate nursing diagnoses if indicated.

4. Screen for vision and hearing deficits in a selected population group (e.g., college students, workers in an industrial setting, clients in a senior citizens' facility). What potential vision or hearing deficits did you identify?

5. Perform a thorough assessment on several individuals with varying sensory–perceptual–neurological deficits (e.g., stroke, head injury, blindness,

deafness). Describe findings. What nursing diagnoses are supported?

6. Using one or more selected pain assessment tools, evaluate a client experiencing acute pain and a client experiencing chronic pain. Compare and contrast the pain experience in each case. What cultural variables influenced the clients' pain experience? What nursing diagnoses are supported for each client?

Recommended Readings

Bondestam, E., Hovgren, F., Johansson, F., Jern, S., Herlitz, J., & Holmberg, S. (1987). Pain assessment by patients and nurses in the early phase of acute M.I. *Journal of Advanced Nursing, 12,* 677–682.

Camp, L.D., & O'Sullivan, P. (1987). Comparison of medical, surgical, and oncology patients' descriptions of pain and nurses' documentation of pain assessments. *Journal of Advanced Nursing, 12,* 593–598.

Hahn, K. (1989). Think twice about sensory loss. *Nursing '89, 19*(2), 97–99.

Kaufman, J. (1990). Assessing the 12 cranial nerves. *Nursing '90, 6,* 56–58.

Kim, S. (1980). Pain: Theory, research, and nursing practice. *Advances in Nursing Science, 2,* 43–59.

Olsson, G., & Parker, G. (1987). A model approach to pain assessment. *Nursing '87, 5,* 52–57.

Reimer, J. (1989). Head injured patients: How to detect early signs of trouble. *Nursing '89, 19*(3), 34–41.

Reizian, A., & Meleis, A.I. (1986). Arab-Americans' perceptions of and responses to pain. *Critical Care Nurse, 6*(6), 30–37.

Stevens, S.A. (1988). A simple, step-by-step approach to neurologic assessment, part 1. *Nursing '88, 18*(9), 53–61.

Stevens, S.A. (1988). A simple, step-by-step approach to neurologic assessment, part 2. *Nursing '88, 18*(10), 51–58.

Wate-Watson, J.H. (1987). Nurses' knowledge of pain issues: A survey. *Journal of Symptom Management, 2,* 207–211.

References

Copp, L.A. (1974). The spectrum of suffering. *American Journal of Nursing, 74,* 491.

Donovan, M., & Girton, S. (1984). *Cancer care nursing.* Englewood Cliffs, NJ: Prentice Hall.

Eland, J. (1981). Pain. In L. Hart, J. Reese & M. Fearing (Eds.), *Concepts common to acute illness,* (pp. 164–196). St. Louis: Mosby.

Flaherty, B., & Grier, M. (1984). Analgesic medication for elderly people post-surgery. *Nursing Research, 33*(6), 369–372.

Geldard, F. (1972). *The human senses* (2nd ed.). New York: Wiley.

Grimes, J., & Burns, E. (1987). *Health assessment in nursing practice* (2nd ed.). Boston: Jones and Bartlett.

Guyton, A. (1987). *Basic neuroscience: Anatomy and physiology.* Philadelphia: Saunders.

Ignatavicius, D., & Bayne, M. (1991). *Medical-surgical nursing: A nursing process approach.* Philadelphia: Saunders.

Jacox, A. (1977). *Pain: A source book for nurses and other health professionals.* Boston: Little, Brown.

Kim, S. (1980). Pain: Theory, research and nursing practice. *Advances in Nursing Science, 2*(2), 43–59.

Kligman, A., Grove, G., & Balin, A. (1985). Aging of human skin. In C.E. Finch & E.L. Schneider (Eds.), *Handbook of the biology of aging.* New York: Van Nostrand Reinhold.

Leslie, D. (1988). Patient assessment: History taking and physical examination. *Nurse Review* (Vol. 1). Bethlehem Pike, PA: Springhouse.

McCaffery, M. (1979). *Nursing management of the patient with pain.* Philadelphia: Lippincott.

Melzack, R., & Wall, P. (1965). Pain mechanisms: A new theory. *Science, 150,* 971.

Melzack, R. (1975). The McGill Pain Questionnaire: Major properties and scoring methods. *Pain, 1,* 272–281.

Metcalf, J. (1988). Sensation: An overview. In P. Mitchell, L. Hodges, M. Muwaswes, & C. Wallach, (Eds.), *AANN's neuroscience nursing* (pp. 359–372). Norwalk, CT: Appleton-Lange.

Miller, C. (1990). *Nursing care of older adults.* Glenview, IL: Scott, Foresman.

Peele, T. (1977). The neuroanatomic basis for clinical neurology (3rd ed.). New York: McGraw-Hill.

Sternback, R.H. (1968). *Pain: A psychological analysis.* New York: Academic Press.

Stevens, S., & Becker, K. (1988). A simple, step-by-step approach to neurological assessment, Part 2. *Nursing, 18*(10), 51–58.

Teasdale, G., & Jennett, B. (1974). Assessment of coma and impaired consciousness: A practice scale. *Lancet, 2,* 81.

16

Activity–Sleep Assessment

OBJECTIVES

Upon completion of this chapter, you should be able to:

◼ Recognize the importance of normal activity–sleep patterns for physiological and psychological well-being.

◼ Discuss the concept of mobility.

◼ Discuss the health effects of activity and sleep.

◼ Describe the effects of inactivity and sleep deprivation on health.

◼ Recognize normal changes in activity–sleep patterns throughout the life cycle.

◼ Collect appropriate subjective and objective data related to activity–sleep patterns.

◼ Individualize the activity–sleep assessment according to age, culture, and health.

◼ Recognize common deviations from normal activity–sleep patterns.

◼ Perform and record an activity–sleep assessment, including history and clinical appraisal.

◼ Develop valid and appropriate nursing diagnoses for clients with alterations in activity–sleep.

There are probably no factors more closely linked to an individual's overall sense of well-being than the ability to move about freely and with purpose, to engage in those activities that are meaningful, and to obtain adequate rest or sleep. Often, clients first recognize and acknowledge that they have a health problem when they begin to have difficulty carrying out their usual daily activities. In fact, alterations in the client's normal patterns of activity and sleep can provide some of the earliest cues that a health problem exists.

People require a balance of activity and sleep to maintain both physiological and psychological well-being. The relative amounts of time needed to maintain this balance vary as an individual grows from infancy to adulthood. Once adulthood is reached, the activity–sleep balance remains relatively constant, with only gradual changes in patterns as the person moves into the later years. Assisting clients to maintain a balance between activity and sleep is based on a thorough understanding of the functions served by the sleep–activity cycle.

KNOWLEDGE NEEDED TO ASSESS ACTIVITY–SLEEP

All individuals need regular physical activity to maintain optimal health. To engage in activity, one needs mobility and an environment that supports activity.

Mobility

Mobility is an extremely complex process that has physiological, psychological, and environmental components (Hollerbach, 1988). Any assessment of mobility must, therefore, consider each of these dimensions.

According to Hodges and Callihan (1988), three elements are essential for mobility. These are "the ability to move (an intact neuromuscular system or compensated movement), the motivation to move, and a free, nonrestrictive environment in which to move" (p. 270). The ability to move refers to the physical dimension of mobility. A number of anatomic elements are necessary for movement to occur. These elements are "the muscles, themselves, their afferent and efferent innervations and the segmental spinal cord connections made by these peripheral nerve fibers" (Hodges & Callihan, 1988, p. 270). Also necessary are the descending motor tracts within the spinal cord. These tracts carry messages from higher brain centers, which influence muscle activity at the segmental level of the spinal cord. The higher centers of the central nervous system involved in the regulation of motor activity include the cerebellum, the basal ganglia, certain brainstem nuclei, and the cerebral cortex (Barr & Keirnan, 1983). Thus, the ability to move is the result of voluntary and automatic coordinated musculoskeletal activity. The musculoskeletal system provides the "structure, support, stability, and protection for movement, and the central nervous system provides the necessary neural innervation" (Hollerbach, 1988, p. 283).

The psychosocial dimension of mobility refers to the motivation to move, to be active, to engage in interactions with others, and to cope with the environment. The ease with which one interacts and copes depends on a number of factors. Each of the following factors should be evaluated carefully when assessing the psychosocial aspects of mobility: "self-perception and self-concept patterns, individual strengths and weaknesses, coping patterns (including independency and dependency needs), available support systems, and emotional and social adjustment" (Hollerbach, 1988, p. 297). The reader is referred to Chapter 12 for a discussion of these aspects. This dimension of mobility is important to an individual's self-image and self-esteem. An individual's self-perception as "healthy" or "sick" often is based on the ability to maintain normal mobility. Motor activity also provides individuals with a means of self-expression and a socially acceptable outlet for aggression and tension. Motor activity is a primary means of expressing emotion, particularly in children, who may show their anger or frustration by hitting or running away. In the adult, selected physical activities, such as running or other forms of vigorous exercise, can provide a way to relieve tension that might otherwise be internalized or manifested in ways that could be harmful to the individual or others, such as drinking or drug use.

The third aspect for consideration is the environmental dimension of mobility. The environment can greatly influence an individual's ability to get around. Older adults who experience age-related changes in vision and hearing may voluntarily limit their mobility out of concern for personal safety. The individual recovering from a total hip replacement will have to adjust if there are stairs at home. To the young child beginning to walk, the home is a new and wonderful world for exploration, but the child lacks the judgment to avoid potentially dangerous obstacles.

Environmental dimensions that should be considered in evaluating an individual's mobility include such aspects as physical barriers or obstacles (both at work and at home), assistive devices, safety factors (including the influence of sensory deficits, mental status, and developmental level), available support systems, financial resources, and community resources (Hollerbach, 1988). The reader is referred to Chapter 9 for a discussion of these aspects.

For an individual to be mobile, all three elements must be present. Movement or mobility would be altered if there were a dysfunction in one of the elements (Hodges & Callihan, 1988). The concept of mobility is basic to any discussion of physical activity, exercise, or physical fitness. Approaching the concept of mobility from a physiological, psychosocial, and environmental perspective offers the nurse a more comprehensive framework within which to evaluate needs and ultimately plan care.

Health Effects of Activity

Regular physical activity is necessary for good health and longevity. In an extensive study of physical activity and longevity, Rose and Cohen (1977) examined 69 factors in lifestyle and characteristics predictive of longevity. In order of decreasing importance, the top factors were: 1) fewer illnesses, 2) younger age appearance at age 40, 3) less smoking, 4) less worry, 5) rural residence, 6) sense of humor, 7) higher occupational level, 8) leisure activity, and 9) physical exercise.

National goals as specified in *Healthy People 2000* place greater emphasis on decreasing inactivity and increasing light to moderate activity (Department of Health and Human Services, Public Health Service, 1990). This report indicates that few Americans are engaged in regular physical activity. The following statistics are offered:

> Currently, only 22% of adults are engaged in at least 30 minutes of light to moderate physical activity 5 or more times a week and only 12% report that they are this active 7 days a week. Less than 10% of the population exercises 3 or more times a week at the more vigorous level to improve cardiorespiratory fitness. Nearly 25% of adults report no leisure-time physical activity, and the prevalence of sedentary behavior increases with advancing age. (p. 55)

According to Caspersen, Powell, and Christenson (1985), "physical activity," "exercise," and "physical fitness" describe different concepts. The terms frequently are confused and often used interchangeably. Physical activity is a broad concept. It refers to bodily movement produced by skeletal muscles that results in the expenditure of energy. Energy expenditure is measured in kilocalories (Kcal). All individuals perform physical activities in order to maintain life. The types of physical activity in which an individual engages are varied. Occupational, household, leisure, sleep, sports, conditioning, and other activities reflect the broad scope performed in daily life. The therapeutic value of physical activity on morale and self-esteem was demonstrated in a nursing study of institutionalized elderly (Goldberg & Fitzpatrick, 1980). Through the intervention of a movement therapy group (use of motion and language to meet therapeutic goals), the experimental subjects exhibited higher morale and more positive attitudes toward their own aging. Similarly, *Walking to Better Health* was the goal of a structured nursing program for improving the quality of life for residents of a skilled geriatric facility (Warner, 1988). Clients in this pilot project demonstrated increased motivation, renewed interest in their environment, increased physical activity, flexibility, alertness, and improved appetite as a result of walking.

"Exercise is a subset of physical activity that is planned, structured, and repetitive and has as a final or an intermediate objective the improvement or maintenance of physical fitness" (Caspersen et al., 1985, p. 126). The benefits of regular physical endurance exercise are well-documented in the literature (see Table 16-1). The normal activities of daily living (with the exception of sleep) also may be considered exercise if they are labor-producing rather than labor-saving in the ways in which they are performed. For physical exercise to have a positive impact on reducing an individual's risk of disease and improving the quality of one's life, it must, ideally, be initiated early in life and maintained as a lifelong habit (Dawber, 1973).

Physical fitness, on the other hand, is a set of attributes or characteristics that people exhibit or work to achieve. Individuals who are physically fit tend to differ from those not physically fit in such aspects as muscular strength and endurance, flexibility, cardiorespiratory endurance, speed, reaction time, and agility. An individual's degree of physical fitness can be measured with specific tests, such as the skinfold pinch test, which measures body composition, the sit-and-reach test, which measures flexibility, and the step test, which measures cardiorespiratory endurance.

Health Effects of Inactivity

Individuals increase their risk for serious health problems when they choose inactive lifestyles or are forced to inactivity by injury or illness. A lack of activity produces systemic and functional effects. No body system is spared from the effects of im-

TABLE 16-1
Benefits of Regular Physical Endurance Exercise

Musculoskeletal Effects
Increased physical work capacity
Improved muscle endurance and
   vigor
Improved agility
Increased flexibility
Increased muscle tone and
   strength
Increased development/mainte-
   nance of bone tissue
Increased strength of connective
   tissue
Increased coordination
Increased lean muscle mass
Increased thickness and mass of
   bone with weight-bearing
   activity

Metabolic Effects
Increased levels of high-density
   lipoproteins (including HDL-
   cholesterol)
Increased glucose use
Increased thyroid function
Increased growth hormone pro-
   duction
Increased tolerance to stress
Decreased chronic catecholamine
   production
Decreased neurohumoral over-
   response
Decreased percentage of body fat
Decreased serum triglyceride level
Decreased blood glucose

Psychological Effects
Improved appearance
Improved self-image
Improved self-confidence
Increased vitality and energy
Improved sense of well-being
Enhanced intellectual and emo-
   tional–interpersonal behaviors
Decreased anxiety and tension
Decreased depression

**Cardiac–Peripheral Vascular
   Effects**
Increased cardiac output
Increased mechanical efficiency
Increased stroke volume
Improved collateral blood supply
Increased cardiac size
Increased venous return
Increased fibrinolysis
Decreased vulnerability to
   arrhythmias
Decreased resting pulse
Decreased cardiac rate with exer-
   tion
Decreased blood pressure
Decreased venous stasis

Elimination Effects
Increased intestinal tone and motility
Increased efficiency in maintaining
   fluid and acid base balance
Increased efficiency in excretion of
   body wastes

Respiratory Effects
Increased functional capacity
Increased exchange of oxygen and
   carbon dioxide
Increased vital capacity
Increased rate and depth

Integumentary Effects
Increased tissue perfusion
Improved turgor, color, and tone

---

mobility or inactivity. When a client's normal activity patterns are altered, the nurse can anticipate certain physiological, psychological, and developmental effects. The extent of these effects will depend on the client's age, overall health, and the degree and duration of the change. The "hazards of immobility" are extensive (Olson, 1967).

Musculoskeletal Alterations

One of the most obvious physiological changes is the loss of muscle tone (hypotonicity), strength (paresis or paralysis), and mass (muscular atrophy). This occurs when the muscle fibers are not being regularly contracted to at least 20 to 30% of their maximal tension. Muscle strength is extremely important to mobility since endurance or tolerance for exercise is directly proportional to the amount of muscle strength. Muscle strength varies

greatly from individual to individual as well as within the same individual.

Muscle tone can be evaluated by palpating the muscles at rest and during passive and active range of motion. Muscle strength can be assessed by asking the client to push against the nurse's hands while the nurse exerts resistance. Loss of muscle mass can be assessed by periodically measuring the girth of the affected muscle body; the assessment is discussed later in this chapter.

Another common physiological change is loss of joint mobility, as when a joint is immobilized with a cast or splint. Connective tissue fibers are deposited in the joint capsule and become dense or fibrotic within as few as 5 days of immobility. Fibrosis limits the extent of movement in the joint. This limitation can be assessed by moving the joint through its range of motion; the assessment is discussed later in this chapter.

Contractures also may develop when fibrosis occurs within a muscle and may cause progressive shortening of that muscle. The contracted muscles pull the joint to which they attach into an abnormal position, which can be easily observed.

If the client is unable to bear weight or place muscular tension on the bones, calcium and phosphorus will be released from the bony matrix to dissolve in the blood. Since mineral deposits are responsible for the hardness of bone, release of these minerals will cause osteoporosis. The term "disuse osteoporosis" is used to describe the condition in which bone formation decreases while the breakdown of bone increases due to the lack of weight-bearing activity (Rubin, 1988). This occurs after 2 to 3 days of immobility, as evidenced by increased urinary levels of calcium. Under these conditions, pathological fractures are more common because the bones lack structural firmness.

Renal–Urinary Alterations

Since the mineral content of the urine is increased by the release of calcium and phosphorus from bone, the client is more likely to develop renal stones, especially if the immobilized client is supine. Gravity interferes with the normal flow of urine through the kidney; it collects in stagnant pools (urinary stasis) from which the minerals precipitate to form stones. Urinary stasis is a prime medium for the growth of bacteria leading to urinary tract infections. In addition, urinary retention commonly occurs if the client is unable to assume an upright position, which facilitates emptying of the bladder. As a result, bladder muscle tone decreases, further contributing to the problem of urinary retention. With retention, clients usually void frequently and in amounts of less than 100 ml.

Gastrointestinal Alterations

Immobility causes decreased muscular activity and lowered metabolism. This results in diminished appetite and altered digestion and use of nutrients (Rubin, 1988). Clients with impaired motor function may experience a variety of gastrointestinal complaints, including difficulty expelling flatus, constipation, and possibly fecal impaction. These may occur because clients are unable to assume a position that eases defecation. Also, they may experience weakness or loss of the abdominal and perineal muscle tone needed for defecation.

Skin Alterations

If clients are unable to change positions frequently by themselves or have sensory impairments that prevent them from feeling pressure, they are at increased risk of developing pressure sores, or decubitus ulcers. Pressure sores occur when unrelieved pressure on skin and subcutaneous tissue results in impaired oxygenation and nutrition to the area. Skin that covers bony prominences of the body is especially vulnerable to breakdown. Moist bed linens from client perspiration, coupled with impaired circulation over bony prominences, create an ideal environment for bacteria to grow on the skin, further increasing the risk of skin breakdown (Rubin, 1988).

The body's defense against infection is decreased as a result of bed rest. The breakdown of immunoglobin G (IgG) doubles. IgG comprises 75% of an individual's normal concentration of antibodies (Rubin, 1988). With fewer antibodies, the individual's susceptibility to infection increases. This occurs because muscle inactivity probably prevents the transport of lymph. The body's ability to resist infection is compromised further by a decrease in the ability of the leukocytes to engage in phagocytosis (Rubin, 1988).

Respiratory Alterations

A decrease in muscle strength and tone may result in reduced respiratory excursion and in decreased efficiency of the cough reflex. Therefore, mucus is much more likely to accumulate and pool in dependent portions of the lungs. Incomplete filling of the lungs occurs as all lung volumes (except tidal volume) decrease (Rubin, 1988). Incomplete filling, coupled with the development of mucus plugs, increases the likelihood of atelectasis. If the client is taking narcotics or sedatives, respiratory depth is compromised further. In addition, lack of activity decreases the usual stimulus to breathe deeply.

When the client is supine, gravity causes mucus to pool in dependent areas, while upper surfaces of the airway may become quite dry. In this situation, the cilia do not function adequately, pooling of secretions increases, and risk of infection and obstruction is increased. The supine client has the added pressure of a bed mattress against the posterior chest, which tends to limit chest expansion. In addition, the pressure of abdominal contents on the diaphragm further limits lung expansion.

The nurse should assess the client's respiratory rate and depth and determine the muscles being used for breathing. The character of the client's cough and mucus also should be observed. Auscultation of the client's lung fields is necessary to assess for fluid accumulation in dependent areas of the lungs. (see chap. 17).

Cardiovascular Alterations

Inactivity and bed rest may rest most of the individual's body, but they do not rest the heart. Cardiac output increases when body position changes from standing to supine, because a large portion of the volume of blood in the vessels of the legs is added to the general circulation. Stroke volume and total workload of the heart also increase because of this redistribution of blood.

Other effects of decreased motor function, especially if bed rest is required, are dependent edema, orthostatic hypotension, and increased potential for thrombus formation. Each of these problems is related to changes in the peripheral vascular system that occur with muscular inactivity.

Dependent edema is caused by dilation of the veins in dependent parts of the body, especially the legs, during muscular inactivity. The muscles do not exert their usual pressure, and blood pools in the dilated veins, increasing pressure so that fluid leaks into the interstitial spaces. In addition, a client who is sitting frequently has pressure exerted on the popliteal vessels by the seat of the chair. This pressure interferes with venous return, increases venous pressure, and forces more fluid into the tissues.

Orthostatic hypotension is a drop in blood pressure associated with a change in position from supine to erect. It is thought to occur because of a failure of the body's normal compensatory response to position changes. Normally, a change from lying to standing causes vasoconstriction of splanchnic and peripheral vessels so that blood pressure is maintained. With inactivity, this mechanism is not used and the body's ability to respond rapidly to position changes decreases. Peripheral and splanchnic vessels fail to constrict, blood pools in the viscera and muscles, and the client experiences weakness and dizziness when rising, owing to a drop in blood pressure.

Thrombi are also more likely to develop because of the stasis of blood in the lower extremities associated with muscular inactivity. The nurse should assess for unilateral changes in temperature and girth, redness, and reports of pain in the extremities.

Decreased Tolerance for Exercise

A decrease in exercise tolerance during and after physical inactivity is a function of cardiovascular effects and decreased muscle strength. Thus, clients who are recovering from major illness or surgery, who have been bedridden for prolonged periods for any reason, or who are recuperating from exacerbations of chronic illness may be expected to experience some activity intolerance as they attempt to resume normal functioning. This is especially true of clients who have cardiovascular or respiratory problems.

Activity prescriptions are often vague and do not give the nurse much guidance regarding the amount and type of activity that would be beneficial. Specific decisions about such orders as "activity as tolerated" are left to the nurse's clinical judgment. Those decisions can be more sound if the nurse can predict which clients are likely to experience a disproportionate response to gradually increasing activity levels and can aid in prompt detection of these signs. Typical responses include chest pain, dyspnea, palpitations, heart rate greater than 120 per minute, and a decrease in systolic blood pressure of more than 10 to 15 mm Hg.

These responses can be predicted more accurately (Gordon, 1976) if the nurse considers such factors as:

> Age
> Health (acute or chronic illnesses)
> Height-to-weight ratio
> Nutritional status
> Pre-illness activity level and current level tolerated
> Current emotional and motivational state
> Cardiovascular and respiratory status and stability
> Resting vital signs (especially rate and rhythm of pulse)
> Hemoglobin and hematocrit levels
> Comfort level (pain)

The type of activity (duration and effort required) and the temperature and humidity in the room are also factors in predicting the client's activity tolerance.

While the client is engaged in activity, it is important to periodically assess pulse rate and rhythm, since these give a fairly decent measurement of the status of the critical organs and also can be easily and reliably measured. The pulse should be checked before, during (if activity is prolonged), and immediately following activity. If there is a change, the nurse should measure at 3, 5, and 10 minutes following the activity to determine the length of time required to return to resting level. A normal heart can double or even triple (in rare instances) its rate during strenuous exercise. Generally, a client on complete bed rest or coronary precautions is not permitted to exceed a 20-per-minute increase (approximately 25%) during or immediately following activity. Within 5 minutes after the activity, the pulse rate should return to baseline. If, at baseline, tachycardia is present or cardiac status is unstable, a 25% increase may be contraindicated. The nurse should monitor any changes in rhythm from regular to irregular. Any arrhythmias that occur at rest should be evaluated carefully (apical pulse preferred) before the client initiates activity. Weakening of pulse strength during the activity may indicate that the client's activity tolerance has been exceeded. Of course, the client's normal response to exercise will be altered if the client is receiving beta blockers or other drugs that suppress the heart rate response to activity. Well-conditioned individuals also will show less deviation from normal during exercise.

Changes in blood pressure before, during, and after activity are also helpful in judging the activity tolerance of a client with myocardial pathology, hypertension, or heart failure. A drop in systolic blood pressure of more than 20 mm Hg indicates vascular dilation and decreased stroke volume. Diastolic values should increase only slightly, if at all.

Additional parameters that should be assessed during the activity are changes in skin color or temperature, postural changes, or disturbances in equilibrium. Client reports of dyspnea, fatigue, muscle heaviness, feelings of tightness, and loss of interest in the activity also may indicate decreasing tolerance.

In healthy clients, the average pulse rate during exercise should not exceed 60 to 75% of the predicted maximal heart rate for their age group. The maximum heart rate is calculated by subtracting the client's age from 220.

Sensory-Perceptual Alterations

The client with altered motor ability frequently is subjected to a decrease in environmental stimulation. This deficit may cause the individual to become even less physically active and, if prolonged, tends to produce certain behavioral changes, such as anxiety, egocentricity, difficulty in solving problems, and changes in body image. Clients immobilized (for extended periods of time without adequate sensory stimulation) can experience visual and auditory hallucinations, as well as numbness in the fingers and toes.

Impaired mobility often forces the individual to become somewhat dependent on others to meet basic needs. If the client must be bedridden because of a health problem, the supine position may compound the feelings of dependency. Clients must look up to other people rather than relating to them at similar eye levels.

During periods of immobility, an individual may experience some disruptions in the normal pattern of sleep. Because sensory stimulation is needed to maintain wakefulness, a decrease or absence of sensory stimulation results in difficulty staying awake. Consequently, the individual dozes and naps frequently during the day. When napping occurs in the late afternoon, the individual begins to approximate the nightly sleep cycle. Consequently, when it is time for the individual to go to sleep, sleeplessness prevails.

Hospital environments are also not conducive to sleep. Noise levels, daily and nightly interruptions, unfamiliar surroundings, intercoms, lighting, and the presence of another person (stranger) in the room are only a few of the factors that interfere with an individual's ability to sleep and sleep well.

Fluid-Electrolyte Alterations

The body begins the process of diuresis during the first day of bed rest. The majority of fluid lost is extracellular (approximately 600 ml by the second day of bed rest according to Rubin [1988, p. 51]). Major shifts in blood volume occur with more fluid shifted to the areas of the trunk and head. In the supine position, nasal mucosa swell as a result of the increased blood flow to the head. As a result, individuals on bed rest often complain of nasal congestion.

Initially, sodium and chloride ions are lost after one day of bed rest. The loss of potassium, however, occurs after an extended period of time on bed rest. The effect of prolonged bed rest is one of reducing the ability of the kidneys to excrete sodium, chloride, potassium, and water (Rubin, 1988).

Metabolic-Hormonal Alterations

Limited mobility or bed rest results in a decrease in the body's basal metabolic rate (BMR). Immobility causes catabolic processes (breakdown of body structures for energy production) to increase while anabolic processes (synthesis of body substances for growth) decrease. A state of negative nitrogen balance will occur if the rate of catabolism exceeds anabolism for an extended period of time. A major consequence of a negative nitrogen balance is the lack of an adequate supply of nitrogen for the synthesis of protein. Protein is essential for healing wounds and rebuilding muscle mass.

After 3 days on bed rest, the body's insulin loses its ability to regulate serum glucose levels. This results from a decline in the function of the pancreas (Rubin, 1988). When a client resumes daily activities, the pancreas functions normally within approximately a week. In addition to insulin, other body hormones demonstrate a 24-hour cyclic pattern (e.g., growth hormone, cortisol, epinephrine, aldosterone, and androgen). Research indicates that the cyclic pattern of these hormones also is altered by bed rest.

Developmental Alterations

Immobility can affect developmental changes through the life span. However, for the young and the elderly, the developmental changes associated with immobility are particularly pronounced. Activity is crucial to the development of gross and fine motor skills in children. Activity also provides an important mechanism for social interaction, communication, and meeting basic needs of clients of all ages. When the client is ill, social inactivity as well as physical inactivity frequently result. For the elderly, immobility can accelerate the functional losses in body systems. As a result of declining ability, the older person grows increasingly dependent. Thus, normal physical and psychosocial development may be altered because of changes in the client's health and activity level. In any situation where mobility is limited, the nurse needs to assess the client's developmental level and determine its appropriateness for the client's chronological age. The reader is referred to chapters 10 and 11 for a discussion of developmental aspects. Careful assessment is the basis for selecting strategies to facilitate maintenance of normal development.

Psychosocial Alterations

Prolonged inactivity can force clients to become dependent on others to meet some or all of their basic needs. Adult clients may experience role changes as other family members take on financial or homemaking responsibilities that previously belonged to the client. These changes can diminish the client's self-esteem and may be manifested as depression, lethargy, and insomnia, or hostile, belligerent, or withdrawn behavior. Coping difficulties are very common for both the immobilized individual as well as the individual's family. Information in the chapters on family assessment (7) and psychosocial assessment (12) will assist the nurse in evaluating the psychosocial impact of immobility on the client.

Health Effects of Sleep

Most people spend about one fourth to one third of their lives sleeping. Sleep is needed daily and in prolonged periods to maintain optimal physiological functioning. Without sleep, humans perform poorly, cannot concentrate for prolonged periods, are irritable and restless, and eventually may exhibit bizarre behavior patterns. Not only does an individual need sleep, but it is needed on a daily basis to maintain well-being.

Cyclic Aspects of Sleep

An invisible pattern or order underlies most of what we assume to be constant in ourselves and in the world around us. Life is in a continual state of change, but that change is not chaotic. Although we cannot see or feel them, we are surrounded by rhythms of gravity, electromagnetic fields, light waves, and sound. As the Earth turns on its axis each day, we experience the alternation of light and darkness. In phase with that daily rotation, animals and plants exhibit a pronounced daily rhythm. Often some rhythmic factor, such as light, stimulates diurnal creatures like humans to be wakeful and active. Even when test subjects are isolated from these usual time cues, they exhibit rhythms that do not deviate much from the 24-hour daily period. This daily rhythm is called "circadian," which means "about a day."

Most living organisms, including humans, show a circadian rhythm of activity and rest. Once about every 24 hours, activity is suspended for a prolonged rest. Sleep and waking also act as synchronizers for many internal functions (Kleitman, 1963). When a person lives on a regular routine of daytime work and nighttime sleep, such physiological functions as hormone levels and vital-sign ranges vary in a related rhythm. When this pattern is upset by illness or environmental changes, the body's patterned functioning is altered, and symptoms result. Some of these alterations are discussed later in this chapter.

Just as sleep is a part of our circadian rhythm of behavior, sleep itself is rhythmic. Its striking rhythmicity first was noticed in infants, who were observed to undergo a quiet sleep followed by an active period of sleep with considerable eye movement. Since that time, considerable research has been devoted to the nature of sleep, and much has been learned.

The cyclical nature of sleep is controlled by two regions in the brainstem. These are the reticular activating system (RAS) and the bulbar synchronizing region (BSR). The RAS maintains wakefulness and alertness through stimulation (e.g., physical activity, thought process, sensory input). As stimulation of the RAS declines, sleep ensues. The BSR is involved in the onset of sleep activity, although its function is not clearly understood.

Sleep has been found to consist of a series of cyclic patterns that recur over the sleep period. These cycles vary in length from 45 to 60 minutes in the newborn and 90 to 100 minutes in the adult. The adult pattern is thought to develop by the time a child is 2 to 3 years old. Each cycle has five stages.

■ Stage I NREM (nonrapid eye movement) or slow wave sleep (SWS) is characterized by the person being somewhat aware of the environment but being in a very relaxed state. Brain activity, as measured on the electroencephalogram (EEG), resembles that of the waking state with small, irregular, rapidly changing waves. People in Stage I may jerk involuntarily and waken in the process. If aroused during this stage, the person will often deny having been asleep, although sleep has actually begun. Muscles retain their tone, although a slow rolling of the eyes takes place.

■ Stage II NREM is characterized by being unaware of surroundings but easily arousable. This stage is marked by the beginning of muscle relaxation, and brain waves gradually become larger with frequent quick bursts, or spindles. Eyes continue to roll slowly from side to side.

■ Stage III NREM consists of deeper sleep, manifested by still more slowing of the brain waves and loss of muscle tone. Some reflexes also diminish.

■ Stage IV NREM is the stage of deepest sleep from which arousal is difficult. It is characterized by very large, slow brain waves. During this stage there is very little body movement, and vital signs (pulse, respiration, and blood pressure) are decreased. The dreams that occur in this stage are realistic, resemble thought processes, and are not likely to be recalled. The need for Stage IV sleep is increased by strenuous activity. Deprivation of this level of sleep causes the individual to become physically uncomfortable. Symptoms commonly encountered include sensations of a tight band around the head, burning eyes, muscle tremors and weakness, and joint pain. Generalized body fatigue is a frequent complaint. Other symptoms of deprivation include withdrawn or depressed behavior. Stage IV sleep is also called obligatory sleep because of its necessity for maintenance of physical health and well-being. When missed, obligatory sleep is recovered during subsequent sleep periods—before REM sleep is recovered (Kales, Beall, Berger, Heuser, Jacobsen, Kales, Parmelee & Walter 1968).

■ The REM (rapid eye movement) stage is characterized by rapid, irregular, small brain waves that resemble the waking stage and by frequent, rapid, horizontal eye movements that can be observed through closed eyelids. In newborns, one can observe slow, rolling eye movements upon which are superimposed occasional rapid eye movements. Infants spend approximately half of their sleeping time in an active sleep state resembling adult REM sleep, whereas adults spend approximately 20 to 25% of total sleep time in REM stage sleep. It is believed that this active state serves as an internal source of stimulation to higher brain centers at a time when external sources are minimized owing to short periods of arousal. In addition to the darting movements through the eyelids, the nurse may observe an infant kicking, making small twitching movements with the fingers, and sucking, smiling, or grimacing during sleep. Slowly this active stage diminishes, and by the time the child is 2 to 3 years old, 20 to 25% of sleep time is spent in the REM phase. This change is thought to be due to maturation of the central nervous system.

Other visible characteristics of the REM stage include complete relaxation of most of the skeletal muscles. The lower jaw is noticeably relaxed. Despite skeletal muscle relaxation, there is heightened autonomic activity, which causes increased gastric secretions, penile erections, and irregular vital signs. For this reason, REM sleep is often called paradoxical sleep. The dreams that frequently take place in REM sleep are vividly detailed, emotionally charged, and much more likely to be recalled than dreams occurring in NREM (non-REM) stages. REM-stage dreams are thought to be essential in the process of psychological and mental restoration. REM-stage sleep is important in helping a person organize, categorize, store, and integrate new information and experiences into the memory.

While vigorous physical activity increases the need for Stage IV sleep, emotional stress or strenuous cognitive activity increases the need for REM sleep. For example, students who are learning large amounts of new material in a short period or hospitalized clients who are facing many new and perhaps stressful experiences can be expected to require more REM sleep. Deprivation of this level of sleep can cause changes in personality and performance. Difficulty concentrating, heightened sensitivity to pain or discomfort, fatigue, more frequent errors, apathy, and poor judgment all may result from REM sleep deprivation. Decreased productivity often occurs, particularly with monotonous or prolonged tasks, such as studying for a final examination, working a double shift in a hospital, or performing routine tasks on an assembly line.

Four to six times during a full sleep period, an adult proceeds through a cycle usually lasting 90 to 100 minutes (see Figure 16-1). During a given cycle, the individual proceeds through Stages I to IV and then passes back through Stages III, II and into a period of REM stage sleep. Following the REM period, the individual begins a second cycle, proceeding back through Stages II to IV. The transition from one sleep stage to another is marked visibly by changes in position. The duration of Stage IV sleep shortens and the REM stage lengthens progressively with each cycle. Therefore, most Stage IV sleep occurs in the early part of the sleep period, and the majority of REM sleep occurs closer to the time of awakening. Thus, an individual who consistently gets 4 to 5 hours of sleep each night may awaken physically rested (sufficient Stage IV sleep), but may have difficulty with optimal performance owing to inadequate REM sleep. Another important factor to consider is that a person awakened during any stage of the sleep cycle must begin again with Stage I when sleep resumes and must repeat the cycle in its entirety. Thus, people whose sleep is interrupted frequently (for example, hospitalized clients) may be expected to become "REM-sleep deprived." Table 16-2 summarizes the stages of the normal sleep cycle.

Age Variables in Sleep Cycles and Requirements

The newborn spends approximately 50% of sleep time in REM-type sleep. By the age of 2 to 3 years, REM sleep decreases to 20 to 25% of total sleep time, which approaches the amount of REM sleep needed in later childhood and in adult years. On the other hand, Stage IV sleep lasts longer in childhood, as shown by the ease with which infants and small children can be picked up, dressed, and diapered without arousing. Stage IV sleep decreases markedly from 10% in young adults to 0 to 4% in the elderly (Kales et. al., 1968). These variations are depicted in Figure 16-2.

Total sleep requirements vary throughout the life span. Generally, total sleep needs decrease as an individual progresses from infancy to adulthood. An exception to this occurs during the rapid growth period of adolescence. Increased fatigue occurs during adolescence because the rapid growth of the musculoskeletal system exceeds the ability of the cardiac and respiratory systems to keep pace. The elderly need the same amount of sleep as other adults. Because they awaken more often and stay awake longer, they may spend more time in bed to get the same amount of sleep. This may lead to the erroneous impression that the elderly sleep more than other adults (Bahr, 1983; Miller, 1990).

A summary of total sleep requirements and age-related variations is depicted in Table 16-3.

Naps

Not much is known about the effects of naps on the major sleep period. It is known, however, that the character of the sleep that occurs during naps differs according to the time of day when the nap occurs. Naps occurring soon after the major sleep period consist primarily of REM sleep. Those occurring later in the day have a preponderance of Stage IV sleep.

Naps seem to be needed during periods when the individual's body is in the process of rapid growth or cellular repair. This is evidenced by the need for naps by infants, toddlers, and by individuals recovering from illness or surgery. Naps also may serve to make up for sleep deficits during the

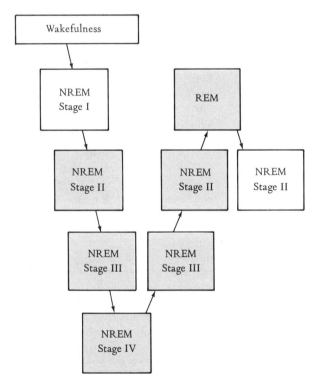

FIGURE 16-1. A Single Normal Sleep Cycle. In the normal nocturnal pattern, shaded cycle is repeated four or five times. Periods of REM sleep generally increase in duration, and periods of deep sleep (Stage IV) progressively decrease as morning approaches. (*Note.* From Taylor, C., Lillis, C., & LeMone, P. (1989). *Fundamentals of Nursing.* Philadelphia: J.B. Lippincott, p. 694.)

TABLE 16-2
The Stages of a Normal Sleep Cycle

Stage	Brain Waves	Behavior and Sensations	Depth of Sleep	Physiologic Changes	Dreams
The threshold of sleep (alpha) and relaxed wakefulness	An even rhythm (the alpha rhythm), 9–12 cycles per second	Serene relaxation, no concentrated thought	Perceptions slowing down		Fragments of thought
. . . the myoclonic jerk	. . . tiny bursts of electrical activity in the brain	. . . a sudden spasm, causing the body to jerk	Momentary arousal		
I	Small and pinched; irregular and rapidly changing	Sometimes a floating sensation, drifting with idle thoughts and dreams	Can still be awakened easily and will insist has not been asleep	Muscles relaxing, pulse growing even, breathing becoming regular, temperature falling	Images and thoughtlike fragments
II	Growing larger, quick bursts, resembling wire spindle	If eyes are open, will not see	May be awakened with a modest sound	Eyes roll slowly from side to side	Some thoughtlike fragments and low-intensity dreams
III	Large, slow waves—one a second	Removed from the waking world	Takes louder noise to awaken	Muscles relaxed, breathing even; heart rate slowed, temperature declining, muscles relaxed, blood pressure dropping	Rarely recalled
IV (Delta)	Very large, slow waves (delta waves) that trace a jagged pattern	Period of beginning sleepwalking, or bedwetting	The deepest sleep, most difficult to awaken	Even breathing, heart rate, blood pressure slowly falling	Poor recall makes this seem a dreamless oblivion most of the time. Rare nightmares.
REM	Irregular and small—resemble those of waking	Rapid eye movements (REMs) as if watching	Hard to bring to the surface and reality	Lies limp, chin muscles slack; penile erections; increased gastric secretions in ulcer patients; fluctuating blood pressure; irregular pulse, respiration; twitching of fingers and toes	Very vivid dreams 85% of the time

The entire cycle is repeated roughly *every 90 minutes,* or about 4 or 5 times in a normal night. Stage IV is most protracted in early part of the night. REM dreams grow more vivid as the night progresses.

Bill Berger/Associates, Inc. for G.G. Luce and J. Segal, 1969, *Insomnia.* Garden City: Doubleday, and Company, pp. 22–23, Reprinted by permission.

major sleep period. Examples of this include night-shift workers, who frequently sleep about 5 hours shortly after working hours and then nap for a period before going to work again the next night (Smith & Wedderburn, 1980), and the elderly individual who naps to compensate for increased awakenings during the major sleep period (Hayter, 1985). Individuals who are undergoing periods of psychological stress also may nap more frequently. In addition, boredom may be a factor in napping and may account for some of the naps taken by inactive or elderly clients.

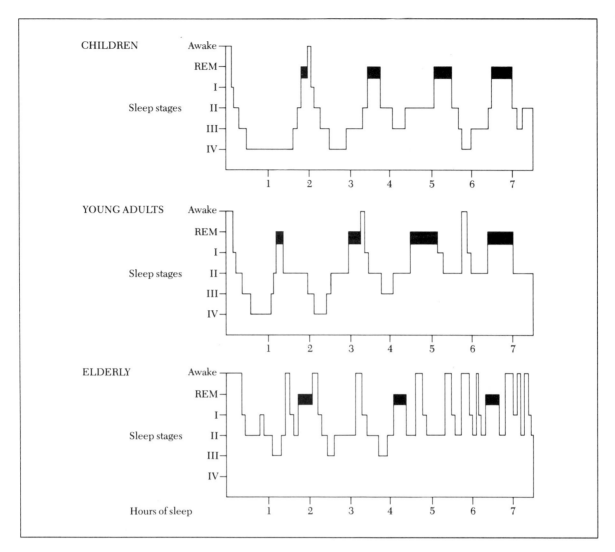

FIGURE 16-2. Sleep Cycles of Normal Subjects. The sleep of children and young adults shows early preponderance of Stages III and IV, progressive lengthening of the first three REM periods, and infrequent awakenings. In elderly adults there is little or no Stage IV sleep, REM periods are fairly uniform in length, and awakenings are frequent and often lengthy. (*Note.* From Kales, A. et al. "Sleep and Dreams: Recent Research in Clinical Aspects." *Annals of Internal Medicine*, 68:1078, May 1968. Reprinted with permission.)

Drug Use and Sleep

The use of drugs for other than medicinal purposes has been increasing in the United States since the early 1960s, when a rather dramatic change in social attitudes toward drug use and toward established norms in general took place. From that time, use of various types of drugs has extended to all socioeconomic and ethnic groups in the United States. Although drug use is more common in urban areas, rural areas also have been affected. Types of drugs used range from central nervous system depressants like alcohol and opiates (morphine, heroin, marijuana, codeine), barbiturates, and hypnotics to such stimulants as amphetamines and cocaine. They may be prescribed, purchased

over the counter, or obtained from illegal sources. Regardless of the source or the reason for taking, many of these drugs can adversely affect normal sleep patterns, and the nurse needs to be cognizant of their effects so that potential alterations can be more adequately assessed.

Many sleeping medications (barbiturates and hypnotics) reduce the duration of REM sleep, as well as stages III and IV of NREM sleep (Pagliaro & Pagliaro, 1986), although the total sleep time may be lengthened. In addition, narcotic analgesics, antidepressants, and some amphetamines alter the proportion of REM sleep to total sleep. Over-the-counter medications such as antihistamines and sleeping medications may produce similar effects, especially if taken indiscriminately. A few medica-

TABLE 16-3
Age Variations in Total Sleep Needs

Age	Total Sleep Needs
Neonate (up to 1 month)	16 to 20 hours
Infant (up to 1 year)	10 to 12 hours plus 2 to 3 naps
Toddler (1 to 3 years)	10 to 12 hours plus 1 to 2 naps
Preschooler (3 to 5 years)	9 to 11 hours plus 1 nap or rest period
School-age child (6 to 12 years)	9 to 11 hours
Adolescent (13 to 18 years)	9 to 11 hours
Adult (over 18 years)	7 to 8 hours

tions, such as sodium pentobarbital (Nembutol), chlordiazepoxide (Librium), glutethimide (Doriden), and high dozes of diazepam (Valium) and chloral hydrate increase Stage IV NREM sleep (Fass, 1971).

Because marijuana and cocaine use continue to be widespread in our society, special consideration of its effects on sleep is warranted. Marijuana is a central nervous system depressant, and tends to produce effects on sleep similar to other central nervous system depressants, particularly barbiturates. These effects have been readily demonstrated in animal studies in which dosage and route of administration can be carefully controlled. Although sedative effects have been demonstrated in humans, the effects are much more variable, because dosages are not exact and route of administration varies. The setting in which the drug is used and the prior experience and expectations of the user also influence its effects. For example, marijuana commonly causes feelings of relaxation and sleepiness if the user is alone, but sleepiness is less pronounced in social situations (Pagliaro & Pagliaro, 1986).

Cocaine and cocaine derivatives are central nervous system stimulants and tend to affect sleep like other central nervous system stimulants (amphetamines). Because of the stimulating effect of these drugs (psychomotor agitation, hypervigilance, euphoria), clients have difficulty sleeping. Usually, both the quality and the quantity of sleep are affected.

Hallucinogenic drugs (PCP) can produce illusions, hallucinations and significant changes in mood. Depending on the individual, reactions to this group of drugs may range from feelings of calmness and oneness with the universe to severe anxiety, feelings of depersonalization, and hyper-

vigilance. People using these drugs may also have marked sleep disturbances.

A client taking any of these drugs should be carefully assessed for altered sleep patterns. In addition, the nurse should be aware that discontinuing any of these medications abruptly may lead to a rebound effect. If this occurs, the individual spends more time in the deprived stage in an attempt to catch up. During this period, the client is likely to experience vivid, frightening nightmares and vague physical discomforts. Careful assessment of the drugs the client is taking is imperative so that abrupt withdrawal can be avoided if at all possible. It is important to remember that drug-dependent clients who are being withdrawn from such drugs as morphine, heroin, meperidine, barbiturates, and hypnotics may experience these symptoms. Careful assessment will also assist the nurse in determining the drug-dependent client's need for supportive medication during withdrawal.

Some foods and beverages that may comprise a part of the client's normal diet also can alter normal sleep. Caffeine-containing foods and beverages, such as coffee, tea, colas, and chocolate, act as stimulants. Taken too close to bedtime, they may make it more difficult to fall asleep. As stated earlier, excessive alcohol consumption depresses the central nervous system and interferes with REM sleep. Thus, the individual who consumes excessive alcohol may fall asleep more quickly but may have difficulty staying asleep.

Sleep Deprivation

The vital relationship between sleep and normal functioning of the human body is clearly illustrated by the various physiological and psychological changes that occur when a person is deprived of sleep. The types of deprivation that have been studied most frequently are total deprivation, REM deprivation, and Stage IV (NREM) deprivation.

After approximately 4 days of total sleep deprivation, healthy individuals begin to exhibit such symptoms as increased fatigue, difficulty concentrating, periods of disorientation, and general irritability. It is common for these individuals to misinterpret events occurring in their immediate environment and to feel paranoid or persecuted. If deprivation continues, symptoms such as auditory or visual hallucinations, confusion, and progressive disorientations to time, place, and person may be experienced. The nature and extent of symptoms exhibited and the amount of deprivation necessary to elicit symptoms vary greatly among individuals. Someone recovering sleep following a period of total deprivation will have an increased percentage of both stage IV (NREM) and REM sleep.

REM deprivation occurs when people are allowed to sleep for only short periods (one hour or less) or when they sleep only a total of three to four hours during a 24-hour period. This situation occurs frequently when clients are critically ill and are being cared for in intensive care units. Some of the changes observed in REM-deprived individuals include:

> Difficulty concentrating
>
> Increased sensitivity to pain or discomfort
>
> Fatigue
>
> More frequent errors
>
> Apathy
>
> Poor judgment
>
> Reduced productivity

Individuals deprived of REM stage sleep may have difficulty coping with stressful experiences. People recovering from missed REM sleep will go into the REM sleep stage more quickly and will remain in it longer than usual. Moreover, it is important to remember that REM sleep is made up only after any missed Stage IV sleep has been recovered.

Stage IV (NREM) deprivation occurs naturally with a few diseases, including untreated hypothyroidism, chronic alcoholism, and depression. It also can occur when individuals are awakened frequently or are totally deprived of sleep. Deprivation of this level of sleep causes the individual to become physically uncomfortable. Symptoms may include:

> Muscle tremors or weakness
>
> Joint pain
>
> A sensation of a tight band around the head
>
> Burning eyes

The individual also may appear withdrawn and depressed. Although physical activity increases the need for and promotes achievement of Stage IV sleep, physical activity should occur no closer than two hours to the time of sleep to achieve the desired effects.

Sleep deprivation can be diagnosed by identifying behavioral and physiological cues as well as by obtaining a history of recent sleep patterns.

Insomnia

Insomnia is the term used to describe difficulty sleeping. Individuals may have difficulty falling asleep, staying asleep, or going back to sleep after awakening. Insomnia may be temporary or it may be a problem that continues for years. Many re-

searchers agree that primary insomnia (actual sleep disorder) is not very common. More frequently, sleep difficulties occur from poor sleep habits or are a symptom of some other problem. For example, anxiety, depression, alcohol use, narcotic analgesics and peptic ulcer disease all may affect sleep. An individual who experiences sleep difficulties usually indicates that the quantity and quality of sleep has diminished.

When the nurse assesses an individual who complains of difficulty sleeping, it is important to determine the specific type of difficulty the client is experiencing. Is the individual having difficulty going back to sleep after awakening, or does the individual take an unusually long time to fall asleep (45 minutes to an hour)? Identifying the exact nature of the sleep difficulty can help to determine the cause of the problem.

There is a group of sleep disorders, known as parainsomnias, associated with specific stages of sleep. Sleep walking or somnambulism occurs during stage III or IV of non-REM sleep. The individual who sleep walks is not aware of the immediate environment and reacts slowly. A second disorder, involuntary urination, or *nocturnal enuresis*, occurs as the individual moves from stage IV sleep into stage II before the onset of REM sleep. This condition appears to be hereditary, with the exact cause unknown.

Sleep apnea and narcolepsy are additional sleep disorders. Sleep apnea is a disordered breathing that occurs during sleep. In the apneic state, the ability of the individual to take in air via the nose or the mouth ceases for at least 10 seconds. It is estimated that a fairly large percentage of the general population experiences some type or degree of this disordered breathing.

Narcolepsy, on the other hand, is a sleep disorder characterized by the sudden onset of sleep. The individual who suffers from narcolepsy falls asleep at inappropriate times. These sleep episodes characteristically are REM stage sleep and are associated with periods of temporary loss of muscle tone.

A careful and thorough assessment of any complaint of sleeping difficulty is necessary in order to determine the exact nature of the problem. A family member, particularly the spouse, is often very helpful in validating the client's sleep difficulties and providing more details.

Variables That Influence Activity–Sleep

It is important for the nurse to be able to collect pertinent data for each client. Because a client's activity–sleep patterns vary throughout the life span and among various cultural groups, including these variables in an assessment of a particular client is necessary to derive an individualized profile of that client. Consideration of the effects of the client's current health on activity–sleep patterns also is needed in a comprehensive assessment.

Age

The nurse needs to assess different factors of activity–sleep patterns depending upon the age of the individual. Age-specific influences on activity-sleep patterns in this chapter will focus on the adult. The reader is referred to chapters 21 to 24 for specific information on the sleep-activity patterns of clients in other age groups.

Early Adulthood. Problems with activity are usually minimal during adulthood except for modifications related to episodic or chronic illnesses. Sleep disturbances, when they occur, frequently are related to failure to allow sufficient time for rest and sleep. Work, social activities, family responsibilities, and educational pursuits may occupy many hours and cause clients in this age group to go for long periods without adequate sleep. Worries about these aspects of life also can interfere with optimal sleep. In addition, work and family demands may reduce the time available for regular exercise. Frequently, adults try to make up this deficit by engaging in strenuous physical activity on weekends or holidays, and this sporadic activity frequently results in muscle strains, other musculoskeletal trauma, or even heart attacks. Lack of regular exercise may contribute to sleep problems, since physical activity enhances Stage IV (NREM) sleep.

Late Adulthood. As age progresses, additional factors may affect the client's ability to remain active. Because of the normal deterioration in the senses, the older client may not see or hear as well, and these limitations may account for reduced activity. The older person may be afraid (or unable) to undertake previously enjoyed activities because of these declining sensory faculties. Inactivity may lead to boredom and depression, which can further limit normal activity.

Transportation available to the elderly also needs to be assessed. The older person may no longer drive and may be dependent on others to continue usual activities outside the home, including seeking health care. What about the crime level in the client's neighborhood? Is the client afraid to walk on the streets?

Finally, safety considerations related to activity need to be considered. The elderly person frequently walks with a shuffling gait, which may make it more dangerous. The elderly individual is much more likely to trip over doorsills and slide on throw rugs. Stiff joints related to the aging process may compound the problem of performing enjoyable activities, such as handwork or gardening.

With age, the quality of sleep declines. It takes longer to fall asleep, the number of nightly awakenings increases, and the amount of time spent in deep sleep diminishes. Consequently, the sleep of older individuals often has been described as fitful.

For the older individual, the total amount of sleep does not occur at night but is distributed throughout the day in short naps (Hayter, 1983 & 1985; Bahr, 1983; Ross, Hare & McPherson, 1985). So while the need for sleep (total hours of sleep) does not change appreciably from earlier adult years, the older person spends more time in bed.

Culture

Modern technology has caused lifestyle changes that have had a direct effect on the activity–sleep patterns of individuals. Until recently, individuals lived in phase with nature—working during the day, resting at night, and traveling only as fast as animals or sails could carry them. Our society is still largely structured around night as the major sleep period. Many businesses close, lights are dimmed, and traffic diminishes during the late evening and night hours. These changes in activity levels during later evening and night may cause problems for those individuals who work during the evening or night. As stated earlier, their sleep patterns frequently are quite different from those of daytime workers, and they may be deprived of REM sleep. Social activities may be limited because they frequently occur during the individual's sleep time. Recently, however, shopping malls, theaters, and television stations are operating longer hours, which helps to meet the needs of these individuals for diversion.

Modern technology also has favored the development of a sedentary lifestyle. It is no longer necessary for each family group to produce its own food, nor do most individuals engage in manual labor to make a living. Some people attribute the increase in disability and death from such chronic disorders as atherosclerosis, obesity, and hypertension at least in part to this gradual decline in physical activity. In our culture, many individuals are making conscious efforts to maintain or improve their physical fitness through regular exercise programs, such as jogging and aerobic exercise. Participation in team sports, like softball, and competitive sports, such as tennis, also is increasing.

Books that describe various individual exercise programs are very popular. Although these books usually caution the reader about seeking medical advice before initiating the specific program, the nurse should evaluate clients' current exercise patterns or programs to see if they are appropriate to the individual's situation. This is especially important for individuals with preexisting health problems, such as joint disease or cardiorespiratory problems. An evaluation of the client's level of physical fitness also is needed to advise about exercise programs.

As mentioned earlier, it is also important to carefully assess the client's usual sleep environment while taking the health history. There is considerable variation among various cultures and subcultures with respect to sleeping arrangements. Awareness of individual sleep preferences will enable the nurse to plan more effectively for maintenance of normal sleep patterns. For instance, a toddler who is used to sleeping in a room with parents may have a great deal of difficulty sleeping in a hospital crib and, in fact, may become quite frightened when placed in the crib alone. Alternative sleeping arrangements, such as allowing for the child to sleep in a hospital bed with the parent, can facilitate sleep.

Some Asian clients may be accustomed to sleeping on futons and may find a hospital bed a strange experience indeed.

Health

Changes in health often alter an individual's normal patterns of activity and sleep. The most obvious example of this alteration is loss or reduction of motor function related to disease or trauma. Since motor function requires intact neurological and musculoskeletal systems, any disease or injury affecting either of these systems may affect mobility. Common examples include cerebrovascular accidents, fractures, arthritis, myasthenia gravis, and certain psychological states, such as catatonia and conversion reactions.

With other health problems, the client is able to move about (systems involved in maintaining motor function are intact), but some restrictions or limitations have been placed on the extent of activity permitted. This commonly occurs when physicians prescribe bed rest, apply casts or traction, or connect clients to various machines, tubes, and other therapeutic devices that mechanically limit mobility.

Other clients who are likely to experience at least temporary alterations in activity–sleep patterns include those who have impaired vision. This includes those clients who will have permanent sensory deficits and those whose interference is temporary (e.g., client with cataracts, both presurgically and postsurgically, since eyes will be patched).

Being placed in a hospital, nursing home, or other health-care facility also will be likely to alter an individual's normal activity and sleep patterns (Closs, 1988; Lukasiewicz-Ferland, 1987). Often, the client is confined to a small space and is subjected to regulations that limit the extent of mobility. Being unfamiliar with the environment and perhaps fearful of getting lost may be other limiting factors. It may also be difficult for the hospitalized client to sleep well because of the unfamiliar surroundings, strange noises, anxieties about the illness or diagnostic process, and separation from significant others or meaningful objects. In addition, customary bedtime routines may be difficult to follow in an unfamiliar setting.

ACTIVITY–SLEEP HISTORY

Most of the information needed to assess a client's activity–sleep patterns can be gathered during the nursing history (see Table 16-4). Questions should focus on the client's usually daily patterns and any alterations in those patterns. It is important to ascertain what a typical day is like for the client. The nurse may find it helpful to proceed from inquiries about usual time of rising to questions about bedtime and sleep habits so that data will be recorded systematically. By asking the client how a typical day is spent, the nurse can learn about the client's occupation; the time spent in that endeavor; the type of activity involved (active or sedentary); how the client usually performs activities of daily living; and what leisure activities the client enjoys.

Careful questioning of the client will help the nurse identify any changes in activity that have occurred as a result of neuromuscular deficits, a lack of motivation to engage in activity or an environment that is unsafe or restricts movement. Any one of these factors can interfere with an individual's ability to be mobile and therefore active in everyday events.

Knowing the client's recreational preferences makes it easier to plan any lifestyle modifications and to suggest appropriate diversionary activities. Pertinent data include amount of time spent daily or weekly in a given activity and the type of activity enjoyed. If the activity involves strenuous physical exercise or stimulating mental activity, it is important to determine the relationships of that activity to bedtime, since either may account for diffi-

TABLE 16-4
Activity–Sleep History

Activity	Sleep
Usual time of arising	Usual bedtime and relationship of activity to bedtime
Activities during a typical day	Sleep environment
In-home activities and outside activities	Light and noise tolerance
Occupation and number of hours worked/shift	Temperature preference
Equipment/prosthesis needed for activity/walking	Equipment needed (pillows, blankets)
(cane, walker, wheelchair, braces, artificial limbs)	Type of bed (size, firmness, position)
Environmental factors influencing mobility	Sleep alone or in a room or bed with others
Physical surroundings (home, neighborhood)	Bedtime rituals/routines/aids to sleep (e.g., reading,
Financial resources	drinking, bathing, eating, watching TV, smoking)
Motivation to be active	Medications/drugs taken (OTC, prescription, street,
Effort made to be active	alcohol, stimulants, depressants)
Enjoyment of activity	Arousals during sleep (number and reason)
Leisure Activities	Difficulty falling or staying asleep
Time spent daily (frequency/regularity)	Naps (number, length, time of day)
Type of activity (sedentary vs. active)	Changes in usual patterns
Exercise patterns (type, frequency, duration, regu-	Difficulties caused by changes in patterns
larity)	Client's perception of adequacy/quality
Special abilities (creative, athletic)	
Past history of activity/exercise; recent change	
Attitudes about exercise and motivation to exercise	
Current exercise/fitness goals	

culty falling asleep if occurring less than two hours before retiring.

To determine total sleep needs, the nurse must collect information about the client's usual time of rising, retiring, and going to sleep, as well as the number, duration, and time of day for any naps. Determining if the client works various shifts is necessary because the body's circadian rhythms, including sleep, are upset by frequent alterations in activity–sleep patterns. Apparently, shift workers adapt to varying hours of work by becoming better at coping with the contradiction between the body's biological "set" for day-time activity and the necessity for working at night. The body clock remains set as before, and hormone production, electrolyte excretion, vital signs, and sleep patterns remain altered for the duration of the night work.

The nurse also should collect information about the client's usual sleep habits and environment, since disruption of the individual's routine can alter sleep patterns. In assessing the client's usual sleep environment, the nurse should ask about tolerance for lights and noise. Many clients are unable to sleep in a lighted room, whereas others sleep better with a night light. Since familiar objects often serve as a stimulus for sleep, especially when associated with rituals, it is important to determine if any such equipment facilitates the client's sleep. Special pillows, blankets, or toys may be very important to maintaining normal sleep

patterns for a young child. Bedtime rituals or routines provide for a transition from wakefulness to sleep and constitute a signal that it is time for sleep. It is important for the nurse to be aware of these habits so that they can be incorporated into plans for maintaining normal sleep patterns. For example, drinking a glass of milk and having a story read may ease an often-resisted bedtime for a toddler. For an adult, reading a book or taking a warm bath may serve the same function.

The nurse also should assess whether the client is accustomed to sleeping alone or in a room or bed with others. It may be customary in some cultures for the infant or small child to sleep with the parents. In these instances, the child might be quite frightened at being placed in a room alone to sleep. On the other hand, a client may be unable to sleep in a room with others if accustomed to sleeping alone. Clients who are used to sleeping with windows open for fresh air may have an especially difficult time sleeping in an artificially heated or cooled environment such as a hospital.

A drug history is needed to determine whether the client is taking any over-the-counter or prescription medications for sleep or any other health problems. Central nervous system depressants, such as narcotic analgesics, barbiturates, hypnotics, and alcohol, may interfere with REM sleep, leading to difficulty staying asleep. Rapid withdrawal of these medications also causes sleep disturbances (see Drug Use and Sleep). Stimulants, such as beverages, foods, or over-the-counter medications containing caffeine, taken too close to bedtime also may disrupt sleep. Some of these items may be part of the client's bedtime ritual, but may actually be causing problems with sleep.

The nurse also should assess how well the client sleeps. Difficulties falling asleep or staying asleep should be determined. If the client is experiencing difficulty falling asleep, additional attention should be focused on the presleep routine and the kind of activity that immediately precedes bedtime. Any activity that stimulates wakefulness (e.g., vigorous exercise, reliving the events of the day, worry, anxiety) can delay the onset of sleep.

If the difficulty is with staying asleep, further assessment is indicated. Areas to be considered include environmental conditions unfavorable to sleep and the possibility of interference by health problems, such as a urinary tract infection, which requires frequent trips to the bathroom or paroxysmal nocturnal dyspnea.

Early morning awakenings and the inability to fall back to sleep can be associated with depression. However, the nurse should not assume that a client is depressed if the client awakens early and has difficulty falling back to sleep. Early morning awakenings need to be thoroughly and carefully assessed.

Finally, it is important to obtain clients' perceptions of the adequacy or quality of their activity and sleep. The nurse should ask if there have been any changes in activity–sleep patterns and whether those changes have caused any interference in the client's usual daily functioning. If there have been changes, the nurse needs to consider, or help the client identify, whether they are due to environmental changes, developmental or situational stressors, health problems, or restrictions imposed by medical treatment. It is important to remember that any health condition associated with pain, anxiety, depression, or fear of death may alter normal activity–sleep patterns. Clients' own perceptions and level of satisfaction regarding their activity and sleep patterns provide one of the most reliable sources of information about adequacy and always should be elicited.

CLINICAL APPRAISAL AND SCREENING

Clinical appraisal of activity consists of a general appraisal followed by specific assessments aimed at determining the function of body structures associated with mobility. These structures include the bones, muscles, and joints (musculoskeletal system)

and their ability to function in a way that allows the client to be mobile. Assessment of mobility also includes an evaluation of those structures that provide the neural innervation (neurological system) for movement, discussed in the previous chapter. The emphasis in this chapter is on assessment of the musculoskeletal system, which provides structure and support for the body and allows for movement by muscle contraction. At the end of this section, a model for the assessment of movement that integrates the two systems will be presented.

General Appraisal

The nurse can collect a great deal of information about the client's level of activity through observation. The client's overall movements can be observed as the history is being taken. Symmetry and a general sense of muscle strength also can be assessed by observing the client move in bed or walk into the room. If the client is ambulatory, the nurse can readily observe balance and gait, noting symmetry, rhythm, arm swing, and alignment.

Information from the nursing history gives the nurse an indication of the functional status of the client. This information will guide and direct the nurse in the examination of the musculoskeletal system. The findings on clinical appraisal will provide objective information about the client's functional status relative to mobility.

The techniques of inspection and palpation are the primary methods used in the clinical appraisal of the musculoskeletal system. The examination should proceed systematically, starting at the head and neck and moving to the upper extremities, then to the lower extremities, and finally to the back. The examination should be done symmetrically: one side of the body should be compared with the other. Individual examiners, however, will vary in their approaches to this exam. For example, one examiner may begin at the fingers and work up to the shoulder, neck, and head. Another examiner may work from the head down. The important point is not so much the order of the examination, as the way in which it is carried out. It should be done systematically to avoid omitting an aspect of the examination. With the client appropriately draped, the area being examined should be adequately exposed and free of any kind of restriction.

Specific Appraisal

The specific appraisal of the musculoskeletal system focuses on the structure and function of bones, muscles, and joints.

Skeletal System[1]

The body is built around a solid skeletal structure. Bone serves as a surface for the attachment of muscles, tendons, and ligaments. While the techniques for examining bone are basically the same for all clients, the nurse focuses on different factors according to the age of the client. For example, the nurse examining an infant would include specific maneuvers to detect congenital hip dysplasia, whereas the nurse examining an older client would inspect for spinal curvature such as kyphosis. Detailed assessments in certain areas are indicated in various age groups to detect and screen for commonly occurring problems that may affect the client's mobility (see chapters 21 to 24).

While inspecting the skeletal system, the nurse considers the normal form and structure of the body as well as the deformities that can occur. During an examination of each anatomic area, the nurse inspects the client from the front, back, and sides. While doing this, the nurse observes for symmetry and the normal curvature of the spine (curved posteriorly in the thoracic region and anteriorly in the cervical and lumbar regions).

Following inspection, the nurse palpates each anatomic area to determine any tenderness (see boxed insert).

The young and the old are at increased risk of injury from falls. Therefore, the nurse should be alert for signs and symptoms of fractures, including pain with extreme tenderness over the fracture site, bruising, edema, and limited movement. Shortening of the extremity also may occur. Any anatomic area about which the client has a subjective complaint should be examined carefully after the nurse has examined the unaffected areas.

Range of Motion

The nurse can determine necessary information about the client's joints and mobility through a systematic assessment of range of motion. Muscle tone and strength also can be determined while the nurse observes the client's muscle movements during range-of-motion activity. The range of motion (ROM) for a particular joint is the extent to which the joint is capable of being moved. The anatomic areas evaluated in a musculoskeletal assessment and their corresponding joint movements are defined in Table 16-5.

Technique for Inspection and Palpation of the Bones

1. Observe client from front, side, and back.
2. Ask client to straighten and hold back shoulders.
3. Ask client to bend over at the waist, and inspect the spine for curvature.
4. Palpate all bones for tenderness, pain.

Note. Adapted from Grimes/Burns: *Health Assessment in Nursing Practice*, Second Edition, © 1987. Boston: Jones and Bartlett Publishers, p. 324.

Range of motion, together with the strength, coordination, and endurance of the surrounding muscles, determines the extent to which the body part can be used in physical activity. The combination and coordination of motions in all parts of the body enable clients to go about their daily activities, whether they consist of housework, manual labor, play, or athletics.

Not everyone has the same range of motion. An individual's range is affected by many factors: genetic makeup, developmental level, the presence

TABLE 16-5
Anatomic Area and Corresponding Joint Movements

Anatomic Area	Joint Movements
Temporomandibular	Open and close jaw
Neck	Flexion and extension; rotation and lateral flexion
Shoulder	Abduction and adduction; flexion and extension; internal and external rotation
Elbow	Flexion and extension; supination and pronation
Wrist	Dorsiflexion (or extension) and palmar flexion; supination and pronation
Fingers	Abduction and adduction; flexion
Thumb	Flexion and extension; opposition
Hip	Flexion and extension; abduction and adduction; internal and external rotation
Knee	Flexion and hyperextension
Ankle	Dorsiflexion and plantar flexion
Foot	Eversion and inversion
Lumbar spine	Flexion and extension; rotation and lateral extension

---

[1]Adapted from Grimes/Burns: *Health Assessment in Nursing Practice*, Second Edition, © 1987. Boston: Jones and Bartlett Publishers.

or absence of disease, and the amount and type of physical activity in which the individual normally engages. Range of motion of all joints is greatest in infancy and gradually lessens throughout childhood to adult ranges. A comparison of the corresponding right and left sides of the body is helpful in assessing deviations in range of motion, as well as comparison with the average ranges described in Figure 16-3. Conditions that may limit motion include the bony changes of arthritis and the muscle abnormalities of spasticity, contractures, and rigidity.

To facilitate uniform recording and interpretation of this information, a standard method of recording joint motion has been developed by the American Academy of Orthopedic Surgeons. This method is based on a neutral zero position. Using this method, the zero point is the extended (anatomic) position of the joint. The range of motion for each joint then can be determined by measuring the number of degrees in each direction that the specific joint moves. The directions of joint movement from neutral zero position are defined in Table 16-6.

To assess range of motion, the nurse should ask the client to move each of the joints through its range of motion. It is helpful for the nurse to place one hand on the joint being assessed so that any swelling, nodules, bony enlargement or deformity, and crepitation, or grating, can be felt as the joint moves. Comparing range of joint movement on right and left sides is helpful in determining limitations of the specific client. The average figures depicted in Figure 16-3 should serve only as a general guide, not as an absolute standard, because many factors may alter a client's normal range. If the client is unable to move the joint, the nurse can move

---

Technique for Inspection and Palpation of the Joints

1. Inspect and palpate:
   Temporomandibular joints
   Neck
   Shoulders
   Elbows
   Interphalangeal, intermetacarpal,
     carpal bones and joints
   Hips
   Patellar areas
   Ankles and feet
   Vertebral column and thoracic cage
2. Range of motion:
   Active
   Passive

Note. Adapted from Grimes/Burns: *Health Assessment in Nursing Practice*, Second Edition, (c) 1987. Boston: Jones and Bartlett Publishers, p. 334.

---

the joint and assess the extent of movement possible. It is important not to force a stiff joint because of the possibility of causing trauma or pain.

If the range of motion is limited, further assessment is needed to determine the presence of:

Fluid in the joint

An irregularity in joint surface

A contracture of the muscles, ligament, or joint capsule

Fragments loose in the joint capsule

Movement of the joint also may reveal hypermobility, which could indicate such conditions as torn supporting ligaments, or an intra-articular fracture.

TABLE 16-6
Joint Movement Terminology

Term	Definition	Term	Definition
Flexion	Bending a joint to form an acute angle; a decrease in angle from neutral position	Rotation	Motion around a central axis
		Internal	Toward midline
		External	Away from midline
Extension	Neutral position	Pronation	Position of hand with palmar side down
Hyperextension	Increase in angle beyond usual arc		
Abduction	Moving arm, leg, finger, or toe away from its neutral position (midline)	Supination	Position of hand with palmar side up
		Inversion	Turning inward
Adduction	Moving arm, leg, finger, or toe toward neutral position (midline)	Eversion	Turning outward
Circumduction	Rotation of one bone around a stationary disk		

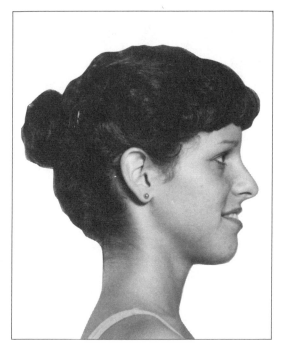

FIGURE 16-3. Location of the Temporomandibular Joint. ROM assessed by having examiner's index fingers in front of the tragus while client opens and closes jaw. (*Note.* From Grimes/Burns: *Health Assessment in Nursing Practice,* Second Edition, © 1987. Boston: Jones and Bartlett Publishers, p. 327.)

Muscle[2]

An assessment of the muscular portion of the musculoskeletal system is done by determining symmetry, muscle size, muscle tone, and muscle strength. Again, it is important for the nurse to compare corresponding muscle groups. Variations can exist among individuals and within the same individual.

Muscle size and symmetry usually are assessed by visually comparing the arms, thighs, and calves for general contour, local landmarks, and abnormal prominences. If a discrepancy in size is observed, use a tape measure to confirm it. It is normal, for example, to observe hypertrophy of certain muscle groups in an individual who lifts weights. In contrast, a malnourished individual may exhibit signs of dehydration and muscle wasting, or atrophy. It is important that all muscle groups, including the fine muscles of the hands, be systematically inspected. Any tremors or fasiculations (involuntary twitching) of the hands should be documented.

Muscle tone is determined by palpating the

muscles at rest (see boxed insert). The tone and consistency of the muscles are documented as either normal, flaccid, or spastic. The muscles also should be palpated during active and passive ranges of motion. Again, the tone and consistency should be recorded. In addition to tone, the strength of each functional group of muscles is tested using resistance: have the client push against your hands. To test the strength of the major muscle groups, have the client initially flex and extend the major joints actively without resistance. This enables the examiner to observe the normal range of motion of the joint before resistance is applied. Any muscle weakness or limitations in movement can be noted and evaluated more specifically during the examination. Next, have the client flex and extend the major joints actively against resistance. Compare the strength of the muscles as the client meets your resistance; observe neck flexion, extension, and rotation, shoulder abduction and adduction, elbow flexion and extension, wrist flexion and extension, finger adduction (grip) and abduction, hip flexion and extension, and ankle plantar flexion and dorsiflexion. Also, compare the distal strength of each extremity (where able) to the proximal strength. Record the muscle strength of all individual muscles or muscle groups using the appropriate scale (see Table 16-7). Examples of assessing the muscle strength of the biceps and triceps are depicted in Figures 16-4 and 16-5.

The procedures just outlined assess the joint motion and muscle strength of each of the major joints. There are two simple screening procedures that can be used to assess the general muscle strength of the upper extremities and the strength of the lower extremities.

To test the strength of the upper extremities,

Technique for Inspection and Palpation of the Muscles

1. Examine both sides of the body.
2. Compare muscle size of arms, thighs, and calves. Measure with tape if discrepancy noted.
3. Examine for tremors: Have client stretch arms in front. To detect fine tremors, place sheet of paper on top of client's hands.
4. Palpate muscles at rest to determine muscle tone.
5. Note condition of muscles when client does active and passive range of motion.
6. Assess client's muscle strength.

Note. Adapted from Grimes/Burns: *Health Assessment in Nursing Practice,* Second Edition, © 1987. Boston: Jones and Bartlett Publishers, p. 318.

---

[2]Adapted from Grimes/Burns: *Health Assessment in Nursing Practice,* Second Edition, © , 1987. Boston: Jones and Bartlett Publishers.

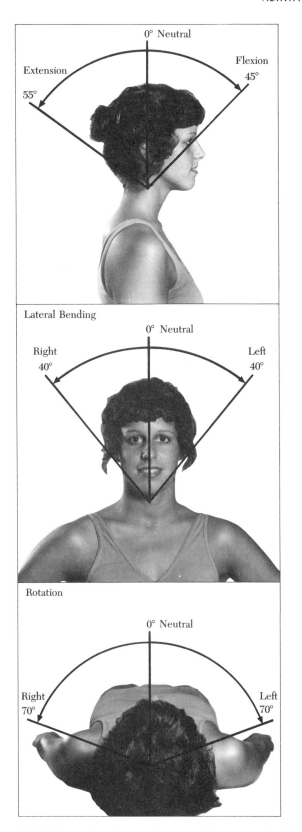

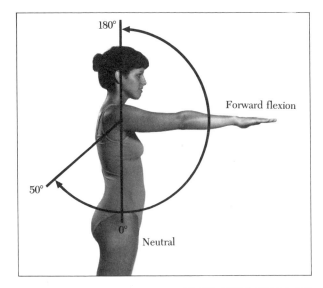

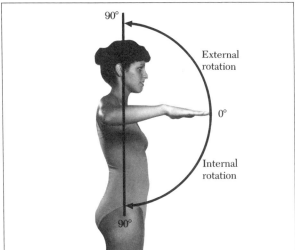

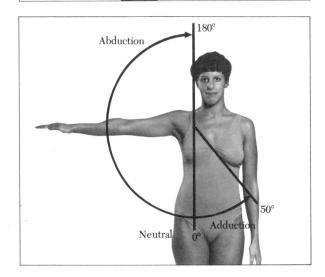

FIGURE 16-3 Continued. Range of Motion for the Neck and the Shoulders.

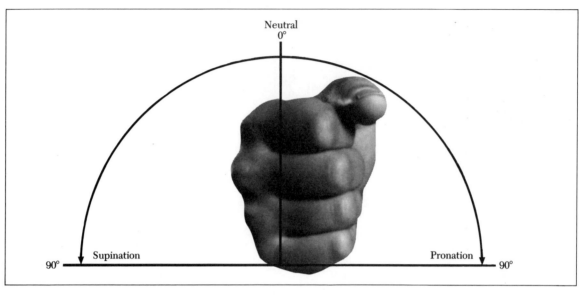

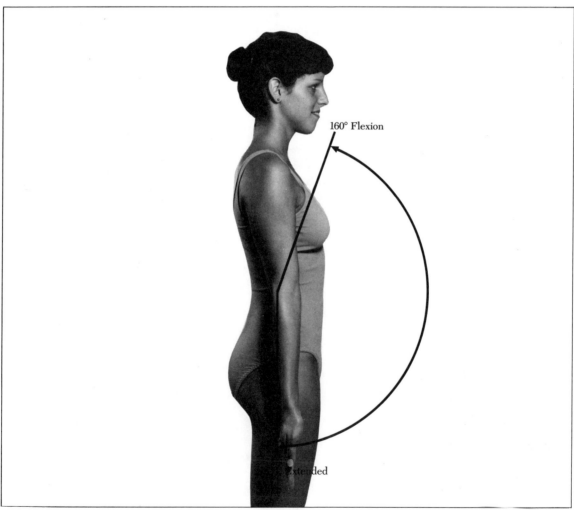

FIGURE 16-3 Continued. Range of Motion for the Elbow.

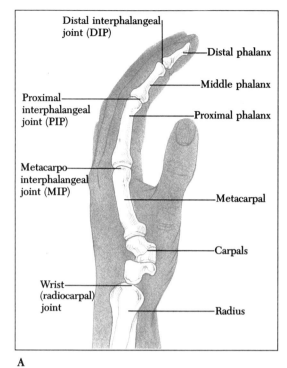

A

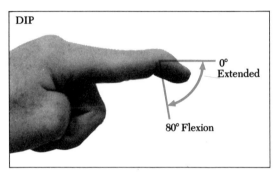

D

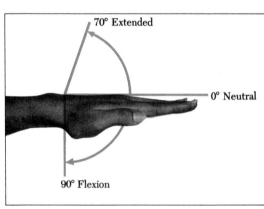

E

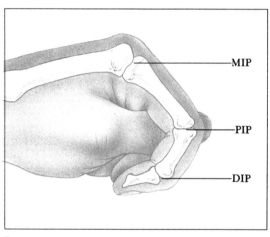

B

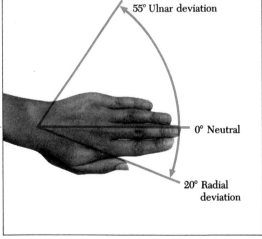

F

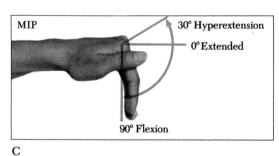

C

FIGURE 16-3 Continued. Location and Range of Motion of the Interphalangeal, Intermetacarpal, and Carpal Joins and Bones. (A) Basic joints of the hand. (B) Normal fist. (C, D, E) Range of movement of finger joints. (F, G) Range of wrist motion.

G

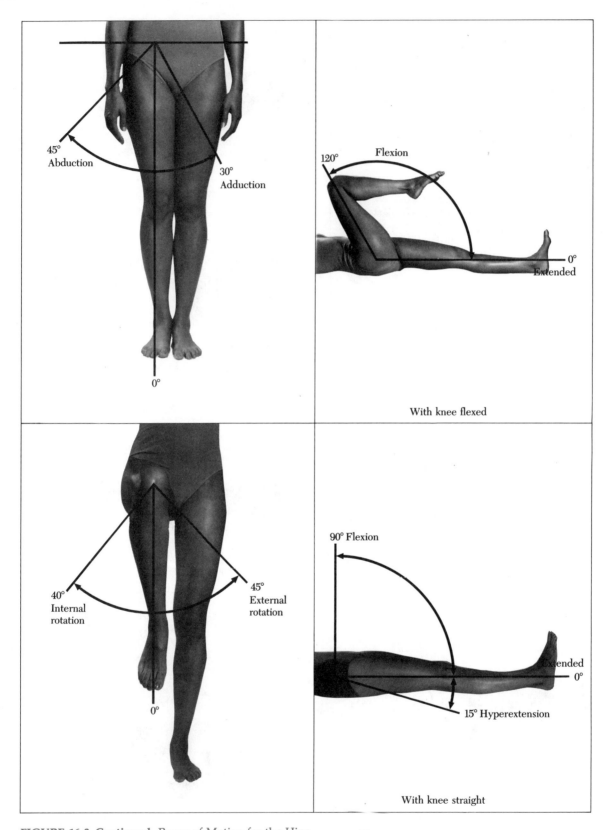

45°
Abduction

30°
Adduction

0°

120° Flexion

0°
Extended

With knee flexed

40°
Internal
rotation

45°
External
rotation

0°

90° Flexion

Extended
0°

15° Hyperextension

With knee straight

FIGURE 16-3 Continued. Range of Motion for the Hips.

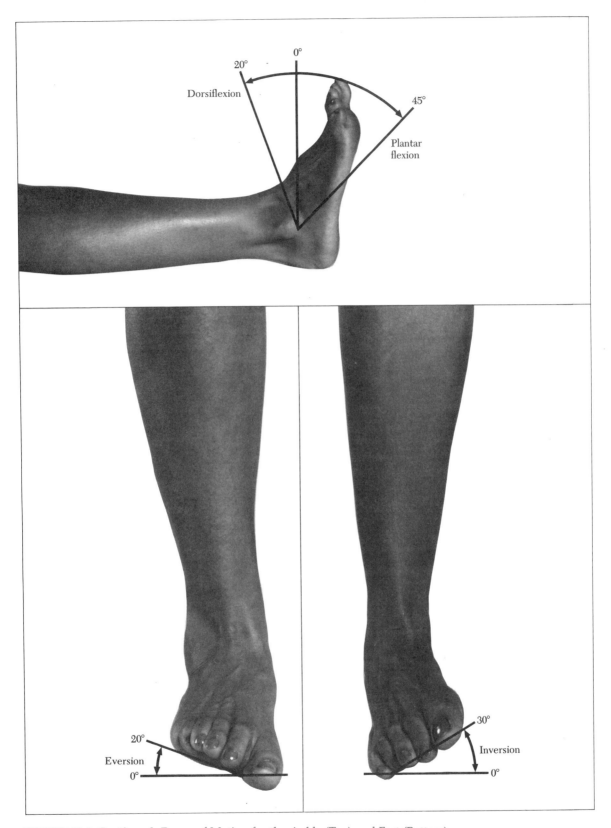

FIGURE 16-3 Continued. Range of Motion for the Ankle (Top) and Feet (Bottom).

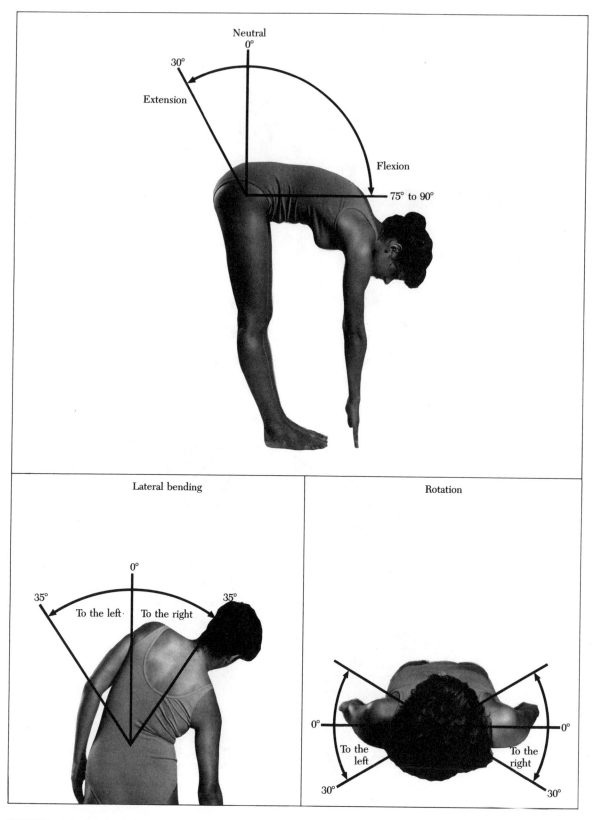

FIGURE 16-3 Continued. Range of Motion for the Spine.

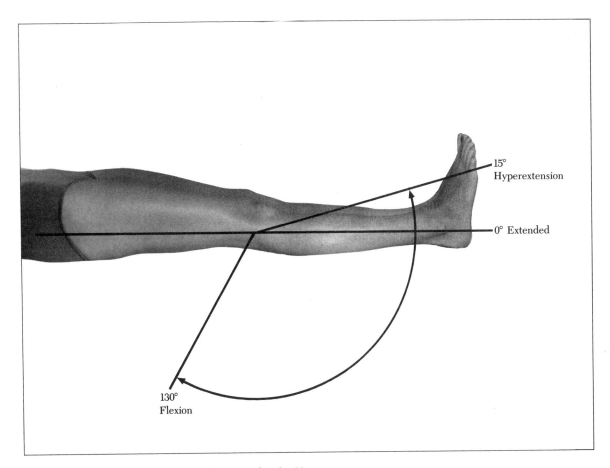

FIGURE 16-3 Continued. Range of Motion for the Knee.

have the client grasp the middle and index fingers of your hands. Instruct the client to resist the movement of your hands in the medial, lateral, upward, and downward positions. To test the strength and joint function of the lower extremities, have the client squat on the floor. Then, stand in front of the client. In this position, the client's hips and knees should be fully flexed. Hold the client's hands to provide balance and instruct the client to stand up. This technique can help determine the strength and joint motion of the lower extremities. A variety of factors, such as age, mental status, and health problems, may prevent an examiner from employing these techniques, requiring individual assessments of muscle groups. However, when appropriate, these procedures provide a quick and valid measure of muscle strength and joint motion in the upper and lower extremities.

Gait

The client's gait is assessed by having the client walk normally across the room and then back again. As the client walks, the nurse observes the two phases of the normal gait, the stance and the swing. In the stance phase the series of movements includes heelstrike, foot flat, midstance, and push-off. The movements in the swing phase include acceleration, midswing, and deceleration. The two phases of the normal gait occur simultaneously, so that when one limb is in the stance phase, the other is in the swing phase.

Integrated Function: Movement

The integrated function of the neurological and musculoskeletal systems enables movement. Mitchell and colleagues (1984) developed a very helpful nursing model that conceptualizes movement and thus provides a framework for assessing the functional ability of the patient with respect to movement (Table 16-8). The focus of the model is on the individual's ability to function in a self-care capacity.

According to this model, there are six integrated functions of movement. These functions are seeing, eating, expressing (facially), speaking, moving, and walking. These functional categories are depicted in Table 16-8 with their anatomical correlates and the specific tests to assess each function. Organizing the assessment in this framework enables the nurse to more comprehensively evaluate the client's mobility, identify dysfunction, and

TABLE 16-7
Scales for Grading Muscle Strength

Letter Scale	Percent Scale	Number Scale	Interpretation
Normal (N)	100%	5	Normal power
Good (G)	75%	4	Muscle can make full normal movement but not against resistance
Fair (F)	50%	3	Muscle cannot move against resistance or make full normal movement but can make normal movement against gravity
Poor (P)	25%	2	Full muscle movement possible with force of gravity eliminated
Trace (T)	10%	1	No movement of limb or joint, but contraction is visible or palpable
Zero (0)	0%	0	Total paralysis

Note. From Grimes/Burns: *Health Assessment in Nursing Practice,* Second Edition, © 1987. Boston: Jones and Bartlett Publishers, p. 320.

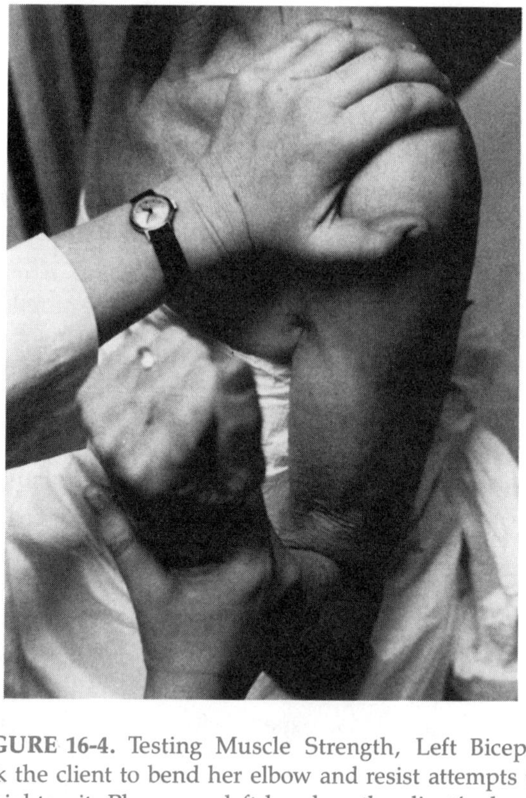

FIGURE 16-4. Testing Muscle Strength, Left Biceps. Ask the client to bend her elbow and resist attempts to straighten it. Place your left hand on the client's shoulder. With your right hand, grasp the client's wrist and attempt to straighten the arm. The degree of resistance is then assessed. If you release the client's wrist suddenly, her fist should not strike the hand on her shoulder. Such an overshooting response occurs in cerebellar disease. (*Note.* From Grimes/Burns: *Health Assessment in Nursing Practice,* Second Edition, © 1987. Boston: Jones and Bartlett Publishers, p. 319.)

determine the effect of dysfunction on the client's daily life (Konikow, 1985). Ultimately, thorough assessment is the basis for making accurate nursing diagnoses and developing appropriate nursing strategies.

Physical Fitness

Methods and procedures developed primarily in physical education programs are used to assess the level of physical fitness. Information from these procedures assists in planning an exercise program that meets the specific needs of the client: cardiovascular conditioning, muscle strengthening, or increasing joint mobility.

Initial baseline information about the client includes age, height, weight, resting pulse and blood pressure, and current health. Laboratory data, such as cholesterol, triglycerides, glucose, and high density lipid (HDL) levels, should be obtained because these measurements are closely related to metabolic or vascular status. The type of program the client needs—and can tolerate physiologically—is likely to be related to the client's percentage of body fat compared with norms for the individual's sex and age. Thus, the first step in determining body fat percentage would be to measure skinfold in the triceps, subscapular, midaxillary, suprailiac, abdominal, and thigh regions as described in Chapter 18. These measurements then are converted to percentage of body fat. These percentages provide helpful information for modifying diet and exercise. Measuring the girth of the client's chest, waist, hips, thigh, calf, ankle, and biceps will help determine what muscle groups a given client can exercise.

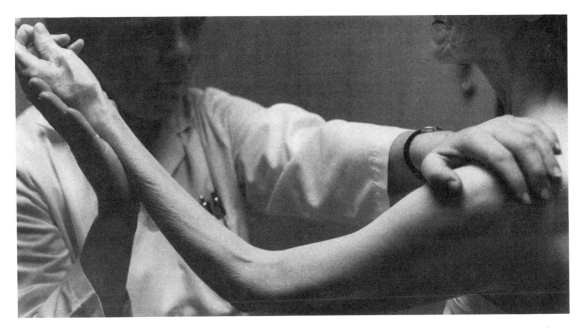

FIGURE 16-5. Testing Muscle Strength, Left Triceps. Ask the client to hold her left arm bent at the elbow. Place your left hand on the client's shoulder. Support the client's wrist with your right hand, and ask the client to straighten her elbow against the resistance of your right hand. (*Note.* From Grimes/Burns: *Health Assessment in Nursing Practice*, Second Edition, © 1987. Boston: Jones and Bartlett Publishers, p. 319.)

Probably the most significant test to determine the need for a cardiovascular conditioning program is the step test, a modified version of the laboratory stress test that can be performed in settings other than the laboratory.

The step test consists of having the client step up and down on a step approximately 17 to 18 inches high. It is recommended that the step height be decreased to 12 to 14 inches if the client is less than 5'3" and increased to 20 inches if the client is 6' or taller. A single step consists of lifting the left foot up, right foot up, left foot down, and right foot down. The client should aim at 24 to 30 steps per minute and continue for 3 minutes. A baseline pulse should be obtained prior to beginning the test. The pulse rate should then be counted:

for 30 seconds immediately following the exercise

for 30 seconds one minute after completion

another 30 seconds two minutes after

another 30 seconds three minutes after the exercise is completed

The apical or carotid pulses and the radial pulse should be used, because the carotid rate can be falsely lower because of the proximity to the vagus nerve, which may lower the pulse rate during exercise. To calculate the recovery index, the pulse rates obtained at 1, 2, and 3 minutes after the exercise should be added; the sum is the recovery index. This value should be compared with normative values for men and women. The step test should be stopped immediately if the client has chest pain, difficulty breathing, dizziness or faintness, or expresses a desire to stop. It is recommended that a physician be available for emergency backup if the client is over 40, obese, or has a history of cardiovascular or respiratory difficulties (Pender, 1982). *It is extremely important to point out here that the assessment of a client's level of physical fitness, like the assessment of any other dimension, must be performed by a knowledgeable and skilled professional.* Nurses are in a prime position to take a leadership role in this area. However, nurses must be specially trained to do this. They should be trained to assess physical fitness as well as to develop programs that assist clients in modifying diet and exercise to achieve a degree of physical fitness appropriate for the client. Nurses do clients a great disservice by pointing out health concerns or risk factors and then not providing them with the education and skills to change their behavior.

Sleep

When the nurse works in any setting in which the client stays for an extended period, it is possible to observe clients as they sleep. The nurse can make some observations about the general character of

TABLE 16-8
Assessment of Movement

Functional Category	Anatomical Correlates	Tests
Head		
Seeing (motor aspects)	oculomotor (III), trochlear (IV), abducens (VI) nerves and brainstem pathways, the cerebellum	extraocular movements
Eating		
chewing	trigeminal (V) and hypoglossal (XII) nerves	chewing, jaw opening, moving tongue
swallowing	glossopharyngeal (IX) and vagal (X) nerves	swallowing
Expressing	hypoglossal (XII) nerve	facial movements (eye closing, smile, frown)
Speaking		
articulating	facial (VII), glossopharyngeal (IX) vagal (X) and hypoglossal (X) nerves and the cerebellum	"ma," "la," "ca"
phonating	vagal (X) nerve	vocal sounds "ah," soft palate elevation

These functions involve 8 of the 12 cranial nerves

Body		
Walking	Cortex, basal, ganglia, pyramidal and extrapyramidal systems, cerebellum	observation of gait—arm swing, rhythm, symmetry, coordination
Activities of daily living	as above	muscle strength testing, assessment of bulk/tone, observation of movement excesses/deficits, (involuntary movements, bradykinesia)
Coordination—essential for normal execution of all voluntary movement	cerebellum	finger-nose, heel-shin, rapid alternating movements, tandem walking, Romberg

Developed by Judy Ozuna, R.N., M.N., CNRN, Clinical Assistant Professor, Dept. of Physiological Nursing, University of Washington, Seattle.

Note. From Konikow, N. (1985). Alterations in movement: Nursing assessment and implications. *Journal of Neuroscience Nursing, 17*(1), 61–65.

the client's sleep. Does the client appear to sleep soundly and quietly, or does the client appear restless and fitful during sleep? The length of time the client sleeps also can be noted. A knowledge of the stages of the sleep cycle can help the nurse assess whether a client is in REM or NREM sleep at certain times of the night. However, this may be difficult due to individual variation. Beyond this, it is difficult to assess the character and quality of an individual's sleep to any specific degree.

Sometimes clients report that they are not getting adequate sleep despite the fact that nurses or family members report that the client is sleeping. When this occurs, the nurse may need to assess the client's total sleep time more thoroughly. The nurse can ask the client to keep a log of daily activities and sleep patterns for several days. The log can provide cues about relationships of physical activity, number and length of naps, and major sleep periods. Asking the client about recent psychological stresses or new experiences will provide infor-

mation indicating any increased need for REM sleep. Any of these may account for the client's perception of having less than adequate sleep. If the client is hospitalized, the nurse can validate the reports of the client and family with hourly observations of the client and recording the time spent sleeping or napping. It is possible that the client is not considering frequent napping when reporting inadequate sleep. In addition, it is important for the nurse to assess these clients more closely for signs of sleep deprivation, which have been discussed earlier.

NURSING DIAGNOSES RELATED TO ACTIVITY–SLEEP

After the nurse has gathered information from the client, the nurse analyzes it to identify any problems related to activity–sleep. The nurse often will discover that if there are problems, they usually are interrelated.

A variety of nursing diagnoses related to activity–sleep is listed in Table 16-9. These nursing diagnoses are categorized in the North American Nursing Diagnosis Association, 1990 (NANDA) Taxonomy I under the human response pattern of "moving." An important diagnosis to consider for any hospitalized client would be the diagnosis of "sleep pattern disturbance." This diagnosis is used to describe the state in which an individual experiences disruption in the quantity or quality of the sleep pattern, thus causing discomfort. To support the diagnosis of a disturbance in the pattern of sleep, data from the nursing history and clinical appraisal may reflect a number of findings. The client most likely would report difficulty falling asleep, staying asleep, or returning to sleep after awakening. The lack of a good night's sleep can cause one to feel fatigued on awakening as well as to experience increased irritability. The client also may indicate napping during the day and that it helped to ease the feelings of tiredness. Physically, the client may complain of headaches and tremors and exhibit dark circles under the eyes. The nurse may have observed that the sleep of the client was fitful and restless and that the total number of hours slept had decreased from previous nights. Based on these defining characteristics, the nurse is able to identify a disturbance in sleep pattern and, through careful questioning of the client, determine the nature of the problem. To support a diagnosis of "impaired physical mobility," the nursing history and clinical appraisal would yield some different defining characteristics. This diagnosis describes the state in which an individual experiences limitations of physical movement because of inability or reluctance. Older adults may demonstrate limitations in physical movement as a result of the musculoskeletal changes associated with aging. Data probably would reflect limited range of motion, decreased muscle strength, and

possibly diminished muscle mass. An older client may be reluctant to be mobile because of such aging changes as diminished visual acuity, decreased depth perception, and difficulty hearing. In this instance, the older client may relate self-imposed restrictions on movement for fear of falling. While the client may exhibit some of the same physical symptoms as the client who limits mobility due to musculoskeletal changes, the cause differs. The nurse who is knowledgeable and skilled in the areas of history-taking and clinical appraisal will be able to distinguish differences and similarities and make the appropriate diagnosis.

When a client exhibits lethargy or listlessness, disinterest in surroundings, impaired ability to concentrate, increase in rest requirements, inability to restore energy even after sleeping and verbalizations of an overwhelming lack of energy, a nursing diagnosis of "fatigue" may be indicated. A variety of factors may be associated with fatigue, among them acute or chronic illness, certain medications, overwhelming role demands, and sleep disorders. Usually, the diagnosis of fatigue is not associated with one specific factor but a number of factors. "Because fatigue is subjective, its identification, extent and impact must be described by the client" (McFarland & McFarlane 1987, p. 374). Because many factors contribute to a diagnosis of fatigue, the nurse must take this into account when conducting the assessment.

The diagnosis of "potential activity intolerance" describes the state in which an individual is at risk of having insufficient physiological or psychological energy to endure or complete required or desired daily activities. Risk factors contributing to potential activity intolerance include such factors as sedentary life-style, chronic or progressive disease, pain, inexperience with activity, weight more than 15% over acceptable standard, expressions of disinterest in activity, or fatigue. This diagnosis deals with the fact that the client is at risk for developing activity intolerance. The nurse must therefore assess the client's current risk factors in order to develop the appropriate diagnosis (McFarland & McFarlane, 1987).

TABLE 16-9
Nursing Diagnosis Related to Activity–Sleep

Activity intolerance, potential for related to sedentary lifestyle or generalized weakness

Activity intolerance related to exertional discomfort or self-management deficit

Diversional activity, deficit related to long term hospitalization or environmental lack of diversional activity

Fatigue related to disrupted sleep or chronic pain

Mobility, impaired physical related to limited range of motion or decreased muscle strength

Sleep pattern disturbance related to hospitalization, emotional stress or nocturia

Chapter Highlights

■   To engage in activity, one needs to have the capacity for mobility (intact neuromuscular system or compensated movement), the motivation to move, and a free, nonrestrictive environment in which to move.

■   The musculoskeletal system provides the structure, support, and protection for movement, and the central nervous system provides the neural innervation.

■　Mobility is important to an individual's self-image and self-esteem, providing a means for self-expression and a socially acceptable outlet for aggression and tension.

■　Environmental aspects, such as physical barriers, assistive devices, safety factors, available support systems, and community resources, must be considered in evaluating an individual's mobility.

■　Physical activity, exercise, and physical fitness describe different concepts, but they often are confused and used interchangeably.

■　When a client's normal activity patterns are altered, the nurse can anticipate that certain physiological, psychological, and environmental effects will occur.

■　Nonrapid eye movement sleep (NREM, Stages I–IV) rests and restores the body while rapid eye movement sleep (REM) appears to be important for coping, memory, and learning.

■　An individual's sleep patterns and total sleep requirements vary throughout the life span.

■　Such factors as health, culture, environment, exercise, naps, drug use, stress, medications, work schedule, and lifestyle can affect an individual's activity–sleep patterns.

■　Inspection and palpation are the primary methods used in the clinical appraisal of the musculoskeletal system.

■　The findings from the history and clinical appraisal enable the nurse to develop appropriate nursing diagnoses related to activity–sleep.

Practice Activities

1. Using the activity–sleep history (Table 16-4), systematically collect data to assess the activity-sleep patterns of another student or family member.
2. Role-play to obtain an activity–sleep history from the following clients:
   a. Mother of an infant who has come for a regular 6-week checkup.
   b. A 26-year-old pregnant woman during her third trimester.
   c. A 75-year-old gentleman who has come for an annual examination.
3. Complete an assessment of activity–sleep patterns on two clients with differing health problems (e.g., rheumatoid arthritis, chronic obstructive pulmonary disease, depression). Compare the two assessments. What nursing diagnoses are indicated?
4. Perform a clinical appraisal on an immobilized client and assess for alterations in the following areas:
   a. muscle strength and tone
   b. joint mobility
   c. bowel and bladder status
   d. skin integrity
   e. sensory and perceptual integrity
   f. respiratory status
   g. cardiovascular status (dependent edema, orthostatic hypotension, and thrombosis)
   h. activity tolerance
   i. psychosocial and developmental changes
5. Using the neutral zero method described in this chapter, measure and record another student's range of motion for the following joints: neck, shoulder, elbow, wrist, fingers, toes, ankle, knee, hip, spine.
6. Document in writing a clinical appraisal of the musculoskeletal system of a client. What conclusions can you draw? Indicate appropriate nursing diagnoses.

Recommended Readings

Clapin-French, E. (1986). Sleep patterns of aged persons in long-term care facilities. *Journal of Advances in Nursing Science, 11*, 57–66.

Dishman, R., Sallis, J., & Orenstein, D. (1985). The determinants of physical activity and exercise. *Public Health Reports, 100*(2), 158–171.

Goodmote, E. (1985). Sleep deprivation in the hospitalized patient. *Orthopedic Nursing, 4*, 33–35.

Jordan-Marsh, N. (1985). Development of a tool for diagnosing changes in concern about exercise: A means of enhancing compliance. *Nursing Research, 34*(2), 103–107.

Kavey, N., & Anderson, D. (1986). Why every patient needs a good night's sleep. *RN, 49*(2), 16–20.

Pressman, N.R., & Fry, M. (1988). What is normal sleep in the elderly? *Clinics in Geriatric Medicine, 4*, 71–81.

Snyder-Halpern, R., & Verran, J. (1987). Instrumentation to describe subjective sleep characteristics in healthy subjects. *Research in Nursing and Health, 10*, 155–163.

Taylor, C., Sallis, J., & Needle, R. (1985). The relationship between physical activity and exercise and mental health. *Public Health Reports, 100*(2), 195–202.

Weaner, T., & Millman, R.P. (1986). Broken sleep. *American Journal of Nursing, 86*(2), 146–150.

References

Bahr, T. (1983). Sleep-wake patterns in the aged. *Journal of Gerontological Nursing, 9*, 534–593.

Barr, M., & Kiernan, J. (1983). *The human nervous system: An anatomical viewpoint* (64th ed.). Philadelphia: Harper & Row.

Grimes, J., & Burns, E. (1987). *Health assessment in nursing practice* (2nd ed.). Boston: Jones and Bartlett.

Caspersen, C., Powell, K., & Christenson, G. (1985). Physical activity, exercise and physical fitness: Definitions and distinctions for health related research. *Public Health Reports, 100*(2), 126–130.

Closs, S.J. (1988). Assessment of sleep in hospitalized patients: A review of methods. *Journal of Advanced Nursing, 13*, 501–510.

Dawber, T.R. (1973). Risk factors in young adults: The lessons from epidemiologic studies of cardio-vascular disease. Framingham, Tecumseh and Evans County. *Journal of the American College of Health Associations, 22*, 84–95.

Fass, G. (1971). Sleep, drugs, and dreams. *American Journal of Nursing, 71*, 2316.

Goldberg, W., & Fitzpatrick, J. (1980). Movement therapy with the aged. *Nursing Research, 29*(6), 339–346.

Gordon, M. (1976). Assessing activity tolerance. *American Journal of Nursing, 76*, 72–75.

Hayter, J. (1983). Sleep behaviors of older persons. *Nursing Research, 32*, 242.

Hayter, J. (1985). To nap or not to nap? *Geriatric Nursing, 6*(2), 104–106.

Hodges, L., & Callihan, C. (1988). Human mobility: An overview. In P. Mitchell, L. Hodges, M. Muwaswes, & C. Wallack (Eds.), *AANN's neuroscience nursing: Phenomena and practice* (pp. 269–281). Norwalk, CT: Appleton and Lange.

Hollerbach, A. (1988). Assessment of human mobility. In P. Mitchell, L. Hodges, M. Muwaswes, & C. Wallack (Eds.), *AANN's neuroscience nursing: Phenomena and practice* (pp. 283–302). Norwalk, CT: Appleton and Lange.

Kales, A., Beall, G., Berger, R.J., Heuser, G., Jacobsen, A., Kales, J., Parmelee, A.H., & Walter, R.D. (1968). Sleep and dreams: Recent research in clinical aspects. *Annals of Internal Medicine, 68*, 1078–1104.

Kleitman, N. (1963). *Sleep and wakefulness.* Chicago: University of Chicago Press.

Konikow, N. (1985). Alterations in movement: Nursing assessment and implications. *Journal of Neurosurgical Nursing, 17*(1), 61–65.

Lukasiewicz-Ferland, P. (1987). When your ICU patient can't sleep. *Nursing 87', 17*(11), 51–53.

McFarland, G., & McFarlane, E. (1987). *Nursing diagnosis and intervention.* St. Louis: Mosby.

Miller, C. (1990). *Nursing care of the older adult.* Glenview, IL: Scott, Foresman.

Mitchell, P., Ozuna, J., Cammermeyer, M., & Woods, N.F. (Eds.). (1984). *Neurological assessment for nursing practice.* Reston, VA: Reston Publishing.

Office of the Assistant Secretary for Health (1990). *Healthy people 2000: National health promotion and disease prevention objectives.* (DHHS Publication No. PHS 91-50213). Washington, DC: U.S. Government Printing Office.

Olson, E. (1967). The hazards of immobility. *American Journal of Nursing, 67*, 779–797.

Pagliaro, A., & Pagliaro, L. (1986). *Pharmacologic aspects of nursing.* St. Louis: Mosby.

Pender, N. (1982). *Health promotion in nursing practice.* Norwalk, CT: Appleton and Lange.

Rose, C.L., & Cohen, M.L. (1977). Relative importance of physical activity for longevity. *Annuals of the New York Academy of Science, 301*, 671–702.

Ross, N.M., Hare, K., & McPherson, M. (1985). When sleep won't come: Helping our elderly clients. *The Canadian Nurse, 82*(9), 14–18.

Rubin, M. (1988). The physiology of bedrest. *American Journal of Nursing, 88*(1), 50–58.

Smith, P., & Wedderburn, Z. (1980). Sleep, body rhythms and shiftwork. *Nursing: The Add-On Journal of Clinical Nursing, 1*, 889–892.

Warner, D. (1988). Walking to better health. *American Journal of Nursing, 88*(1), 64–66.

17

Oxygenation Assessment

CHAPTER OUTLINE

- Knowledge Needed to Assess Oxygenation
  Structures of the Respiratory System
  Structures of the Cardiovascular System
- Variables That Influence Oxygenation
  Age Race Health Status
- The Oxygenation History
- Clinical Appraisal and Screening
  Inspection Palpation Percussion Auscultation Laboratory Data
- Nursing Diagnoses Related to Oxygenation

OBJECTIVES

Upon completion of this chapter, you should be able to:

- Describe the purposes and essential components of the oxygenation assessment.
- Collect subjective information related to oxygenation using the nursing history.
- Perform a clinical appraisal of a client's oxygenation.
- Use the results of selected laboratory and diagnostic screening tests to validate the oxygenation assessment.
- Modify the assessment of oxygenation according to the client's age and health, and with consideration of racial differences.
- Formulate valid and appropriate nursing diagnoses for clients with actual or potential alterations in oxygenation.

Oxygenation is a dynamic process involving the transportation of oxygen to all body parts and the removal of carbon dioxide. Atmospheric oxygen enters the lungs, where it is picked up by the blood and carried throughout the body by a complex and extensive vascular network. The heart serves as the pump that propels the blood throughout the vascular system and through the lungs, where the actual oxygen–carbon dioxide exchange occurs.

Although the assessment of all body systems is essential to competent nursing practice, the value of the ability to assess oxygenation cannot be overstated. In no other area does the nurse's ability to observe, examine, synthesize information, and intervene effectively have such great potential influence on life or death.

One purpose of oxygenation assessment is to determine the client's ability to maintain adequate oxygen levels throughout the body. Understanding the physiological basis of oxygenation is essential to thorough assessment of oxygenation. The nurse also systematically assesses oxygenation to detect any actual or potential interferences that may compromise the client's well-being and place the client at risk for disability or death.

KNOWLEDGE NEEDED TO ASSESS OXYGENATION

Oxygenation is accomplished by the combined functions of the pulmonary and cardiovascular systems. The functions of the pulmonary system consist of (1) ventilation, the mechanical and physical process by which oxygen moves from the atmosphere into the lung (alveolar) spaces, and (2) diffusion of oxygen across the alveolar membrane into the pulmonary capillary network. At this point the circulatory system takes over. The diffused oxygen binds with hemoglobin to form oxyhemoglobin and is transported in this form by the red blood cells (erythrocytes) throughout the vascular network of the body. Successful completion of this task requires adequate numbers of viable blood cells; patent, elastic vessels; and a reliable pumping mechanism. Each of these factors is discussed in greater detail later.

At the cellular level, an additional diffusion process takes place. Oxygen leaves the red blood cells by dissociating from the hemoglobin and crosses into the body cells, where it provides energy to support cellular and tissue functions. The elimination of carbon dioxide (CO_2) is accomplished by the same diffusion process, only in reverse. The carbon dioxide diffuses from the body cells into the venous capillary network. Some CO_2 dissolves in the plasma, other amounts react with water to form carbonic acid, and some enters the red blood cells. Within the red blood cells, carbon dioxide either dissolves and forms carbamine compounds, or when catalyzed by carbonic anhydrase, forms bicarbonate and hydrogen ions.

The bicarbonate formed by catalysis then exchanges with chloride ions in the plasma, thus increasing the amount of carbon dioxide transported in some form by the plasma. Sixty percent of all carbon dioxide in the blood is transported in the plasma as bicarbonate (Guyton, 1990). Carbon dioxide then is transported to the pulmonary capillaries, where it diffuses in gaseous form through the alveolar membrane and is propelled by expiration from the lung spaces through the respiratory airway into the atmosphere.

Structures of the Respiratory System

Ventilation can be accomplished only when the respiratory structures are intact. Structures of the upper airway include the nasal passages, nasopharynx, and pharynx, which opens into the trachea, or windpipe. The functions of the upper airway include warming and humidifying inspired air by means of secretions from the mucous membranes. Fine hairlike cilia that line these passages filter particulate matter from the air.

Air then passes through the oropharynx and enters the larynx, which is constructed of cartilage and contains the vocal chords. The larynx is capped by the epiglottis, which covers the larynx during swallowing to prevent the aspiration of food. The epiglottis, tonsils, and vocal cords also assume great importance in the assessment, as they are primary sites of respiratory obstructive conditions—especially in the young. Below the larynx, the trachea—a slender tubular structure constructed of C-shaped cartilaginous rings—extends downward and branches into the right and left main bronchi. These in turn carry air into the right and left lungs. Smaller segmental bronchi carry this air through smaller and smaller bronchioles until it reaches the alveolar sacs, where oxygen–carbon dioxide exchange takes place. The structures of the trachea and bronchi often are called the tracheobronchial tree.

Respiration is regulated by the respiratory center, located in the medulla oblongata. This center is triggered by the concentration of CO_2 in the arterial circulation. Excess amounts of CO_2 stimulate chemoreceptors that proportionally increase the respiratory rate to "blow off" the CO_2. Peripheral receptors in the aortic and carotid bodies respond to drops in O_2 levels by stimulating the glossopharyngeal, vagus, and phrenic nerve fibers that innervate the diaphragm, thus increasing alveolar ventilation.

Structures of the Cardiovascular System

The cardiovascular system carries oxygen from the alveolar exchange site to the areas of cellular exchange. Several mechanisms interrelate to facilitate this process. The heart serves as the pump, and circulation maintains blood pressure and supports the viability of blood components.

With the pumping action of the heart, blood circulates through two distinct circulatory systems—the systemic circuit and the pulmonary circuit. Movement through both of these circuits is essential to the pickup of available oxygen and its subsequent delivery to peripheral tissues.

The heart is a four-chambered organ with two atria and two ventricles. The contraction of the two ventricles supplies the force to push blood through both the pulmonary and the systemic systems. Venous blood returns from the systemic circuit via the inferior and superior vena cavae and empties into the right atrium, subsequently passing into the right ventricle. With contraction, the blood then is pumped into the main pulmonary artery and into the pulmonary circulation. Oxygenated blood from the pulmonary exchange is returned to the left atrium via the pulmonary veins. It then passes into the left ventricle and with contraction flows into the aorta and throughout the systemic circulation.

The period of time from the end of one contraction to the end of the next is called the cardiac cycle. The spontaneous generation of an action potential in the sinoatrial (SA) node initiates the cycle. This impulse then travels to the atrioventricular (AV) node, stimulating ventricular contraction. A slight delay between atrial and ventricular stimulation enables the ventricles to fill with blood from the atria prior to their contraction.

The phase of contraction, when blood is sent into the systemic circulation, is called the systolic phase; the phase of relaxation, or period of ventricular filling, is called the diastolic phase.

During the cardiac cycle, the heart produces sounds, which when heard through a stethoscope take on the characteristic lupp-dupp sound. The relationship between the heart sounds and the electrocardiogram (EKG) is depicted in Figure 17-1. The first heart sound (S_1 or lupp) is heard at the onset of systole and represents the closing of the mitral and tricuspid valves. While the mitral valve closes slightly before the tricuspid valve, S_1 usually is heard as one sound (Figure 17-1).

The second heart sound is caused by the closing of the aortic and pulmonic valves and represents the beginning of ventricular diastole (Figure 17-1). Because the events on the right side of the heart are slightly slower than those on the left side, the aortic valve closes slightly before the pulmonic valve. Usually, this too is heard as one sound (S_2 or dupp). During inspiration, however, the closing of both valves may be audible (physiological split S_2), due to the changes in pressure gradient between the right and left sides of the heart.

A third heart sound (S_3) occurs early in diastole shortly after S_2 (Figure 17-1). This sound is produced by rapid ventricular filling when the volume of early filling is increased or there is a decrease in the compliance of the ventricles. A physiological S_3 commonly is found in children and young adults. It may be heard until the age of 40. It is also a common finding during the last trimester of pregnancy. However, when it is heard in the adult over 40, it usually is pathological. In this instance, S_3 also is referred to as the ventricular gallop.

A fourth heart sound (S_4) occurs late in diastole just before S_1 (Figure 17-1). This sound is caused by the final ejection of blood from the atria into a noncompliant ventricle. It occasionally is heard in a normal individual, especially an older person. However, it usually is seen in individuals who have some degree of cardiomyopathy such as in hypertension. In this instance S_4 is referred to as the atrial gallop.

These four sounds form the basic four heart sounds of which S_1 and S_2 are the most audible and distinct. Additional sounds, known as extra sounds, may be found on cardiac examination. Some are made by the opening of valves (which usually open noiselessly) as in the case of an opening snap (audible opening of the mitral valve). Inflammation of the pericardial sac can produce a pericardial friction rub, which can easily be mistaken for a heart sound. A further type of extra sound is a murmur. A murmur is indicative of some disruption of blood flow in the heart. The sound of a murmur is prolonged compared with that of a heart sound. A murmur can occur in systole, diastole, or both (*timing,* see p. 535). A systolic murmur may or may not be pathological. For example, the so-called innocent murmur is a functional murmur that does not present a problem for the client. Diastolic murmurs always are pathological and should, therefore, be evaluated.

In addition to timing, murmurs are described according to location, radiation, pitch, quality and loudness or intensity. *Location* refers to the area of the precordium where the murmur is heard. Some murmurs are confined to a specific area. Others are

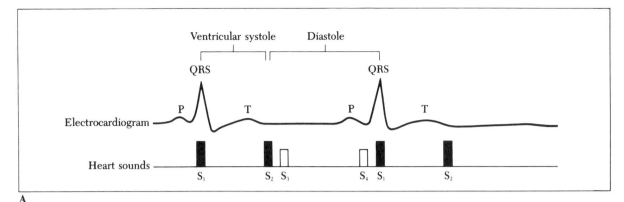

A

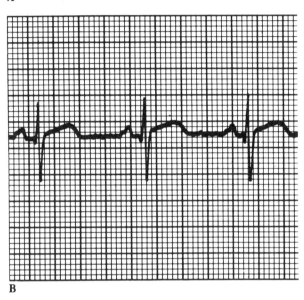

B

FIGURE 17-1. (A) Heart Sounds in Relation to the Cardiac Cycle. (B) The Electrocardiogram (EKG).

more diffuse and heard over the entire precordium. Murmurs may radiate to other areas such as the carotids (murmur of mitral stenosis) or to the axilla (murmur of mitral regurgitation).

The *quality* of a murmur describes such characteristics as musical, harsh, or blowing. The velocity or force of the blood flow determines the *pitch* of a murmur. Murmurs that are high pitched have a greater velocity and those that are low pitched have a lower velocity.

The *intensity* of a murmur describes the loudness of the murmur. The use of the following six-point grading scale is helpful in documenting intensity (Grimes & Burns 1987, p. 269):

I Is difficult to hear; experienced examiner and quiet environment are needed

II Is not readily heard upon laying stethoscope on chest; examiner must listen closely to hear

III Requires no effort to hear and is readily heard when stethoscope is placed on chest

IV Is accompanied by a thrill (vibration); loud enough that there is no question of its presence

V Can be heard with stethoscope held an inch away from chest; thrill present

VI Does not require use of stethoscope to hear; thrill present

The heart is innervated by both sympathetic and parasympathetic nerves. These nerves, according to Guyton (1990), affect cardiac pumping in two ways: by changing the heart rate and by changing the strength of the contraction of the heart. Stress, physical exertion, and chemical changes throughout the body affect heart action by these mechanisms.

The heart rate of an adult at rest averages 70 to 75 beats per minute. The amount of blood pumped from the ventricles with each beat (stroke volume) ranges from 70 to 80 ml. By multiplying the stroke volume by the number of beats per minute (i.e., 80 ml $\times$ 72 bpm = 5,760 ml), it is possible to determine the volume of blood pumped into the systemic circulation per minute. An equal amount is simultaneously pumped into the pulmonary circuit. These two amounts together comprise the total per minute cardiac output.

With each pumping action of the heart a pulsation or vascular expansion occurs in arteries throughout the body because of the expansion and rebound of these blood vessels. This expansion and rebound is called the pulse and may be palpated at varying locations throughout the body (see chap. 14).

The volume of blood within the circulatory system usually remains fairly constant and exerts a force against the walls of the vessels that carry it. This internal vascular pressure, referred to as the blood pressure, will vary with the strength of the heartbeat. During ventricular systole there is a marked rise in pressure that is called the systolic pressure. It is normally equal to 120 mm Hg at its maximum. During ventricular diastole this pressure falls to a lower diastolic pressure. This diastolic pressure represents the constant intravascular pressure and approximates 80 mm Hg (see chap. 14).

According to Grollman (1974), five important factors are responsible for maintaining normal arterial blood pressures:

1. *Heart action*, which influences cardiac output as well as the resulting energy supply

2. *Blood volume*, since blood pressure is directly proportional to the volume

3. The *peripheral resistance* or frictional resistance of the vessels through which blood passes.

4. The *physical properties* of the walls of large blood vessels

5. The *viscosity* of the blood—the greater the viscosity the more resistance to the flow.

VARIABLES THAT INFLUENCE OXYGENATION

Because a client's age, race, and health can influence oxygenation, it is important to collect pertinent information on these aspects in a comprehensive assessment.

Age

The nurse needs to consider the influence of age on the client's oxygenation. Age-specific influences on oxygenation in the adult are detailed in this chapter. The reader is referred to chapters 20 to 23 for specific information on oxygenation of clients in other age groups.

By adulthood, the organs involved in oxygenation have achieved their maximum growth. The issues then become those of maintaining adequate functioning in spite of physical changes and environmental influences. Smoking has been linked strongly to cardiovascular disease as well as to lung cancer. A diet high in saturated fats may lead to premature degenerative diseases in the blood vessels and may predispose the client to obesity, another high risk factor for heart problems. The work environment also may contribute to chronic changes in respiratory tissue, especially if the client works in an industrial or highly polluted area. These influences should be noted by the nurse.

As the adult becomes older the lungs change again. Efficiency in expelling air is lost, which results in incomplete emptying of the lungs and a reduced vital capacity. The chest wall also loses some of its elasticity, limiting its expansion and thereby decreasing the ability of the lung to exchange gases.

Although very little change is seen in the heart itself, the coronary arteries narrow because of increased fatty deposits. This reduces blood flow to the heart muscle, thereby increasing the possibility of a myocardial infarction. Research has shown that sedentary older individuals demonstrate a 19 to 20% greater decline in maximum oxygen uptake than do individuals of the same age who remain active (Wei & Gersh, 1987). A variety of factors, including inactivity, can contribute to physical deconditioning and thus place an individual at increased risk of poor cardiovascular functioning (Miller, 1990).

It is important to consider that the maximum level of respiratory performance in the middle and older adult years is greatly influenced by the maximum level of respiratory performance reached during the second decade of life (Sparrow & Weiss, 1988). If the maximum level was high, then the older individual can tolerate a "greater degree of age-related changes and risk factors before experiencing respiratory dysfunction" (Miller, 1990, p. 336). In contrast, if the maximum level was low, respiratory symptoms may appear with only minimal evidence of age-related changes (Miller, 1990).

Race

Clients who are dark-skinned may require certain modifications in the oxygenation assessment, since skin color is a major indicator of oxygenation. These modifications are discussed in detail in Chapter 14.

In addition, clients of certain racial groups are statistically at risk for specific health problems that directly interfere with oxygenation. In particular, black clients are at risk for sickle cell disease, an inherited autosomal recessive defect of the red blood cells (RBCs) that alters oxygen-carrying capability. Instead of the typical smooth circular shape, the RBCs are changed under conditions of low oxygen tension, acidosis, and dehydration into rigid crescent-shaped cells (Guyton, 1990). These "sickle" cells have a much shorter life expectancy than normal cells. Because of their shape, they move poorly through the vascular network, causing localized obstruction with oxygen deprivation and pain.

Sickle cell disease is found almost exclusively in blacks and is manifested in one of two variations, either sickle cell trait or sickle cell disease (Rooks & Pack, 1983). It is very important that carriers of the sickle cell trait be identified so that the risk associated with their having children can be considered carefully. To help accomplish this, screening programs have been initiated in community settings and massive public education programs have been instituted.

Various tests exist to help screen the population for this condition. A blood smear may reveal sickle cells or, if the smear is deprived of oxygen by means of a cover slip, sickling may be precipitated. In the Sickledex test, anticoagulated blood is suspended in a solution. If sickled hemoglobin is present, the solution turns cloudy. Since this is a simple and quick procedure, usually accomplished by a fingerstick, it is probably the most commonly used screening measure. Both of these procedures are screening measures only and are not used to actually diagnose the carrier or disease. Hemoglobin electrophoresis is the most accurate method of diagnosing abnormalities in hemoglobin. This procedure usually is reserved for use with those clients who have a positive blood smear or Sickledex test, since hemoglobin electrophoresis actually diagnoses the disease.

Any black child who is brought to a health-care facility with reported random joint and abdominal pain, fever, anorexia, general weakness, and small stature should be tested immediately for sickle cell disease.

Health Status

A number of health problems may affect oxygenation status. Hypertension, ischemic heart disease, and chronic obstructive pulmonary disease are among the leading health problems.

Hypertension

Hypertension menaces 20 to 25 million Americans, producing premature sickness, disability, and death. It is a massive health threat, with as many as 50 percent of those affected being undiagnosed and untreated. In screening for hypertension the recommendations of the American Heart Association should be utilized. These guidelines recommend an age-related definition of hypertension. For persons under the age of 40 years a pressure of 140/90 or greater is indicative; for those over the age of 40 years, 160/95 or greater. The World Health Organization also indicates 160/90 mm Hg as the upper limit of normal. One high blood pressure reading does not necessarily indicate hypertension. Situational stress, drugs, or physical activity can cause significant variations and elevations. However, any significant elevation should have a follow-up check.

Long, Winslow, Scheuhing and Callihan (1976) developed guidelines a number of years ago that are still used to document actual hypertension:

> Take blood pressure with the client in a sitting position on three different occasions at least one week apart.

Reevaluate as an outpatient any normotensive hospitalized client suspected of having elevated pressure, because bedrest reduces blood pressure.

Consider any hospitalized client hypertensive if three out of four diastolic pressures are greater than 100 mm Hg on two consecutive days.

Reevaluate pregnant women 6 weeks after delivery.

Reevaluate women suspected of hypertension while taking birth control pills after they have used some other form of contraception for from 4 to 6 months, because oral contraceptives may elevate blood pressure.

The presence of other risk factors such as smoking, obesity, excessive use of sodium, presence of concurrent diabetes or hyperlipidemia, and high stress in the hypertensive client should be screened for as well. Hypertension, at present, is more prevalent in males and members of the black race although figures for women are increasing.

The National Task Force on Nursing in High Blood Pressure Control emphasized some years ago that "since nursing provides the greatest percentage of direct care given to consumers, [nurses] have frequent opportunities for case finding, for educating consumers to maximize participation in their own health care and for assuring followup and continuity. . . ." (Robinson 1976, p. 779). Although many parts of the country have implemented very active screening programs since then, it is strongly suggested that *nurses, in whatever health care setting, check the blood pressure of each and every client no matter for what reason health care is sought.*

Ischemic Heart Disease

If blood vessels are narrowed due to age or existing vascular disease, the oxygen-carrying capacity is subsequently reduced. This reduction in oxygen is called *ischemia*. The most common causes of ischemia are arteriosclerosis and atherosclerosis. In arteriosclerosis the vessels become narrowed and thickened by calcium deposits, thereby decreasing elasticity and oxygen-carrying capacity. This condition is commonly associated with the peripheral vessels.

Atherosclerosis on the other hand, is usually associated with a buildup of adherent fat within the lumen of the vessels. This may eventually cause obstruction and primarily affects the coronary vessels and the aorta. Adults with elevated cholesterol and triglyceride levels are more at risk for ischemic heart disease.

If the causes of ischemia are not held in check, arterial disease may result. Coronary artery disease persists as the number one killer of adults in the United States. If the coronary arteries are temporarily obstructed, cutting off blood flow to the myocardium, the oxygen deprivation causes an intense crushing chest pain that may radiate to the left neck, jaw, and arm. The client may also experience a choking feeling. This pain, known as *angina pectoris*, is relieved by the sublingual administration of nitroglycerin.

Total occlusion of a coronary artery results in a myocardial infarction. Tissue anoxia and necrosis result, causing a disruption in the electrical functioning of the heart. A myocardial infarction produces a similar crushing substernal chest pain, also radiating predominantly to the left arm, but is not relieved by nitroglycerin. The client is pale, diaphoretic, and dyspneic. Intense activity usually accompanies and compounds the other symptoms. The damage to the myocardium weakens the contractile force of the heart, leading to increased heart rate and decreased blood pressure as a compensatory measure.

In assessing for a myocardial infarction the nurse should be aware of several additional signs. EKG changes and elevations in blood enzyme levels such as SGOT, LDH, and CPK are indicative of tissue damage and should be continuously monitored during the initial infarction period and for several days afterward. The erythrocyte sedimentation rate and white blood cell count may also rise because of tissue destruction.

Peripheral arterial disease may take several forms but usually demonstrates some measure of local ischemia. Arteriosclerosis may produce obstruction in the extremities. Symptoms that indicate arteriosclerotic obstruction include coldness of the extremities, diminished peripheral pulses, pallor, and cyanosis of the extremities. Pain and muscle cramping, especially at night, may also occur.

In young women, spasms of the arteries, called Raynaud's disease, may cause blanching and numbness in the extremities. In young men, Buerger's disease (thromboangiitis obliterans) causes inflammation of the arteries and veins resulting in localized ischemia. Coldness, numbness, and tingling of the extremities are usually present. Muscle cramps occurring after exercise (intermittent claudication) are due to the ischemia and are relieved by rest.

Chronic Obstructive Pulmonary Disease

Chronic obstructive pulmonary disease (COPD) is the most common chronic pulmonary disease. The term refers to a group of progressive, debilitating lung conditions. COPD is common in residents of highly polluted urban areas, and those from low socioeconomic classes. The lung pathology of COPD is characterized by lower airway obstruction and resistance to air flow. Cigarette smoking is considered highly contributory.

Chronic bronchitis is an inflammation of the bronchi due to infection or chronic irritation. A cough, thought to be a smoker's cough, may be the first symptom noted. There is also a concomitant history of frequent upper respiratory infections. With progression of the disease, coughing becomes more frequent and is associated with expectoration of larger and larger amounts of sputum, especially in the early morning and at night. Symptoms also intensify in cold, damp air. Eventually extensive pulmonary insufficiency develops.

Emphysema is an enlargement of the alveoli related to destructive changes in the alveolar walls impairing gas diffusion. It is a physiologic response to recurrent infection and inflammation, with edema, exudate release, and ultimate fibrosis of lung tissue. These destructive responses cause narrowing of the air passages with air trapping and hyperinflation. Symptoms include dyspnea on exertion and breathlessness. In more advanced stages, anorexia and weight loss are common. It is commonly seen in the older age group. Respiratory tract infections are common.

In assessing the client with suspected COPD the nurse should pay special attention to the history of coughing and should elicit information regarding the amount, type, and consistency of the sputum. Fatigability needs to be ascertained as well as the ability for self-care in activities of daily living. The amount of respiratory compromise can be assessed by acquiring information related to respiratory effort and presence of wheezing. The past history of the client's health status should include a family history of respiratory conditions such as asthma and hay fever. Data should be collected regarding smoking habits as well as possible occupational exposures to irritants, allergens, and pesticides.

The client should be observed for a barrel-shaped chest. Are accessory muscles being used, or does the expiratory phase seem prolonged? In advanced COPD, clubbing of the fingers may be present, and pursed-lip breathing is common. The client may lean forward with hands propped to assist respiratory effort.

Chest x-rays reveal hyperinflation, prominent pulmonary artery markings, and in the later stages, right ventricular hypertrophy. Sputum is thick and tenacious, with bacteria present during recurrent infections. Pulmonary function studies will show an increase in lung capacity and residual volume, and a decrease in vital capacity and forced expiratory volume. Arterial blood gases reflect a normal PaO_2 at rest which falls somewhat with exertion. $PaCO_2$ is normal at rest, elevating as the airways become more obstructed.

Many acute and chronic illnesses have varying effects on the oxygenation status of the body. If the nurse is alert and applies appropriate assessment techniques, many of these can be detected early in their course and treated effectively. The history is the vital tool to identify these conditions and lead to initiation of planning appropriate care.

THE OXYGENATION HISTORY

The oxygenation assessment is to a great extent dependent upon the quality of the information obtained from the nursing history. The nurse can begin with a question to elicit the client's perceptions about cardiovascular and respiratory functioning. For example, the nurse may ask, "Tell me about your breathing." If the client identifies a problem, the nurse can gather more detailed information with more specific questions such as, "How often do you experience wheezing?" and, "What do you do to help alleviate the problem?" If the client says there are no problems, the nurse should systematically review with the client any potential areas for concern.

A thorough respiratory history should include documentation of any past or current respiratory problems:

Has the client experienced any breathing difficulties, such as changes in respiratory rate, depth, or character?

What factors precipitate breathing difficulties?

What does the client do to alleviate the problem (e.g., rest, positioning, medications)? For example, how many pillows does the client use for sleeping?

Does the client use a vaporizer or humidifier?

More specifically, the nurse should ascertain if the client has experienced any shortness of breath (dyspnea), wheezing, stridor, or retractions (use of accessory muscles). Has the client ever had asthma, croup, bronchitis, pneumonia, tuberculosis, or other major respiratory illnesses?

The nurse also should ask about the number of colds or respiratory infections, including otitis media, that the client has had within the past year. How were these treated? Did they linger or respond rapidly to treatment? The presence of a cough should be noted, as well as time of occurrence. Is it productive or nonproductive of sputum? If productive, what type of sputum is produced? Sputum color and consistency should be noted. Is the cough high-pitched or low? Can it be characterized as harsh, or croupy and barky? Is it accompanied by pain? Has the client experienced any hemoptysis (blood in the sputum)?

The nurse should also ask if the client has ever had a chest x-ray and its results (if known).

Environmental factors that may contribute to respiratory problems are important components of the history.

Does the client smoke? If so, what (cigarettes, cigars, pipe, marijuana)? For how many years? How much (e.g., number of packs per day)?

Do other family members smoke?

Is the client routinely (or seasonally) exposed to airborne allergens, such as pollen, or industrial air pollution?

Does the client's occupation increase the likelihood of respiratory difficulty; for example, coal mining, painting, or building construction? Such occupational experiences may compromise oxygenation through prolonged exposure to chemicals or particular inhalants.

The oxygenation history (see Table 17-1) should include questions related to cardiac and circulatory function. Any previous or existing cardiovascular problems, such as hypertension or arrhythmia, should be noted, including prescribed treatment and the client's response. Does the client follow the prescribed regimen? If not, what reasons for noncompliance can the client identify (knowledge deficit, unacceptable effect on lifestyle, economic reasons)?

Has the client ever experienced episodes of chest or epigastric pain? The client should be asked to describe the pain according to quality, location, and intensity. Does the client ever experience palpitations or cyanosis? If so, when do these occur? Are any of these episodes (pain, palpitations, cyanosis) precipitated by eating, exercise, exertion, or emotional stress? What does the client do to alleviate these manifestations?

Vascular problems, such as varicosities, a history of thrombophlebitis, or severe headaches, should be noted. In addition, the nurse should inquire whether the client has ever experienced anemia or prolonged bleeding episodes. Does the client bruise easily or tire quickly?

Because a number of hereditary and lifestyle factors may increase the client's risk for impaired

TABLE 17-1
Oxygenation History

Client's Usual Pattern of Respiration
  Character of breathing pattern
  Presence of allergies?
    Type
    Symptoms
    Frequency of occurrence
    Occurrence of wheezing

Does the Client Smoke or Chew Tobacco?
  Number of years of smoking
  Number of packs or amount chewed per day

Recent Changes in Breathing Pattern?
  Symptoms
  Onset (sudden or gradual)
  Associated with any other symptoms?
  What helps to ease the problem?
  What makes it worse?
  Is breathing painful?

Past History of Respiratory Problems
  Infections
    Type
    Frequency
    Treatment

Cough
  Recent or longstanding (how long)?
  How often and how much?
  Character of the cough (dry, hacking, wet)
  Is the cough productive or nonproductive of sputum?
  Character of the sputum
    Color

  Viscosity (fluid, thick or tenacious)
  Amount of sputum (estimate)
  Presence of odor

Shortness of Breath (Dyspnea)
  Continual or intermittent?
  Associated with activity?
  What helps to ease the problem?
  What makes it worse/better?
  Occurrence of any other symptoms?
  Affected by different positions?

Stress
  Perception of level of stress?
  Usual method of coping with stress?
  Perception of coping abilities?

Medication
  Current listing of prescription and over-the-counter
    drugs
  Purpose for use
  Length of time taking medication
  Observed side effects

Pulmonary Risk Factors
  Family history of hypertension, lung cancer, or
    other cardiopulmonary conditions
  Client history of hypertension, lung cancer, or other
    cardiopulmonary conditions

Environmental Influences
  Work setting (use of chemicals or gases)
  Air pollution
  Exposure to radiation

oxygenation, the nurse should inquire about them. Among these risk factors are:

> Middle age or older
>
> Family history of heart disease, hypertension, cerebrovascular accident
>
> Overweight or obesity
>
> Diet high in saturated fats
>
> Elevated serum cholesterol or triglycerides
>
> Sedentary lifestyle
>
> Smoking

In addition to the above factors, people who have a "Type A" personality are considered at risk for oxygenation interferences (see chap. 11). This personality type has been characterized as driven and competitive; Type As are said to be achievers who work, more often than not, under intense pressures. The nursing history, therefore, should include information about how the client handles stress. Many stressful situations, if the client has not learned techniques for handling them, may cause cardiovascular manifestations such as hyperventilation, nervousness, tremors, diaphoresis, elevated blood pressure, tachycardia, and palpitations. Information about precipitating events and the client's response is helpful in making a valid assessment.

The client's rest pattern also should be ascertained (see chap. 16). Occasional wakefulness may be caused by situational stress, but occurrences of sudden nighttime dyspnea or the inability to sleep in a reclining position may indicate compromised oxygenation.

A careful medication history may provide key information concerning the client's oxygenation. The nurse should inquire whether the client takes (or has previously taken) such prescription medications as antihypertensives, digoxin, anticoagulates, diuretics, or antiarrhythmic drugs. If so, the specific drugs, their dosage, frequency, and the client's response, including side effects, should be ascertained. It is especially important to elicit the client's understanding of why the medication has been prescribed and how it is to be taken. Caffeine consumption should be noted because of its cardiovascular effects. The client should be asked about daily use of coffee, tea, chocolate, and caffeine-containing soft drinks. Use of over-the-counter medications containing caffeine, such as some headache remedies, should be noted as well. Many clients are not aware that one or two tablets of some popular analgesic compounds contain more caffeine than a cup of coffee.

Information about health should not only include data about physical status and relevant family history but should deal with psychosocial issues as well. For example, individual and family stressors, such as illness, separation or divorce, unemployment, and alcoholism, may increase the client's risk of cardiovascular problems. It is not uncommon for clients to be undergoing multiple stressors: for example, a divorced woman who had recently moved to take a job, lost the job and concurrently learned that one of her children had end-stage renal failure. Such things as a client's perception about state of well-being, personal strengths and weaknesses, and ability to care for self and provide an environment conducive to good health practices also need to be explored. When this information has been obtained, the nurse is ready to move on to an in-depth clinical appraisal of oxygenation.

CLINICAL APPRAISAL AND SCREENING

Before beginning the clinical appraisal, the nurse should review the anatomical landmarks for assessment of the thorax, lungs, and heart (Figure 17-2). These landmarks will be helpful in describing the location of physical findings. For the purpose of organizing this examination, the thorax and lungs are examined first. The examination begins with the posterior thorax and then proceeds to the anterior thorax. After the examination of the lungs, the nurse proceeds to examine the heart and then the peripheral vascular system (see chap. 14). While the thorax and lung exam and the cardiac exam are discussed together under the various techniques of physical examination, the approach to the assessment of each system is presented separately in two boxed inserts.

Inspection

A careful and comprehensive period of observation should initiate any examination. This may be accomplished to some extent during the process of obtaining the history. For example, the client's mood and general appearance should be noted. Is the client's demeanor calm or anxious? The client's mental status should be assessed briefly for alertness and orientation to surroundings. Disturbances in level of consciousness may indicate impairment of oxygen supply to the vital centers of the brain.

The nose should be inspected for structural deviations, type and amount of secretions, and the color and condition of mucous membranes. Nasal polyps create the potential for nasal passage obstruction and often are associated with excessive use of nasal decongestant solutions. The pharynx should be inspected for enlarged tonsils, which may be a source of upper respiratory obstruction. The neck should be observed well to determine any distention or pulsation in the neck vessels. The trachea should lie in the midline. What is the color of the skin and of the buccal and pharyngeal mucous membranes? The earlobes, nail beds, and mouth should be inspected for cyanosis. If present, its location and severity should be noted. Is it intensified upon exertion? Examination of the structures of the upper respiratory system (nose, sinuses, mouth, and trachea) is an important component of the assessment. If the nurse were doing a complete physical examination, these structures normally would be assessed during the examination of the head and neck. If an examination of the head and neck is not to be performed on the client, then the structures of the upper respiratory system must be examined during the clinical appraisal of the thorax and lungs.

While the thyroid gland is not a structure of the upper respiratory system, it also must be examined. The thyroid gland lies at the lower pole of the thyroid cartilage and the upper trachea. The thyroid is inspected for gross enlargement (goiter).

The client's breathing should be noted—is it fast or slow, easy or labored? If chest retractions are present, they indicate some degree of bronchial obstruction. The use of accessory chest or abdominal muscles also suggests respiratory compromise. Are accessory muscles being used to assist respiratory effort? Is the client breathing through pursed lips? Do respirations appear to be costal or abdominal? Abdominal respiration is normal in the young child. After the age of 7, respiration is usually abdominal in males and costal in females. The chest wall should be carefully observed for visible pulsations (Figure 17-3) in the following areas: the suprasternal notch, the second right intercostal space, the second left intercostal space, the third left intercostal space, and the fifth left intercostal

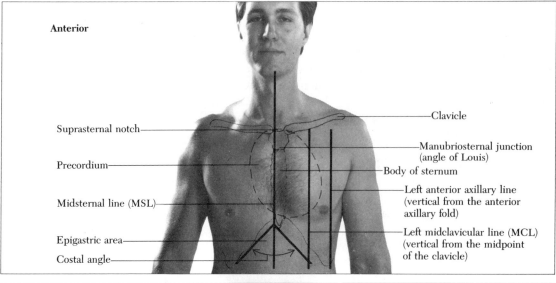

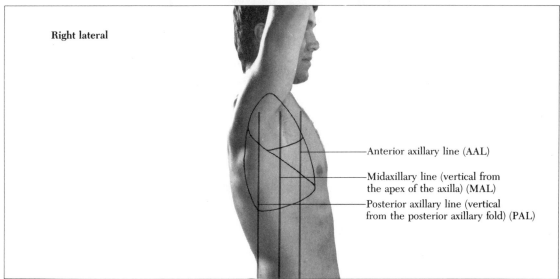

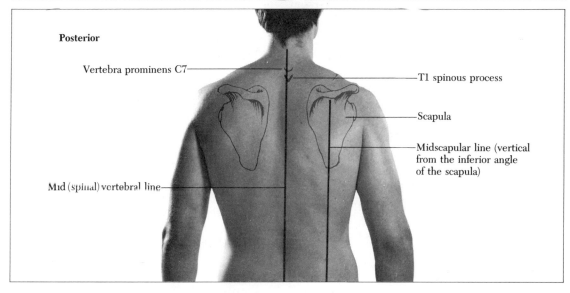

FIGURE 17-2. Topographic Landmarks for Physical Assessment of the Chest and Respiratory System. (*Note.* From Grimes/Burns: *Health Assessment in Nursing Practice,* Second Edition, © 1987. Boston: Jones and Bartlett Publishers, pp. 236–237.)

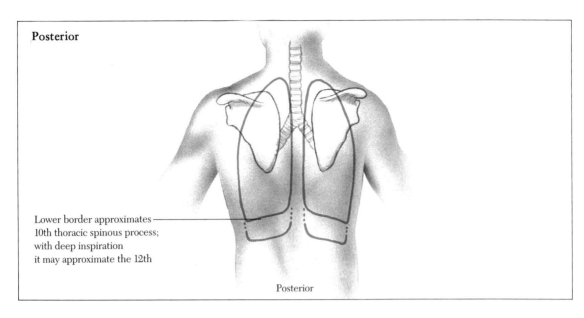

Posterior

Lower border approximates 10th thoracic spinous process; with deep inspiration it may approximate the 12th

Posterior

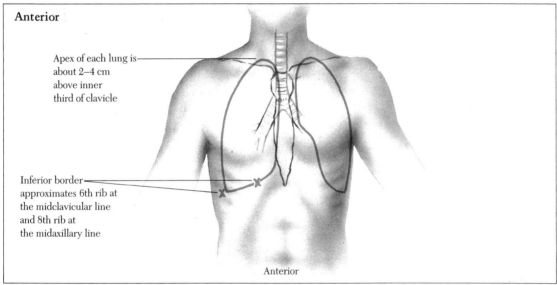

Anterior

Apex of each lung is about 2–4 cm above inner third of clavicle

Inferior border approximates 6th rib at the midclavicular line and 8th rib at the midaxillary line

Anterior

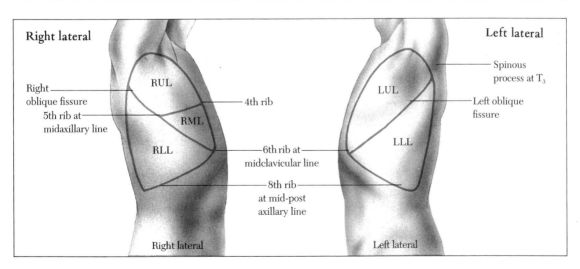

Right lateral

Right oblique fissure

5th rib at midaxillary line

RUL

RML

RLL

4th rib

6th rib at midclavicular line

8th rib at mid-post axillary line

Left lateral

Spinous process at T₃

Left oblique fissure

LUL

LLL

Right lateral

Left lateral

FIGURE 17-2. Continued.

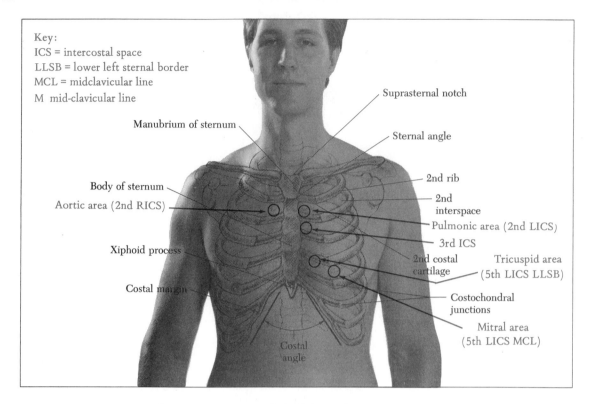

Key:
ICS = intercostal space
LLSB = lower left sternal border
MCL = midclavicular line
M mid-clavicular line

Suprasternal notch
Sternal angle
Manubrium of sternum
2nd rib
2nd interspace
Body of sternum
Pulmonic area (2nd LICS)
Aortic area (2nd RICS)
3rd ICS
2nd costal cartilage
Tricuspid area (5th LICS LLSB)
Xiphoid process
Costal margin
Costochondral junctions
Mitral area (5th LICS MCL)
Costal angle

FIGURE 17-3. Anatomy of the Chest. (*Note.* Adapted from Grimes/Burns: *Health Assessment in Nursing Practice,* Second Edition, © 1987. Boston: Jones and Bartlett Publishers, p. 234.)

spaces at the lower left sternal border and mitral area. The apical impulse (fifth left intercostal space midclavicular line) may or may not be visible.

The forceful contractions of the ventricles under conditions of stress can produce what is known as a heave or lift, the visible thrusting (pulsation) of the ventricle against the chest wall observed in the tricuspid and mitral areas. The nurse also should observe for retractions in the intercostal spaces. Normally, the precordium is quiet and pulsations, heaves, or retractions usually are not noted. However, activity in the precordium can be observed, for example, in children, very thin individuals, and in those individuals who are in a hypermetabolic state. The configuration of the thorax should be observed carefully. A client with a normal rib cage is shown in Figure 17-4. Such congenital abnormalities as a pectus excavatum or pectus carinatum, if severe, can cause some degree of respiratory compromise. In cases of cardiac enlargement there may be a change in chest configuration characterized by a bulge in the area of the left sternal border. Those clients who have respiratory conditions characterized by air trapping and expiratory air flow problems (e.g., emphysema) may exhibit an increase in anteroposterior diameter, giving the chest a barrel-like shape. The nurse always should

note whether respiratory movements are bilaterally symmetrical.

If respiratory distress is apparent, is it worse on inspiration or expiration? Intensification on inspiration indicates the possibility of an upper airway obstruction. Symptoms that intensify during expiration indicate a lower airway problem involving the smaller bronchi and bronchioles (e.g., asthma or emphysema).

The internal jugular veins should be observed for pulsations and distention. The jugular venous pressure (JVP) indicates the pressure in the right atrium. A great deal of inaccuracy exists in measuring the JVP, so it is not a precise indicator of venous pressure. It would be more accurate to document the degree of neck vein distention in relation to the jaw line with the client sitting upright.

Palpation

The sinuses should be palpated for tenderness by applying gentle pressure slightly above the orbit of the eye (Figure 17-5). The maxillary sinus may be palpated by applying gentle pressure to the maxillary area just lateral to the nasal opening. Pain in the sinus region, accompanied by redness or edema, may indicate sinusitis.

Sequence of Respiratory Assessment

Inspection
- Respiration: rate, rhythm, use of accessory muscles
- Configuration of thorax: symmetry, anterioposterior diameter
- Skin and nail beds: color, temperature, configuration
- Spine: curvature, prominences, deformities

Palpation
- Tenderness: spinous processes, paravertebral muscles and scapula; clavicle, sternum, and anterior thorax.
- Respiratory excursion
- Tactile fremitus
- Trachea
- Frontal and maxillary sinus
- Nose

Percussion
- Total lung field
- Diaphragmatic excursion (posteriorly)

Auscultation
- Total lung field

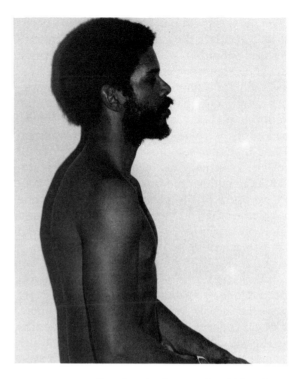

FIGURE 17-4. The client's rib cage should be observed for deformities or an increase in the anterio-posterior diameter. The rate, rhythm, and depth of the client's breathing should also be noted. This client's rib cage is normal.

Sequence of Cardiovascular Assessment

Cardiac

Inspection
- Precordium: pulsations, retractions, heaves or lifts
- Chest wall: configuration

Palpation
- Thrills: aortic, pulmonic, tricuspid, and mitral areas
- Point of maximum impulse (PMI) or apical impulse

Percussion
- Left cardiac border (not done routinely)

Auscultation
- Areas: aortic, pulmonic, tricuspid, and mitral areas

Peripheral Vascular

Inspection
- Jugular veins
- Carotid Arteries
- Abdominal aorta

Palpation
- Peripheral pulses
- Abdominal aorta
- Inguinal nodes
- Temperature
- Edema
- Varicosities

Auscultation
- Abdominal aorta
- Renal, iliac, and femoral arteries

The nurse should palpate the trachea to determine its position in the midline, and the surrounding tissues should be palpated for any crepitation or crackling sounds (crepitus) that might indicate extravasation of air into the subcutaneous tissues.

The thyroid is palpated for consistency, the presence of nodules, and to detect enlargement. Palpation of the thyroid gland can be performed with the examiner standing behind or in front of the client. Whichever technique is used, it is important to remember the following principles: adequate exposure of the gland, comparison of one side with the other, and the movement of the gland through the fingertips.

To palpate the thyroid, the nurse should press gently on one side of the gland to displace the larynx and trachea laterally. The opposite side then is well exposed for palpation. While the nurse lightly palpates the thyroid, the client is asked to swallow. This motion moves the gland past the fingertips while the nurse feels for the presence of nodules and enlargement. The nurse then repeats this technique to palpate the other side. Following the examination of the thyroid, the nurse begins to observe respiratory status.

Palpation of the thoracic area is done to determine tenderness of the bony structures (both anteriorly and posteriorly), respiratory excursion, and fremitus. The examiner should place the palms of the hands over the lower thoracic region and feel the expansion that occurs with each respiration (Figure 17-6). This excursion should be equal bilaterally. Fremitus is the vibration that can be felt through the chest wall when the client vocalizes. The nurse can ask the client to speak a phrase, such as "blue moon" or "ninety-nine." The force of the vibrations should be more intense at the apex of the lungs and weaken as the examiner moves toward the base, always comparing one side with the other (Figure 17-7).

The point of maximal impulse (PMI) at the apex of the heart should be palpated. In young children this usually is located in the fourth left intercostal space close to the midclavicular line. In adults it is lower and usually is found in the fifth left intercostal space toward the midclavicular line. Displacement of the apical impulse (or PMI) to the left is indicative of cardiac enlargement. Thrills may be palpated over the major palpatory and auscultatory areas (Figure 17-2). The examiner will feel a sensation akin to the purring of a kitten. Thrills are abnormal and may indicate congenital heart conditions, such as a patent ductus arteriosis or ventricular septal defect, or acquired defects such as mitral stenosis in the older child or adult. Thrills

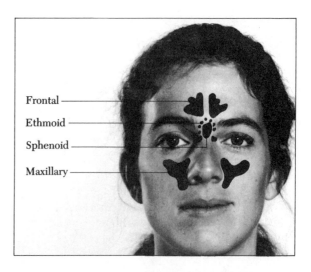

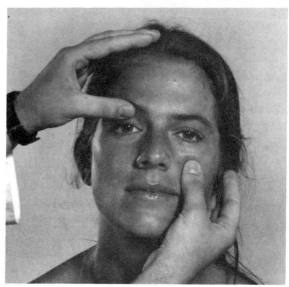

FIGURE 17-5. Palpation of the Sinuses. (*Note.* From Grimes/Burns: *Health Assessment in Nursing Practice,* Second Edition, © 1987. Boston: Jones and Bartlett Publishers, p. 220.)

in the aortic region may indicate aortic stenosis or hypertension.

All pulses of the neck and extremities should be palpated bilaterally for rate, rhythm, and quality (see chap. 14). The nurse should remember that the pulse is an early and consistent indicator of potential alterations in cardiovascular status. Tachycardia is an early sign of stress or impending heart failure, whereas bradycardia may indicate an overdose of cardiac medication or an alteration in electrical impulse conduction. In young children the nurse always should compare the radial pulse to the femoral. A time lag or decrease in force may indicate coarctation of the aorta.

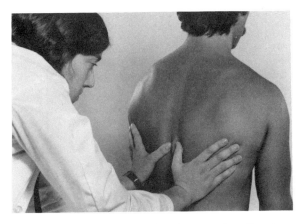

FIGURE 17-6. Technique for Determining Respiratory Expansion. (*Note.* From Grimes/Burns: *Health Assessment in Nursing Practice*, Second Edition, © 1987. Boston: Jones and Bartlett Publishers, p. 241.)

Percussion

Percussion of the thorax is performed after the completion of palpation. The technique of percussion is described in Chapter 3. The intercostal spaces of the thorax are percussed rather than the ribs as this would elicit dullness (Stevens & Becker, 1988). The thorax is percussed systematically, from the apex to the base, comparing one side with the other (Figure 17-8). The normal percussion notes on the anterior and posterior chest are depicted in Figure 17-9. Descriptions of the various percussion notes and their defining characteristics are listed in Table 17-2. The normal percussion note of the lungs is that of resonance. Individuals who have chronic obstructive pulmonary disease may exhibit an increased anterioposterior diameter and lungs that percuss hyperresonantly due to overinflated alveoli.

Percussion of the left cardiac border usually is not done on routine examination. This technique is a gross estimate of cardiac size and a chest x-ray can easily be done to determine the exact size. If the examiner does wish to percuss the left cardiac border, the technique is illustrated in Figure 17-10. By percussing from the left anterior axillary line in the third, fourth, and fifth intercostal spaces toward the midline (sternum), the examiner can outline the left border of the heart. The examiner will hear the percussion note changing from one of resonance over the lung to dullness over the heart. As the nurse outlines the left cardiac border, in the appropriate interspaces, the left cardiac border is measured from the midsternal line. The normal measurements of cardiac size are approximately 4, 7, and 10 cms, respectively, in the third, fourth,

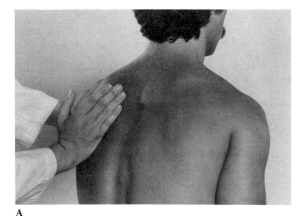

A

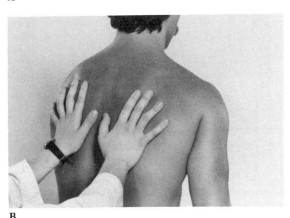

B

FIGURE 17-7. Palpation Technique for Fremitus. (A) Ulnar. (B) Palmar. (*Note.* From Grimes/Burns: *Health Assessment in Nursing Practice*, Second Edition, © 1987. Boston: Jones and Bartlett Publishers, p. 242.)

and fifth left intercostal spaces. This assessment technique is difficult to do accurately if the client is very obese, muscular, or has large breasts. However, it is helpful to know this technique as some measurement of cardiac size can be obtained if the option of a chest x-ray is not readily available.

Auscultation

Auscultation of the respiratory system involves listening with a stethoscope over the posterior, anterior, and lateral chest walls for variations in breath sounds that may indicate the presence of an obstruction or a disease process (see Figure 17-11).

Moving the stethoscope systematically, the examiner listens to ascertain the normality or abnormality of breath sounds. Normal breath sounds are those created by the movement of air in the tracheobronchial tree with each inspiration and expiration. These sounds generally are classified according to three types:

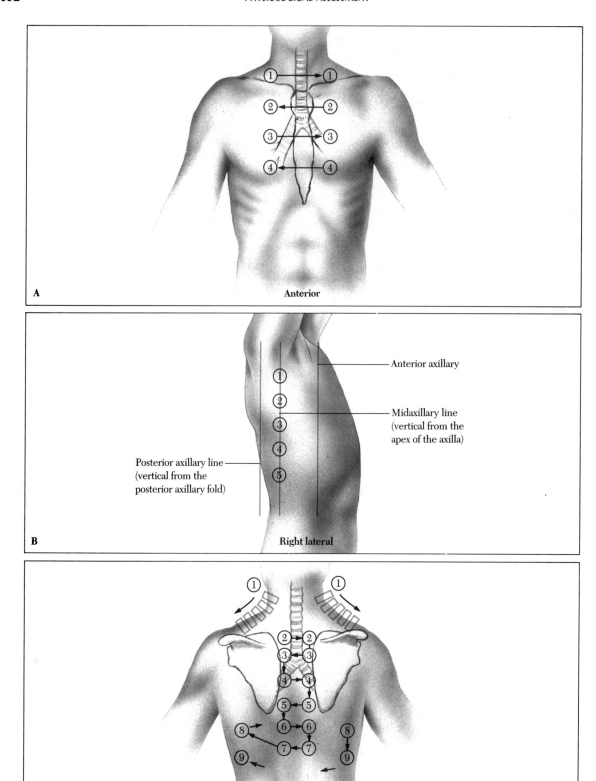

FIGURE 17-8. Method of Thoracic Percussion. (A) Percussion of anterior thorax. (B) Right lateral percussion. (C) Percussion of posterior thorax. (*Note*. From Grimes/Burns: *Health Assessment in Nursing Practice,* Second Edition, © 1987. Boston: Jones and Bartlett Publishers, p. 243.)

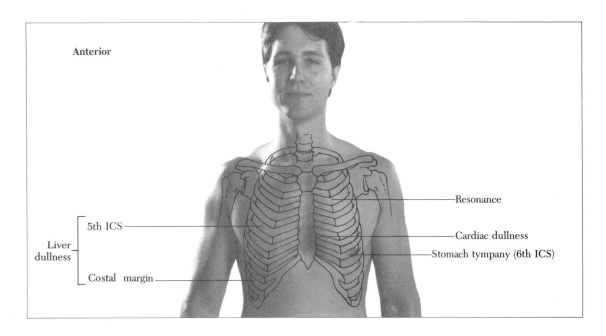

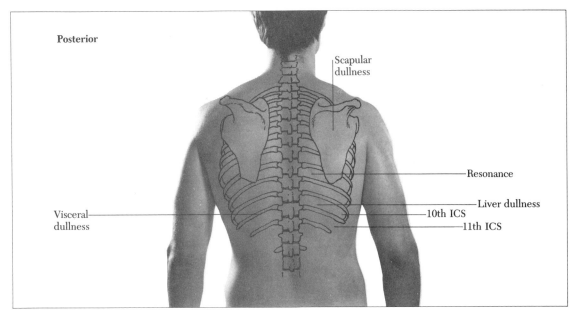

FIGURE 17-9. Normal Percussion Notes on the Anterior and Posterior Chest. (*Note.* From Grimes/Burns: *Health Assessment in Nursing Practice,* Second Edition, © 1987. Boston: Jones and Bartlett Publishers, p. 244.)

Vesicular sounds are soft swishing sounds with a prolonged inspiratory phase and a shorter expiratory phase. These usually are heard over all open lung areas.

Bronchovesicular sounds have a more moderate intensity, and the inspiratory–expiratory ratio is approximately equal. Bronchovesicular sounds normally are heard over the mediastinum at the bifurcation of the main bronchi.

Bronchial sounds are more harsh and are heard over the trachea. The inspiratory phase is about half the length of the expiratory phase.

If these sounds are auscultated in regions other than those delineated they usually indicate some form of lung pathology.

Adventitious sounds are abnormalities in breath sounds. They usually are classified as follows:

TABLE 17-2
Description of Percussion Notes

Note	Intensity	Pitch	Duration	Quality	Normal location
Flatness	Soft	High	Short	Extreme dullness	Thigh
Dullness	Soft	High	Moderate	Thudlike	Liver
Resonance	Moderate to loud	Low	Long	Hollow	Peripheral lung
Hyperresonance	Very loud	Very low	Very long	Booming	Child's lung
Tympany	Loud	High	Moderate	Musical, drumlike	Air-filled stomach

Note. From Grimes/Burns: *Health Assessment in Nursing Practice*, Second Edition, © 1987. Boston: Jones and Bartlett Publishers, p. 244.

Rales are fine crackly sounds heard most often on inspiration and usually indicate lower airway pathology.

Rhonchi are more coarse, harsh, louder sounds heard best on expiration. Rhonchi usually indicate upper airway problems.

Wheezes are squeeky, musical sounds indicative of bronchial constriction and usually are heard on expiration.

Friction rubs are the sounds emitted when the lubricant beneath the pleural membrane (pulmonary surfactant) is decreased, allowing the lung and pleura to rub with each respiration.

If the nurse percusses or auscultates abnormal sounds during the examination of the lungs, additional techniques should be performed. Otherwise, these techniques usually are not done. The three techniques are bronchophony, whispered pectoriloquy, and egophony. Whispered pectoriloquy and bronchophony will assist in determining consolidation of the lungs. Egophony is a type of bronchophony and is used to assess the presence of fluid in the lung. The higher pitched sound of fluid will alter the pattern of the spoken word. The use of these techniques is described in the boxed insert.

Auscultation of the cardiovascular system involves listening with a stethoscope over specified areas on the precordium, the auscultatory areas. These include the aortic area (second right inter-

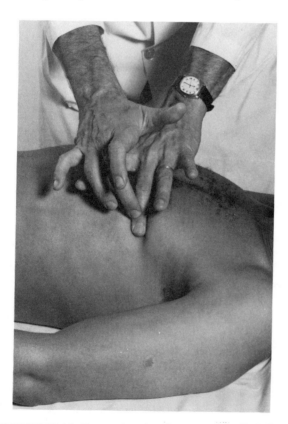

FIGURE 17-10. Percussing the Contour of the Left Cardiac Border. (*Note.* From Grimes/Burns: *Health Assessment in Nursing Practice*, Second Edition, © 1987. Boston: Jones and Bartlett Publishers, p. 273.)

Special Assessment Techniques of the Lungs

1. *Bronchophony:* Place diaphragm of stethoscope over abnormal area of lung field. Ask client to softly repeat "one-two-three." *Normal finding: "one-two-three" sounds muffled.* Presence of bronchophony is pathologic. Finding in bronchophony is clearly transmitted "one-two-three."

2. *Egophony:* Place diaphragm of stethoscope over abnormal area of lung field. Ask client to say "eeeeeee." *Normal finding: "eeeeeee" sound maintained.* Presence of egophony is pathological and is reflected by the change of "eeeeee" to an "aaaaayyh" sound.

3. *Whispered Pectoriloquy:* With the diaphragm of the stethoscope over an abnormal area of the lung, ask the client to whisper "one-two-three." *The normal finding is a muffled, whispered "one-two-three."* The pathological presence of whispered pectoriloquy is reflected by sharp/distinct, clear transmission of the whispered "one-two-three."

Note. Adapted from Grimes/Burns: *Health Assessment in Nursing Practice*, Second Edition, © 1987. Boston: Jones and Bartlett Publishers, p. 252.

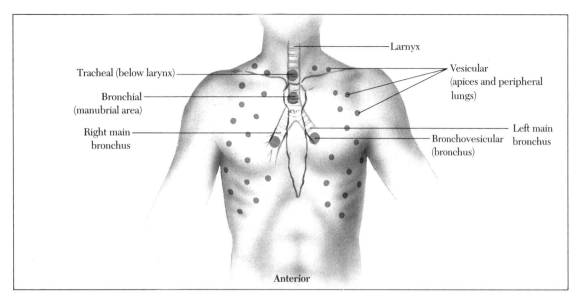

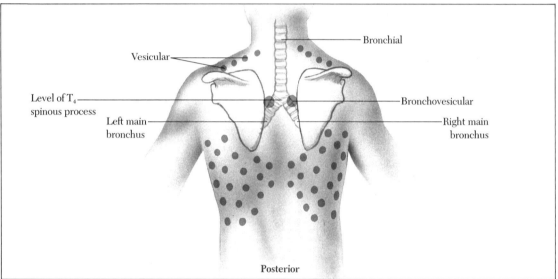

FIGURE 17-11. Locations of Normal Breath Sounds of the Neck and Thorax (all small circles are vesicular). (*Note.* From Grimes/Burns: *Health Assessment in Nursing Practice,* Second Edition, © 1987. Boston: Jones and Bartlett Publishers, p. 248.)

costal space), pulmonic area (second left intercostal space), third left intercostal space, tricuspid (fifth left intercostal space, lower left sternal border) and mitral (fifth left intercostal space, midclavicular line) areas. Both the diaphragm and bell are used to listen to heart sounds. Because the diaphragm is better at picking up high pitched sounds, it should be used when listening for S_1 and S_2. Low pitched sounds are best heard with the bell of the stethoscope. Therefore, the bell should be used when listening for S_3 and S_4.

As the nurse begins the auscultatory segment of the cardiac exam, the concept of timing as it relates to the cardiac cycle becomes important. The nurse must be able to distinguish sounds heard in systole from those heard in diastole in order to document physical findings. Several tips: The loudest of the two heart sounds at the base is S_2. This heart sound usually is the dominant heart sound heard over the entire precordium with the exception of the mitral area, where the sound of S_1 is loudest. Knowing this enables the nurse to determine when systole and diastole are occurring. Any sounds heard during the interval between S_1 and S_2 would be systolic and those heard occurring between the interval of S_2 and S_1 are diastolic in origin.

A second way to determine timing is palpation of the point of maximum impulse. This is helpful if neither of the sounds at the base is louder. The up-stroke (felt beat) of the PMI or the apical impulse is synchronous with S_1. So, while auscultating with the stethoscope, the nurse feels the pulse that is synchronous with the sound. This then, is the first heart sound, S_1. If no apical impulse can be felt, the nurse can palpate the carotid artery. The up-stroke (felt beat) of the carotid is approximately synchronous with S_1 and the onset of systole. This serves as a third method for determining the timing of the cardiac cycle.

The nurse may begin to auscultate the heart at either the base or the apex. Listening to heart sounds is done first with the diaphragm of the stethoscope and then with the bell. While listening first at the base, for example, the nurse should concentrate on one sound and follow that sound throughout the precordium. Note how the sound changes in the different auscultatory areas. The nurse then should listen again to the same sound and follow it throughout the precordium. This should be followed by listening with the bell in each of the auscultatory areas. It is important that the nurse listen carefully, concentrating on the sounds and the cardiac events being auscultated.

Answers to the following questions will help the nurse describe cardiac findings. Are S_1 and S_2 audible and distinct? Is any additional sound heard? Does the sound occur in systole or diastole? Does the extra sound appear similar to a heart sound or a murmur? Where is the sound the loudest? Does the sound radiate down the left sternal border, for example, or to the axilla, or does the sound remain concentrated in one auscultatory area? Does the sound change in intensity if the client's position changes? Does the sound radiate to the carotids? The beginning student of physical assessment should take every opportunity to have physical findings validated. Also critical to developing comfort and proficiency with physical assessment skills is practice.

Auscultation of heart sounds to identify abnormalities or underlying cardiac pathology is an advanced skill requiring specialized preparation and intense practice. Sessions with an experienced practitioner and the use of a heart sound simulator are ways in which the nurse can develop increased expertise. If the nurse is able to distinguish between S_1 and S_2 and determine the timing of events in the cardiac cycle, the nurse has acquired a very critical skill of cardiac assessment. Knowing this, the nurse is able to describe what is heard, alert care providers to the findings, and document that there are changes or distinctly different sounds without necessarily putting the exact diagnosis on the findings. This ability takes time and practice and is not expected of the beginning student of physical assessment.

Following auscultation of heart sounds, the nurse also should auscultate the neck vessels for the presence of bruits (harsh blowing sounds in the region of the carotid artery). These may indicate a vascular abnormality.

The assessment of blood pressure is mandatory to complete the oxygenation assessment. This procedure is an extremely important screening device to detect blood pressure abnormalities in all age groups. The most significant abnormality is hypertension, which often is completely asymptomatic except for the elevation in blood pressure reading. Chapter 14 describes the correct techniques for measuring blood pressure.

All extremities should be checked for skin color, bruising, petechiae, purpura, or the presence of edema. If edema is present in the lower extremities, it is usually of cardiac origin. Edema that pits on pressure from the thumb (pitting edema) may indicate congestive heart failure. Edema usually is described on a four-point scale of 1+ to 4+, with the higher number indicating more severe edema. Clubbing of fingers and toes indicates a state of chronic oxygen deprivation. Clubbing is discussed in Chapter 14.

Laboratory Data

The ability to interpret laboratory data is an essential assessment skill that should be continuously reinforced throughout the professional development of any nurse. There are numerous laboratory tests that are of importance in assessing and validating any client's oxygenation (Mulligan, 1986; Westra, 1986).

Hematological Studies

Blood studies are generally performed on all clients when they enter the health-care system (Table 17-3). Several specific determinations that are a part of this survey pertain directly to oxygenation. Since hemoglobin (Hgb) is so essential to oxygen transport, its measurement provides an accurate index of oxygen-carrying capability. If the Hgb level is below normal, the oxygenation level is proportionally reduced.

The hematocrit (Hct) is an estimate of the volume of blood cells as compared with the total blood volume. If the red blood cell volume is significantly reduced, the hemoglobin content of the blood is also reduced.

Platelets are an important factor in the blood

TABLE 17-3
Clinical Laboratory Values of Relevant Blood Studies

Studies	Norms	
Hematologic		
Hemoglobin (Hgb)	Females	12 to 16 g/100 ml
	Males	13 to 18 g/100 ml
Hematocrit (Hct)	Females	37 to 48%
	Males	45 to 52%
Platelets	150,000 to 350,000/mm³	
Erythrocyte sedimentation rate (ESR)	Males	1 to 13 mm/hr
	Females	1 to 20 mm/hr
Chemistries		
Serum cholesterol	120–220 mg/100 ml	
Serum triglycerides	40–150 mg/100 ml	

Note. Adapted from Tilkian, S.M., Conover, M.B., & Tilkian A.G., (1987). *Clinical implications of laboratory tests.* St. Louis: Mosby.

clotting mechanism. If their numbers are diminished, this may be indicative of a variety of diseases that affect the bone marrow. The cardiovascular significance of platelets lies in their necessity for blood coagulation.

The erythrocyte sedimentation rate (ESR) is the rate at which red blood cells settle out of a suspended blood sample. An elevation or increase in the sedimentation rate takes place in acute myocardial infarctions or in the presence of an inflammatory disease such as rheumatic fever.

Blood Chemistry Tests

The level of many substances in the blood serves as a sensitive barometer to changes that have the potential to become problematic. Of these, two tests stand out as having particular ramifications for oxygenation.

The serum cholesterol level is a determination of the amount of circulating cholesterol in the blood. Elevations of cholesterol indicate the potential for arteriosclerotic changes in the vessel walls. The serum triglyceride level is a determination of circulating simple lipids in the blood. Here again, elevations indicate a potential for vascular changes such as those seen in arteriosclerotic heart disease. Since these vascular changes may place the client at risk for thrombosis and coronary artery occlusion, they always should be noted by the nurse as part of the oxygenation assessment.

Arterial Blood Gases

Over the last several decades the use of arterial blood gases has become prevalent in assessing oxygenation. Venous blood sometimes is used, but arterial samples are considered a much better index of oxygen exchange throughout the body.

The oxygenation saturation (O_2 Sat) is the measure of oxygen carried in the blood by the hemoglobin. Normally arterial blood is almost fully saturated with an O_2 saturation of 95% to 99%. The partial pressure of oxygen in the arterial blood (PaO_2) is a measure of pulmonary transport function. The partial arterial carbon dioxide level ($PaCO_2$) measures the CO_2 level in the circulating blood and is an index of alveolar ventilation. Elevation of $PaCO_2$ usually indicates hypoventilation and the existence of respiratory acidosis. A decrease in the $PaCO_2$ indicates hyperventilation and potential respiratory alkalosis. The bicarbonate HCO_3—and base excess measures also reflect metabolic acidosis or alkalosis. The actual acid-base status of the blood finally is reflected in the pH. Acidity will result from an excess of hydrogen (H+) ions, alkalinity from too few. If lung function is altered and CO_2 is exhaled, as in hyperventilation, there is a decrease in H+ ions, and respiratory alkalosis ensues. Table 17-4 lists the clinical norms of arterial blood gases and their implications. Table 17-5 presents a systematic assessment of arterial blood gases that is very helpful in evaluating arterial blood gas values.

Pulmonary Function Studies

Pulmonary function studies document the presence of a functional impairment in oxygenation resulting from respiratory disease (Table 17-6). They also often are used to evaluate the therapeutic response and progression of disease. If an oxygenation deficit is suspected, the nurse should be alert to the findings of these studies.

The volume of air, either inhaled or exhaled, is measured by a spirometer. The vital capacity (VC) is a measure of the total volume of air exhaled after

TABLE 17-4
Arterial Blood Gases

Term	Normal Value	Definition—Implications
pH	7.35–7.45	Reflects H^+ concentration; acidity increases as H^+ concentration increases (pH value decreases as acidity increases) ■ pH < 7.35 (acidosis) ■ pH > 7.45 (alkalosis)
$PaCO_2$	38–42 mm Hg	Partial pressure of CO_2 in arterial blood ■ When <38 mm Hg, hypocapnia is said to be present (respiratory alkalosis) ■ When >42 mm Hg, hypercapnia is said to be present (respiratory acidosis)
PaO_2	80–100 mm Hg (decreases with age)	Partial pressure of O_2 in arterial blood ■ Any reading above 80 mm Hg (on room air) is considered acceptable ■ In adults <60 yr (on room air) <80 mm Hg indicates mild hypoxemia <60 mm Hg indicates moderate hypoxemia <40 mm Hg indicates severe hypoxemia ■ Somewhat lower levels are accepted as normal in aged persons because there is some loss of ventilatory function with advanced age
Standard HCO_3	22 mEq–26 mEq/liter	HCO_3 concentration in plasma of blood that has been equilibrated at a $PaCO_2$ of 40 mm Hg, and with O_2, in order to fully saturate the hemoglobin
Base excess (BE)	−2 mEq– + 2mEq/liter	Reflects metabolic (nonrespiratory) body disturbances, which may be primary or compensatory in nature Always negative in metabolic acidosis (deficit of alkali or excess of fixed acids) Always positive in metabolic alkalosis (excess of alkali or deficit of fixed acids) Arrived at by multiplying the deviation of standard HCO_3 from normal by a factor of 1.2, which represents the buffer action of red blood cells

Note. From Metheny, N. (1987). *Fluid and electrolyte balance.* Philadelphia: Lippincott, 109.

a complete inspiration and forced expiration. The forced expiratory volume (FEV) is the volume of air expired in one second. The residual volume is that amount of air that remains in the lungs after forced expiration. And, the total lung capacity (TLC) indicates the total volume of air within the lungs following a maximal inspiration. (See Table 17-16 for clinical norms.)

Radiological Studies

Various radiological examinations can be used to complete a thorough assessment of oxygenation. Among the most common are chest x-rays, bronchograms, and angiograms. Both posterioanterior (PA) and lateral chest films are used to delineate the cardiac outline and pulmonary vascular structures. Pulmonary lesions and areas of fluid accumulation and consolidation also may be seen. The bronchogram is a radiological procedure that enables the viewer to study the bronchial structures. A radiopaque substance is instilled into the airway passages by means of a catheter. The substance is distributed as the client assumes a variety of positions. X-rays are taken throughout the manipulations. Angiograms are used to study intracardiac and pulmonary vascular structures. A catheter is inserted into the venous system and threaded through the chambers of the heart into the pulmonary circulation. An individualized amount of radiopaque material is injected and filmed as it disperses.

Direct Visualization Techniques

Laryngoscopy involves visualization of the larynx, either indirectly or directly. In the indirect method, a mirror is placed in the back of the throat to reflect the laryngeal area to the eye of the examiner. The direct method is done using sedation or anesthesia. The larynx is directly visualized by inserting a laryngoscope. The direct method is preferred if a tissue biopsy is to be taken.

Bronchoscopy involves the direct visualization

TABLE 17-5
Systematic Assessment of Arterial Blood Gases

The following steps are recommended to evaluate arterial blood gas values. They are based on the assumption that the average values are

$$pH = 7.4$$
$$PaCO_2 = 40 \text{ mm Hg}$$
$$HCO_3 = 24 \text{ mEq/liter}$$

I. *First, look at the pH.* It can be high, low, or normal as follows:

$$pH > 7.4 \text{ (alkalosis)}$$
$$pH < 7.4 \text{ (acidosis)}$$
$$pH = 7.4 \text{ (normal)}$$

A normal pH may indicate perfectly normal blood gases, or it may be an indication of a *compensated* imbalance. A compensated imbalance is one in which the body has been able to correct the pH by either respiratory or metabolic changes (depending on the primary problem). For example, a patient with primary metabolic acidosis starts out with a low bicarbonate level but a normal carbon dioxide level. Soon afterward, the lungs try to compensate for the imbalance by exhaling large amounts of carbon dioxide (hyperventilation). Another example, a patient with primary respiratory acidosis starts out with a high carbon dioxide level; soon afterward, the kidneys attempt to compensate by retaining bicarbonate. If the compensatory maneuver is able to restore the bicarbonate : carbonic acid ratio back to 20 : 1, full compensation (and thus normal pH) will be achieved.

II. *The next step is to determine the primary cause of the disturbance. This is done by evaluating the $PaCO_2$ and HCO_3 in relation to the pH.*

pH > 7.4 (alkalosis)

1. *If the $PaCO_2$ is <40 mm Hg,* the primary disturbance is respiratory alkalosis. (This situation occurs when a patient hyperventilates and "blows off" too much carbon dioxide. Recall that carbon dioxide dissolved in water becomes carbonic acid, the acid side of the "carbonic acid : base bicarbonate" buffer system.)

2. *If the HCO_3 is >24 mEq/liter,* the primary disturbance is metabolic alkalosis. (This situation occurs when the body gains too much bicarbonate, an alkaline substance. Bicarbonate is the basic, or alkaline side of the "carbonic acid–base: bicarbonate buffer system.")

pH < 7.4 (acidosis)

1. *If the $PaCO_2$ is >40 mm Hg,* the primary disturbance is respiratory acidosis. (This situation occurs when a patient hypoventilates and thus retains too much carbon dioxide, an acidic substance.)

2. *If the HCO_3 is <24 mEq/liter,* the primary disturbance is metabolic acidosis. (This situation occurs when the body's bicarbonate level drops, either because of direct bicarbonate loss or because of gains of acids such as lactic acid or ketones.)

III. *The next step involves determining if compensation has begun.*
This is done by looking at the value other than the primary disorder. If it is moving in the same direction as the primary value, compensation is underway. Consider the following blood gases:

Example:

	pH	$PaCO_2$	HCO_3
(1)	7.20	60 mm Hg	24 mEq/liter
(2)	7.40	60 mm Hg	37 mEq/liter

The first set (1) indicates acute respiratory acidosis without compensation (the $PaCO_2$ is high, the HCO_3 is normal). The second set (2) indicates chronic respiratory acidosis. Note that compensation has taken place; that is, the HCO_3 has elevated to an appropriate level to balance the high $PaCO_2$ and produce a normal pH.

Note. From Metheny, N. (1987). *Fluid and electrolyte balance.* Philadelphia: Lippincott, 109.

of the tracheobronchial tree by means of a broncho-scope passed through the mouth. This is usually done under anesthesia (local for adults and general for children). This examination assists in evaluating disease and facilitates the aspiration of specimens for laboratory examination.

Electrocardiography

The electrocardiogram (EKG or ECG) is a graphic record of the electrical activity of the myocardium. Electrodes are placed on the skin to detect the elec-trical currents. These patterns then are transmitted to an oscilloscope or to graph paper for recording (Figure 17-1). Because cardiac changes become more prevalent with the aging process, an EKG is recommended as part of a periodic health checkup after maturity is reached.

Throat and Sputum Cultures

Throat cultures of secretions in the nasopharynx are obtained when the presence of an infecting or-ganism is suspected. In particular, the throat cul-

TABLE 17-6
Normal Pulmonary Function Tests

Test	Age 20–39	Age 40–59	Age 60+
VC (liters)			
Men	3.35–5.90	2.72–5.30	2.42–4.70
Women	2.45–4.38	2.09–4.02	1.9–3.66
FEV$_1$ (liters)			
Men	3.11–4.64	2.45–3.98	2.09–3.32
Women	2.16–3.65	1.60–3.09	1.30–2.53
FEV% (FEV$_1$/VC%)			
Men	77	70	60
Women	82	77	74
Residual volume (liters)			
Men	1.13–2.32	1.45–2.62	1.77–2.77
Women	1.00–2.00	1.16–2.20	1.32–2.40
Total lung capacity (liters)			
Men	4.80–7.92	4.50–7.62	4.35–7.32
Women	3.61–6.18	3.41–6.02	3.31–5.86

FEV = forced expiratory volume
VC = vital capacity

Note. From Tilkian, S.M., Conover, M.B., Tilkian, A.G. (1987). *Clinical implications of laboratory tests* (4th ed.). St. Louis: Mosby, 221.

ture is used to differentiate a viral sore throat from one caused by group A betahemolytic streptococci. The tongue is depressed with a tongue blade while the posterior nasopharynx is swabbed with a sterile cotton swab. The swab then is placed in a special test tube and sent to the laboratory for culturing.

Sputum cultures are obtained and examined to identify the presence of causative organisms in respiratory conditions. The client is asked to cough and expectorate into a small sputum container. The sample should be processed immediately to ensure maximum accuracy. Early morning specimens are preferred. If the specimen is difficult to obtain, percussion and postural drainage may assist in loosening secretions. Tracheal aspiration also may be used if necessary. Occasionally, especially in suspected pulmonary tuberculosis, the process of gastric washing must be used to obtain samples of sputum from the stomach. This is always done early in the morning prior to breakfast. This procedure requires the insertion of a nasogastric tube and aspiration of gastric secretions. These secretions then are examined for swallowed sputum.

Tuberculin Test

The tuberculin test is the most commonly used screening tool for the detection of pulmonary tuberculosis. As a general rule, it is a recommended part of any child's or adult's routine health appraisal. Many school systems require this test prior to admission. If a client has been infected by the organism, a positive reaction will develop to products of the organism. The most commonly used tuberculin tests are the purified protein derivative (P.P.D.) and the Tine Test. The P.P.D. has higher accuracy. However, in mass screening, the Tine, or multipuncture, test has proved to be a valuable and less expensive alternative. The tuberculin is planted or injected intercutaneously on the inner aspect of the forearm and then observed at 48 to 72 hours for evidence of reaction. A positive reaction is easily observable and consists of an enlarged reddened area about the injection site. The area of induration should be measured. A measurement of 10 mm or more of induration indicates a positive reaction. Further screening by chest x-ray and sputum examination is indicated.

NURSING DIAGNOSES RELATED TO OXYGENATION

Following careful analysis and synthesis of assessment data, the nurse makes appropriate nursing diagnoses. Several nursing diagnoses related to oxygenation are listed in Table 17-7. These nursing diagnoses are categorized in the North American Nursing Diagnosis Association, 1990 (NANDA) Taxonomy I under the human response pattern "exchanging." The diagnosis of "ineffective breathing pattern related to pain," for example, is a diagnosis that may be seen in persons suffering from acute pain. Data that would support such a diagnosis would reflect changes in the client's rate and depth of respiration. Tachypnea would be evident as well as shortness of breath. Shallow respiration and the use of accessory muscles also may be observed. The client most likely will appear to be restless and very anxious. If the respiratory distress is prolonged, the client can exhibit abnormal arterial blood gases.

A nursing diagnosis of "ineffective airway clearance related to chronic debilitation," for example, can be observed in the client with cancer who is extremely cachectic. Such a client would exhibit marked weight loss and muscle wasting. As a result, the effort to breathe is markedly increased. Such a client would exhibit signs and symptoms similar to the client in acute pain. However, in ad-

TABLE 17-7
Nursing Diagnoses Related to Oxygenation

Airway clearance ineffective, related to surgical anesthesia or chronic debilitation.

Aspiration, potential for, related to generalized weakness or diminished gag reflex.

Breathing pattern, ineffective, related to postoperative pain, anxiety, or upper airway obstruction.

*Cardiac output, decreased, related to alterations in rate or conduction.

*Gas exchange, impaired, related to ineffective ventilation.

*Tissue perfusion, altered in: cardiopulmonary, related to vascular changes associated with aging.

*These are collaborative diagnoses and often require medical interventions.

---

ditio , the nurse may observe ineffective coughing due to extreme debilitation, cyanosis, diaphoresis, and possibly substernal retraction. In this situation, the nurse would observe the client spending a great deal of energy and effort on the work of breathing.

A number of the diagnoses that fall in this category pose some problems for nursing because of their medical orientation. Inherent in the ability to make a nursing diagnosis is the ability to treat the problem independently. Therefore, confusion can arise when the nature of the problem the nurse is treating is more medical than nursing. In such situations, the independent role of the nurse shifts to one that is more collaborative. Nurses need to be aware of these situations and acknowledge the dilemma. Nurses also must continue to evaluate these diagnoses in an effort to bring clarity to the issue.

Chapter Highlights

■ Although the assessment of all body systems is essential to competent practice, in no other area does the nurse's ability to observe, examine, synthesize information, and intervene effectively have such great potential influence on life or death.

■ Oxygenation is accomplished by the combined functions of the pulmonary and cardiovascular systems.

■ A variety of factors, such as age, race, health, and environment, can influence a client's oxygenation.

■ The oxygenation assessment is to a great extent dependent upon the quality of the information obtained from the oxygenation history.

■ An oxygenation history should review the following aspects of respiratory function: cough, wheezing, shortness of breath, exposure to environmental elements, pain, allergies (type and frequency), respiratory tract infections (type and frequency), existing cardiovascular problems, medication, stress, and cardiopulmonary risk factors.

■ The ability to interpret laboratory data is an essential assessment skill that should be reinforced continuously throughout the professional development of any nurse.

■ Clinical appraisal of oxygenation involves physical assessment of the client's circulatory and respiratory capabilities as well as careful evaluation of relevant laboratory data.

■ The techniques of inspection, palpation, percussion, and auscultation are used in the clinical appraisal of a client's oxygenation.

■ Appropriate nursing diagnoses related to oxygenation are based on an analysis and synthesis of the information found in the oxygenation history, clinical appraisal, and laboratory findings.

Practice Activities

1. Practice obtaining an oxygenation history from a colleague, classmate, or family member. Perform a clinical appraisal of the individual. What laboratory data or other laboratory studies would be useful for validating the findings of your assessment? What nursing diagnoses are supported by the data you collected?

2. Conduct a complete oxygenation assessment of at least two of the following clients. Formulate appropriate nursing diagnoses.
   a. An immobilized adult.
   b. A client with hypertension.
   c. An adult with a history of chronic obstructive lung disease or ischemic heart disease.
   d. An elderly client.

3. Review the health record of a client hospitalized with an interference in oxygenation. What laboratory data appear in the record to validate impaired oxygenation?

4. Analyze your own family history and lifestyle, including environmental factors, in terms of their effect on your own oxygenation. Which factors can

be modified to reduce the long-term health risk in relation to oxygenation?

Recommended Readings

Birdsall, C. (1987). How do you measure transcutaneous oxygen? *American Journal of Nursing, 87*(8), 1273.

Carroll, P. (1988). Cyanosis. *Nursing 88, 18*(3), 50.

Dennison, R. (1986). Cardiopulmonary assessment. *Nursing, 16*(4), 34–39.

Ingersoll, G.L. (1989). Respiratory muscle fatigue research: Implications for clinical practice. *Applied Nursing Research, 2*(1), 6–15.

Miller, V. (1984). The ABCs of blood gases. *Emergency Medicine, 16*, 36.

Moldovanyi, C. (1988). Fruity breath odor: Two major implications. *Nursing 88, 18*(3), 65–69.

Nuracle, V. (1986). Anatomy of a murmur. *Nursing, 16*(7), 26–31.

Openbrier, D.R., & Corey, M. (1987). Ineffective breathing pattern related to malnutrition. *Nursing Clinics of North America, 22*, 225–246.

Stevens, S., & Becker, K. (1988). How to perform picture-perfect respiratory assessment. *Nursing 88, 18*, 57–63.

Ward, J.J. (1989). Lung sounds: Easy to hear, hard to describe. *Respiratory Care, 34*, 17–19.

References

Grimes, J., & Burns, E. (1987). *Health assessment in nursing practice* (2nd ed.). Boston: Jones and Bartlett.

Grollman, S. (1974). *The human body: Its structure and physiology* (3rd ed.). New York: MacMillan.

Guyton, A.C. (1990). *Textbook of medical physiology* (8th ed.). Philadelphia: Saunders.

Miller, C. (1990). *Nursing care of older adults.* Glenview, IL: Scott, Foresman.

Mulligan, J. (1986). Diagnostic tests: Patient teaching and nursing care. *Nurse Review.* Springhouse, PA: Springhouse.

Robinson, A.M. (1976). Detection and control of hypertension: Challenge to all nurses. *American Journal of Nursing, 76*, 779.

Rooks, Y., & Pack, B. (1983). A profile of sickle cell disease. *Nursing Clinics of North America, 18*(1), 131–138.

Sparrow, D., & Weiss, S.T. (1988). Pulmonary system. In J.W. Rowe and R.W. Besdine (Eds.), *Geriatric medicine.* Boston: Little, Brown.

Stevens, S.A., & Becker, A.L. (1988). How to perform a picture-perfect respiratory assessment. *Nursing, 18*(1), 57–63.

Wei, J.Y., & Gersh, B.J. (1987). Heart disease in the elderly. *Current Problems in Cardiology* 12, 1–65.

Westra, B. (1986). Diagnostic studies: Patient teaching, preparation, and nursing care. *Nurse Review.* Springhouse, PA: Springhouse.

18

Nutritional Assessment

CHAPTER OUTLINE

- Purposes and Scope of the Nutritional Assessment
- Whose Nutrition Should Be Assessed
- Knowledge Needed to Assess Nutritional Status
  Standards Used to Determine Dietary Needs
- Variables Influencing Nutritional Requirements
  Environmental Influences   Influence of Age
  Influence of Illness and Surgery   Illnesses
  Affecting Nutrition   Influence of Drugs
- The Nutritional History
  Nutritional History Obtained by Interview
  Dietary Intake Assessment   Analyzing Dietary
  Intake
- Clinical Appraisal and Screening
  Anthropometric Measurements   Biochemical
  Measurements
- Nursing Diagnoses Related to Nutrition

OBJECTIVES

Upon completion of this chapter, you should be able to:

- Explain the purposes and scope of nutritional assessment.
- Describe a framework for organizing information from a nutritional assessment.
- Identify clients at increased risk for nutrition-related problems.
- Recognize results from a nutritional screening that indicate the need for more in-depth assessment.
- Collect information needed to evaluate a client's nutrition.
- Use nutritional assessment techniques appropriate for a client's age, cultural background, and health.
- Compare and contrast methods for evaluating dietary intake.
- Analyze nutritional assessment data using appropriate norms for comparison.
- Formulate appropriate nursing diagnoses for clients with actual or potential alterations in nutrition.

Nutrition is one of the most critical factors affecting health today. The maxim "You are what you eat" oversimplifies the importance of nutrition but diet always has had a vital influence on health. Nutritional deficiency diseases have diminished, replaced in large part by diseases of dietary excess, overconsumption, and imbalance—problems that now contribute to the leading causes of illness and death in the United States. According to the Office of the Surgeon General, these problems touch the lives of most Americans and generate substantial health-care costs [U.S. Department of Health and Human Services (HHS), 1988].

A client's nutrition has a significant impact on health and disease. For the healthy client, optimum nutrition helps maintain health, promotes normal growth and development, and protects against disease. For the ill client, optimum nutrition reduces the risks of complications and death, hastens recovery, decreases health-care costs, lessens the severity of symptoms, decreases the need for medication, delays progression of disease, increases stamina, and improves outlook. Good nutrition is an essential part of quality care. Nurses are involved not only in providing nutritional care but also in nutritional research.

Malnutrition, which can be defined as less than optimal nutrition, is to some extent a product of today's fast-paced yet sedentary way of living. From a global perspective, malnutrition or lack of adequate food is the major health problem (Williams, 1990). In the United States, well-advertised and easily accessible nutrient-empty snack foods, as well as many meals, are eaten on the run. In addition, inadequate income, inflation and unemployment, ignorance of or confusion about nutritional principles, lack of interest, lack of food preparation skills, and food fads are contributing factors to this nationwide problem. General classification of malnutrition is described in Table 18-1.

The results of several national nutrition surveys indicate widespread obesity, retarded growth and development, iron-deficiency anemia, and dental caries. The Surgeon General's Report (HHS, 1988) noted that 5 of the 10 leading causes of death in the United States have been associated scientifically with diet (coronary heart disease, some types of cancer, stroke, diabetes mellitus, and atherosclerosis) and another three (cirrhosis of the liver, accidents, and suicides) have been associated with excessive alcohol intake. Many studies report that protein–calorie malnutrition is widespread (30–50%) in hospitalized clients (Fournet, 1988; Grant & Kennedy-Caldwell, 1988). Protein–calorie malnutrition has been called the skeleton in the hospital closet.

Little can be done to improve an individual's nutrition unless the specific problem and its cause can be identified. Nutritional assessment is an essential part of promoting health, preventing disease, and restoring health. The nurse already gathers much of the information necessary for nutritional assessment in the health history, the clinical appraisal, and developmental screening tests. With a few additional tools, the nurse can identify clients at nutritional risk, evaluate nutrition, and make nursing diagnoses of nutritional problems.

PURPOSES AND SCOPE OF THE NUTRITIONAL ASSESSMENT

Nurses assess nutrition for a variety of reasons:

- To identify areas where nutritional intervention is required to promote health, prevent, or treat disease.
- To identify a client's self-care deficits related to nutrition.
- To evaluate the client's response to nutritional instruction and treatment.
- To provide a baseline for later evaluation of a client's progress.
- To provide an opportunity for the client to ask questions about nutrition and eating practices.

As important as nutritional assessment is to the health of the individual, it unfortunately is not an easy, one-step process. *Optimal nutrition* is defined as nutrition that maximizes health potential. Nutrition experts, however, do not agree on what constitutes optimal nutrition. *Adequate nutrition* may be defined as the intake by an individual of quantities of nutrients sufficient to prevent clinical or subclinical deficiency or excess of one or more nutrients. The quantity of each nutrient needed for adequate nutrition is determined by each individual's body, its activity, and health at a given time. No one set of signs defines good versus poor nutrition because various subclinical levels of malnutrition exist before signs of overt deficiency appear. An individual can be deficient or oversupplied in one nutrient or many (for example, intake may be deficient in vitamin C and/or excessive in calories). The deficiency or excess of each nutrient affects the body in different ways, thus causing different observable signs. Many signs of malnutrition may have other causes. For example, weight in excess of

TABLE 18-1
General Classification of Malnutrition

Type		Description
Specific		The crisis is frequently associated with clinical diseases which may mask the underlying nutrient deficiency or excess.
Long-Standing		There is a latent period between nutritional deficiency or excess and clinical appearance, brought about by a long period of poor eating habits. Chronic undereating may lead to protein–calorie malnutrition. Chronic over-eating may lead to obesity.
Sudden		Marked changes in food intake following traumatic events such as surgery, illness, or bereavement cause a sudden problem.
Recurrent		Severe malnutrition follows worsening cycle of illness and poor nutrient intake contributing to poor nutritional status.

Note. Adapted from Davies, L. (1988). Practical nutrition for the elderly. *Nutrition Reviews, 46,* 85.

published norms may be caused by excess fat, which is considered unhealthy, or by excess muscle secondary to exercise, which is considered healthy.

Another difficulty with nutritional assessment is that many of the norms or standards are being questioned. For example, how does one determine ideal or desirable weight? Some recommended weight tables are based on statistical norms and percentiles, whereas others are based on weights of individuals with the lowest mortality rates. What is best for good health? Many standards are based on statistics from only one segment of the population. For example, skinfold thickness standards used in assessing obesity are based primarily on measurements of Caucasian Americans. Therefore, differences among races or other groups must be interpreted cautiously.

WHOSE NUTRITION SHOULD BE ASSESSED

Nutritional screening and assessment are aspects of total (holistic) health assessment of individuals and should be part of periodic health evaluations. Increased attention should be given to identifying and assessing clients at increased risk for nutritional problems. At certain stages of the life cycle and under certain circumstances, people are at increased risk. Table 18-2 identifies clients who are likely to benefit from nutritional assessment.

All of the clients listed in Table 18-2 should have a nutritional assessment. If evaluation indicates no nutritional problem, these individuals should be reevaluated at predetermined intervals or whenever new risk factors occur. If assessment discloses abnormal findings, however, further in-depth evaluation and intervention by the nurse or nutritionist should follow. Abnormal findings include:

- Diet pattern or content that appears unusual, repetitive, excessive, or inadequate.
- Overt clinical signs of a nutritional deficiency or excess.
- Obesity or underweight.
- Anemia, hypercholesterolemia, or any other abnormal laboratory value related to nutrition.

As an example, if a client's diet indicates that the intake of protein is below the recommended dietary allowance (RDA), the nurse looks for supporting evidence of protein malnutrition from the client's history and profile, anthropometrics, physical examination, and biochemical tests.

If a nutritionist is available, the specific role of the nurse in nutritional assessment is not always clear. The agency or institution may have clear guidelines, but if not, a team decision may avoid duplication and undermining of efforts. In many situations, the nurse is responsible for nutritional screening. If a specific nutritional problem is identified, the nurse may counsel the client or may refer the client to the dietitian or nutrition specialist for more quantitative and in-depth studies and counseling. In other places, a nutritionist reviews all data collected by nurses and determines who would benefit from the professional services of a clinical nutritionist or dietitian.

TABLE 18-2
Clients Who Benefit from Nutritional Assessment

Pregnant women, especially

Pregnant teenagers

Those with inadequate or excessive weight gain, anemia, pregnancy-induced hypertension, or such chronic health problems as diabetes or heart disease

Those with a history of premature birth, low birth weight, stillbirth, or spontaneous abortions

Those who smoke, or who use alcohol or drugs

Those with low income

Infants and children especially

Low-birth-weight or premature infants

Those under 2 years of age

Those who are underweight or overweight for age, stature, and gender

During puberty

Those who have specific health problems, such as dia-

betes, anemia, cystic fibrosis, or congenital heart disease

Those with physical or mental disabilities that affect feeding

Those with low income

Elderly persons, especially those who

Live alone

Have reduced incomes

Have ill-fitting dentures or no dentures

Clients with chronic disorders, such as diabetes, hypertension, atherosclerosis, obesity, alcoholism, drug abuse, depression, neuromuscular disease, renal disease, and gastrointestinal disorders

Hospitalized clients (illness, surgery, trauma)

Clients who live in poverty or who are homeless

KNOWLEDGE NEEDED TO ASSESS NUTRITIONAL STATUS

Quality nursing care is guided by knowledge. Nurses must assume professional responsibility for obtaining and updating their educations. High quality nutritional care for clients requires a knowledge of facts, principles, and concepts related to nutrition, an ability to use concepts from behavioral sciences, an ability to identify the need for nutritional care, skill in using tools and resources for identifying and providing nutritional care, and a commitment to the professional role.

The nurse, who has more time with the client than any other health professional, is in a unique position to assess nutrition. Knowledge and skills enable the nurse to make sound assessments, but the importance the nurse places on nutritional assessment will be affected by the nurse's beliefs and values.

The nurse also must determine the level or depth of the nutritional assessment if this determination has not been made by agency protocols. There is no universal agreement among health professionals about the level of assessment. Dietary assessment frequently is confused with the more holistic nutritional assessment. The role of the professional nurse in doing in-depth nutritional assessment sometimes is questioned by the nutrition professional; however, all agree that nutrition-related care is a vital component of holistic nursing. In providing nutritional care, the nurse frequently functions in an independent and interdependent role with other health professionals. Nurses use nutritional screening to identify clients with nutritional problems and then perform a more in-depth nutritional assessment to determine the cause of the problem. Whether screening or completing an in-depth nutritional assessment, the nurse should analyze specific nutritional factors to formulate a nursing diagnosis with the client. Thus, to complete a nutritional assessment, the nurse needs a broad education in the applied and behavioral sciences, as well as nursing, health, and nutrition, along with beliefs and values that support quality nutrition care. In addition to knowledge and skills in using the nursing process, in performing a clinical appraisal, and obtaining a health history, the nurse needs specific knowledge of dietary needs, caloric intake and expenditures, growth and development, environmental factors affecting nutrition, and the impact of alterations in health on nutrition.

Standards Used to Determine Dietary Needs

The nurse must know the standards used to evaluate dietary intake and the information that can be obtained when these standards are used. The following discussion of the most commonly used standards will provide the nurse with basic information.

The Basic Food Groups

In comparing intake with food groups, the basic food groups found in the Cooperative Extension Service's *Guide for Healthy Food Choices* (Table 18-3) or an adaptation of it usually is used. This method of analysis is simple and can point out weaknesses in the diet, but the nurse should recognize that within each group, the foods listed are not equal in the nutrients they supply. Comparison with the basic food groups does not assure adequate intake of necessary nutrients. For example, when the diet of a child under age 6 contains recommended servings of the basic food groups, the Recommended Dietary Allowance for iron most likely is not met. Use of the basic food groups is only an approximate measure of the adequacy of the diet. Also, the basic food groups are difficult to use when the diet contains items that are combinations of foods; for example, lasagne contains food from four food groups. A list of nutrient sources is helpful to the nurse in assessing dietary intake and is often used in combination with the basic food groups (Table 18-4).

Dietary Guidelines

In addition, the basic food groups do not aid the nurse in assessing diet for compliance with the recommendations issued in 1989 by the Committee on Diet and Health of the National Research Council. These guidelines, listed in Table 18-5, are aimed at reducing the dietary risks associated with chronic diseases.

These guidelines, like the basic food groups, are intended for healthy American adults and children. They are aimed at maintaining health, considering what is known about the relationship between diet and prevention of such health problems as heart attacks, high blood pressure, strokes, dental caries, diabetes, and some forms of cancer.

To use these guidelines in conjunction with the basic food groups in evaluating a client's diet, the nurse must consider the fat, starch and fiber, sugar, sodium, and alcohol content of foods. Evaluating the diet for most of these items requires a record of eating patterns over several days. The nurse may keep eating patterns in mind, however, when reviewing a 24-hour recall.

Dietary Exchange Lists

A more precise tool for evaluating nutritional intake (calories, carbohydrates, protein, and fat) is

TABLE 18-3
A Guide for the Healthy Person's Food Choices.

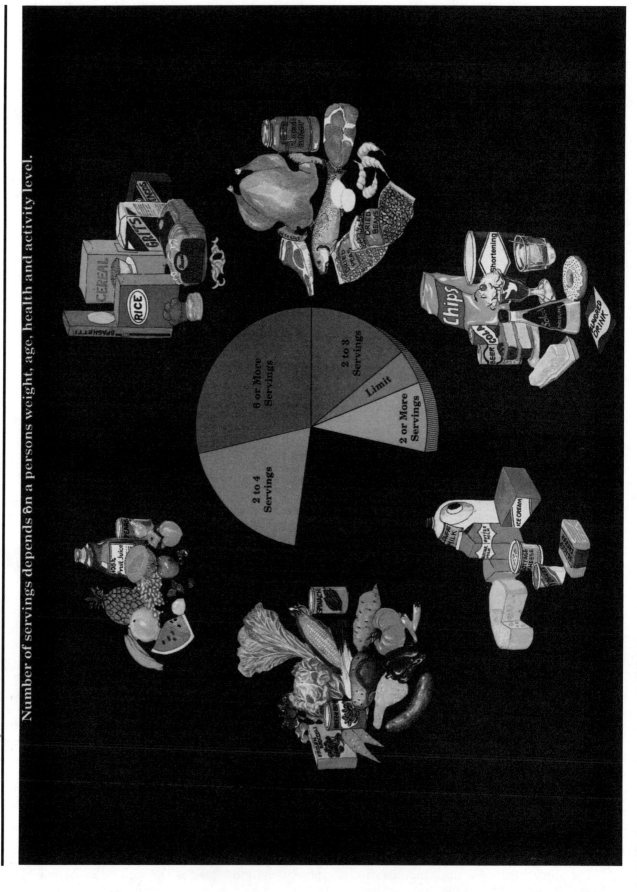

Number of servings depends on a persons weight, age, health and activity level.

TABLE 18-3 (Continued)

Food Group	Servings per Day	Count as a Serving
Breads, Cereals, and Grains	6 or more	1 slice of whole-grain bread, 1/2 hamburger bun, 1 small roll, biscuit, or muffin; 4–6 crackers; 1/2 cup cooked cereal, rice, grits, spaghetti, macaroni, or 1 cup of ready-to-eat cereal. Eat a variety of foods from this group. Make at least one-half of your servings whole grain.
Fruits	2 to 4	1 fresh, medium-size piece of fruit, such as an apple, banana, orange, grapefruit half, or melon wedge; 1/2 cup of juice; 1/2 cup cooked, canned, or frozen fruit; or 1/4 cup dried fruit. Eat a variety of foods from this group. (Eat raw fruits as often as possible).
Vegetables	3 to 5	1/2 cup cooked or raw vegetables or 1 cup leafy raw vegetables, such as cabbage or spinach. Eat a variety of foods from this group. (Eat raw vegetables as often as possible).
Meat, Poultry, and Fish	2 to 3 Pregnancy 3 Breast-Feeding 4	A serving of lean meat, poultry, or fish is 3 ounces. Serving sizes will differ. A piece of meat the size and thickness of the palm of a woman's hand is about 3–5 ounces; a man's palm, 5–7 ounces. Count 1 egg, 1/2 cup cooked dried beans and peas, or 2 tablespoons peanut butter as 1 ounce of meat. Eat a variety of foods from this group.
Milk, Cheese, and Yogurt	Adults 2 Children (6–10 yrs) 3 Teens (11–18 yrs) 4 Pregnancy 4–6 Breast-feeding 4–6	1 cup of buttermilk, skim, low-fat, or whole milk; 1 cup of plain or low-fat yogurt; 1 1/2 ounces of cheese; 2 slices of packaged cheese; 2 cups of low-fat cottage cheese; 1 3/4 cups of ice cream or frozen yogurt. Eat a variety of foods from this group.
Fats, Sweets, Sweetened Drinks, and Alcoholic Beverages	Limit	Limit fats, sweets, sodas, and other sweetened beverages. Choose liquid vegetable oil more often than solid fats and shortenings. Limit bacon and other high fat meats such as sausage and luncheon meats. If you drink alcohol, do so in moderation.

Note. From Clemson University Cooperative Extension Service and the South Carolina Department of Health and Environmental Control, Office of Public Health Nutrition. (1988). *A guide for healthy food choices.* Clemson: Author.

TABLE 18-4
Nutrients: Sources and Functions

Nutrient	Important Sources	Build and Maintain Body Cells	Regular Body Processes
Protein	Meat, Poultry, Fish Dried Beans and Peas Egg Cheese Milk	Constitutes part of the structure of every cell, such as muscle, blood, and bone; supports growth and maintains healthy body cells.	Constitutes part of enzymes, some hormones and body fluids, and antibodies that increase resistance to infection.
Carbohydrate	Cereal Potatoes Dried Beans Corn Bread Sugar	Supplies energy so protein can be used for growth and maintenance of body cells.	Unrefined products supply fiber—complex carbohydrates in fruits, vegetables, and whole grains—for regular elimination. Assists in fat utilization.
Fat	Shortening, Oil Butter, Margarine Salad Dressing Sausages	Constitutes part of the structure of every cell. Supplies essential fatty acids.	Provides and carries fat-soluble vitamins (A, D, E, and K).
Vitamin A (Retinol)	Liver Carrots Sweet Potatoes Greens Butter, Margarine	Assists formation and maintenance of skin and mucous membranes that line body cavities and tracts, such as nasal passages and intestinal tract, thus increasing resistance to infection.	Functions in visual processes and forms visual purple, thus promoting healthy eye tissues and eye adaptation in dim light.
Vitamin C (Ascorbic Acid)	Broccoli Orange Grapefruit Papaya Mango Strawberries	Forms cementing substances, such as collagen, that hold body cells together, thus strengthening blood vessels, hastening healing of wounds and bones, and increasing resistance to infection.	Aids utilization of iron.
Thiamin (B$_1$)	Lean Pork Nuts Fortified Cereal Products		Functions as part of a coenzyme to promote the utilization of carbohydrates. Promotes normal appetite. Contributes to normal functioning of nervous system.
Riboflavin (B$_2$)	Liver Milk Yogurt Cottage Cheese		Functions as part of a coenzyme in the production of energy within body cells. Promotes healthy skin, eyes, and clear vision.
Niacin	Liver Meat, Poultry, Fish Peanuts Fortified Cereal Products		Functions as part of a coenzyme in fat synthesis, tissue respiration, and utilization of carbohydrates. Promotes healthy skin, nerves, and digestive tract. Aids digestion and fosters normal appetite.
Calcium	Milk, Yogurt Cheese Sardines and Salmon	Combines with other minerals within a protein framework to give structure and strength to	Assists in blood clotting. Functions in normal muscle contraction and relaxation,

TABLE 18-4 (Continued)

Nutrient	Important Sources	Build and Maintain Body Cells	Regular Body Processes
	with Bones Collard, Kale, Mustard, and Turnip Greens	bones and teeth.	and normal nerve transmission.
Iron	Enriched Farina Prune Juice Liver Dried Beans and Peas Red Meat	Combines with protein to form hemoglobin, the red substance in blood that carries oxygen to and carbon dioxide from the cells. Prevents nutritional anemia and its accompanying fatigue. Increases resistance to infection.	Functions as part of enzymes involved in tissue respiration.

Note. From *Guide to Good Eating,* 4th edition, Courtesy of National Dairy Council® .

the Food Exchange Lists jointly developed by the American Diabetes Association and American Dietetic Association (1986). Although originally developed to aid clients with diabetes in making appropriate food selections, the lists can be used to determine the nutritional quality of any client's dietary intake. Foods are grouped into six exchange categories: milk, vegetables, fruits, breads, meat (lean, medium fat, or high fat), and fats. Table 18-6 outlines the nutrient and caloric values of each of the six exchange groups.

Once the client's daily energy (caloric) needs are known (Table 18-7), the nurse can consult the Food Exchange Lists (Table 18-6) to determine an appropriate balance of the six exchange groups equal to the client's recommended caloric intake. The recommended distribution of protein, fats, and carbohydrates in a daily diet is protein—10 to 20%, fats—25 to 30%, and carbohydrates—50 to 60%.

A client's sample daily dietary intake then may be compared with the recommended exchanges needed to achieve the client's correct caloric intake.

TABLE 18-5
The Recommendations of the Committee on Diet and Health

- Reduce total fat intake to 30% or less of calories. Reduce saturated fatty acid intake to less than 10% of calories, and the intake of cholesterol to less than 300 mg daily. The intake of fat and cholesterol can be reduced by substituting fish, poultry without skin, lean meats, and low- or nonfat dairy products for fatty meats and whole milk dairy products; by choosing more vegetables, fruits, cereals, and legumes; and by limiting oils, fats, egg yolks, and fried and other fatty foods.

- Every day eat five or more servings[1] of a combination of vegetables and fruits, especially green and yellow vegetables and citrus fruits. Also, increase intake of starches and other complex carbohydrates by eating six or more daily servings of a combination of breads, cereals, and legumes.

- Maintain protein intake at moderate levels.

- Balance food intake and physical activity to maintain appropriate body weight.

- The committee does not recommend alcohol consumption. For those who drink alcoholic beverages, the committee recommends limiting consumption to the equivalent of less than 1 ounce of pure alcohol in a single day. This is the equivalent of two cans of beer, two small glasses of wine, or two average cocktails. Pregnant women should avoid alcoholic beverages.

- Limit total daily intake of salt (sodium chloride) to 6 g or less. Limit the use of salt in cooking and avoid adding it to food at the table. Salty, highly processed salty, salt-preserved, and salt-pickled foods should be consumed sparingly.

- Maintain adequate calcium intake.

- Avoid taking dietary supplements in excess of the RDA in any one day.

- Maintain an optimal intake of fluoride, particularly during the years of primary and secondary tooth formation and growth.

[1]An average serving is equal to a half cup for most fresh or cooked vegetables, fruits, dry or cooked cereals and legumes, one medium piece of fresh fruit, one slice of bread, or one roll or muffin.

Note. Reprinted with permission from *Diet and Health: Implications for Reducing Chronic Disease Risk,* © 1989 by the National Academy of Sciences. Published by National Academy Press, Washington, DC.

TABLE 18-6
Exchange Lists

Exchange List	Carbohydrate (grams)	Protein (grams)	Fat (grams)	Calories
Starch/ Bread	15	3	trace	80
Meat				
Lean	—	7	3	55
Medium fat	—	7	5	75
High fat	—	7	8	100
Vegetable	5	2	—	25
Fruit	15	—	—	60
Milk				
Skim	12	8	trace	90
Low fat	12	8	5	120
Whole	12	8	8	150
Fat	—	—	5	45

Table 18-8 illustrates the recommended exchanges for a typical 1,800 kcal diet. Table 18-9 lists sample foods in each of the dietary exchange groups and their exchange equivalents.

Recommended Dietary Allowances (RDAs)

If precise food intake information has been obtained and a more specific assessment of the intake of individual nutrients and/or calories is desired, the diet can be compared to the standard well-known to most Americans, the Recommended Dietary Allowances (RDA) of the Food and Nutrition Board of the National Academy of Sciences/ National Research Council (Table 18-10). Much controversy surrounded the 1980 RDAs. New guidelines were due in 1985 but nutrition experts could not agree about requirements and about the format for releasing new RDAs; the RDAs were not released until 1989. One of the major questions

TABLE 18-7
Median Heights and Weights and Recommended Energy Intake

Category	Age (years) or Condition	Weight (kg)	Weight (lb)	Height (cm)	Height (in)	REE[a] (kcal/day)	Multiples of REE	Average Energy Allowance (kcal)[b] Per kg	Average Energy Allowance (kcal)[b] Per day[c]
Infants	0.0–0.5	6	13	60	24	320		108	650
	0.5–1.0	9	20	71	28	500		98	850
Children	1–3	13	29	90	35	740		102	1,300
	4–6	20	44	112	44	950		90	1,800
	7–10	28	62	132	52	1,130		70	2,000
Males	11–14	45	99	157	62	1,440	1.70	55	2,500
	15–18	66	145	176	69	1,760	1.67	45	3,000
	19–24	72	160	177	70	1,780	1.67	40	2,900
	25–50	79	174	176	70	1,800	1.60	37	2,900
	51+	77	170	173	68	1,530	1.50	30	2,300
Females	11–14	46	101	157	62	1,310	1.67	47	2,200
	15–18	55	120	163	64	1,370	1.60	40	2,200
	19–24	58	128	164	65	1,350	1.60	38	2,200
	25–50	63	138	163	64	1,380	1.55	36	2,200
	51+	65	143	160	63	1,280	1.50	30	1,900
Pregnant	1st trimester								+0
	2nd trimester								+300
	3rd trimester								+300
Lactating	1st 6 months								+500
	2nd 6 months								+500

[a]Calculation based on Food & Agriculture Association (FAO).

[b]In the range of light to moderate activity, the coefficient of variation is ±20%

[c]Figure is rounded.

Note. From the National Research Council. (1989). *Recommended dietary allowances* (10th ed.). Washington, DC: National Academy Press.

TABLE 18-8
Total Food Exchanges in an 1800 kcal Diet

Food List	Number of Exchanges	Protein (g)	Carbohydrate (g)	Fat (g)	kcal*
Nonfat milk	2	16	24	0	160
Vegetables	3	6	15	0	75
Fruits	4	0	60	0	240
Bread	9	27	135	0	630
Meat, lean	5	35	0	15	330
Fat	8	0	0	40	360
TOTAL	31	68	234	55	1,830

*Calories are obtained by using the following equivalence: 1 g protein = 4 kcal
1 g of carbohydrate = 4 kcal
1 g of fat = 9 kcal
The above meets the ADA recommendations of 30% fat, 15% protein, and 50–60% carbohydrate.

concerns calcium. Most nutrition experts agree that calcium intake for women needs to be increased to 1,000–1,500 mg. To use the RDAs the nurse first must compare the foods listed in a diet recall or food diary with a food composition table to determine the approximate amount of a given nutrient in the diet. Tables most commonly used are those from the U.S. Department of Agriculture, *Nutritive Value of American Foods* (1985) and those in Bowes and Church's *Food Values of Portions Commonly Used* (Pennington & Church, 1985). Milligrams or units of a nutrient are totaled for each day and averaged for the week. The daily average then is compared with the RDA for the client's age group, sex, weight, and height. These calculations are done either by hand or computer.

The nurse must be careful when using nutrition tables to be sure portion sizes consumed by the client are comparable to those in the tables. For example, the listed vegetable serving sizes often are larger than what most people usually eat. Also, many clients use convenience and combination foods that make it difficult to use the tables. It may be necessary to contact the food manufacturer or to obtain the food packages and check the labels.

For research purposes, samples of all foods consumed can be weighed and analyzed by a chemist for a precise evaluation of nutrient intake. Laboratory analysis is particularly useful when there is little variety in the diet, as with certain fad diets emphasizing a single nutrient, such as "the grapefruit diet" and the "liquid protein diet." Clients on these diets usually have deficiencies in certain other nutrients, and such deficiencies should be evaluated. Obese clients often use such diets for short periods, so questions in the history should be directed at eliciting information about past diets.

Comparing nutrients consumed with RDAs has some limitations. By definition, Recommended Dietary Allowances "are the levels of intake of essential nutrients considered . . . on the bases of available scientific knowledge, to be adequate to meet the known nutritional needs of practically all healthy persons" (National Research Council, Food and Nutrition Board, 1980, p. 1). These allowances are neither minimum requirements nor lists of what is necessary for an ideal diet. They are intended for estimating dietary needs of groups of healthy people, for example, for developing food programs. Individual needs vary with height and weight, energy expenditure, use of nutrients (which can be affected by food and medication interactions, form of the nutrient, and similar factors), climate, and health. Each allowance (except calories) includes a "margin of safety" that varies with each nutrient. Thus, if the calculated intake of a given nutrient for an individual is lower than the RDA of that nutrient, one cannot assume that the diet is deficient. The converse also is true. If the individual being assessed is healthy, has a normal stress level, and lives in a temperate climate, and if there are no clinical or biochemical signs of deficiency, an intake slightly lower than the RDA may be acceptable. However, according to the National Research Council (1980), "if nutrient intake is insufficient to meet requirements for a prolonged period, the ability to respond to trauma and illness may ultimately be lessened, and depletion and deterioration may eventually occur" (p. 7). Even though RDAs are high enough to cover those with high average requirements, the nurse must consider individual variations in evaluating the adequacy of intake.

As with the basic food groups of the Cooperative Extension Service, the RDAs can be used to

TABLE 18-9
Sample Food Exchanges

	Amount Equal to One Exchange		Amount Equal to One Exchange
Milk Exchanges		Mango	1/2 small
Skim or nonfat milk	1 cup	Melon—cantaloupe	1/3 melon
2% lowfat milk (includes 1 fat exchange)	1 cup		or 1 cup
Whole milk (includes 2 fat exchanges)	1 cup	watermelon	1 1/4 cup
Buttermilk made from skim milk	1 cup	Nectarine	1 small
Plain yogurt made from skim milk	1 cup	Orange	1 small
Dry nonfat milk	1/3 cup	Orange juice	1/2 cup
		Papaya	1 cup
Vegetable Exchanges		Peach	1 medium
Asparagus	1/2 cup	Pear	1 small
Bamboo shoots, canned	1 cup	Persimmon	2
Bean sprouts, raw	1 cup	Pineapple	3/4 cup
Bok choy, cooked	1 cup	Pineapple juice	1/2 cup
Beets	1/2 cup	Plums, prunes	3 medium
Broccoli	1/2 cup	Prune juice	1/3 cup
Brussel sprouts	1/2 cup	Raisins	2 tbsp.
Cabbage or Chinese cabbage (cooked)	1/2 cup	Strawberries	1 1/4 cup
Carrots	1/2 cup	**Bread Exchanges**	
Cauliflower	1/2 cup	(includes bread, cereal, pasta, and starchy vegetables)	
Greens (spinach, kale, collards, chards, mustard, turnip)	1/2 cup	*Bread*	
Green beans	1/2 cup	White, refined, French, Italian, Challah	1 slice
Eggplant	1/2 cup	Whole wheat, rye, pumpernickel	1 slice
Lotus root	1/2 cup	Raisin	1 slice
Miso	1 tbsp.	Bagel or biale, small	1/2
Mushrooms (cooked)	1/2 cup	English muffin	1/2
Dried black mushrooms	1/4 cup	Plain roll	1
Okra	1/2 cup	Frankfurter or hamburger bun	1/2
Sauerkraut	1/2 cup	Pita bread	1
Snow peas	1/2 cup	Tortilla, 6″	1
Squash (summer, zucchini)	1/2 cup	*Cereal/Pasta*	
Taro root	1/4 cup	Dry, unsweetened	3/4 cup
Tomatoes	1 large	Cooked cereal	1/2 cup
Tomato juice	1/2 cup	Cellophane noodles, cooked	1/2 cup
Turnips	1/2 cup	Fried rice (includes 1 fat exchange)	1/2 cup
Water chestnuts	1/2 cup	Grits, cooked	1/2 cup
		Barley, cooked	1/2 cup
Fruit Exchanges (fresh or no sugar added)		Rice	1/3 cup
Apple	1 small	Pasta, cooked	1/2 cup
Apple juice	1/2 cup	Popcorn (popped, no fat added)	3 cups
Applesauce, unsweetened	1/2 cup	Mungbean noodles	1/2 cup
Apricots (medium, raw)	4	*Crackers*	
Banana	1/2	Animal Crackers	8
Berries (blackberries, blueberries)	3/4 cup	Arrowroot	3
Raspberries	1 cup	Graham	3
Carambola (starfruit)	1	Matzoh	3/4 oz.
Cherries	12 large	Oyster	24
Grapefruit	1/2	Pretzels (small stick)	25
Grapefruit juice	1/2 cup	Saltines	6
Grapes	15 small	*Dried Beans, Peas, Lentils*	
Grape juice	1/3 cup	Beans, peas, lentils, cooked	1/3 cup
Guava	1 small	Garbanzo beans	1/3 cup
Kiwi fruit	1 large		
Kumquats	4		

TABLE 18-9 (Continued)

	Amount Equal to One Exchange		Amount Equal to One Exchange
Baked beans, canned (no pork)	1/4 cup	grated parmesan,	2 Tbsp.
		diet cheeses* [with less than 55 calories per ounce])	1 oz.
Starchy Vegetables		Other	
Corn	1/2 cup	(95% fat-free luncheon meat,	1 oz.
Lima beans	1/2 cup	egg whites,	3 whites
Parsnips	2/3 cup	egg substitutes with less than 55	1/4 cup
Peas, canned or frozen	1/2 cup	calories per 1/4 cup)	
Potato	1 small		
Mashed potatoes	1/2 cup	*Medium-Fat Meat and Substitutes*	
Potato knish, 3" round	1	*(One exchange is equal to any one of the following items.)*	
Winter squash, pumpkin	3/4 cup	Beef (Most beef products fall into this	1 oz.
Yams, sweet potatoes	1/3 cup	category. Examples are: all ground	
		beef, roast [rib, chuck, rump], steak	
Prepared Foods		[cubed, Porterhouse, T-bone], and	
Biscuit, 2" (includes 1 fat exchange)	1	meatloaf.)	
Corn bread, 2" (includes 1 fat exchange)	1	Pork (Most pork products fall into this	1 oz.
		category. Examples are: chops, loin	
French fries (medium size) (includes 1 fat exchange)	10	roast, Boston butt, cutlets.)	
		Lamb (Most lamb products fall into	1 oz.
Potato or corn chips (includes 2 fat exchanges)	15	this category. Examples are: chops, leg, and roast.)	
Matzoh balls, 2"	1	Veal (cutlet [ground or cubed, un-breaded])	1 oz.
Pancake or waffle (includes 1 fat exchange)	1	Poultry (chicken [with skin], domestic	1 oz.
		duck or goose [well-drained of fat],	
Refried beans (includes 1 fat exchange)	1/3 cup	ground turkey)	
		Fish	
Meat Exchanges		(tuna* [canned in oil and drained],	1/4 cup
Lean Meat and Substitutes		salmon* [canned])	1/4 cup
(One exchange is equal to any one of the following items.)		Cheese (skim or part-skim milk cheeses, such as:	
Beef (USDA Good or Choice grades of	1 oz.	ricotta,	1/4 cup
lean beef, such as round, sirloin,		mozzarella,	1 oz.
and flank steak; tenderloin; and		diet cheeses* [with 56–80 calories	1 oz.
chipped beef)*		per ounce])	
Pork (lean pork, such as fresh ham;	1 oz.	Other	
canned, cured or boiled ham*; Ca-nadian bacon*, tenderloin)		(86% fat-free luncheon meat,	1 oz.
Veal (All cuts are lean except for veal	1 oz.	egg [high in cholesterol, limit to 3	1
cutlets [ground or cubed]. Examples of		per week],	
lean veal are chops and roasts.)		egg substitutes with 56–80 calories	1/4 cup
Poultry (chicken, turkey, Cornish hen	1 oz.	per 1/4 cup,	
[without skin])		tofu [2 1/2 in. × 2 3/4 in. × 1 in.],	4 oz.
Fish		liver, heart, kidney, sweetbreads	1 oz.
(all fresh and frozen fish;	1 oz.	[high in cholesterol])	
crab, lobster, scallops, shrimp, clams	2 oz.		
[fresh or canned in water*];		*High-Fat Meat and Substitutes*	
gefilte fish	1 oz.	*Remember, these items are high in saturated fat, choles-*	
oysters	6 medium	*terol, and calories, and should be used only three (3)*	
tuna* [canned in water];	1/4 cup	*times per week.*	
herring [uncreamed or smoked];	1 oz.	*(One exchange is equal to any one of the following items.)*	
sardines [canned];	2 medium	Beef (most USDA Prime cuts of beef,	1 oz.
lox [smoked salmon])	1 oz.	such as ribs, corned beef*)	
Wild Game	1 oz.	Pork (spareribs, ground pork, pork	1 oz.
(venison, rabbit, squirrel,		sausage* [patty or link])	
pheasant, duck, goose [without	1 oz.	Lamb (patties [ground lamb])	1 oz.
skin])		Fish (any fried fish product)	1 oz.
Cheese			
(any cottage cheese,	1/4 cup		

(continued)

TABLE 18-9 (Continued)

	Amount Equal to One Exchange		Amount Equal to One Exchange
Cheese (all regular cheeses*, such as American, blue, cheddar, Monterey, Swiss)	1 oz.	of those items that have a specific serving size. Be sure to spread them out through the day.	
Other (luncheon meat*, such as bologna, salami, pimento loaf;	1 oz.	*Drinks* Bouillon*** or broth without fat Bouillon, low-sodium	
sausage*, such as Polish, Italian;	1 oz.	Carbonated drinks, sugar-free	
knockwurst, smoked;	1 oz.	Carbonated water	
bratwurst*;	1 oz.	Club soda	
frankfurter* [turkey or chicken];	1 frank (10/lb.)	Cocoa powder, unsweetened Coffee/Tea	1 Tbsp.
peanut butter [contains unsaturated fat])	1 Tbsp.	Drink mixes, sugar-free Tonic water, sugar-free	
Count as one high-fat meat plus one fat exchange:		*Nonstick pan spray*	
frankfurter* (beef, pork, or combination)	1 frank (10/lb.)	*Fruit* Cranberries, unsweetened	1/2 cup
		Rhubarb, unsweetened	1/2 cup
Fat Exchanges		*Vegetables (raw, 1 cup)*	
Butter or margarine	1 tsp.	Cabbage	
Margarine, diet	1 Tbsp.	Celery	
Avocado, 4"	1/8	Chinese cabbage**	
Oils (corn, cottonseed, sesame, safflower, soy, sunflower, peanut, olive)	1 tsp.	Cucumber Green onion	
Olives	5 large or 10 small	Hot peppers Mushrooms	
		Radishes	
Nuts and seeds:		Zucchini**	
Almonds, dry roasted	6 whole	*Salad greens*	
Cashews, dry roasted	1 Tbsp.	Endive	
Pecans	2 whole	Escarole	
Peanuts	20 small or 10 large	Lettuce Romaine	
Walnuts	2 whole	Spinach	
Other nuts	1 Tbsp.	*Sweet substitutes*	
Seeds, pine nuts, sunflower (without shells)	1 Tbsp.	Candy, hard, sugar-free Gelatin, sugar-free	
Pumpkin seeds	2 tsp.	Gum, sugar-free	
Bacon	1 strip cooked & drained	Jam/Jelly, sugar-free Pancake syrup, sugar-free	2 tsp. 1–2 Tbsp.
Chicken or bacon fat	1 tsp.	Sugar substitutes (saccharin, aspartame)	
Cream (half & half or sour)	2 Tbsp.	Whipped topping	2 Tbsp.
Heavy cream	1 Tbsp.	*Condiments:*	
Cream cheese	1 Tbsp.	Catsup	1 Tbsp.
Salad dressings	1 Tbsp.	Horseradish	
Mayonnaise	1 tsp.	Mustard	
Mayonnaise, reduced calorie	1 Tbsp.	Pickles***, dill, unsweetened	
Lard	1 tsp.	Salad dressing, low-calorie	2 Tbsp.
Salt pork	3/4" cube	Taco sauce	1 Tbsp.
		Vinegar	

Free Foods

A free food is any food or drink that contains less than 20 calories per serving. You can eat as much as you want of those items that have no serving size specified. You may eat two or three servings per day

Seasonings can be very helpful in making food taste better. Be careful of how much sodium you use. Read

TABLE 18-9 (Continued)

	Amount Equal to One Exchange		Amount Equal to One Exchange
the label, and choose those seasonings that do not contain sodium or salt.		Lemon	
		Lemon juice	
Basil (fresh)		Lemon pepper	
Celery seeds		Lime	
Cinnamon		Lime juice	
Chili powder		Mint	
Chives		Onion powder	
Curry		Oregano	
Dill		Paprika	
Flavoring extracts (vanilla, almond, walnut, peppermint, butter, lemon, etc.)		Pepper	
		Pimento	
		Spices	
Garlic		Soy sauce***	
Garlic powder		Soy sauce, low sodium ("lite")	
Herbs		Wine, used in cooking	1/4 cup
Hot pepper sauce		Worcestershire sauce	

Combination Foods

Much of the food we eat is mixed together in various combinations. These combination foods do not fit into only one exchange list. It can be quite hard to tell what is in a certain casserole dish or baked food item. This is a list of average values for some typical combination foods. This list will help you fit these foods into your meal plan. Ask your dietitian for information about any other foods you'd like to eat. The *American Diabetes Association/American Dietetic Association Family Cookbooks* and the *American Diabetes Association Holiday Cookbook* have many recipes and further information about many foods, including combination foods. Check your library or local bookstore.

Food	Amount	Exchanges
Casseroles, homemade	1 cup (8 oz.)	2 starch, 2 medium-fat meat, 1 fat
Cheese pizza***, thin crust	1/4 of 15 oz. or 1/4 of 10″	2 starch, 1 medium-fat meat, 1 fat
Chili with beans**, *** (commercial)	1 cup (8 oz.)	2 starch, 2 medium-fat meat, 2 fat
Chow mein**, *** (without noodles or rice)	2 cups (16 oz.)	1 starch, 2 vegetable, 2 lean meat
Macaroni and cheese***	1 cup (8 oz.)	2 starch, 1 medium-fat meat, 2 fat
Soup:		
Bean**, ***	1 cup (8 oz.)	1 starch, 1 vegetable, 1 lean meat
Chunky, all varieties*	10-3/4 oz. can	1 starch, 1 vegetable, 1 medium-fat meat
Cream*** (made with water)	1 cup (8 oz.)	1 starch, 1 fat
Vegetable*** or broth***	1 cup (8 oz.)	1 starch
Spaghetti and meatballs*** (canned)	1 cup (8 oz.)	2 starch, 1 medium-fat meat, 1 fat
Sugar-free pudding (made with skim milk)	1/2 cup	1 starch
If beans are used as a meat substitute:		
Dried beans**, peas**, lentils**	1 cup (cooked)	2 starch, 1 lean meat

Foods for Occasional Use

Moderate amounts of some foods can be used in your meal plan, in spite of their sugar or fat content, as long as you can maintain blood-glucose control. The following list includes average exchange values for some of these foods. Because they are concentrated sources of carbohydrate, you will notice that the portion sizes are very small. Check with your dietitian for advice on how often and when you can eat them. [*Note:* Specifically for diabetic individuals.]

(continued)

TABLE 18-9 (Continued)

Food	Amount	Exchanges
Angel food cake	1/12 cake	2 starch
Cake, no icing	1/12 cake, or a 3″ square	2 starch, 2 fat
Cookies	2 small (1 3/4″ across)	1 starch, 1 fat
Frozen fruit yogurt	1/3 cup	1 starch
Gingersnaps	3	1 starch
Granola	1/4 cup	1 starch, 1 fat
Granola bars	1 small	1 starch, 1 fat
Ice cream, any flavor	1/2 cup	1 starch, 2 fat
Ice milk, any flavor	1/2 cup	1 starch, 1 fat
Sherbet, any flavor	1/4 cup	1 starch
Snack chips***, all varieties	1 oz.	1 starch, 2 fat
Vanilla wafers	6 small	1 starch, 1 fat

*400 mg or more of sodium per exchange

**3 grams or more of fiber per serving

***If more than one serving is eaten, these foods have 400 mg. or more of sodium

partially evaluate the diet. Allowances for calories, fiber, fluid, some trace elements, and saturated versus unsaturated fats are not given.

Caloric Intake and Energy Expenditure

Calorie standards usually are given in terms of age, sex, height, and weight. Several formulas can be used by the nurse to estimate caloric needs. The most widely used is the Basal Energy Expenditure Formula shown in Table 18-11.

Other Dietary Recommendations

Various federal, professional, and health organizations have published dietary recommendations for healthy Americans that focus on the relationship of diet to health and risk of disease. Cronin and Shaw (1988) summarize these recommendations, and many are reflected in the general guidelines in Table 18-5. Several organizations recommend that the caloric content of our diet come from 55–60% carbohydrates, 15–20% protein, and 25–35% fat. Specific recommendations may be used to assist the nurse in analysis of nutrient adequacy, body weight, fats, cholesterol, carbohydrates (starch, fiber, and refined sugars), sodium, and alcohol. Not all professionals agree with all these recommendations. For example, the American Academy of Pediatrics (AAP) states that children should consume approximately 30 to 40% of calories from fat for optimal growth and development, rather than 27 to 35% recommended for healthy Americans in most guidelines (AAP, 1986).

VARIABLES INFLUENCING NUTRITIONAL REQUIREMENTS

Some modifications in approach will be necessary, depending on the client's environment, age, and health. Health problems may be treated with drugs. Nutrient–drug interactions may influence nutrition, and nutrition may influence the body's response to certain drugs.

Environmental Influences

Environmental factors affect nutrition. Many of these factors affect dietary intake and affect anthropometric and biochemical measurements, clinical appraisal, and history. The nurse needs to assess cultural and religious influences on nutrient intake as well. It is also important to assess food availability, sanitation, economics, and education. These environmental factors could influence the plans and interventions suggested by the nurse. If these areas are not assessed, the nurse may never determine why the nursing care plan failed to achieve the desired results.

Racial, ethnic, and religious practices frequently influence nutrition. The nurse practicing in an area serving many members of minority groups needs to consider practices dictated by tradition or religious law that influence the food consumed and the nutritional values of the foods related to preparation methods. For example, the person who eats fresh spinach would be getting many more water-soluble vitamins compared to

TABLE 18-10
Recommended Dietary Allowances (RDA), 1989[a]

Age (years)	Weight (kg)	(lb)	Height (cm)	(inches)	(g) Protein	(μg RE) Vitamin A	(μg) Vitamin D	(mg α-TE) Vitamin E	(μg) Vitamin K	(mg) Vitamin C	(mg) Thiamin	(mg) Riboflavin	(mg NE) Niacin	(mg) Vitamin B6	(μg) Folate	(μg) Vitamin B12	(mg) Calcium	(mg) Phosphorus	(mg) Magnesium	(mg) Iron	(mg) Zinc	(μg) Iodine	(μg) Selenium
Infants																							
0.0–0.5	6	13	60	24	13	375	7.5	3	5	30	0.3	0.4	5	0.3	25	0.3	400	300	40	6	5	40	10
0.5–1.0	9	20	71	28	14	375	10	4	10	35	0.4	0.5	6	0.6	35	0.5	600	500	60	10	5	50	15
Children																							
1–3	13	29	90	35	16	400	10	6	15	40	0.7	0.8	9	1.0	50	0.7	800	800	80	10	10	70	20
4–6	20	44	112	44	24	500	10	7	20	45	0.9	1.1	12	1.1	75	1.0	800	800	120	10	10	90	20
7–10	28	62	132	52	28	700	10	7	30	45	1.0	1.2	13	1.4	100	1.4	800	800	170	10	10	120	30
Males																							
11–14	45	99	157	62	45	1,000	10	10	45	50	1.3	1.5	17	1.7	150	2.0	1,200	1,200	270	12	15	150	40
15–18	66	145	176	69	59	1,000	10	10	65	60	1.5	1.8	20	2.0	200	2.0	1,200	1,200	400	12	15	150	50
19–24	72	160	177	70	58	1,000	10	10	70	60	1.5	1.7	19	2.0	200	2.0	1,200	1,200	350	10	15	150	70
25–50	79	174	176	70	63	1,000	5	10	80	60	1.5	1.7	19	2.0	200	2.0	800	800	350	10	15	150	70
51+	77	170	173	68	63	1,000	5	10	80	60	1.2	1.4	15	2.0	200	2.0	800	800	350	10	15	150	70
Females																							
11–14	46	101	157	62	46	800	10	8	45	50	1.1	1.3	15	1.4	150	2.0	1,200	1,200	280	15	12	150	45
15–18	55	120	163	64	44	800	10	8	55	60	1.1	1.3	15	1.5	180	2.0	1,200	1,200	300	15	12	150	50
19–24	58	128	164	65	46	800	10	8	60	60	1.1	1.3	15	1.6	180	2.0	1,200	1,200	280	15	12	150	55
25–50	63	138	163	64	50	800	5	8	65	60	1.1	1.3	15	1.6	180	2.0	800	800	280	15	12	150	55
51+	65	143	160	63	50	800	5	8	65	60	1.0	1.2	13	1.6	180	2.0	800	800	280	10	12	150	55
Pregnant					60	800	10	10	65	70	1.5	1.6	17	2.2	400	2.2	1,200	1,200	320	30	15	175	65
Lactating																							
1st 6 mo					65	1,300	10	12	65	95	1.6	1.8	20	2.1	280	2.6	1,200	1,200	355	15	19	200	75
2nd 6 mo					62	1,200	10	11	65	90	1.6	1.7	20	2.1	260	2.6	1,200	1,200	340	15	16	200	75

[a]The allowances are intended to provide for individual variations among most normal, healthy people in the United States under usual environmental stresses. They were designed for the maintenance of good nutrition. Diets should be based on a variety of common foods in order to provide other nutrients for which human requirements have been less well defined.

Note. From National Academy of Sciences (1989). *Recommended dietary allowances* (10th ed.). Washington, DC: National Academy Press.

the person who eats spinach that has been cooked for one to two hours in an open pot. The American Dietetic Association (1976) developed a booklet entitled *Cultural Food Patterns in the U.S.A.*, which a nurse can use for looking at characteristic food patterns and making suggestions for better nutrition and economy.

General awareness of what foods normally are included and excluded from diets of various cultures helps the nurse direct assessment toward food groups and nutrients that often are lacking or deficient. For example, there are a number of types of vegetarianism. Individuals who adhere to a lacto-ovo vegetarian diet include milk, milk prod-

ucts, and eggs in their diets. They have less difficulty achieving balanced diets than do strict vegetarians (vegans) such as Zen macrobiotics followers. The macrobiotic diet includes food only from specified plant sources and is likely to be deficient in essential amino acids unless the diet is well-planned. Some vitamins also may be lacking because the diet eschews "nightshade" plants, including potatoes, tomatoes, and peppers. At particular risk of protein malnutrition are pregnant and lactating women. Another nutrient lacking in diets containing no animal foods is vitamin B_{12}. Children who do not consume milk or milk products, most probably need calcium supplements.

TABLE 18-11
Basal Energy Expenditure (BEE)

MEN — BEE = 66 + (13.7 × W) + (5 × H) – (6.8
           × A)
WOMEN — BEE = 655 + (9.6 × W) + (1.7 × H) –
              (4.7 × A)

W = actual weight in Kg
H = height in cm
A = age in years

The nurse should be careful, however, not to make assumptions about what is included in the diet of a particular group.

The nurse should learn the names of foods common to various cultures and the nutrients they provide in order to assess a 24-hour recall or food record and to make up food frequency lists. For example, Zen macrobiotic staples include miso and tofu, soy products that are protein sources. Since these and many other cultural or foreign foods are not listed in standard food tables, evaluating intake may be difficult.

Lactose intolerance is a problem found more commonly in certain ethnic groups, especially those of African-American, Jewish, Chinese, Thai, Filipino, and Vietnamese descent. Diets of those with lactose intolerance must be assessed for adequacy of calcium intake since such individuals frequently avoid dairy products. Calcium intake is especially important during pregnancy and lactation and, with special planning, some of these individuals may eat small amounts of certain dairy foods.

Some cultural/religious groups still practice days of fasting. For example, Roman Catholics may fast prior to certain holy days. Jews traditionally fast on Yom Kippur, the "Day of Atonement." Food records and 24-hour recalls need to take this into consideration.

In assessing anthropometric and biochemical data of individuals from ethnic groups, population-specific standards should be used if they are available. Garn and Clark (1966) found significant differences between African-Americans and Caucasians in height (African-Americans are taller), development as determined by postnatal ossification centers and tooth emergence (African-Americans show earlier development), and hemoglobin levels (African-Americans had a 1.0 g/100 ml lower average in income-matched groups).

A dietary practice that deserves special attention here is pica. Pica refers to compulsive ingestion of non-food substances such as clay or dirt, laundry starch, paint, and plaster chips. Pica is prevalent among African-American women of rural southern heritage, particularly during pregnancy (Committee on Nutrition of Mother and Preschool Child, National Research Council, 1982). Lewis (1986) discusses the incidence, etiology, detrimental effects, and interventions. Usual assessment techniques may not detect pica so it is important to ask questions that are both open-ended ("Do you crave anything in particular?") and straight-forward ("Do you eat ice, laundry starch, clay, coffee grounds?"). If pica is detected, the specific type and amount of substance being consumed and the duration of the practice should be determined. Nutrient deficiencies may result because pica may displace nutritious foods in the diet or may interfere with absorption of nutrients. Lead poisoning is likely to occur from ingestion of lead-based paints or plaster or dirt containing lead. Clients who eat clay are at increased risk for intestinal parasites and fecal impactions. Clay also may contain potassium, which can produce life-threatening hyperkalemia in some clients (Lewis, 1986). If pica is detected, interventions should be geared toward preventing harmful effects and guiding the client toward a self-directed solution.

Influence of Age

The age of the client provides clues to particular nutritional problems that warrant screening. The age-related findings of the *Ten-State Nutrition Survey* (Staff, 1972), a detailed study of the nutritional status of 40,000 people conducted from 1968 to 1970, are especially helpful. Also, techniques for collecting information vary according to the age of the client. Table 18-12 offers cues for minimal assessment of various age groups.

A more in-depth discussion of the nutritional needs and assessment for various age groups may be found in the chapters focusing on specific age groups (pregnant women, newborns, infants and children, and adolescents).

Early Adulthood

Although nutritional intake in early adulthood more adequately meets needs, nutritional problems still exist. The *Ten-State Nutrition Survey* found obesity to be particularly prevalent in adult women, especially African-Americans (Staff, 1972). Snacks are a significant part of food intake because of busy schedules. Although it is difficult to reverse obesity, the influence of parents' eating patterns on obesity in their children makes nutritional assessment and attempts at modifying patterns of diet and exercise worthwhile.

TABLE 18-12
Minimal Assessment of Nutritional Status

Age Group	Anthropometric Measurements	Biochemical Evaluation	Clinical History and Appraisal	Dietary Assessment
Infants	Weight Length Overall pattern of growth Head circumference	Hematocrit Hemoglobin	Birth weight Length of gestation Skin color, turgor Malformations	Bottle- or breast-fed Supplemental feedings (fluids, solids, method of preparation, weaning, self-feeding) Source of iron Vitamin supplements
Children	Weight Height Arm circumference Overall pattern of growth	Hematrocrit Hemoglobin BUN	Birth weight Chronic/recent illness Physical activity Skin color, turgor Muscle tone Subcutaneous fat Dental caries	Food intake* Appetite Feeding jags, pica Snacking habits Vitamin/mineral supplements Arrangements for eating away from home
Adolescents	Weight Height Recent weight changes	Hemoglobin Urine protein Blood sugar	Medical history/allergies Socioeconomic data Physical activity Family history Medications General appearance of hair, skin, eyes Muscle tone Subcutaneous fat Dental caries	Food intake* (assess for excessive salt or sugar) Where and when foods are eaten Snacking habits Fad diets (especially females) Vitamin/mineral supplements Alcohol intake
Adults	Weight Height Recent weight changes	Hemoglobin Urine protein Blood sugar Urinary pH	Medical history Age Number in family Socioeconomic data Physical activity Family history Medications General appearance and maintenance of hair, skin, eyes, muscles Dental caries Blood pressure	Food intake* (assess for saturated fat, cholesterol, sugar, salt; iron and calcium in females) Snacking habits Vitamin/mineral supplements Alcohol intake
Elderly People	Weight Height Recent weight changes	Hemoglobin Blood sugar Urinalysis Feces	Chronic illness or disability Use of tobacco, alcohol, drugs Source of income; amount for food Any physical changes (bleeding, bowel/urinary patterns, fainting, headaches) Skin color, pallor Blood pressure Dentition	Food intake* and patterns Supplements (protein, vitamins, minerals) Who purchases and prepares food Changes in food habits Taste changes Dietary restrictions

*Question about the frequency of use of the basic food groups.

Women taking oral contraceptives may show deficiencies in pyridoxine (vitamin B_6), vitamin C, and folic acid and should be assessed for these, particularly if dietary intake is inadequate.

Middle Adulthood

Clients in the middle years of adulthood need fewer calories to maintain their body weights because physical growth is complete, basal metabolic rate is decreasing, and energy expenditure usually is less than it was in the early adult years. Consequently, middle-aged adults must reduce their caloric consumption or increase their energy expenditure through exercise if they are to avoid excessive weight gain. Overweight and obesity are common health problems in this age group and may contribute to other health problems, such as atherosclerosis and diabetes mellitus.

Busy work schedules and demands may interfere with intake of essential nutrients. Increased affluence at this age, especially among middle and upper class Americans, may have a negative influence on nutrition. For instance, use of automobiles, modern appliances, elevators, frequent dining out, and increased alcohol consumption all may contribute to decreased energy expenditure and increased intake of calories, protein, fats, and sodium.

Thus, it is important to assess the middle-aged client's dietary intake, eating habits, exercise patterns, lifestyle, caffeine and alcohol consumption, and sodium intake to determine nutritional excesses or deficiencies.

Older Adulthood

Low intake of calories, protein, calcium, and iron commonly is found in elderly people, although obesity also occurs. In interviewing and observing the elderly client, the nurse should ask about problems that can lead to undernutrition, such as:

- Difficulty chewing (missing or loose teeth, poorly fitted dentures)
- Poor appetite secondary to diminished taste, smell, and sight, medications, eating alone
- Indigestion
- Modified diet required for treatment of a chronic illness
- Low income and restricted access to shopping (impaired mobility, lack of transportation)
- Fad diets believed to increase vigor.

Many elderly people use mineral oil as a laxative, increasing the likelihood that fat-soluble vitamins will be absorbed poorly. During the health history, the nurse should ask about the use of mineral oil and other laxatives and should assess for fat-soluble vitamin deficiencies if mineral oil is used. Also, the diet should be evaluated for intake of fiber and fluids, since gastrointestinal motility decreases with age. Thus, the elderly client needs to be assessed for supplement use and for nutrient deficiencies. A recent study by Hartz and colleagues (1988) found that 55% of women and 45% of men older than 60 reported vitamin/mineral supplement use; however, users and nonusers had comparable percentages of deficiencies.

A change in the elderly client's mental status that actually is related to poor nutrition may be incorrectly attributed to senility. Because of this possibility, nutritional assessment of the elderly is especially important.

If the aged client has poor recall, the nurse may need to interview a caretaker or obtain a food diary to provide more accurate data. Jenkins (1988) reviews the nutritional problems associated with aging and offers suggestions for the nurse in assessing nutrition.

Influence of Illness and Surgery

The same data need to be collected and assessed whether a client is well or ill. Some information may be more easily obtained when the client is ill, especially if hospitalized. For example, biochemical test results and a clinical review of systems already may be on the client's record because of the illness that precipitated hospitalization. Dietary intake information is obtained more easily in a health-care facility, since food offered and refused can be directly observed and measured, although unfortunately often is not. Some data may be more difficult to obtain—anthropometric measurements if the client is immobilized in traction, or diet history if the client is comatose. Nevertheless, all categories of information discussed previously in this chapter need to be obtained and reviewed. Modifications in assessment during illness are concerned principally with intake and differences in nutritional needs. Nutritional assessment reference cards for several diseases have been developed by Bell (1987) to assist the nurse or nutritionist in assessing nutrition.

Amount of Intake

Ill and hospitalized clients often have a poor level of nutrition, although this too often is not observed by health personnel. The nurse needs to note how much a client eats, especially during illness and before and after surgery. An order for "nothing by mouth" or "clear liquids" over a period of time without adequate nutrition by other means can lead to malnutrition. This is not uncommon when tests or surgery are scheduled, cancelled, and rescheduled. When intake is poor, the nurse needs to determine why the client is not eating well. Anxiety, loneliness, nausea, pain, or the disease itself may be responsible and should be discussed with the client.

Oral intake may be supplemented or replaced by intravenous infusion of glucose, water, and electrolytes, parenteral hyperalimentation, or gastrointestinal tube feedings. Volume and specific nutrients must be determined to assess dietary intake. Commercial products usually provide this information on their labels, and hospital dietary or pharmacy personnel should be able to provide information about hospital-prepared formulas.

Adequacy of Intake

Burns, stress, surgery, and many illnesses increase the body's need for protein, calories, and other nutrients. It is not possible to determine the specific requirement for each nutrient for every client, but the nurse must be aware of changes in nutritional needs resulting from illness, trauma, or surgery, and must work to assure adequate intake.

Calorie/Energy Needs. Most illnesses result in some decrease in activity level, but the disease itself may increase the basal metabolic rate and also caloric needs. Such illnesses include pneumonia, trauma, and hypermetabolic diseases such as hyperthyroidism. Fever increases basal metabolic caloric needs by about 7% for each degree over normal. Increased energy needs for various health problems are shown in Figure 18-1. The nurse should add these energy needs to basal needs when determining total energy needs for a client with a health problem. A normal man at rest may burn only 1,500 calories a day, and a woman only 1,000 calories. Caloric needs may increase to 2,500 to 4,000 calories per day for a client immediately after surgery. Ten thousand calories may be required by burned or severely septic patients (Salmond, 1980). It is not uncommon for those in greatest need of calories to receive almost starvation levels of calories; one liter of 5% dextrose provides only 170 calories. Intravenous dextrose solutions cannot provide total daily caloric needs, since the volume needed to assure adequate calories would be prohibitive. Guidelines for estimating calories in parenteral solutions are outlined in Figure 18-2.

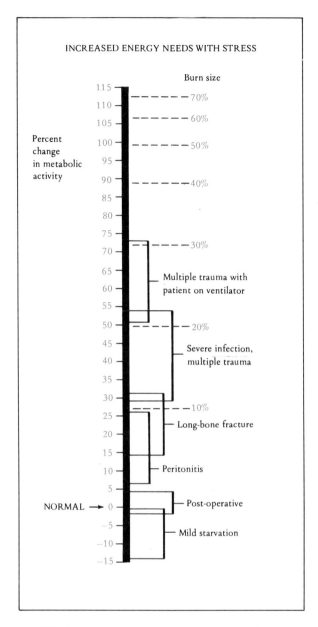

FIGURE 18-1. Increased Energy Needs with Stress. (*Note.* Courtesy of Mead Johnson, Evansville, Indiana. Reprinted by permission from *Dialogues in Nutrition* 3:1–12, 1979. Adapted from Wilmore, D. [1977]. *The Metabolic Management of the Critically Ill.* New York: Plenum Medical Book Co., 1977.)

Protein Requirements. When the basal metabolic rate increases, protein needs also increase. In addition, surgery places the body in a state of catabolism, resulting in a loss of protein from muscles and a loss of body fat. Inadequate caloric and protein intake also can lead to body use of protein stores. Clients admitted to the hospital in good nutrition who are given mainly non-nitrogen calories often deplete their body protein levels, but fre-

Glucose or amino acid* solutions:

$$\text{Milliliters of solution} \times \frac{\text{Concentration of nutrient in solution}}{} = \frac{\text{Grams of glucose or amino acid infused}}{}$$

$$\text{Grams of nutrient} \times \frac{\text{Physiological fuel factor}}{} = \text{Kilocalories}$$

Sample calculations:

To determine the number of kilocalories per gram in 3000 cc of D_5W:

$$3000 \text{ cc} \times \frac{5 \text{ mg of glucose}}{100 \text{ cc}} = 150 \text{ gm of glucose} \times \frac{3.4 \text{ kcal}}{\text{gm}} = 510 \text{ kcal}$$

To determine the number of kilocalories per gram in 3000 cc of 3.5 percent amino acid solution:

$$3000 \text{ cc} \times \frac{3.5 \text{ gm of amino acid}}{100 \text{cc}} = 105 \text{ gm of amino acids (or protein)}$$

$$70 \text{ gm of amino acid} \times \frac{4 \text{ cal}}{\text{gm}} = 280 \text{ kcal/gm}$$

To calculate the number of kilocalories for fat emulsions: 1 ml of 10 percent fat emulsion provides 1.1 kcal.

Number of milliliters $\times$ 1.1 = Number of kilocalories provided

In simpler terms, the number of milliliters of fat emulsion roughly equals the number of kilocalories provided.

*While the amount of protein supplied is important to determine adequacy, the number of calories from protein is normally unimportant because protein is usually given in minimal amounts to support protein synthesis and anabolism.

FIGURE 18-2. Estimating Kilocalories in Parenteral Solutions. (*Note.* From Burtis, G., Davis, J., & Martin, S. [1988] *Applied nutrition and diet therapy.* Philadelphia: Saunders, 398.)

quently are not recognized as malnourished until clinical signs are observed. In such clients, height, weight, skinfold thickness, and mid-upper-arm muscle circumferences may be within normal limits, but dietary assessment, along with serum albumin and transferrin levels, will indicate the poor protein status being created. A thorough nutritional assessment is indicated.

Conditions that increase protein requirements include sepsis, fever, wound healing, surgery, hemorrhage, fractures, burns, infections, and cancer. Conditions such as hepatic coma and acute and chronic renal failure dictate a *lower* intake of protein. Protein requirements may increase from 0.5 to 1 g/kg/day in healthy people to 1.0 to 3.5 g/kg/day in certain ill clients. Measurements of total serum protein and serum albumin will aid the nurse in assessing adequacy of protein nutrition. Mid-upper-arm circumference measurements also will be useful in assessing loss of muscle mass.

Vitamin and Mineral Requirements. The Recommended Dietary Allowances for vitamins and minerals are based on the needs of healthy individuals. Many medical and surgical conditions increase the needs for some of these nutrients. For example, vitamin C is needed in the healing of burns and for tissue formation. The burned client may need 100 times the RDA of vitamin C. By being aware of the functions of each nutrient and the effects of various health problems, the nurse can judge which nutrients should be evaluated specifically for each client. The blood levels of many minerals are measured routinely in hospitalized clients, but laboratory tests for most vitamins will have to be requested specifically. Many medications interfere with nutrient availability in the body in addition to the obvious influence on intake of anorexia, nausea, and vomiting secondary to medications.

Illnesses Affecting Nutrition

Certain illnesses affect nutrition directly and place the client at nutritional risk. These include conditions that affect:

- ingestion (e.g., mouth or esophageal disorders)
- digestion (e.g., cystic fibrosis)
- absorption (e.g., diarrhea)
- transportation (e.g., shock)
- metabolism (e.g., diabetes mellitus) and
- excretion (e.g., renal disease).

Alcoholism affects nutrition in multiple ways. Clients with these conditions should receive thorough nutritional assessments.

Influence of Drugs

Interactions of drugs and foods (nutrients) are common. The two basic results of interaction mechanisms are:

- altered nutrition
- altered drug effects.

Drugs can interact with the nutrients to alter nutrition, or a person's diet can interact with drugs to affect the function of the drug in the body.

Drugs may alter nutrition by:

- increasing appetite and weight gain (examples: Periactin, Librium, Valium, Thorazine, Elavil, steroids)
- decreasing appetite (example: amphetamines)
- changing taste and smell (examples: cocaine, Benzocaine, chemotherapeutic agents, Amphotericin B, Ampicillin, tetracyclines, Clofibrate)
- inducing nausea and vomiting (examples: chemotherapeutic agents such as Methotrexate, Adriamycin, and cardiac glycosides and digitalis if used in large amounts)
- increasing absorption (example: cimetidine (Tagamet) increases absorption of protein and carbohydrate)
- decreasing absorption (examples: Colchicine can cause vitamin B_{12} deficiency; Neomycin decreases fat and fat-soluble vitamin absorption.)
- increasing renal excretion (example: diuretics may increase excretion of sodium, potassium, magnesium, zinc)
- altering metabolism (examples: monoamine oxidase inhibitors interact with certain foods to cause sometimes fatal reactions; coumadin derivatives interfere with action of vitamin K and reduce formation of several clotting factors).

Foods (nutrients) may interact with drugs by:

- increasing absorption (example: food increases absorption of Darvon, Lithium, Valium, Propranolol)
- delaying absorption (examples: fatty foods delay absorption of most drugs; food delays absorption of Theophylline).
- decreasing absorption (examples: milk interferes with absorption of tetracyclines when taken together; food decreases absorption of many antibiotics such as Amoxicillin, Cloxacillin, Lincomycin, penicillin)
- affecting drug distribution and metabolism.

The above examples are only a few of the nutrient–drug interactions. The nurse must carefully assess each client's medications (both prescription and nonprescription) to determine nutrient–drug interactions and instruct the client accordingly.

THE NUTRITIONAL HISTORY

In assessing nutrition, the nurse looks at the total person and uses a variety of methods for collecting information. The nurse completes a nutrition history, collects information on dietary intake, and completes a clinical appraisal that includes a physical exam and collection of anthropometric and biochemical measurements. A helpful mnemonic (see boxed insert) for remembering the framework for nutritional assessment is the "ABCDEF Method." Each aspect of the nutritional assessment will be discussed, but not necessarily in the order specified in the ABCDEF method. Usually a history is taken, followed by a physical examination. The order in which the other data are obtained depends on the philosophy and approach of the nurse performing the nutritional assessment. The mnemonic is merely a helpful device for remembering the components of a nutritional assessment.

Abnormal or deficient findings in any one of these areas do not indicate malnutrition per se. Data from each area must be evaluated in light of the total findings. That is, assessment of the total person is essential. As discussed in Chapter 3, the various types of information collected during assessment (subjective and objective, current and historical) when combined and interpreted, provide a complete basis for determining a nursing diagnosis.

Nutritional History Obtained by Interview

It is important not to duplicate efforts if one is to make wise use of time and benefit the most people. Much information obtained by interview already may be available. If the client already is receiving health care and has a record, the nurse should re-

---

**Framework for Nutrition Assessment
ABCDEF Method**

Anthropometrical measurements
Biochemical measurements
Clinical history & physical exam
Dietary evaluation
Environmental, economic, educational history
Fluid assessment

view it before spending time (the nurse's and the client's) in this area. Much of the information in the record relates to assessing nutrition.

Knowledge of basic interviewing techniques is particularly important when assessing nutrition. Nutrition and eating practices often have heavy emotional significance, especially in regard to dietary intake. The nurse should be conscious of emotional factors when asking any questions related to nutrition. A judgmental approach may provoke outright hostility or may cause the client to withhold information for fear of the nurse's disapproval.

Throughout the interview, the nurse should be alert to the client's spoken or unspoken perception of his or her nutritional needs, as well as the client's motivation to change nutritional practices. Intervention or plans based on the nurse's perception of the client's needs are unlikely to bring about change if they conflict with the client's attitudes and goals.

The nutrition history is outlined in Table 18-13.

The client's race, ethnic/cultural group, and religious affiliation may indicate the need to modify the evaluation of dietary intake as discussed in

Chapter 8. Financial status, especially the client's ability to meet living expenses, and the educational level of the household's food purchaser and preparer are important to consider. Some surveys show increasing evidence of malnutrition and retarded growth as levels of income and education decline. High levels of education and adequate finances, however, are no guarantee against poor food choices and unwise use of money. Obesity is more commonly found in children from high income families; anorexia nervosa is found more often in middle and upper income groups. Participation in such programs as Food Stamps, School Breakfast Program, and the Special Supplemental Food Program for Women, Infants, and Children (WIC), should be considered in evaluating income. The client's age also should be considered in nutritional assessment.

The nurse must know the client's living environment. Does the client live in an urban, suburban, or rural area? This is important in order to be aware of risk factors common in certain communities, to determine resources available for improving nutrition, and for evaluating dietary intake more accurately. For example, milk that has not been for-

---

TABLE 18-13
Nutritional History

Client's Profile
  Age, sex and race:

Client/Family Data
  Number and ages of people living in household
  Race, ethnic, and cultural background
  Religious affiliations that affect food
  Educational level
  Financial status (money available for food)
  Gatekeeper of food (who purchases, prepares, and/or serves food)
  Participation in food/nutrition planning, preparation, and consumption
  Motivation to eat balanced meals
  Family composition
  Recent changes in family

Environmental Data
  Place of residence—urban, suburban, rural, geography, climate, and other factors affecting food availability
  Occupation (place and work schedule, availability of food, snacks, changes in nutrient needs due to occupational environment and activities)
  Hobbies and leisure activities (that may influence nutrient needs or actual food intake)
  Home and neighborhood facilities for purchase, storage, preparation, and serving foods

Health History
  Present height, usual weight, and current weight
  Recent changes in weight or health
  Recent attempts in changing nutrient intake
  Health habits affecting nutrient intake, such as alcohol and medications (prescription and over-the-counter)
  Usual bowel habits
  Use of laxatives
  Past and present exercise patterns
  Health problems, physical handicaps, or surgery

Dietary History
  Usual intake of foods and fluids with types and amounts
  Food preferences and aversions
  Number, frequency, and time of meals and snacks
  Appetite changes
  Lifestyle habits affecting dietary intake
  Vitamin, mineral, and nutrition supplements used
  Changes in dietary intake
  Use of dentures
  Chewing or swallowing difficulties
  Food allergies and symptoms
  Problem foods that cause gas, diarrhea, or indigestion

tified with vitamin D is readily available in some rural areas at a lower cost than fortified milk. The fluoride content of drinking water varies by locality. Snack foods may be more readily available in some communities, as with curbside vendors in large cities. Inadequate kitchen facilities for storing and preparing food in the client's home may contribute to such poor dietary practices as lack of fresh vegetables in the diet or over-reliance on packaged foods.

Certain aspects of the psychosocial and sociocultural history may bring out factors relating to nutrition. For example, the client may indicate that educational or job demands on family members leave little time for purchasing food and preparing it. Also, a parent may indicate that because a child spends much time in day care, only partial dietary intake information is available. Assessment of individual and family stressors and coping mechanisms may reveal factors related to significant weight loss or gain or poor eating habits.

The client's past health history, especially recent illnesses, often is significant in evaluating nutrition. Illnesses, such as diseases or surgery of the gastrointestinal tract and inborn metabolic and endocrine diseases, affecting ingestion, absorption, use, or excretion of nutrients are especially relevant. Diseases that are indirectly related to poor nutrition because of lowered resistance, such as tuberculosis, may be noted in the history. Clients who are obese actually may be undernourished because of poorly balanced intake or because of repeated weight loss/gain cycles ("yo-yo syndrome") related to fad diets.

Abnormalities of intestinal absorption are common in bulimics. Loss of weight may be secondary to chronic illnesses such as congestive heart failure or emphysema, and the approach to dealing with the weight loss must take this into consideration. Knowledge of food allergies and reactions is important in planning nutritional counseling when essential nutrients are found to be deficient in the diet.

Health habits, such as alcohol consumption and use of tobacco, are known to affect nutrition, as are medications, whether prescription or over-the-counter. Drugs may interact with or interfere with nutrients and decrease their absorption, decrease appetite (as with mouth soreness), cause nausea and vomiting or diarrhea, affect the individual's rate of metabolism, or affect intestinal bacterial flora necessary for using certain nutrients.

If the client participates in regular exercise, particularly if very strenuous, the nutritional need for calories, vitamins C and B-complex, water, and

salt may be affected. Physical handicaps also may influence nutrition, especially when they interfere with independence in feeding.

Family health history information should be assessed for nutritional significance. Obesity, diabetes mellitus, atherosclerotic heart disease, and anemia may have familial links. Dietary evaluation provides the nurse with information related to actual food intake. Additional tools may be used to guide the nurse in collecting and assessing data. Fluid assessment is part of dietary assessment, but to assist the nurse in focusing on the importance of fluid, a separate assessment is included. The reader is referred to Chapter 19.

Dietary Intake Assessment

Food intake is an important part of total nutritional assessment. Some of this information may be obtained as part of the complete health history in the elimination section.

The major purpose of assessing dietary intake is to provide a baseline for determining whether the individual's diet contains deficient or excessive amounts of calories or one or more nutrients and to determine whether intervention is needed. A secondary purpose is to allow an opportunity for the client or parent (caretaker) to ask questions about nutritional concerns.

The information obtained provides only presumptive evidence of nutritional problems, because each of the available methods of data collection has its limitations. The time period selected for assessment may not be typical of usual intake; the client may consciously or unconsciously improve the diet while recording intake, perhaps because of greater awareness of what foods are lacking or in excess. If the latter is the case, the client will have gained at least a perception of the need for improvement. However, the client who is aware of and perhaps embarrassed by poor dietary habits may change them only temporarily. This is one of the most serious limitations of available dietary intake methods. In the case of children, if there are multiple providers (as with children spending time at day care centers) or if the child is old enough to obtain food independently (preschoolers and older), the parent honestly may not know what the child has eaten. Once children reach school age, they probably know more about their diets than their parents. School-age children often swap lunches with their friends, meaning that what parents report their child eats at school may not always be accurate. Some school-age children and adolescents also pocket the money intended for lunch tickets and go without lunch. Children 5 to 6 years of age probably can describe accurately food eaten away from home and between meals.

As mentioned, basic interviewing techniques play a special role here because there is such an emotional overlay to family nutrition and eating. It is important to have accurate information, but also it is important not to make the client feel defensive. The client must feel at ease with the interviewer before information will be shared. Mothers, especially, may feel threatened by questions about their children's diets because food is so much a part of the motherly role. Obese people tend to feel very defensive when discussing nutrition with a health professional, often with good reason. Many health professionals sound and act extremely judgmental when interviewing obese and overweight clients.

Methods of Determining Dietary Intake

The primary methods of determining dietary intake that are useful to the nurse are diet recall, food diary, and dietary history.

Diet Recall. The diet recall method generally covers a 24-hour period and therefore usually is called the "24-hour recall." The diet recall is a fairly simple method of obtaining dietary intake data. One need not be a nutrition specialist to administer it, so it is probably the dietary screening tool used most often by nurses. In a period of 15 to 20 minutes the nurse can ask questions of the client (or parent) to determine (in portion sizes) the entire intake for the prior 24-hour period. The interview need not be lengthy.

Since it relies on the client's memory and cooperation, this method provides only a rough estimate of food intake. Moreover, the prior day may not be representative of usual intake because of day-to-day variations in diet. Therefore, the 24-hour recall alone is not a reliable tool for evaluating the adequacy of an individual's diet.

The nurse may improve reliability by using the following techniques:

■ Providing props that will help the client estimate portion sizes:

    Ordinary household measuring cups and spoons
    Cups, mugs, glasses, and dishes in a variety of sizes
    A ruler

■ Ask specifically about use of seasonings and garnishes that the client may overlook otherwise. These are usually additions to foods already recorded:

Fats such as butter, margarine, peanut butter, mayonnaise, lard, meat drippings, or cheese spreads:
    Used on toast, breads, rolls, buns, cookies, crackers, sandwiches?
    Used on vegetables?
    Used on potatoes, rice, noodles?
    Used on other foods?
Sugars, such as jam, jelly, honey, and syrup. Also artificial sweeteners:
    Used on breads, cereals, sandwiches, vegetables, fruit?
    Used in coffee, tea, other beverages?
Condiments, such as catsup, mustard, relish, soy sauce (Orientals), chiles, jalapenos (Mexican-Americans).
Beverage "lighteners" such as cream, half and half, milk, artificial lighteners.
Gravies and sauces:
    Used on bread, biscuits, meat, potatoes, or other vegetables, rice, noodles?
Mayonnaise and salad dressings:
    Used on vegetables, salads, sandwiches?
Chocolate or other flavoring in milk, such as Quick, Bosco.

■ Ask about preparation. For example:
Eggs—fried? scrambled? boiled?
Meat, poultry, fish—fried? boiled? stewed? roasted? baked? broiled?
Major ingredients of mixed dishes such as tuna fish and noodles? Macaroni and cheese? Pasta and sauce? Chili?
Special preparation—strained? chopped?

■ Ask about special additional details, such as
Kinds of milk—whole? lowfat? skim? powdered? chocolate?
Kinds of carbonated beverages—regular? low-calorie? caffeine content?
Kinds of fruits—canned? frozen? fresh? dried? cooked with sugar added?
Kinds of fruit juices, fruit drinks, or juice substitutes.

■ Ask about the day's activities to help the client recall what was eaten by associating meals or snacks with them. "Did you eat while you were at your job? Did you have a break and eat then? Did you go out to eat? To a party or sports activity?"

■ Let the client talk without interruption.

■ Use general terms to ask about probable omissions, such as a beverage with a meal: "What did you drink with lunch?" Do not suggest correct answers. For example, do not ask, "Did you eat an egg for breakfast?" Ask, "When was the first time you ate today? What did you eat?"

- Do not show approval or disapproval.
- Do not expect the client to recall every detail. Put the client at ease when difficulty is experienced in remembering.

Another, less frequently used form of diet recall is the food frequency list. A detailed list of specific foods, arranged by major foods groups, is presented, and the client is asked to state how often each day the food is eaten. An example of a food frequency form (along with many other forms for collecting dietary intake information) can be found in *Nutrition Assessment: A Comprehensive Guide for Planning Intervention* (Simko, Cowell, & Gilbride, 1984, p. 123). The food frequency method is particularly useful if the nurse suspects a deficiency in a specific nutrient. A list of food sources of that nutrient can be developed by the nurse to determine frequency of intake.

Food Diary (Food Intake Record). Although food diaries usually are interpreted by professional nutritionists, the nurse may be involved in obtaining the information from the client and occasionally may evaluate for specific nutrients or calories. The client (or the nurse in a hospital) is asked to record all food and beverages consumed for a specified period of time, usually three or seven days. It is difficult to gain client cooperation for longer periods, and day-to-day intake variations make three days about the shortest period for reliability. A three-day period is recommended for those with little variation in diet (infants, school-age children, most adults). A seven-day period should be used if there is more variation in day-to-day intake (toddlers, preschoolers, adolescents, clients with eating problems like anorexia or obesity).

A useful form for recording three- to seven-day intake information is shown in Figure 18-3. Additional instructions include:

- Asking the client to carry the record throughout the day so that intake may be recorded immediately. This means taking it to the office, for example.
- Specifying the food type in the "how prepared" column, such as canned or fresh fruit, skim or whole milk.
- Asking that recipes of mixed dishes be attached.
- Reminding the client that vitamin and mineral supplements are considered intake.
- Telling a parent who is recording for a child that the amount consumed can be determined by measuring portions offered and the amount refused and recording the difference.

- Asking clients to record with whom they ate and their feelings at the time, if the food diary is being used to evaluate an eating problem such as overeating or anorexia. A code such as A—Anxious, B—Bored, C—Tired, D—Depressed, E—Angry, F— _____, G— _____ may be suggested.

Review the record with the client when it is returned so that the client can clarify any ambiguities, especially in preparation method, serving sizes, and form of food used. These details often are omitted even when the client is instructed to include them.

A very precise modification of this method is the *weighed intake method*, in which all food intake is weighed by the client or a trained person. This method is very time-consuming and is rarely used except in research.

Analyzing Dietary Intake

Once dietary intake has been recorded, it must be analyzed by comparing it with recommended amounts of nutrients or calories. The method of evaluation used depends on the specificity of information collected and the type of information desired (see boxed insert). Sometimes the diet will be compared with the basic food groups. At other times more specific information is desired, and intake of specific nutrients is calculated and compared with a standard table. Comparing a client's nutrient intake to a standard table is important when the client is under- or overweight, or if the source of a certain food appears on the client's record only occasionally.

Dietary Analysis

I. Dietary Intake
   Diet recall
   Food diary
   Food frequency
   Diet history

II. Analysis of Intake by Comparison to Standards
   Comparison to standards
   Basic food guide
   Exchange lists
   Dietary goals & guidelines
   Guidelines for cancer prevention
   Guidelines for healthy heart

III. Determining Needs
   RDA
   Formulas

INSTRUCTIONS

1. Record *all* food or beverages immediately *after* they are eaten or drunk.

2. Measure the amounts of each food carefully in terms of standard measuring cups and spoons. Record meat portions in ounces or as fractions of pounds, for example: 8 ounces of milk; one medium egg; 1/4 pound of hamburger; one slice of bread, white; 1/2 small banana.

3. Indicate method of preparation, for example: medium egg, fried; 1/2 cup baked beans with two-inch slice salt pork; four ounces steak, breaded.

4. Be sure to include any condiments, gravies, salad dressings, butter, margarine, whipped cream, relishes, etc., for example; 1/4 cup mashed potatoes with 3 tablespoons brown gravy; 1/4 cup cottage cheese salad with two olives; 1/2 cup cornflakes with 1 teaspoon sugar and 1/3 cup 2% milk.

5. Be sure to include all between meal foods and drinks, for example: coffee with 1 ounce of cream; 12 ounces of cola; four sugar cookies; one 10¢ candy bar (list brand).

6. If you eat away from home, please put a little symbol beside the foods.

Date _____

Weight _____

Day of week _____

Time	Food	Amount	How prepared

FIGURE 18-3. Seven-Day Food Record. (*Note.* Adapted from Pipes, P. [1981]. Assessing food and nutrient intake. In M. C. Powell (Ed.), *Assessment and management of developmental changes and problems in children* [2nd ed.]. St. Louis: Mosby).

CLINICAL APPRAISAL AND SCREENING

Physical signs and symptoms of poor nutrition provide vital supporting evidence for a diagnosis of a nutritional problem. The physical examination also can identify chronic medical conditions that may be related to nutritional insufficiency such as congenital heart disease.

Physical clues may be derived from casual observations while interviewing a client. A hand-shake can indicate muscle tone. A compliment generates a smile and shows the nurse the client's teeth. Attention to posture, body size, activity level, and appearance of hair and skin can aid in easily confirming a nutritional problem.

A nurse who is skilled in techniques for physical examination can review the body systematically to obtain further information. In addition, the client should be examined for edematous extremities, heart murmurs, thyroid enlargement, hepatomegaly, and splenomegaly to diagnose chronic conditions influencing nutritional and non-nutritional causes of growth failure or weight loss.

Care must be taken in evaluating signs and symptoms. Observations of hair, eyes, tongue, skin, and nails tend to be subjective. Hair that appears dull to one nurse may appear normal to another.

There are limitations to using physical signs and symptoms to confirm nutritional problems. For example, physical manifestations often do not appear until the deficiency is fairly severe. Another problem is that signs and symptoms sometimes are associated with deficiency of more than one nutrient. Hyperpigmentation of the skin may be related to vitamin B_{12}, folic acid, or niacin deficiency. Signs associated with poor nutrition can be caused by non-nutritional factors; for example, food stains on teeth may be mistaken for fluorosis (mottled enamel) caused by excess fluoride, and skin dryness may be caused by overexposure to wind or sun. Some signs may be related to medical conditions as well as nutritional problems. For example, anemia may be caused by iron deficiency or blood loss.

A review of systems is beneficial because an abnormal sign may indicate the need for a more thorough physical examination, evaluation of dietary intake, and biochemical and anthropometric measurements. Abnormal signs are clues, not diagnoses.

Although the nurse's observations are colored by values, past experiences, and expectations, the clinical appraisal is a useful technique for providing data about specific tissues that might exhibit physical signs suggesting less than optimal nutrition. The signs of good and poor nutrition are outlined in Table 18-14.

It is desirable to observe the client's general appearance and then progress to specific areas. When it isn't possible to conduct a head-to-toe assessment, observations can be made informally. Make a careful and descriptive record of observations in the client's clinical record. According to Suitor and Crowley (1984), the tissues of the mouth are one of the first areas to exhibit signs of nutritional deficiencies, so observe carefully.

Anthropometric Measurements

Anthropometric measurements (see boxed insert) are useful in assessing nutrition, especially protein and calorie intake. Normal body growth is directly related to caloric intake.

Undernutrition will cause weight loss and, in children, may interfere with normal growth and development. Overnutrition will lead to excess weight gain and thus increase the risk of developing heart disease, hypertension, diabetes, certain types of cancer, gall bladder disease, and other problems. Anthropometric measurements are crude compared to laboratory tests, but they are useful and objective measures that are simple and cost-effective. Measurements can be compared to the population as a whole and repeated measurements over time can provide an index to changes in the person's nutrition and/or health. To minimize the margin of error, the nurse must gain skill through careful practice. To obtain useful data the nurse should:

- Select and maintain proper equipment
- Select measurements appropriate to the age of the client
- Obtain the client's cooperation
- Use appropriate technique
- Record data directly on the client's record
- Analyze data with appropriate standards for sex and age
- Consider body build of the client.

Weight and Height

Weight and height measurements should be part of any nutritional assessment. Comparison of these measurements with a height–weight table (for adults), pregnancy weight gain grid (for pregnant women), or percentile standards (for children) provides data for identifying under- or over-nutrition. Actual standards for height (length) and weight, and directions for measurements are discussed in chapters 14 and 20 to 23.

The height and weight tables most frequently used are the 1983 Metropolitan Height and Weight Tables for Adults. These tables were based on approximately four million insurance policy holders. Only healthy subjects were included and the sample may not be representative of the population as

---

Anthropometric Measurements

Height
Weight
Skinfold thickness
Mid-arm circumference
Body frame size—wrist, elbow
   % weight of individual body parts
   % weight loss ($\geq$ 10%)

TABLE 18-14
Clinical Signs of Nutritional Status

Body Area	Signs of Good Nutrition	Signs of Poor Nutrition
General appearance	Alert, responsive	Listless, apathetic, cachexic
Weight	Normal for height, age, body build	Overweight or underweight (special concern for underweight)
Posture	Erect, arms and legs straight	Sagging shoulders, sunken chest, humped back
Muscles	Well developed, firm, good tone, some fat under skin	Flaccid, poor tone, undeveloped, tender, "wasted" appearance, cannot walk properly
Nervous control	Good attention span, not irritable or restless, normal reflexes, psychological stability	Inattentive, irritable, confused, burning and tingling of hands and feet (paresthesia), loss of position and vibratory sense, weakness and tenderness of muscles (may result in inability to walk), decrease or loss of ankle and knee reflexes
Gastrointestinal tract function	Good appetite and digestion, normal regular elimination, no palpable organs or masses	Anorexia, indigestion, constipation or diarrhea, liver or spleen enlargement
Cardiovascular function	Normal heart rate and rhythm, no murmurs, normal blood pressure for age	Rapid heart rate (above 100 beats/min. tachycardia), enlarged heart, abnormal rhythm, elevated blood pressure
General vitality	Endurance, energetic, sleeps well, vigorous	Easily fatigued, no energy, falls asleep easily, looks tired, apathetic
Hair	Shiny, lustrous, firm, not easily plucked, healthy scalp	Stringy, dull, brittle, dry, thin and sparse, depigmented, can be easily plucked
Skin (general)	Smooth, slightly moist, good color	Rough, dry, scaly, pale, pigmented, irritated, bruises, petechiae
Face and neck	Skin color uniform, smooth, healthy appearance, not swollen	Greasy, discolored, scaly, swollen, skin dark over cheeks and under eyes, lumpiness or flakiness of skin around nose and mouth
Lips	Smooth, good color, moist, not chapped or swollen	Dry, scaly, swollen, redness and swelling (cheilosis), or angular lesions at corners of the mouth or fissures or scars (stomatitis)
Mouth, oral membranes	Reddish pink mucous membranes in oral cavity	Swollen, boggy oral mucous membranes
Gums	Good pink color, healthy, red, no swelling or bleeding	Spongy, bleed easily, marginal redness, inflamed, gums receding
Tongue	Good pink color or deep reddish in appearance, not swollen or smooth, surface papillae present, no lesion	Swelling, scarlet and raw, magenta color, beefy (glossitis), hyperemic and hypertrophic papillae, atrophic papillae
Teeth	No cavities, no pain, bright, straight, no crowding, well-shaped jaw, clean, no discoloration	Unfilled caries, absent teeth, worn surfaces, mottled (fluorosis), malpositioned
Eyes	Bright, clear, shiny, no sores at corner of eyelids, membranes moist and healthy pink color, no prominent blood vessels or mound of tissue or sclera, no fatigue circles beneath	Eye membranes pale (pale conjunctivae), redness of membrane (conjunctival injection), dryness, signs of infection, Bitot's spots, redness and fissuring of eyelid corners (angular palpebritis), dryness of eye membrane (conjunctival xerosis), dull appearance of cornea (corneal xerosis), soft cornea (keratomalacia)
Neck (glands)	No enlargement	Thyroid enlarged

TABLE 18-14 Continued

Body Area	Signs of Good Nutrition	Signs of Poor Nutrition
Nails	Firm, pink	Spoon shape, (koilonychia), brittle, ridged
Legs, feet	No tenderness, weakness, or swelling; good color	Edema, tender calf, tingling, weakness
Skeleton	No malformations	Bowlegs, knock-knees, chest deformity at diaphragm, beaded ribs, prominent scapulas

Note. From Williams, S.R.: Nutrition assessment and guidance in prenatal care. In Worthington-Roberts, B.S., & Williams, S.R.: *Nutrition in pregnancy and lactation*, ed. 4, St. Louis, 1989, Times Mirror/Mosby College Publishing. Reprinted with permission.

a whole. The weights are those associated with the lowest mortality. Height measurements should be taken at regular intervals on pediatric and geriatric clients rather than relying on the client's recall. Height decreases with age after middle age because of osteoporosis, curvature of spine, and inability to stand straight. After ages 65 to 70, body weight usually decreases because of decreasing lean body mass (Grant & DeHoog, 1985). A quick method for estimating ideal body weight of the adult is shown in Table 18-15.

The height and weight data for adults can be used to evaluate "body mass index" (BMI). For BMI, record weight (W) in kilograms and height (H) in meters. BMI is equal to W/H^2. The desirable range for men is 20 to 25 and the desirable range for women is from 19 to 24 (Simko et al., 1984, p. 85).

With loss of body parts, estimation of body weight becomes more difficult. Figure 18-4 shows the approximate percent of adult body weight contributed by various body parts. These figures can be used as a guide for adjusting ideal body weight. A change in weight may be significant in the adult. To determine the percent of weight change, use the formula (Burtis, Davis, & Martin, 1988, p. 369):

% Weight Change =

$$\frac{\text{Usual weight} - \text{current weight}}{\text{Usual weight}} \times 100$$

Weight and height measurements that usually indicate the need for more in-depth assessment to determine a nutritional or other cause include:

- Sudden or unexplained weight loss of 5% or more of body weight in a month or 10% in a six-month period
- Rapid weight loss of more than 2 pounds per week
- Significant change in weight after age 25
- Height for age above the 10th percentile, but weight for height less than the 5th percentile for children
- Excess weight for height (greater than the 95th percentile) in children.

When weight for height for a child is greater than the 90th percentile or when any adult's weight for height and age is 15 to 20% greater than the standard norm on a weight chart, differentiation between obesity and overweight should be made. Fat and muscle contribute to overall weight. Muscular athletes may weigh more than the norm, but not because of fatness secondary to excess caloric intake. Inactive, handicapped individuals with poor muscle tone may have an unhealthy excess ratio of fat to muscle, but may have a weight in the desirable range.

TABLE 18-15
Rule of Fives and Sixes for Determining Ideal Body Weight

Build	Adult Women	Adult Men
Medium	100 lb for first 5 feet of height, plus 5 lb/inch for each inch over 5 feet	Allow 106 lb for first 5 feet of height, plus 6 lb for each inch over 5 feet
Small	Subtract 10%	Subtract 10%
Large	Add 10%	Add 10%

Note. Adapted from *Nutrition Guide for Professionals: Diabetes Education and Meal Planning.* Copyright © 1988 by the American Diabetes Association, Inc., and the American Dietetic Association. Reprinted with permission.

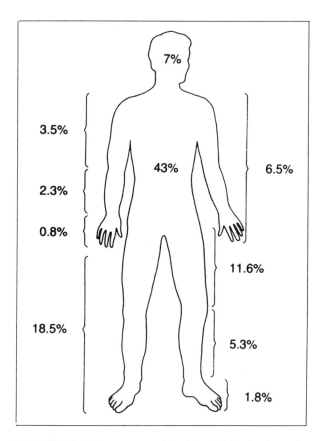

7%

3.5%

2.3%

0.8%

43%   6.5%

11.6%

18.5%

5.3%

1.8%

FIGURE 18-4. Percentage of Total Body Weight Contributed by Individual Body Parts. (*Note.* From Grant, A., & DeHoog, S. [1991]. *Nutritional assessment and support* [4th ed.]. Seattle, WA: Author, p. 20.)

Determining Frame Size

To use weight/height measurements as an index for evaluating a client's weight, frame size must be determined. Several methods are available for determining an adult's frame size. Grant and DeHoog (1985) outlined the following procedure for estimating frame size using wrist circumference and height:

1. Select the client's right wrist for measurement.

2. Place a soft measuring tape around the smallest part of the wrist distal (towards the fingers) to the styloid process of the radius and ulna ("wrist bone") (Figure 18-5). If the measuring tape is calibrated in centimeters, divide by 2.54 to get wrist circumference in inches.

3. After obtaining height and wrist circumference (both in inches), determine the client's frame type using the Body Frame Type chart (Figure 18-6).

Elbow breadth is reported to be a reliable indicator of frame size that is not affected by obesity or

greatly affected by age (Frisancho, 1981). To determine frame size using elbow breadth:

1. Have the client extend his or her right arm in front and bend the forearm upward at a 90° angle. The inside of the wrist should face the body (Figure 18-7).

2. Place your thumb and index finger of one hand on the two prominent bones on either side of the client's elbow and measure the distance between the bones (in inches) with a ruler or tape measure.

3. Obtain the client's height without heels.

4. Compare results with Tables 18-16 and 18-17 to identify a medium frame. Larger values indicate a large frame and smaller values indicate a small frame.

Simko, Cowell, and Gilbride (1984) report that irrespective of height, a person with a thick chest and broad shoulders and pelvis should be classified as having a large frame. Conversely, a person with a thin chest and narrow shoulders and pelvis should be classified as having a small frame. Those in between should be considered to be of medium frame. Glove size is sometimes a useful guide. Women wearing gloves smaller than size 6 and men smaller than size 8 are generally of small frame. Women wearing gloves larger than size 7 and men larger than size 9 are generally of large frame.

Measuring Body Fat

Since obesity can be defined as a condition in which the amount of fat in the body is excessive in relation to total body weight, and since diagnosis of obesity is so important from a nutritional and general health standpoint, it is desirable to obtain a measure of fat in the body. Measurement of a fold of skin and subcutaneous fat, usually in the triceps or subscapular areas, provides an indirect but well-correlated estimate of total fatness. A rough measurement, illustrated in Figure 18-8, can be made by "pinching" a fat fold on the back of the arm or side of the lower chest. A fold greater than 1 inch probably indicates obesity, while a fold that is less than half an inch probably indicates too little subcutaneous fat.

When the abdominal girth equals or exceeds the girth of the chest, excess abdominal fat is present. The adage "The longer the belt line, the shorter the life line," probably has something to do with obesity. The Ruler Test to evaluate excess abdominal fat is described by Simko, Cowell, and Gilbride (1984). However, other causes of abdominal enlargement might include accumulation of

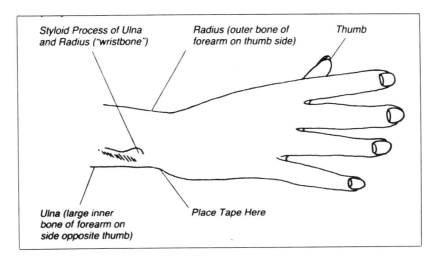

FIGURE 18-5. Determination of Wrist Circumference. (*Note.* From Grant, A., & DeHoog, S. [1991]. *Nutritional assessment and support* [4th ed.]. Seattle, WA: Author, p. 13.)

fluid, tumor formation, enlarged organs, intestinal distention (gas), or pregnancy.

A more sophisticated and standardized measurement can be made with calibrated skinfold calipers such as the Lange or Harpenden calipers. These measurements are useful for detecting fat excess or deficit as well as for differentiating between an overweight or overly fat client. Measurements of skinfold thickness may be made at triceps, subscapula, suprailiac, and/or thigh (Figure 18-9).

The triceps skinfold (TSF) measurement is the most common, easily measured, and best indicator of percentage of body fat in children and women. Subscapular and suprailiac skinfold measurements are a better indicator of total body fat in boys and men.

To obtain a TSF measurement:

1. Use the client's nondominant arm.

2. Have the client bend the arm at a right angle with hand across abdomen.

3. Locate the midpoint between acromial process and the olecranon process.

4. Mark the midpoint with a marking pencil.

5. Have the client stand, hanging the arm loosely.

6. Use your thumb and forefinger to grasp a vertical pinch of the client's skin and subcutaneous fat about 1 to 2 cm above the previously marked midpoint.

7. Pull the skinfold gently away from underlying muscle (if you are in doubt about muscle, have the client contract and relax the muscle).

8. Place the caliper on the skinfold at the previously marked midpoint while maintaining your grasp of the client's skin.

9. Read the measurement within 2 to 3 seconds after releasing the caliper extender.

10. Record the measurement in millimeters.

11. For increased accuracy, repeat steps 7, 8, and 9 to obtain 3 measurements and use the mean

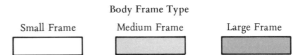

The wrist is measured distal to styloid process of radius and ulna at smallest circumference. Use height without shoes and inches for wrist size to determine frame type from this chart

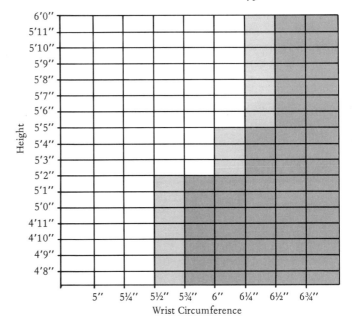

FIGURE 18-6. Body Frame Type. (*Note.* From Grant, A., & DeHoog, S. [1991]. *Nutritional assessment and support* [4th ed.]. Seattle, WA: Author, p. 14.)

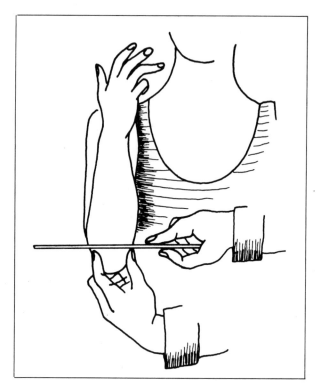

FIGURE 18-7. Measurement of Elbow Breadth. (*Note. From Grant, A., & DeHoog, S. [1991]. Nutritional assessment and support [4th ed.]. Seattle, WA: Author, p. 16.*)

or average of the three measurements. (Do not release the pinch between readings.)

12. Compare to reading standards. (Tables 18-18 and 18-19).

Measures below the 5th percentile indicate depletion of fat. Measures above the 95th percentile indicate excessive body fat.

To obtain subscapular skinfold thickness (SSF):

1. Use the left side of the client's body.

2. Just below the midpoint of the scapula, grasp a skinfold as with TSF.

3. Place the caliper jaws on a downward and lateral axis.

4. Read, record, and repeat in same manner as described for TSF.

To obtain mid-upper arm circumference (MAC):

1. At the midpoint used in determining TSF, measure the circumference of the client's arm with a nonstretchable centimeter tape.

2. While the arm is relaxed and hanging at the client's side, secure the tape snugly, but not tight enough to make an indentation.

3. Read and record the measurement to the nearest 0.1 centimeter.

4. Compare it to norms in Table 18-20.

Mid-upper arm muscle circumference (MAMC) is an indirect measure of the body's skeletal muscle mass, a sensitive index of the body protein reserves.

To calculate MAMC:

1. Convert TSF mean value from millimeters to centimeters (divide millimeter value by 10).

2. Calculate MAMC: MAMC (cm) = MAC (cm) − [3.14 × TSF (cm)]

3. Convert value to millimeters (multiply centimeter value by 10) and compare it as a percentage of the standard in Table 18-20.

Measurements of MAMC are only estimates because the formula assumes the arm is perfectly round and the thickness of the humerus is included. The measurement also is affected by sex, degree of obesity, and age. Fat is more easily compressed in females, the obese, and all individuals over age 40.

Norms for anthropometric measurements for people over 50 and non-Caucasians are not available. Also, measurements on very young children

TABLE 18-16
Elbow Breadth for Men with Medium Frame Size

Height* (in.)	Height* (cm)	Elbow Breadth (in.)	Elbow Breadth (mm)
5'1" to 5'2"	155.0 to 157.5	2½ to 2⅞	63.5 to 73.0
5'3" to 5'6"	160.0 to 167.6	2⅝ to 2⅞	66.7 to 73.0
5'7" to 5'10'	170.2 to 177.8	2¾ to 3	69.8 to 76.2
5'11" to 6'2"	180.3 to 188.0	2¾ to 3⅛	69.8 to 79.4
6'3"	190.5	2⅞ to 3¼	73.0 to 82.5

*Without shoe heels

Note. Adapted from Metropolitan Life Insurance Company tables in Grant, A., & DeHoog, S. (1991). *Nutritional assessment and support* (4th ed.). Seattle, WA: Author, 16.

TABLE 18-17
Elbow Breadth for Women with Medium Frame Size

Height* (in.)	Height* (cm)	Elbow Breadth (in.)	Breadth (mm)
4'9" to 4'10"	144.8 to 147.3	2¼ to 2½	57.1 to 63.5
4'11" to 5'2"	150.0 to 157.0	2¼ to 2½	57.1 to 63.5
5'3" to 5'6"	160.0 to 167.6	2⅜ to 2⅝	60.3 to 66.7
5'7" to 5'10"	170.1 to 177.8	2⅜ to 2⅝	60.3 to 66.7
5'11"	180.3	2½ to 2¾	63.5 to 69.8

*Without shoe heels

Note. Adapted from Metropolitan Life Insurance Company tables in Grant, A., & DeHoog, S. (1991). *Nutritional assessment and support* (4th ed.). Seattle, WA: Author, 17.

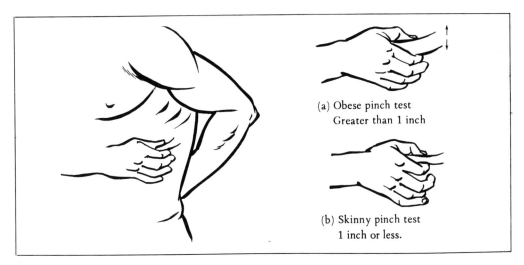

(a) Obese pinch test
Greater than 1 inch

(b) Skinny pinch test
1 inch or less.

FIGURE 18-8. The Pinch Test. (*Note.* From Simko, M.D., Cowell, C., & Gilbrid, J.A. [1984]. *Nutrition assessment.* Rockville, MD: Aspen Systems, p. 368. Source: Jolliffe, N. *Reduce and stay reduced.* Copyright 1952, 1957 by Normal Jolliffe, M.D. Reprinted by permission of Simon & Schuster.)

are difficult to assess. The nurse needs to use discretion in interpreting measurements in these individuals. If the client is in a balanced state of nutrition, height, and weight, skinfold thickness and body circumferences should fall within norms on standard tables.

Biochemical Measurements

Biochemical data obtained through laboratory studies (see boxed insert) provide objective and precise supporting evidence of nutritional problems. The nurse does not usually decide what tests are to be administered, except perhaps cholesterol, glucose, hemoglobin, and hematocrit measurements as routine screening procedures for selected groups. The nurse uses studies already ordered by the physician, or the nurse can recommend that particular studies be done, depending on the facility's capabilities.

Laboratory tests can be helpful in detecting subclinical or marginal deficiencies, such as anemia, when clinical signs are not yet evident, and in confirming a suspicion of a deficiency based on dietary or clinical evaluation.

Laboratory studies for nutritional assessment usually are obtained from blood or urine. The parameters most often measured are levels of nutrients and their metabolites, levels of enzymes associated with the nutrient, and sometimes compounds clearly related to the nutrient under consideration. Serum cholesterol measurements also are useful in assessing nutrition. The National Cholesterol Educational Program is a cooperative, nationwide effort to reduce the prevalence of high blood cholesterol. It recommends that adults with total blood cholesterol greater than 200 mg/dl begin a dietary intervention program (Ernst, Cleeman, Mullis, Sooter-Bochenek, & Van Hern, 1988). For in-depth nutritional assessments, it is possible to measure directly or indirectly the levels of most vitamins and minerals.

Several diagnostic tests used to evaluate nutrition, specifically protein levels and metabolism, include:

- *Serum albumin,* which is a late indicator of protein–calorie malnutrition. A low serum albumin level (<3.4 mg/dl) is a very specific indicator of

---

Biochemical Evaluation

General
  Hemoglobin, hematocrit
  Cholesterol, lipid profile
  Glucose

Visceral Protein Status
  Serum albumin, prealbumin
  Serum transferrin
  Total iron binding capacity

Immune Function
  Total lymphocyte count

Cellular Immunity (Skin Testing)
  PPD, mumps, Candida, streptokinase—streptodornase

Nitrogen Metabolism
  Creatinine—CHI
  Urea nitrogen—urine (24-hour), blood

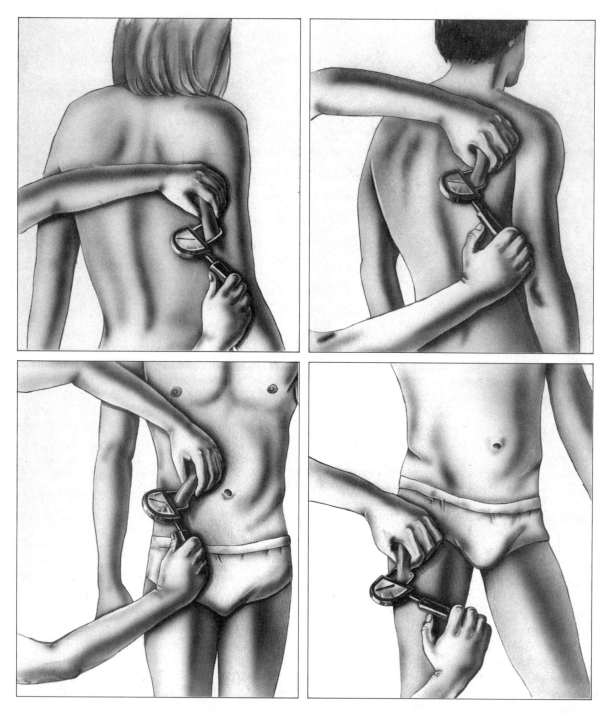

FIGURE 18-9. Measurement of Skinfold Thickness with Calipers. Skinfold sites: triceps, subscapula (top, left and right), suprailiac and thigh (bottom, left and right).

poor nutrition in the absence of other known causes. The half life of albumin is 14 to 21 days; thus, levels fall and recover slowly.

- *Serum prealbumin* is more responsive to dietary changes. Response time is 2 to 3 days. Levels decrease with stress, inflammation, restrictions of protein and/or calories, liver disease, trauma, and infection, and levels are increased with renal dis-

ease. Depletion of protein will interfere with healing.

- *Hemoglobin and hematocrit* values frequently are used. It has been said that iron deficiency anemia is one of the most common nutritional problems, and anemia frequently is associated with malnutrition. Values are lower in the elderly and in African-Americans.

TABLE 18-18
Triceps Skinfold Percentiles (mm) for Males

Age	5th	10th	25th	50th	75th	90th	95th
1–2	6	7	8	10	12	14	16
2–3	6	7	8	10	12	14	15
3–4	6	7	8	10	11	14	15
4–5	6	7	8	10	11	14	15
5–6	6	6	8	9	11	12	14
6–7	6	6	8	9	11	14	15
7–8	5	6	7	8	10	13	16
8–9	5	6	7	9	12	15	17
9–10	5	6	7	8	10	13	16
10–11	6	6	7	10	13	17	18
11–12	6	6	8	10	14	18	21
12–13	6	6	8	11	16	20	24
13–14	6	6	8	11	14	22	28
14–15	5	5	7	10	14	22	26
15–16	4	5	7	9	14	21	24
16–17	4	5	6	8	11	18	24
17–18	4	5	6	8	12	16	22
18–19	5	5	6	8	12	16	19
19–25	4	5	6	9	13	20	24
25–35	4	5	7	10	15	20	22
35–45	5	6	8	12	16	20	24
45–55	5	6	8	12	16	20	23
55–65	6	6	8	12	15	20	25
65–75	5	6	8	11	14	19	22
75–80	4	6	8	11	15	19	22

Note. Adapted from Frisancho, A. (1981). New norms of upper limb fat and muscle areas for assessment of nutritional status. *American Journal of Clinical Nutrition, 34*, 2540, in Grant, A., & DeHoog, S. (1991). *Nutritional assessment and support* (4th ed.). Seattle, WA: Author, 45.

TABLE 18-19
Triceps Skinfold Percentiles (mm) for Females

Age	5th	10th	25th	50th	75th	90th	95th
1–2	6	7	8	10	12	14	16
2–3	6	8	9	10	12	15	16
3–4	7	8	9	11	12	14	15
4–5	7	8	8	10	12	14	16
5–6	6	7	8	10	12	15	18
6–7	6	6	8	10	12	14	16
7–8	6	7	9	11	13	16	18
8–9	6	8	9	12	15	18	24
9–10	8	8	10	13	16	20	22
10–11	7	8	10	12	17	23	27
11–12	7	8	10	13	18	24	28
12–13	8	9	11	14	18	23	27
13–14	8	8	12	15	21	26	30
14–15	9	10	13	16	21	26	28
15–16	8	10	12	17	21	25	32
16–17	10	12	15	18	22	26	31
17–18	10	12	13	19	24	30	37
18–19	10	12	15	18	22	26	30
19–25	10	11	14	18	24	30	34
25–35	10	12	16	21	27	34	37
35–45	12	14	18	23	29	35	38
45–55	12	16	20	25	30	36	40
55–65	12	16	20	25	31	36	38
65–75	12	14	18	24	29	34	35

Note. Adapted from: Frisancho, A. (1981). New norms of upper limb fat and muscle areas for assessment of nutritional status. *American Journal of Clinical Nutrition, 34*, 2540, in Grant, A., & DeHoog, S. (1991). *Nutritional assessment and support* (4th ed.). Seattle, WA: Author, p. 45.

■ *Serum transferrin* is increased with iron deficiency, and it changes rapidly in response to changes in protein nutrition. Serum transferrin levels lower than 200 indicate visceral protein depletion. The half life is 8 to 10 days.

■ *Twenty-four hour urine tests for creatinine excretion and urea nitrogen.* Levels of creatinine excretion in urine are considered a reasonable index of lean body mass in the absence of altered renal function and rapid muscle catabolism. With protein malnutrition, creatinine excretion decreases.

■ *Lymphocyte count.* Malnutrition is associated with depressed immune competence and a lymphocyte count of less than 2,000 per cubic millimeter. A decreased total lymphocyte count contributes to impaired ability to fight infection.

■ *Skin testing for delayed sensitivity to common recall antigens, such as mumps, Candida, purified protein derivative of tuberculin (PPD), and streptokinase-streptodornase (SKSD).* The presence of one positive test at 24 hours (greater than 5 mm) indicates intact immunity. In a malnourished client there may be no response or a delayed response because of a slowing in the synthesis of antibodies and a slowing in antibody response to stimulation.

All of these tests may be affected by many different factors, such as the client's hydration, health, and disease, the presence of stress and trauma, and even body position, so care must be taken in interpreting test results.

NURSING DIAGNOSES RELATED TO NUTRITION

After gathering data from the client, the next step is to analyze it to identify any nutrition-related health problems. If a problem exists, there frequently are interrelationships among different assessment parameters. When analysis is completed, nursing diagnoses can be used to develop a plan of care.

The nursing diagnoses for nutritional problems shown in Table 18-21 are categorized under

TABLE 18-20
Percentiles of Upper Arm Circumference (mm) and Estimated Upper Arm Muscle Circumference (mm) for Whites of the United States Health and Nutrition Examination Survey I of 1971 to 1974

Age Group	Arm Circumference (mm)							Arm Muscle Circumference (mm)						
	5	10	25	50	75	90	95	5	10	25	50	75	90	95
Males														
1–1.9	142	146	150	159	170	176	183	110	113	119	127	135	144	147
2–2.9	141	145	153	162	170	178	185	111	114	122	130	140	146	150
3–3.9	150	153	160	167	175	184	190	117	123	131	137	143	148	153
4–4.9	149	154	162	171	180	186	192	123	126	133	141	148	156	159
5–5.9	153	160	167	175	185	195	204	128	133	140	147	154	162	169
6–6.9	155	159	167	179	188	209	228	131	135	142	151	161	170	177
7–7.9	162	167	177	187	201	223	230	137	139	151	160	168	177	190
8–8.9	162	170	177	190	202	220	245	140	145	154	162	170	182	187
9–9.9	175	178	187	200	217	249	257	151	154	161	170	183	196	202
10–10.9	181	184	196	210	231	262	274	156	160	166	180	191	209	221
11–11.9	186	190	202	223	244	261	280	159	165	173	183	195	205	230
12–12.9	193	200	214	232	254	282	303	167	171	182	195	210	223	241
13–13.9	194	211	228	247	263	286	301	172	179	196	211	226	238	245
14–14.9	220	226	237	253	283	303	322	189	199	212	223	240	260	264
15–15.9	222	229	244	264	284	311	320	199	204	218	237	254	266	272
16–16.9	244	248	262	278	303	324	343	213	225	234	249	269	287	296
17–17.9	246	253	267	285	308	336	347	224	231	245	258	273	294	312
18–18.9	245	260	276	297	321	353	379	226	237	252	264	283	298	324
19–24.9	262	272	288	308	331	355	372	238	245	257	273	289	309	321
25–34.9	271	282	300	319	342	362	375	243	250	264	279	298	314	326
35–44.9	278	287	305	326	345	363	374	247	255	269	286	302	318	327
45–54.9	267	281	301	322	342	362	376	239	249	265	281	300	315	326
55–64.9	258	273	296	317	336	355	369	236	245	260	278	295	310	320
65–74.9	248	263	285	307	325	344	355	223	235	251	268	284	298	306
Females														
1–1.9	138	142	148	156	164	172	177	105	111	117	124	132	139	143
2–2.9	142	145	152	160	167	176	184	111	114	119	126	133	142	147
3–3.9	143	150	158	167	175	183	189	113	119	124	132	140	146	152
4–4.9	149	154	160	169	177	184	191	115	121	128	136	144	152	157
5–5.9	153	157	165	175	185	203	211	125	128	134	142	151	159	165
6–6.9	156	162	170	176	187	204	211	130	133	138	145	154	166	171
7–7.9	164	167	174	183	199	216	231	129	135	142	151	160	171	176
8–8.9	168	172	183	195	214	247	261	138	140	151	160	171	183	194
9–9.9	178	182	194	211	224	251	260	147	150	158	167	180	194	198
10–10.9	174	182	193	210	228	251	265	148	150	159	170	180	190	197
11–11.9	185	194	208	224	248	276	303	150	158	171	181	196	217	223
12–12.9	194	203	216	237	256	282	294	162	166	180	191	201	214	220
13–13.9	202	211	223	243	271	301	338	169	175	183	198	211	226	240
14–14.9	214	223	237	252	272	304	322	174	179	190	201	216	232	247
15–15.9	208	221	239	254	279	300	322	175	178	189	202	215	228	244
16–16.9	218	224	241	258	283	318	334	170	180	190	202	216	234	249
17–17.9	220	227	241	264	295	324	350	175	183	194	205	221	239	257
18–18.9	222	227	241	258	281	312	325	174	179	191	202	215	237	245
19–24.9	221	230	247	265	290	319	345	179	185	195	207	221	236	249
25–34.9	233	240	256	277	304	342	368	183	188	199	212	228	246	264
35–44.9	241	251	267	290	317	356	378	186	192	205	218	236	257	272
45–54.9	242	256	274	299	328	362	384	187	193	206	220	238	260	274
55–64.9	243	257	280	303	335	367	385	187	196	209	225	244	266	280
65–74.9	240	252	274	299	326	356	373	185	195	208	225	244	264	279

Note. Frisancho, A. R. (1981). New norms of upper limb fat and muscle areas for assessment of nutritional status. *American Journal of Clinical Nutrition, 34,* 2542. © *American Journal of Clinical Nutrition,* American Society for Clinical Nutrition.

TABLE 18-21
Common Nursing Diagnoses for Nutritional Problems

Body image disturbance, related to obesity or anorexia

Feeding self-care deficit, related to inability to bring food to the mouth

Altered nutrition, less than body requirements, related to swallowing difficulties or anorexia or inability to procure food

Altered nutrition, more than body requirements, related to imbalance of intake versus energy expenditure

Altered nutrition, potential for more than body requirements, related to excessive vitamin intake

the North American Nursing Diagnosis Association's (NANDA 1990) Taxonomy I under the human response pattern of "exchanging." To support the diagnosis of "altered nutrition," data from the nursing history and clinical appraisal should reflect a lack or of an excess of nutrients or a problem related to ingestion, digestion, absorption, metabolism, or elimination of nutrients.

A single cause or many factors may contribute to altered nutrition. The diagnosis "altered nutrition: less than body requirements," may be related to chewing or swallowing difficulties, anorexia, or difficulty or inability to procure food or metabolize nutrients. The assessment should reveal intake less than the recommended amount of one or more nutrients or that actual or potential metabolic needs for one or more nutrients exceed intake. The client may or may not have an actual weight loss. If caloric intake is less than body requirements over time, the client will exhibit weight loss.

If calories are adequate or excessive but intake of protein is inadequate, the client actually may gain weight due to fluid retention. This protein deficiency (without calorie deficit) is referred to as kwashiorkor and is found frequently in some Third World countries. A less severe type of protein deficiency is observed in many hospitalized patients who exhibit a decreased serum albumin, prealbumin, serum transferrin or iron-binding capacity. Analysis of dietary intake will reveal a diet deficient in foods containing protein. If the protein deficiency is long-term, a decrease in muscle mass will be observed. The protein deficiency can delay the healing process and contribute to or cause other complications.

This diagnosis also may be used to describe the situation of a client who is having difficulty consuming the recommended amounts of nutrients because of problems related to medical interventions or treatments, such as surgery, chemotherapy, wired jaw, or inadequate absorption of nutrients because of medication side effects. Other contributing factors could arise from situational or maturational problems such as inadequate finances for purchasing food, depression, nausea and vomiting, allergies, use of crash or fad diets, ethnic or religious eating patterns, congenital anomalies, anorexia nervosa or an altered sense of taste. Nutritional assessment techniques may identify problems related to inadequate nutrition before these problems cause pathological changes in the body. Nursing assessment, early diagnosis, and appropriate interventions may prevent the need for medical intervention.

The diagnosis, "altered nutrition: more than body requirements," describes the situation wherein an individual experiences weight gain associated with an intake in excess of metabolic requirements. The person's body weight is 10% or more than the ideal weight for frame and height and the triceps skinfold is greater than 15 mm in men and 25 mm in women. The problem is related either to a lack of energy expenditure or excess intake or both. With early assessment and intervention the nurse may diagnose "altered nutrition: potential for more than body requirements," describing the state wherein an individual is at risk of experiencing an intake of nutrients that exceeds metabolic needs. The nurse may collect data that reveal a family history of obesity, rapid transition across growth percentiles, use of food for reward or comfort, or dysfunctional eating patterns.

"Feeding self-care deficit" illustrates the state in which an individual experiences impaired ability to perform or complete activities related to feeding. This diagnosis may be used in the situation of a client who is unable to bring food to his or her mouth or is unable to cut the food. Illness and age-related changes may result in self-care deficits. An older client with Parkinson's disease, for example, may have difficulty holding a fork or spoon because of hand tremors, and thus require assistance with feeding. The visual changes associated with aging (see chap. 24) may make it difficult for a client to cut food.

The diagnosis of "body image disturbance" is a disruption in the perception one has of one's body image. Defining characteristics may include nutritional fads and distress about changes in body structure or function. Preoccupation with being thin, for example, may lead to nutritional fads such as crash diets or fasting, which can result in possible health risks. Weight gain associated with illness and immobility also may result in a disturbance in body image that challenges coping abilities. Through careful assessment, the nurse can determine whether the client has the ability to adjust to a change in self-perception.

NANDA-approved nursing diagnosis statements are for identifying clients' responses to health problems. Nurses should not only identify problems but also support clients in attaining or maintaining optimal health. Therefore, nursing diagnosis statements related to good health might include "optimal nutritional status," or "nutrition: adequate to meet or maintain body requirements," or "nutritional intake: effective for optimal growth." The diagnosis of optimal nutritional status could indicate that the client consumes the ideal diet, that body measurements, both anthropometric and biochemical, are within normal range and that all findings related to nutrition from the clinical exam are normal. In other words, this client is the picture of nutritional health and adheres to all dietary recommendations for improving health.

In assessing and using nursing diagnoses related to nutrition, the nurse should strive to assist the client in identifying positive and negative factors affecting health. The overall goal is to assist the client in developing a healthy lifestyle within the context of his or her environment.

Chapter Highlights

- Nutrition is a critical factor in health.

- Nutritional assessment is an integral part of quality nursing care.

- To assess nutrition, the nurse uses a multifaceted approach for collecting data including anthropometric measurements, biochemical measurements, clinical history and exam, dietary and fluid intake, and environmental assessment.

- Nutritional assessment information is obtained by interview, appraisal, and examination of biochemical data.

- Once data related to nutritional assessment are collected, the nurse compares them to selected norms and standards to determine the individual's nutritional status.

- An abnormal finding in any one area does not necessarily indicate a nutritional problem. An abnormality leads the nurse to do a more thorough assessment to find additional evidence.

- Although the types of data needed for nutritional assessment are the same for all clients, cer-

tain modifications are appropriate for the client's environment, age, and health.

- Certain nutritional problems are more common in particular age groups, ethnic/cultural/religious groups, and during illnesses.

- The findings from the nutritional history and clinical appraisal enable the nurse to develop appropriate nursing diagnoses related to nutrition.

Practice Activities

1. Critique at least one dietary history section of a health history form used by a local health agency and at least one dietary history section of a nursing history form of a local hospital. What changes and/or additions would you recommend?

2. Using a case history, role-play with another student or colleague, obtaining data by interview to evaluate nutrition.

3. Collect and evaluate interviews, clinical appraisal, and anthropometric data from an adult client for the purpose of assessing nutrition.

4. Review the record of one hospitalized client and record all data that relate to nutrition. What additional information should be obtained for a complete nutritional assessment?

5. Obtain a 24-hour dietary recall from another student and evaluate it by comparing it with the basic food groups and the ADA Exchange Lists. Using the same data, evaluate the dietary intake of two nutrients (for example, iron and vitamin A), using the Recommended Dietary Allowances. Was the 24-hour recall information adequate for making a comparison with the RDAs?

6. Select an ethnic group in your locality that has food customs different from your own. Visit a food store serving this group to learn about the nutritional values of food items commonly used by them.

7. Record dietary intake, including intake offered as medications, of one hospitalized client for 24 hours, and evaluate the intake of protein, calories, and any one vitamin or mineral. Describe the effects of the client's health and activity level on nutritional requirements and compare this with the client's actual intake.

8. Review the chart of a client who has been hospitalized for 2 weeks or more and has had intravenous intake for at least 5 days. What biochemical data are recorded on the chart that are helpful in assessing nutrition?

Recommended Readings

Carruth, B. R. (1988). Nutritional assessment: A guide for nutrition education. *Journal of Nutrition Education, 20,* 280–288.

Cassell, J. A. (Ed.). (1987). Nutrition assessment. *Topics in Clinical Nutrition, 2*(4).

Chernoff, R., Mitchell, C., & Lipschitz, D.A. (1984). Assessment of the nutritional status of the geriatric patient. *Geriatric Medicine Today, 3*(5), 129–141.

Cockran, D., & Kaminski, M. V. (1986). Current concepts in nutritional assessment. *Nutritional Support Services, 6*(5), 14–15.

Horner, R., Lackey, C., Kolsa, K., & Warren, K. (1991). Pica practices of pregnant women. *Journal of the American Dietetic Association, 91*(1), 34–38.

Laffrey, S. C. (1986). Normal and overweight adults: Perceived weight and health behavior characteristics. *Nursing Research, 35*(6), 173–177.

Leninger, M. (1988). Transcultural eating patterns and nutrition: Transcultural nursing and anthropological perspectives. *Holistic Nursing Practice, 3*(1), 16–25.

Miller, I. J. (1988). Human taste bud sensitivity across adult age groups. *Journal of Gerontology: Biological Sciences, 43*(1), B26–30.

Morgan, J. (1984). Nutritional assessment of critically ill patients. *Focus on Critical Care, 11*(3), 28–34.

Suter, C. B., & Att, D. B. (1984). Maternal and infant nutrition recommendations: A review. *Journal of the American Dietetic Association, 84,* 572.

References

American Academy of Pediatrics, Committee on Nutrition. (1986). Prudent life style diet for children: Dietary fat and cholesterol. *Pediatrics, 78,* 521–525.

American Diabetes Association & American Dietetic Association. (1986). *Exchange lists for meal planning.* Alexandria, VA and Chicago: Author.

American Dietetic Association. (1976). *Cultural food patterns in the U.S.A.* Chicago: Author.

Bell, L. R. (1987). Disease-specific nutrition assessment reference cards. *Topics in Clinical Nutrition, 2*(4), 27–37.

Burtis, G., Davis, J., & Martin, S. (1988). *Applied nutrition and diet therapy.* Philadelphia: Saunders.

Committee on Nutrition of the Mother and Preschool Child, National Research Council. (1982). Alternative dietary practices and nutritional abuses in pregnancy. *Proceedings of a Workshop* (pp. 44–96). Washington, DC: National Academy Press.

Cronin, F. J., & Shaw, A. M. (1988). Summary of dietary recommendations for healthy Americans. *Nutrition Today, 23*(6), 26–34.

Ernst, N. D., Cleeman, J., Mullis, R., Sooter-Bochenek, J., & Van Hern, L. (1988). The national cholesterol education program: Implications for dietetic practitioners from the adult treatment panel recommendations. *Journal of the American Dietetic Association, 88,* 1401–1408.

Fournet, R. M. (1988). A preoperative nutritional assessment for determining postoperative complications. *Topics in Clinical Nutrition, 3*(4), 27–35.

Frisancho, A. R. (1981). New norms of upper limb fat and muscle areas for assessment of nutritional status. *American Journal of Clinical Nutrition, 34,* 2542.

Garn, S. M., & Clark, D. C. (1966). Problems in nutritional development of black individuals. *American Journal of Public Heath, 80,* 922–924.

Grant, A., & DeHoog, S. (1985). *Nutrition assessment and support.* Seattle, WA: Author.

Grant, J. A., & Kennedy-Caldwell, C. (1988). *Nutritional support in nursing.* Philadelphia: Grune and Stratton.

Hartz, S. C., Otradovex, C. L., McGandy, R. B., Russell, R. M., Jacob, R. A., Sahyown, N., Peters, H., Abrams, D., Scura, L. A., & Whinston-Perry, R. A. (1988). Nutrient supplement use by healthy elderly. *Journal of the American College of Nutrition, 7,* 119.

Jenkins, C. H. (1988). *Nutrition and the older adult: Nursing update.* Princeton, NJ: Continuing Professional Education Center.

Lewis, C. M. (1986). *Nutrition and nutritional therapy in nursing.* Norwalk, CT: Appleton-Century-Crofts.

Medlin, C. & Skinner, J. (1988). Individual dietary intake methodology: A 50-year review of progress. *Journal of American Dietetic Association, 88,* 1250–1257.

National Dairy Council. (1987). *How to eat for good health.* Rosemont, IL: Author.

National Research Council, Food and Nutrition Board. (1980). *Recommended dietary allowances* (9th ed.). Washington, DC: National Academy of Sciences.

National Research Council, Food and Nutrition Board. (1989a). *Recommended dietary allowances* (10th ed.). Washington, DC: National Academy Press.

National Research Council. (1989b). *Diet and health: Implications for reducing chronic disease risk.* Washington, DC: National Academy Press.

Pennington, J. A., & Church, H. N. (1985). *Bowes and Church's food values of portions commonly used.* Philadelphia: Lippincott.

Salmond, S. W. (1980). How to assess the nutritional status of acutely ill patients. *American Journal of Nursing, 80,* 922–924.

Simko, M. D., Cowell, C., & Gilbride, J. A. (1984). *Nutrition assessment: A comprehensive guide for planning intervention.* Rockville, MD: Aspen Systems.

Staff. (July, 1972). Highlights of the ten-state nutrition survey. *Nutrition Today, 7,* 4–11.

Suitor, C. W., & Crowley, M. F. (1984). *Nutrition principles and application in health promotion.* Philadelphia: Lippincott.

U.S. Department of Agriculture. (1985). *Nutritive value of American foods: Handbook no. 8.* Washington, DC: U.S. Government Printing Office.

U.S. Department of Health and Human Services. (1988). *The Surgeon General's report on nutrition and health: Summary and recommendations* (PHS Publication No. 88–50211). Washington, DC: U.S. Government Printing Office.

Williams, S. R. (1990). *Essentials of nutrition and diet therapy.* St. Louis: Times Mirror/Mosby.

19

Fluid–Electrolyte and Elimination Assessment

OBJECTIVES

Upon completion of this chapter, you should be able to:

■ Describe the mechanisms that regulate fluid–electrolyte balance and elimination.

■ Discuss the factors that affect fluid–electrolyte balance and elimination patterns.

■ Explain the purposes and parameters of the fluid–electrolyte and elimination assessment.

■ Modify the fluid–electrolyte and elimination assessment according to the client's age, cultural background, and health.

■ Collect subjective and objective data concerning a client's fluid–electrolyte balance and elimination patterns.

■ Use appropriate laboratory findings to validate fluid–electrolyte and elimination assessment.

■ Accurately assess clients with potential or actual alterations in fluid–electrolyte and acid-base balance.

■ Formulate valid and appropriate nursing diagnoses for clients with alterations in fluid–electrolyte balance and elimination patterns.

Fluids and electrolytes are essential for homeostasis. Optimal cellular functioning, necessary for survival, depends on the availability of an adequate supply of nutrients (see chap. 18), body fluids, electrolytes, and acid-base balance and the ability to eliminate waste materials from the body. These waste materials are eliminated primarily through the bowel and bladder as well as through the less obvious routes of the integumentary and respiratory systems.

Any alteration that impairs the functioning of the body's delicate fluid and electrolyte balance or alters elimination patterns will, at minimum, cause social inconvenience and psychological and physical discomfort for the client. At worst, these alterations may be life-threatening.

In a healthy client, or a client newly admitted to a hospital or long-term care facility, the primary purpose of assessing fluid–electrolyte and elimination status is to identify the client's usual patterns of ingestion and elimination and the balance between fluid intake and output. A secondary purpose is to detect actual or potential alterations in fluid–electrolyte balance or elimination patterns.

KNOWLEDGE NEEDED TO ASSESS FLUID–ELECTROLYTE BALANCE AND ELIMINATION

To maintain optimal health, the body's finely tuned homeostatic mechanisms must be functioning optimally.

Fluid Balance

The greatest proportion of body mass is fluid, approximately 50 to 60%, (Figure 19-1), and it varies with age (Table 19-1), sex, and body fat. The percentage of body fluid is inversely proportionate to age: the younger the client, the greater the percentage of body fluid. Women have a lower percentage of body fluid than men because of women's greater proportionate amounts of adipose tissue and smaller muscle mass. Obese people have a lower percentage of body fluid compared with those who are not overweight. Body fluid is divided between intracellular and extracellular spaces. Intracellular fluid (ICF), sometimes called cellular fluid, is the fluid contained within the cells of the body. Extracellular fluid (ECF) is the fluid found in the interstitial spaces, plasma, bone, connective tissue and within the gastrointestinal tract, brain and cerebrospinal fluid (Hui, 1985; Martof, 1985a).

In an adult, two-thirds of the body fluid exists within cells, primarily skeletal muscle. The remaining one third exists outside of the cell, specifically between cells and in the plasma (Metheny, 1987). The essential functions of body fluid are maintaining blood volume, influencing body temperature, providing a medium for cell metabolism, transporting both nutrients and waste products to and from cells, and functioning as the solvent for the solutes essential for cell function (Guyton, 1990).

In the course of a day, the average adult processes from 2.5 to 3.0 liters of water. Basic mechanisms control the intake and output of water. These mechanisms are thirst and drinking and hormonal controls. Thirst and drinking regulate intake by complex interactions involving the hypothalamus and hormonal influence. Hormonal controls in the form of vasopressin and aldosterone regulate renal water elimination (Williams & Worthington, 1988).

Electrolyte Balance

In addition to water, body fluid is composed of electrolytes, substances that develop an electrical charge when dissolved in water. These electrically charged particles (ions) conduct electrical current, allowing cellular excitability. Ions that carry a positive charge, such as potassium (K^+), are referred to as cations. Ions that carry a negative charge are known as anions.

Electrolytes serve major functions in the body, including regulating hydrogen–ion balance, maintaining membrane excitability, maintaining body

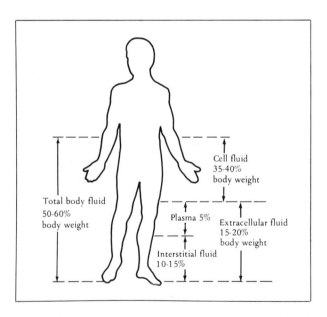

FIGURE 19-1. Total body fluid represents 50% to 60% of body weight of a normal adult. (*Note.* From Taylor, C., Lillis, C., & LeMone, P. [1989]. *Fundamentals of nursing.* Philadelphia: J.B. Lippincott, p. 945.)

TABLE 19-1
Percentage of Body Water by Age*

Age	Percentage of Water
Early human embryo	95 to 97%
Newborn	75
Older infant	65 to 70
Child	60 to 65
Adult male	57
Adult female	55
Elderly adult	45 to 50

*As age increases, the proportion of body water decreases.

TABLE 19-2
Daily Loss of Water (Adults)

	Normal Temperature	Hot Weather	Prolonged Heavy Exercise
Insensible loss:			
Skin	350 ml	350 ml	350 ml
Respiratory tract	350 ml	250 ml	650 ml
Sensible loss			
Urine	1,400 ml	1,200 ml	500 ml
Sweat	100 ml	1,400 ml	5,000 ml
Feces	100 ml	100 ml	100 ml
Total	2,300 ml	3,300 ml	6,600 ml

Note. From Guyton, A. (1991). Textbook of medical physiology. Philadelphia: Saunders, 275.

fluid–osmolality, and moving body fluid between body fluid compartments. While the electrolyte content of extracellular fluid differs from that of intracellular fluid, the total number of cations and anions within the body and within each fluid compartment must be equal.

The movement of water and particles between intracellular and extracellular spaces is essential in the balance and regulation of fluid and electrolytes. The regulation of fluid and electrolytes occurs through several mechanisms. The exchange of water occurs through osmosis and filtration while the exchange of particles occurs through diffusion, filtration, or active transport. The homeostatic mechanisms of a number of systems (kidneys, lungs, heart, blood vessels, adrenal glands, parathyroid gland, and pituitary gland) maintain the composition volume of body fluid within normal, but narrow limits (Metheny, 1987).

In healthy individuals, the balance of fluids ingested and those formed from metabolic processes in a 24-hour period is approximately equal to fluids excreted in that same 24-hour period. Table 19-2 shows the approximate amounts of fluid loss in a 24-hour period for a healthy adult, as well as the changes that occur in a healthy individual in hot weather or after heavy exercise. These norms are helpful in evaluating daily fluid balance in clients.

Homeostasis is not only a function of fluid balance but also a function of intracellular and extracellular electrolytes and of a balance of the ratio of bicarbonate to hydrogen ion concentration in the blood known as acid-base balance. The primary extracellular electrolyte is sodium (Na^+), and the primary intracellular electrolyte is potassium (K^+).

Sodium

Water balance and extracellular sodium (NaCl) concentration are closely related, since sodium has the principal responsibility for osmosis, the movement of water between intracellular and extracellular compartments. When an individual is in good health and normal environmental conditions prevail, serum sodium is regulated by the kidneys, and a balance is struck between sodium ingested and that excreted. When necessary, the kidneys are capable of conserving sodium. If increased environmental temperature or heavy exercise causes excessive perspiration, sodium depletion may occur in proportion to water depletion (Guyton, 1990). Ingesting large amounts of water alone will not prevent sodium depletion; therefore, fluids containing sodium (e.g., Gatorade) must be consumed, or some other source of sodium (e.g., high sodium food) must accompany fluid replacement.

The client who has an alteration in gastrointestinal function should be monitored for a potential sodium deficit (hyponatremia). Consistent loss of sodium through vomiting, diarrhea, or nasogastric drainage may lead to sodium depletion. As sodium deficiency occurs, compensation first takes place in the kidneys, where both increased secretion of aldosterone and antidiuretic hormone (ADH) enhances the amount of sodium and water reabsorbed in the renal tubule (Metheny, 1987). A shift of sodium from interstitial to intravascular compartments also occurs. Eventually, if these compensatory mechanisms are insufficient and the serum sodium level drops, vascular collapse occurs. It is not difficult to see that symptoms of sodium depletion are similar to those of fluid volume deficit. Such signs and symptoms as apprehension, weakness, fatigue, dizziness, lowered blood pressure, and abdominal cramps may indicate a sodium deficit. The nurse should be especially alert for these subjective and objective cues in clients at risk for sodium depletion, as with clients losing gastrointestinal secretions through nasogastric tubes or vomiting, or those who engage in heavy exercise in hot weather.

Hypernatremia (sodium excess) is an equally

serious problem and is indicative of a serious stress placed on the body's adaptive mechanisms. Any condition that leads to decreased intake or increased output of water may lead to hypernatremia. Conversely, increased intake or decreased output of sodium also may lead to hypernatremia. Metheny and Snively (1979) cite several pertinent examples: the erroneous use of salt rather than sugar when preparing baby formulas, profuse watery diarrhea where water loss is greater than sodium loss, salt water drowning, or respiratory problems that lead to an increase in insensible loss of water. Clients' manifestations that may indicate hypernatremia include neurological irritation ranging from agitation to convulsions; dry, sticky mucous membranes; and edema manifesting itself as firm, rubbery tissue turgor or pitting edema.

These manifestations are similar to those seen in fluid volume depletion or overload. This should not be surprising, since sodium is the major electrolyte associated with water balance.

Potassium

The potassium level is determined by measuring its extracellular plasma volume concentration. These measurements may not reflect the true level of potassium in the body, since its major concentration is intracellular. In a state of optimal health, most persons' bodily needs for potassium are met through normal dietary intake. Potassium is lost through urine, perspiration, gastrointestinal secretions, and feces. The body does not have the same ability to conserve potassium as it does sodium. Therefore, hypokalemia (low potassium concentration) is a frequent problem for clients with a decreased intake, such as a client who is not eating and not receiving intravenous replacement. The nurse should remember that potassium depletion is a common problem for clients undergoing diuretic therapy. Nasogastric drainage and diarrhea can also contribute to potassium depletion. The human body is very vulnerable to small changes in the extracellular concentration of potassium. Since potassium plays a vital role in cell membrane depolarization (that is, in the transmission of action potentials), any deficit in potassium leads to nonspecific symptoms of muscle weakness and increased tiredness. With a continued deficit, further objective cues develop, such as abdominal distention and impaired respiratory function. Potassium levels must be monitored closely in the vulnerable client. The cardiac muscle (the myocardium) is particularly responsive to changes in potassium levels. Hypokalemia may cause a weak, irregular pulse and certain electrocardiogram (EKG) changes, specifically a flattened T wave.

A client who is neither eating nor drinking will need 40 to 50 mEq of potassium daily to replace the usual urinary excretion of 40 to 50 mEq per day. If additional potassium loss is occurring as a result of diarrhea, diuretic therapy, or other means, the client's replacement needs increase accordingly.

As noted above, potassium is primarily an intracellular electrolyte with total body stores estimated at 4,000 mEq. Normally, the kidneys excrete any excess potassium that is ingested. Thus potassium excess usually is related to trauma that causes extensive injury to cells (Martof 1985b); as in severe burns or crushing-type injuries. Such injury causes intracellular potassium to enter the extracellular fluid. Extraordinarily high potassium intake may cause potassium excess, however, as may impaired renal function. Excess potassium, as with depleted potassium, may cause gastrointestinal disturbances and skeletal muscle weakness and paralysis. Because the myocardium is particularly vulnerable to hyperkalemia, cardiac arrest can result. On electrocardiogram the T wave will peak and, in fact, the EKG changes, rather than the serum potassium, are the critical measurement of the effect of potassium on the myocardium. It is important then that a client with altered serum potassium be carefully monitored for electrocardiogram changes. It is also essential that potassium levels be monitored when a client is on digitalis. In this instance, if the client becomes hypokalemic while taking digitalis, the client is prone to digitalis toxicity.

Acid-Base Balance

Another facet of homeostatic regulation is acid-base balance, defined essentially as the maintenance of the 20:1 ratio of base bicarbonate to carbonic acid in the body. The measurement of serum pH in arterial blood reflects this balance. Normal serum pH falls within the narrow range of 7.35 to 7.45. Since pH is the negative log of hydrogen ion concentration, as the pH goes up, hydrogen ion concentration decreases, with a concomitant increase in bicarbonate. As the pH decreases, hydrogen ion concentration increases or, in other words, the carbonic acid ratio increases (Guyton, 1990).

Arterial blood gas measurement provides specific information concerning the possible source of acid-base alterations: whether the alteration is metabolic or respiratory in origin. For example, if normal serum pH is 7.35 to 7.45, then a client with a pH of 7.31 is in a state of acidosis; alternately, a client with a pH of 7.48 is in a state of alkalosis. Loss of hydrochloric acid from gastric drainage or from severe persistent vomiting, especially if there is pyloric obstruction and the drainage is purely gastric, leads to a decrease in hydrogen ion concentration and a resultant metabolic alkalosis. Renal dysfunction that causes increased output of hydrogen ion, or a potassium deficiency resulting from diuretics, also contributes to a metabolic alkalosis.

Loss of large quantities of sodium through small-bowel or large-intestinal contents results in metabolic acidosis. The kidneys attempt to compensate by excreting hydrogen ions or conserving bicarbonate, and the respiratory system will respond with hyperventilation to rid the body of excess carbon dioxide. Hyperventilation in turn increases insensible loss through the lungs.

It is necessary to monitor clients carefully for early signs of acid-base imbalance. Table 19-3 compares the clinical manifestations of metabolic acidosis and metabolic alkalosis.

Clearly, there is a strong interrelationship between fluid and electrolyte status and acid-base balance. Any change that occurs in one may lead to a concomitant change in the other. Frequently, a change in fluid and electrolyte status or serum pH is a result of an alteration in a client's elimination functions. Because many of the clinical manifestations that are indicative of acid-base imbalance are nonspecific, skilled observation by the nurse is essential. Clinical observations may be validated by checking results of laboratory tests and through ongoing assessment of the client.

Table 19-4 summarizes fluid and electrolyte balance and imbalance.

Normal Elimination

The structures and functions of the gastrointestinal tract (specifically the intestines) and the kidneys are involved in the elimination of waste materials from the body.

Peristaltic movement propels the contents of the small intestines (chyme) toward the anus. Contents pass slowly, taking anywhere from 3 to 10 hours to move from the stomach to the large intestines. The action of pancreatic enzymes, intestinal secretions, and bile carry out the work of digestion. The major portion of digestion is accomplished in the small intestines, as is 90% of the absorption of nutrients.

The passage of chyme in the large intestines is also slow, taking about 12 hours for contents to move to the rectum. Electrolytes, water, and bile salts are reabsorbed predominantly in the ascending colon. The colon has the ability to absorb six to eight times more fluid than it normally does. Approximately 100 ml of fluid is contained in the fecal material that is evacuated regularly. The reflex to defecate occurs when fecal material enters the rectum from the sigmoid colon. This action initiates the transmission of afferent impulses to the spinal cord and results in reflex impulses transmitted back to the colon, sigmoid, and rectum. These reflex impulses cause relaxation of the anal sphincter, enabling defecation.

While thirst is the major control of fluid intake, the kidney is the major organ controlling output. Through a number of control mechanisms, the kidney is able to regulate the volume and osmolality of body fluids. The osmolality of body fluids is primarily determined by sodium and its associate anions. Water and sodium balance is maintained through the glomerular filtration rate (GFR), antidiuretic hormone (ADH) and the aldosterone-renin–angiotensin system.

The process of micturition (voiding or urination) is largely an involuntary reflex that occurs when stretch receptors in the bladder are stimulated as the urine collects. However, control of micturition can be learned. Multiple factors, such as developmental level, food and fluid, medications, illness, psychological variables, and lifestyle can affect micturition, as well as bowel elimination.

TABLE 19-3
Clinical Manifestations of Metabolic Acidosis
and Alkalosis

Metabolic Acidosis	Metabolic Alkalosis
Decreased alertness	Confusion
Headache	Dizziness
Hyperventilation	Hypoventilation
Respirations deeper	Numbness and tingling
Acetone breath odor	Tetany
Disorientation	Convulsions
Stupor	
Coma	

VARIABLES THAT INFLUENCE FLUID–ELECTROLYTE BALANCE AND ELIMINATION

Differences in patterns of elimination may be a function of the client's age, culture, or health. To accurately assess client's fluid–electrolyte and elimination status and derive valid nursing diagnoses, the nurse needs to be aware of these differences.

TABLE 19-4
Summary of Fluid and Electrolyte Balance and Imbalance

Fluid/ Electrolyte	Normal Findings	Predisposing Factors	Manifestations of Deficit	Manifestations of Excess
Extracellular fluid	*Infant:* 29% of body weight *Adult:* 15% of body weight	*Deficit:* Insufficient fluid intake, vomiting, diarrhea *Excess:* Excessive administration or intake of fluid with NaCl	Weight loss, dry skin and mucous membranes, thirst, oliguria, low blood pressure, plasma pH above 7.45, urine pH above 7.0	Weight gain, edema, puffy eyelids, high blood pressure
Bicarbonate (HCO_3^-)	Plasma bicarbonates 21–29 mEq/L, urine pH 4.6–8.0, plasma pH 7.35–7.45 (arterial blood)	*Deficit:* Uncontrolled diabetes mellitus, starvation, severe infectious disease, renal insufficiency *Excess:* Loss of Cl^- and H^+ through vomiting, gastric suction, hyperadrenalism, prolonged ingestion of alkali	Metabolic acidosis, disorientation, weakness, shortness of breath, sweet fruity odor to breath, plasma pH below 7.35, HCO_3^- below 25 mEq/L	Metabolic alkalosis, slow and shallow respirations, tetany, hypertonic muscles, plasma pH above 7.45, HCO_3^- above 30 mEq/L
Carbonic acid (H_2CO_3)	Pa_{CO_2} 35–45 mm. Hg, plasma pH 7.35–7.45 (arterial blood)	*Deficit:* Oxygen lack, fever, anxiety, pulmonary infections, hyperventilation *Excess:* Hypoventilation, chronic asthma, emphysema, barbiturate poisoning	Respiratory alkalosis, deep and rapid breathing, unconsciousness, plasma pH above 7.45, low Pa_{CO_2}	Respiratory acidosis, disorientation, shallow respirations, plasma pH below 7.35, high Pa_{CO_2}
Sodium (Na^+)	135–145 mEq/L (plasma)	*Deficit:* Excessive perspiration, gastrointestinal suction, diarrhea *Excess:* Inadequate water intake	Apprehension, abdominal cramps, rapid and weak pulse, oliguria, plasma sodium below 135 mEq/L	Dry and sticky mucous membranes, fever, thirst, firm rubbery tissue turgor, plasma sodium above 145 mEq/L
Potassium (K^+)	3.6–5.0 mEq/L (plasma)	*Deficit:* Diarrhea, vomiting, some kidney disease, diuretic therapy, increased stress *Excess:* Renal failure, burns, excessive administration	Muscle weakness, abnormal heart rhythm, anorexia, abdominal distention	Oliguria, intestinal colic, irritability, irregular pulse, diarrhea
Calcium (Ca^{2+})	4.3–5.3 mEq/L (plasma)	*Deficit:* Removal of parathyroid glands, excessive loss of intestinal fluids, massive infections *Excess:* Overactive parathyroid gland, excessive ingestion of milk	Muscle cramps, tingling in the fingers, tetany, convulsions	Relaxed muscles, flank pain, kidney stones, deep bone pain
Chloride (Cl^-)	98–108 mEq/L	*Deficit:* Increased HCO_3^-, loss through vomiting, excessive	See sodium	See sodium

TABLE 19-4 (Continued)

Fluid/ Electrolyte	Normal Findings	Predisposing Factors	Manifestations of Deficit	Manifestations of Excess
		ECF loss through intestinal fistula		
		Excess: Increased Na$^+$, excessive fluid loss through kidneys, severe dehydration		

Note. From *Fundamentals of Nursing: Concepts and Procedures,* 2nd ed., by B. Kozier and G. Erb. Copyright © 1983 by Addison-Wesley Publishing Company. Reprinted by permission.

Age

Because of the physiological changes associated with aging, the assessment of elimination patterns and practices requires some modifications. Vulnerability to fluid and electrolyte imbalances may be caused by many things, among them age. Infants (see chap. 22) and older individuals are far more vulnerable to variations in fluid volume than are healthy older children and adults.

Elderly individuals are particularly vulnerable to dehydration because of the changes in renal function and the decreased renal reserve that occur with aging. Renal blood flow and glomerular filtration rate decrease by 50% by the time a person reaches 90 years of age. Maximum specific gravity also decreases; therefore, the kidneys are less able to concentrate urine (see chap. 24). Older persons must excrete more fluid via the kidney to rid themselves of all metabolic wastes. The problems of fluid balance in the elderly are complicated further if they suffer from physical disabilities or urinary incontinence. Physical disabilities may limit their access to fluids. Urinary incontinence may cause them to voluntarily restrict their intake.

Whenever older individuals suffer either a decrease in fluid intake or an increase in either sensible or insensible loss, they must be monitored closely for signs of dehydration. Since their fluid needs are proportionately greater, dehydration may have especially ominous consequences.

Daily weights are a particularly significant indicator of the degree of dehydration experienced by the older individual:

A weight loss of 2 to 4% indicates mild dehydration.

A weight loss of 5 to 9% indicates moderate dehydration.

A loss of 10% or more of body weight (in fluid) places the client in danger of circulatory collapse and death.

With a 10% weight loss in water, the eyes recede.

Table 19-5 lists the signs of dehydration (fluid depletion). It is especially important to remember that in older people the early signs of dehydration may be misleading, since a decrease in skin turgor may be due to the loss of skin elasticity that normally occurs with aging.

Measuring output from any source is especially important when fluid balance is precarious. Fluid replacement needs must be calculated precisely to lessen the risk of further dehydration and to avoid overhydration.

Culture

American culture is very bathroom-oriented. The amount of money that is spent on bathrooms in residences reflects this fact. Bathrooms are beautified, virtually beatified, in modern American life. Although there is great willingness to discuss bathroom decor, there is little willingness to discuss bodily functions that take place there. In fact, there is general reluctance to discuss bowel and bladder habits. To obtain accurate data about a client's elimination patterns nurses must first overcome their own taboos regarding this subject, and must then acknowledge the embarrassment and fear clients may experience when the topic is brought up.

This cultural conditioning is evident in many of the nurse's encounters with clients. Elimination is a private activity that takes place behind the closed doors of our homes. During illness or hospitalization, this formerly private activity suddenly may be exposed for all to discuss, possibly view, and perhaps even worse, for others to smell. The client's privacy during elimination must be protected if the client's self-esteem is to be preserved.

The early emphasis on toilet training in American culture is a further example of cultural conditioning. Parents often place an emphasis on their children's elimination patterns well into adolescence. Thus, another bathroom-oriented generation of people is perpetuated.

Another factor the nurse must recognize is that many clients' home environments differ from the sanitized, flushing-toilet version portrayed on television commercials and with which most nurses are familiar. Many rural areas of the United States still do not have indoor toilet facilities but rely on the outhouse. When hospitalized, clients from rural areas may be unfamiliar with and even fearful of indoor plumbing. On the other hand, the nurse should never assume that because clients reside in rural areas they do not have indoor plumbing facilities. The nurse should tactfully query the client about toileting facilities in the home to be certain.

Clients from foreign countries may have totally different experiences with bathroom facilities, and the values they place on them may vary. Non-flush indoor toilets are common in some parts of Western Europe, for example. In addition, different cultural groups may use special words or phrases to describe toileting functions. For example, "make" is used to refer to elimination in the Jewish culture.

Nurses care for clients from many cultures and subcultures. Some clients, depending on their past experiences and ages, will need more privacy than others. Some may be unfamiliar with modern plumbing. In other instances, nurses may visit homes and see bathroom facilities very different from those the nurse is used to in terms of functioning or cleanliness. Nurses should recognize that cultural variations in elimination practices exist and need to be assessed in order to plan appropriate nursing interventions.

TABLE 19-5
Clinical Manifestations of Fluid Imbalance

Fluid Overload	Fluid Depletion
Shortness of breath	Thirst
Increased urine output	Oliguria
Weight gain	Weight loss
Elevated blood pressure	Lowered blood pressure
Diluted urine	Concentrated urine
Low urine specific gravity	High urine specific gravity
Venous filling time less than 3 seconds	Venous filling time more than 5 seconds
Engorged neck and hand veins	Collapsed neck and hand veins
Edema—pedal, sacral, scrotal	Poor skin turgor
Increased abdominal girth	Pallor
"Wet" respiration	Sunken eyeballs (sunken fontanel in infants)
	Dry mucous membranes

Health

Any change in health may alter the client's fluid and electrolyte balance and elimination patterns.

Increased Insensible Loss

The nurse needs to be alert for conditions that can cause increased insensible fluid loss. One such condition is fever. For every degree Fahrenheit of temperature elevation, a client loses an extra 50 to 75 ml of fluid in a 24-hour period. The increased metabolism associated with fever increases fluid loss. Fever also increases the respiratory rate and may increase sensible fluid loss in the form of perspiration. A client with a temperature of 39.5 °C (103 °F) will have approximately a 300 ml daily increase in insensible fluid loss.

An increased respiratory rate is yet another source of increased insensible loss. Normally, the greatest amount of insensible fluid loss is through the lungs. This loss is in direct proportion to the increase in rate. If the respiratory rate doubles, then insensible fluid loss is doubled. Children frequently quadruple their respiratory rate when ill. This increase in insensible loss may cause serious dehydration.

Diarrhea and Constipation

When considering the problems of constipation and diarrhea, it is important to differentiate between frequency of defecation and consistency of the stool. Individuals vary in the frequency of their bowel movements. Although it is not necessary to have a bowel movement every day, many people expect to, and they will report that they are constipated if a day goes by without a bowel movement. The consistency of the stool is of greater concern than is the frequency.

Keane and Miller (1987) define diarrhea as the rapid movement of fecal matter through the intestine resulting in poor absorption of water, nutritive elements, and electrolytes, and producing abnormally frequent evacuation of watery stools.

Diarrhea varies in its severity from causing discomfort and inconvenience to creating a severe life-threatening situation. The seriousness of the situation will be affected by such factors as age, health, and the actual amount of fluids and electrolytes lost. The nurse must thoroughly assess the severity of the diarrhea and identify those clients at risk, in particular infants and the elderly.

With diarrhea, the usual 100 ml of fluid lost daily in the stool will increase. If the diarrhea is severe enough to place the client at risk for dehydration, the volume should be measured. Any increase in the number of stools or change in consistency should be recorded.

A client suffering from diarrhea is also at great risk for developing potassium depletion. Each liter of diarrhea contains 25 mEq of potassium. With severe diarrhea a person may lose up to 75 mEq in 24 hours. Even mild diarrhea can cause a severe potassium deficiency. The client with diarrhea must be closely observed for signs of potassium depletion (depressed respirations, muscle weakness, lethargy, cardiac arrhythmias, diminished peristalsis).

The color of diarrhea stools also should be noted. Green, watery diarrhea usually indicates infection. White, colorless diarrhea indicates bile duct obstruction. The presence of blood and mucous in the stools may be significant for certain diseases. Explosive diarrhea may indicate enterocolitis.

The client with diarrhea may complain of gas pains, and the nurse may note increasing abdominal girth indicating abdominal distention. Distention occurs when gas and fluid accumulate in the bowel. In healthy states most of the 7 to 10 liters of gas formed in the large intestine is reabsorbed, with an average of 0.6 liter expelled. Diarrhea may cause an increase in expelled flatus since the increased motility of the gastrointestinal tract does not allow time for the gas to be reabsorbed.

Certain environmental conditions are known to cause diarrhea. Therefore, the nurse should assess the client's home environment for crowding and inadequate sanitation or refrigeration, which may lead to food and water contamination.

If too much fluid is absorbed from the large bowel, constipation occurs. Constipation is defined as difficulty in passing a hard, dry stool, a decrease in the frequency of stools, or a total cessation of bowel movements (Battle & Hanna, 1980). If the client reports constipation, further assessment is needed. Contributory factors such as a decrease in dietary bulk, a change in meal regularity, a decrease in fluid intake, a reduction in exercise, or other factors should be identified (Battle & Hanna, 1980). Sedatives, tranquilizers, and narcotics all can decrease gastrointestinal motility, so the nurse should inquire about medications the client is taking. For example, a football player on bed rest after suffering a knee injury has markedly decreased his exercise (Rubin, 1988). At the same time, he is receiving morphine for pain, and he ignores the urge to defecate because he is uncomfortable about using the bedpan. All three factors (immobility, morphine, and lack of privacy) contribute to constipation.

When assessing clients with altered elimination patterns, the nurse must be alert for symptoms indicating abdominal obstruction, such as colicky abdominal pain, nausea, and vomiting, abdominal distention, and constipation. Distention occurs as gas and fluid accumulate above the level of the obstruction. Increased abdominal distention may be assessed by measuring abdominal girth with a tape measure around the abdomen at the level of the umbilicus. Progressive obstruction can lead to large amounts of fluid and electrolyte loss with resultant electrolyte imbalance and dehydration. Close assessment of the client is imperative.

Vomiting and Nasogastric Output

If the upper gastrointestinal tract becomes irritated or overdistended, the stomach may empty itself through vomiting. The strongest stimulus to vomit comes from distention or overstimulation of the stomach or duodenum. Vomiting also may be caused by certain medications—for example, many chemotherapeutic drugs—or by motion (airplane or car sickness).

The nurse should measure the amount of emesis when possible and also should note the color and consistency of the vomitus. It is especially important to note if any "coffee grounds" material, which may mean bleeding in the upper gastrointestinal tract, is present. The nurse should try to determine what factors precipitated the vomiting, such as drugs, food intolerance, or emotional upset.

The client who is vomiting persistently may have a nasogastric tube inserted to relieve the discomfort of vomiting. Clients who are suffering from gastrointestinal disturbances or those who have had abdominal surgery will frequently have nasogastric tubes in place. The nurse should specifically note the source of the drainage or emesis so that the electrolyte content of the output can be estimated. Drainage or emesis due to a pyloric obstruction is acid in nature and places the client at risk for developing metabolic alkalosis. Drainage or emesis resulting from obstruction in the small intestine may be neutral because of equal losses of acid and base electrolytes. This occurs because vomitus (emesis) is acidic, while contents of the lower intestine are alkaline. In this instance large amounts of fluids and electrolytes are lost, resulting in dehydration but maintaining acid-base balance. Drainage from an obstruction lower in the intestine is more alkaline in character and places the client at risk for developing metabolic acidosis. The client with extensive intestinal obstruction may become more and more constipated and may vomit less. If the obstruction is unrelieved, however, vomiting may become fecal in character. This is believed to be due to reverse peristalsis. The nurse must remember that a client with a paralytic ileus should be producing nasogastric output. If the client is not, the tube probably is obstructed.

The color, consistency, and amount of nasogastric drainage should be noted. Gastric drainage is pale, yellow-green. Intestinal drainage is dark green to brown. The type of nasogastric tube used serves as a clue to the type of drainage expected. Levine and Anderson tubes are inserted into the stomach. Tubes such as the Miller-Abbott or Cantor tube are designed to drain the small intestine. Table 19-6 describes the expected drainage from the various types of tubes and catheters.

Urinary Catheter Output

For a variety of reasons, a client may require a catheter be inserted into the bladder to drain urine. Usually this is done using a Foley catheter, a two-way catheter inserted into the bladder through the urethra. Some clients may have a drainage tube inserted directly into the bladder via a suprapubic catheter. Urine may also drain through catheters inserted into the ureter or the renal pelvis. These are known, respectively, as ureterostomy and nephrostomy tubes.

Urinary drainage catheters should be carefully and regularly inspected for patency. A urinary catheter should drain at least 50 ml/hour to achieve a 24-hour output of 1,200 to 1,500 ml (Table 19-6). An output of less than 30 ml per hour may indicate dehydration or renal disease. The urine in the drainage tubing and collection bag should be examined for appearance, noting its color, consistency, and presence of sediment. It is crucial that urinary drainage systems remain closed to prevent ascending infections of the urinary tract.

Ostomies

Certain factors specific to physiological, psychological, and social functioning must be assessed when a client has had an intestinal or urinary diversion performed.

To manage a stoma, the client or significant

TABLE 19-6
Expected Drainage from Selected Tubes and Catheters (Adults)

Device	Substance	Daily Drainage	Color	Odor	Consistency
Foley catheter	Urine	500 to 700 ml for first 2 post-op days; 1,500 to 2,500 ml normal	Clear, yellow	Ammonia	Watery
Gastrostomy tube	Gastric	Up to 1,500 ml	Pale, yellow-green	Sour	Watery
Hemovac	Wound drainage	Varies with procedure	Varies with procedure	Like wound dressing	Variable
Ileal conduit	Urine	500–2,500 ml	Clear, yellow	Ammonia	Watery (with mucus and blood initially)
Ileostomy	Small bowel contents	Up to 4,000 ml in first 24 hr; then less than 1,000 ml	Brown	Sour, fecal	Initially serous with mucus; brown liquid stool when peristalsis resumes
Miller-Abbott tube	Intestinal contents	Up to 3,000 ml	Dark green or brown	Neutralized acid; fecal	Thick
Nasogastric tube	Gastric contents	Up to 1,500 ml	Pale, yellow-green	Sour	Watery
T tube	Bile	500 ml	Bright yellow to dark green	Acrid	Thick
Suprapubic catheter	Urine	500–2,500 ml	Clear, yellow	Ammonia	Watery
Ureteral catheter	Urine	250–1,250 ml	Clear, yellow	Ammonia	Watery

Note. Adapted from Croushore, T.M. "Postoperative Assessment: The Key to Avoiding the Most Common Nursing Mistakes." *Nursing 79*, 9:48 (April 1979), Copyright © 1979, Intermed Communications, Inc., Horsham, PA 19044. Reprinted with permission.

other must be able to assume responsibility for self-care. Therefore, it is important to assess the client's age, intellectual ability, and psychomotor skills to determine the client's self-care ability. The nurse should determine also if there are significant others who can offer support to the client undergoing such a major change in body image and function. Exploration of the client's lifestyle, hobbies, occupation, and physical limitations is necessary to determine what adaptations the ostomy will require of the client. The nurse should note the client's willingness to look at and touch the stoma, since self-care management necessitates the client's acceptance of the stoma's presence.

The nurse should be familiar with the particular type of ostomy and the drainage expected from it. An *ileostomy*, which is formed from a section of ileum, will drain liquid material. This type of ostomy cannot be regulated, so the client must wear a continuous drainage appliance. Postoperatively, drainage from an ileostomy ranges from an initial high of up to 4,000 ml in 24 hours to less than 1,000 ml per day (Table 19-6).

While the drainage from a continent ileostomy is initially liquid, after the client begins eating solids, the drainage thickens. A catheter is inserted into a nipple valve to drain the continent ileostomy. If the drainage becomes too thick, a problem may develop. If this happens, the client's fluid intake should be assessed, as it may need to be increased. The presence of undigested fibrous foods such as corn, nuts, lettuce, celery, peas, and oranges in the drainage should be noted.

Gas pains may cause a problem for the client with an ostomy. The client's diet should be assessed for intake of gas-producing foods such as dried beans, cabbage, broccoli, onions, peppers, and sauerkraut. Odor is often a continual source of embarrassment to the client with an ostomy. Gas-forming foods also may be a source of odor.

A *colostomy* excretes more solid fecal matter. As fecal matter descends in the large colon, more water is absorbed and digestive enzymes are neutralized. The type of colostomy, which is formed from segments of the colon, determines the nature of the fecal output. Fecal output from a right-sided transverse colostomy has a high percentage of water, and the stool is usually soft, mushy, and unformed. Stool from a left-sided transverse colostomy contains less water, and is therefore semisolid. A colostomy formed from the sigmoid colon usually produces solid stool that enables the client to regulate the colostomy with daily irrigation.

Postoperatively, the stoma of an ostomy will initially be edematous. Stomal shrinkage, which is expected to occur as healing takes place, should be noted. As the stoma shrinks, the size of the appliance may need to change. Clients are not fitted for permanent drainage appliances until shrinkage is complete. Skin irritation is a major problem for the client with an ostomy, particularly if digestive enzymes are present (as is the case with an ileostomy). Conscientious, careful, and regular inspection of the periostomal skin is an integral part of the nursing assessment.

Urinary output may be diverted via a *cutaneous ureterostomy*, where the ureters are directly implanted on the skin. Two openings are usually present if both ureters are diverted. In the early postoperative period, catheters will be inserted into the renal pelvis. (See Table 19-6 for expected drainage from ureteral catheters). It is crucial that these catheters remain patent. Once the catheters are removed, the nurse must carefully monitor urine output since these stomas are very susceptible to stricture.

A more common type of urinary diversion is an *ileal conduit*, in which a section of the ileum is isolated from the small intestines and fashioned into a stoma. The ureters then are implanted in the ileal pouch, which functions as a conduit for urine output. Since the conduit is not designed to serve as a urinary reservoir, urine drainage will be continuous (Table 19-6). Immediately after the surgery, the urine will contain blood. The stoma should be observed for edema, since this could dangerously obstruct the flow of urine. If the urine is foul smelling, the client may have a urinary tract infection. The urine should be cultured to determine the presence and type of infecting organism. Mucus normally is secreted by the ileum and is an expected constituent of urine drained from an ileal conduit.

The client with a urinary diversion is susceptible to the same skin breakdown and body image problems as are clients with intestinal diversions.

Incontinence

In our society, those who suffer from bowel or bladder incontinence often experience a serious threat to their sense of self-control and may suffer a significant decrease in self-esteem. Indeed, it is common for such individuals to feel a strong sense of powerlessness. Incontinent clients require complete physical and psychological assessment so that if the incontinence cannot be solved, at least steps can be instituted to salvage the client's self-esteem.

The causes of bowel and bladder incontinence are many and vary with both age and health. Trauma to, or disease of, the spinal cord may result in incontinence at any age.

The elderly are particularly suspectible to problems with bowel and bladder control. Studies from England and the United States (Thomas, 1980) indicate that 50 to 80% of geriatric admissions suffer incontinence. The elderly pay a very high psychological price for this, suffering simultaneous loss of self-esteem and self-control (Wells & Brink, 1988). When this inner sense of control is lost, a sense of powerlessness develops, and the total health of the elderly client is affected. Incontinence of either bowel or bladder may cause the client to withdraw and become psychologically and socially isolated.

Assessing the effect that incontinence has on the client's body image and self-esteem is crucial. If institutionalized elderly clients are not participating in activities, is it because of disinterest or because of fear of embarrassment if they soil themselves? The elderly client at home frequently refuses to go out because of such fears. A vicious cycle can develop. The client is anxious, which causes loss of control. The loss of control generates a sense of irritation in the staff or family. This leads to avoiding the client, which causes increased anxiety and increased incontinence. It is the responsibility of the nurse to determine if such a cycle of behavior has developed and then work with the client to manage the problem.

Urinary Incontinence. Women are particularly at risk for developing urinary incontinence. When obtaining the health history, the nurse should note any contributing factors, such as pregnancy, childbirth, gynecological surgery, and old age. Special attention should be paid to any psychological and social problems that may have resulted from the incontinence.

There are several types of urinary incontinence. With *urgency incontinence*, the client reports that once the urge is felt, it cannot be controlled. To assess for this, the client should be asked whether urination begins immediately after or simultaneously with perception of the urge to void.

Clients who experience *stress incontinence* report a release of urine when laughing, coughing, or sneezing. Straining at stool or stooping also may produce a loss of urine. Stress incontinence commonly occurs during the last trimester of pregnancy.

To assess for stress incontinence, the client should be asked whether urination occurs when changing position from sitting to standing or standing to sitting. If the answer is affirmative, the client is experiencing stress incontinence. Such clients also may report a feeling of increased pressure when the bladder is full. They report almost complete relief after voiding.

A frequent cause of incontinence in obese women is "girdle choke" from a too-tight girdle. Thus, female clients should be asked if they wear a tight girdle since a looser girdle may provide immediate relief.

Women are more susceptible to cystitis than men, and infection also may precipitate incontinence.

As men age they develop enlarged prostates with resultant hesitancy, frequency, nocturia, and decreased force of stream. Later in the course of prostatic hypertrophy, obstructive symptoms of dribbling and overflow incontinence may occur.

Incontinence in the elderly may be due to urgency during the day and frequency at night (Wells & Brink, 1988).

Various neurological injuries may contribute to urinary incontinence. One of these is *neurogenic bladder*, which is caused by spinal cord or brain stem damage. The signals that inhibit urination are interrupted, and sacral reflex centers become very excitable. Clients with neurogenic bladders suffer from frequent and uncontrollable urination. Even small quantities of urine stimulate the micturition reflex.

In the *atonic bladder*, the sensory nerve fibers from the bladder to the spinal cord are destroyed. There is loss of all bladder control. Overflow dribbling becomes a problem since the bladder fills to capacity and then continually overflows a few drops at a time. With an atonic bladder, no reflex contractions are present. The client who has suffered a crushing injury to the spinal cord should be observed for signs of an atonic bladder.

Another variation is the *autonomic bladder*. This usually results from an injury to the spinal cord above the sacral region. Since the sacral region is still intact, the micturition reflex still occurs. Voluntary control by the brain cannot be achieved, but the client can be taught to control urination by alternative means.

Once the type of incontinence is determined, appropriate interventions designed to relieve the client from embarrassment and loss of self-esteem can be employed.

Bowel Incontinence. Once bowel control has been mastered, the healthy child and adult usually maintain this function throughout their lifetimes. As with urinary incontinence, many factors may contribute to an inability to control bowel function. Any problem that causes loss of anal sphincter tone, a decrease in voluntary control, or spinal cord damage can lead to fecal incontinence. Fecal incontinence increases with aging and presents a particular problem for the institutionalized elderly suffering from long-term disabilities. Problems in the elderly such as confusion, which affects perception of rectal fullness, and neurological changes that affect the functioning and tone of the anal sphincter, may contribute to bowel incontinence.

If a client is experiencing fecal incontinence, a thorough assessment of the client and the environment will assist the nurse in developing a plan of care for this client.

The client's mental status should be assessed first:

Is the client confused?

Does the client have a decreased awareness and perception of events?

Is there a pattern to the incontinence? For instance, does it occur every morning after breakfast?

Does the client have adequate privacy?

Can the client discern if on the toilet or commode?

Is the client comfortable using the bedpan or bedside commode? Can another means be provided?

Can the client reach the toilet and manage the clothing?

Is a call bell readily available and answered promptly?

The solution to the client's incontinence may well be found in the answers to these questions. The anal sphincter should be examined to determine its tone. To further assess for fecal stasis and impaction, a digital examination may be performed. Rectal sensation and reflex activity should be noted as well. If rectal sensation and reflex activity are present, incontinence may be handled by providing the person with manageable clothing and readily accessible toileting facilities.

For other clients, assessment of their individual elimination patterns may assist them in controlling their incontinence. A bowel management program then may be developed for such clients.

The client who experiences urinary or bowel incontinence is at great risk for skin breakdown. The perineal and rectal areas should be inspected regularly for any signs of excoriation. This becomes especially important for the client who cannot achieve any degree of elimination control.

THE FLUID–ELECTROLYTE AND ELIMINATION HISTORY

As with other areas of the nursing assessment, the nurse should elicit data concerning the client's elimination patterns and any interferences or potential problems with these (Table 19-7). To assess elimination, data from a review of several systems must be obtained, in particular the integumentary, gastrointestinal, and urinary systems. In addition, data from the oxygenation assessment, especially respiratory function, should be considered, since insensible fluid loss occurs with exhalation. Such data become especially important if the client is experiencing a significant increase in respiratory rate or has other alterations in respiratory status that may increase insensible fluid loss.

Additional questions related to gastrointestinal functioning should focus on the client's usual bowel and urinary elimination habits. These patterns are highly individual and often involve ritualistic behaviors, a common and normal characteristic associated with elimination. Elimination rituals are begun in infancy and are learned from the family and cultural group. Infants quickly learn to associate parental responses of pleasure, distaste, or disgust with their elimination routines. Toddlers are very ritualistic about their elimination habits as they begin to learn bowel and bladder control. Any disruptions in the toddler's routine may diminish the child's sense of control and mastery.

Many of the elimination rituals and practices learned in childhood persist into adult life and then are transmitted to the next generation. The need for privacy and reading in the bathroom are prominent examples of rituals common in our society.

Because maintenance or restoration of a client's elimination patterns is important for the client's optimal functioning, the nurse should ask about usual elimination routines, including any special words used to refer to urine or stool. It is especially common for children and people of varying ethnic origins to have special words for urination and defecation.

Fluid and Electrolyte Balance

The nursing history should include questions that yield information related to the client's fluid and electrolyte balance. What is the client's average daily fluid intake (amount, types, frequency)? (See Table 19-8 for age-appropriate daily fluid intake.) Does the client have a particular health problem that may interfere with fluid and electrolyte balance, such as a history of congestive heart failure or chronic diarrhea?

Is the client taking medications that may disrupt fluid and electrolyte balance or that have been prescribed to maintain fluid and electrolyte balance, such as diuretics or electrolyte supplements?

TABLE 19-7
The Fluid–Electrolyte and Elimination History

Describe usual pattern of fluid intake.
  Average number of cups (4 ozs) or glasses (8 ozs) con-
    sumed in a 24-hour period:
    Coffee, tea, soda (caffeinated, or decaffeinated)
    Water
    Other fluid (specify)
  Average number of ounces consumed per week:
    Beer
    Wine
    Hard liquor
  Any recent changes in frequency, type, or amount of
    fluid consumed?
  Current weight and height
  Any recent change in weight?
  How stable is client's weight?

Describe usual pattern of urinary elimination.
  Frequency
  Approximate amount
  Color
  Odor (if present)
  Other characteristics
  Explore any specific bathroom rituals
  Does client experience discomfort or pain with urina-
    tion?
  Any recent changes in the pattern of urinary elimina-
    tion?
  Any changes in health that would indicate additional
    fluid loss, such as vomiting, diarrhea, draining

    wound, excessive perspiration?
  Client's perception of the adequacy of intake and out-
    put?

Describe usual pattern of bowel elimination.
  Frequency
  Approximate amount
  Color
  Odor (if present)
  Other characteristics
  Explore any specific bathroom rituals
  Does client experience any discomfort or pain with
    bowel elimination?
  Does client have any current problem with bowel elim-
    ination?
    Nature and symptoms of the problem
    Sudden or gradual onset
    Frequency of the problem
    Severity
    Measures used to remedy the problem
  Does client use anything to facilitate bowel elimina-
    tion, such as laxatives, enemas, or natural products
    (bran cereal)?
  Does client eliminate through an artificial orifice, such
    as a colostomy, ileostomy, or ileal conduit?
    What is client's normal routine?
    Does client have any difficulty managing the urinary
    or bowel diversion?

Are there any dietary restrictions that may upset fluid and electrolyte balance? The client's understanding of medications and dietary restrictions should be assessed to identify potential inaccuracies in adhering to the prescribed regimen.

Has the client recently experienced any changes in health that may indicate an interference with fluid and electrolyte balance? Such changes may include:

Increased thirst	Weight loss or gain
Excessive perspiration	Nausea
Increased or decreased urinary output	Vomiting
	Anorexia
	Cramps
Chronic diarrhea	Muscle tremors or twitches
Weakness	
Dizziness	Hyperventilation (or hypoventilation)
Fatigue	Fever
Irritability	Palpitations

Questions about the frequency or precipitating factors associated with these manifestations should be

included in the history. Methods used for relief of symptoms, such as nausea, vomiting, diarrhea, and cramps, also should be noted.

Several additional factors influence an individual's fluid and electrolyte requirements (Table 19-9). It is important to assess such factors during the nursing history or clinical appraisal.

Urinary Elimination

To collect information about urinary functioning, the nurse should ask about the client's daytime and nighttime voiding patterns, including any problems such as nocturia or enuresis. Frequency of urination will vary with the client's age, fluid intake, and the availability of bathroom facilities. Any increase in the frequency of voiding, especially if the client reports that the amounts of urine at each voiding are small, may indicate bladder irritability or infection. Problems such as hesitancy, urgency, dribbling, burning, or pain—including character, location, and duration—should be assessed. The client should be asked to describe the color, clarity, and volume of the urine output. (Table 19-10 lists average daily urine output by

TABLE 19-8
Average Daily Water Requirements by Age and Weight

Age	ml	ml/kg Body Weight
3 days	250 to 300	80 to 100
1 year	1,150 to 1,300	100 to 130
2 years	1,350 to 1,500	100 to 120
4 years	1,600 to 1,800	90 to 110
10 years	2,000 to 2,500	60 to 85
18 years	2,200 to 2,700	30 to 50
Adult	2,400 to 2,600	20 to 30

age.) Any changes in urinary color or clarity, including such abnormalities as blood or pus, or any noticeable increase or decrease in volume, should be identified. The client also should be asked how other health problems, such as pregnancy, an enlarged prostrate, recent surgery, or a vaginal infection, affect urination.

Bowel Elimination

Questions about the client's bowel routines should focus on the frequency and usual time of day of bowel movements. Clients should also be asked about the consistency and color of the stool. Terms such as soft, hard, loose, watery, runny, pasty, or seedy may be suggested to the client to describe the stool's consistency. Terms that describe the stool's color include brown, yellow, green, black, tarry, and blood-tinged. Any changes in the client's bowel habits should be noted, including increased or decreased frequency, changes in consistency, bloody stools, excessive flatulence, abdominal cramping, or straining during a bowel movement.

It is especially important to ask the client to identify any practices that help maintain regular bowel habits, as well as any particular questions or concerns the client may have about elimination habits. For example, does the client routinely use laxatives or stool softeners? If so, which ones? How often? Usual dose? Usual response? Are fruit juices or bran part of the client's daily routine? Does regular exercise or lack of it affect the client's bowel patterns? Does the client believe his or her usual patterns are "normal"? Bowel regularity is often a major concern of adults in our society—a concern that is fostered by the many television and magazine advertisements for laxatives and antacids. The nurse should explain that there are wide variations in "normal" and that the consistency and color of the stool are better indicators of bowel function than the frequency of bowel movements.

Any anal or rectal problems should be noted,

TABLE 19-9
Factors That Influence Fluid and Electrolyte Requirements

Body Surface Area
In general, the younger the client is, the greater the surface area in proportion to body weight. Because body surface area is difficult to measure, tables have been developed to correlate body surface with the client's height and weight. Daily fluid requirements per square meter (m^2) of body surface area are 1,500 ml/m^2, regardless of age.

Percentage of Body Fat
The greater the percentage of body fat, the smaller the percentage of body fluid there is. Thus, females and obese people have a lower proportionate daily fluid requirement.

Body and Environmental Temperatures
Higher internal or external temperatures increase insensible and sweat loss of fluids and electrolytes.

Exercise
Exercise, especially heavy exercise, increases insensible fluid and electrolyte losses from the skin and lungs. Sweating also contributes to loss of fluids and electrolytes, such as sodium chloride, urea, and potassium.

Health
Many health problems cause or contribute to fluid and electrolyte imbalances, such as burn injuries, diabetes, renal failure, vomiting, diarrhea, surgery. Also, certain medications may upset fluid and electrolyte balance, including diuretics, prednisone, and barbiturates.

such as hemorrhoids, fissures, pain on defecation, or pruritus. If the client has a colostomy or ileostomy, the nurse should ask about the daily functioning and maintenance of the ostomy. The nurse might ask:

What is your daily routine?

When do you evacuate?

What kind of appliance do you use?

Do you have any problems with the stoma or surrounding skin?

Are you concerned about odor? What methods do you use to control it?

What are your special dietary needs?

Most important, the nurse should assess the client's psychosocial adjustment to having an ostomy.

CLINICAL APPRAISAL AND SCREENING

A thorough, objective clinical appraisal includes an abdominal examination and an assessment of fluid and electrolyte status as well as observation

TABLE 19-10
Average Daily Urine Output

Age	Amount
Newborn	15 to 300 ml
Infant	400 to 500 ml
1 to 3 years	500 to 600 ml
3 to 6 years	600 to 700 ml
6 to 9 years	700 to 1,000 ml
9 to 15 years	800 to 1,400 ml
15 years through adult	1,200 to 1,500 ml
Older adult	1,500 ml or less

and measurement of urinary and gastrointestinal output.

Fluid and Electrolytes

To assess a client's fluid status, the nurse not only uses the history as previously described but also collects objective data to verify the history (see boxed insert). The first step in this process is a thorough inspection, beginning with the skin, or integument.

The client's skin should appear full and well hydrated (see chap. 14). Given a normal environmental temperature of 21°C (70°F) and moderate humidity, little obvious perspiration should be evident. Palpation of the client's skin will allow the nurse to evaluate skin turgor and determine the presence of perspiration. Skin turgor is a reliable indicator of hydration in infants, children, and young and middle-aged adults. To assess skin turgor, the skin on the abdomen or thighs should be pinched and quickly released. Well-hydrated skin is elastic and quickly will return to normal, without indentations. If poorly hydrated, the client's skin will appear "doughy," with the skin folds slow to return to an unpinched state. If the client is elderly, skin turgor may not be as reliable an index of hydration because elasticity of the skin decreases with aging.

The eyes should be examined for their appearance. They should appear alert and the eyes should be moist. Any deviations such as sunken eyes or periorbital edema may indicate fluid imbalance.

Dependent parts of the client's body, such as the lower extremities, should be free of edema. The nurse should assess for pitting edema, characterized by indentations of the skin that persist after pressure from the nurse's thumb or finger. Vital signs also furnish important information.

Assessment of plasma volume serves as a reliable guide to the client's general hydration. Plasma

Assessment of Fluid–Electrolyte Status

- Comparison of total intake and output of fluids.
- Urine volume and concentration.
- Skin and tongue turgor.
- Degree of moisture in oral cavity.
- Body weight.
- Thirst.
- Tearing and salivation.
- Appearance and temperature of skin.
- Facial appearance.
- Edema.
- Temperature, pulse, and respiration.
- Blood pressure.
- Neck vein filling.
- Hand vein filling.
- Central venous pressure.
- Neuromuscular irritability.
- Other signs.

Note. From Metheny, N. (1987). *Fluid and electrolyte balance.* Philadelphia: Lippincott, 13.

volume may be assessed by elevating the client's hand and forearm. Normally the hand veins empty in 3 to 5 seconds. When lowered, the veins should refill in approximately the same time. In a volume-depleted state, the veins take longer than 5 seconds to fill, whereas in an overhydrated state they take longer than 5 seconds to empty. Neck vein filling, an indicator of overall venous pressure, also should be evaluated (see chap. 17). Clients in heart failure may exhibit neck vein engorgement due to volume overload, whereas clients who are volume depleted exhibit diminished filling of the neck veins.

The oral cavity should be thoroughly inspected. Normally, the mucous membranes will appear pink and moist. Pallor or dryness may indicate dehydration.

Other cues should be noted. Is the client drinking adequate amounts of fluids? Is the client urinating regularly? Is there any evidence of behavioral changes, such as restlessness or lethargy?

The appearance of the urine and stool are also important indicators of the individual's state of hydration. In a well-hydrated person, the urine should be yellow or straw-colored, neither too dilute nor too concentrated. The stool should be firm and well-formed, not loose, watery, or hardened.

A particularly precise measure of fluid balance is daily weighing of the client. It is indeed considered one of the most accurate indices of the daily variations in fluid balance. However, weighing a client daily can provide meaningful data or can become a meaningless routine. The nurse can make the difference by ensuring that accurate weight measurements are obtained. The client must be weighed on the same accurately balanced scale each time, at the same time of day (preferably before breakfast), and with the same amount of clothing each time. Any alterations in this routine will render the data useless. Even more serious, an inaccurately obtained weight can affect the accuracy and appropriateness of drug dosage, fluid replacement, or prescribed diet, and may be responsible for any number of other errors.

One question that may arise is how changes in fluid balance can be differentiated from changes related to alterations in the client's nutrition. A malnourished person loses approximately one-half to one pound each day, assuming that kidney function remains normal. A fluctuation above or below this range (of one-half to one pound), then, is a reflection of over- or underhydration. Every two pounds lost or gained reflects approximately a liter of fluid. For example, if a client who is eating a diet that meets caloric needs gains 4 pounds in a 24-hour period, the nurse may estimate that the client has a 2-liter fluid overload. If the same client loses 4 pounds, then a 2-liter fluid deficit has occurred. If the same client had lost 4 pounds while NPO for diagnostic tests, the nurse would estimate 1 pound lost as a result of lost caloric intake and 3 pounds from fluid depletion, or a 1500 ml deficit.

Observation of the client for any deviations that may indicate dehydration, overhydration, or electrolyte imbalance is critical to the overall assessment of fluid/electrolyte and elimination status.

Dehydration may be a mild alteration or may cause serious consequences for a client. As noted earlier, such observations as dry skin and a decrease in skin turgor may indicate dehydration. Other observations that serve as clues that a client may be suffering from dehydration include:

Dry mucous membranes

Sunken eyes

Increased thirst

Decreased blood pressure

Elevated pulse rate

Oliguria

Increased urine specific gravity

Loss of weight

Collapsed neck and hand veins

Laboratory analysis may show an elevated blood urea nitrogen (BUN).

On the other hand, edema is usually a cue that the client is experiencing fluid overload. Edema is seen most often in dependent body parts, such as the legs and feet, the sacral area, and in males, the scrotum. Periorbital edema also may be present. Other observations that may indicate fluid overload include:

Elevated blood pressure

Low urine specific gravity

Dilute urine (pale color)

Sudden weight gain

Decreased venous filling time

Engorged neck and hand veins

Some clients may develop ascites or pleural effusion. If fluid overload is severe, pulmonary edema may develop, with dyspnea, frothy sputum, and moist noisy respiration audible to the unassisted ear. If less pronounced, pulmonary edema may be detected by auscultation of the lungs, in which case moist rales will be noted. Table 19-5 offers a comparison of clinical manifestations of fluid depleted and overhydrated states. Table 19-11 compares degrees of severity of fluid excess and deficit.

Acid-Base Balance

Through chemical buffering mechanisms, the lungs and the kidneys, the body maintains a narrow plasma pH between 7.35 and 7.45. "The best way to evaluate acid-base balance is by measurement of arterial blood gases," according to Metheny (1987, p. 109). Arterial blood gases, their normal values, helpful guidelines for interpretation and implications are presented in Chapter 17.

Abdominal Examination

As the nurse prepares to examine the client's abdomen, it is helpful to picture mentally the structures that will be assessed during the examination. Dividing the abdomen into sections by using imaginary lines is a useful technique that assists in identifying abdominal organs and structures.

One of the most common methods used is one that divides the abdomen into four segments (Figure 19-2). The structures contained within each of the four quadrants are listed in Table 19-12. Placement of the organs within the four quadrants is shown in Figure 19-3. A second method divides

TABLE 19-11
Degree of Fluid Deficit and Excess

Severity	Magnitude of Deficit or Excess (liters)	% of Body Water Deficit or Excess	Serum Na+ (mEq/liter)*	Serum Osmolality* (mOsm/kg)
Fluid Deficit				
Mild	1.5–2.0	3.0–4.5%	149–151	294–298
Moderate	2.0–4.0	4.5–10	152–158	299–313
Severe	4.0–6.0	10–15	159– 166	314–329
Very severe	>6.0	>15	>166	>330
Fluid Excess				
Mild	1.5–4.0	3–8	139–132	275–262
Moderate	4.0–6.0	8–13	131–127	261–251
Severe	6.0–10.0	13–22	126–118	250–233
Very severe	>10.0	>22	<118	<233

*Normal serum Na+ is 144 mEq/L and normal serum osmolality is 285 mOsm/kg.

Note. Adapted from Harvey, A.M.; Johns, R.J.; McKusick, V.A.; Owens, A.H.; and Ross, R.S. *The Principles and Practice of Medicine* 22nd ed., pp. 689, 691. Copyright © 1988, Appleton & Lange, Norwalk, Connecticut. Reprinted with permission.

the abdomen into nine regions (Figure 19-4). For consistency, the four quadrant method of identifying abdominal structures will be used in this text.

The abdomen is a very sensitive area, and the client may be nervous or feel uncomfortable about being examined. Therefore, it is important that the client be relaxed for the examination. An explanation of the procedure and proper positioning (client supine with arms at side or folded across chest) will help to accomplish this purpose. If an individual is particularly tense, the nurse can put a pillow under the client's slightly flexed knees. This position helps to decrease the tension on the abdominal muscles. Good lighting and full exposure of the abdomen are also necessary for the examination. Having the client void before the examination will promote comfort and enable adequate palpation of the lower quadrant areas.

The sequence of the examination is modified for the abdomen with auscultation being performed after inspection, followed by percussion and then palpation (see boxed insert). This is done because auscultatory sounds may be noticeably different after percussion and palpation. The four techniques of examination can be reviewed in Chapter 3.

Inspection

The nurse begins the examination by inspecting the abdomen. The nurse inspects the skin for scars, striae, dilated veins, rashes, and lesions. The umbilicus is inspected for contour, location, hernias, and inflammation. The contour of the abdomen is noted (Figure 19-5), as is the symmetry. The nurse also observes for the presence of any en-

larged organs or masses. Peristalsis may be noticeable in thin individuals and the pulsations of the aorta frequently may be visible in the epigastric area. It is helpful to inspect the abdomen at an angle when inspecting for peristalsis or pulsations. An angle is also helpful when observing for symmetry and contour.

Auscultation

After inspecting the abdomen, the nurse listens with a stethoscope for bowel sounds and vascular abnormalities. Auscultation of bowel sounds is an important part of the clinical appraisal, especially for clients who are experiencing problems with elimination, such as diarrhea or constipation. In addition, postoperative clients, especially those who have had abdominal surgery, should be assessed frequently for the return of bowel sounds. The resumption of bowel sounds is usually used to determine when the postoperative client may begin taking fluids by mouth.

Clients who are at risk for developing bowel complications (e.g., paralytic ileus, obstruction, and peritonitis) also should be assessed frequently. Clients who have undergone surgery, the client who has suffered a serious burn, and immobilized clients are especially likely to develop such complications.

In addition, clients who present with interferences in elimination such as gastroenteritis, ulcerative colitis, persistent vomiting, obstruction, or fecal impaction need frequent assessment of bowel sounds.

Peristaltic sounds vary in frequency, intensity, and pitch. Normal bowel sounds may be gurgling,

Sequence of Abdominal Assessment

Inspection

- Skin
  - Scars
  - Striae
  - Dilated veins
  - Rashes and lesions
- Umbilicus
  - Contour
  - Location
  - Inflammation
  - Hernias
- Contour
- Symmetry
- Enlarged organs
- Masses
- Peristalsis
- Pulsations

Auscultation

- Bowel sounds

- Bruits
  - Aorta
  - Renal arteries
  - Iliac arteries
  - Femoral arteries

Percussion

- General
- Liver
- Spleen
- Kidneys

Palpation

- Light
- Deep
  - Masses
  - Tenderness
  - Liver
  - Spleen
  - Kidneys

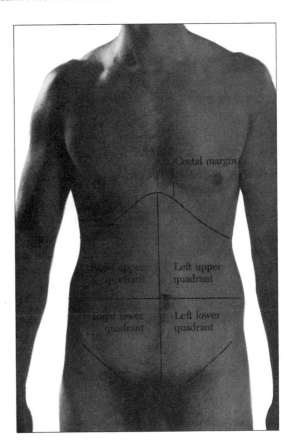

FIGURE 19-2. Four Divisions of the Abdomen. (*Note.* From Grimes/Burns: *Health Assessment in Nursing Practice,* Second Edition, © 1987. Boston: Jones and Bartlett Publishers, p. 244.)

bubbling, trickling, rumbling, or gulping. Sounds may be quite loud, especially when the client is hungry or NPO, or they may be quiet. They also may be continuous or intermittent, depending upon the phase of digestion.

Abnormalities in bowel sounds include absence or high-pitched tinkling, both of which may indicate bowel obstruction. It is important to auscultate each abdominal quadrant for a full minute before concluding that bowel sounds are absent.

Auscultation of bowel sounds is done by placing the diaphragm of a warmed stethoscope lightly on the abdominal wall. The nurse then proceeds to listen in all four quadrants for bowel sounds and notes their character and frequency. Bowel sounds usually are heard as gurgles or clicks. They are irregular and occur from 5 to 35 per minute. The nurse also should listen with the diaphragm for bruits (high-pitched sounds) in each of the four quadrants over the renal, iliac, and femoral arteries and in the epigastric area over the aorta. The sequence should be repeated using the bell of the stethoscope to detect any low pitched sounds (Figure 19-6).

Percussion

Percussion is performed to detect the presence of a mass, the enlargement of any organ, or the presence of abdominal distention. The percussion note heard over the abdomen is one of tympany. Tym-

pany normally is percussed throughout the abdomen except for the areas over the spleen, liver, and the symphysis pubis bone. General percussion of the abdomen is done initially in all four quadrants. Following this, the nurse may percuss (if appropriate to the situation) the liver span in the right midclavicular line and the spleen slightly posterior to the left midaxillary line. The technique for percussion of the liver span and the spleen are outlined in the boxed insert, and the techniques for determining shifting dullness and measuring fluid wave appear in Figure 19-7. Whether the nurse incorporates these aspects in the abdominal examination depends on the clinical situation, the purpose of the examination, and the nurse's skill level.

Palpation

The client's abdomen should be palpated lightly to detect the presence of pain or masses and then deeply palpated to assess abdominal organs. If palpation is difficult due to obesity or muscular resistance, the nurse may use a bimanual technique

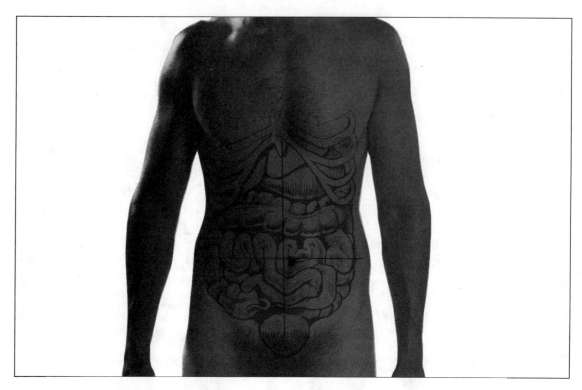

FIGURE 19-3. Placement of Organs Within the Four Divisions of the Abdomen. (*Note*. From Grimes/Burns: *Health Assessment in Nursing Practice*, Second Edition, © 1987. Boston: Jones and Bartlett Publishers, p. 295.)

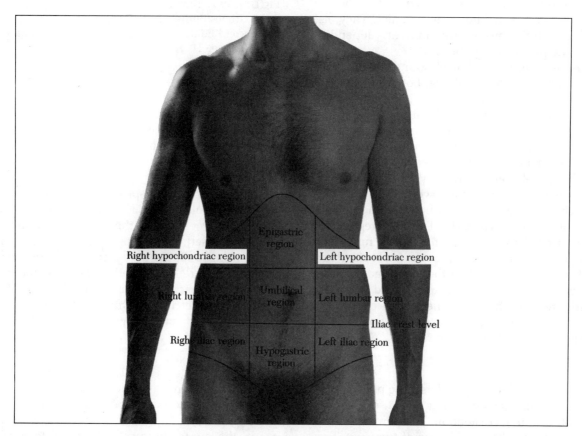

FIGURE 19-4. Nine Divisions of the Abdomen. (*Note*. From Grimes/Burns: *Health Assessment in Nursing Practice*, Second Edition, © 1987. Boston: Jones and Bartlett Publishers, p. 295.)

TABLE 19-12
Abdominal Contents Within the Four Quadrants of the
Abdomen

Quadrant	Contents
Right upper	Liver Gallbladder Duodenum Pancreas Right kidney and right adrenal gland Hepatic flexure of the colon
Left upper	Stomach Spleen Left kidney and left adrenal gland Pancreas Splenic flexure of the colon
Right lower	Cecum Appendix Right ovary and tube (female) Bladder (if distended) Uterus (female—if enlarged) Right spermatic cord (male) Right ureter
Left lower	Sigmoid colon Left ovary and tube (female) Bladder (if distended) Uterus (female—if enlarged) Left spermatic cord (male) Left ureter
Midline of lower abdomen	Bladder Uterus (female)

Note. From Grimes/Burns: *Health Assessment in Nursing Practice,*
Second Edition, © 1987. Boston: Jones and Bartlett Publishers.

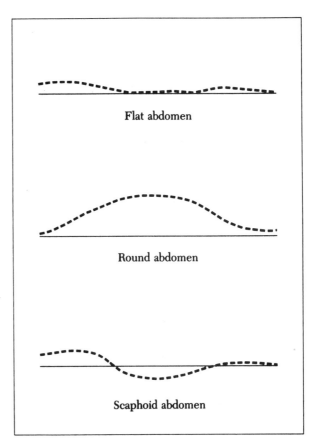

FIGURE 19-5. Contours of the Abdomen. (*Note.* From
Grimes/Burns: *Health Assessment in Nursing Practice,* Second Edition, © 1987. Boston: Jones and Bartlett Publishers, p. 296.)

with one hand on top of the other. In this technique, pressure is exerted with the top hand while the bottom hand palpates the underlying structures. The nurse should palpate the abdomen in all four quadrants moving systematically from quadrant to quadrant. The normal abdomen is soft, palpable, and nontender. It is important for the nurse to periodically observe the client's facial expression during the abdominal examination. Nonverbal behavior, such as wincing or holding one's breath when in pain, provides cues that can validate physical findings. Nonverbal behavior also can cue the examiner in to the general comfort level of the client during the exam.

If a mass is felt on palpation, specific characteristics should be noted: location, shape, size, tenderness, pulsations, mobility, and movement with respiration. It is most helpful for the beginning student in physical assessment to have clinical findings validated by an experienced examiner in order to distinguish normal structures and findings from

abnormal findings. For example, it is not unusual to palpate a descending colon filled with stool in an individual who is very constipated. What may appear to be an abdominal mass in the left lower quadrant in this instance would be hardened fecal material. Knowing what might usually be found on clinical examination will assist the nurse in distinguishing normal from abnormal findings.

Additionally, any areas where the client complains of pain or tenderness should be examined last. This minimizes client discomfort and allows the nurse to palpate all other areas first.

Following light and deep palpation of the abdomen, the nurse may palpate the liver, spleen, and kidneys if this is appropriate to the clinical situation. The techniques for palpating these organs are outlined in the boxed insert, and the examinations are demonstrated in Figures 19-8, 19-9, and 19-10. These techniques require additional skill and may not be used routinely by a nurse. The presence of any tenderness of the kidneys is determined by striking the costalvertebral angle (CVA) on the left and on the right with the heel of the right hand or a closed fist (Figure 19-11).

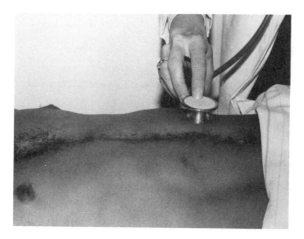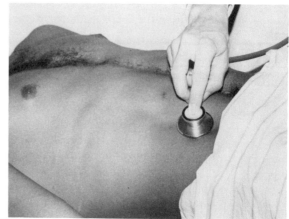

FIGURE 19-6. The nurse should auscultate bowel sounds using both the stethoscope's bell for low-pitched sounds (*left*) and diaphragm for high-pitched sounds (*right*). All four abdominal quadrants should be auscultated as well as either side of the umbilicus.

Daily measurement of abdominal girth (circumference) assists in determining an increase or decrease of abdominal distention. This should be done at the same place on the body each day. Causes of abdominal distention include gastrointestinal obstruction and fluid accumulation in the abdominal cavity (ascites). Increased abdominal girth also may indicate an abdominal mass, such as a tumor.

Measurement of Intake and Output

Measuring and recording intake and output (I&O) are essential in assessing a client's fluid balance. Intake and output indicate the total amount of fluid taken in and lost, and the relationship between the two. An intake and output record should be initiated for any client with an actual or potential fluid and electrolyte problem. It is not necessary to wait for a physician's order.

Intake should include all fluids taken into the body: oral fluids, foods that are liquid at room temperature, intravenous fluids, subcutaneous fluids, fluids instilled into drainage tubes as irrigants, tube feeding solutions, water given through feeding tubes, even enema solutions in patients requiring strict fluid intake recordings, such as those suffering from renal failure.

Output should include urine, vomitus, diarrhea,

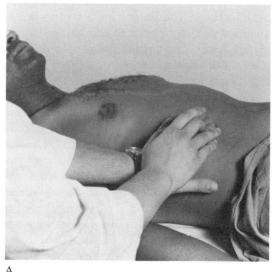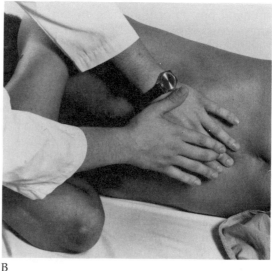

A   B

FIGURE 19-7. Technique of Shifting Dullness. (A) With patient supine, percuss from umbilicus to flank until dullness is heard. (B) Repeat percussion with client on side. (*Note.* From Grimes/Burns: *Health Assessment in Nursing Practice*, Second Edition, © 1987. Boston: Jones and Bartlett Publishers, p. 303.)

Technique for Percussion of the Abdomen

1. Have client remain in comfortable position.
2. Percuss entire abdomen lightly in all four quadrants.
3. *Liver:*
   a. Percuss down right MCL to upper border of liver dullness.
   b. Percuss upward from a level below the umbilicus to the liver to determine the lower border of liver dullness.
   c. Measure span of liver dullness vertically at the right MCL.
4. *Spleen*
   a. Percuss downward behind the left MAL between 8th and 11th ICS.
   b. Measure the vertical span of splenic dullness.
   c. Percuss lowest left ICS at point between AAL and the MCL. Note presence or absence of tympany.
5. Percuss gastric air bubble.
6. Decision-making: Employ techniques for detection of shifting dullness and fluid wave in the presence of abdominal distention.

   a. Technique for shifting dullness
      1. Client supine.
      2. Begin percussion at umbilicus and move toward nearest flank.
      3. Mark point of dullness.
      4. Have client turn on side.
      5. Repeat percussion from umbilicus downward.
      6. Note whether level of dullness has shifted.
   b. Technique for measuring fluid wave
      1. Place palm of one hand on client's flank.
      2. Have third person or client place ulnar edge of hand firmly into middle of client's abdomen.
      3. Examiner strikes opposite flank with free hand.
      4. In the presence of ascites, the blow will be transmitted by the fluid moving across the abdomen and will be felt against the palm of the hand pressed on the opposite flank.

Key: MCL—midclavicular line
MAL—midaxillary line
ICS—intercostal space
AAL—anterior axillary line

Note. Adapted from Grimes/Burns: *Health Assessment in Nursing Practice,* Second Edition, © 1987, Boston: Jones and Bartlett Publishers, p. 303.

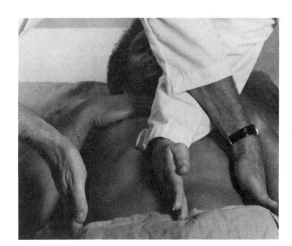

FIGURE 19-7. Continued. Production of Fluid Wave. (*Note.* From Grimes/Burns: *Health Assessment in Nursing Practice,* Second Edition, © 1987. Boston: Jones and Bartlett Publishers, p. 304.)

drainage from fistulas, drainage from suction apparatus, drainage from lesions (noted and estimated) and perspiration (noted and estimated). (Metheny, 1987, p. 13)

If intake and output are to have any clinical significance, the measuring and recording of fluid intake and output must be accurate. The variations in volumes of different containers used in different agencies may make measurements of intake and output questionable. Therefore, the nurse should be certain that a list showing the volumes of fluid in the various containers is at hand for easy reference. Whenever there is doubt about the amount of fluid a container holds, the amount should be measured using a calibrated graduate. Many times a problem arises with fluid measurement when a client can take only small sips. Using a calibrated medicine cup or placing a premeasured amount of fluid in a small cup will ensure accuracy.

The most common source of other than oral intake is intravenous solutions, including blood, plasma, and total parenteral nutrition (hyperalimentation) fluids. In addition, clients may be receiving intravenous medications that often are

Techniques for Palpation of the Liver, Spleen, and Kidneys

After entire abdomen has been lightly palpated with fingertips, begin deep palpation of abdominal organs:

a. *Liver*
   1. Place right hand below lower right costal margin and point fingers toward client's right shoulder.
   2. Push fingers deeply into abdomen while moving up toward the right costal margin.
   3. Ask client to take deep breath.
   4. Continue deep palpation to under the rib cage.

b. *Spleen*
   1. Stand at right side of supine client.
   2. Place left hand under the client's left flank at level of 11th and 12th ribs.
   3. Push right hand gently under left anterior costal margin.

4. Decision-making: If suspicious of splenomegaly, have client lie on right side and repeat technique described above.
5. Remember to palpate gently.

c. *Kidneys*
   1. Right—place right hand on anterior abdomen in MCL next to umbilicus.

      Place left hand under client's left flank. Ask client to take deep breath while applying pressure with examining hand.
   2. Left—difficult to feel left kidney but palpation can be tried using same technique described above.
   3. CVA tenderness—strike CVA with heel of hand or closed fist on left and right sides.

Key: MCL—midclavicular line
       CVA—costal vertebral angle

Note. Adapted from Grimes/Burns: *Health Assessment in Nursing Practice*, Second Edition, © 1987. Boston: Jones and Bartlett Publishers.

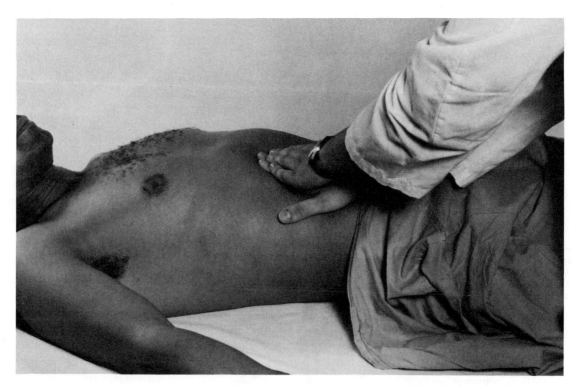

FIGURE 19-8. Palpation of the Liver. (*Note.* From Grimes/Burns: *Health Assessment in Nursing Practice*, Second Edition, © 1987. Boston: Jones and Bartlett Publishers, p. 306.)

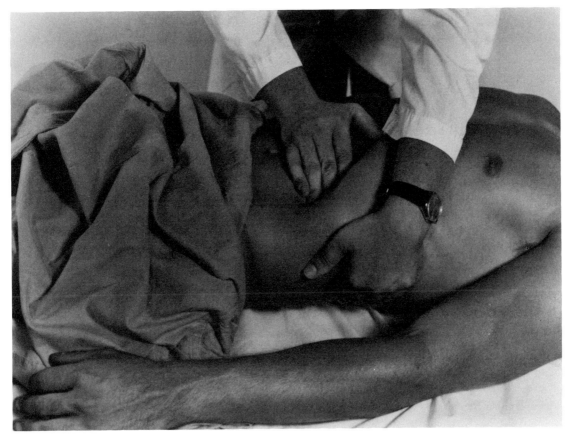

FIGURE 19-9. Palpation of the Spleen. (*Note.* From Grimes/Burns: *Health Assessment in Nursing Practice,* Second Edition, © 1987. Boston: Jones and Bartlett Publishers, p. 306.)

administered in 50 to 100 ml of solution as often as every 2 to 3 hours. A little quick arithmetic shows that a client receiving one medication every 4 hours in 100 ml of fluid and another medication every 6 hours in 50 ml of fluid is receiving 800 ml of fluid daily with medications alone! It is essential that this additional fluid intake not be overlooked when recording daily fluid intake.

In clients with actual or potential fluid alterations, urine output should be accurately measured with a calibrated graduate. The time and amount of voiding also should be recorded. The color and clarity of the urine should be noted. Vomitus should be measured, if at all possible, and its color, consistency, and frequency noted. Bowel movements are noted and described, but usually are not measured unless diarrhea is present. Output from other sources also should be measured and described. Accurate measurement of fluid output is crucial because fluid replacement needs usually are calculated on the basis of these measurements and the client's body weight. In addition, when the source of fluid output is known, an estimation of

its electrolyte content can be determined in order to calculate replacement needs.

There are many common errors in measuring intake and output. Some examples involving both intake and output include failing to communicate to all the staff which patients require I&O monitoring, failing to explain I&O to the patient and family, and guessing at the amount because it takes less time than measuring it (Metheny, 1987). Errors related to intake can involve overestimating fluid volume when given as ice chips, assuming that all of the fluids on a client's tray were consumed by the client, and failing to remember that parenteral fluids usually contain more than the specified amount (a 1,000 ml bottle may actually contain 1,100 ml). Errors related to output can include failing to estimate fluid lost as wound exudate or liquid feces, not using a calibrated device to measure small amounts of urine, failing to estimate the amount of incontinence (by indicating amount of bed linen and clothing saturated with urine), and failing to estimate amount of perspiration. In regard to this last point, Metheny (1987) indicates that perspira-

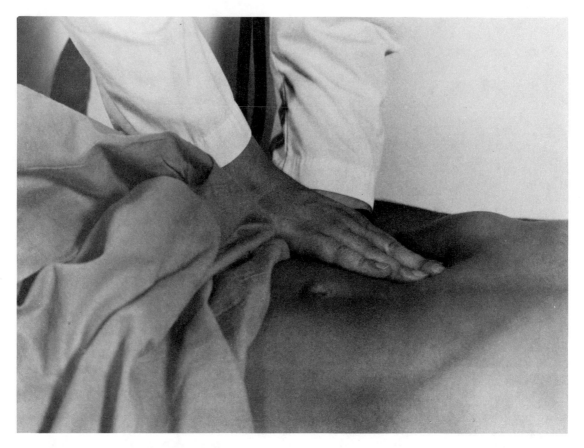

FIGURE 19-10. Palpation of the Kidney. (*Note.* From Grimes/Burns: *Health Assessment in Nursing Practice,* Second Edition, © 1987. Boston: Jones and Bartlett Publishers, p. 307.)

tion can be assessed either by describing the amount of clothing or bed linen soaked with perspiration or using a plus system to represent degree (+ indicates sweating that is just visible to + + + + that indicates profuse sweating).

Stool Examination

As noted previously, the observation, recording, and measuring, when necessary, of stool is a critical part of the elimination assessment.

The stool itself is examined for shape, color, and consistency. Normal stool is a formed, semisolid, cylindrical mass. Its usual brown color is caused by bilirubin derivatives. Certain foods and medications, red gelatin, spinach (especially in infants), and ferrous sulphate, may change its color. It is usually odiferous, but the specific odor will vary depending on the type of normal flora present and the type of food the individual has eaten. Any changes in shape, color, or consistency of the stool may be indicative of some alteration in gastrointestinal functioning. For example, diarrhea may indicate viral or bacterial gastroenteritis.

Within the last several years, examination of the stool for occult blood has become an important mechanism in screening for colorectal cancer. Laboratory examination of the stool also is performed to determine the presence of ova and parasites, occult blood (associated with conditions other than cancer), and bacterial cultures.

The normal characteristics and composition of feces are summarized in Tables 19-13 and 19-14.

A stool specimen for culture or ova and parasites should be collected in the early morning. The specimen (approximately one inch of formed stool) should be placed in a clean container and immediately sent to the laboratory. If, for any reason, it is not possible to obtain a stool specimen, a rectal swab may be used to swab the anus, although this method is not as effective. To collect a specimen for pinworms, clear cellophane tape is placed over the client's anal area. It is then immediately removed and fixed to a slide. This specimen should be collected in the morning before the client has bathed or had a bowel movement. Pinworms usually move toward the anal area during the night and then move back into the rectal canal during the day.

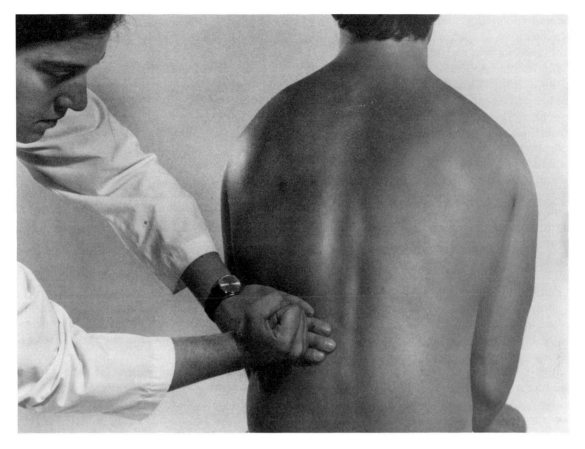

FIGURE 19-11. Blunt Percussion for CVA Tenderness. (*Note.* From Grimes/Burns: *Health Assessment in Nursing Practice,* Second Edition, © 1987. Boston: Jones and Bartlett Publishers, p. 309.)

TABLE 19-13
Normal Characteristics of Feces

Parameter	Expected Findings
Appearance:	Formed, cylindrical, soft to firm but neither mushy nor hard, malleable.
Color:	Brown
Blood:	Absent
Mucus:	Absent
Pus:	Absent
Parasites:	Absent
Fat:	Colorless, neutral fat 18%; also fatty acids and crystals.
Undigested foods and fibrins:	Absent
pH:	Weakly alkaline
Occult blood:	Negative

TABLE 19-14
Usual Composition of Feces

Constituent	Percentage of Feces	Percentage of Solid Constituents
Water	75%	
Solid Materials		
Dead bacteria		30%
Fat		10 to 20%
Inorganic matter		10 to 20%
Protein		2 to 3%
Undigested roughage and dried constituents of digestive juicies (e.g., bile pigment and sloughed epithelial cells)		30%

Adapted from Guyton, A.C. (1990). *Human physiology and mechanisms of disease* (8th ed.). Saunders, 735.

There are many important factors to remember when collecting stool specimens. If the specimen is to be collected for ova and parasites, it should be warm. A specimen obtained to look for pathogens should be examined immediately or refrigerated because the pathogens may be destroyed on standing by coliform bacteria. If mucus and blood are present in the stool, they should be sent with the specimen because parasites are more likely to be found there.

A bedpan or commode may be used when a stool specimen is to be collected. Needless to say, the client should be afforded privacy. The client should be instructed to urinate first and to wait for the urine to be discarded before defecating. The bismuth from paper towels and toilet paper may interfere with the tests, so paper products should not be placed in the bedpan.

As previously stated, stool specimens frequently are tested for occult blood. A test for occult blood may be done in the laboratory or with the use, for example, of a Hema-Chek Slide Pak (Ames, 1990). A thin smear from a stool specimen is placed on the slide. Then, two drops of developing solution are placed on the development area. The Pak also contains a control area that also is tested with developing solution. If the specimen area turns blue, it is considered positive for occult blood. Red meat in the client's diet may interfere with the test's accuracy and should be limited for 3 days prior to the specimen collection.

There are a number of factors that can affect the consistency, shape, odor, and color of stool (Table 19-15).

When a client experiences difficulties with elimination, a focused assessment should be performed to obtain more detailed information.

Urinalysis

Urinalysis is a common screening exam performed during periodic health visits and on all admissions to the hospital. Data obtained from a urinalysis can provide information about renal function and about the body's metabolic state. Many times people suffer from undetected urinary tract infections. Damage to the urinary tract can occur unbeknown to the individual. Routine screening of the urine can identify such problems before permanent damage to the kidneys and such sequelae as hypertension or renal failure develop. Normal characteristics of urine are summarized in Table 19-16. Every time a urine specimen is collected from a client, it should be assessed for clarity, color, odor, and the presence of sediment. For certain clients, the specific gravity and pH will be determined, along with the presence of any abnormal findings such as glucose, protein, bacteria, or ketones.

TABLE 19-15
Abnormalities in the Appearance of Feces

Abnormalities	Assessment
Increase in fluid content—diarrhea	Assess for presence of mucus, blood, or pus. Check history for change in diet or presence of anxiety and tension. Note volume and frequency of stool. Check for abdominal pain or cramps. Assess for signs of dehydration and electrolyte imbalance.
Decrease in fluid content—constipation, hard stools	Assess for change in diet, exercise, decrease in fluid intake. Assess for psychological factors. Check for availability of bathroom facilities.
"Pasty" stools	May indicate an increased fat content. Assess and describe the specific appearance of the stool.
Narrow or ribbon-like stools	Assess for signs of obstruction.
Odor	Note any unusual odor and describe.
Color: Yellow, yellow-green, or green	Associated with diarrhea. Assess for infection and dehydration. Check for contaminated milk and water or other source of contamination. Check history for diet high in green vegetables.
Obvious blood	Associated with gastrointestinal bleeding below stomach.
Color: Black	Associated with medication, specifically iron or gastrointestinal bleeding at level of stomach or higher.

TABLE 19-16
Normal Urine Characteristics

Parameter	Expected Findings
Color	Straw or golden yellow
Consistency	Clear, transparent
Odor	Slightly aromatic
pH	4.5 to 7.0 (usually slightly acidic)
Specific gravity	1,010 to 1,025 (normal fluid intake)
Glucose	None
Protein	None
Sediment	<1 to 3 RBCs
	<1 to 3 WBCs
	Occasional cast
Sterility	No microorganisms

When collecting urine specimens, certain factors must be considered. The urine should be fresh so that accuracy of the test is not compromised. If urine is allowed to stand, the urine pH becomes alkaline, and casts and white blood cells are destroyed. Glucose is consumed by bacteria if the urine is not tested when fresh. A clean, dry container should be used to collect a routine specimen, and the specimen should be sent to the laboratory as quickly as possible.

To screen for urinary tract infections and to identify the causative organisms, urine cultures are obtained. If the client does not have a catheter in place, the specimen is usually a midstream, clean-catch specimen. Normal urine is sterile, but the anterior urethra of men and women is contaminated with bacteria. To successfully obtain a midstream urine for culture, the client's cooperation is essential. That purpose of a clean-catch urine specimen is to decrease the contamination from the urethra, vagina, labia, foreskin, and surrounding skin. To obtain a clean-catch specimen, the client first cleanses the area around the urethra, then begins voiding, after which a sterile container is put in position to collect the midstream urine. Careful attention should be paid to assure that neither the edges nor the lid of the container are touched, as this would contaminate the specimen. To obtain a clean-catch specimen from an uncircumcised man, retract the foreskin and cleanse the head of the penis. With the foreskin retracted, the client begins to void and then slips a sterile container under the stream to collect the specimen. Urine obtained in this manner is believed to be most characteristic of the urine produced by the body. After the client has voided, the foreskin is replaced.

At times, it may be necessary to catheterize a client to obtain a specimen for culture. This should only be done when absolutely necessary since catheterization increases the risk of introducing organisms into the urinary tract. Consultation with the physician and a physician's order are needed before catheterizing a client to obtain a specimen. A client with an indwelling catheter in place should have the specimen taken from the catheter port with a sterile syringe. Most indwelling catheters have self-seal ports or openings for collecting a urine specimen. This should be cleansed before the specimen is obtained. The integrity of the closed urinary drainage system should not be interrupted since this increases the risk of ascending infection. A urine specimen for culture should never be obtained from the drainage bag. If a culture needs to be obtained from an ileoconduit, the stoma may be catheterized.

If a culture has been obtained via clean catch, a colony count of 1,000 to 10,000/ml is considered normal. Only if the count is higher than 100,000/ml is an infection diagnosed. A colony count of 10,000 to 100,000/ml may indicate contamination of the specimen. In this instance, a new specimen should be obtained for a repeat culture. With a specimen obtained from a urinary catheter, a count of 10,000/ml indicates infection. The urine should be stored in the refrigerator at 39°F (4°C) if the urine cannot be cultured within an hour. At room temperature, organisms can breed in the urine, doubling in 20 to 30 minutes, and thereby cause false bacterial readings.

Many substances can be detected in the urine with dipsticks. A variety is on the market, and they allow the client's home or the hospital utility room to function as a mini-laboratory. The sticks are impregnated with chemicals that react with substances in the urine. Depending on the type of test desired and type of stick used, the dipsticks measure sugar and acetone, protein, hemoglobin, urobiligen, and urine pH. Each type and brand has its own instructions and a color chart against which comparisons must be made. The instructions should be read carefully and the specifics as to time of reading followed. Color comparisons should be matched precisely.

Urine glucose also may be measured by the reducing tablet Clinitest. This, too, has specific instructions and a color comparison chart. There are two Clinitest methods, the two-drop and the five-drop. It is important that the instructions and color chart be appropriate for the particular method being employed. Previously, results of Clinitest measurements were reported as 1+, 2+ and so on, but this has been replaced by reporting the percent of glucose present in the urine. In this way, there is less danger of error if a client changes testing methods. One problem with the Clinitest measurement is that it is not specific for glucose, but measures other sugars as well. Therefore, false positives may occur. Many drugs, especially antibiotics, cause false positives and some false negatives, depending on the testing method used. The nurse always must know what medications a client is taking in order to know which test will yield an accurate reading. For example, ascorbic acid (vitamin C) may cause a false negative reading in the presence of a small amount of glucose (75–125 mg/dl) with Ames Multistixs (Ames, 1990).

Acetone can be measured with a dipstick that contains a test for ketone bodies or with an Acetest tablet. Here again, the exact specifications must be followed, and the color changes compared to the appropriate color chart.

Urine may be collected for a variety of other purposes. A double voided specimen, commonly used to indicate glucose level in the urine, is obtained to determine the next dose of insulin. For this procedure, the patient is asked to void approximately one-half hour before the specimen is to be obtained. The client is encouraged to drink fluids before the "second voided" specimen is collected. The urine obtained for the second specimen more accurately reflects the body's glucose level. Certain tests require the collection of a 24-hour urine specimen. If the nurse must collect a 24-hour specimen from a client, certain important points should be remembered (Fischbach, 1987):

The client should be asked to void: the urine is discarded.

The exact time of voiding should be noted.

All urine that is voided thereafter is placed in the container, which should be labeled with the client's name and identification, the time the test started, the time it will be completed, and the name of the test.

The client should void at the end of 24 hours, adding that urine to the bottle, completing the 24-hour collection.

All urine must be saved or the test results may be inaccurate.

The client and family should be carefully instructed about the urine collection, so they do not inadvertently disrupt the specimen collection.

Some 24-hour urine tests require refrigeration; others have a special preservative in the bottle. The exact procedure for the test ordered should be checked with the laboratory personnel or the procedure manual before the collection is begun.

There are many tests to measure renal func-tion. However, two commonly ordered blood tests have particular relevance in the assessment of elimination. These are tests that measure serum creatinine and blood urea nitrogen (BUN) levels.

Protein is metabolized into amino acids and nitrogenous wastes. These end products of protein metabolism are found in the circulating blood and are excreted in the urine. The normal blood urea nitrogen (BUN) is 8 to 20 mg/ml. The BUN functions as a secondary tool in the evaluation of renal function. The BUN level is affected by factors other than kidney function. As previously noted, dehydration can lead to an elevated BUN because the decreased circulation to the kidney decreases the glomerular filtration rate (GFR). An increase in protein intake or gastrointestinal bleeding may also cause the BUN to rise.

Creatinine is a nitrogenous waste product produced by muscle metabolism. Since it is unaffected by nutritional or fluid intake, it can serve as a primary tool in assessing renal function. Creatinine is excreted in direct proportion to the amount produced. Its normal serum level is 0.6 to 1.2 mg/ml. Changes in glomerular filtration rates do not cause significant changes in creatinine.

The BUN and creatinine levels are most useful when viewed in unison. Specifically, if the BUN rises and the creatinine level remains stable, then the likely culprits are poor renal perfusion, dehydration, or an increase in protein metabolism. An elevated BUN provides useful information when assessing fluid volume and the adequacy of urine output.

Creatinine more accurately reflects renal function. The serum creatinine level elevates with any renal disease that destroys more than 50% of the renal nephrons (Tilkian, Conover, & Tolkian, 1987). At 50% destruction, the creatinine level doubles; at 75%, it quadruples from the 50% level; and if 90% of the nephrons are destroyed, the serum creatinine level reaches 10 mg/ml (Metheny, 1987). If a client's creatinine level is elevated, the nurse will be able to approximate the amount of renal damage the client has suffered. It is important to realize that, unlike other norms, which are individual norms, the norms for creatinine are population norms. Thus, if a woman is admitted with an 0.6 creatinine level and a week later is 1.2, she has suffered a 50% nephron loss. The level of 1.2 is not normal for this client if the original level was 0.6. The nurse must know the client's original creatinine level in order to determine if the current level represents an increase or decrease. Clients with impaired renal function have difficulty concentrating urine and therefore need to put out a greater volume of urine in order to excrete metabolic wastes.

A variety of factors may cause a change in the appearance of urine (Table 19-17). There are a number of physiological conditions, as well as medications, that can alter the color of urine. A careful history and recheck by the nurse should be done to determine if urine color change is due to a drug.

NURSING DIAGNOSES RELATED TO FLUID–ELECTROLYTE BALANCE AND ELIMINATION

The nurse analyzes the data from the assessment of the client's fluid, electrolyte, and elimination status and then formulates appropriate nursing diagnoses (Table 19-18). The nursing diagnoses for fluid, electrolyte, and elimination problems are classified under the North American Nursing Diagnosis Association (NANDA) 1990 Taxonomy I human response pattern of "exchanging."

To support the diagnosis of "fluid volume deficit" due to fever, for example, data from the nursing history, clinical appraisal, and laboratory values should reflect an individual who experiences or is at risk of experiencing an alteration in body fluids resulting in dehydration. Defining characteristics would include such indicators as increased temperature, diminished skin turgor, decreased blood pressure and urine output, and decreased venous filling. The client also would exhibit thirst, generalized weakness, and dry skin and mucous membranes.

In contrast, the client with a nursing diagnosis of "fluid volume excess" due to excessive fluid or sodium intake, for example, would experience or be at risk of experiencing an excess of body fluids. Defining characteristics, in this instance, would in-

dicate an intake that is greater than the output. Also the client may exhibit edema, abnormal breath sounds (rales or crackles due to the presence of fluid in the alveoli), possibly an S_3 heart sound, oliguria, weight gain, restlessness, and anxiety.

When an individual's pattern of elimination is characterized by decreased frequency of stool passage, abdominal distention, painful defecations, and a dry hard stool, a nursing diagnosis of "colonic constipation" may be indicated. The client who is immobilized as a result of a car accident or the client with metastatic cancer who is receiving frequent narcotics for pain are examples of clients at risk for developing constipation.

In contrast, a nursing diagnosis of "diarrhea" would describe the pattern of elimination of a client who exhibits loose liquid stools, increased urgency and frequency, anal irritation, and change in stool color and odor. Factors such as stress, anxiety, change in dietary intake, infection, and cathartic abuse can produce diarrhea.

A diagnosis of "total incontinence" describes the state in which a client experiences an unpredictable and continuous loss of urine. Defining characteristics may include continuous or nearly continuous flow of urine, lack of awareness of incontinence, and no regular cycle of bladder emptying. Surgical procedures that damage nerves or the bladder sphincter, neurological diseases that affect body functioning, and congenital anomalies may all cause total incontinence.

To support the diagnosis of "urinary retention" related to prostatic enlargement, for example, data should reflect an individual who experiences incomplete emptying of the bladder. Defining characteristics would include indicators such as sensation of bladder fullness, decrease in force of stream, inability to start stream of urine, intake greater than out-

TABLE 19-17
Abnormalities in Appearance of the Urine

Appearance	Cause	Assessment
Colorless	Dilute urine Low specific gravity	Assess for causes of increased fluid output, i.e., diuretic therapy, increased fluid intake, varying disease states. Depending on cause, client may show signs of overhydration or dehydration.
Dark urine	Concentrated High specific gravity	Assess for signs of decreased fluid intake or increased insensible loss. Check BUN and creatinine levels. Check for hematuria.
Strong-tea colored	May indicate urobiligen in urine.	Check skin and sclera for jaundice. Check for clay-colored (acholic) stool.
Orange	May be caused by medications.	Check for drugs a client is taking, specifically Pyridium.
Red	Medications or blood.	May be drug related, but check for blood.

TABLE 19-18
Nursing Diagnoses Related to Fluid–Electrolyte Balance and Elimination

Constipation, colonic, related to, for example, malnutrition, narcotics (codeine, morphine), immobility, or fear of rectal or cardiac pain.

Constipation, perceived, related to, for example, central nervous system deterioration, obsessive-compulsive disorders, or cultural/family health beliefs.

Diarrhea, related to stress and anxiety, change in dietary intake and cathartic abuse.

Fluid volume deficit, related to, for example, fever, infection, diarrhea, nausea/vomiting, climate, exposure (extreme heat/sun), or excessive use of diuretics.

Fluid volume deficit potential, related to, for example, extremes of age, increased metabolic rate, altered mental status, or excessive drainage through artificial orifices, wounds, or drainage tubes.

Fluid volume excess, related to, for example, the effects of pregnancy or medications, excessive fluid or sodium intake, or low protein intake.

Incontinence, functional, related to, for example, loss of sphincter control, progressive dementia, inflammatory bowel diseases, or depression.

Incontinence, reflex, related to, for example, cord injury, tumor, or infection.

Incontinence, total, related to, for example, diabetic neuropathy, trauma, post-indwelling catheters, inability to communicate needs, or confusion.

Incontinence, urge, related to, for example, urethritis, parkinsonism, general or spinal anesthesia, or loss of perineal tissue (recent substantial weight loss).

Tissue, perfusion, altered: renal, related to hypotension, dehydration, or hypothermia.

Urinary elimination, altered patterns of, related to, for example, urinary tract infection, spinal cord injury, or incontinence.

Urinary retention, related to, for example, strictures, prostatic enlargement, diagnostic instrumentation, pregnancy, decreased attention to bladder cues, or environmental barriers to bathroom.

---

put, and frequent voiding of small amounts. Psychosocial or environmental problems can also contribute to urinary retention. "Lack of privacy, inability to assume a usual voiding position, timing difficulties, or the use of different receptacles (bedpans, urinals) are potential contributors to this problem" (McFarland & McFarlane 1989, p. 323). It is therefore important for the nurse to consider all information obtained from the client when identifying the cause of an elimination problem.

Chapter Highlights

■ Optimum cellular functioning, necessary for survival, depends on the availability of an adequate supply of nutrients, body fluids, electrolytes and acid-base balance, and the ability to eliminate waste materials from the body.

■ Knowledge and consideration of the client's cultural background and home facilities are important for determining whether elimination patterns and practices are within normal parameters.

■ The percentage of body fluid is inversely proportional to age: the younger the client, the greater the percentage of body fluid.

■ The essential functions of body fluid are maintaining blood volume, influencing body temperature, providing a medium for cell metabolism, transporting both nutrients and waste products to and from cells, and functioning as the solvent for the solutes essential for cell function.

■ Electrolytes serve the major functions of regulating hydrogen-ion balance, maintaining membrane excitability, maintaining body fluid osmolality, and moving body fluid between body fluid compartments.

■ Fluid and electrolyte requirements are influenced by body surface area, percentage of body fat, body and environmental temperature, exercise, and health.

■ Accurate measurement of fluid output is crucial because fluid replacement needs usually are calculated on the basis of these measurements and the client's body weight.

■ Common errors in measuring intake and output include failing to inform all staff as to which patients require I&O monitoring, failing to explain I&O to the family, and guessing at the amount instead of measuring it because it takes less time.

■ The body has the amazing ability to maintain the pH of the plasma within the narrow normal range of 7.35 to 7.45 by means of the lungs, kidneys, and chemical buffering system.

■ The best way to evaluate acid-base balance is by measuring arterial blood gases.

■ Clinical appraisal of elimination, and fluid and electrolyte balance, yields objective data via observation, inspection, palpation, and auscultation.

■ Laboratory data, such as urinalysis, stool exam, and serum electrolytes are useful in screening clients for potential health problems and in validating the findings of the history and clinical appraisal.

■ Data obtained from the nursing history, clinical appraisal, and selected laboratory findings should be analyzed to formulate appropriate nursing diagnoses related to a client's fluid–electrolyte balance and elimination.

Practice Activities

1. Examine your own elimination habits and practices (routine; facilities available; rituals, such as privacy, bathroom reading, etc.; effects of such temporary interferences as diarrhea on your lifestyle.)

2. Interview at least one healthy adult about his or her usual elimination patterns and practices.

3. Obtain a history and perform a clinical appraisal of at least one hospitalized client with an alteration in bowel elimination and at least one hospitalized client with an alteration in urinary elimination. Validate your findings, including laboratory data, and formulate appropriate nursing diagnoses. Record your findings.

4. Perform a history and clinical appraisal of an elderly client with an actual or potential alteration in fluid and electrolyte balance. Validate your assessment with appropriate laboratory findings, and formulate appropriate nursing diagnoses.

5. Interview clients from different socioeconomic and cultural backgrounds about their elimination practices and attitudes. What different attitudes and practices can be identified in the different groups?

Recommended Readings

Aberman, A. (1982). The ins and outs of fluids and electrolytes. *Emergency Medicine, 14*, 121.

Becker, L.B., & Stevens, S.A. (1988). Performing in-depth abdominal assessment. *Nursing, 18*(6), 59–63.

Didich, J.M. (1981). Gauging abdominal girth accurately. *Nursing, 11*(7), 32–33.

Folk-Lighty, M. (1984). Solving the puzzles of patients' fluid imbalances. *Nursing, 14*(2), 34–41.

Grant, M., & Kubo (1975). Assessing a patient's hydration status. *American Journal of Nursing, 75*(8), 1306–1311.

Mager, O'Connor, E. (1984). How to assess and remove fecal impaction. *Geriatric Nursing, 5*(3), 158–161.

Martof, M. (1985a). Fluid balance, Part 1. *Journal of Nephrology Nursing, 2*(1), 10–18.

Martof, M. (1985b). Electrolyte balance, Part 2. *Journal of Nephrology Nursing, 2*(2), 49–55.

McConnell, E.A. (1985). Assessing the bladder for bladder distension. *Nursing, 15*(11), 44–46.

McShane, R.E., & McLane, A.M. (1985). Constipation: Consensual validation and empirical validation. *Nursing Clinics of North America, 20*(4), 801–808.

Pflaum, S. (1979). Investigation of intake–output as a means of assessing body fluid balance. *Heart and Lung, 8*(3), 495–498.

Romanski, S. (1986). Interpreting ABGs in four easy steps. *Nursing, 16*(9), 58–64.

Schwartz, M.W. (1987). Potassium imbalances. *American Journal of Nursing, 87*(10), 1292.

Voith, A.M., & Smith, D.G. (1985). Validation of the nursing diagnosis of urinary retention. *Nursing Clinics of North America, 20*(4), 723–729.

Yu, L.C. (1987). Incontinence stress index: Measuring psychological impact. *Journal of Gerontological Nursing, 13*(7), 18–25.

References

Ames Division, Miles Laboratories. (1990). Ames product insert for Multistixs. Insert. Elkhart, IN: Miles Laboratories.

Ames Division, Miles Laboratories (1990). Hema-Check Slide Pak. Elkhart, IN: Miles Laboratories.

Battle, E.H., & Hanna, C.E. (1980). Evaluation of a dieting regimen for chronic constipation. *Journal of Gerontological Nursing, 6*, 527.

Fischbach, F.A. (1987). *Manual of laboratory diagnostic tests*. Philadelphia: Lippincott.

Guyton, A.C. (1990). *Textbook of medical physiology* (8th ed.). Philadelphia: Saunders.

Hui, Y.H. (1983). *Human nutrition and diet therapy*. Monterey, CA: Wadsworth.

Keane, C., & Miller, B. (1987). *Encyclopedia and dictionary of medicine, nursing and allied health* (4th ed.). Philadelphia: Saunders.

Martof, M. (1985a). Fluid balance, Part 1. *Journal of Nephrology Nursing, 2*(1), 10–18.

Martof, M. (1985b). Electrolyte balance, Part 2. *Journal of Nephrology Nursing, 2*(2), 49–55.

McFarland, G., & McFarlane, E. (1989). *Nursing diagnosis and intervention*. St. Louis: Mosby.

Metheny, N. (1987). *Fluid and electrolyte balance*. Philadelphia: Lippincott.

Metheny, N., & Snively, W.D. (1979). *Nurses' handbook of fluid balance* (3rd ed.). Philadelphia: Lippincott.

Rubin, M. (1988). The physiology of bed rest. *American Journal of Nursing, 88*(1), 50–58.

Thomas, B. (1980). Problem solving urinary incontinence in the elderly. *Journal of Gerontological Nursing, 6*, 533.

Tilkian, S.M., Conover, M.B., & Tilkian, A.G. (1987). *Clinical implications of laboratory tests.* St. Louis: Mosby.

Wells, T., & Brink, C. (1988). Elimination: Urinary. In Burnside, I. (Ed.), *Nursing and the aged.* New York: McGraw-Hill.

Williams, S., & Worthington, B. (1988). *Nutrition throughout the life cycle.* St. Louis: Times Mirror/ Mosby College.

PART VI

Nursing Assessment of Special Clients

Assessment of the Pregnant Woman

OBJECTIVES

Upon completion of this chapter, you should be able to:

■ Describe physiological changes experienced by the pregnant woman in antepartum, intrapartum, and postpartum periods.

■ Delineate normal emotional changes during the woman's transition to parenting.

■ Demonstrate an understanding of the impact of pregnancy on physical integrity, activity–sleep patterns, oxygenation, fluid–electrolyte balance and elimination patterns, role acquisition, attachment, sexuality, and family/culture.

■ Use the antepartal nursing history to assess the client's health.

■ Perform designated procedures to clinically appraise the health of the pregnant woman and her fetus.

■ Analyze assessment information to formulate valid and appropriate nursing diagnoses.

The pregnant woman provides a unique opportunity for comprehensive assessment of two separate though interrelated clients. While physiological research of human reproduction reveals that a fetus is a separate rather than parasitic being, recent legal decisions suggest a trend toward treating the mother and her dependent fetus as one (Johnson, 1987). Emotional changes during childbearing are the subject of many studies of both individual and family adaptation. Recent anthropological research looks at birth practices that are in harmony with beliefs, values, culture, and the environment (Choi & Hamilton, 1986).

While scholars from many disciplines contribute to a better understanding of pregnancy, nurses are concerned with the interrelatedness of physiological, emotional, social, and environmental factors and their impact on health during pregnancy. In an era of multiple technological advances to enhance assessment, the nurse must have broad knowledge to deliver competent care that can affect the quality of life at its very beginning.

A brief overview of the reproductive process serves as a foundation for nursing assessment of the pregnant woman, including biophysical changes in the woman and her fetus, and psychosocial adaptations common to childbearing.

KNOWLEDGE NEEDED TO ASSESS THE PREGNANT WOMAN

Pregnancy is a significant biological, psychosocial, and cultural event. Because of the unique changes that occur during pregnancy, the pregnant woman and her developing fetus require special consideration during the nursing assessment. To effectively assess and diagnose the pregnant woman's responses to pregnancy and childbearing, nurses must have knowledge of the biophysical and psychosocial changes that occur during this special event in a woman's life.

Biophysical and Psychosocial Changes Following Conception

Intercourse during the fertile phase of a woman's menstrual cycle may lead to conception if contraceptive measures have not been used. As millions of ejaculated sperm ascend toward the fallopian tubes, they are aided by the slightly alkaline cervical secretions that accompany ovulation. Because the ovum is fertilized by a single sperm, the product of conception combines the genetic characteristics of each parent. After 7 days of rapid cell change, the zygote implants in the upper third of the uterine endometrium.

Rapid changes follow. Cell differentiation results in thickening of the endometrium (now called the decidua) and the beginning formation of placental tissue. The zygote–embryo develops fetal membranes, the chorion and the amnion, that provide a protective environment filled ultimately with about 1,000 ml of clear amniotic fluid. As the embryonic cells multiply and divide, chorionic villi become embedded in the uterine wall, which has a rich capillary network to complete the placental exchange system. By the third week after conception, this rudimentary placenta secretes several hormones. One of these, human chorionic gonadotropin (HCG), seems to prevent loss of the embryo. Detection of HCG is possible in maternal serum at this time; identification of its presence in urine takes somewhat longer.

During the critical first trimester (3 months) of the usual 38 to 42 weeks of gestation, the embryonic structures for organ development form from differentiated cell layers. A specialized circulatory system provides for fetal needs and returns waste products to the placenta through the umbilical cord's two arteries and one vein.

By the third month of pregnancy, the placenta and embryo–fetus are a tightly knit unit. The placenta, through indirect exchange with the embryo-fetus, provides for the respiration, nutrition, elimination, and endocrine needs of the unborn child. While the placenta serves as a selective barrier to certain substances, many viruses, toxins, and some antigens can reach the fetus.

The fetus is active within the uterine environment and responds to noise, touch, and light. Movements are evident by about 3 months, although the woman may not perceive quickening (fetal movement) until 4 or 5 months of gestation. As the fetus grows, pressure within the uterus and on maternal pelvic organs increases. While there is less space as pregnancy advances, the well-oxygenated fetus continues to be active, kicking and turning frequently.

Rapid bone growth occurs in the developing fetus. Viability, the point at which the fetus theoretically can exist outside of the uterine environment, occurs after 20 weeks of development. However, lung maturity is poor until sufficient surfactant lines the alveoli. Survival of a preterm newborn depends on availability of technological resources and a skilled health-care team.

As the fetus develops, many biophysical changes occur within the pregnant (gravid) woman. During the antepartal period, uterine muscle fibers change to prepare for later function. The uterus enlarges to accommodate the growing fetal–placental unit. In response to increased levels of estrogen, secreted initially by the corpus luteum and subsequently by the placenta, the uterus and cervix soften. Vaginal secretions increase in a slightly acidic environment. Expanded blood supply to the reproductive organs and perineum further prepare the woman's body for birth.

Other hormones contribute to antepartal adaptation. Progesterone production by the placenta prevents premature uterine contraction and appears critical in maintaining the pregnancy. Human placental lactogen (HPL) affects the woman's insulin production and seems to influence fetal development (Greenspan & Forsham, 1988).

Circulatory and excretory adaptations occur in response to fetal needs. Cardiac output and circulating volume increase dramatically to provide for approximately 600 ml of placental blood flow per minute. The pregnant woman's kidneys filter waste products at an increased rate to maintain fluid balance.

Mammary tissue changes as the milk duct system prepares for lactation. Fat deposits increase in response to hormones. Colostrum, an early form of breast milk, is secreted by the 10th week.

During the last trimester, uterine contractions cause little discomfort. These Braxton-Hicks contractions differ from the productive contractions of labor. At some time prior to birth, the uterus drops into the pelvic cavity in a process called lightening. The blood-tinged mucous plug that blocks the cervix throughout pregnancy is dislodged just before or during labor.

The intrapartal period, or time of labor and birth, begins with the onset of true labor. This is marked by the onset of regular contractions and cervical changes. While the combination of factors that stimulate labor is not well understood, it is believed that both maternal and fetal influences contribute to the onset of labor.

Increasingly regular uterine contractions stimulate dilation and thinning (effacement) of the cervix and promote expulsion of the fetus. During the first labor stage, from the onset of true labor until birth, the fetus contributes to progress by its position. The optimal situation finds the head presenting with the fetus engaged in the true pelvis. Ideally, the fetal membranes remain intact until shortly before delivery, ensuring a protective environment.

Through a series of movements, the fetus adapts to the labor process, descends, and rotates. With the assistance of bearing down efforts by the woman, the force of uterine contractions, and perhaps surgical episiotomy, the fetus leaves the womb and enters the extra-uterine environment. This second stage of labor is a critical adaptive period for the fetus–newborn.

Shortly after delivery, the placenta separates from the uterine lining and is expelled with a contraction. Following this third labor stage, the uterus contracts firmly and descends to just above the symphysis pubis.

The critical adaptive period for the woman is the first hour following delivery. Massive physiological changes occur as intra-abdominal pressure shifts, fetal–placental needs cease, and hormones respond to the altered state. As estrogen and progesterone levels drop suddenly, prolactin is secreted. With stimulation of the breast by a sucking newborn, oxytocin is released by the posterior pituitary to enhance secretion of breast milk.

The uterus remains palpable for about the first 2 weeks of the postpartal period. It then descends into the pelvic cavity. New endometrial tissue develops rapidly; however, healing at the placental site takes several weeks. The uterus returns to normal size by 6 weeks postpartum as the muscle fibers diminish in size. A vaginal discharge, or lochia, containing blood and decidua, persists for about 3 weeks. Cervical tissue heals rapidly. Vaginal mucosa regains tone but may remain atrophic for many weeks.

While psychosocial adaptations to childbearing vary with the individual, such factors as developmental level, cognitive preparation, economic stressors, support systems, and cultural variables contribute to the woman's emotional state. Certain psychosocial responses occur during each trimester of pregnancy. The usual pattern of responses is delineated in Table 20-1. The unique situation of each pregnant woman affects her specific emotional responses.

Nurse researchers have contributed much to knowledge of common psychosocial alterations during and following childbirth. It is generally accepted that birth is a developmental and situational crisis for women. Rubin (1967, 1984) has studied pregnancy and postpartal adaptation extensively, identifying specific tasks that must be resolved for each phase. According to Rubin, ambivalence is common during the first weeks after conception, with the reality of pregnancy. For example, the woman may be delighted at the possibility she will become a mother, yet unsure if this is the "best time" for her to do so.

The pregnant woman views the fetus as a separate being during the second trimester as the

TABLE 20-1
Psychosocial Responses to Pregnancy

| Parameters | Trimester | | |
	First	Second	Third
Focus	Self	Baby	Labor and delivery; safety of self and baby
Response to being pregnant	"Am I pregnant?" "Is there a pregnancy?"	"I am pregnant!" "Pregnancy is wonderful!"	"No doubt about it, I'm pregnant and I'm tired of it; I don't want to be pregnant again."
Affective response	Waiting, unsure, scared, moody	Pride, joy, pleasure, looks good, feels good	Despairing, fearful, vulnerable, trapped; becomes angry and hostile
Baby	Not there	Baby and self are one	Baby and self are one; begins to separate from pregnancy; wants baby in outside world
Weight	Not much weight gain; disappointed because weight gain would help verify pregnancy	Weight gain means baby is growing/thriving; she's a good mother	Too much; baby is too big; "I'm fat, too big."
Time	Time is empty	Time is present	Time is unbearable, time is running out
Space	Begins to become introverted so she examines own body to determine whether she is pregnant	Introversion, inward focus; restricts social sphere; attention on mothers and children	Introversion further restricts space because of vulnerability

Note. From Auvenshine/Enriquez: *Comprehensive Maternity Nursing*, Second Edition, © 1990. Boston: Jones and Bartlett Publishers, p. 227.

baby's movements are felt. The expected baby often is visualized with specific characteristics and the desired gender.

As the time for birth approaches, the woman prepares for delivery with excitement and some fear. She often feels that her body is large and clumsy and worries about the unknown aspects of labor.

Following delivery, the new mother integrates the experience into her own life. Rubin (1967, 1984) describes the patterns of "taking in," "taking hold," and "letting go" as typical. Once the woman's physical needs are met and she is comfortable, she can begin to take care of her newborn.

Hormonal changes may lead to brief periods of "postpartum blues" during the first weeks after delivery. Common emotional responses such as weepiness and fatigue rarely interfere with normal function. Should the woman be unable to carry out usual daily activities, psychological consultation may be indicated.

Prenatal classes provide an opportunity for the pregnant woman and her partner to better understand antepartal health and the birth process. In addition, a childbirth educator can encourage sharing of fears and concerns that couples may not have discussed. Classes for siblings and grandparents may help prepare family members for the anticipated birth.

Physiological Effects of Pregnancy

The assessment of the childbearing woman builds on the knowledge of normal adaptations to pregnancy. The competent nurse caring for the antepartal or postpartal client in a clinic, office, hospital, or the home must be able to make relevant observations, ask pertinent questions, and organize data to determine the pregnant woman's responses to normal pregnancy or health alterations that may occur during pregnancy. Using the conceptual framework of this text, the impact of pregnancy on health patterns is discussed for the antepartal, intrapartal and postpartal periods.

Physical Integrity

Changes in the integument are characteristic of pregnancy. Vital sign changes and weight gain reflect physiological adaptations as the woman's body responds to the demands of the developing fetus.

Skin. Many antepartal changes in skin integrity occur during pregnancy. The influence of hormones such as estrogen and progesterone cause characteristic alterations in pigmentation. *Striae,* or stretch marks, may occur on the abdomen, thighs, or breasts. A dark line (*linea nigra*) may appear on the abdominal wall. The mask of pregnancy, *chloasma,* may be evident as a darkened area near the eyes. Nipple areolae darken. These skin changes are less evident following delivery.

Mucous membranes respond to estrogen changes. For example, edema of the nasal membranes may cause stuffiness. Gum tenderness is common for many pregnant women. Vaginal mucosa becomes increasingly stretchable in preparation for birth. Following delivery, lacerations and the repaired episiotomy heal rapidly as hormone levels drop sharply.

Vital Signs. Changes in vital signs during pregnancy reflect vascular adaptations. Maternal pulse rate increases slightly, while blood pressure remains fairly constant despite a slightly higher aldosterone level, fluid changes, and postural edema.

During the intrapartal period, little change in vital signs is evident in the healthy client. Postpartally, the pulse rate slows in response to massive fluid volume shift. While the blood pressure usually remains stable, body temperature may rise slightly due to an inflammatory response. Excluding delivery day, the client's body temperature should remain below 100.4° F.

Weight. Antepartal weight gain reflects embryo–fetal growth patterns. The usual weight curve shows minimal change during the first trimester, but with consistent week-to-week gains during the latter part of pregnancy. The average fetus weighs close to seven pounds at term; the placenta, breasts, and amniotic fluid account for several pounds. Intracellular fluid and increasing circulating blood volume also add weight. Figure 20-1 depicts weight gain during pregnancy.

Following delivery, initial weight loss is about 10 pounds. Additional reduction of stored fat takes at least several weeks and may require caloric modification.

Activity–Sleep Patterns

Biophysical and psychological changes during pregnancy alter the usual activity and rest patterns for many women. Fatigue, caused by high estrogen levels, is common in the first trimester. Some pregnant women report the need for several naps daily. Usual energy levels are restored after the 12th week, and many clients continue to lead active lives until close to term.

Previously established exercise patterns may be continued as tolerated. Because the growing embryo–fetus may be harmed by maternal dehydration or elevated body temperature, warming up, cooling down, and rest periods are particularly important during active exercise. The pregnant woman should not begin a new or strenuous exercise program without approval from her primary health care provider. The nurse should advise the client to pay attention to her body's responses, such as pain, fatigue, or joint weakness. Pulse rate should not exceed 140/minute during exercise. Adequate fluids and a balanced diet should be part of any fitness program during pregnancy.

Research has found no ill effects of continued exercise during pregnancy if adequate nutrition is maintained (Slavin, 1986). However, the pregnant woman should avoid straight leg raises, hot tubs or saunas, and attempts to exercise to lose weight. Long distance running and prolonged jogging may contribute to temperature elevation or jarring of the uterus and could harm the fetus.

Swimming and rapid walking are healthy activities during pregnancy. For maximum benefit, the exercise should be maintained for at least 15 minutes three times weekly.

Because the environment in which the woman exercises or works affects her health, exposure to pollutants can change an activity from a healthy behavior to one that increases risk. Such hazards can damage the fetus during critical growth periods. Among the hazards that affect embryo-fetal development are passive smoke, radiation, vinyl chloride, and other toxic chemicals. The potential risks of exposure to video display terminals are being studied. Since research shows that more than one million babies are born each year to employed women, the National Council to Prevent Infant Mortality, formed in 1988, actively is seeking the cooperation of employers in increasing the benefits provided to pregnant women, including a healthy and safe work environment (Greenspan & Forsham, 1988).

During labor, walking promotes comfort and is preferred by many women to remaining in bed. If there are no contraindications such as leaking amniotic fluid or bleeding, the client can remain active. The force of gravity may shorten the labor process. Studies of giving birth in the squatting po-

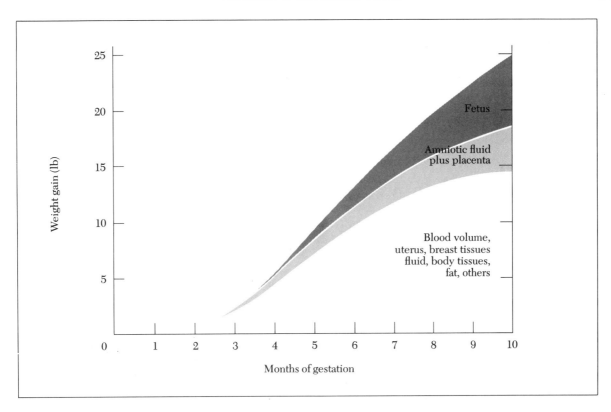

FIGURE 20-1. Weight Gain During Pregancy. (*Note.* Hui, H.Y., *Human Nutrition and Diet Therapy*. Monterey, CA Wadsworth Health Sciences, 1983, p. 327. Used with permission.)

sition confirm that this is more natural and less uncomfortable.

Throughout the usual 8 to 14 hours of labor, rest between contractions maintains the woman's energy. A quiet environment and the presence of a supportive coach or consistent caregiver can enhance rest. Applying previously learned breathing techniques and exercises often promotes relaxation.

During the immediate postpartal period, exhilaration may interfere with rest. Although very tired from the birth, many women experience some insomnia for a day or two. This is thought to be a response to hormone shifts. With the trend of early discharge, newborns' needs often prevent new mothers from getting a full night's sleep at home. Napping may help to restore some energy during the first weeks. Delegation of some child care responsibilities to other adults or older children may provide free time for the new mother.

Early walking has benefits for both elimination and oxygenation. While physicians differ on recommendations for postpartal exercise programs, Kegel (perineal) exercises strengthen the pelvic floor muscles and may be performed shortly after delivery. The nurse should suggest that while void-

ing, the client briefly stop the stream of urine, then release the sphincter. Low impact aerobics may be resumed as tolerated.

Oxygenation

Changes in cardiac output and circulating volume lead to hemodilution during pregnancy. However, hemoglobin levels usually remain stable, depending on preconception health and adequate iron intake. In the third trimester, a hemoglobin of 11 and a hematocrit of 34 are considered normal (Pritchard, MacDonald, & Gant, 1985). The risk of thrombus formation is slightly higher for the pregnant woman than for other young adults. However, clotting factors remain unbalanced. After delivery, these factors are not as well regulated and may contribute to clot formation in the inactive woman. Hematological changes during pregnancy are outlined in Table 20-2.

During the last trimester of pregnancy, the increasing size of the fetus may displace the diaphragm upward. Normal breathing patterns may be compromised and the pregnant woman may experience shortness of breath. This is especially likely to occur if she assumes a reclining position or

---

TABLE 20-2
Hematological Changes During Pregnancy

Lab Indicator	Nonpregnant Value	Pregnant Value
Hematocrit (average)	41.7	37
Hemoglobin	12–16 g/dl	>10 g/dl
Red blood cell (RBC) volume	1355 ml	1790 ml
White blood cells (WBC)	5,000–10,000/μl	5,000–12,000/μl 25,000/μl during labor
Plasma protein	4.0–4.5 g/dl	3.0–3.5 g/dl
Fibrinogen	200–400 mg/dl	300–600 mg/dl
Platelets	150,000–400,000/μl	150,000–400,000/μl

Note. From Auvenshine/Enriquez: *Comprehensive Maternity Nursing*, Second Edition, © 1990. Boston: Jones and Bartlett Publishers, p. 204.

following exertion, such as walking up a flight of stairs or getting from a sitting to a standing position. For some women, comfortable breathing may be possible only while sitting in a chair. The effects of pregnancy on the respiratory system are depicted in Table 20-3.

Faintness is experienced by some women in response to sudden position changes. This light-headedness diminishes if the woman rises slowly from a reclining or sitting position. Sleeping on her side relieves uterine pressure on the aorta and vena cava, thus improving oxygen delivery to the placenta and fetus.

Fetal gas exchange is dependent on healthy cardiovascular function of the mother. Normal blood pressure maintains optimum circulation to the placenta and allows for oxygen delivery and carbon dioxide removal. Optimal placental–fetal oxygenation is reflected in rising maternal estriol levels and a normal fetal growth pattern. Since fetal activity is a good indicator of adequate placental oxygenation, recent technological developments have improved the assessment of fetal–placental status. For example, the nonstress test is a measure of the frequency of fetal activity and fetal heart rate response to that movement. Periodic timing of fetal

kicking by the pregnant woman is a simple assessment of fetal well-being. Since this involves tuning in to her unborn child's activity patterns, early attachment is facilitated as well.

The effects of nicotine and carbon monoxide from smoking by either parent reduces available oxygen to the fetus. Placental gas exchange also is compromised by maternal use of alcohol, cocaine, and other drugs.

During labor and delivery, the stress of contractions produces a vagal response that reduces the fetal heart rate, thus conserving oxygen. Since less blood is available, shunting to vital organs occurs. Additionally, the fetus extracts more oxygen from the blood during labor. Thus, the stress of uterine contractions of normal intensity helps prepare the fetus for adaptation to extra-uterine life. During the relaxation phase following a contraction, normal gas exchange occurs (Simkin, 1986).

Maternal blood loss during the intrapartal stage is usually less than 500 ml. Increased fluid volume compensates for this loss. Following separation and expulsion of the placenta, uterine contraction prevents excessive blood loss at the placental site. Administration of oxytocic drugs enhances this adaptation.

TABLE 20-3
Effects of Pregnancy on the Respiratory System

No change	Increase	Decrease
Respiratory rate	Tidal volume	Functional residual capacity
Maximum breathing capacity	Minute ventilatory volume	Residual volume
Vital capacity	Minute O_2 uptake	Arterial pO_2
	Arterial pO_2	
	Gradient between alveolar and arterial pO_2	

Note. From Auvenshine/Enriquez: *Comprehensive Maternity Nursing*, Second Edition, © 1990. Boston: Jones and Bartlett Publishers, p. 205.

During the postpartal period, hematocrit levels remain low for one to two days. As the cardiac output increases once again, excessive fluids no longer needed for placental circulation are eliminated. Vaginal bleeding following delivery may continue for 3 weeks. Lochia changes from bright red to serous in a few days; passage of clots is not unusual. Supplemental iron can restore hemoglobin to normal levels.

Nutritional Requirements

During pregnancy and lactation, the need for nearly every nutrient increases (see Table 20-4). Daily energy requirements increase about 300 kcal during pregnancy and by 500 to 800 kcal during lactation.

In order for the embryo–fetus to develop normally, the expectant mother must provide essential nutrients. An additional 30 mg of protein during pregnancy is needed for fetal bone growth and

TABLE 20-4
Nutritional Requirements During Pregnancy and Lactation

Daily Dietary Allowance*	Pregnancy (after 1st trimester)	/	Lactation (1st 6 months)
Calories	+300	/	+500
Protein	0	/	+15
Vitamin A	0	/	+500
Vitamin D	+5	/	+5
Vitamin E	+2	/	+4
Vitamin C	+10	/	+35
Thiamin	+0.4	/	+0.5
Riboflavin	+0.3	/	+0.5
Niacin	+2	/	+5
Vitamin B6	+0.6	/	+0.5
Folate	+220	/	+100
Vitamin B12	+0.2	/	+0.6
Calcium	+400	/	+400
Phosphorus	+400	/	+400
Magnesium	+20	/	+150
Iron	+15**	/	0**
Zinc	+5	/	+7
Iodine	+25	/	+50
Selenium	+10	/	+20

*Recommendations reflect increases over normal requirements for age (see chap. 18).

**The increased requirement during pregnancy cannot be met by iron content of habitual American diets nor by the existing iron stores of many women; therefore the use of 30 to 60 mg of supplemental iron is recommended. Iron needs during lactation are not substantially different from those of nonpregnant women, but continued supplementation of the mother for 2 to 3 months after parturition is advisable in order to replenish stores depleted by pregnancy.

Note. Reprinted with permission from *Recommended Dietary Allowances*, 9th edition, © 1980 by the National Academy of Sciences. Published by National Academy Press, Washington, DC.

brain development. Caloric intake of at least 2,400 kcal each day is required, depending on the trimester (Greenspan & Forsham, 1988). Increased amounts of calcium (400–600 mg daily), vitamin D, and phosphorous also should be added to the diet. If the pregnant woman is an adolescent, her own growth needs require even higher levels of these nutrients.

Since iron is stored in the fetal liver for several months after birth, adequate dietary intake of iron (30–60 mg) is essential during the third trimester. Use of an iron supplement, taken with food or a glass of orange juice, may be advised.

Selected vitamins and minerals contribute to the health of the mother and her unborn child. Some physicians suggest that the pregnant woman take a multiple vitamin tablet daily after the 20th week to ensure adequate intake of vitamins B, C, and D. Folic acid supplements may be recommended if a deficiency is evident or the woman is expecting twins or triplets.

Overuse of vitamin A may lead to fetal damage. For this reason, the pregnant woman is advised to avoid high doses of this or any other vitamin. Medications that are prescribed for acne treatment may contain retinol. Women who plan to become pregnant should avoid this preparation as it has been known to cause birth defects (Vitamin A Supplementation, 1987).

Two nutritional problems common in pregnant and lactating women include anemia related to low dietary intake of iron, and inadequate protein consumption. Clinical and biochemical signs of iron and protein deficiency should be evaluated during pregnancy (see chap. 18).

Morning sickness and heartburn may require dietary modifications. Some women find that eating small meals or dry foods on arising diminishes discomfort. Later in the day, when nausea passes, a well-balanced diet containing sufficient roughage promotes elimination. Foods high in fiber include whole grains, raw fruits, and vegetables.

Changing carbohydrate metabolism results in breakdown of some fats during pregnancy, causing occasional periods of hyperglycemia and ketosis. In the healthy woman, this is not a problem since insulin (which does not cross the placenta) balances the higher blood sugar levels.

Studies of caffeine use during pregnancy have been inconclusive. Selected herbal teas may cause diarrhea, vomiting, and behavior changes.

Ingestion of non-nutritive substances, such as clay or starch, is common among pregnant women in some cultural groups. This practice, *pica*, can lead to bowel obstruction, parasitic intestinal disease, or lead poisoning.

During labor, the woman may experience some nausea as the cervix dilates. Fasting during the intrapartal stage reduces the danger of aspiration. Intravenous fluids may be used to supplement oral intake.

Following delivery, hunger and thirst are adaptive responses to replenish energy expended during labor and the birth. Unless general anesthesia has been administered, food and fluids are provided as desired. During the postpartal period, a well-balanced diet meets the restorative needs of the new mother. Supplemental vitamins and iron usually are continued for 2 to 3 months after delivery. The breast-feeding mother's needs for protein are approximately 20 grams more per day than the nonlactating mother. She also needs greater amounts of nearly every vitamin and mineral, especially vitamins A, C, and D, plus calcium and iron (see Table 20-4). Supplemental vitamins and iron generally are recommended for the breast-feeding mother during the period of lactation.

Fluid–Electrolyte Requirements

The pregnant or breast-feeding woman needs 6 to 8 glasses of fluids daily to provide for circulatory volume changes or lactation, respectively. Electrolyte deficit or excess may need to be assessed in some women. For example, the client who has excessive vomiting may experience sodium depletion. A pregnant woman with elevated blood pressure and edema may need to be advised to restrict the use of table salt.

During the intrapartal stage, reduced oral intake, excessive IV fluids, or the administration of ritodrine for preterm labor may cause hypokalemia. Close assessment for signs of hypokalemia is essential. Slowing the IV infusion rate or adding potassium to the fluids can correct this deficit. The nurse also must be alert to symptoms of respiratory alkalosis resulting from hyperventilation, especially during the transition phase of labor. Slow, deep breathing into a paper bag or cupped hands can correct the problem before it affects the fetus.

Following an uncomplicated birth, electrolyte imbalance is seldom a problem. Adaptive thirst, ingestion of sufficient oral fluids, and a balanced diet, including fruits, maintains health.

Lactation

The woman who plans to breast-feed can prepare her nipples for nursing by avoiding soaps, and by towel drying vigorously after showering. She also may wish to apply a lanolin cream daily.

During pregnancy, prolactin levels stimulate the secretion of colostrum. Immediately after the placenta is expelled, a drop in estrogen further stimulates increased release of prolactin. This hormone acts to stimulate milk production. When the newborn is placed to breast, ideally immediately following delivery, the sucking response triggers the release of oxytocin. The resulting let-down reflex ejects milk from the breast (see Figure 20-2). However, when the mother is tense, anxious, or insecure when breast-feeding her infant, the let-down reflex and milk production may be inhibited (see Figure 20-3).

Engorgement of the breasts commonly occurs approximately 48 hours after delivery. The breasts become tender as they fill with lymphatic fluid, blood, and milk, a normal physiological response. The mother should continue to nurse regularly. Using a pump may promote comfort after the infant has fed.

Elimination Patterns

The pressure of the growing fetus and uterus on the urinary bladder causes urinary frequency during the first and third trimesters. Since hormonal changes lead to reduced bladder capacity, the pregnant woman should empty her bladder frequently to prevent overdistention, discomfort, and susceptibility to urinary tract infection.

Normal bowel elimination depends on adequate hydration and fiber intake. Constipation and hemorrhoids are common during pregnancy due to increasing uterine weight and slowing peristalsis. The active woman may be too busy to take a break in her schedule to eliminate regularly. Use of cathartics to stimulate defecation is potentially harmful to the fetus and should be avoided.

During the intrapartal stage, emptying the bladder regularly promotes comfort and eases fetal descent. An enema may be given in early labor to facilitate bowel evacuation.

Elimination patterns gradually return to normal during the postpartal stage. Initially, the woman may not feel the urge to urinate due to edema of the trigone muscle from fetal pressure. Most new mothers are able to void if assisted to the bathroom. Urinary output usually is measured to ensure that the bladder is emptied completely. Catheterization is seldom necessary following a normal delivery; however, the nurse should be aware of oral and IV fluid intake and the time lapse since delivery.

Postpartal bowel elimination is facilitated by intake of fluids and high fiber foods. Physicians often prescribe a stool softener to ease stool passage. If the episiotomy is quite swollen, sitz baths can pro-

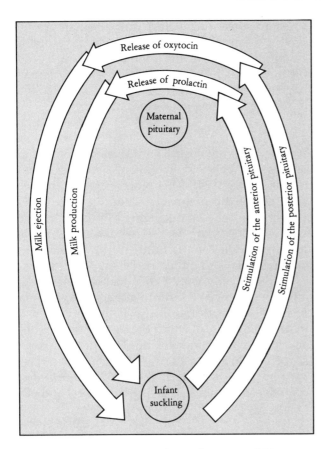

FIGURE 20-2. Lactation: Milk Production and Ejection. (*Note.* From Auvenshine/Enriquez: *Comprehensive Maternity Nursing*, Second Edition, © 1990. Boston: Jones and Bartlett Publishers, p. 440.)

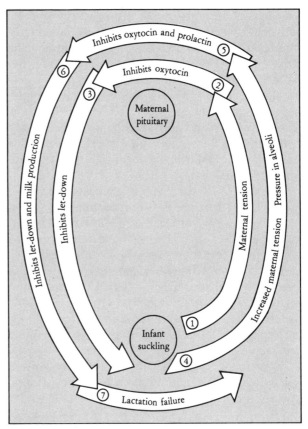

FIGURE 20-3. The Effect of Maternal Tension on Lactation. (*Note.* From Auvenshine/Enriquez: *Comprehensive Maternity Nursing*, Second Edition, © 1990. Boston: Jones and Bartlett Publishers, p. 440.)

mote comfort and reduce edema. If these measures are not helpful, an enema may be administered.

Psychosocial Effects of Pregnancy

Pregnancy has a profound influence on psychosocial well-being. In particular, pregnancy affects the woman's sexuality and self-concept, her relationships with others (especially her partner), and her role behaviors, including maternal role acquisition and attachment.

Sexuality

There is little research on sexuality and the pregnant woman. Most studies focus on the couple's relationship. Bernhard and Dan (1986) suggest that a woman's sexuality might be defined as an awareness of her whole body based on her unique experiences and feelings. Biophysical changes during pregnancy often affect the woman's sexual self-concept (see chap. 13). Breast and abdominal enlargement alter her body image, may affect her

perception of her attractiveness to her partner and may decrease her sexual desire.

Fetal and uterine growth often cause discomfort during intercourse. Hormonal changes lead to periods of diminished or heightened sexual desire. The expectant father may be confused by these fluctuations and is sometimes fearful that lovemaking will harm his unborn child. Expressions of the couple's feelings and concerns related to sexual practices should be encouraged. Within a group setting, or in private, couples need to know that sexual concerns during pregnancy are normal.

Modifications of positions for intercourse may increase comfort as pregnancy advances. Unless there are problems, such as bleeding or leaking amniotic fluid, the couple may continue sexual intercourse throughout pregnancy. The only restriction is oral-genital sexual activity that involves blowing air into the vagina, which may lead to an air embolus.

Labor and delivery is a time of enhanced emotional and physical intimacy. Couples who have prepared together for the birth experience a unique closeness. The nurse must respect their need for privacy and allow the couple to use relaxation techniques they have practiced. For example, the woman may be comfortable squatting, using her spouse's shoulders as an anchor. The partner may stroke her thighs or lower abdomen frequently (effleurage) to promote relaxation. Sensitivity to the client's feelings and needs allows the nurse to work with the couple as labor progresses. The father's participation in birth enhances the couple's intimacy (Figure 20-4).

Postpartally, the healing process affects the new mother's sexuality. An episiotomy or laceration requires several weeks to heal. After a restorative period of several weeks, the couple may be encouraged to resume sexual relations when they desire to do so. However, vaginal secretions are diminished, and atrophic changes may cause painful intercourse for several months. The unpredictable newborn's needs often interfere with spontaneity, and fatigue limits the energy available for couple interaction.

The nurse working with new parents should encourage open communication between partners, so that expressions of love and affection are not limited to sexual intercourse. To reduce discomfort during sexual intercourse, the use of a water-soluble lubricating jelly is helpful. The couple's knowledge of contraception should be reinforced so that an unplanned pregnancy does not occur.

Maternal Role Acquisition

Antepartal psychological and developmental adaptations are believed to enhance role transition (Rubin, 1967, 1984). This process begins with acceptance of the pregnancy, continues with birth preparation, and is heightened by early contact with the newborn. As the woman takes on the mothering role, she is influenced by family and cultural variables and her social support systems.

Rubin's early work (1975) focused on women after they had given birth to a first child. In more recent research, Rubin looks at the formation of maternal identity, in which the woman defines herself in relation to her infant. This process is described in Table 20-5.

The maternal role is complex, comprised of cognitive elements, caregiving behaviors, and em-

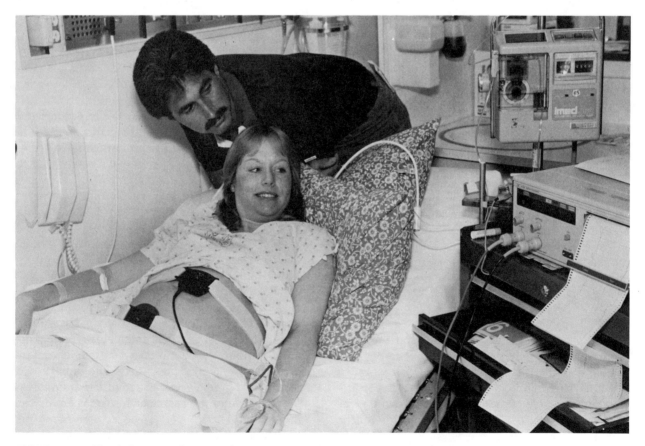

FIGURE 20-4. The father provides a comforting presence for the laboring woman. (*Note.* From Auvenshine/Enriquez: *Comprehensive Maternity Nursing*, Second Edition, © 1990. Boston: Jones and Bartlett Publishers, p. 808.)

TABLE 20-5
Maternal Identity Tasks

	Trimester		
	First	Second	Third
Safe passage	Concern about self. Alerted, something is "not there." "Am I sick or am I pregnant?"*	Concern about baby. Care of and for baby. "Is my baby all right?"*	Concern about self and baby. Seeking delivery care. "Will I and my baby safely go through labor and delivery?"*
Securing acceptance	Works on acceptance of herself as pregnant.	Works on acceptance of her baby. Task not as important because of own pleasure in pregnancy.	Works on acceptance of this baby, as it is.
Giving	Cost analysis: "What do I have to give up?" "Can I give up all that I have to?"*	Works on meaning of giving. What does gift symbolize? Care/love. Learns to give by being given to.	Feels "given out." Feels she cannot give any more. Extracts gifts from others.
Binding-in	Binds in to idea of self as pregnant. Baby is not real.	Attachment to baby. Secret, romantic love between self and baby. Feels good—attributes it to baby. Seeks messages from baby.	Carries a valuable treasure. Becomes fearful—what one treasures/possesses can be taken away. Hates being pregnant but wants her baby.

*Examples in quotations have been added for clarification.

Note. Adapted from Rubin, R. (1975). Maternal tasks in pregnancy. *Maternal-Child Nursing Journal, 4*(3), 143–153.

pathic interaction. Mercer (1985) suggests that the woman who has attained the maternal role is "competent." During the brief postpartal hospitalization, the new mother has an opportunity to learn caregiving skills and to gain confidence in handling her baby. Empathy, however, seems to be a developmental achievement rather than a behavior that can be taught.

Reciprocity in the mother–newborn relationship contributes to a smooth role transition. The baby who has a pleasant temperament and is responsive elicits positive mothering behaviors.

Tomlison (1987) notes many problems for women who are beginning a commitment to parenthood and urges study of changes in both parents from pregnancy through parenting. Inequity in dividing tasks seems to be a common cause of tension. Changes in marital satisfaction after the birth of a first child may reflect role strain.

Perceptions of support are explored in many studies. McBride (1988) suggests that outside employment, single parenting, poverty, and abusive situations contribute to the high stress of many young mothers. She recommends further longitudinal studies on the effects of stress during role transition.

Some mothers have unique problems during role transition. The adolescent, still struggling with her developing identity, may have great difficulty attaining the role of a nurturing parent (M. Young, 1988). Women from other cultures often discover that their expectations of a mother's behavior are in conflict with those of mainstream America (Hollingsworth, Brown, & Brooten, 1980). The mobility-impaired woman may find few resources available to assist her during adaptation to parenthood (Kopala, 1989).

Maternal Attachment

During the past 20 years, definitions of bonding and attachment have changed. Early research on newborns separated from their mothers differentiated between these two terms. Attachment was identified as the child's tie to the parent, which was seen as critical to survival. Bonding was defined as the relationship of the parent to the infant. Today, attachment includes parental affectional ties to the offspring. The terms bonding and attachment often are used interchangeably (Hans, 1986).

Earliest attachment occurs during pregnancy and has been studied by many researchers. Typically, the pregnant woman talks to her unborn child, often calling it by name. She may stroke her abdomen and respond with pleasure when the fetus moves.

Early contact with the newborn contributes to attachment. The mother who holds the newborn immediately after birth is able to look into its eyes during the alert first hour of life. She begins to explore the baby, hold it close, talk quietly and, perhaps, breast-feed. The LeBoyer gentle birth method promotes such early contact in a controlled environment.

Affectional ties begin to develop in birthing rooms or family-centered maternity settings, which permit prolonged family contact after birth. Rooming-in provides an opportunity for the mother to tune in to her newborn's cues and to begin to identify the unique characteristics of her baby. Early discharge from the hospital or birth center reduces the opportunity for nurses to witness the beginning of the reciprocal mother–newborn relationship. However, observing the mother as she holds or touches the infant, and as she notes the infant's unique characteristics helps identify signs of attachment prior to early discharge.

Family and Cultural Considerations

The family's adaptation to pregnancy depends on the type of family and stages in the family life cycle. The usual interaction patterns and roles of each member also influence the part that is played by the pregnant woman, her partner, and other family members. Realistic expectations for involvement vary with the parents' ages and number of other children in the family. An adolescent may find that her mother continues to make decisions for her during pregnancy, while a 35-year-old woman with several school-age children may have to learn to balance antepartal health visits with car-pooling. The opportunity to discuss family members' participation in childbearing may arise in antepartal classes or during nurse–client interactions during antepartal care visits or postpartum recovery.

Culture often dictates the roles of the partner and other family members during pregnancy. Shared symptoms, such as morning sickness or labor pains (known as couvade syndrome), are common among expectant fathers in some cultures (Fawcett & York, 1986; Strickland, 1987). In other groups, it is rare for the partner to be involved in the pregnancy; his expected role is to provide economic support.

A number of studies have investigated the presence of physical and psychological symptoms in male spouses or partners of pregnant women. Fawcett and York (1986) studied pregnant women and their spouses in early and late pregnancy and during the postpartum period. They found that both spouses experienced minor physical discomforts, such as nausea and vomiting, heartburn, food cravings, backache, fatigue, skin irritations, and urinary frequency. Women reported a higher incidence of physical symptoms than men, most notably during the third trimester of pregnancy. There were no significant differences among men according to their spouses' stage of pregnancy.

Strickland (1987) surveyed expectant fathers during early, middle, and late pregnancy and found greater numbers of psychological and somatic symptoms in men who were African-American or working-class, or in the case of unplanned pregnancy. In contrast to Fawcett and York's (1986) findings, symptoms experienced by white expectant fathers increased throughout pregnancy, whereas African-American expectant fathers reported a decrease in symptoms in later pregnancy.

Each partner brings a different perspective to childbearing, based on personal past experiences in the family of origin. Pregnancy may present a first opportunity for the couple to examine their perceptions of the parenting role. They may decide to follow family cultural patterns closely, to blend the traditions of both families, or to establish new ways of sharing childbearing. The latter is common among immigrant couples eager to adopt customs of their new country.

The single mother from any cultural heritage depends on her extended family. In many situations, these kin are directly involved in antepartal care, labor coaching and child care. Kopala (1989) notes that the sensory- or mobility-impaired woman uses existing support systems or develops new networks among childbearing women with similar disabilities. Older children also may be involved in helping.

Participation in the birth is influenced by cultural values, beliefs, and attitudes. Customs vary with the way in which people of a particular culture view the world, life, and death. Among some groups, rich symbolism and imagery pervade the birth environment.

While it is quite common for the American father to be present during the typical birth in a medically controlled environment, women in traditional cultures often prefer birth in the home setting attended by a woman. A comfortable, familiar chair or bed for delivery may be ideal. If the woman from a traditional culture must deliver in a hospital, environmental adaptations may contribute to a positive experience.

Rituals for cutting the cord, disposing of the placenta, and bathing the newborn may be important for a harmonious birth in some cultural groups. After delivery, the woman may desire some time in seclusion or wish to be surrounded by many family members. Rituals for swaddling the newborn may be prescribed by either cultural or family preference. Spiritual beliefs often include ceremonies for the woman and her child.

Sibling participation in newborn care may be expected in some cultures (Figure 20-5), while in others older children continue with their own lives, helping out now and then. Some degree of ambivalence toward the newborn is often evident among American siblings. An older child may express delight over the new baby, but show embarrassment over the mother's breast-feeding.

As the new family develops, sources of strain may emerge from close living arrangements. In dual career families, the mother often assumes all child care responsibilities. Inequity in sharing tasks may be cultural or the result of prior relationship patterns. Needs of older children reduce opportunities for the couple to enjoy each other. Marital satisfaction may diminish. Extended family members may assist young parents in coping with these

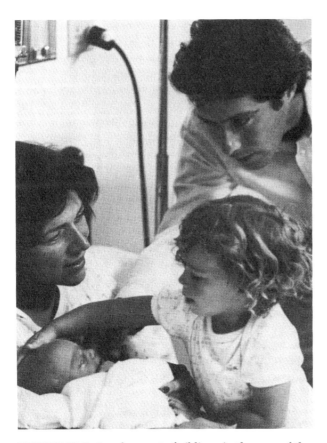

FIGURE 20-5. Involvement of siblings in the care of the newborn helps increase their acceptance of the family newcomer. (*Note.* From Auvenshine/Enriquez: *Comprehensive Maternity Nursing,* Second Edition, © 1990. Boston: Jones and Bartlett Publishers, p. 611.)

stresses. Role models who have managed pregnancy and infant care are helpful and often provide a support network.

Nurses who work with clients from varied cultural and ethnic backgrounds should learn more about the traditions of their clients, so that assessments of variations lead to correct analyses. Recent anthropological and nursing studies contribute much to the knowledge of culture and birth. LaDu (1985) identifies cultural influences on childbearing among Hmong women. Jordan (1987) compares high technology and traditional birth customs in four diverse cultural groups. Interactions between American and Korean mothers and their infants have been described by Choi and Hamilton (1986).

THE NURSING HISTORY

The ideal time to begin antepartal care is very early in pregnancy to ensure continued good health patterns for the woman and the embryo–fetus. However, whether the first antepartal visit occurs in the 4th or 30th week of pregnancy, the client should be made to feel welcome and cared for. It is the woman who decides when to confirm her suspicion that she is pregnant. Patterson, Freese, and Goldenberg (1986) studied the process of self-diagnosis of pregnancy and ways women who believe they are pregnant attempt to reduce the uncertainty associated with self-diagnosis. They conclude that, as is typical in Western cultures, women rely on laboratory or professional confirmation to legitimize their own diagnosis. The authors found, however, varying levels of tolerance for uncertainty among the subjects, which influenced how soon they sought confirmation. Patterson and colleagues (1986) further conclude that a woman's self-diagnosis of pregnancy generally is accurate and suggest that to remove autonomy from the decision to seek care may diminish shared participation.

Gathering accurate and pertinent data on reproductive health can be time-consuming. Since many questions are of a sensitive nature, a trusting relationship must be established first. Privacy during the assessment and clinical appraisal is essential, although the woman may wish to have her partner or another significant person with her. The nurse should ascertain the client's wishes in this matter.

While initial interview forms are useful guides, the nurse often may have to vary the question sequence in response to information provided by the client. A woman may offer information on her family situation or prior birth experiences before she is asked. Or, responding to the question, "How many times have you been pregnant?" a client may offer, "Twice. But the first baby died of a congenital heart problem." The interview focus should change at this point, allowing the woman to express her feelings and perhaps to discuss what she believes caused the problem. Table 20-6 provides a sample nursing history for the pregnant woman.

Pregnancy necessitates some additions and changes in the data to be obtained for nutritional assessment. Not only the mother's health but also the health of the unborn child is affected by the mother's nutritional practices. In addition to the usual nutritional questions asked when taking a history, the nurse should determine:

> The mother's age, because there is a higher risk of nutritional problems during adolescence when greater nutritional needs are already a factor.
>
> Birth weights of the mother's previous children, since a history of low birth weight may indicate nutritional problems.
>
> Maternal weight patterns during previous pregnancies, and weight changes (gain or loss) during this pregnancy.
>
> Interconceptual period, because the mother may have deficient nutritional reserves with repeated pregnancy and lactation and also with the use of steroid contraceptives during the interim.

Weight gain as a single indicator, however, may be misleading. For example, overweight pregnant clients should be assessed carefully for the quality of their diets since they may be consuming high calorie but low nutrient foods. Underweight pregnant clients are especially at risk of delivering premature or low birth weight infants. Women who are underweight may need to be encouraged to gain more weight than the recommended amount.

When evaluating dietary intake, the nurse should determine food loss from vomiting during the first trimester of pregnancy as well as loss of appetite related to nausea. Pica (ingestion of nonnutritive substances) and cravings also should be considered. Determining the presence of pica is important not only because essential nutrients may be replaced by nonfood items but also because of the frequent existence of iron deficiency anemia with pica. Luke (1977) recommends straightforward questioning, for example, "Do you eat cornstarch, laundry starch, ice, paraffin, coffee grounds?" (p. 99). A more open-ended question also should be asked: "Do you crave anything in particular?" (Luke, 1977, p. 99).

Assessment of the pregnant woman's attachment to her unborn baby is also a critical factor that should be noted in the nursing history. How often does the expectant mother talk about her baby? Do her references reveal that she perceives the fetus as a unique individual: "He is the most active baby! I can just imagine what a handful he'll be!" Gaffney's (1988) review of the literature suggests that other indicators of prenatal maternal attachment include consideration of a name for the baby, projecting the child's future, engaging in "conversations" with the fetus, especially in response to fetal movements, decorating the baby's room, seeking information about fetal and child development, and attending childbirth education classes.

It is also important to assess continued attachment of the mother to the infant during the postpartum period. The postpartum nursing history should include assessment of the mother's perceptions of herself as a parent and her perceptions of her infant, as these may change over time. Walker, Crain, and Thompson (1986) studied postpartum maternal role attainment and identity at 1 to 3 days after delivery and then again at 4 to 6 weeks postpartum. They found that mothers felt more positive about themselves in their maternal role over time, but less positive about their infants. The latter finding perhaps could be attributed to the transition the new mother must make from the ideal to the real infant. The researchers also found that multiparas had more positive attitudes about themselves and their infants than primiparas. Implications for the postpartum nursing history include ascertaining new mothers' perceptions of themselves and their babies and the degree of confidence they have about caring for the infant. Expressions of concern or lack of confidence can alert the nurse to look for other cues of maternal attachment and maternal role identity and to detect problems early so appropriate nursing interventions can be designed and implemented.

The expectant or new mother's stressors, coping styles, and available social support also should be asked about during the nursing history. Life stressors have been shown to have a negative effect in pregnant women. Norbeck and Tilden (1983) studied the impact of stress and social support on pregnant women's emotional health and on the incidence of perinatal complications. They found that high life stress and low social support significantly increased the incidence of maternal and neonatal complications. Cranley (1982) found a strong positive association between adequate social support systems and prenatal attachment of the mother to her fetus.

Brown (1986) studied factors related to expectant parents' health and found that social support

TABLE 20-6
Nursing History—The Pregnant Woman

Age (birth date)
Marital status
Indicators of current pregnancy (missed menstrual period, nausea, breast tenderness, results of home pregnancy
  test, other)

Reproductive History
  Gravida, para, aborta
  Onset of menses; usual menstrual cycle; use of pads vs. tampons; problems, how treated
  Use of contraceptives (type, length of use, problems or concerns)
  Date of last menstrual period (LMP); was pregnancy planned?
  Fertility problems (difficulty conceiving); how treated
  Previous pregnancies:
    number, outcomes (live, full-term births, premature or stillbirths, miscarriages or abortions)
    health during previous pregnancies; antepartal care; problems, how treated
  Blood type; if Rh negative, previous administration of RhoGam
History of sexually transmitted disease (STD)—self, partner(s)

Cultural-Environmental History
  Beliefs about pregnancy and childbirth
  Special diet or care during pregnancy and childbirth important to cultural group
  Health hazards (home, workplace)—chemicals, radiation, noise, high temperatures, smoke, physical barriers,
    heavy work (lifting, climbing)
  Immunization history; history of childhood illnesses; especially communicable or infectious diseases
  Use of tobacco, alcohol, other potentially harmful substances
  Medication history—current and previous use (prescription, over-the-counter); IV drug use (self or partner)
  High-risk sexual activity (anal intercourse, bisexual partner)
  Recent exposure to viral illness
  Home environment—living arrangements, facilities (plumbing, heat, refrigeration)
  Economic status—income, health insurance, financial problems
  Health care—major provider, frequency of use; problems with accessibility

Psychosocial-Family History
  Feelings about current pregnancy
  Relationship with partner (satisfaction, problems, how handled)
  Sexuality concerns—impact of pregnancy on sexual relationships, perceptions of self as a sexual person; body
    image changes resulting from the pregnancy; fears or concerns about sex and pregnancy
  Relationships with children, other family members—how current pregnancy has changed or may change these;
    availability of and satisfaction with social support
  Actual or anticipated role changes as a result of this pregnancy
  Perceptions of prenatal attachment to the infant, the self as a parent, parenting knowledge and skills
  Temperament—usual temperament; usual response to stressful situations; recent changes in mood/affect; usual
    coping strategies, effectiveness
  Knowledge about pregnancy, childbirth, and health needs during pregnancy (nutrition, exercise, rest/sleep, health
    hazards)

Physiological History
Physical Integrity
  Usual weight; recent weight gain or loss
  Personal hygiene habits
  Skin changes or problems (acne, chloasma, linea nigra, striae, dryness, rash)
  Allergies—food, medications
  Recent illnesses, fever

Activity–Sleep
  Usual sleep patterns; recent interferences with sleep
  Typical daytime activity patterns; exercise—type, frequency
  Changes in activity/exercise with pregnancy
  Limitations that interfere with activity/exercise

Oxygenation
  Breathing problems
  History of anemia, high blood pressure, varicose veins, headaches, dizziness
  Bleeding or spotting during pregnancy

(continued)

TABLE 20-6 (Continued)

Nutrition
   Typical daily diet; changes in nutritional habits since becoming pregnant
   Special cravings since becoming pregnant; intake of non-nutritive substances (pica)
   Problems that interfere with nutrition—nausea, lack of money, use of foods high in fat, sodium
Fluids–Electrolytes & Elimination
   Daily fluid intake—amounts, types of fluids
   Urinary elimination—frequency, changes since becoming pregnant, problems (urgency, stress incontinence)
   Bowel elimination patterns—changes since becoming pregnant; problems with constipation, hemorrhoids
   Excess perspiration
   Fluid retention—swelling of feet, hands, or face

from the partner and significant others contributed positively to both mothers' and fathers' well-being. However, expectant mothers showed evidence of relying on both partner support and support from others, whereas partner support was more important than support from others to expectant fathers. The nurse should inquire about the presence and quality of partner support as well as support from others, and ascertain the pregnant woman's degree of satisfaction with her social support system. Absence of or dissatisfaction with social support systems may indicate a woman at risk for emotional disequilibrium or physiological complications who will require special nursing attention.

The initial nursing history should be expanded upon in subsequent visits as the client describes changes in comfort levels, new concerns, or sudden problems. An opportunity to discuss feelings should be provided at each antepartal visit, as the woman adapts to her advancing pregnancy. The client's adoption and maintenance of health habits also should be assessed with each visit. Table 20-7 outlines health habits that contribute to optimal pregnancy outcomes. Collaboration of client, nurse, and physician can be enhanced by teaching the pregnant woman about certain changes that should be reported immediately. These changes are delineated in Table 20-8.

CLINICAL APPRAISAL AND SCREENING

During the initial antepartal visit, the nurse should note the client's general appearance and affect. The clinical appraisal (Table 20-9) usually focuses first on confirming the pregnancy, and second on the woman's physiological and psychosocial responses to the event.

Confirmation of Pregnancy

At the initial visit, the nurse should note the client's general appearance. While the woman may have performed a pregnancy test at home, this pro-

cedure should be repeated. The presence of HCG in maternal urine can be detected about 10 days after a missed menstrual period. A positive pregnancy test, the cessation of menses, and onset of morning sickness are not, however, considered definitive signs of pregnancy. Diagnosis is not confirmed until fetal outline or movement is detected by the examiner. Visualizing the fetus with ultrasound, hearing the fetal heart beat, or palpating fetal parts are definitive signs that the client is pregnant.

The nurse can estimate the woman's delivery date using Naegele's Rule. The expected date of confinement (EDC) is calculated by subtracting 3 months and adding 7 days from the first day of the last regular menstrual period (see boxed insert). If the woman is unsure of the exact time of her last period, application of the rule is more difficult. The anticipated birth date is a rough estimate given in the range of plus or minus one week. As preg-

TABLE 20-7
Positive Health Habits During Pregnancy

- Keeps antepartal appointments
- Adheres to professional recommendations
- Increases daily calcium, protein, vitamin, and mineral intake
- Eats balanced meals with sufficient fluids
- Rests in left lateral position
- Exercises at least 3 times weekly for 15 minutes
- Modifies work/home environment to reduce hazards
- Avoids alcohol, tobacco, drugs and over-the-counter medications
- Reports all problems to health-care provider
- Maintains adequate personal and dental hygiene
- Uses social support networks
- Collaborates with health-care provider in making decisions that affect own health and that of embryo–fetus

TABLE 20-8
Changes to Be Reported to Nurse or Physician Immediately

- Excessive first trimester vomiting
- Prolonged vomiting past third month
- Headache or visual changes
- Edema of the hands or face
- Epigastric pain
- Bleeding or spotting at any time
- Leaking amniotic fluid
- Change in fetal activity
- Increased personal/family stress
- Infection
- Trauma

nancy progresses, uterine and fetal growth may alter estimation of the due date.

Weight Changes

Weight patterns before conception provide baseline data for assessments during pregnancy. Weights at the initial and monthly antepartal visits are compared to those expected in each trimester. The woman's stature, body frame, nutrition, exercise patterns, and general health influence the desired weight gain for her. Weight changes should be plotted on a prenatal weight gain chart on an ongoing basis (see Figure 20-1). Expected weight gain in a pregnant American woman is 24 to 29 pounds (Table 20-10). The recommended weight gain is for women of normal prepregnancy weight or those who were overweight prior to pregnancy. Weight gain should occur in a smooth, progressive fashion: little weight gain during the first trimester followed by a gradual, steady increase.

Ideal weight patterns are evaluated individu-

Naegele's Rule

Subtract 3 months from first day of last regular menstrual period, then add 7 days.

Example:
First day of last menstrual period — August 12th
Subtract 3 months — May 12th
Add 7 days — May 19th

May 19th (of the subsequent year) is the woman's "due date."

TABLE 20-9
Clinical Appraisal of the Pregnant Woman

Confirmation of pregnancy
Weight changes
Vital signs/oxygenation
  Blood pressure
  Rollover test
  Fetal heart tones
Skin integrity
Nutritional status
Elimination (urinalysis)
Abdominal assessment
  Measurement of fundal height
  Ballottement
  Leopold's maneuvers
  Palpation of uterine contractions
Lactation and breast-feeding
  Milk production
  Breast-feeding process
Maternal role acquisition and attachment behaviors

ally. For instance, if the client conceives while underweight, advice for total weight gain may vary from the usual 24 to 29 pounds. A sudden change in weight from one visit to the next, even though it may be within the usual range for the trimester, should be evaluated further. For example, a gain in excess of two pounds in one week, accompanied by proteinuria and altered reflex responses, may be an early indication of pregnancy-induced hypertension.

If a poor weight gain pattern is observed, the client should be asked about protein intake, deliberate weight reduction, or purging (use of emetics or laxatives to evacuate the stomach or bowel). Inadequate maternal nutrition increases the risk of a low birth weight newborn or adverse effects on fetal brain development. Repeating the 24-hour diet recall may be indicated. Diagnostic tests for fetal growth may be indicated.

The pregnant woman should be examined during each antepartal visit for evidence of fluid retention. While the presence of postural edema of the feet and ankles is common during pregnancy, swelling of the hands and face is never normal. Such edema commonly accompanies sudden weight gain and generally indicates complications requiring medical intervention.

Vital Signs and Oxygenation

Assessment of vital signs at the initial visit provides baseline data. Pulse rate generally remains stable during pregnancy, fluctuating with activity

TABLE 20-10
Distribution of Weight Gain During Pregnancy

Component	Approximate Weight (lb)
Fetus	7½ (5–10)
Placenta	1½
Amniotic fluid	2
Uterus	2
Mother's tissue fluid	3
Blood volume	4
Breasts*	½
Fat and other reserve+	3½
Total	24

*The increase is much greater in some women and is considered as reserve.

+In some women, fat reserve may be as high as 8 lb.

Note. From Hui: *Human Nutrition and Diet Therapy,* © 1983. Boston: Jones and Bartlett Publishers.

and rest patterns. A slight increase in heart and respiratory rates is common as the uterus displaces the diaphragm. Body temperature should remain normal. Any elevation should be reported immediately.

Comparison of blood pressure to preconception and earlier antepartal measurements should be performed at each visit. While blood pressure may decrease slightly during the second trimester, little change is expected in the healthy client. The blood pressure should be taken in both arms; if it is elevated, it is repeated in a left lateral position. A rising diastolic pressure is of greater concern than systolic changes. Generally, a 15 mm or more rise in the diastolic, a 30 mm or more increase in the systolic, or an overall rise to 140/90 or higher is cause for concern (Pritchard et al., 1985).

The *rollover test* is used between the 28th and 32nd weeks of pregnancy as a predictive assessment for pregnancy-induced hypertension (preeclampsia). While the test is not highly accurate, an abnormal result is helpful in identifying risk. This test is performed by measuring the client's blood pressure while she rests in the left lateral position. She then is assisted in rolling over to her back. Blood pressure is measured again while she is supine. If there is an increase of more than 20 mm, the test is considered positive, and the client is evaluated more frequently for signs of pregnancy-induced hypertension.

As pregnancy advances, the thoracic cage widens at the base and the diaphragm is displaced toward the lungs. During the second and third trimesters, an increased respiratory rate and short-

ness of breath are common. When the uterus settles into the pelvis at lightening, the diaphragm returns to normal position.

It is common to hear a systolic murmur over the pulmonary valve at the second left intercostal space. This finding is normal and is related to fluid volume shift. Additional murmurs may be heard at the mitral and tricuspid valves.

Fetal Heart Tones

Fetal heart tones may be measured with an electronic device as early as the 10th week of pregnancy. The client should be positioned on her back, with knees slightly flexed. The clear, rapid beat is heard at the fetal back. A slower, whistling sound indicates the flow of uterine blood through the placenta. When the nurse is in doubt, the maternal radial pulse is compared to the apparent fetal rate. The expected fetal heart rate is between 120 and 160 beats per minute.

At subsequent visits, the nurse should use a fetoscope or a doppler to assess the fetal heart tones (see Figures 20-6 and 20-7). As the fetus grows, its outline may be palpated more easily through the abdominal wall. In order to determine the point of maximum intensity for the fetal heart rate, the fetal back, arms, legs, and head are located. *Leopold's maneuvers,* illustrated in Figures 20-8 to 20-11 facilitate assessment of fetal presentation and position closer to term. With the woman resting on her back, the nurse gently palpates the abdomen in four movements. After locating the fetal back, the nurse should listen to the heart beat for one full minute. Often the fetus responds to this stimulation by kicking and moving away from the examiner.

Late in pregnancy, a nonstress test may be indicated to electronically monitor fetal heart rate responses to activity. Adequacy of placental oxygen is evaluated by a fetal heart rate increase with movement. In a high risk pregnancy, an oxytocin challenge test or a contraction stress test may be necessary. Since dilute pitocin is administered to induce mild uterine contractions, this test is performed in a hospital. Fetal heart rate responses to contractions are noted. A normal fetal heart rate pattern during contractions indicates adequate placental function.

During labor, fetal heart rate may be assessed by intermittent or continuous use of an electronic fetal monitor. A pattern of bradycardia, tachycardia, or deceleration (a drop in heart rate) not con-

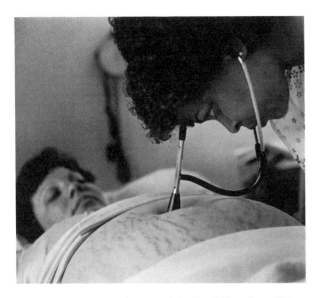

FIGURE 20-6. Auscultation of the Fetal Heartbeat Using the Fetoscope. (*Note.* From Auvenshine/Enriquez: *Comprehensive Maternity Nursing,* Second Edition, © 1990. Boston: Jones and Bartlett Publishers, p. 362.)

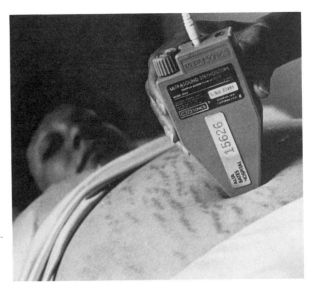

FIGURE 20-7. A Doppler Used for Fetal Heart Rate Assessment. (*Note.* From Auvenshine/Enriquez: *Comprehensive Maternity Nursing,* Second Edition, © 1990. Boston: Jones and Bartlett Publishers, p. 363.)

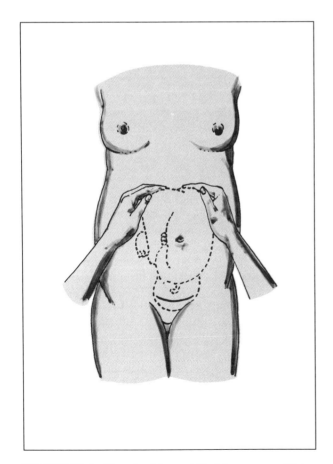

FIGURE 20-8. Step 1 of Leopold's Maneuvers. (*Note.* From Auvenshine/Enriquez: *Comprehensive Maternity Nursing,* Second Edition, © 1990. Boston: Jones and Bartlett Publishers, p. 326.)

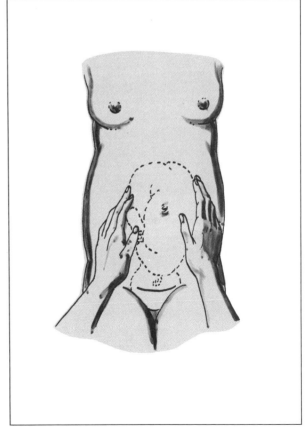

FIGURE 20-9. Step 2 of Leopold's Maneuvers. (*Note.* From Auvenshine/Enriquez: *Comprehensive Maternity Nursing,* Second Edition, © 1990. Boston: Jones and Bartlett Publishers, p. 326.)

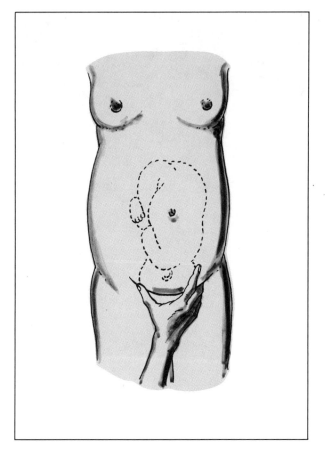

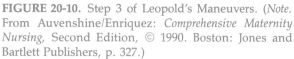

FIGURE 20-10. Step 3 of Leopold's Maneuvers. (*Note.* From Auvenshine/Enriquez: *Comprehensive Maternity Nursing,* Second Edition, © 1990. Boston: Jones and Bartlett Publishers, p. 327.)

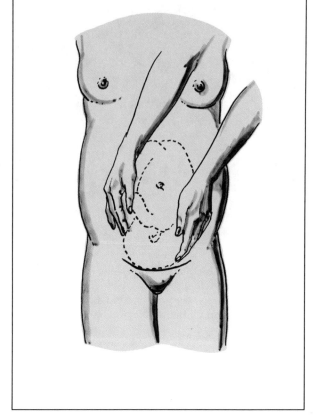

FIGURE 20-11. Step 4 of Leopold's Maneuvers. (*Note.* From Auvenshine/Enriquez: *Comprehensive Maternity Nursing,* Second Edition, © 1990. Boston: Jones and Bartlett Publishers, p. 327.)

current with uterine contractions is a sign of fetal distress. The client should be turned to the left side, given oxygen, and assessed further. In some situations, a Caesarean delivery is performed as a fetal life-saving measure.

Skin Integrity

Palpation and inspection of skin integrity is an essential part of antepartal assessment. The nurse should note skin color, dryness, tone, hygiene, and the presence of a rash, acne, or angiomas. Many women notice increased perspiration during pregnancy. Pigmentation changes around the eyes, *chloasma*, appears as mottling. Swelling around the eyes is not normal and may be related to hypertension.

Swelling and bleeding of the gums and the appearance of small nodules are quite common and related to estrogen levels. However, inflammation also may indicate vitamin deficiency. Nasal membranes may appear slightly swollen, and the client may report stuffiness. Slight thyroid enlargement is common during pregnancy.

Breast changes prepare the woman for lactation. Enlargement, nodules, and prominent veins on the breasts are characteristic of advancing pregnancy. After the initial visit, palpation of the breasts for masses is deferred because of pregnancy-associated tenderness. Secretion of colostrum may be noted after the 10th week. Advice from health-care providers varies about the hand expression of colostrum during pregnancy. While gentle stimulation probably is not harmful, vigorous massage may lead to preterm labor. Women with identified risk conditions are advised not to express colostrum.

Striae or stretch marks may be evident on breasts, thighs, and abdomen (see Figure 20-12). In the dark skinned woman, changes in skin appearance may be less apparent.

During the postpartum period, inspection of the healing episiotomy or repaired perineal lacera-

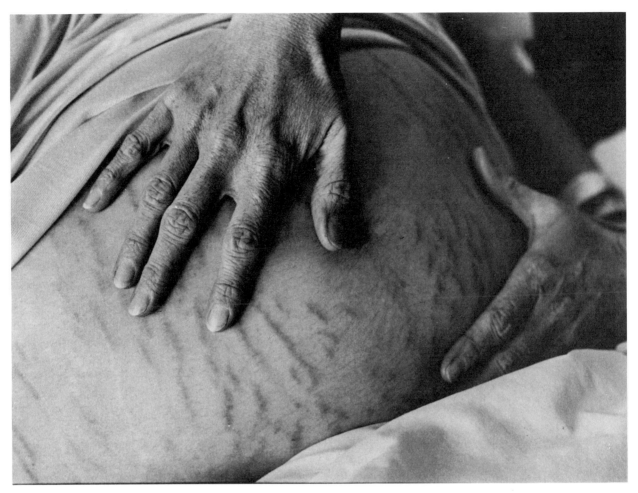

FIGURE 20-12. Abdominal striae should be noted. (*Note.* From Auvenshine/Enriquez: *Comprehensive Maternity Nursing,* Second Edition, © 1990. Boston: Jones and Bartlett Publishers, p. 324.)

tion should be performed during hospitalization and following discharge. Bruising, swelling, drainage, or poor approximation of wound edges should be noted. Inflammation usually subsides within one week, although tenderness to touch may continue for several weeks. The response of the episiotomy to a heat lamp or sitz baths should be noted as these may enhance healing.

Lower extremities are assessed for swelling, redness, or tenderness. A negative Homan's sign indicates absence of thrombophlebitis. With the client resting in the supine position, toes are flexed toward her head. She should experience no pain with this movement.

Postpartum vaginal discharge occurs as the outer layer of the uterine endometrial lining is sloughed off. This discharge, known as *lochia*, should be assessed as a reliable indicator of normal involution (return of the uterus to a nonpregnant state). Table 20-11 delineates the changing characteristics of lochia when involution progresses as expected.

Skin discolorations, such as chloasma and linea nigra, gradually fade and disappear within 6 to 8 weeks following delivery. The purplish color associated with striae (stretch marks) of the abdomen changes to silver-white within a few months. Stretch marks themselves, however, do not disappear.

Abdominal Assessment

Uterine and fetal growth are estimated by measuring fundal height. This palpation assessment is performed after the client empties her bladder. There is a gradual rise of the fundus as fetal growth occurs (see Table 20-12 and Figure 20-13). The level of the fundus is usually at the umbilicus at about 20 weeks. By the 38th week, the fundal height is at the xiphoid process. The use of McDonald's rule (the height of the fundus × 8/7 = duration of pregnancy in weeks) provides an estimate of appropriate fetal growth.

Abdominal palpation also includes *ballotte-*

TABLE 20-11
Characteristics of Lochia

Type of Lochia	Color	Duration	Composition
Rubra	Red	1–3 days	Blood, fragments of decidua and mucus
Serosa	Pink or brown-tinged	3–10 days	Blood, mucus, and leukocytes
Alba	White	10–14 days May last for 6 weeks	Predominantly mucus; leukocyte count high

ment, in which the examiner feels the resistance and rebounding of fetal body parts in the amniotic fluid. Occasionally, uterine fibroids may be identified. Gas pockets may be evident as peristalsis slows.

The pregnant woman may report feeling fetal movements around the 18th week of pregnancy. The nurse may observe such activity during physical appraisal. Braxton-Hicks uterine contractions may be palpated during the third trimester, as the uterus tightens and relaxes.

Tissue changes in reproductive organs are evident on pelvic examination. The lower uterine segment softens (*Hegar's sign*), as does the cervix (*Goodell's sign*). A bluish discoloration is evident on the vulva and cervix (*Chadwick's sign*).

Extremities should be palpated for the presence of edema. While leg and ankle swellings are normal late in the day for pregnant women, puffiness of hands and fingers is abnormal and should be brought to the attention of the health-care provider.

Clinical appraisal of the postpartal client includes inspection and palpation of the abdomen. The uterus should be firm and well-contracted. Fundal height descends about one finger breadth daily, until it is barely evident (see Figure 20-14). A

slight separation of the rectus muscles may be noted while palpating the abdomen. During the assessment, the client should relax on her back with knees flexed, then raise her head and shoulders slightly. Any separation is measured in finger breadths.

Assessment of Lactation and Breast-Feeding

The breasts of the lactating mother should be assessed postpartum. Nipples should be inspected for cracks, redness, or soreness. The breasts fill gradually, becoming engorged or distended on the second or third day. Discomfort is usually present

TABLE 20-12
Fundal Heights and Estimated Gestation

Fundal Height	Weeks
At level of symphysis pubis	12
Halfway between symphysis pubis and umbilicus (usually about 4 fingerbreadths above symphysis pubis)	16
1–2 fingerbreadths below umbilicus	20
1–2 fingerbreadths above umbilicus	24
One-third of distance between umbilicus and xiphoid process	28–30
Two-thirds of distance between umbilicus and xiphoid process	32
1–2 fingerbreadths below xiphoid process	36–38
2–3 fingerbreadths below xiphoid process if lightening occurs	40

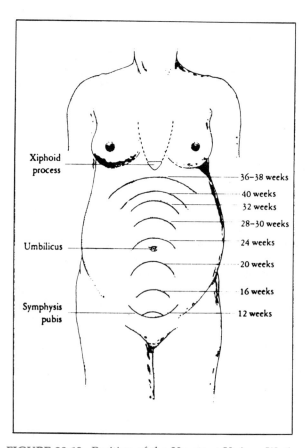

FIGURE 20-13. Position of the Uterus at Various Weeks of Gestation. (*Note.* From Auvenshine/Enriquez: *Comprehensive Maternity Nursing,* Second Edition, © 1990. Boston: Jones and Bartlett Publishers, p. 325.)

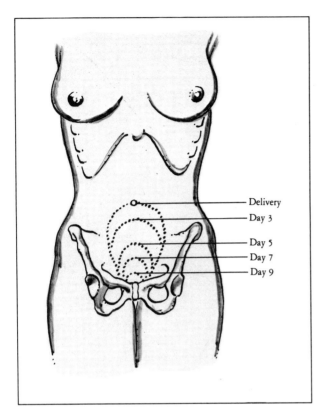

FIGURE 20-14. Involution of the Uterus. (*Note*. From Auvenshine/Enriquez: *Comprehensive Maternity Nursing*, Second Edition, © 1990. Boston: Jones and Bartlett Publishers, p. 424.)

and may be relieved by using warm compresses prior to breast-feeding. In order to produce sufficient milk to satisfy a newborn, the lactating mother should empty both breasts with each feeding.

While assessment of milk production is difficult, the woman may be observed during breast-feeding. An assessment guide such as shown in Table 20-13 may be helpful. The nurse should observe the mother's initiation of breast-feeding, the infant's position on the breast, and the mother's ability to take the baby off the breast correctly.

Feeding on both breasts should begin with five-minute periods, gradually increasing the time over the next several feedings. The mother should be advised to sit in a comfortable chair with arm rests, so that she can relax during feeding. The newborn's mouth should cover the nipple areola completely (see Figures 20-15 through 20-21). Usually the sucking infant obtains sufficient volume to satisfy hunger in the first 20 minutes of feeding. If the newborn sucks vigorously, the volume produced can exceed 800 ml daily. This natural food provides sufficient nutrition for the first several months of life. Because medications taken by the mother may pass through breast milk, the woman

must be aware of and minimize all possible risks of over-the-counter and prescription drugs. Sucking needs beyond that needed to empty the breasts may be met with a pacifier. Gradual newborn weight gain and a contented baby indicate adequate lactation.

Role Acquisition and Attachment

Assessment of role acquisition and attachment is difficult without consistent contact with the mother during pregnancy and following delivery. Behaviors observed on the delivery day or the first day after birth may be affected by pain, fatigue, or treatment (Hans, 1986). Prior losses, birth of a child different from the desired sex, and lack of resolution of her own developmental tasks may result in the mother's initial indifference to her newborn. Goodness-of-fit in the parent–infant dyad is critical (Mercer, 1985).

Patterns of interaction over time reflect satisfaction in the mothering role (see Figure 20-22). A contented baby whose behavior indicates a sense of trust reflects nurturing parenting. Competence in the maternal role may be assessed by patterns of compliance with clinic appointments, safe handling of the infant, and adequate care given to the infant during illness. Table 20-14 summarizes positive indicators of antepartal and postpartal attachment to the infant.

The community health or clinic nurse usually has an opportunity to assess maternal–infant attachment. During a visit the nurse should observe the mother's reaction to the baby and the infant's response. Statements about pleasurable and bothersome tasks of parenting contribute to the assessment.

Tools for assessing maternal–infant interactions are available and have been used widely. With early postpartum discharge, the nurse's opportunity to observe behaviors over time is limited.

Palisin (1981) suggests that nurses carefully observe the mother and infant during contact in the delivery room, postpartal unit, and clinic. She believes that a nurse–client relationship based on open communication may be more valuable than completing a detailed assessment during a single observation. Young (1982) provides a list of potential indicators to assess parent–infant problems (Table 20-15).

NURSING DIAGNOSES RELATED TO THE PREGNANT WOMAN

Analysis of data leads to individualized nursing diagnoses that form the basis of a care plan. Since there are so many normal variations in a healthy

TABLE 20-13
A Breast-Feeding Assessment Tool

Needs or Problems	Need or Problem Active	Need Met or Problem Resolved
Supportive needs		
1. Early initiation of breastfeeding (note when baby first breastfed).		
2. Correct position is being used (observed twice).		
3. Baby is feeding on a demand schedule.		
4. Baby is receiving no supplements. (If so, state reason.)		
5. Let-down reflex is present.		
6. Mother makes positive statements about her feeding skills.		
7. Support is present after mother goes home.		
Teaching needs		
1. Advantages and disadvantages of breastfeeding (usually done prenatally).		
2. Knowledge of breasts and their function.		
3. Breast care.		
Wash once daily with no soap.		
Air dry for 10–15 minutes after feedings.		
Knowledge of lubricants and their use.		
Use of both breasts at each feeding.		
Knowledge of how to take baby off the breast.		
Inverted or retracted nipples—use of breast cups (may have been done prenatally).		
4. Diet for breastfeeding.		
5. How to tell if baby is getting enough.		
6. Growth spurts.		
7. Infant feeding behavior.		
8. Normal infant stool patterns.		
9. Additional reading sources.		
Breastfeeding problems (hospital/home/well-baby visit)		
Possible hospital problems:		
1. Engorgement		
2. Sore nipples		
3. Difficult attachment		
Later problems:		
4. Colicky baby		
5. Mastitis		
6. Slow weight gain		
7. Other		

Note. From Auvenshine/Enriquez: *Comprehensive Maternity Nursing,* Second Edition, © 1990. Boston: Jones and Bartlett Publishers, p. 442.

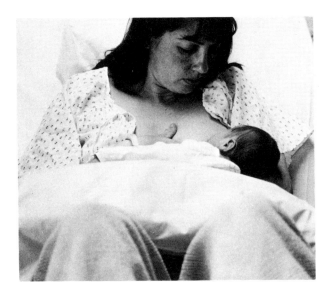

FIGURE 20-15. A Comfortable Breast-Feeding Position with Pillows Placed Between Bent Knees of Mother and Baby. (*Note.* From Auvenshine/Enriquez: *Comprehensive Maternity Nursing,* Second Edition, © 1990. Boston: Jones and Bartlett Publishers, p. 443.)

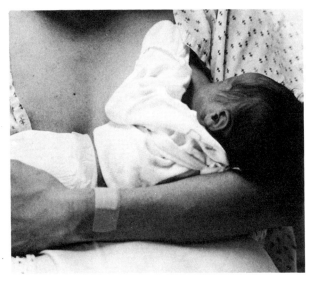

FIGURE 20-16. Infant Placed Across Abdomen with Head in Mother's Anecubital Fossa. Infant entirely faces the mother. (*Note.* From Auvenshine/Enriquez: *Comprehensive Maternity Nursing,* Second Edition, © 1990. Boston: Jones and Bartlett Publishers, p. 443.)

pregnancy, the nurse may experience difficulty in separating expected adaptations, potential problems, and actual deviations.

Nutrition, exercise patterns, and lifestyle affect metabolism and elimination. The most common alterations are noted during the third trimester as the uterus enlarges to accommodate the developing fetus. Peristalsis diminishes and the potential for

constipation exists even though adequate fluids and fiber-rich foods are included in the daily diet. This expected change in late pregnancy should be assessed and, if present, a nursing diagnosis of "constipation" should be made as a basis for nursing care planning.

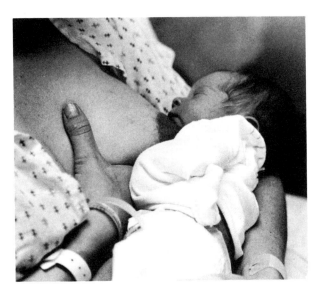

FIGURE 20-17. The thumb is placed on the upper breast and the fingers and hand under the breast to give the breast good support. (*Note.* From Auvenshine/Enriquez: *Comprehensive Maternity Nursing,* Second Edition, © 1990. Boston: Jones and Bartlett Publishers, p. 443.)

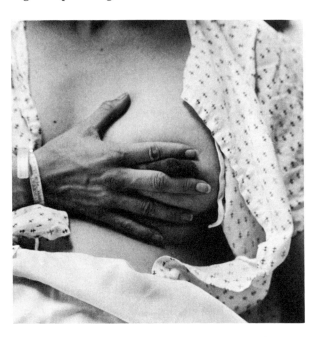

FIGURE 20-18. The cigarette hold is frequently recommended for breastfeeding; however, having thumb and fingers spread is more effective. (*Note.* From Auvenshine/Enriquez: *Comprehensive Maternity Nursing,* Second Edition, © 1990. Boston: Jones and Bartlett Publishers, p. 443.)

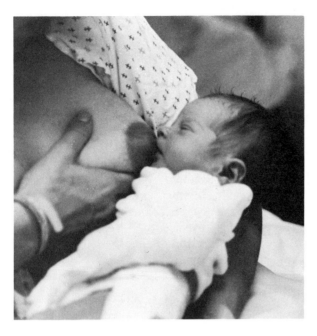

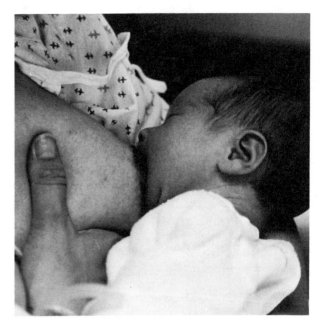

FIGURE 20-19. The mother tickles the infant's upper lip with her nipple. (*Note.* From Auvenshine/Enriquez: *Comprehensive Maternity Nursing*, Second Edition, © 1990. Boston: Jones and Bartlett Publishers, p. 444.)

FIGURE 20-20. If the mother will wait patiently, the infant will open widely. (*Note.* From Auvenshine/Enriquez: *Comprehensive Maternity Nursing*, Second Edition, © 1990. Boston: Jones and Bartlett Publishers, p. 444.)

Increased uterine size also affects urinary bladder function, as noted earlier in this chapter. If the client reports frequency in voiding, with no reported burning or dysuria, the problem generally

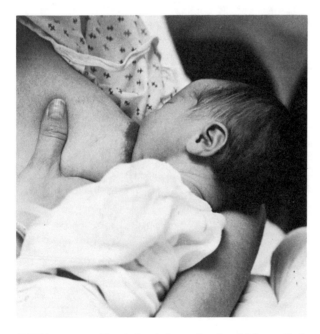

FIGURE 20-21. The infant's buttocks should be pulled toward the mother's torso. (*Note.* From Auvenshine/Enriquez: *Comprehensive Maternity Nursing*, Second Edition, © 1990. Boston: Jones and Bartlett Publishers, p. 444.)

is related to fetal pressure. A urine specimen should be obtained and analyzed to rule out the presence of infection. Any pattern of "altered urinary elimination" should be diagnosed, with the appropriate statement based on the client's reported symptoms and confirming findings.

As the woman's figure changes in response to fetal growth, she sees herself differently than before her pregnancy. During the second trimester, both expectant parents often view the physical changes positively. During the third trimester, however, mobility is reduced and backaches increase as the abdomen enlarges. It is common for the pregnant woman to express her feelings about bodily changes and to wish impatiently for the pregnancy to end. Self-concept is altered as weight is gained and body dimensions enlarge. The nurse should be alert for behaviors that indicate the client is seriously disturbed about her appearance or that she becomes careless in grooming. Even in the absence of such negative observations, a nursing diagnosis of "body image disturbance" may be indicated based on verbalized feelings about normal pregnancy adaptations.

Normal variations in skin integrity and mucous membranes usually are related to hormonal changes in pregnancy. A nursing diagnosis of "altered oral mucous membrane" should be made if swelling and bleeding of the gums are noted, even though this is an expected change of pregnancy.

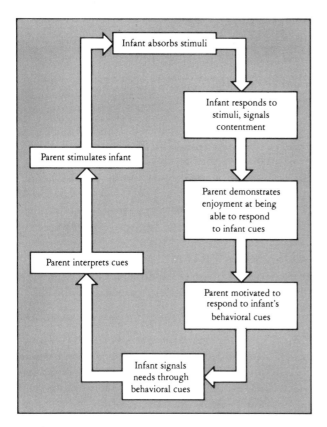

FIGURE 20-22. Response to Stimulation: Reciprocal Responses of Parent and Infant. (*Note.* From Auvenshine/Enriquez: *Comprehensive Maternity Nursing,* Second Edition, © 1990. Boston: Jones and Bartlett Publishers, p. 632.)

However, pain, discharge, and excessive bleeding from oral mucous membranes are abnormal, and the client should be referred to a dentist for further evaluation. Inadequate mouth care or malnutrition may be contributing factors.

Every woman in labor experiences some discomfort during labor and delivery. Pain perception is affected by a variety of factors, including fetal presentation and position, length of labor, maternal pain tolerance, and culturally conditioned responses. A nursing diagnosis of "pain" is commonly made as part of the intrapartal nursing care plan. However, the nurse should identify the specific etiological factors and the woman's ability to cope with the discomfort, as well as her responses to pain-relieving measures, including pharmacological agents.

Should an episiotomy be necessary to facilitate delivery, healing of the site should be assessed carefully. In the absence of infection, inspection of the area should reveal an intact surgical incision, free of redness with minimal swelling. The client may experience some discomfort in walking, depending on the type of episiotomy performed. A nursing diagnosis of "impaired skin integrity" is appropriate until healing of the episiotomy is complete.

When the mother is experiencing success in breast-feeding her infant, a diagnosis of "effective breast-feeding" related to, for example, adequate knowledge, family support, maternal confidence, or a healthy infant may be indicated. This positively stated nursing diagnosis allows the nurse to emphasize an area of strength as the mother adapts to her maternal role. Clinical signs in this instance indicate that breast-feeding is a positive and satisfactory process for both mother and infant.

A diagnosis of "ineffective breast-feeding" may be indicated when the mother is experiencing difficulty in achieving successful breast-feeding of her newborn. Factors that may contribute to this diagnosis include maternal anxiety or ambivalence about breast-feeding, insufficient knowledge about breast-feeding, or an unsupportive partner or family. Premature infants often have poor sucking re-

TABLE 20-14
Positive Indicators of Role Taking/Attachment

The Pregnant Woman	The New Mother
Accepts responsibility for health management	Attaches to the newborn ("en face" position, touches baby, etc.)
Resolves identity crisis	Eager to learn about infant development
Maintains an intimate relationship with significant other	Has realistic expectations of newborn needs
Sees the fetus as a separate, dependent being	Gives safe care
Prepares for the childbirth experience	Conveys empathy to infant (responds to distress cues appropriately)
Bonds to the fetus (refers to the baby as "he" or "she," pleased by fetal movements, "talks" to baby, etc.)	Nurtures (cuddles, soothes, talks to baby)
Plans for parenting responsibilities	

Note. Adapted from "Parenting during middle-adolescence: A review of developmental theories and parenting behaviors," by M. Young, *Maternal-Child Nursing Journal* (Vol. 17, Spring 1988, pp. 1–12; published at the University of Pittsburgh), with permission of the editor and the author.

TABLE 20-15
Potential Problem Indicators in Parent–Infant Interaction

1. Does not have fun with or enjoy the baby.
2. Is disappointed over the sex of the child.
3. Sees the infant as ugly or unattractive.
4. Avoids direct eye contact with the infant.
5. Is annoyed at having to change the infant's diapers.
6. Is disgusted by the infant's drooling.
7. Is upset by vomiting, but may also seem fascinated by it.
8. Is preoccupied by the odor, consistency, and number of stools.
9. Lets the infant's head dangle, without support or concern.
10. Holds the infant away from the body, avoiding close cuddling and skin-to-skin contact.
11. Does not talk or coo with the infant.
12. Thinks that the infant does not love her (or him).
13. Is jealous of the infant and will not allow others to care for him or her.
14. Either underfeeds or overfeeds the infant.
15. Plays with infant roughly after feeding, even though it makes the infant vomit.
16. Expects the infant to respond as an older child would.
17. Leaves the infant in the crib alone, most of the time.
18. Constantly demands reassurance for self and the infant.
19. Does not know how to comfort the infant.
20. Does not find pleasure in caring for the infant.

Note. From Young, R.K. (1982). *Community Nursing Workbook.* Norwalk, CT: Appleton-Century-Crofts, p. 180. Reprinted by permission.

flexes and thus may contribute to breast-feeding difficulties.

When the new parents begin to care for their infant at home, many adaptations occur. Feeding schedules require adjustments in social activities, sleep and meal times, and couple interaction. Fatigue and loss of energy commonly are reported by new mothers. If the mother's hemoglobin is within normal range and there are no problems such as excessive bleeding, a diagnosis of "sleep pattern disturbance" should be made. Insomnia, depression, or severe mood changes accompanying fatigue should be reported.

In some childbearing women, obvious deviations from normal adaptations may occur. For example, postural edema during evening hours is an expected change in the third trimester of pregnancy. Should the pregnant woman experience edema accompanied by hypertension and pro-

teinuria, the actual problem of "fluid volume excess" may be related to arteriospasm and vasoconstriction. Manifestations should be noted at each visit. Responses to therapy may indicate that the problem is resolved. Edema of the hands and face should alert the nurse that the actual problem has worsened and warrants referral.

Nurses are beginning to focus on clients' strengths as well as actual or potential problems, especially in healthy clients. Stolte (1986) advocates this approach for maternity clients, so that strengths as well as problems are identified. Such emphasis is particularly appropriate when the data suggest positive maternal role transition or adaptive coping. For example, the client who uses support systems appropriately, adapts to stress with exercise or practiced relaxation, and modifies risk behaviors to maintain health during pregnancy is coping positively with her pregnancy and soon-to-

TABLE 20-16
Nursing Diagnoses Related to the Pregnant Woman

Body image disturbance related to physical changes of pregnancy

Ineffective breast-feeding related to maternal anxiety, premature infant, knowledge deficit, or nonsupportive partner/family

Constipation related to advancing pregnancy, pressure of growing fetus on lower colon, inadequate dietary fluids and fiber, or inadequate exercise and activity

Fluid volume excess related to effects of pregnancy

Altered oral mucous membrane related to effects of pregnancy or inadequate oral hygiene

Pain related to uterine contractions during labor or episiotomy incision

Altered sexuality patterns related to knowledge deficit about effects of pregnancy on sexuality

Impaired skin integrity related to effects of pregnancy or episiotomy incision

Sleep pattern disturbance related to minor discomforts of pregnancy or demands of caring for newborn infant

Altered urinary elimination related to uterine pressure during first or third trimester

change roles. A nursing diagnosis of "effective coping" acknowledges the client's successful adaptation to pregnancy and the maternal role.

Stevens (1988) expresses optimism for a changing approach to nursing diagnoses in the childbearing care environment. Simple changes in terminology may enable nurses to build on clients' existing strengths. Using positive descriptors, rather than primarily negative, problem-oriented terms, focuses on healthy processes. When health alterations are evident, Stevens suggest a dual approach to organizing data. Thus, the childbearing woman's health record may indicate several positive diagnoses based on adaptations in addition to several more traditional problem-oriented diagnostic statements. During the course of antepartal care, changes in diagnostic statements may reflect resolution of problems or successful attainment of the maternal role.

Table 20-16 summarizes commonly identified nursing diagnoses for the pregnant woman.

Chapter Highlights

■ Knowledge of the biophysical and psychosocial changes associated with pregnancy serves as a basis for nursing assessment of the pregnant woman.

■ The impact of pregnancy and childbirth on the woman's skin integrity, activity–sleep patterns, oxygenation, nutritional requirements, fluid–electrolyte balance, and elimination patterns should be assessed carefully.

■ The pregnant woman and her embryo–fetus are susceptible to numerous health hazards in the environment, which should be assessed for specific risk factors.

■ Assessment of the impact of pregnancy and childbearing on the woman's sexuality, role enactment, and role acquisition is essential.

■ Family and cultural beliefs, customs, and values play a significant role in the pregnancy–childbearing experience and should be assessed in order to identify unique needs or problems.

■ The nursing history of the pregnant woman should be adapted to incorporate patterns and responses unique to pregnancy and childbearing.

■ Clinical appraisal of the pregnant woman should include confirmation of the pregnancy; use of special techniques for assessing vital signs, fetal heart tones, and palpation of the abdomen; and attention to observable indicators of health during pregnancy.

■ Postpartum assessment should include appraisal of lactation and breast-feeding, involution, and behavioral cues of maternal role acquisition and attachment.

■ The findings of the nursing assessment should be analyzed and interpreted to formulate nursing diagnoses unique to the pregnant woman and her childbearing experience.

Practice Activities

1. Obtain a complete nursing history (see Table 20-6) from three pregnant women: one in her first trimester of pregnancy, one in her second trimester, and one in her third trimester. Analyze the data and formulate appropriate nursing diagnoses. Compare and contrast the data and the nursing diagnoses for each of the three clients. What are the similarities? differences?

2. Perform a complete nutritional assessment on a woman who is in her third trimester of pregnancy and, if possible, a breast-feeding mother during the first six weeks postpartum (see Chapter 18 for guidelines). Analyze the data and formulate appropriate nursing diagnoses.

3. Interview three pregnant women from different ethnic/cultural backgrounds concerning the values, beliefs, and customs associated with pregnancy and childbirth in their respective cultural groups (see Chapter 8 for suggested approaches). Compare and contrast their responses. What are the implications for nursing interventions?

4. Interview a woman during her first pregnancy using the following questions as a guide:
   a. Describe your baby. What do you expect your baby to be like?
      What hopes do you have for your baby? What are you doing to prepare for your baby's arrival?
   b. Describe yourself as a mother. What kind of parent do you think you will be? What qualities or skills do you think are important for new mothers to have?

Analyze her responses for evidence of prenatal maternal attachment and prenatal maternal role attainment and identity. What conclusions can you draw?

5. Conduct a clinical appraisal of two pregnant women of different races for skin integrity changes. Compare and contrast your findings.

6. Perform Leopold's maneuvers on a full-term pregnant woman, and auscultate fetal heart tones using a fetoscope and a doppler. Compare findings with maternal pulse rate. What conclusions can you draw about fetal position and fetal heart rate?

7. Interview a pregnant woman about potential or actual health hazards in her home and work environments. What are the risks to the mother and to the fetus? What modifications are suggested?

8. Observe the interaction between a breast-feeding mother and her infant and between a bottle-feeding mother and her infant. Identify behaviors in both that indicate attachment, and compare your findings.

Recommended Readings

Affonso, D.D. (1987). Assessment of maternal postpartum adaptation. *Public Health Nursing, 4*(1), 9–20.

Barbour, B.C. (1990). Alcohol and pregnancy. *Journal of Nurse Midwifery, 35,* 78–85.

Brown, M. (1986). Social support, stress and health: A comparison of expectant mothers and fathers. *Nursing Research, 35*(2), 72–76.

Cronenwett, L. (1985). Network structure, social support, and psychological outcomes of pregnancy. *Nursing Research, 34*(2), 93–99.

Engstrom, J.L (1988). Measurement of fundal height. *Journal of Obstetric, Gynecologic, and Neonatal Nursing, 17,* 172–178.

Gaffney, K.F. (1988). Prenatal maternal attachment. *Image: Journal of Nursing Scholarship, 20,* 106–109.

Horner, R.D., Lackey, C.J., Kolasa, K. & Warren, K. (1991). Pica practices of pregnant women. *Journal of the American Dietetic Association, 91*(1), 34–38.

Lewallen, L.P. (1989). Health beliefs and health practices of pregnant women. *Journal of Obstetric, Gynecologic, and Neonatal Nursing, 18,* 245–246.

Moleti, C. (1988). Caring for socially high-risk pregnant women. *MCN: The American Journal of Maternal-Child Nursing, 13*(1), 24–27.

Patterson, E.T., Freese, M.P., & Goldenberg, R.L. (1986). Reducing uncertainty: Self-diagnosis of pregnancy. *Image: Journal of Nursing Scholarship, 18,* 105–109.

Stevens, K. (1988). Nursing diagnosis in wellness childbearing settings. *Journal of Obstetric, Gynecologic, and Neonatal Nursing, 17*(5), 329–335.

Stolte, K. (1986). Nursing diagnosis and the childbearing woman. *MCN: The American Journal of Maternal-Child Nursing, 11*(1), 13–15.

Walker, L., Crain, H., & Thompson, E. (1986). Maternal role attainment and identity in the postpartum period: Stability and change. *Nursing Research, 35*(2), 68–71.

References

Bernhard, L., & Dan, A. (1986). Redefining sexuality from women's own experience. *Nursing Clinics of North America, 21*(1), 125–136.

Brown, M.A. (1986). Social support, stress and health: A comparison of expectant mothers and fathers. *Nursing Research, 35,* 72–76.

Choi, E., & Hamilton, R. (1986). The effects of culture on mother-infant interaction. *Journal of Obstetric, Gynecologic, and Neonatal Nursing, 15*(3), 256–260.

Cranley, M.S. (1982). *Social support in the development of parents' attachment to their unborn.* Paper presented at Nursing Roundtable on Social Support and Families of Vulnerable Infants, University of Washington, Seattle.

Davis, B., Holtz, N., & Davis, J. (1985). *Conceptual human physiology.* Columbus, OH: Merrill.

Drife, J., & MacNab, G. (1986). Mineral and vitamin supplements. *Clinics in Obstetrics and Gynecology, 13*(2), 253–267.

Fawcett, J., & York, Y. (1986). Spouses' physical and psychological symptoms during pregnancy and postpartum. *Nursing Research, 35,* 144–148.

Gaffney, K.F. (1988). Prenatal maternal attachment. *Image: Journal of Nursing Scholarship, 20,* 106–109.

Greenspan, F., & Forsham, P. (1988). *Basic and clinical guidelines for perinatal care* (pp. 193–196). Washington, DC: American Academy of Pediatrics and American College of Obstetricians & Gynecologists.

Hans, A. (1986). Postpartum assessment: The psychological component. *Journal of Obstetric, Gynecologic, and Neonatal Nursing, 15*(1), 49–51.

Hollingsworth, A.O., Brown, L.A., & Brooten, D.A. (1980). The refugees and childbearing: What to expect, Part 3. *RN, 43,* 44–49.

Johnson, D. (1987). A new threat to the pregnant woman's autonomy. *Hastings Center Report, 14*(4), 33–40.

Jordan, B. (1987). The hut and the hospital: Information power and symbolism in the artifacts of birth. *Birth, 14*(1), 36–39.

Kopala, B. (1989). Mothers with impaired mobility speak out. *MCN: The American Journal of Maternal-Child Nursing, 14,* 115–119.

LaDu, E. (1985). Childbirth care for Hmong families. *MCN: The American Journal of Maternal-Child Nursing, 10*(6), 382–385.

Luke, B. (1977). Understanding pica in pregnant women. *MCN: The American Journal of Maternal-Child Nursing, 2,* 99.

McBride, A. (1988). Mental health effects of women's multiple roles. *Image: The Journal of Nursing Scholarship, 20*(1), 41–47.

Mercer, R. (1985). The process of maternal role attachment over the first year. *Nursing Research, 34*(4), 198–204.

National Commission to Prevent Infant Mortality. (1988, July). *NAACOG Newsletter, 15,* p. 1.

Norbeck, J.S., & Tilden, V.P. (1983). Life stress, social support and emotional disequilibrium in complications of pregnancy: A prospective multivariate study. *Journal of Health and Social Behavior, 24,* 30–36.

Palisin, H. (1981). The Neonatal Perception Inventory: A review. *Nursing Research, 30*(5), 285–299.

Patterson, E., Freese, M., & Goldenberg, R. (1986). Reducing uncertainty: Self-diagnosis of pregnancy. *Image: Journal of Nursing Scholarship, 18*(3), 105–109.

Pritchard, J., MacDonald, P., & Gant, N. (1985). *Williams' obstetrics* (17th ed.). Norwalk, CT: Appleton-Century-Crofts.

Rubin, R. (1967). Attainment of the maternal role: 1. Processes. *Nursing Research, 16,* 237–245.

Rubin, R. (1975). Maternal tasks in pregnancy. *MCN: The American Journal of Maternal-Child Nursing, 4*(3), 145.

Rubin, R. (1984). *Maternal identity and the maternal experience.* New York: Springer.

Simkin, P. (1986). Stress, pain and the catecholamines in labor. *Birth, 13*(4), 227–232.

Slavin, J. (1986). The expectant exerciser. *Sports Nutrition News, 5*(2), 1–4.

Stevens, K. (1988). Nursing diagnosis in wellness childbearing settings. *Journal of Obstetric, Gynecologic, and Neonatal Nursing, 17*(5), 329–335.

Stolte, K. (1986). Nursing diagnosis and the childbearing woman. *MCN: The American Journal of Maternal-Child Nursing, 11*(1), 13–15.

Strickland, O.L. (1987). The occurrence of symptoms in expectant fathers. *Nursing Research, 36,* 184–189.

Tomlison, P. (1987). Spousal differences in marital satisfaction during transition to parenthood. *Nursing Research, 36*(4), 239–242.

Walker, L.O., Crain, H., & Thompson, E. (1986). Maternal role attainment and identity in the postpartum period: Stability and change. *Nursing Research, 35,* 68–71.

Vitamin A supplementation during pregnancy. (1987). Bulletin #52. American College of Obstetricians & Gynecologists (Opinion).

Young, M. (1988). Parenting during mid-adolescence: A review of developmental theories and parenting behaviors. *Maternal-Child Nursing Journal, 17*(1), 1–12.

Young, R.K. (1982). *Community nursing workbook.* Norwalk, CT: Appleton-Lange.

Assessment of the Neonate

OBJECTIVES

Upon completion of this chapter, you should be able to:

- Explain the physiological changes that occur as the neonate adapts to extra-uterine life.

- Interpret the neonate's behavioral responses during the periods of reactivity and sleep that occur during the first 12 hours of life.

- Explain the characteristics and functioning of the healthy newborn in the following areas: physical growth, vital signs, integument, immune system, sensory–neurological status, activity–sleep patterns, oxygenation, nutrition, fluid balance, elimination patterns, external genitalia, and behavioral responses.

- Describe factors that should be taken into account when conducting the clinical appraisal of the newborn.

- Describe the following tools or measures for evaluating the newborn's health: the Neonatal Perception Inventories I and II, APGAR scoring system, gestational age assessment, Silverman-Andersen Index, standardized growth charts, and the Brazelton Neonatal Behavioral Assessment Scale.

- Obtain and record a neonatal nursing history from the parents of a newborn.

- Conduct a systematic clinical appraisal of the newborn, using the techniques of observation, inspection, palpation, and auscultation.

- Analyze the findings of the newborn appraisal to formulate valid and appropriate nursing diagnoses.

Dramatic changes occur in the infant during the initial days and weeks of life. The first four weeks following birth are referred to as the *newborn period*, during which the infant is known as a *neonate*. Because of their immaturity, neonates are at risk of suffering adverse consequences as they respond to the complex demands of the extra-uterine environment. Neonatal mortality is highest in the first 24 hours of life, although the vast majority of infants adapts readily to life outside the womb. Despite their immaturity, healthy newborns have unique capabilities that facilitate their adjustment to a world in which they must breathe on their own and adapt to a variety of new and such previously unknown stimuli as light, variations in environmental temperature, gravity, odors, and acute sounds.

Careful and comprehensive nursing assessment of the newborn is essential to the neonate's successful adaptation to extra-uterine life. The focus of the newborn assessment is to form the most complete and accurate picture possible of the neonate's health in the first moments, hours, and days of life. While advances in technology permit sophisticated monitoring of the fetus and newborn, no technology can take the place of first-hand observation of the neonate's unique responses. For example, appraisal of sucking and swallowing responses, reactions to breast- or bottle-feeding, and level of alertness depends on direct observations of the newborn's behaviors. These observations are critical components of a comprehensive assessment, which form the basis for clinical judgments or specific nursing diagnoses and the subsequent plan of care. Careful and ongoing evaluation of the newborn permits early detection of problems and lessens the likelihood of neonatal morbidity or mortality.

All newborns should be assessed thoroughly within the first 24 hours of life, preferably within the first several hours, whether birth has occurred in a hospital or an alternative setting such as a birthing center or the home. Nurses are ideally suited to perform such assessments. Identification of specific nursing diagnoses leads to a plan of nursing care, whereas detection of problems requiring medical attention can be referred to the physician.

Portions of this chapter have been adapted from Auvenshine/Enriquez: *Comprehensive Maternity Nursing*, Second Edition, © 1991. Boston: Jones and Bartlett Publishers.

KNOWLEDGE NEEDED TO ASSESS THE NEONATE

Understanding the neonate's physiological capabilities and limitations is essential for conducting a comprehensive assessment. Most newborns adapt to the stressors of extra-uterine life without obvious difficulty. For some neonates, however, the adjustment is compromised and requires intervention to assist the transition.

Assessment of the infant's physiological and behavioral responses to extra-uterine life assists in the detection of problems that may interfere with successful adaptation. In most instances, nurses are the ones who care for the neonate in the immediate postbirth period and therefore are most likely to conduct the initial newborn assessment.

Many important observations and judgments about the neonate's adaptation to extra-uterine life must be made within the first minutes of life, including the presence of visible congenital anomalies, skin color, heart rate, respirations, and reflex response. A more comprehensive assessment, including measurements of physical growth, cardio-pulmonary functioning, characteristics of the integument, and elimination patterns, can be conducted later, when the newborn is quiet. Assessment, and the clinical judgments or nursing diagnoses that emerge, is guided by knowledge of the many unique characteristics of the neonate.

Adaptation to Extra-uterine Life

Phenomenal changes occur in the first minutes and hours of life. Throughout the prenatal period, the fetus is dependent on the mother for oxygenation, nutrition, elimination, and protection from infection. Within a matter of seconds, the neonate must perform these functions independently.

Respiratory Adaptation

The neonate's first breath marks the beginning of extra-uterine life. Mechanical, sensory, and chemical factors interact to both stimulate and permit independent breathing (see Table 21-1). The first breath typically is a gasp, followed by up to five more gasps. A sustained rhythmic yet irregular respiratory pattern usually is established within 20 to 30 seconds after birth.

To establish independent ventilation, the infant must have (1) an intact and functioning respiratory center to regulate the rate of breathing, (2) an intact nervous system to transmit messages to the respiratory muscles in the chest, (3) sufficient energy to contract the respiratory muscles, and (4) a clear airway. Respiration is relatively stable in the newborn

TABLE 21-1
Factors That Establish Independent Respiration
in Neonates

Mechanical
Rupture of membranes
Uterine contractions (compress thorax and expel lung fluid)
Chest compression during final stage of delivery
Change from intrauterine to extra-uterine pressure

Sensory
Temperature (room temperature colder than intra-uterine temperature)
Touch
Light
Sound
Gravity

Chemical
Surfactant production
Transient asphyxia
Medications administered to mother during labor

TABLE 21-2
Transition From Fetal to Postnatal Circulation

Fetal Circulation
Oxygen needs are met by the placenta.
A well-oxygenated blood supply to the vital organs (brain, heart, liver) is maintained.
Ductus venosus shunts freshly oxygenated blood from the placenta to the inferior vena cava.
Ductus arteriosus and *foramen ovale* shunt blood to bypass lungs.
Lungs are fluid-filled, which maintains vascular resistance in the pulmonary vascular bed.
A small amount of blood is circulated to the lungs to maintain tissue integrity.

Postnatal Circulation
Placental circulation ceases as the lungs begin to function.
Increased pressure in left side of heart closes the foramen ovale.
Increased oxygen concentration in lungs stimulates the ductus arteriosus to constrict and become nonfunctional within 15 hours of birth.
With clamping of the umbilical cord, the ductus venosus becomes nonfunctional. Fibrosis occurs within 3 to 7 days.

period. Factors that sustain breathing include clamping of the umbilical cord, acidosis, hypoxia, CO_2 retention, some degree of pain or discomfort, cold, touch, and noise.

In the first 15 to 30 minutes of life, the respiratory rate may be as high as 80 breaths per minute. This period is one of intense activity for the healthy newborn. Following the second period of reactivity (periods of reactivity are discussed later in this chapter), the neonate's respiratory rate slows to an average of 40 breaths per minute. The neonate's chest wall is thin, and the rib cage is flexible. Breathing is diaphragmatic, and slight sternal retractions may be evident.

Circulatory Adaptation

Clamping of the umbilical cord establishes independent circulation. Many circulatory changes occur simultaneously (see Table 21-2). Placental circulation ceases as the newborn's lungs begin to function. With the first breath, a large amount of blood is returned to the heart and lungs, increasing the pressure in the left atrium and closing the *foramen ovale* (a fetal structure that permits blood to bypass the lungs).

As the oxygen concentration in the blood increases, the *ductus arteriosus* (a fetal structure that shunts blood from the pulmonary artery to the aorta) constricts. Functional closure of the ductus is complete by 15 hours of age, although anatomical closure (fibrosis) is not complete until 3 weeks of age. The *ductus venosus*, a third fetal structure, which connects fetal portal circulation with the in-

ferior vena cava, becomes fibrosed within 1 week of birth.

During neonatal life, the heart is large in proportion to total body size and lies at a transverse angle. Several changes also occur in the hematologic system during the transition to extra-uterine life. Normal hematologic laboratory values for the newborn are summarized in Table 21-3.

Thermoregulation

Regulation of body temperature in the extra-uterine environment is difficult for the neonate because control mechanisms have not yet matured. This is particularly exaggerated in preterm and low birth weight infants. The newborn has the capacity for reasonably effective heat production, but is highly susceptible to heat loss. This susceptibility is related to several factors: (1) large body surface area in relation to weight, (2) lower metabolic rate, (3) a thinner layer of subcutaneous fat, and (4) poor vasomotor control. Body temperature is highly unstable for the first 12 to 24 hours of life (Figure 21-1). Hypothermia is common and may threaten the neonate's physiological stability. On the other hand, hyperthermia may occur in response to high environmental temperatures because the neonate's sweat mechanisms are not fully developed.

The thermal environment plays a major role in

TABLE 21-3
Common Neonatal Laboratory Values

Value	Age/Gender	Normal Ranges
Bilirubin, serum	Cord	<2 mg/dl
	0–2 days	<8 mg/dl
	2–5 days	<12 mg/dl
	Thereafter	<1 mg/dl
Hematocrit	3 days	45–75%
	1 month	30–44%
Hemoglobin	3 days	14–22.5 gm/dl
	1 month	10–14 gm/dl
RBC count	3 days	4.0–6.5 million/mm³
	1 month	3.0–5.5 million/mm³
WBC count	3 days	8,000–32,000/mm³
	1 month	5,000–20,000/mm³
Platelet count		84,000–450,000
PO_2	birth	8–24 mm Hg
	1 day	55–95 mm Hg
	1 month	80–108 mm Hg
PCO_2		27–40 mm Hg
pH (blood)		7.33–7.45
Urine		
pH		5–7
specific gravity		1.005–1.025
BUN		3–12 mg/dl
Glucose (blood)		30–90 mg/dl

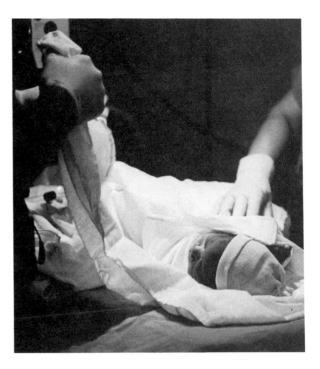

FIGURE 21-1. Body temperature is highly unstable for the first 12 hours of life. The newborn infant should be wrapped in a warm blanket and the head covered with a cap to prevent heat loss. (*Note.* From Auvenshine/Enriquez: *Comprehensive Maternity Nursing*, Second Edition, © 1990. Boston: Jones and Bartlett Publishers, p. 408.)

regulating the neonate's body temperature. When the environment is too cold or too warm, the newborn's metabolic demands and oxygen consumption increase and adaptive capacities are strained. A neutral thermal environment, one that allows the neonate to maintain an axillary temperature of 96.8° F to 97.7° F, is essential to conserve body heat and prevent heat loss (Perez, 1981).

Heat Conservation and Production. The primary mechanisms by which the newborn is able to conserve and produce body heat include vasomotor control, thermal insulation, shivering and muscle activity, and metabolic thermogenesis. Vasoconstriction occurs in response to heat loss and enables the newborn to conserve body heat. Thermal insulation varies in proportion to the amount of fat deposits, which account for approximately 11 to 17% of body weight in full-term neonates. Fat deposits provide insulation and permit the body to act as a heat reservoir. Muscle activity and body movement help produce heat. However, unlike adults, newborns do not shiver (except in response to extreme cold) and therefore cannot rely on shivering to produce heat. Metabolic thermogenesis is probably the most effective and consistent mecha-

nism of heat production in the newborn (Perez, 1981). The brain, liver, and possibly skeletal muscle are the major thermogenic organs. Another source of heat production is brown fat, which makes up about 1.5% of body weight and is found between the scapulae, behind the sternum, in the axilla, and around the neck, head, heart, great vessels, kidneys, and adrenal glands. Norepinephrine, which is released in response to cold, stimulates chemical activity in these subcutaneous deposits of brown fat, thus increasing body heat.

Heat Loss. Mechanisms of heat loss in the newborn include radiation, conduction, convection, and evaporation. Radiant heat loss is believed to be the major mechanism of heat loss in the neonate (Perez, 1981). Heat is transferred from the newborn to a cooler, solid environmental surface, such as a wall or isolette surface. When the newborn's skin comes into direct contact with a cooler surface, such as a bassinet wall, heat loss occurs by conduction. Both the thermal conductivity and the temperature of the surface affect the amount of heat lost. Convective heat loss involves the transfer of body heat from the body's surface to the cooler surrounding air. The temperature and velocity of air (such as drafts) influence the amount of heat lost in this manner. Finally, the newborn may lose body heat through evaporation of insensible water or fluid (such as amniotic fluid) from the skin, as well as moisture released from the respiratory tract during exhalation. Evaporative heat loss is greater when the environment is dry.

Metabolic Adaptation

The abrupt termination of a continuous intra-uterine supply of glucose and calcium requires the neonate to make profound adaptations in the metabolic process. Rapid changes occur in plasma glucose and calcium during the first days of life. Blood glucose at birth is normally 60 to 70% of the maternal level. Blood glucose then falls over the next 1 to 2 hours and stabilizes at a minimum of 35 to 40 mg/dl, rising to 60 mg/dl by 6 hours of age.

Serum calcium also drops during the first 24 to 48 hours after birth, then stabilizes at 9.0 to 10.9 mg/dl. Hypocalcemia (serum calcium less than 7 mg/dl) is most likely to occur during the first 2 days or between 6 and 10 days of age. Hypocalcemia and hypoglycemia both may cause irritability, jitteriness, listlessness, hypothermia, apnea, and seizures.

Another metabolic change involves the liver, which becomes the chief organ for breaking down and excreting bilirubin. As the liver begins this important function, it relinquishes its function as the chief organ of blood formation. The bone marrow becomes the chief site of blood cell production postnatally. Because the newborn's liver produces insufficient quantities of glucuronyl transferase, an enzyme needed to convert indirect bilirubin to direct (excretable) bilirubin, *physiological jaundice* may result. Physiological jaundice occurs in response to high levels of indirect bilirubin, which can cause *kernicterus* (bilirubin staining of brain tissue) and result in brain damage. Approximately half of all newborns become visibly jaundiced by 48 hours of age. Jaundice appears once the bilirubin level reaches 7 mg/dl. Asian and native American newborns have higher initial bilirubin levels (10 to 14 mg/dl) than white, African-American, and Hispanic neonates (Locklin, 1987). Jaundice typically appears head-to-toe and diminishes toe-to-head. As long as the bilirubin level does not exceed 12 mg/dl, there is little danger to brain tissue.

Periods of Reactivity

The first 12 hours of life have been termed a *transitional period* for the newborn infant. These first hours are characterized by rapid change and adaptation. Two periods of reactivity in the immediate postbirth period occur within the first half day of life. These two periods are separated by a period of sleep. Figure 21-2 depicts these reactivity and sleep periods and illustrates what changes occur in the neonate during the critical first 6 hours of life. Individual variations in the length of each period depend on the length and difficulty of the birth process, maternal medication and anesthesia, and the amount of stress experienced by the fetus.

First Period of Reactivity

The first period of reactivity is characterized by heightened responsiveness and intense activity (Figure 21-3). Approximately the first 40 minutes of life are spent in this quiet, alert state. The infant is active and the eyes may be open. Parent–neonate interaction should be initiated during this period. Research has shown that the response characteristics of the newborn influence parent–infant interactions and that the quiet alert period is most conducive to helping parents become acquainted with their infant's behavioral style (Als & Brazelton, 1981).

Characteristic responses during the first period of reactivity include nasal flaring or "sniffing" unrelated to respiratory difficulty; movements of the head from side to side; spontaneous startles and the Moro reflex; grimacing; sucking; swallowing; pursing and smacking the lips; tremors of the extremities and mandible; opening and closing the eyes; short, rapid, jerky movements of the eyeball; sudden outcries; and abrupt cessations of crying (Klaus & Fanaroff, 1979). During this period, body temperature decreases and muscle tone and activity increase. Responses in the first period of reactivity are governed predominantly by the sympathetic nervous system.

Sleep Period

Following the first period of reactivity, the neonate enters a phase characterized by diminished responsiveness and sleep. Respirations may be rapid, while the heart rate slows. General skin color improves and *acrocyanosis* (cyanosis of the hands and feet) lessens. During sleep, spontaneous jerks and twitches often occur. Abdominal peristaltic waves and small amounts of clear mucus at the lips may be observed. This period begins approximately 1 hour after birth and lasts up to 6 hours.

Second Period of Reactivity

During the second period of reactivity, the neonate exhibits an exaggerated responsiveness character-

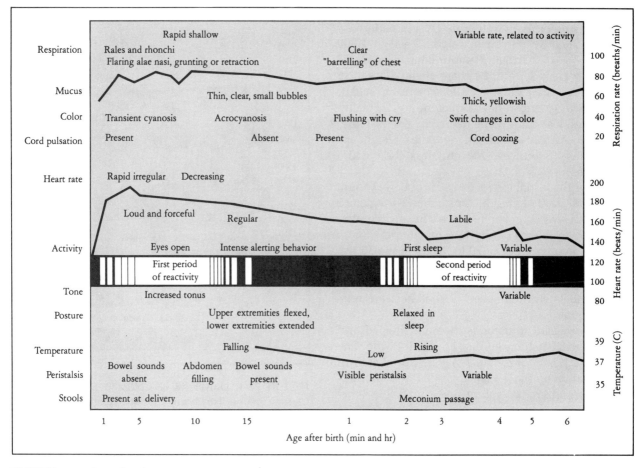

FIGURE 21-2. Periods of Reactivity and Sleep. (*Note.* From Arnold, H.W., Putnam, N.J., Barnard, B.L., Desmond, M.M., & Rudolph, A.J. Transition to extrauterine life. Copyright 1965 American Journal of Nursing Company. Reprinted from *American Journal of Nursing,* 1965, *65*[10], 78. Used with permission. All rights reserved.)

ized by marked swings in intensity of activity. This period may be brief or continue for several hours. The heart rate fluctuates, with episodes of tachycardia and bradycardia. Skin color remains pink and reflects improved vasomotor tone. Respirations vary from 30 to 60 breaths per minute and remain irregular. Oral secretions thicken, and gagging or regurgitation is common. The first stool, *meconium,* is passed during this period. Toward the end of this period, the infant is ready for the first feeding.

Physical Growth and Integrity

The infant's physical integrity depends on intrauterine growth, gestational age, and birth weight (Lubchenco, 1981), as well as the maturity of the integument. The neonate's vital signs also attest to the infant's general physiological integrity.

Physical Growth

Intrauterine growth is influenced by a host of genetic and environmental factors: height and weight

of parents; racial characteristics; the mother's health and nutrition; and possibly intrauterine insults such as infection, radiation, smoking, and maternal drug or alcohol use. The infant's birth

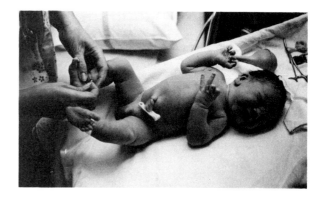

FIGURE 21-3. The first period of reactivity immediately after birth is characterized by heightened responsiveness and intense activity. (*Note.* From Auvenshine/Enriquez: *Comprehensive Maternity Nursing,* Second Edition, © 1990. Boston: Jones and Bartlett Publishers, p. 416.)

weight in relation to gestational age provides a general measure of the intrauterine growth pattern.

The healthy newborn weighs 2,500 to 4,300 grams (5½ to 9½ lbs) and is approximately 45 to 53 cm (18 to 21) in length. Boys are slightly larger on the average than girls. African-American, Asian, and native American newborns tend to be smaller and weigh less than white neonates. For example, full-term African-American neonates weigh approximately 8 ounces (200 gm) less than white newborns.

After the initial loss of 5 to 10% of body weight in the first days of life, the typical newborn gains 5 to 7 ounces weekly. The neonate's head circumference is 32 to 37 cm (12½ to 14½ in) compared with a chest circumference of 30 to 33 cm (12 to 13 in). Head circumference is generally 2 to 3 cm (1 in) larger than chest circumference. The anterior-posterior and lateral diameters of the chest are relatively equal.

The anterior fontanel is diamond-shaped and may range from 2.5 to 4.0 cm (1 to 1¾ in) wide. The triangular posterior fontanel may be closed at birth or should be no more than 1 cm (0.4 in) wide. Immobile, rigid cranial suture lines indicate premature closure or fusion, which can compromise brain development and neurological functioning.

Gestational age influences the newborn's capacity for successful extra-uterine adaptation. Full-term infants are those born between 38 and 42 weeks of gestation (measured from the date of the mother's last menstrual period). Preterm infants are those of fewer than 38 weeks' gestation; postterm infants are born after 42 weeks' gestation. Neonates who are born prematurely are at risk for respiratory and cardiac difficulty, thermoregulatory problems, and digestive and neurological complications.

Comparison of the newborn's gestational age with birth weight is used to categorize the infant as appropriate for gestational age (AGA), small for gestational age (SGA), or large for gestational age (LGA). The relationship of gestational age and birth weight to neonatal mortality risk is depicted in Figure 21-4. Note that mortality risk is inversely proportional to gestational age and birth weight. However, preterm infants who are large for gestational age are at greater risk of death than full-term infants who are small for gestational age. Thus, gestational age seems to be the more significant factor.

Vital Signs

Of all the vital signs, temperature is probably the most significant for successful extra-uterine adap-

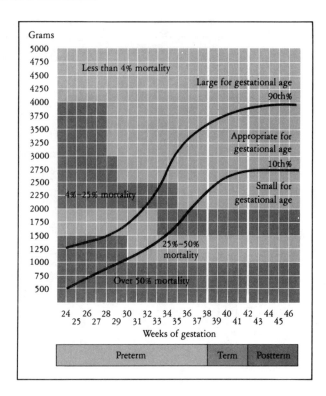

FIGURE 21-4. University of Colorado Medical Center Classification of Newborns by Birth Weight, Gestational Age, and Neonatal Mortality Risk. (*Note.* From Battaglia, F.C., & Lubchenco, L.O. [1967]. A practical classification of newborn infants by weight and gestational age. *Journal of Pediatrics, 71,* 161.)

tation of the newborn. Axillary temperature is typically 36.5° to 37° C (97.7°–98.6° F). Crying may increase body temperature as will warmer environmental temperatures. Sleep and cool environmental temperatures can lead to hypothermia.

After the initial periods of reactivity, the neonate's resting apical heart rate averages 120 to 140 beats per minute, although the range can vary widely depending on the infant's state. While sleeping, the pulse can drop as low as 80 beats per minute, whereas intense crying or fever can cause the pulse to rise as high as 220 beats per minute. Respiratory rates vary as well, ranging from 30 to 80 breaths per minute, with an average rate 35 to 40 breaths per minute.

The newborn's systolic blood pressure gradually rises throughout the first month of life. Mean systolic and diastolic pressures at 1 day of age are 73/55 for boys and 65/55 for girls. At the end of the newborn period, mean blood pressure is 86/52 for boys and 84/52 for girls.

Integument

At birth, the neonate's skin is soft, edematous (caused by pressure), velvety, and covered by varying amounts of *vernix caseosa*, a greasy, yellowish-white sebaceous material. Immediately after birth, the newborn's hands and feet may be cyanotic (acrocyanosis) due to poorly developed peripheral circulation. Forceps marks may be evident. These marks are red or purple discolorations, usually over the temporal and parietal areas of the scalp as well as the cheeks, caused by the pressure used during a forceps-assisted delivery. They typically disappear within several days.

Several hours after birth, the skin develops an intense red color. By the second to third day, the neonate's skin is pink, dry, and flaky. Skin color is influenced by the infant's racial and familial characteristics. White infants are pinkish red, whereas African-American infants appear pinkish brown or yellowish brown. Hispanic neonates have an olive or yellowish brown skin color, and native American infants vary from light pink to rosy brown.

In general, the newborn's skin is thinner and more sensitive to trauma than that of older children and adults. The nails tend to be thin and peel easily. Hair on the scalp is soft and fine and may be sparse or quite thick. Hair color depends on genetic factors and may lighten or darken as the infant gets older.

There are many common variations in the neonate's skin, which may be evident at birth or appear within the first weeks of life. Variations include mottling, birthmarks, the presence of vernix caseosa or lanugo, erythema toxicum, jaundice, and milia. These variations and their assessment are described in Table 21-7 later in this chapter.

Immune System

The neonate's immune system is immature, placing the infant at some risk for contracting infectious disease. Infants lack the capacity to produce their own gamma globulins until the second month of life. The neonate receives immunoglobulin G (IgG) through placental transfer during the final weeks of gestation. Through IgG, neonates receive passive immunity for the majority of childhood communicable diseases (e.g., measles, rubella, polio, diphtheria, and infectious hepatitis) if the mother has produced antibodies to these diseases.

Newborns do not receive immunoglobulins A (IgA) or M (IgM) from the mother, so they are susceptible to many viral and bacterial organisms, particularly gram-negative infections. However, breast-fed newborns acquire certain agglutins and IgA from colostrum and breast milk, which help defend against gram-negative organisms. Because of the immaturity of the immune system, the newborn's response to infection is often unclear and unspecific.

Sensory–Neurological Functioning

The sensory-neurological capacities of the newborn are remarkably well developed. Neonates exhibit the ability to organize and habituate to stimuli in their environment. They are able to attend to and process a variety of visual, auditory, olfactory, gustatory, and tactile stimuli; maintain muscle tone and coordinate certain motor behaviors (for example, bringing hand to mouth); and demonstrate protective responses to stressors, such as the ability to inhibit a startle response or withdraw from a painful stimulus.

Sensory Processes

The neonate has the capacity to alert to, turn the eyes and head to follow, and fixate on an object held 8 to 12 inches from the face (Fanaroff & Martin, 1983). Newborns have been found to prefer human faces to inanimate objects (Goren, Sarty, & Wu, 1976) (Figure 21-5). Limited color vision is

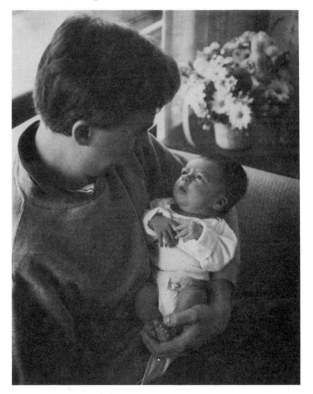

FIGURE 21-5. The neonate has the capacity to fixate on an object 8 to 12 inches from the face. Neonates prefer human faces to inanimate objects. (*Note.* From Auvenshine/Enriquez: *Comprehensive Maternity Nursing,* Second Edition, © 1990. Boston: Jones and Bartlett Publishers, p. 811.)

present at birth since the cones of the retina are not fully matured. The amount of vision present at birth and in the newborn period is not precisely known, but visual acuity probably ranges from 20/300 to 20/600. Corneal and blink reflexes in response to touch are present, and the pupils react readily to light. *Nystagmus*, involuntary spasmodic movements of the eyes, and *strabismus*, an imbalance of the eye muscles, which causes the eyes to appear deviated or cross-eyed, are common and considered normal for the first few months of life.

Newborns are capable of responding to sound whether awake or asleep. When awake, neonates will turn their eyes and head toward the sound. Sleeping newborns react to sound with a start, blink and open their eyes, and they breathe irregularly. Low frequency sounds tend to soothe the infant whereas high frequency sounds may cause distress responses, such as increased heart rate and crying (Fanaroff & Martin, 1983).

The sense of smell is present at birth. When presented with a noxious smell, such as ammonia or alcohol, the newborn responds with nasal flaring, blinking, and sometimes sneezing. The smell of milk elicits rooting and sucking reflexes. Newborns respond to sweet or pleasurable tastes with sucking movements and show aversion to bitter, salty, and sour tastes.

Touch is the most highly developed sense at birth (Figure 21-6). The premature infant at 28 weeks' gestation can differentiate touch, which increases alertness and motor activity, from pain, which results in withdrawal and crying. At 35 to 36 weeks' gestation, the infant will rapidly turn the head away from a pinprick over the side of the face (Avery, 1981). Touch is especially well-developed in the facial area, as evidenced by the newborn's rooting and sucking behaviors in response to stimulation. Newborns also respond positively to being stroked, bundled, and held. Soothing, gentle touch often elicits quieting behavior. The newborn responds in a generalized way and cannot determine precisely the area of cutaneous stimulation, but the ability to discriminate improves as the touch receptors mature and multiply.

Pain Responses

The ability of newborns to discriminate and respond to pain is difficult to measure because of their limited cognitive development. Newborns do experience pain, although their pain threshold tends to be higher than that of older children and adults (Jones, 1989). Further, the incomplete myelination of the neonate's nerve tracts results in a delayed response to a painful stimulus. Behavioral

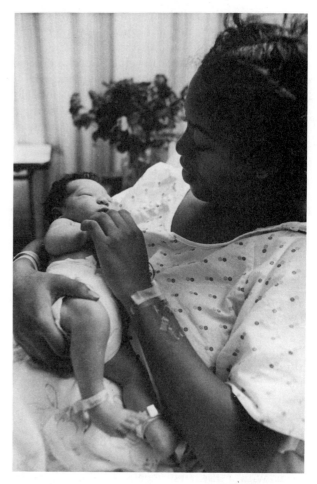

FIGURE 21-6. Touch is the most highly developed sense at birth. Newborns respond positively to being bundled, held, and stroked. (*Note.* From Auvenshine/Enriquez: *Comprehensive Maternity Nursing,* Second Edition, © 1990. Boston: Jones and Bartlett Publishers, p. 493.)

cues that indicate a newborn is experiencing pain include fussiness, crying, grimacing, restlessness, increased respiration and heart rate, sleeplessness, rigid posture, and whimpering (Jones, 1989).

Neurological Functioning

The newborn infant's neurological capabilities are largely reflexive. Absence of certain reflexes may indicate neurological impairment. Reflexes may be *localized,* such as blinking, sucking, rooting, extrusion, grasp, and Babinski reflexes, or *generalized,* such as Moro, startle, tonic neck, and stepping reflexes. Neonatal reflexes and their assessment are described in Table 21-10 later in this chapter.

Activity–Sleep Patterns

The skeletal system of the newborn infant is incompletely ossified. The bones are pliable and porous. The muscles, however, are essentially completely formed in full-term neonates. Muscle growth thereafter is due to hypertrophy.

The healthy neonate's posture and spontaneous movements are symmetrical. Resting posture is one of complete flexion of the head and extremities. The newborn holds the head to a preferred side, except when crying, at which time a midline position is assumed. The fingers are curled into a fist. The trunk tends to lean toward the preferred side (the side to which the head is turned). The newborn's hips are flexed and rotated externally, with knees slightly flexed. Full range of motion is present in all joints. Muscle tone is equal bilaterally. The newborn can turn the head from side to side when prone and usually is able to hold the head erect momentarily when held in a sitting position.

Following the periods of reactivity and sleep during the first hours after birth, the neonate's activity–sleep levels are categorized by state. Brazelton (1973) categorizes the newborn's state on a six-point scale:

1. Deep sleep
2. Light sleep
3. Drowsy
4. Quiet alert
5. Agitated alert
6. Vigorous crying

The newborn's state influences every physiological and neurosensory function (see Table 21-4).

While the fetus is still in utero, a sleep/wake cycle is established. This cycle is disrupted almost immediately after birth. The newborn stays awake for longer periods of time, with periods of quiet alertness alternating with periods of activity. By the fifth day of life, the state cycles have stabilized (Fanaroff & Martin, 1983).

The neonate's wake/sleep patterns are influenced by several variables, including gestational age, behavioral characteristics, and the environment. For example, preterm infants spend more hours sleeping than full-term infants (Dubowitz & Dubowitz, 1981). Individual differences in behavioral characteristics often are reflected in the neonate's sleep/wake patterns. "Easy" newborns tend to spend more time in sleep or quiet, alert states than "difficult" neonates, who spend more time in active alert and crying states (Brazelton, 1973). Keefe (1987) found significant differences in neonatal nighttime sleep/wake patterns between newborns in nursery versus rooming-in environments. Neonates who slept in their mother's room had significantly more quiet sleep and cried less than those who stayed in the nursery at night.

During the first week the healthy neonate spends only 8 to 16% of the day in a quiet, alert state, with the remaining time spent in quiet or active sleep. Approximately 50% of sleep time is active (REM) sleep. Healthy newborns tend to awaken at 2- to 4-hour intervals.

Oxygenation

As mentioned earlier, neonates breathe diaphragmatically. Because of the close proximity of the soft palate and the epiglottis, newborns are obligatory nose breathers, which enables them to feed without distress. The rate and depth of inhalation tend to be irregular. The chest is barrel-shaped, the chest wall is thin, and the rib cage is narrow, cylindrical, and flexible. Slight sternal retractions are not unusual.

The newborn's heart is large in proportion to

TABLE 21-4
Effects of State on Body Functions

Body Functions	State		
	Quiet Sleep	Active Sleep	Awake/Crying
Heart rate	Regular	Irregular	Irregular
Respiration	Regular	Irregular and faster; apnea and periodic breathing may occur	Irregular and faster
O_2 consumption	Lower	Higher	Higher (especially if crying)
Transcutaneous pO_2	Higher	Lower	
Blood pressure	Lower	Variable	Higher
Endocrine			Cortisol secretion increases with increasing arousal

Note. From Auvenshine/Enriquez: *Comprehensive Maternity Nursing*, Second Edition, © 1990. Boston: Jones and Bartlett Publishers, p. 575. Adapted from Fanaroff, A., & Martin, R.J. (1983). *Behrman's neonatal-perinatal medicine* (3rd ed.). St. Louis: Mosby.

total body size and lies at a transverse angle. The apex is located between the fourth and fifth intercostal space, lateral to the left sternal border. The newborn's hematocrit ranges from 44 to 70%, and the hemoglobin averages 17 grams/dl. Newborns tend to have poor blood coagulation because they lack the normal intestinal flora needed to synthesize vitamin K.

Nutritional Requirements

While in utero, the nutritional needs of the fetus are met through the placenta. At birth, the healthy newborn is able to independently ingest, digest, absorb, and metabolize food and fluids to meet nutritional needs.

The normal newborn is equipped with reflexes to permit competent feeding. The neonate has coordinated sucking and swallowing reflexes as well as a rooting reflex that causes the infant to turn toward and open its mouth in response to a stimulus, such as stroking the cheek.

Oral feedings usually are begun within about 6 hours of birth. Delayed feelings can compromise the neonate's well-being because glycogen stores are limited. The newborn needs water, protein, carbohydrates, fat, vitamins, and minerals for adequate nutrition. Approximately 120 calories per kg per day are required to meet growth needs. Gastrointestinal enzymes are sufficient to digest proteins and simple carbohydrates, but insufficient production of pancreatic amylase impairs the newborn's ability to digest complex carbohydrates. In addition, a deficiency of pancreatic lipase limits the absorption of fats.

Fluid Balance

Weight loss of 5 to 10% of body weight is typical in the first days of life. Weight loss can be attributed to fluid lost through elimination and insensible routes and to the fact that feeding is not begun until approximately 6 hours of age.

The newborn infant's renal system is immaturely developed, so the ability to regulate fluid balance may be precarious. The neonate's kidneys do not concentrate urine effectively, requiring proportionately more water to excrete wastes.

The newborn's body is 75% water, compared to 55% in adults. A greater percentage of the neonate's fluid volume remains in the extracellular compartment (40% compared to 20% in adults). Therefore, newborns must ingest and excrete proportionately more fluid in a 24-hour period. Newborns require 80 to 100 ml per kg of body weight, much higher than the 20 to 30 ml per kg of body weight required by adults.

Elimination Patterns

Although the fetus ingests amniotic fluid in utero, normally no stool is passed before birth. Bowel sounds are present within a few hours after birth, and the first stool, *meconium*, is passed within 24 to 36 hours. Meconium in the amniotic fluid of newborns delivered in positions other than breech is considered a sign of fetal distress. The first meconium stool is greenish-black, tarry, and odorless.

During the first few days of life, newborns pass what are known as *transitional stools*. These appear after feeding has begun, usually within 2 to 4 days after birth. Transitional stools are loose and have a pasty consistency, changing from greenish brown to greenish yellow to yellowish brown. Milk curds may be present, and the stools have a slightly sour odor.

By the fourth day, a typical *milk stool* is passed. The character of the milk stool will vary depending on the feeding method. Stools of the formula-fed baby usually are harder, have a yellowish brown color, and an offensive odor. The stools of the breast-fed infant are more numerous, of softer consistency, are golden yellow, and smell like slightly sour milk. The frequency of the stool pattern is highly individual and usually well-established within the first month of life.

Usually, the normal newborn voids within the first 24 hours following birth. During the first 48 hours of life, approximately 30 to 60 ml of urine is voided. By the end of the first week, daily urine output is 150 ml. The normal newborn voids an average of 15 to 20 times daily. The urine is usually odorless and colorless, although in the first week of life the urine may contain protein and large amounts of urates, the latter causing pink staining of the diaper.

External Genitalia

The external genitalia of both male and female newborns are enlarged due to transfer of maternal estrogen across the placenta. The breasts also may be enlarged and may secrete a white fluid resembling milk. Genital hypertrophy and breast engorgement disappear within two weeks as the maternal hormones are excreted by the neonate.

In girls, the labia minora appear relatively prominent in relation to the labia majora, and the clitoris may be enlarged. The urethral meatus is visible below the clitoris. A white mucoid vaginal discharge, sometimes blood-tinged, may be evident. A hymenal tag may protrude from the vagina. Both the vaginal discharge and the hymenal tag disappear within several weeks.

The penis of the normal male neonate is 3 to 4

cm long and 1 to 1.3 cm wide. The *prepuce* (foreskin) is usually adherent to the glans. *Smegma*, a white cheese-like substance, is often present beneath the foreskin. The urethral meatus should be located at the tip of the glans. The scrotum usually is enlarged, pendulous, and covered with rugae. In term infants, the testes have descended fully into the scrotal sac. Reflexive erections of the penis are common.

Circumcision is a choice made by the infant's parents and usually is performed within the first 2 days of life unless the family's religious practices dictate otherwise. For example, Jewish male infants usually are circumcised by a rabbi in a special ceremony, a *bris*. Approximately 80 to 90% of newborn boys in the United States are circumcised, although those born at home or in alternative birth settings are less likely to be (Harris, 1986). Harris (1986) recommends that parents be encouraged to follow cultural norms when deciding whether to permit circumcision. For instance, white middle and upper middle class families accept newborn male circumcision as a cultural norm, whereas Southern blacks, Hispanics, and native American Indians do not.

Behavioral Responses

The newborn is in the first stage of the sensorimotor phase of cognitive development, responding reflexively to most stimuli. The neonate quiets in response to a human voice, cries to show displeasure or discomfort, makes small throaty sounds, and coos. Many newborns smile vaguely. Toward the end of the neonatal period infants begin to exhibit a distinct temperament, patterned responses, and unique personality characteristics, all of which are shaped by the dynamic and reciprocal interaction that occurs between the infant and the environment.

THE NEONATAL HISTORY

The neonatal nursing history should include information concerning prenatal, perinatal, and postnatal periods. Information usually is obtained from the mother, although the father, other close relative, or the mother's health record may serve as secondary sources.

The history should include information about the neonate's natural parents, specifically their ages, blood types, and general health, as these factors influence the infant's well-being. For example, if the mother's blood type is Rh negative and the neonate is Rh positive, the infant is at risk for hemolytic disease caused by Rh incompatibility. Infants of mothers who are under 17 years of age or over 35 are at greater risk for health complications. The mother's parity (gravida, para, aborta) also should be determined. First pregnancy or more than five pregnancies increase the risk to the fetus.

The frequency and quality of prenatal care also influence fetal well-being and should be ascertained. Other prenatal factors that should be assessed include the mother's nutrition, use of medications, and exposure of the fetus to potential hazards, such as infection, smoking, alcohol, caffeine, recreational drugs, and radiation. Tests of fetal well-being, such as amniocentesis, ultrasonography, and nonstress testing, often are conducted during the prenatal period, and findings should be noted.

Factors in the perinatal period that should be obtained from the history include the onset and length of labor, fetal presentation, use of analgesia or anesthesia, type of delivery (spontaneous, forceps, Caesarean), and complications, such as premature labor, pregnancy-induced hypertension, placenta previa, abruptio placenta, fetal distress, or anoxia. The neonate's APGAR scores at 1 and 5 minutes of age (see "APGAR Scoring System" later in this chapter); birth weight, length, and head circumference; and any injuries or anomalies detected at birth should be noted.

The mother's choice of infant feeding method (breast or bottle) usually is ascertained during the antepartal history. Postnatally, it is important to determine the mother's readiness to initiate infant feedings. For instance, does the mother know how to get the baby on and off the breast? Does she understand how to prepare infant formula?

Other information important to assess as a basis for care of the infant can be obtained during the early postnatal period. If the neonate is a boy, the nurse should inquire whether the parents plan to circumcise the infant. The nurse also should assess the parents' knowledge of the newborn's capabilities and need for sensorimotor stimulation, their knowledge of or previous experience with basic infant care (feeding, bathing, safety), resources available to the family (adequate income, health insurance, living facilities), the parents' hopes and expectations for this baby, and the responses of family members to the infant's birth. Any special cultural or religious beliefs and practices related to newborn care also should be determined. For instance, a Vietnamese mother is expected to have her newborn with her at all times, although her mother-in-law helps with the actual care (Hollingsworth, Brown, & Brooten, 1980). Many cultures ritualize the bathing and dressing of the newborn. For example, the Mexican-American newborn is tightly swaddled, and a belly band, or *fajita*, is placed around the mid-abdomen to prevent the umbilicus from bulging (Zepeda, 1982).

The parents' perceptions of the neonate are a critical part of the nursing history. It is necessary for the parents to make the transition from the fantasized infant anticipated throughout the pregnancy to the real infant. If discrepancies between the fantasy newborn and the real newborn are too great, parent–infant attachment may be at risk. The Neonatal Perception Inventory (NPI) provides a means for assessing the mother's perceptions of her new infant compared to her image of an "average" infant (Broussard, 1979). Broussard suggests that the mother needs to perceive her new infant as better than the average infant and that failure to do so can lead to alterations in parenting. The NPI I and II are illustrated in Figure 21-7.

The mother should be asked to complete the NPI I during the final weeks of pregnancy or within 1 to 2 days of the infant's birth. The NPI I is useful in detecting potential problems in parental expectations and the parent–child relationship. Guidance early in the neonatal period can assist parents in making a successful transition to the parental role and to being able to respond appropriately to their infant's needs. The NPI II should be administered when the newborn is approximately 1 month old. The Neonatal Perception Inventory II is particularly significant since it has been shown to predict childhood adjustment problems (Broussard, 1979).

The essential elements of the neonatal nursing history are outlined in Table 21-5.

APPROACHES TO ASSESSING THE NEWBORN

Assessment of the newborn infant involves the same techniques—observation, inspection, palpation, percussion, and auscultation—as any other nursing assessment. Because of their unique characteristics, however, newborns require special consideration and handling during the assessment process. Certain factors can influence the neonate's responses to the assessment. These include:

1. Timing of assessment in relation to feedings.
2. Temperature of the environment.
3. The neonate's state of arousal.
4. Gestational age.
5. Health.

Generally, the optimum time for performing a newborn appraisal is approximately midway between feedings. The temperature of the environment should be thermoneutral to prevent hypothermia, which can result in a depressed response, or hyperthermia, which may cause irritability. The newborn should be in a quiet, alert state for the most effective assessment. Gestational age can influence the infant's responses and physical appearance and should be kept in mind when examining the newborn. Finally, the neonate's health will influence the findings of the assessment. A healthy, stable newborn should exhibit effective adaptive responses in extra-uterine life. Abnormal findings usually indicate the neonate is having difficulty adapting to the demands of the extra-uterine environment and require immediate attention.

Prior to beginning the assessment, the nurse should gather equipment, including pen light, tape measure, tongue depressor, stethoscope, and the health record for recording findings. The room should be free of drafts and well-lighted. The newborn's bassinet, the mother's bed, or a padded counter top or exam table may be used. Of utmost importance is assuring the infant's safety during the assessment. Newborns *should never be left unattended during the assessment* unless they are in a bassinet or crib with side rails.

The newborn assessment provides an excellent opportunity to acquaint parents with their infant and teach them about the unique characteristics and capabilities of the newborn (Figure 21-8). The assessment can be conducted at the mother's bedside or the parents may be invited to the nursery (using appropriate handwashing and gowning techniques). When the assessment is conducted at the mother's bedside, it may be possible to involve other family members, such as older siblings or grandparents, who often are eager to get to know the newest addition to the family.

When assessing the neonate, the nurse should proceed systematically, appraising the infant from the head to the toes. The nurse's hands should be clean and warm, soothing voice tones should be used, and motions should be confident, smooth, and unhurried. Sudden, abrupt movements may startle the infant. Intrusive measures, such as taking a rectal temperature or examining the mouth, should be performed after less intrusive ones, such as the skin assessment. The nurse should begin the assessment when the infant is sleeping or in a quiet, alert state.

Before disturbing the infant, the nurse should listen to the heart rate and observe the breathing pattern. The nurse should note skin color and thickness, amount of subcutaneous tissue, resting posture, and alertness. Preferably, the infant

Neonatal Perception Inventory I and II*

Average Baby

How much crying do you think the average baby does?

| a great deal | a good bit | moderate amount | very little | none |

How much trouble do you think the average baby has in feeding?

| a great deal | a good bit | moderate amount | very little | none |

How much spitting up or vomiting do you think the average baby does?

| a great deal | a good bit | moderate amount | very little | none |

How much difficulty do you think the average baby has in sleeping?

| a great deal | a good bit | moderate amount | very little | none |

How much difficulty does the average baby have with bowel movements?

| a great deal | a good bit | moderate amount | very little | none |

How much trouble do you think the average baby has in settling down to a predictable pattern of eating and sleeping?

| a great deal | a good bit | moderate amount | very little | none |

*Parents are requested to fill in the Inventory about the average baby and their own baby twice, once during pregnancy and again during the neonatal stage.

Neonatal Perception Inventory I*

Your Baby

How much crying do you think your baby will do?

| a great deal | a good bit | moderate amount | very little | none |

How much trouble do you think your baby will have feeding?

| a great deal | a good bit | moderate amount | very little | none |

How much spitting up or vomiting do you think your baby will do?

| a great deal | a good bit | moderate amount | very little | none |

How much difficulty do you think your baby will have sleeping?

| a great deal | a good bit | moderate amount | very little | none |

How much difficulty do you expect your baby to have with bowel movements?

| a great deal | a good bit | moderate amount | very little | none |

How much trouble do you think your baby will have settling down to a predictable pattern of eating and sleeping?

| a great deal | a good bit | moderate amount | very little | none |

Neonatal Perception Inventory II*

Your Baby

How much crying has your baby done?

| a great deal | a good bit | moderate amount | very little | none |

How much trouble has your baby had feeding?

| a great deal | a good bit | moderate amount | very little | none |

How much spitting up or vomiting has your baby done?

| a great deal | a good bit | moderate amount | very little | none |

How much difficulty has your baby had in sleeping?

| a great deal | a good bit | moderate amount | very little | none |

How much difficulty has your baby had with bowel movements?

| a great deal | a good bit | moderate amount | very little | none |

How much trouble has your baby had in settling down to a predictable pattern of eating and sleeping?

| a great deal | a good bit | moderate amount | very little | none |

Degree of Bother Inventory**

Crying	a great deal	somewhat	very little	none
Spitting up or vomiting	a great deal	somewhat	very little	none
Sleeping	a great deal	somewhat	very little	none
Feeding	a great deal	somewhat	very little	none
Elimination	a great deal	somewhat	very little	none
Lack of a predictable schedule	a great deal	somewhat	very little	none
Other (specify):	a great deal	somewhat	very little	none
_____	a great deal	somewhat	very little	none
_____	a great deal	somewhat	very little	none
_____	a great deal	somewhat	very little	none
_____	a great deal	somewhat	very little	none

**This Inventory is used to summarize the presence of potential or actual problem areas.

FIGURE 21-7. Neonatal Perception Inventories I and II. (*Note.* From Further considerations regarding maternal perceptions of the first born, by E.R. Broussard and M.S. Hartner. In J. Hellmuth [Ed.], *Exceptional infant: Studies in abnormalities*, Vol. 2, pp. 442–443. Copyright © 1971 by Brunner/Mazel. Reprinted by permission.)

TABLE 21-5
The Neonatal History

Prenatal Period

Maternal age, parity, health, nutrition, blood type

Paternal age, health, blood type

Family history of genetic or chromosomal abnormalities

Prenatal care—when begun, frequency, provider

Complications (e.g., pregnancy-induced hypertension, diabetes, heart disease, bleeding) during pregnancy

Mother's use of medications (over-the-counter or prescription) during pregnancy

Exposure to infectious disease (e.g., rubella, toxoplasmosis) or other hazards (alcohol, caffeine, smoking, recreational drugs, radiation)

Perinatal Period

Onset (spontaneous, induced; premature, term, postmature) and length of labor

Fetal presentation (vertex, breech, tranverse lie, footling)

Use of analgesia, anesthesia

Type of delivery (spontaneous, forceps, Caesarean)

Complications during L&D (fetal distress, hypoxia/ anoxia, placenta previa, abruptio placenta, uterine inertia)

Postnatal Period

Birth weight, length, head circumference

APGAR scores at 1 and 5 minutes of age

Birth injuries or anomalies

Feeding method (breast or bottle)

Circumcision (boys)

Infant's name(s)

Parental responses to newborn

Sibling responses to newborn

Family resources (health insurance, living arrangements, income)

Parents' knowledge of and previous experience with child care (bathing, diapering, feeding, safety, cord care, growth and development)

Parents' hopes and expectations for infant; parents' perceptions of neonate (Neonatal Perception Inventories I and II)

Special cultural or religious beliefs related to newborn care (cord care, skin care, dressing, visitors, mother's role, father's role, family involvement)

---

should be unclothed and in a supine position. While undressing the infant, the nurse should observe general muscle tone and response to external stimuli.

CLINICAL APPRAISAL AND SCREENING

Careful monitoring of the fetus during the mother's labor and delivery provides clues to fetal well-being. For instance, auscultation or monitoring of fetal heart tones enables assessment of the fetus's responses to the stress of labor. Actual clinical appraisal of the neonate begins at the moment of delivery when the infant makes its initial contact with the extra-uterine environment. The clinical appraisal should include assessments that help determine how well the neonate is adapting to extra-uterine life. The first assessment performed usually is APGAR scoring.

APGAR Scoring System

Once the neonate has established respiration and the airway is clear, an initial assessment of the infant using the APGAR scoring system should be done. This system of evaluating the newborn's initial adaptation to the extra-uterine environment was developed by Dr. Virginia Apgar (1966) as a simple system for rating the infant at 1 and 5 minutes of age. A total score ranging from 0 to 10 is assigned, with 10 the optimal score.

The neonate is assessed on five parameters:

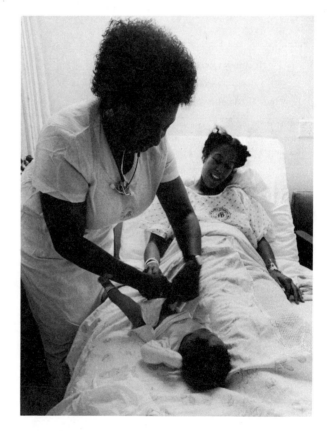

FIGURE 21-8. Conducting the newborn appraisal in the mother's presence provides an excellent opportunity for her to become acquainted with her infant. (*Note.* From Auvenshine/Enriquez: *Comprehensive Maternity Nursing,* Second Edition, © 1990. Boston: Jones and Bartlett Publishers, p. 498.)

A—appearance (skin color)

P—pulse (heart) rate

G—grimace (reflex response)

A—activity (muscle tone)

R—respiratory effort

For each parameter, the newborn receives a score of 0, 1, or 2. The five scores for each parameter are added for a total APGAR score. The 1-minute APGAR score indicates whether the infant needs resuscitation to assist the transition to extra-uterine life. A score of 8, 9, or 10 indicates the newborn is adapting successfully and requires only nasal or oral suctioning, drying, and warmth. Lower scores require varying degrees of additional intervention, ranging from oxygen therapy and vigorous back-rubbing to cardiopulmonary resuscitation.

The 5-minute APGAR has been shown to be closely related to neurological status at 1 year of age. APGAR scores can be affected by analgesics or anesthetics administered to the mother during labor, low birth weight, and neonatal asphyxia. The APGAR scoring chart is depicted in Figure 21-9.

Measuring Vital Signs

After determining the neonate's 1- and 5-minute APGAR scores, the nurse should continue to monitor the infant closely. Ongoing assessment of vital signs (see Table 21-6) provides an important measure of the newborn's adaptation and stability. The American Academy of Pediatrics recommends monitoring the newborn's vital signs once every hour until they are stable for 2 hours, then every 8 hours thereafter.

The first priority in assessing and caring for the neonate is to establish a clear airway and initiate respiration. A large amount of mucus, amniotic fluid, blood, and possibly meconium is present in the nasopharynx at birth and is suctioned by the nurse midwife or physician as soon as the neonate's head emerges during delivery. After delivery, the nurse should suction the infant's mouth before suctioning the nose to prevent the infant from aspirating the large amount of fluid in the mouth. While clearing the air passages, the nurse should observe the infant closely for adequate respiration. The respiratory rate should range from 30 to 80 breaths per minute, and skin color should be reddish pink, although acrocyanosis may be present. Crying increases the respiratory rate, whereas sleeping causes the respiratory rate to drop.

The thorax should be inspected for shape and symmetry. Breathing should be diaphragmatic and may be irregular. Breath sounds should be clear (crackles may be present for the first few hours after birth) and equal bilaterally. Tachypnea (respiration above 80 breaths per minute), bradypnea (below 30 breaths per minute), repeated apneic spells, nasal flaring, retractions, grunting, and diminished or unequal breath sounds indicate respiratory distress and require immediate attention.

The Silverman-Andersen Index (Silverman & Andersen, 1956), a tool for evaluating respiratory status of the neonate, provides guidelines for continued monitoring after the initial APGAR scores are obtained. Using this index, the neonate is evaluated on five criteria:

- chest lag
- intercostal retraction
- xiphoid retraction
- nares dilation
- expiratory grunt

A score of 0, 1, or 2 is assigned for each of these criteria, and the scores are totaled. An optimal score of 0 indicates no respiratory distress, a sign that the neonate is achieving successful respiratory adaptation and functioning. A score of 10 indicates severe respiratory distress. The Silverman-Andersen Index is depicted in Figure 21-10.

The neonate's heart rate should be measured apically with a stethoscope. The apical impulse usually is palpable over the fourth to fifth intercostal space and lateral to the left sternal border. The

Assessment Parameter	Score		
	0	1	2
A Appearance (color)	Absent	Slow, below 100	Above 100
P Pulse (heart) rate	Absent	Slow; irregular weak cry	Good strong cry
G Grimace (reflex response)	Flaccid	Some flexion of extremities	Well flexed
A Activity (muscle tone)	No response	Grimace	Cry, reflexive withdrawal
R Respiratory effort	Blue, pale, dusky	Body pink, extremities blue	Completely pink

FIGURE 21-9. APGAR Scoring System

TABLE 21-6
Vital Signs—Neonatal Norms

Axillary Temperature
36.5°–37.0° C (97.9°–98.6° F)

Heart Rate

Sleeping	80–140 beats/minute
Quiet awake	100–180 beats/minute
Exercise, crying, fever	120–220 beats/minute

Respiratory Rate '

Sleeping or resting	30–40 breaths/minute
Exercise, crying, illness	40–80 breaths/minute

Blood Pressure (averages)

1 day (boys)	73/55
1 day (girls)	65/55
1 month (boys)	86/52
1 month (girls)	84/52

point of maximal impulse (PMI) is often visible. Both S_1 and S_2 sounds should be auscultated. S_2 is typically sharper and higher pitched than S_1. Sinus arrhythmia is a common finding in neonates. Murmurs (common in newborns), thrills, persistent cyanosis, and displacement of the apex may indicate cardiac abnormalities and should be referred for further evaluation. Femoral pulses should be palpated for presence, strength, and quality.

Blood pressure is best measured using the doppler method. Both upper arm and thigh measurements should be obtained. A newborn blood pressure cuff may be used to measure the blood pressure. The flush method typically is used to determine systolic pressure (the pressure at which the arm or leg distal to the cuff "flushes"). Systolic pressures in the upper arm and thigh should be relatively equal. A difference of more than 10 mm Hg requires further evaluation. Systolic pressures should be no greater than 100 mm Hg or less than 40 mm Hg.

The infant's axillary temperature should be monitored frequently in the early neonatal period. Axillary temperatures are preferred because of the trauma a rectal thermometer can cause to the fragile rectal mucosa (Schiffman, 1982). The neonate's axillary temperature should be between 36.5° and 37°C. Chilling or overheating may cause the body temperature to drop or rise, respectively, and should be corrected immediately.

Assessment of Gestational Age

Assessment of gestational age is a critical measure of the neonate's maturity and is important because of its relationship to infant morbidity and mortality. There are a number of methods for estimating gestational age.

The neonate's gestational age may be estimated by calculating the number of weeks since the mother's last menstrual period. However, numerous factors can reduce the accuracy of this method, including the reliability of the mother's recall, irregularity of the mother's menstrual cycle, interval since last pregnancy, breast-feeding, and postconceptual bleeding. Gestational age also can be ascertained by obstetric methods, including measurement of the height of the uterine fundus, quickening date, auscultation of fetal heart tones, sonography, and amniotic fluid analysis. The latter two methods are considered highly reliable indicators of gestational age; however, they are not employed routinely in all pregnancies.

The most widely used method of assessing gestational age is the Dubowitz scoring system (Dubowitz, Dubowitz, & Goldberg, 1970). This method is based on an examination of the neonate within the first few hours of life, using 11 physical characteristics as assessment parameters. Ten more neurological characteristics are measured after the first 24 hours to confirm the initial gestational age assessment. The advantages of the Dubowitz scoring system are its:

- ease of use by staff not trained in neonatal neurology
- simple recording method
- reliability
- completion time of less than 15 minutes
- application to preterm, full-term, and postterm infants

Many newborn-nursery nurses use only 5 of the characteristics: breasts, ears, genitals, sole creases, and posture, which have been shown to determine correct gestational age in almost all neonates (Sullivan, Foster, & Schreiner, 1979). The neonate's gestational age (maturity rating) is considered accurate within plus or minus 2 weeks of the infant's true age. The Dubowitz scoring system is illustrated in Figure 21-11 and discussed in the boxed insert.

Measuring Physical Growth

Parameters of physical growth include weight, length, and head circumference. When measuring the neonate's physical growth, consistency of technique and measurement tools (e.g., weight scale, tape measure) is important to ensure the validity and reliability of findings.

Weight should be measured while the neonate is nude. A calibrated and balanced infant scale should be used to assure accuracy of measurement and the safety of the infant. While in the hospital,

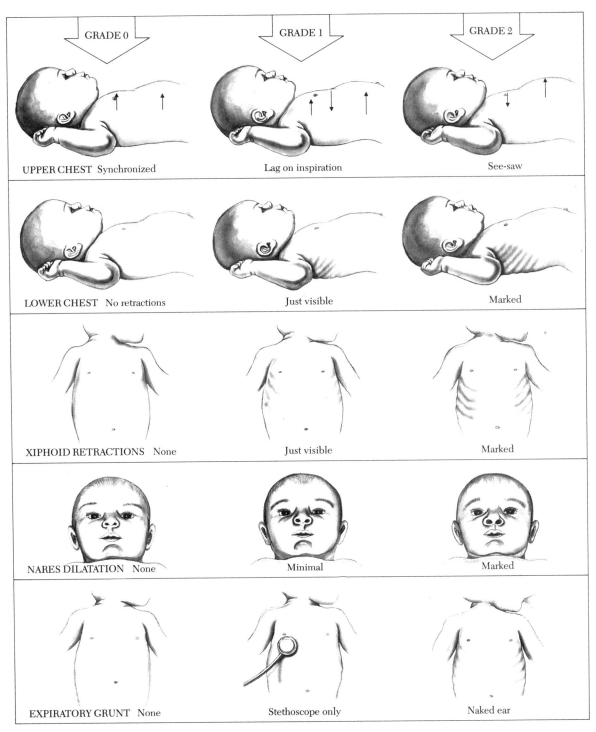

FIGURE 21-10. The Silverman-Andersen Index. This index is designed to provide a continued evaluation of the infant's respiratory status. An index of respiratory distress is determined by grading each of the five arbitrary criteria: chest lag, intercostal retraction, xiphoid retraction, nares dilatation, and expiratory grunt. The "retraction score" is computed by adding the values (0, 1, or 2) assigned to each factor that best describes the infant's manifestation at the time of a single observation. *A score of 0 indicates no respiratory distress; a score of 10 indicates severe respiratory distress.* (*Note.* From "Evaluation of Respiratory Status: Silverman and Andersen Index," by W.A. Silverman and D.H. Andersen, *Pediatrics, 17,* 1, 1956. Copyright American Academy of Pediatrics. Reprinted by permission.)

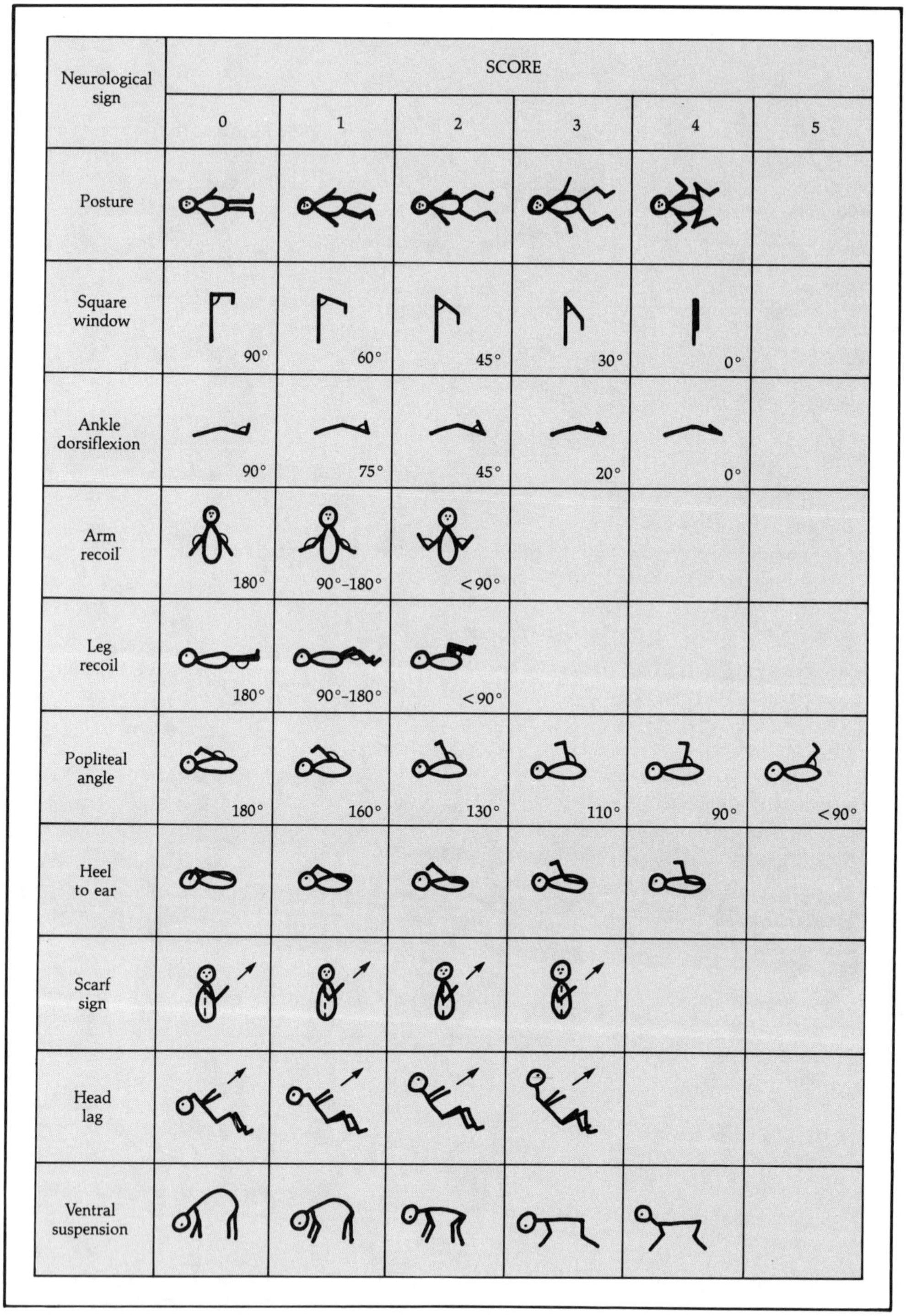

Neurological sign	SCORE					
	0	1	2	3	4	5
Posture						
Square window	90°	60°	45°	30°	0°	
Ankle dorsiflexion	90°	75°	45°	20°	0°	
Arm recoil	180°	90°–180°	<90°			
Leg recoil	180°	90°–180°	<90°			
Popliteal angle	180°	160°	130°	110°	90°	<90°
Heel to ear						
Scarf sign						
Head lag						
Ventral suspension						

FIGURE 21-11. The Dubowitz Scoring System for Clinical Estimation of Gestational Age. (*Note.* From Dubowitz, L., Dubowitz, V., & Goldberg, C. [1970]. Clinical assessment of gestational age in the newborn infant. *Journal of Pediatrics, 77*[1], 1–10.) (Figure continues on page 672.)

Some Notes on Techniques of Assessment of Neurologic Criteria
(for use in conjunction with Fig. 21-11)

Posture: Observed with infant quiet and in supine position. Score 0: Arms and legs extended; 1: Beginning of flexion of hips and knees, arms extended; 2: Stronger flexion of legs, arms extended; 3: Arms slightly flexed, legs flexed and abducted; 4: Full flexion of arms and legs.

Square window: The hand is flexed on the forearm between the thumb and index finger of the examiner. Enough pressure is applied to get as full a flexion as possible, and the angle between the hypothenar eminence and the ventral aspect of the forearm is measured and graded. (Care is taken not to rotate the infant's wrist while doing this maneuver.)

Ankle dorsiflexion: The foot is dorsiflexed onto the anterior aspect of the leg, with the examiner's thumb on the sole of the foot and other fingers behind the leg. Enough pressure is applied to get as full a flexion as possible, and the angle between the dorsum of the foot and the anterior aspect of the leg is measured.

Arm recoil: With the infant in the supine position the forearms are first flexed for 5 seconds, then fully extended by pulling on the hands, and then released. The sign is fully positive if the arms return briskly to full flexion (Score 2). If the arms return to incomplete flexion or the response is sluggish, it is graded as score 1. If they remain extended or are only followed by random movements, the score is 0.

Leg recoil: With the infant supine, the hips and knees are fully flexed for 5 seconds, then extended by traction on the feet, and released. A maximal response is one of full flexion of the hips and knees (Score 2). A partial flexion scores 1, and minimal or no movement scores 0.

Popliteal angle: With the infant supine and his pelvis flat on the examining couch, the thigh is held in the knee-chest position by the examiner's left index finger and thumb supporting the knee. The leg is then extended by gentle pressure from the examiner's right index finger behind the ankle and the popliteal angle is measured.

Heel to ear maneuver: With the baby supine, draw the baby's foot as near to the head as it will go without forcing it. Observe the distance between the foot and the head as well as the degree of extension at the knee. Grade according to diagram. Note that the knee is left free and may draw down alongside the abdomen.

Scarf sign: With the baby supine, take the infant's hand and try to put it around the neck and as far posteriorly as possible around the opposite shoulder. Assist this maneuver by lifting the elbow across the body. See how far the elbow will go across and grade according to illustrations. Score 0: Elbow reaches opposite axillary line; 1: Elbow between midline and opposite axillary line; 2: Elbow reaches midline; 3: Elbow will not reach midline.

Head lag: With the baby lying supine, grasp the hands (or the arms if a very small infant) and pull him slowly toward the sitting position. Observe the position of the head in relation to the trunk and grade accordingly. In a small infant the head may initially be supported by one hand. Score 0: Complete lag; 1: Partial head control; 2: Able to maintain head in line with body; 3: Brings head anterior to body.

Ventral suspension: The infant is suspended in the prone position, with examiner's hand under the infant's chest (one hand in a small infant, two in a large infant): Observe the degree of extension of the back and the amount of flexion of the arms and legs. Also note the relation of the head to the trunk. Grade according to diagrams (Fig. 21-11).

If score differs on the two sides, take the mean.

Note. From Dubowitz, L., Dubowitz, V., & Goldberg, C. [1970]. Clinical assessment of gestational age in the newborn infant. *Journal of Pediatrics, 77*[1], 1–10.

the breast-fed neonate should be weighed before and after breast-feedings to determine fluid intake.

The neonate's length should be measured with the infant in a supine position (recumbent length). The infant's head should be placed against a stationary board, the legs extended, and the crown-to-heel length measured with a tape measure (see Figure 21-12).

The size, shape, symmetry, and general appearance of the head should be carefully evaluated. The head often shows pronounced effects from la-

bor and delivery. The most common variation of the head is molding (see Figure 21-13), which disappears within 72 hours of birth. The head should be inspected and palpated for the presence of two fairly common neonatal conditions: caput succedaneum and cephalohematoma (see Figures 21-14, 21-15, and 21-16). Caput succedaneum is edema of the soft tissue of the scalp due to pressure during labor and delivery. Suture line margins are poorly defined and difficult to palpate because of the generalized edema. Cephalohematoma is a subperios-

External sign	Score				
	0	1	2	3	4
Edema	Obvious edema of hands and feet; pitting over tibia	No obvious edema of hands and feet; pitting over tibia	No edema		
Skin texture	Very thin, gelatinous	Thin and smooth	Smooth; medium thickness; rash or superficial peeling	Slight thickening; superficial cracking and peeling especially of hands and feet	Thick and parchmentlike; superficial or deep cracking
Skin color	Dark red	Uniformly pink	Pale pink; variable over body	Pale; only pink over ears, lips, palms, or soles	
Skin opacity (trunk)	Numerous veins and venules clearly seen, especially over abdomen	Veins and tributaries seen	A few large vessels clearly seen over abdomen	A few large vessels seen indistinctly over abdomen	No blood vessels seen
Lanugo (over back)	No lanugo	Abundant; long and thick over whole back	Hair thinning especially over lower back	Small amount of lanugo and bald areas	At least 1/2 of back devoid of lanugo
Plantar creases	No skin creases	Faint red marks over anterior half of sole	Definite red marks over > anterior 1/2; indentations over < anterior 1/3	Indentations over > anterior 1/3	Definite deep indentations over > anterior 1/3
Nipple formation	Nipple barely visible; no areola	Nipple well defined; areola smooth and flat, diameter < 0.75 cm	Areola stippled, edge not raised, diameter < 0.75 cm	Areola stippled, edge raised, diameter > 0.75 cm	
Breast size	No breast tissue palpable	Breast tissue on one or both sides, < 0.5 cm diameter	Breast tissue both sides; one or both 0.5 to 1.0 cm	Breast tissue both sides; one or both > 1 cm	
Ear form	Pinna flat and shapeless, little or no incurving of edge	Incurving of part of edge of pinna	Partial incurving whole of upper pinna	Well-defined incurving whole of upper pinna	
Ear firmness	Pinna soft, easily folded, no recoil	Pinna soft, easily folded, slow recoil	Cartilage to edge of pinna, but soft in places, ready recoil	Pinna firm, cartilage to edge; instant recoil	
Genitals Male	Neither testis in scrotum	At least one testis high in scrotum	At least one testis right down		
Female (with hips 1/2 abducted)	Labia majora widely separated, labia minora protruding	Labia majora almost cover labia minora	Labia majora completely cover labia minora		

FIGURE 21-11 (Continued). (*Note.* From Dubowitz, L., Dubowitz, V., & Goldberg, C. [1970]. Clinical assessment of gestational age in the newborn infant. *Journal of Pediatrics, 77*[1], 1–10).)

The scores for each of the newborn's neurological and external signs should be totaled. A maximum score of 70 is possible. The infant's total score should be compared to the weeks of gestation listed below. An estimate of gestational age is accurate within 2 weeks.

Score	Weeks of Gestation
0–9	26
10–12	27
13–16	28
17–20	29
21–24	30
25–27	31
28–31	32
32–35	33
36–39	34
40–43	35
44–46	36
47–50	37
51–54	38
55–58	39
59–62	40
63–65	41
66–69	42

FIGURE 21-11. (Continued). (*Note.* From Dubowitz, L., Dubowitz, V., & Goldberg, C. [1970]. Clinical assessment of gestational age in the newborn infant. *Journal of Pediatrics,* 77[1], 1–10.)

teal hemorrhage secondary to the trauma of labor and delivery. The edema is localized and suture line margins are well-defined.

The neonate's head circumference should be measured over the supraorbital and occipital prominences (see Figure 21-12). In addition, the anterior

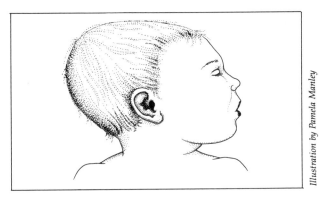

FIGURE 21-13. Molding of a Newborn Head. (*Note.* From Servonsky/Opas: *Nursing Management of Children,* © 1987. Boston: Jones and Bartlett Publishers, p. 96.)

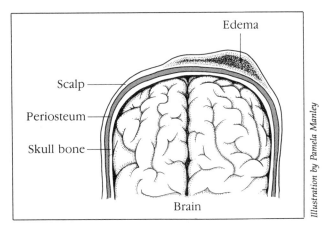

FIGURE 21-14. Caput Succedaneum: Swelling of the Soft Tissues of the Scalp (*Note.* From Servonsky/Opas: *Nursing Management of Children,* © 1987. Boston: Jones and Bartlett Publishers, p. 96.)

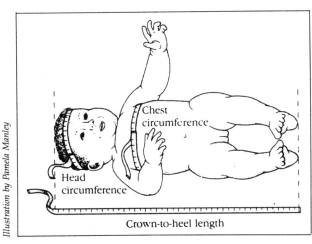

FIGURE 21-12. Neonatal Physical Growth Measurements. (*Note.* From Servonsky/Opas: *Nursing Management of Children,* © 1987. Boston: Jones and Bartlett Publishers, p. 93.)

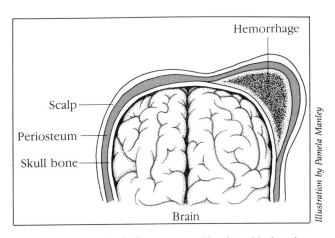

FIGURE 21-15. Cephalhematoma: Bleeding Under the Periosteum, Causing It to Separate from the Bony Plate. (*Note.* From Servonsky/Opas: *Nursing Management of Children,* © 1987. Boston: Jones and Bartlett Publishers, p. 96.)

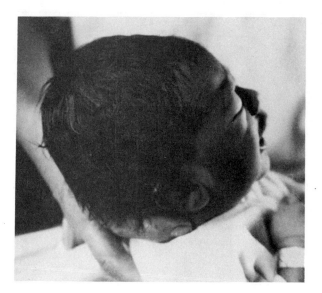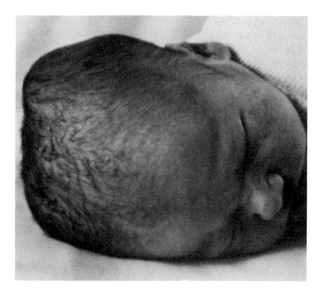

FIGURE 21-16. Caput succedaneum (*left*) is a diffuse, generalized swelling of the scalp, not sharply defined. Cephalhematoma (*right*), subperiosteal hemorrhage, is usually well defined by suture lines. (*Note.* Courtesy of Mead Johnson Laboratories, Evansville, Indiana.)

and posterior fontanels should be gently palpated and their placement noted. The diameter of the fontanel openings should be measured and compared with norms. The anterior fontanel is soft and pulsates with the infant's heartbeat. When the infant is quiet and held in an upright position, the fontanel is slightly depressed. The anterior fontanel is palpated at the junction of the coronal, frontal, and sagittal sutures (see Figure 21-17). The posterior fontanel is palpated at the junction of the sagittal and lambdoidal sutures.

The chest circumference should be measured during inspiration, using the breast nipples as a point of reference. Weight, length, and head circumference should be plotted on a standardized growth chart (see Figures 21-18, 21-19, 21-20, and 21-21). The newborn's measurements should fall between the 5th and 95th percentiles and should be within one standard deviation of each other. If any of the measurements is more than one standard deviation different from the others, further evaluation is warranted. Variables that can influence physical growth and should be taken into account when interpreting growth measurements include hereditary factors (family characteristics, race, gender), maternal nutrition, insults during fetal development, and health deviations. Current growth charts are based on a fairly broad sample of North American children, but may not provide accurate norms for certain groups, such as immigrant children from non-Western cultures. Furthermore, within-group norms (e.g., norms for black chil-

dren) may vary considerably from those used for standardized growth charts.

Neonatal measurements provide a baseline for ongoing evaluation of subsequent physical growth, and therefore are important indices of an infant's general health.

Integumentary Assessment

The skin of newborns is thinner and more sensitive to trauma than that of older children and adults.

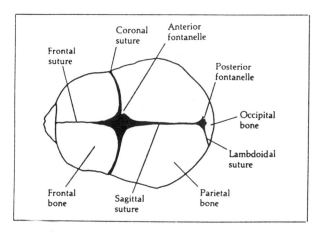

FIGURE 21-17. Locations of Sutures and Fontanels. (*Note.* From Auvenshine/Enriquez: *Comprehensive Maturnity Nursing: Perinatal and Women's Health,* Second Edition, © 1990. Boston: Jones and Bartlett Publishers, p. 555.

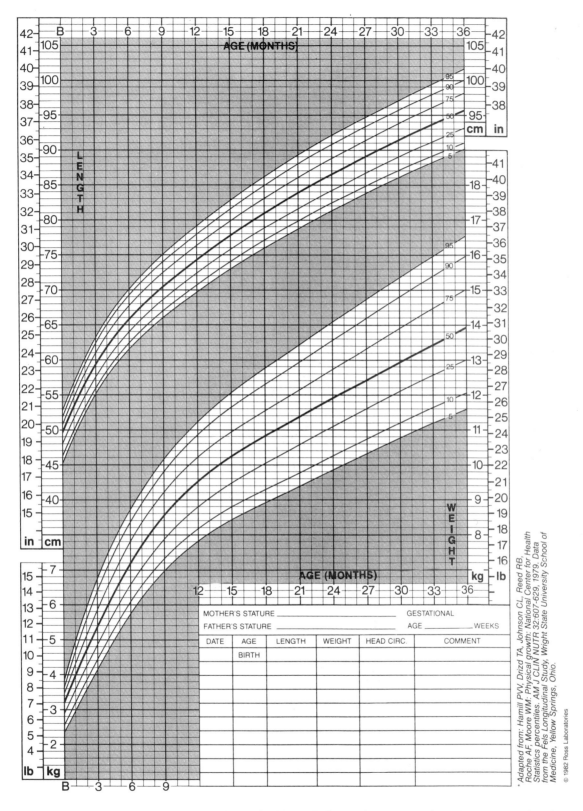

FIGURE 21-18. Standardized Height and Weight Chart: Girls—Birth to 36 Months. (*Note.* Reprinted with permission from Ross Laboratories, Columbus, Ohio. Adapted from Hamill, P.V.V., Drizd, T.A., Johnson, C.L., Reed, R.B., Roche, A.F., Moore, W.M.: Physical growth: National Center for Health Statistics percentiles. *American Journal of Clinical Nutrition* 32: 607–629, 1979. Data from the Fels Longitudinal Study, Wright State University School of Medicine, Yellow Springs, Ohio. © 1982 Ross Laboratories.)

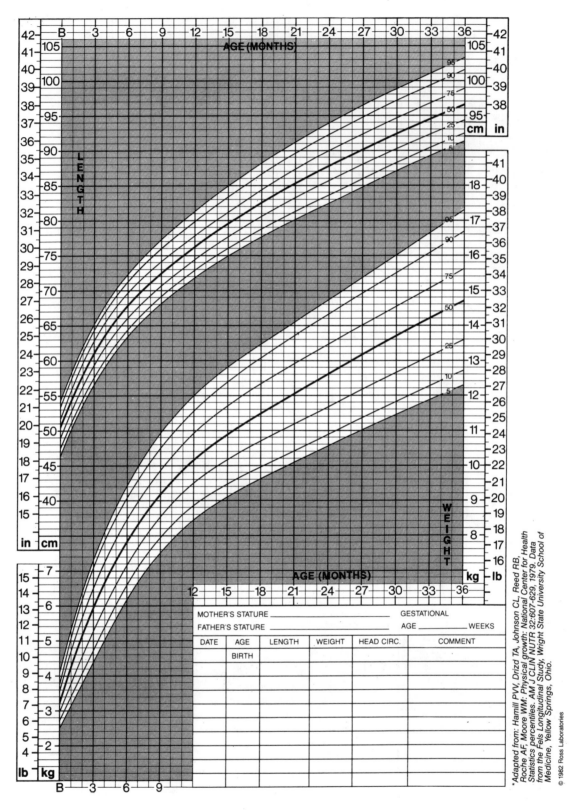

FIGURE 21-19. Standardized Height and Weight Chart: Boys—Birth to 36 Months. (*Note.* Reprinted with permission from Ross Laboratories, Columbus, Ohio. Adapted from Hamill, P.V.V., Drizd, T.A., Johnson, C.L., Reed, R.B., Roche, A.F., Moore, W.M.: Physical growth: National Center for Health Statistics percentiles. *American Journal of Clinical Nutrition,* 32: 607–629, 1979. Data from the Fels Longitudinal Study, Wright State University School of Medicine, Yellow Springs, Ohio. © 1982 Ross Laboratories.)

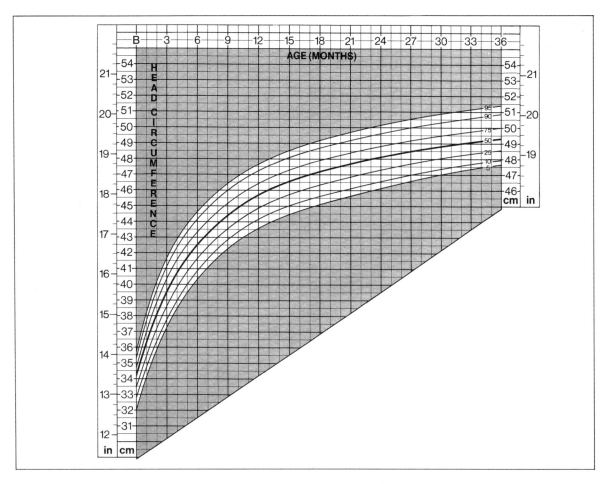

FIGURE 21-20. Standardized Head Circumference Chart: Girls—Birth to 36 Months. (*Note.* Reprinted with permission from Ross Laboratories, Columbus, Ohio. Adapted from Hamill, P.V.V., Drizd, T.A., Johnson, C.L., Reed, R.B., Roche, A.F., Moore, W.M.: Physical growth: National Center for Health Statistics percentiles. *American Journal of Clinical Nutrition* 32: 607–629, 1979. Data from the Fels Longitudinal Study, Wright State University School of Medicine, Yellow Springs, Ohio. © 1982 Ross Laboratories.)

The nails tend to be thin and peel easily. When assessing the neonate, the nurse should handle the infant carefully to prevent injury to delicate skin tissue.

The newborn's skin should be inspected carefully, using a systematic head-to-toe, right-to-left approach. Adequate lighting is essential.

The color and appearance of the skin should be evaluated. The skin should be pink although acrocyanosis may be present. Ruddiness or pallor may indicate complications of the perinatal period such as delayed clamping of the umbilical cord, anemia, or hypotension. Jaundice is the most likely color change to be noted. To assess for the presence of jaundice, the skin over the bony prominences of the frontal bone and cartilage of the nose should be blanched. In nonwhite newborns, the nurse should inspect the mucous membranes of the mouth. A yellowish hue of the skin or mucous membranes indicates jaundice. The sclera of the eyes also may appear yellow.

Jaundice that occurs within the first 24 hours of life always is considered abnormal. The more common physiological jaundice typically appears within 48 to 72 hours of birth and tends to be greater in breast-fed infants (Osburn, Reiff, & Bolus, 1984). The presence of jaundice requires prompt evaluation of serum bilirubin levels.

Because many newborns are discharged from the hospital or birthing center within the first 48 hours of life, it is important to arrange for a home visit by the nurse or a return visit by the mother and baby to ensure careful assessment for jaundice. In addition to inspecting the skin, mucous membranes, and sclera, the nurse may use a noninvasive bilirubinometer to screen for elevated bilirubin levels. Brucker and MacMullen (1987) screened 20 newborns with this device and found significant correlations between serum bilirubin levels and meter readings.

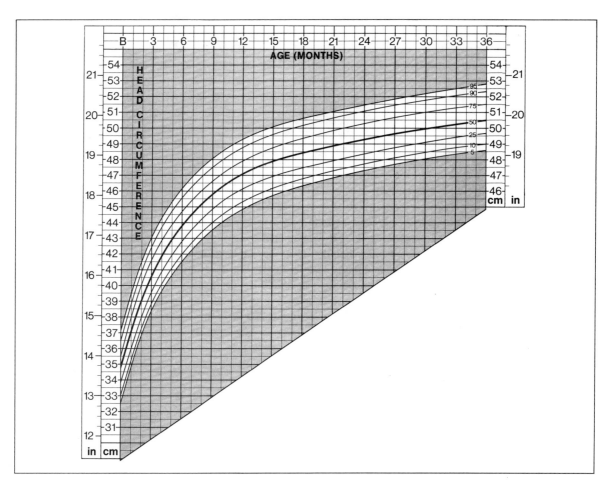

FIGURE 21-21. Standardized Head Circumference Chart: Boys—Birth to 36 Months. (*Note.* Reprinted with permission from Ross Laboratories, Columbus, Ohio. Adapted from Hamill, P.V.V., Drizd, T.A., Johnson, C.L., Reed, R.B., Roche, A.F., Moore, W.M.: Physical growth: National Center for Health Statistics percentiles. *American Journal of Clinical Nutrition* 32: 607–629, 1979. Data from the Fels Longitudinal Study, Wright State University School of Medicine, Yellow Springs, Ohio. © 1982 Ross Laboratories.)

The umbilical cord should be inspected for the presence of three blood vessels (two arteries, one vein). The cord should be dry with no bleeding or discharge evident. The skin around the umbilicus should be examined for redness, edema, or chafing. The umbilical cord, which is bluish white at birth, begins drying within hours. It becomes yellowish brown, then brownish black, and drops off within 7 to 14 days.

There are numerous common variations in the skin of newborn infants. Skin variations often disappear within a period of days or weeks but some may persist throughout life, such as cafe-au-lait spots or port wine stain birthmarks. Common neonatal skin variations are described in Table 21-7 and several are depicted in the accompanying photographs (see Figure 21-22). The nurse should document the location, size, color, and special characteristics of visible skin variations.

Assessment of Sensory Functioning

Assessment of sensory functioning involves a gross evaluation of the newborn's vision and hearing. Smell and taste also may be assessed. Inspection of the eyes, ears, nose, and mouth is an important part of the neonatal sensory assessment.

Eyes

The neonate's eyes should be examined for symmetry, edema, and redness. The eyes usually are round, although epicanthal folds are present in Asian infants, causing the eyes to appear almond-shaped. Conjunctivitis may be evident due to instillation of antibacterial agents, which are used to prevent ophthalmia neonatorum, a gonococcal or chlamydial infection of the eye that may be contracted by the infant during delivery.

The neonate should be observed, in a dimly lit

TABLE 21-7
Common Skin Variations in Neonates

Variation	Description
Acrocyanosis	Cyanosis of the hands and feet within first 12–24 hours of life; abnormal thereafter
Birthmarks	Single brown or reddish colorations; flat or slightly raised; remain throughout life
Cafe-au-lait	Flat, irregular, light brown colorations (dark brown in dark-skinned infants); remain throughout life
Cutis marmorata	Mottling of skin caused by cool environmental temperatures; disappears with warming
Desquamation	Peeling of skin within first few days of birth; especially pronounced in postmature neonates
Ecchymosis	Bruising of face, neck, and head (or other presenting body part) caused by pressure during birth process
Erythema toxicum	Pinkish red papular rash on the trunk, abdomen, and buttocks; appears within first 24 hours of life and resolves within several days
Lanugo	Fine, downy hair covering the body in varying amounts; especially prominent over the shoulders and forehead; sheds within the first few weeks of life
Milia	Pinpoint pearly white or yellow papules on the nose, chin, forehead, and gingivae or palate (Epstein's pearls); disappear by end of neonatal period
Mongolian spots	Flat, bluish colorations of the buttocks and lower back; seen primarily in African-American, Asian, and Hispanic newborns; fade with increasing age
Port wine stain (nevus flammeus)	Flat, irregular, reddish purple coloration; usually confined to one side of the body; remains throughout life
Stork bites	Flat, purplish pink areas usually located above the nose and on the back of the neck; fade with increasing age
Strawberry mark	Slightly raised capillary hemangioma 2 to 3 cm in diameter; usually found on face, scalp, or back of neck; usually disappears with increasing age
Vernix caseosa	White cheesy substance that covers the skin at birth; absorbed or cleansed away within 24 to 48 hours of birth

room, to determine if the eyes open spontaneously (the eyes should never be forced open). Observation of ocular activity is most reliable when the infant is being held quietly or is nursing. The presence of a red reflex and pupil size, symmetry, and reaction to light should be noted. In dark-skinned infants—native American, Hispanic, African-American—the reflex is pale instead of orange-red. The iris of white newborns is dark blue-gray, while African-American, Asian, native American and Hispanic newborns have brown-gray irises. The sclera of all newborns is bluish-white. The cornea should be transparent and shiny. Tear ducts are not functional at birth, but tears usually are produced by 2 weeks of age in term infants. The presence of discharge from the eyes or subconjunctival hemorrhage should be noted. The latter appears as a red, crescent-shaped area in the sclera next to the iris and is absorbed within two weeks. It is related to pressure exerted on the fetus during the birthing process.

Eye movement also should be assessed for the presence of strabismus (see Figure 21-23) or nystagmus, both of which are considered normal. The neonate should be able to fixate (stop sucking, watch intently) momentarily on an object held 8 to 12 inches from the face and should be able to follow the object to midline. Newborns tend to fixate longer on human faces, complex patterns, and bright colors.

Ears

The newborn's ears should be examined for shape, symmetry, position in relation to the eyes, and presence of cartilage. The top of the pinna should be level with the outer canthus of the eye. The pinna should be palpated for firmness and elasticity (see section on gestational age assessment). The surfaces around the ear and the outer portion of the ear canal should be inspected by gently pulling the pinna up and back. The outer ear canal should be clear.

The neonate's responses to sound may be assessed by ringing a bell held laterally and posteriorly to the ear. The infant should respond attentively. A sudden moderate to loud noise, such as clapping the hands, should elicit a startle. Hearing screening is not performed routinely during the newborn period. Neonates at risk of hearing impairment, however, such as premature infants,

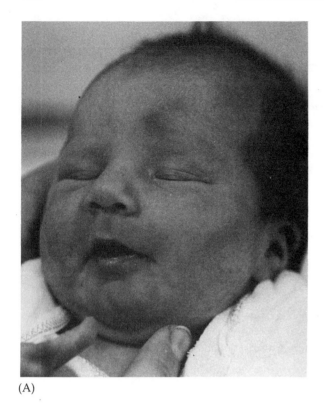

(A)

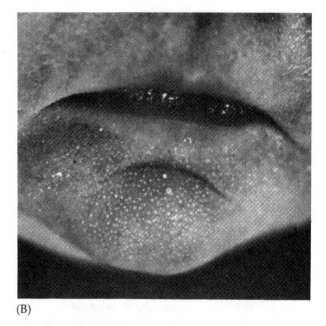

(B)

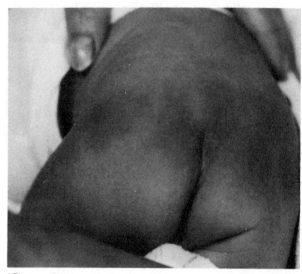

(C)

FIGURE 21-22. Common Neonatal Skin Variations. (A) Facial ecchymosis due to forceps delivery. (B) Milia. (C) Mongolian spots. (*Note.* A from Auvenshine/Enriquez: *Comprehensive Maternity Nursing: Perinatal and Women's Health,* Second Edition, ©. Boston: Jones and Bartlett Publishers, p. 553. B and C courtesy of Mead Johnson Laboratories, Evansville, Indiana.)

those exposed to rubella during the first months of fetal development, or those with family histories of congenital deafness, should be screened using impedance audiometry. A qualified audiologist should conduct the screening.

Nose and Mouth

The size and shape of the nose, the presence of nasal discharge, and any obstruction of nasal breathing should be noted. The nose should be examined for patency. Thin, clear or whitish mucus and sneezing are common. The newborn will demonstrate an aversion to noxious smells, such as an alcohol wipe or ammonia vial, by turning the head away and possibly sneezing.

The mouth can be inspected most easily when the infant is crying. The frenum of the upper lip and frenulum of the tongue are short and tight. The size, shape, and color of the tongue should be noted. Using a tongue depressor and light, the nurse should examine the palate and mucous membranes. The soft and hard palates should be inspected and palpated to confirm that they are intact. Salivation should be minimal in the newborn. *Epstein's pearls,* pinpoint-size white cysts, may be visible on the gum margins and along the midline of the hard palate in approximately half of all newborns. *Natal teeth,* usually soft incisors, may be present at birth. A sucking blister or callus may be present on the midportion of the upper lip after feeding.

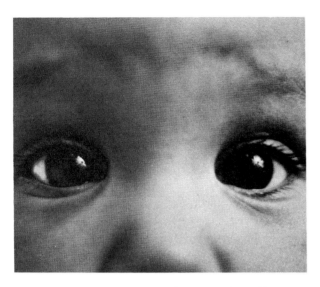

FIGURE 21-23. Neonatal Strabismus. (*Note.* Courtesy Mead Johnson Laboratories, Evansville, Indiana.)

Using a pacifier or finger, the nurse should assess the strength of the neonate's sucking reflex. Full-term infants tend to suck vigorously, whereas the sucking strength of preterm newborns is weaker (Medoff-Cooper, Weininger, & Zukowsky, 1989).

The mucous membranes should be inspected for color and hydration. They should be pink and moist. *Candidiasis* (thrush) may appear within the first few days or weeks as white adherent patches on the tongue, palate, and buccal mucosa. Thrush is a yeast infection (Candida albicans) that the neonate may contract from the mother's vagina during the birthing process. The cheeks should appear full and symmetrical. Accumulations of fat on the inner aspect of the cheeks, *sucking pads*, develop soon after birth.

The neonate's sense of taste can be assessed by offering glucose water and sterile water and noting the newborn's responses. The infant should accept the glucose water readily and seem less interested in the sterile water.

Assessment of Neurological Functioning

Assessment of neurological functioning should incorporate an evaluation of neonatal reflexes and the infant's response to painful stimuli. Neurological functioning often is assessed in conjunction with the gestational age assessment.

Neonatal Reflexes

Many reflexes are present in the healthy newborn. Absence of these reflexes may indicate an abnormality of central or peripheral motor functions. As the infant matures, the neonatal reflexes disappear in a predictable sequence. Persistence of these reflexes generally indicates a developmental delay or lesions of the central nervous system (Behrman & Vaughn, 1983).

Neonatal reflexes that should be assessed are identified in Table 21-8 and depicted in Figure 21-24. The method of eliciting each reflex, and normal and abnormal responses are described.

Responses to Pain

To assess the newborn's response to painful stimuli, the nurse should apply a light pinprick (5 to 10 times) to the infant's hands and feet in succession. A normal response is withdrawal of the pricked extremity and a facial grimace or cry. This maneuver tests the intactness of peripheral pain fibers and pain pathways to the level of the thalamus (Behrman & Vaughn, 1983).

The newborn's response to other painful stimuli, such as heel sticks, vitamin K injection, or circumcision, should be observed for behavioral cues that indicate the infant may be experiencing pain. Such cues include a facial startle, grimacing, and crying. Crying may be intermittent or sustained.

Activity–Sleep Assessment

During the first 12 hours of life, the neonate's level of alertness, general activity, and sleep behavior should be observed and documented. Brazelton's (1973) six states provide an excellent framework for categorizing the newborn's level of consciousness. The nurse may observe the newborn and compare findings (breathing pattern, eye [open or closed, movement], motor activity, and responses to stimuli) with descriptors for each state (see Table 21-9). The infant's responses to stimuli should be interpreted within the context of the infant's state of arousal.

The neonate's posture and spontaneous movements should be observed for symmetry while the infant is in a quiet state. The preferred side to which the newborn holds the head and the degree of flexion of the extremities should be noted.

Muscle Tone

Muscle tone is evaluated by determining the amount of resistance the infant offers to passive movement. Muscle tone of the limbs, trunk, neck, and head should be assessed. The nurse should observe the newborn's ability to lift the head while prone. Preterm infants and those with certain neurological impairments, such as Down syndrome,

TABLE 21-8
Neonatal Reflexes

Reflex	Method of Eliciting Reflex from Infant	Normal Response	Abnormal Response
Rooting	Stroke cheek near corner of mouth.	Head turns toward side being stroked and sucking movements appear.	Persistence beyond 12 months.
Sucking	Place examiner's finger or nipple in infant's mouth.	Rhythmic sucking movements; usually disappears 3–4 months; best noted in a hungry infant.	Persistence as a reflex beyond 12 months.
Extrusion	Touch tip of tongue.	Tongue pushes out of mouth.	Persistence beyond 4 months.
Grasp			
Palmar	Place examiner's finger in palm of infant's hand.	Fingers flex around examiner's hand; becomes voluntary about 6 months.	Persistence beyond 6 months as an involuntary response.
Plantar	Place examiner's finger on sole of infant's foot at base of toes.	Toes flex towards examiner's finger.	Absent in defects of lower spine (meningomyelocele); persistence beyond 8–12 months.
Stepping (dancing)	Hold infant in vertical position with soles of feet lightly touching firm surface.	Flexion and extension of alternate legs as though to simulate walking movements.	Persistence beyond 6 weeks.
Babinski	With fingertip, stroke lateral aspect of sole of foot from midpoint at heel, forward and across the ball of the foot to the great toe.	Great toe flexes dorsally while remaining toes fan outward.	Persistence beyond 12–18 months.
Tonic neck	Quickly turn head to (L) or (R).	Extension of arm and leg on side to which face is turned. Opposite arm and leg flex.	Continuous posturing; persistence beyond 4–6 months.
Moro	Hold in supine position. Permit head to fall back about 3 inches, taking care not to cause too great an extension.	Extension and abduction of arms. Extension and fanning of fingers except thumb and forefinger, which form a "C" shape. Legs flex and adduct.	Persistence beyond 4 months.
Startle	Clap hands loudly.	Arms abduct and flex at elbows; hands are clenched.	Persistence beyond 4 months.
Landau	Suspend in horizontal prone position with head raised actively or passively.	Appears about 4–6 months; lifts head, extends legs and spine.	Absence may signify cerebral palsy; exaggerated in hypertonic infants; persistence beyond 12–24 months.
Parachute	Hold under armpits in vertical position. Move body downward at head first angle.	Appears about 7–9 months. Arms extend in a protective motion.	Absence may signify cerebral palsy.

*One unsuccessful attempt at eliciting the reflex does not mean the reflex is not present. Absence, depression, or asymmetry of response may signal neurological deficit.

may exhibit varying degrees of hypotonia. Hyperflexion of the extremities and extreme resistance to passive movement may indicate cerebral palsy. Hyperextension of the head and neck and arching of the back indicate the need for more comprehensive evaluation.

Several specific measures for evaluating muscle tone can be employed. Specific indicators of muscle tone include arm and leg recoil, scarf sign, head lag, and the infant's response to extension of the heel of the foot to the head (heel-to-ear maneuver) and to ventral suspension. These measures are fully explained earlier in this chapter with the discussion of gestational age assessment.

Physical Mobility

A critical component of the newborn assessment is evaluating the infant for actual or potential impairment of physical mobility. There are several musculoskeletal abnormalities that can be detected during the routine newborn assessment, including *congenital clubfoot* (equinovarus deformity) and *congenital hip dysplasia*.

Congenital clubfoot is characterized by an inversion of the forefoot (varus deformity) and the toes positioned lower than the heel (equinus). It may be unilateral or bilateral. At birth, the neonate's feet may appear to be deformed because of malpositioning in utero. Such positional deformities can be distinguished from a true clubfoot by the ease with which the foot can be moved passively to a corrected position. In addition, if the deformity is positional, scratching or stroking the foot can cause it to assume a normal position. A true deformity, however, cannot be moved into a corrected position and will not respond to scratching or stroking.

Congenital hip dysplasia occurs six to eight times more commonly in girls than boys and three times more often in the left hip. Congenital hip dysplasia should be suspected if there is difficulty diapering the infant due to tight adductor muscles. The abnormality can be detected in the newborn in three ways:

Allis's Sign. The nurse should check leg length by placing the infant's feet flat on the bed with knees flexed and observe the height of the knees. With a unilateral dislocation, one knee will be lower than the other. (Figure 21-26).

Ortolani's Maneuver. This is the most reliable test for a dislocated hip. To do this, the nurse should place the middle fingers over the infant's greater trochanter and the thumbs on the inner aspect of the upper thigh, flex the infant's knees, and abduct the hips until the lateral aspect of each knee touches the bed. A newborn should have 160 to 175° hip rotation. A dislocated hip may be present if there is resistance to having the leg rotated, if the extent of rotation is limited, or if a click can be heard or felt. This click is due to the femur slipping into or out of the acetabulum. (Figure 21-27).

Barlow Test. The infant should be placed in a prone position and the legs extended and compared. When hip dysplasia is present, the leg on the affected side appears shorter and the major gluteal folds are asymmetrical (see Figure 21-28).

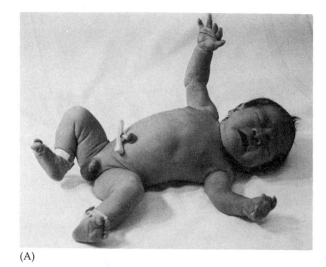

(A)

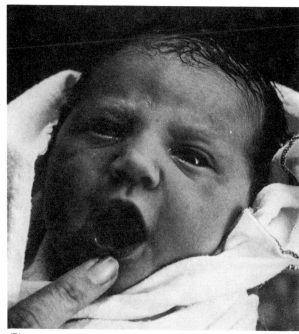

(B)

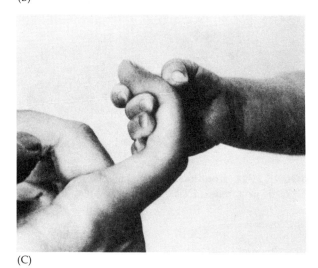

(C)

FIGURE 21-24. Neonatal Reflexes. (A) Moro reflex. (B) Rooting reflex. (C) Palmar grasp reflex.

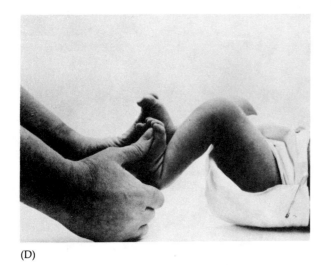

(D)

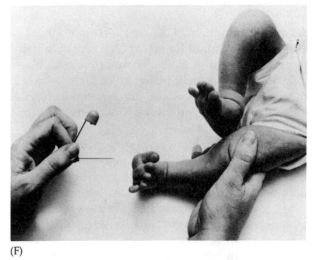

(F)

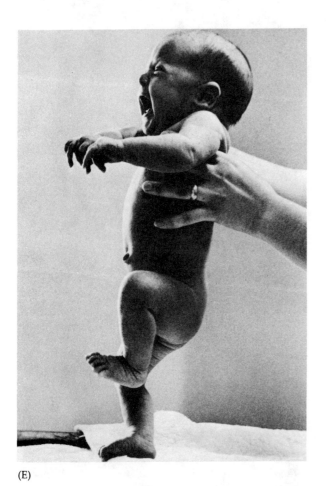

(E)

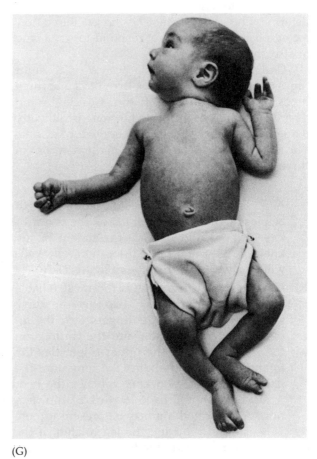

(G)

FIGURE 21-24. Continued. Neonatal Reflexes. (D) Plantar grasp reflex. (E) Stepping (dance) reflex. (F) Babinski reflex. (G) Tonic neck reflex. (*Note.* Courtesy of Mead Johnson Laboratories, Evansville, Indiana.)

TABLE 21-9
Assessment of the Neonate's Activity–Sleep State

State	Behavior	Duration
1. Deep sleep	Regular breathing Eyes closed; no eye movements No spontaneous activity Occasional startles or jerky movements Delayed startle response to external stimuli Rapid suppression of startles	4–5 hr/day; 10–20 min of each sleep cycle
2. Light sleep	Irregular breathing Eyes closed; rapid eye movements observable Minimal activity Occasional muscular twitching or startle response Sucking, whimpering, or groaning may occur	12–15 hr/day; 20–45 min of each sleep cycle
3. Drowsy	Eyes open or closed with eyelids fluttering Mild startle responses Responds to sensory input, but response may be delayed External stimuli may lead to state change Movements are smooth	Varies
4. Quiet alert	Eyes open with bright look Focuses attention on a particular stimulus, such as an object or auditory input Competing stimuli may capture attention after some delay Minimal motor activity	2–3 hrs/day
5. Agitated alert	Eyes open Considerable motor activity with thrusting movements of the extremities Immediate startle in response to external stimuli May whimper or begin to cry Respiration and pulse rate increase	1–3 hrs/day
6. Vigorous crying	Intense crying Uncoordinated thrashing of extremities Decreased responsiveness to external stimuli	Several minutes up to 2 hours

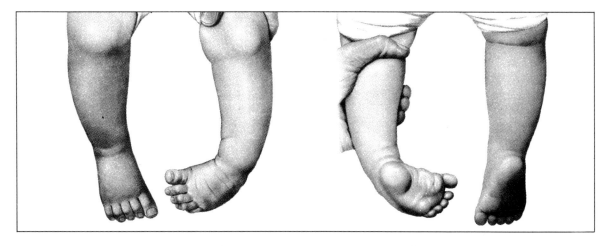

FIGURE 21-25. A true congenital clubfoot (talipes equinovarus) must be differentiated from a positional deformity caused by in utero positioning. A positional deformity can be passively moved into an overcorrected position while a true clubfoot cannot. (*Note.* Courtesy of Ross Laboratories, Columbus, Ohio.)

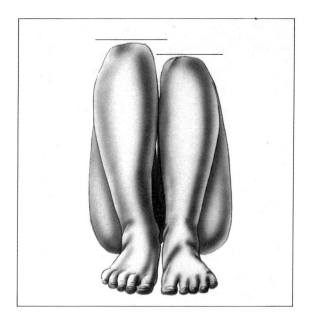

FIGURE 21-26. Allis's Sign Seen in Congenital Hip Dysplasia.

The newborn also should be assessed for evidence of injury to the musculoskeletal system during birth. One of the most common birth injuries is fracture of the clavicle, caused by traction on the shoulder during delivery. The newborn should be observed for decreased range of motion of the shoulder. Each shoulder should be rotated and abducted and the infant's response noted. Crying or grimacing may indicate a fracture. The clavicle also can be palpated for obvious deformity.

Nutritional Assessment

The neonate's physical growth and general appearance provide a general index of nutrition. In addition, the neonate's nutritional intake should be monitored, including type of feeding, amount, frequency, and any feeding difficulties, such as weak suck reflex, regurgitation, or disinterest, noted. Daily intake should be recorded and compared with caloric and fluid needs for optimal growth.

The parents' ability to feed the infant also should be assessed (Figure 21-29). The nurse should observe the parent's interaction with the infant during feeding, how the parent holds the infant and initiates the feeding (getting the infant on the breast correctly or introducing the bottle nipple appropriately), frequency of burping, and the parent's responsiveness to feeding difficulties or the infant's cues to cease feeding.

Five rather distinct phases of feeding behavior have been identified (O'Grady, 1971). These phases include:

- *prefeeding behavior*, which reflects the infant's level of arousal and degree of hunger and is evidenced by crying or fussiness
- *approach behavior*, the infant's attempt to initiate feeding, such as sucking or rooting
- *attachment behavior*, the infant's behavior from initial contact with the nipple until grasping and sucking occur
- *consummatory behavior*, indicated by the infant's coordinated sucking and swallowing, and
- *satiety behavior*, noted when the infant exhibits behavior that indicates hunger has been satisfied, such as falling asleep or losing interest in the nipple.

The healthy neonate has the capacity to feed successfully and should exhibit the above behaviors. The nurse can use these phases as a guide for observing the feeding process to determine whether the infant is feeding successfully or experiencing feeding problems.

Assessment of Elimination and the External Genitalia

The newborn's urinary and bowel elimination patterns should be noted and recorded. In boys, the foreskin of the penis should be retracted and the position of the urinary meatus observed. The urethral meatus in girls should be visible below the clitoris. The forcefulness of the urinary stream should be observed during voiding and the color and clarity of the urine noted.

The anus and rectum should be inspected for irritation, patency, and the presence of fissures. The initial temperature measurement should be obtained with a well-lubricated rectal thermometer to assess for anal or rectal obstruction. The passage of the first meconium stool is an almost certain indication of patency of the lower bowel and rectum. The nurse should observe and document the frequency, color, and consistency of the neonate's stools.

The external genitalia of the newborn should be examined carefully for any evidence of ambiguity. The genitalia should be readily distinguishable as male or female. Ambiguous genitalia should be referred for further evaluation.

In full-term boys, the penis and scrotal sac should be inspected for visible abnormalities. The ease with which the foreskin can be retracted should be determined. The scrotal sac should be covered with rugae and appear deep red. It should be examined for the presence of a *hydrocele*, a fluid-filled sac common in newborns. To differentiate a

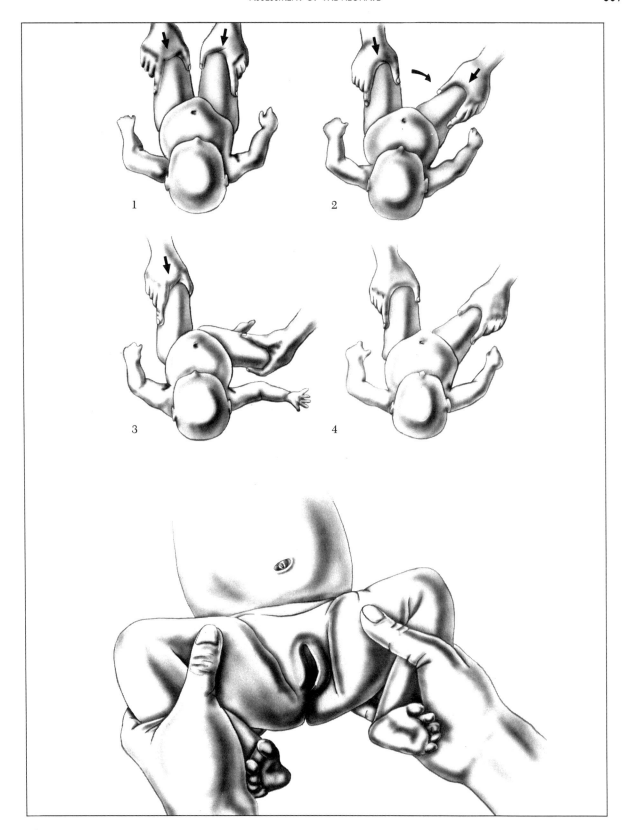

FIGURE 21-27. Ortolani's Maneuver to Detect Congenital Hip Dysplasia.

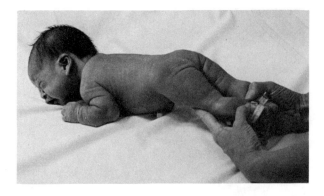

FIGURE 21-28. Barlow Test to Assess Symmetry of Gluteal Folds. (*Note.* Courtesy of Mead Johnson Laboratories, Evansville, Indiana.)

hydrocele from an inguinal hernia, the room should be dimmed and the scrotal sac transilluminated with a pen light. A hydrocele will transilluminate whereas an inguinal hernia will not. The scrotal sac should be palpated gently. Both testes should be well descended.

The external genitalia of the female neonate should be inspected for color and size of the labia. The size and position of the clitoris should be noted. The vagina should appear as a distinct orifice. The color and consistency of any vaginal discharge should be described.

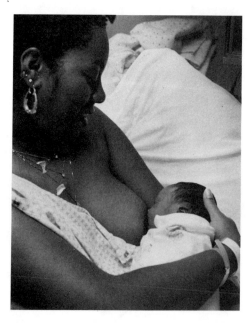

FIGURE 21-29. The parent's ability to feed the newborn should be assessed through observation of the infant's feeding behaviors and the parent's responsiveness to the infant. (*Note.* From Auvenshine/Enriquez: *Comprehensive Maternity Nursing*, Second Edition, © 1990. Boston: Jones and Bartlett Publishers, p. 610.)

Behavioral Assessment

The newborn has been found to have distinct behavior patterns. Research done in the 1950s and 1960s shows that neonates have far greater capabilities for responding to and influencing their environments than previously imagined. Neonates have a repertoire of behavioral responses that allow them to interact in active and patterned ways to various stimuli. The neonate's behavioral capabilities influence parent–child interaction and the infant's subsequent development (Figure 21-30).

The Brazelton Neonatal Behavioral Assessment Scale (BNBAS) was developed by T. Berry Brazelton and associates to evaluate the newborn's interactive behavior (Brazelton, 1973). The scale must be administered by examiners who have been trained in its use. The scale takes approximately 20 minutes to administer and another 10 minutes to score. The BNBAS may be used to evaluate the newborn's habituation, response to environmental stimuli, motor maturity, and interactive capacities through identification of 27 behavioral responses.

The 27 items can be grouped into 4 behavioral dimensions: interactive capacities, motor capacities, organization of state control, and physiological organization (Nugent, 1981).

1. *Interactive capacities.* These items assess the infant's capacity to attend to and process various stimuli. Can the infant follow a stimulus with a bright-eyed, alert look? How responsive is the infant to the environment?

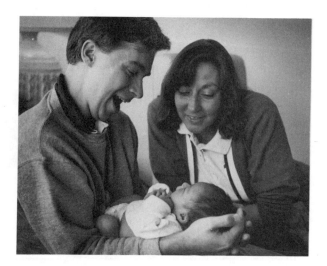

FIGURE 21-30. The neonate's behavioral capabilities influence parent–child attachment and interaction. (*Note.* From Auvenshine/Enriquez: *Comprehensive Maternity Nursing*, Second Edition, © 1990. Boston: Jones and Bartlett Publishers, p. 637.)

2. *Motor capacities.* These items assess the infant's ability to maintain tone, control motor behavior, and coordinate motor activity using smooth movements. Can the infant bring hand to mouth? How does the infant respond to having vision occluded?

3. *Organization of state control.* These items assess the infant's ability to organize and modulate state, control irritability, and habituate. How well can the infant shut out disturbing or overwhelming stimuli? How well can the infant maintain a calm state despite increased input? How smoothly can the infant move from one state to another?

4. *Physiological organization.* These items assess the infant's stability in response to stress. Physical symptoms associated with handling and dressing are observed. How quickly does the infant recover good skin color in stressful situations? How well is the infant able to inhibit startles or tremors in order to attend to social or inanimate stimuli?

Administration of the BNBAS should begin with observation of the infant's initial state, followed by presentation of visual and auditory stimuli. While the infant is still wrapped and quiet (state 1, 2, or 3), a flashlight is used as a visual stimulus, and the degree of response is noted. Next, using a rattle or, if the infant is in an alert state, a bell, the examiner notes the infant's response to auditory stimuli. The infant should then be uncovered, and any reactions to change should be recorded—for example, a change in skin color or movement from a quiet to an agitated state. While the infant is still quiet (state 1, 2, or 3), response to a light pinprick should be tested. While the infant is still dressed, clonus (ankle), foot grasp, and Babinski responses should be determined.

When the infant assumes an awake-alert state, the order of administration of test items can vary. The infant can be undressed and observed, again, for state change, skin color, and response to maneuvers. In the alert state the infant can be pulled to sitting. Standing, walking, and placing reflexes can then be tested. Incurvation, body tone across the hand, and prone responses are assessed next. The newborn's responses to a cloth placed on the face, the tonic neck reflex, and the Moro reflex are tested last. Since these are disturbing to the infant, the infant's self-quieting and consolability can be assessed after these tests.

Table 21-10 delineates the steps to follow when administering the BNBAS. The scale and behavior scoring sheet are shown in Table 21-11.

TABLE 21-10
Steps to Follow When Administering the Brazelton Neonatal Behavioral Assessment Scale (BNBAS)

1. Observe infant for 2 min—note state.
2. Flashlight (3–10 times) through closed lids.
3. Rattle (3–10 times).
4. Bell (3–10 times).
5. Uncover infant.
6. Light pinprick (5 times).
7. Ankle clonus.
8. Plantar grasp.
9. Babinski response.
10. Undress infant.
11. Passive movements and general tone.
12. Orientation, inanimate: visual and auditory.
13. Palmar grasp.
14. Pull to sit.
15. Standing.
16. Walking.
17. Placing.
18. Incurvation.
19. Body tone across hand.
20. Crawling-prone reflex.
21. Pick up and hold.
22. Glabella reflex.
23. Tonic deviation and reflex.
24. Orientation, animate: visual; auditory; visual and auditory.
25. Cloth on face.
26. Tonic neck response.
27. Moro response.

The scale yields a profile of neonatal behavioral functioning rather than a single score. The BNBAS is concerned primarily with assessing the neonate's ability to integrate and organize a variety of complex activities. It has been useful in facilitating parent–infant attachment by demonstrating the behavior of the newborn to teach parents what the infant contributes to the developing parent-child relationship.

NURSING DIAGNOSES RELATED TO THE NEONATE

Initial and ongoing assessment of the newborn infant provides a data base for identifying an infant's strengths or specific nursing diagnoses, which then lead to a plan of nursing care. Because nurses provide most of the initial and continuing care during the first days of life, they are able to carefully monitor the neonate's adaptation to extra-uterine

TABLE 21-11
Brazleton Neonatal Behavioral Assessment Scale (BNBAS)

Behavioral and Neurological Assessment Scale

Infant's name	Date	Hour
Sex Age	Born	
Mother's age Father's age	Father's S.E.S.	
Examiner(s)	Apparent race	
Conditions of examination:	Place of examination	
Birthweight	Date of examination	
Time examined	Length	
Time last fed	Head circ.	
Type of delivery	Type of feeding	
Length of labor	Apgar	
Type, amount and timing of medication given mother	Birth order	
	Anesthesia?	
	Abnormalities of labor	

Initial state: observe 2 minutes

1	2	3	4	5	6
deep	light	drowsy	alert	active	crying

Predominant states (mark two)

1	2	3	4	5	6

Elicited Reponses

	O*	L	M	H	A†					
						Descriptive paragraph (optional)				
Plantar grasp		1	2	3		Attractive	0	1	2	3
Hand grasp		1	2	3		Interfering variables	0	1	2	3
Ankle clonus		1	2	3		Need for stimulation	0	1	2	3
Babinski		1	2	3						
Standing		1	2	3		What activity does he/she use to quiet self?				
Automatic walking		1	2	3		hand to mouth				
Placing		1	2	3		sucking with nothing in mouth				
Incurvation		1	2	3		locking onto visual or auditory stimuli				
Crawling		1	2	3		postural changes				
Glabella		1	2	3		state change for no observable reason				
Tonic deviation of head and eyes		1	2	3						
Nystagmus		1	2	3		COMMENTS:				
Tonic neck reflex		1	2	3						
Moro [reflex]		1	2	3						
Rooting (intensity)		1	2	3						
Sucking (intensity)		1	2	3						
Passive movement		1	2	3						
Arms R		1	2	3						
L		1	2	3						
Legs R		1	2	3						
L		1	2	3						

O* = response not elicited (omitted)
A† = asymmetry

Note. From Brazelton, T.B. (1973). *Neonatal behavioral assessment scale.* Philadelphia: Lippincott, 114.

TABLE 21-11 (Continued)

Behavior Scoring Sheet

Initial state _____

Predominant state _____

Scale (Note State)	1	2	3	4	5	6	7	8	9
1. Response decrement to light (1,2)									
2. Response decrement to rattle (1,2)									
3. Response decrement to bell (1,2)									
4. Response decrement to tactile stimulation of foot (1,2)									
5. Orientation—inanimate visual (4,5)									
6. Orientation—inanimate auditory (4,5)									
7. Orientation—inanimate visual and auditory (4,5)									
8. Orientation—animate visual (4,5)									
9. Orientation—animate auditory (4,5)									
10. Orientation—animate visual and auditory (4,5)									
11. Alertness (4 only)									
12. General tonus (4,5)									
13. Motor maturity (4,5)									
14. Pull-to-sit (4,5)									
15. Cuddliness (4,5)									
16. Defensive movements (3,4,5)									
17. Consolability (6 to 5,4,3,2)									
18. Peak of excitement (all states)									
19. Rapidity of build-up (from 1,2 to 6)									
20. Irritability (all awake states)									
21. Activity (3,4,5)									
22. Tremulousness (all states)									
23. Startle (3,4,5,6)									
24. Lability of skin color (from 1 to 6)									
25. Lability of states (all states)									
26. Self-quieting activity (6,5 to 4,3,2,1)									
27. Hand-to-mouth facility (all states)									
28. Smiles (all states)									
29. Alert responsiveness (4 only)									
30. Cost of attention (3,4,5)									
31. Examiner persistence (all states)									
32. General irritability (5,6)									
33. Robustness and endurance (all states)									
34. Regulatory capacity (all states)									
35. State regulation (all states)									
36. Balance of motor tone (all states)									
37. Reinforcement value of infant's behavior (all states)									

Note. From Brazelton, T.B. (1973). *Neonatal behavioral assessment scale.* Philadelphia: Lippincott, 115.

life. Monitoring the newborn's responses enables the nurse to make clinical judgments about the effectiveness of the infant's adaptive capabilities as a basis for nursing care.

Knowledge of the unique capabilities and needs of newborn infants helps the nurse narrow the field when searching for cues to validate certain common diagnoses that are likely to occur. For instance, the newborn's susceptibility to heat loss suggests that newborns are at risk for "ineffective thermoregulation" related to cool environmental temperatures. This nursing diagnosis can be validated or refuted by monitoring the neonate's body temperature and response to exposure to cooler temperatures when, for example, the infant is unclothed for bathing or examination. A drop in body temperature under these circumstances confirms the diagnosis, and appropriate nursing actions should be instituted. However, if the neonate is able to maintain body temperature within safe ranges (no less than 96.8° F), the diagnosis would not be appropriate.

Newborn infants are at risk of "ineffective airway clearance" or "ineffective breathing pattern" related to the large amount of mucus, amniotic fluid, and other secretions present in the nasopharynx at birth. Also, the infant's respirations may be depressed as a result of anesthesia or medications administered to the mother during labor or delivery. The neonate's ability to clear the airway and breathe effectively also may be compromised by prematurity. Newborns whose gestational age is less than 37 weeks have an immature respiratory system. Factors such as inadequate surfactant production (necessary for alveolar expansion), weak respiratory muscles, weak cough and gag reflexes, and immaturity of the respiratory center in the brain can lead to hypoventilation and even apnea.

Because of their developmental immaturity, newborns are unable to protect themselves from injury. Therefore, they are at risk of aspiration ("potential for aspiration"), suffocation ("potential for suffocation"), and accidental injury ("potential for trauma"), such as falls, auto accidents, or burns caused by bath water that is too hot. If the newborn's parents do not have adequate knowledge of newborn safety needs, the infant becomes especially high risk for injury or death. Bottle-propping, incorrect positioning after feeding (flat on back), failure to use an auto safety restraint (or improper use), hanging a pacifier around the infant's neck, and too much bedding in the infant's crib place the newborn in jeopardy. Thus, identification of these nursing diagnoses ensures that a plan of care is developed to address the newborn's need for protection from injury, suffocation, and aspiration.

Because the neonate's skin is thinner and more fragile than that of older children and adults, "potential impairment of skin integrity" is another nursing diagnosis likely to be formulated for many newborn infants. Chafing, blisters such as postfeeding sucking blisters, redness, dryness, and specific lesions such as erythema toxicum are examples of defining characteristics that support this diagnosis.

Finally, a nursing diagnosis of "pain" may be indicated for neonates subjected to short-term painful procedures such as venipuncture or circumcision. Observable cues that validate a diagnosis of pain include increased respiration and heart rate, fussiness, crying, rigid posture, and grimacing.

Table 21-12 lists the diagnoses approved by the North American Nursing Diagnosis Association (NANDA) commonly identified for newborns. Specific defining characteristics and related factors for each of these diagnoses may be found in Chapter 6 (color-highlighted pages).

Once formulated and validated, the nursing diagnoses for a particular newborn provide the basis for developing specific nursing goals and interventions to assist the neonate in adapting successfully to extra-uterine life. Working with the family, the nurse should devise a plan of care that addresses the newborn's unique needs with consideration for the family's cultural beliefs and practices and economic resources.

TABLE 21-12
Common Nursing Diagnoses for Newborn Infants

Airway clearance, ineffective, related to excess mucus and tracheobronchial obstruction

Aspiration, potential for, related to propped bottle or incorrect positioning after feeding

Breathing pattern, ineffective, related to tracheobronchial obstruction or impaired lung expansion

Breastfeeding, ineffective, related to poor sucking reflex, inability to attach to nipple, or maternal knowledge deficit

Pain related to circumcision or venipuncture

Skin integrity, potential impaired, related to fragility of integument, limited physical mobility, or pressure

Suffocation, potential for, related to pacifier hung around neck, or pillows or bedding in crib

Thermoregulation, ineffective, related to immature control mechanisms, fluctuating environmental temperatures, or inadequate clothing

Trauma, potential for, related to developmental immaturity and environmental risk factors.

Chapter Highlights

■ Assessment of the newborn infant's physiological and behavioral responses to extra-uterine life assists in the detection of problems that may compromise successful adaptation.

■ Careful and ongoing evaluation of the newborn permits early detection of problems and lessens the likelihood of neonatal morbidity or mortality.

■ Despite their immaturity, healthy newborns have unique capabilities that facilitate their adjustment to a world in which they must breathe on their own and adapt to a variety of new and previously unknown stimuli.

■ The first 12 hours of life are characterized by two distinct periods of reactivity, separated by a period of sleep.

■ Successful transition to extra-uterine life involves immediate adaptation of the respiratory, circulatory, thermoregulatory, and metabolic systems.

■ The infant's physical growth depends on intrauterine development and well-being, gestational age, and birth weight.

■ Newborns exhibit distinct temperaments, patterned responses, and unique personality characteristics, all of which are shaped by the dynamic and reciprocal interaction of the infant and the environment.

■ The neonatal history, usually obtained from the mother, should include information about prenatal, perinatal, and postnatal periods, as well as the mother's perceptions of her infant, to provide as complete a picture as possible of favorable and risky health factors.

■ Clinical appraisal of the newborn involves the same techniques as any assessment but newborns require special consideration and handling during the assessment process because of their unique characteristics.

■ The newborn assessment provides an excellent opportunity to acquaint parents and family members with their new infant.

■ Initial assessments, completed at birth or within the first hours of life, help determine how well the neonate is adapting to extra-uterine life and include APGAR scoring, measuring vital signs, assessing gestational age, and measuring physical growth.

■ A systematic assessment of the newborn's skin, sensory–neurological functioning, activity–sleep patterns, oxygenation, nutrition, elimination patterns, external genitalia, and behavioral responses should be performed within the first 48 hours of life.

■ Common nursing diagnoses related to the newborn include "ineffective airway clearance," "ineffective breathing pattern," "potential or actual impaired skin integrity," "ineffective thermoregulation," "potential for trauma," and "pain," and form the basis for nursing care planning.

Practice Activities

1. Obtain a neonatal history from parents of two newborns from different ethnic/cultural groups. Compare and contrast your findings. What are the implications for nursing care for each of these newborns and their families?

2. Administer the Neonatal Perception Inventory I to a mother of a 1- to 3-day-old newborn. Administer the NPI II to the mother when her infant is 1 month old. Analyze your findings. What nursing diagnoses are suggested by the data? How can you further validate your impressions?

3. Observe the initial care of a newborn immediately following delivery. Evaluate the newborn at 1 and 5 minutes of age using the APGAR scoring system. Compare your scores with those obtained by the nurse caring for the infant. Ask the nurse to explain any discrepancies between your scores.

4. With at least two infants in the newborn nursery:
   a. estimate gestational age using the Dubowitz scoring system.
   b. evaluate respiratory status using the Silverman-Andersen Index.
   c. measure physical growth (weight, length, head and chest circumference), plot findings on a standard growth chart, and interpret your findings.
   d. assess state of consciousness, recording the behaviors that led to your conclusions.
   e. examine each infant for common skin variations, and document your findings.

5. Examine the differences in stool patterns among 1-, 2-, and 3-day-old newborns. Note the differences between breast-fed and bottle-fed infants.

6. Observe the feeding process of one breast-fed and one bottle-fed newborn. Are the five stages of feeding behavior evident? What cues did you observe to validate your assessment? What feeding

difficulties (if any) did either mother–infant pair experience? What are the implications for planning nursing care?

7. Observe at least two newborn infants during a painful procedure (e.g., circumcision, venipuncture). What responses to pain did the infants exhibit? What measures were successful in comforting the infants?

8. Conduct a head-to-toe clinical appraisal of at least one newborn. Record and analyze your findings. What nursing diagnoses are suggested?

Recommended Readings

Harris, C.C. (1986). Cultural values and the decision to circumcise. *Image: Journal of Nursing Scholarship, 18,* 98–104.

Jones, M.A. (1989). Identifying signs that nurses interpret as indicating pain in newborns. *Pediatric Nursing, 15,* 76–79.

Judd, J.M. (1985). Assessing the newborn from head to toe. *Nursing 85, 15*(12), 34–41.

Keefe, M.R. (1987). Comparison of neonatal nighttime sleep-wake patterns in nursery versus rooming-in environments. *Nursing Research, 36,* 140–144.

Kiernan, B.S., & Scoloveno, M.A. (1986). Assessment of the neonate. *Topics in Clinical Nursing, 8,* 1–10.

Lieber, M.T., & Taub, A.S. (1988). Common foot deformities and what they mean for parents. *MCN: The American Journal of Maternal-Child Nursing, 13,* 47–50.

Locklin, M. (1987). Assessing jaundice in full-term newborns. *Pediatric Nursing, 13*(1), 15–19.

Maloni, J.A., Stegman, C.E., Taylor, P.M., & Brownell, C.A. (1986). Validation of infant behavior identified by neonatal nurses. *Nursing Research, 35,* 133–138.

Medoff-Cooper, B., Weininger, S., & Zukowsky, K. (1989). Neonatal sucking as a clinical assessment tool: Preliminary findings. *Nursing Research, 38,* 162–165.

Scharping, E.M. (1983). Physiological measurements of the neonate. *MCN: The American Journal of Maternal-Child Nursing, 8,* 70–73.

Wandel, J.C. (1991). Pain perception in the neonate: Implications for circumcision. *Journal of Professional Nursing, 7*(3), 188–195.

References

Als, H., & Brazelton, T.B. (1981). A new model of assessing the behavioral organization of preterm and fullterm infants. *Journal of the American Academy of Child Psychiatry, 20,* 238–242.

Apgar, V. (1966). The newborn (Apgar) scoring system. *Pediatric Clinics of North America, 13,* 640–645.

Arnold, H.W., Putnam, N.J., Barnard, B.L., Desmond, M.M., & Rudolph, A.J. (1965). Transition to extrauterine life. *American Journal of Nursing, 65*(10), 77–84.

Auvenshine, M.A., & Enriquez, M.G. (1990). *Comprehensive maternity nursing: Perinatal and women's health* (2nd ed.). Boston: Jones and Bartlett.

Avery, G.B. (1981). *Neonatology: Pathophysiology and management of the newborn* (2nd ed.). Philadelphia: Lippincott.

Battaglia, F.C., & Lubchenco, L.O. (1967). A practical classification of newborn infants by weight and gestational age. *Journal of Pediatrics, 71,* 159–163.

Behrman, R.E., & Vaughn, V.C. (Eds.). (1983). *Nelson's textbook of pediatrics* (12th ed.). Philadelphia: Saunders.

Brazelton, T.B. (1973). *Neonatal behavioral assessment scale.* Philadelphia: Lippincott.

Broussard, E.R. (1979). Assessment of the adaptive potential of the mother-infant system: The Neonatal Perception Inventories. *Seminars in Perinatology, 3*(1), 91–100.

Brucker, M.C., & MacMullen, N.J. (1987). Neonatal jaundice in the home: Assessment with a noninvasive device. *Journal of Obstetric, Gynecologic, and Neonatal Nursing, 16,* 355–358.

Dubowitz, L., & Dubowitz, V. (1981). *The neurological assessment of the preterm and fullterm newborn infant.* Philadelphia: Lippincott.

Dubowitz, L., Dubowitz, V., & Goldberg, C. (1970). Clinical assessment of gestational age in the newborn infant. *Journal of Pediatrics, 77*(1), 1–10.

Fanaroff, A., & Martin, R.J. (1983). *Behrman's neonatal-perinatal medicine* (3rd ed.). St. Louis: Mosby.

Goren, C.G., Sarty, M., & Wu, P.Y.K. (1976). Visual following and pattern discrimination of facelike stimuli by newborn infants. *Pediatrics, 56,* 544–549.

Harris, C.C. (1986). Cultural values and the decision to circumcise. *Image: Journal of Nursing Scholarship, 18,* 98–104.

Hartner, M.S., & Broussard, E.R. (1971). Further considerations regarding maternal perceptions of the first born. In J. Hellmuth (Ed.), *Exceptional infant: Studies in abnormalities* (Vol. 2, pp. 442–443). New York: Brunner/Mazel.

Hollingsworth, A.O., Brown, L.A., & Brooten, D.A. (1980). The refugees and childbearing: What to expect, Part 3. *RN, 43,* 44–49.

Jones, M.A. (1989). Identifying signs that nurses interpret as indicating pain in newborns. *Pediatric Nursing, 15,* 76–79.

Keefe, M.R. (1987). Comparison of neonatal nighttime sleep-wake patterns in nursery versus rooming-in environments. *Nursing Research, 36,* 140–144.

Klaus, M.H., & Fanaroff, A.A. (1979). *Care of the high-risk neonate* (2nd ed.). Philadelphia: Saunders.

Locklin, M. (1987). Assessing jaundice in full-term newborns. *Pediatric Nursing, 13,* 15–19.

Lubchenco, L.O. (1981). Assessment of weight and gestational age. In G.B. Avery (Ed.), *Neonatology: Pathophysiology and management of the newborn* (2nd ed., pp. 205–224). Philadelphia: Lippincott.

Medoff-Cooper, B., Weininger, S., & Zukowsky, K. (1989). Neonatal sucking as a clinical assessment tool: Preliminary findings. *Nursing Research, 38,* 162–165.

Nugent, J.K. (1981). The Brazelton neonatal behavioral assessment scale: Implications for intervention. *Pediatric Nursing, 7*(3), 18–21.

O'Grady, R. (1971). Feeding behavior in infants. *American Journal of Nursing, 71*(4), 736–739.

Osburn, L.M., Reiff, M.I., & Bolus, R. (1984). Jaundice in the full-term neonate. *Pediatrics, 73,* 520–525.

Perez, R.H. (1981). *Protocols for perinatal nursing practice.* St. Louis: Mosby.

Schiffman, R.F. (1982). Temperature monitoring in the neonate: A comparison of axillary and rectal temperatures. *Nursing Research, 31,* 274–277.

Silverman, W.A., & Andersen, D.H. (1956). Evaluation of respiratory status: Silverman and Andersen Index. *Pediatrics, 17,* 1.

Sullivan, R., Foster, J., & Schreiner, R.I. (1979). Determining the newborn's gestational age. *MCN: The American Journal of Maternal-Child Nursing, 4*(1), 38–45.

Zepeda, M. (1982). Selected maternal-infant care practices of Spanish-speaking women. *Journal of Obstetrical, Gynecological, and Neonatal Nursing, 11,* 371–374.

Assessment of the Infant and Child

OBJECTIVES

Upon completion of this chapter, you should be able to:

■ Explain how the nursing assessment differs for infants and children compared with that for adults.

■ Delineate the health problems confronting children in contemporary society.

■ Trace the changes in physical growth, the immune system, vital signs, sensory–neurological functioning, pain responses, activity–sleep patterns, oxygenation, nutritional requirements, dentition, fluid requirements, and elimination patterns that occur during infancy and childhood.

■ Modify the approach used to obtain the child health history and perform a clinical appraisal, taking into consideration the characteristics of infants and children of various ages.

■ Modify the clinical appraisal for use with infants and children.

■ Screen infants and children for vision, hearing, and speech/language deficits, using age-appropriate techniques and documenting findings accurately.

■ Perform a comprehensive assessment of infants, toddlers, preschoolers, and school-age children, analyzing findings to formulate valid and appropriate nursing diagnoses.

Infants and children have characteristics and needs that require special attention during the nursing assessment. Once viewed as "miniature adults," society has come to recognize that infants and children differ dramatically from adults in several ways. In addition to the obvious differences in size and physical characteristics, children also differ in their cognitive and language abilities, social behavior, and responses to stress and illness.

Nursing assessment and diagnosis with children differ from their use with adults in two major ways: the knowledge base for assessing the child, and the need for family involvement. The knowledge needed to assess children includes an understanding of their anatomical and physiological characteristics, developmental capabilities, and behavioral patterns. Because of the young infant and child's dependence on adult caregivers, family involvement in the assessment process is of utmost importance. Much of the information needed for the nursing assessment often must be obtained from the child's parent or other caregiver who knows the child well. Any resulting plan of care also will depend on the family's ability to implement prescribed treatments or recommendations. Only by understanding these important differences is the nurse prepared to conduct a comprehensive assessment of an infant or child.

That children have special needs and require special services is clearly spelled out in the United Nations Declaration of the Rights of the Child (see boxed insert). Nurses who work with children should be familiar with this document and practice within its framework to ensure that children receive the optimum care to which they are entitled.

Infants and children in the United States and Canada are healthier today than in any previous era. Advances in technology, improved nutrition, widespread immunization, higher standards of living, and better understanding of child development have contributed positively to the health of children in contemporary society. Government-sponsored programs also have improved the health of children, particularly those from low income families and those with disabilities. For example, the Child Health Assessment Program (CHAP), authorized under Medicaid funding, provides comprehensive assessment services, including Early Periodic Screening, Diagnosis and Treatment (EPSDT), for large numbers of poor children. The Special Supplemental Food Program for Women, Infants, and Children (WIC) provides nutrition education for low income women and nutritious food for their infants and children up to age 5. The National School Lunch Program and the Child Care Food Program provide nutritious meals for children in day care centers, Head Start programs, and public schools. Public Law 94–142 (1975) requires that children with disabilities receive comprehensive public school education in the "least restrictive" environment at no cost to their families.

These improvements in society's care for its children have resulted in significant declines in infant and child morbidity and mortality since the early 1900s. Despite these improvements, however, there is still cause for concern about the health of today's infants and children. Among 25 countries with the lowest rates of infant mortality, the United States ranks 21st, behind 20 other developed countries, including Japan, which has the lowest infant mortality rates, and Canada, which ranks 5th (Wegman, 1989). Nonwhite children are 50% more likely to die than their white counterparts. The teen pregnancy rate is higher in the United States than in 28 other developed countries, resulting in twice as many low birth weight infants as those born to older mothers. Increasing numbers of today's children are reared in single parent homes; more than one fifth live in poverty (two fifths of nonwhite children live in poverty) (Figure 22-1).

Other health concerns that confront today's infants and children and may result in illness or death include congenital anomalies, malnutrition, accidents, chronic illness, child abuse and neglect, learning disabilities, substance abuse, suicide, and homicide (see Table 22-1). In nearly all cases, nonwhite children and those reared in poverty are at greater risk for disease and death. Illnesses that result from such behavioral and environmental factors as family dysfunction, poverty, illiteracy, and social isolation have been termed "pediatric social illnesses" (Withrow & Fleming, 1983). High risk children have been identified as those who are (1) from low income families, (2) from single parent families, (3) nonwhite, (4) male, and (5) 7 to 14 years of age (Goldberg, Roghman, McInerny, & Burke, 1984). Children with poor reading skills, high rates of school absences, and those who have chronic physical complaints are especially at risk for pediatric social illnesses.

The major cause of illness among children is infectious disease, accounting for 80% of all childhood illness. Respiratory infections are the most common. Nonfatal accidental injuries also are a leading cause of childhood morbidity. Millions of children are injured seriously enough each year to require medical treatment—30,000 of whom are permanently disabled (Division of Injury Control, 1990). Guyer and Gallagher (1985) estimate that 37% of children are injured seriously enough each

UNITED NATIONS DECLARATION OF THE RIGHTS OF THE CHILD

Preamble

Whereas the people of the United Nations have, in the Charter, reaffirmed their faith in fundamental human rights, and in the dignity and worth of the human person, and have determined to promote social progress and better standards of life in larger freedom,

Whereas the United Nations has, in the Universal Declaration of Human Rights, proclaimed that everyone is entitled to all the rights and freedoms set forth therein, without distinction of any kind, such as race, color, sex, language, religion, political or other opinion, national or social origin, property, birth or other status,

Whereas the child, by reason of his physical and mental immaturity, needs special safeguards and care, including appropriate legal protection, before as well as after birth,

Whereas the need for such special safeguards has been stated in the Geneva Declaration of the Rights of the Child of 1924, and recognized in the Universal Declaration of Human Rights and in the statutes of specialized agencies and international organizations concerned with welfare of children,

Whereas mankind owes to the child the best it has to give

Now therefore the general assembly proclaims

This Declaration of the Rights of the Child to the end that he may have a happy childhood and enjoy for his own good and for the good of society the rights and freedoms herein set forth, and calls upon parents, upon men and women as individuals and upon voluntary organizations, local authorities and national governments to recognize these rights and strive for their observance by legislative and other measures progressively taken in accordance with the following principles:

Principle 1

The child shall enjoy all the rights set forth in this Declaration. All children, without any exception whatsoever, shall be entitled to these rights, without distinction or discrimination on account of race, color, sex, language, religion, political or other opinion, national or social origin, property, birth or other status, whether of himself or of his family.

Principle 2

The child shall enjoy special protection, and shall be given opportunities and facilities, by law and by other means, to enable him to develop physically, mentally, morally, spiritually and socially in a healthy and normal manner and in conditions of freedom and dignity. In the enactment of laws for this purpose the best interests of the child shall be the paramount consideration.

Principle 3

The child shall be entitled from his birth to a name and a nationality.

Principle 4

The child shall enjoy the benefits of social security. He shall be entitled to grow and develop in health; to this end special care and protection shall be provided both to him and to his mother, including adequate pre-natal and post-natal care. The child shall have the right to adequate nutrition, housing, recreation and medical services.

Principle 5

The child who is physically, mentally or socially handicapped shall be given the special treatment, education and care required by his particular condition.

Principle 6

The child, for the full and harmonious development of his personality, needs love and understanding. He shall, wherever possible, grow up in the care and under the responsibility of his parents, and in any case in an atmosphere of affection and of moral and maternal security; a child of tender years shall not, save in exceptional circumstances, be separated from his mother. Society and the public authorities shall have the duty to extend particular care to children without a family and to those without adequate means of support. Payment of state and other assistance toward the maintenance of children of large families is desirable.

Principle 7

The child is entitled to receive education, which shall be free and compulsory, at least in the elementary stages. He shall be given an education which will promote his general culture, and enable him on a basis of equal opportunity to develop his abilities, his individual judgment, and his sense of moral and social responsibility, and to become a useful member of society.

The best interests of the child shall be the building principle of those responsible for his education and guidance; that responsibility lies in the first place with his parents.

The child shall have full opportunity for play and recreation, which shall be directed to the same purposes as education; society and the public authorities shall endeavor to promote the enjoyment of this right.

Principle 8

The child shall in all circumstances be among the first to receive protection and relief.

Principle 9

The child shall be protected against all forms of neglect, cruelty and exploitation. He shall not be the subject of traffic, in any form.

The child shall not be admitted to employment before an appropriate minimum age; he shall in no case be caused or permitted to engage in any occupation or employment which would prejudice his health or education, or interfere with his physical, mental or moral development.

Principle 10

The child shall be protected from practices which may foster racial, religious and any other form of discrimination. He shall be brought up in a spirit of understanding, tolerance, friendship among peoples, peace and universal brotherhood and in full consciousness that his energy and talents should be devoted to the service of his fellow men.

year to restrict their activities for at least one day. Between the ages of 6 and 16 years, children miss 14 million school days annually due to accidental injury (Collins, 1985). The majority of infants and children, however, are relatively healthy and grow to adulthood without serious health problems.

To work effectively with infants and children, a nurse must be knowledgeable of their special characteristics and apply this knowledge when working with them. Specifically, a nurse should be ever mindful of the physical, developmental, and behavioral qualities that characterize children of varying ages and modify the nursing assessment accordingly. Modifications include how the nurse approaches, interacts with, and examines the child client.

The previous chapter focuses on nursing assessment of the neonate. The next chapter considers the special assessment needs of pubescent and adolescent clients. This chapter is concerned

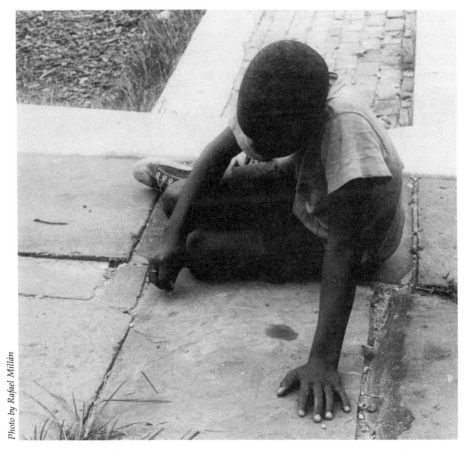

Photo by Rafael Millán

FIGURE 22-1. Children reared in poverty are at greater risk for disease and death. (*Note.* From Lee/Estes: *The Nation's Health*, Third Edition, © 1990. Boston: Jones and Bartlett Publishers, p. 294.)

TABLE 22-1
Deaths and Death Rates for the 10 Leading Causes of Death in Childhood: United States, 1988

Rank Order[1]	Cause of Death	Number	Rate
	Under 1 Year[2]		
———	All causes	38,910	995.3
1	Congenital anomalies	8,141	208.2
2	Sudden infant death syndrome	5,476	140.1
3	Disorders relating to short gestation and unspecified low birth weight	3,268	83.6
4	Respiratory distress syndrome	3,181	81.4
5	Newborn affected by maternal complications of pregnancy	1,411	36.1
6	Accidents and adverse effects	936	23.9
7	Newborn affected by complications of placenta, cord, and membranes	907	23.2
8	Infections specific to the perinatal period	878	22.5
9	Intra-uterine hypoxia and birth asphyxia	777	19.9
10	Pneumonia and influenza	641	16.4
———	All other causes	13,294	340.0
	Ages 1–4 Years[3]		
———	All causes	7,429	50.9
1	Accidents and adverse effects	2,858	19.6
	Motor vehicle accidents	1,005	6.9
	All other accidents and adverse effects	1,853	12.7
2	Congenital anomalies	913	6.3
3	Malignant neoplasms, including neoplasms of lymphatic and blood-forming tissues	542	3.7
4	Homicide	381	2.6
5	Diseases of heart	352	2.4
6	Pneumonia and influenza	186	1.3
7	Certain conditions originating in the perinatal period	129	0.9
7	Meningitis	129	0.9
9	Human immunodeficiency virus infection[4]	114	0.8
10	Septicemia	89	0.6
———	All other causes	1,736	11.9
	Ages 5–14 Years[3]		
———	All causes	8,925	25.8
1	Accidents and adverse effects	4,215	12.2
	Motor vehicle accidents	2,423	7.0
	All other accidents and adverse effects	1,792	5.2
2	Malignant neoplasms, including neoplasms of lymphatic and blood-forming tissues	1,096	3.2
3	Congenital anomalies	499	1.4
4	Homicide	459	1.3
5	Diseases of heart	324	0.9
6	Suicide	243	0.7
7	Pneumonia and influenza	127	0.4
8	Chronic obstructive pulmonary diseases and allied conditions	103	0.3
8	Benign neoplasms, carcinoma in situ, and neoplasms of uncertain behavior and of unspecified nature	103	0.3
10	Cerebrovascular diseases	72	0.2
———	All other causes	1,684	4.9

[1]Rank based on number of deaths.

[2]Rates per 100,000 live births.

[3]Rates per 100,000 population in age group.

[4]Expected to become one of top five leading causes of death in the 1- to 4-year-old age group by 1992 (Novello, 1989).

with assessing infants and children whose chronological ages place them between the neonatal and adolescent periods of development—those between 1 month and 12 years of age.

Nursing assessment of the infant and child varies more in approach and focus than in technique. Generally, a nurse uses the same assessment techniques (interview, observation, inspection, palpation, percussion, and auscultation) used with adult clients. However, the way in which the nurse employs these techniques, as well as what is looked for, varies according to the child's age and developmental level, the child's health, and the particular context in which the assessment is conducted, such as primary care setting, hospital, or home.

KNOWLEDGE NEEDED TO ASSESS THE INFANT AND CHILD

Typically, childhood is divided into four stages: infancy, toddlerhood, preschool years, and school-age. Sometimes, the toddler and preschool years are called early childhood and the school-age years middle childhood. Children in each of these age groups share certain physical, cognitive, and social qualities that distinguish them from each other. Table 10-7 in Chapter 10 summarizes the various developmental characteristics of children in each age group. These characteristics should be taken into account when assessing infants and children. In addition, a nurse must be cognizant of the physiological differences of children that influence the nursing assessment.

Physical Integrity

Physical integrity undergoes dramatic changes throughout infancy and childhood, including changes in physical growth, skin integrity, immune system functioning, and vital signs.

Physical Growth

Infancy is characterized by rapid growth, which slows as the child gets older. Growth is both cephalocaudal and asynchronous (see chap. 10). Physical growth occurs head to toe as illustrated by early fetal development of the head and central nervous system, followed by elongation of the torso during infancy, and lengthening of the legs during childhood. Body organs and systems also mature at different rates. For example, the maturation of the central nervous system predominates during fetal and infant periods, whereas the musculoskeletal and cardiorespiratory systems mature rapidly during adolescence.

Physical growth is influenced by numerous factors, including prenatal influences (such as heredity and maternal nutrition), birth weight, nutritional intake, and general health. Children who were malnourished in utero tend to be small for their ages throughout childhood (Metcoff, Bentle, & Bodwell, 1981). Peck and colleagues (1987) found that the growth of low birth weight Navajo infants never caught up with that of Navajo children whose birth weight was greater than 2500 gm (5 lbs 8 oz).

Physical growth is the primary indicator of a child's health and nutritional status. Poor nutrition during childhood can result in retarded growth patterns and lead to other health problems, such as chronic infections and anemia. Children from different ethnic and geographic backgrounds, such as Asia, Africa, the Middle East, and Latin America, often exhibit growth delays or retardation (Isaacs, 1989). However, their retarded growth patterns are attributable to low socioeconomic status, and the consequent poor nutrition, rather than their ethnic or geographic origin.

During infancy, growth is rapid. Infants typically double their birth weight by 6 months of age and triple it by one year of age. Birth length increases by 50% during the first year. At one year of age the average infant weights 21.5 pounds (9.75 kg) and is 29 inches (74 cm) long. Head circumference is one third greater at age one than at birth, averaging 18 inches (46 cm) at 12 months of age. The posterior fontanel closes by 6 to 8 weeks of age, with the anterior fontanel fusing by 12 to 18 months of age. Head circumference is greater than chest circumference until age 1 when head and chest circumferences become relatively equal. By age 2, chest circumference is greater than head circumference and shortly thereafter exceeds abdominal circumference.

During early childhood, the rate of growth slows considerably. Each year a child gains 4 to 6 pounds (1.8 to 2.7 kg) and grows 2.5 to 3 inches (6.75 to 7.5 cm) in height. Increased height is primarily attributable to lengthening of the legs. The toddler typically has a squat, bow-legged, swayback, potbellied appearance. As young children gain height, their posture becomes more erect, body fat diminishes, and they appear thinner. Preschoolers may be knock-kneed.

School-age children grow at a slow and steady pace, increasing 2 inches (5 cm) per year in height and 4.5 to 6.5 pounds (2 to 3 kg) annually in weight. Between the ages of 6 and 12, children double their weight. Boys generally are taller and heavier than girls. The typical school-age child has a slim, long-legged appearance.

Of particular note is the school-age child's changing facial structure. The face grows faster than the skull, deciduous teeth are lost, and permanent teeth erupt, giving the child a characteristically large-toothed appearance until the growth of the face and jaw catch up. Childhood trends in height and weight gain are summarized in Table 22-2.

Integumentary Changes

During infancy, the skin becomes capable of regulating body temperature effectively. The shivering mechanism matures, and peripheral capillaries respond to changes in environmental temperatures. The development of additional adipose tissue protects the infant from heat loss. During infancy and early childhood, the skin is relatively fragile and therefore more susceptible to bacterial invasion, inflammation, and trauma. As the child grows, the skin becomes functionally mature, thereby increasing the child's resistance to infection and protecting against skin disruptions and fluid loss.

The child's skin produces little sebum, often resulting in dry skin. Although eccrine glands are functional, the child rarely sweats in response to hot weather.

Impairments of skin integrity are common in infancy and childhood. "Cradle cap," an accumulation of excess sebaceous secretions on the scalp, occurs in some infants. Diaper dermatitis (diaper rash) occurs frequently in infants in response to irritation from urine, feces, detergents, or lotions. During early childhood, other skin disorders are common, including contact dermatitis, eczema, fungal and bacterial infections, and insect stings and bites.

Hair growth is minimal during infancy, and scalp hair remains fine and often curly. Throughout childhood, the hair becomes thicker, coarser,

TABLE 22-2
Height (Length) and Weight Gains During Childhood

Age	Weight*	Height*
Infants		
Birth–6 months	Weekly gain: 140–200 g (5–7 oz)	Monthly gain: 2.5 cm (1 inch)
	Birth weight doubles by end of first 6 months	
6–12 months	Weight gain: 85–140 g (3–5 oz)	Monthly gain: 1.25 cm (½ inch)
	Birth weight triples by end of first year	Birth length increases by approximately 50% by end of first year
Toddlers	Birth weight quadruples by age 2½	Height at age 2 is approximately 50% of eventual adult height
	Yearly gain: 2–3 kg (4½–6½ lb)	Gain during second year: about 12 cm (4¾ inches)
		Gain during third year: about 6–8 cm (2⅜–3¼ inches)
Preschoolers	Yearly gain: 2–3 kg (4½–6½ lb)	Birth length doubles by age 4
		Yearly gain: 5–7.5 cm (2–3 inches)
School-age children	Yearly gain: 2–3 kg (4½–6½ lb)	Yearly gain after age 7: 5 cm (2 inches)
		Birth length triples by about age 13
Pubertal growth spurt		
Females—10–14 years	Weight gain: 7–25 kg (15–55 lb)	Height gain: 5–25 cm (2–10 inches); approximately 95% of mature height achieved by onset of menarche or skeletal age of 13
	Mean: 17.5 kg (38⅛ lb)	Mean: 20.5 cm (8¼ inches)
Males—11–16 years	Weight gain: 7–30 kg (15–65 lb)	Height gain: 10–30 cm (4–12 inches); approximately 95% of mature height achieved by skeletal age of 15 years
	Mean: 23.7 kg (52⅛ lb)	Mean: 27.5 cm (11 inches)

*Yearly height and weight gains for each age group represent averaged estimates from a variety of sources.

Note. From Whaley, L.F., & Wong, D.L. (1991). *Nursing care of infants and children* (4th ed.). St. Louis: Mosby-Year Book, p. 113.

straighter, and usually darker. However, until the onset of puberty, the child's body is relatively hairless, except for fine hair on the arms and legs, which becomes more abundant and darker during middle childhood.

Immune System Changes

During infancy, the immune system remains immature. Immunity received from the mother declines gradually during the first months of life. The infant's system begins to synthesize IgG and IgM, reaching adult levels by toddlerhood (see boxed insert for description of immunoglobulin functions). Mature levels of IgA, IgD, and IgE are not achieved until later childhood, thus increasing the young child's susceptibility to microorganisms.

Lymphatic tissues generally are well developed at birth and reach adult proportions by 6 years of age. These tissues, including lymph nodes, thymus, spleen, tonsils, adenoids, and lymphocytes, continue to grow until pubescence, then shrink throughout adolescence until they once again reach adult size.

Lymph nodes collect and filter bacteria and other foreign matter for the circulatory system. Small (1 cm or less in diameter), cool, mobile, not tender, palpable lymph nodes are common in children up to age 12. Lymph nodes that are enlarged, warm, and tender when palpated usually indicate an infection or inflammation.

Vital Signs

Body temperature is less well regulated in infants and children because control mechanisms have not yet matured. Infants have high heat loss in comparison to heat production because they have a large surface area relative to body mass, a thinner layer of subcutaneous tissue, and a lower metabolic rate (Eoff & Joyce, 1981; Eoff, Meier, & Miller, 1974) than adults. Body temperature declines gradually throughout childhood (see Table 22-3), reflecting decreased heat production as the child grows older. Temperature fluctuations are not uncommon, and usually are caused by changes in environmental temperature, crying, emotional distress, exercise, and illness, particularly infections. Stable body temperatures are achieved during puberty.

There are greater individual variations in pulse (see Table 22-4) and respiratory rates (Table 22-5) in infants and children than among adults. Factors that influence pulse and respiratory rates include the child's weight, body temperature, activity level (sleeping, resting, awake, moving, exercising), and health. There is an inverse relationship between

---

Description of Immunoglobulin Functions

IgM	Largely responsible for primary antibody response; does not cross placenta; found in vascular compartment; produced by plasma cells; antibody to blood-group antigens; provides protection from gram-negative bacteria and viruses
IgG	Produced by cells after IgM production is finished; largest immunoglobulin class; crosses placental barrier; provides antitoxin protection (as with diphtheria, tetanus, botulism, snake venoms)
IgA	Primary immunoglobulin found in secretions (tears, breast milk, saliva, and mucous secretions of respiratory, genitourinary, and gastrointestinal tracts); also found in serum; often activated with antigen contact; protection against viruses; does not cross placenta
IgE	Responsible for allergic reactions; capable of attaching to tissue cells (such as skin); heat labile
IgD	Importance and function not understood at this time

Note. From Servonsky/Opas: *Nursing Management of Children,* © 1987. Boston: Jones and Bartlett Publishers, p. 975.

TABLE 22-3
Average Body Temperatures in Children

Age	Temperature (Fahrenheit/Centigrade)
1 month	99.5 (37.5)
6 months	99.5 (37.5)
1 year	99.7 (37.6)
2 years	99.4 (37.4)
4 years	98.6 (37.0)
6 years	98.4 (36.9)
8 years	98.2 (36.8)
10 years	98.0 (36.7)
12 years	98.0 (36.7)

TABLE 22-4
Average Pulse Rates by Age

Age	Average	Range
Infant	120	80–160
2 years	110	80–130
4 years	100	80–120
6 years	95	75–115
8–10 years	90	70–110
12 years	85	70–110

TABLE 22-5
Respiratory Rates by Age

Age	Range of Normal
1–6 months	30–80
6 months to 1 year	25–45
2 years	20–35
4 years	20–30
6–10 years	18–26
12 years	15–25

TABLE 22-6
Normal Blood Pressure Values by Age

Age	Average	Range
1 month	84/52	65–105/35–68
6 months	90/53	72–110/36–70
1 year	90/54	72–110/38–71
2 years	90/56	72–110/40–73
4 years	92/56	73–112/40–73
6 years	96/57	77–115/40–74
8 years	99/60	80–118/43–76
10 years	102/62	83–121/45–79
12 years	107/64	88–126/48–82

Note. From Second Task Force on Blood Pressure Control in Children. (1987). Bethesda, MD: National Heart, Lung and Blood Institute.

the child's age and the pulse and respiratory rates: *the older the child, the lower the pulse and respiratory rates.*

Conversely, there is a direct relationship between the child's age and blood pressure—*the older the child, the higher the blood pressure.* Both systolic and diastolic pressures gradually increase throughout infancy and childhood, reaching adult norms by late adolescence. Ranges of normal blood pressure readings (see Table 22-6) have been established, but are based primarily on white children. There are little data available on blood pressure norms for native American, Hispanic, or Asian children. African-American children, especially after puberty, tend to have consistently higher blood pressures than white children (Lieberman, 1978).

Sensory–Neurological Functioning

Children depend on the intact sensory processes of vision, hearing, touch, smell, and taste to become aware of, interact with, adapt to, and learn about their internal processes and the external world. Children must have intact sensory–neurological systems in order to develop physically, cognitively, emotionally, and socially.

Sensory–perceptual processes develop sequentially throughout infancy and early childhood. Children learn to detect distinctive features of objects and people in the environment and develop the ability to process increasingly larger amounts of stimuli at a time. In early infancy, perceptual abilities are confined primarily to simple detection of stimuli and distinctions between two stimuli. For example, although a 1-month old infant cannot determine precise areas of cutaneous stimulation, the baby reacts positively by quieting in response to stroking. By 12 to 16 months of age, the touch receptors have matured and multiplied so that toddlers are able to identify where they are being stroked.

A progressive increase in the ability to discriminate occurs with sensorineural development and

learning. Thus, the older infant or toddler is able to recognize a form or pattern as familiar: a parental voice or face is recognized as distinct from all other voices and faces, a cat becomes a thing that has fur and a tail while a bird has wings and flies. Random exploration becomes progressively more systematic, selective, and exclusive, and the older preschool and school-age child develops the capacity to attend to and manipulate identified forms, such as letters, numbers, and words.

Sensory Development

Visually, the 1-month old can fixate on the parent's face or a moving object within 90°. Tear glands begin to function at 1 month of age. Intermittent strabismus and nystagmus may be present up to 3 months of age. Visual acuity progresses from 20/300 at 1 month of age to 20/20 by 4 years of age. Recent evidence, however, indicates that children may achieve 20/20 visual acuity as early as 12 months of age based on tests of visually evoked cortical responses (Lewis & Thompson, 1986). Typically, children do not test at this level using the Snellen eyecharts until at least 4 years of age. Depth perception develops in late infancy, as does the ability to distinguish strangers from significant others. Complete binocular vision is established by one year of age, and accommodation (the ability of the eyes to focus) is well developed by 3 years of age. Table 22-7 outlines visual development in childhood.

Although the structures of the ear are developed at birth and the infant can discriminate among sounds, the incomplete myelination of the central nervous system prevents the infant from responding in a specific, discrete way to auditory stimuli, hence the infant's generalized body response to loud noises. The infant's ability to dis-

TABLE 22-7
Major Characteristics of Visual Development

Birth

Eyes move independently.

Can fixate on moving object in range of 45°.

Blinks, squints, or may sneeze when exposed to bright lights.

Eye and head movements not coordinated (doll's eye reflex present).

Farsighted due to immaturity of eyeball (visual acuity approximately 20/300).

Large-angle strabismus at birth: should be evaluated immediately.

1 Month (4 Weeks)

Can fixate on large moving object in range of 90°.

Watches parents intently when they speak.

Fixates on face.

Tear glands start to function.

Intermittent strabismus may be present.

Binocular vision begins at about 6 weeks.

2 Months (8 Weeks)

Peripheral vision of 180°.

Convergence on near objects begins at 6 weeks.

Follows moving object with eyes; movement may be jerky.

3 Months (12 Weeks)

Regards hand; however, blind infants do same.

Convergence should be well established.

Doll's eye reflex has disappeared.

Can follow moving object from side to side (range of 180°).

Briefly able to fixate on near objects.

4 Months (16 Weeks)

Visual acuity 20/80 as measured by visual evoked cortical response (VECP).

Binocular vision fairly well established.

Fixates on 1-inch cube.

Recognizes familiar objects, e.g., feeding bottle or breast.

Observes mirror images.

If strabismus continues, referral should be made by 4–6 months of age.

6 Months (24 Weeks)

Visual acuity 20/20–20/40 as measured by VECP.

Adjusts position to view objects.

Watches falling toy.

Eye-hand coordination is developing.

Smooth-following eye movements in all directions.

9 Months (36 Weeks)

Depth perception developing.

Attentive to environment.

Observes activities of people and animals within distance of 10–12 ft. with sustained interest for several minutes.

1 Year (12 Months)

Visual acuity 20/20 as measured by VECP.

Follows rapidly moving objects.

Recognizes familiar people at 20 ft. or more.

1¹/₂ Years (18 Months)

Convergence well established.

Fixates on small objects.

Sees and points to distant interesting objects outdoors.

2 Years (24 Months)

Fixates on small object for 60 seconds.

Accommodations well developed.

Recognizes fine details in picture books.

3 Years (36 Months)

Visual acuity is 20/20 as measured by VECP, although may test less with Snellen.

Copies geometric designs, circles, cross.

Convergence smooth.

4 Years (48 Months)

Visual acuity 20/20.

High risk for amblyopia.

5 Years (60 Months)

Visual acuity 20/20.

Depth perception fully developed.

Eye achieves full globe size between 5 and 7 years.

Note. New techniques devised for assessing visual acuity are based on optokinetic nystagmus, visually evoked cortical potentials, and preferential looking. These methods indicate an infant's acuity to be much better than previously reported.

Note. From Lewis, K.D., & Thomson, H.B. (1986). *Manual of school health.* Menlo Park, CA: Addison-Wesley, pp. 20–22.

criminate among sounds is shown by the different prelingual responses and nonverbal behaviors that various sounds elicit. Infants show a special sensitivity to the human voice, with the higher-pitched female voice commanding particular attention. Fine discrimination among and responses to sounds increase with maturity. Thus, the ability to hear affects language development and the child's learning to speak normally. Hearing development in childhood is outlined in Table 22-8.

The infant and young child's eustachian tubes are shorter, straighter, and wider than the adult's, which increases children's susceptibility to infectious organisms and may lead to otitis media (middle ear infection). Otitis media is a major cause of temporary hearing impairment in young children and can result in irreversible hearing loss if undetected or untreated.

The ability to respond to tactile stimulation develops in utero and progresses in a cephalocaudal,

TABLE 22-8
Milestones in the Development of Hearing Responses

Age	Hearing Responses
Newborn	Exhibits a startle response to sudden or loud sounds. Arouses from sleep state to loud sounds in the environment. Responds to the human voice more readily than other sounds. Soothed by low frequency sounds.
3 months	Turns head and eyes to side to locate sound. Awakens or quiets in response to mother's voice.
6 months	Locates sound by turning head to side or in an arc. Imitates sounds.
9 months	Responds to own name or familiar sounds (telephone ring, doorbell, opening door). Controls own response to sound, such as listening for repetition of sound or ignoring sound. Understands "No" and "Bye-bye."
12 months	Exhibits differential responses to a variety of sounds, such as frowning or crying when scolded or told "No!," babbling in response to human voice, quieting when familiar person appears. Understands simple commands when accompanied by gesture, such as "Give Daddy the ball" or "Wave bye-bye." Says two or three words; "talks" during play.
18 months	Responds to simple commands, such as "Get your blanket" or "Point to the truck." Identifies body parts.
24 months*	Localizes sound at all angles. Speaks simple sentences ("Me go home," "See doggie").

*Steady gains in speech and language development are reliable indicators of normal hearing. By four years of age, hearing can be tested with an audiometer.

proximodistal direction. This sense is highly developed at birth, particularly in the facial area. In the child, superficial sensations flow from skin receptors to spinal nerves and onto a specific segment of the spinal cord. Pain and temperature sensations pass directly to the thalamus for immediate reaction. Touch, a more complex sensation, follows a route through the thalamus to the cerebral cortex for higher interpretation. This higher level of cortical interpretation also enables the child to distinguish or identify familiar objects simply by touching them (called *stereognosis*).

Smell is the least well developed sense in children. The olfactory receptors are located deep within the nose. They alert the child quickly to an odor, but within one second olfactory awareness decreases about 50%. Thus, the child's awareness of strong odors disappears within a few seconds.

By 2 to 3 months of age, the infant's sense of taste is acute. Infants accept sweet tastes readily, even eagerly. Sour and bitter tastes are aversive to infants and young children. However, taste changes as the child grows. The child's taste preferences and responses are linked closely to cultural and family food practices and also are influenced by sight, smell, and texture of various foods and fluids.

Pain Responses

The child's responses to painful stimuli change with age and the intensity of the pain (see Table 22-9) and are influenced by the child's previous experiences with pain (McGrath, 1989). Situational, behavioral, and emotional factors also play a significant role. For example, the child's anticipation of pain and the child's control over the painful event (situational factors), the child's coping strategies and the parents' responses to the child's pain (behavioral factors), and the child's emotional responses to pain—anger, fear, or depression (emotional factors)—contribute to the meaning a painful event has for the child (McGrath, 1989). These factors also influence children's ability to communicate with others about their pain.

Physiological responses that indicate the presence of pain in children include increases in blood pressure, pulse, and respiration, restlessness, and sweating. However, such responses may be unreliable indicators of persistent acute pain or chronic pain (Mills, 1989). Responses that indicate specific pain sites, including pulling at the ears, holding or rubbing a body part, or flexing the legs, also may occur. Dale (1986) investigated the pain responses of young infants 6 weeks to 6 months of age to DPT

TABLE 22-9
Infants' and Children's Responses to Pain

Infants	School-Age Child
No anticipatory awareness of an impending painful stimulus (e.g., needle)	Avoidance behaviors ("Wait a minute")
Loud crying	Crying (depends on cultural norms)
Thrashing of arms and legs	Rigidity, clenched fists, clenched jaw, tightly closed eyes
Facial expressions: furrowed brow, closed eyes	Denial of pain to avoid "getting a shot" or to appear brave
Easily comforted after painful stimulus is removed	Verbal expressions of "Is it going to hurt?," "Are you almost done?," "Hurry up!," "Stop now!"
Unresponsive to comfort measures (holding, rocking) if pain is internal (e.g., colic, earache, etc.) and continuous	Facial expressions: grimacing, furrowed brow, closed eyes, tear-filled eyes
Altered sleeping and eating behaviors	Altered sleep pattern (increased or decreased)

Toddler/Preschooler	All Ages
Anticipatory awareness of impending painful event	Increased pulse and respiratory rates; elevated blood pressure
Loud crying or screaming	Sweating
Aggression: hitting, kicking, biting	Restlessness and irritability (continuing pain)
Verbal expressions of "Stop!," "Don't!," "Ouch!," "It hurts!," "Help!"	Guarding or rubbing affected body part
Clinging to parent or nurse; whining	Flexing legs (abdominal pain)
Altered sleep pattern (increased or decreased)	

injections. Their responses included crying, increased heart rate, arm waving, and kicking.

While infants under 6 months of age may not be able to remember painful experiences and associated events, infants older than 6 months do seem able to recall such experiences. Anticipatory fear of pain occurs as early as 6 months of age and becomes more pronounced as the child develops the cognitive ability to remember, and thus anticipate, painful events (Mills, 1989). The older infant also becomes more adept at localizing the source of pain or irritation and defending against a painful external stimulus, such as withdrawing the foot from a needle stick or the hand from a hot object. As with touch, localization becomes even more specific during the toddler period when the child may attempt to hold or rub a painful body part.

Preschool children are able to identify the source of pain by pointing to it and can use simple, familiar words such as "funny," "hurt," "poking," or "bad" to describe the sensation. In response to painful experiences, preschool children may exhibit behaviors that include attempts at self-control, verbal expression (yelling, crying, or pleading), aggressive behavior (hitting, pushing, or biting), avoidance (hiding, pulling away, or excessive sleeping), and dependency (whining, clinging, requests to be held or helped, and fear of being alone) (Figure 22-2).

School-age children are better able to describe painful sensations, using appropriate terminology such as "aching," "shooting," or "throbbing."

They also exhibit less fear and aggression. Typically, school-age children try to appear brave and may hold rigidly still or clench their teeth and fists during painful procedures. Nonverbal cues, such as grimacing, tensing of muscles, tear-filled eyes, and protective responses may contradict the child's assertion of feeling "okay."

Older children learn and exhibit culturally conditioned responses to pain, which accounts for the increasing variation in pain responses as children grow and develop. Infants from different cultural backgrounds respond in similar ways to a painful stimulus, whereas school-age children tend to exhibit responses that are characteristic of their family or cultural group.

The environment can influence the child's pain responses significantly. Older infants and toddlers are especially vulnerable to separation from parents and the presence of unfamiliar people. Often, these factors may aggravate or be more significant to the child than the pain itself. Conversely, the presence of familiar people may calm a child's responses to pain.

Neurological Development

The brain appears early in fetal development. By the end of the first month, a neural tube, which subsequently becomes the central nervous system has developed. The upper part of the neural tube widens to become the brain, while the lower tube develops into the spinal cord. In the second

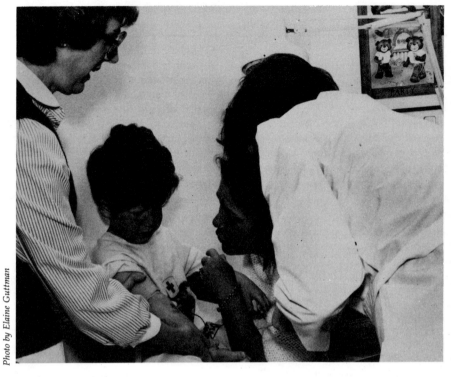

Photo by Elaine Guttman

FIGURE 22-2. Children's responses to pain include crying, grimacing, and attempts to avoid a painful stimulus. They often need help holding still during a painful procedure. (*Note.* From Servonsky/Opas: *Nursing Management of Children,* © 1987. Boston: Jones and Bartlett Publishers, p. 930.)

month, the cerebral hemispheres become visible; cerebellar development occurs during the third month of gestation.

Neurons of the brain undergo mitosis (division) only during the fetal period and the first few months after birth. However, brain tissue grows and differentiates dramatically during the first year of life. Myelination begins in the fetal period and continues until about age 10, although most of the major tracts of the central nervous system are complete by 2 years of age.

The brain and neural tissues grow at a much faster rate than other body tissues during the fetal period, infancy, and early childhood. The brain reaches 75% of adult size by age 2 and 90% by age 4, when cortical development is complete. Ultimate differentiation of the brain is usually complete by age 18.

Neonatal and infant reflexes are reviewed in Chapter 21. These reflexes disappear as the cortical centers of the brain achieve prominence. Most reflexes disappear by 3 months of age. Development of motor abilities is cephalocaudal, proximodistal, and general to specific, facilitating the child's movement from a reflexive being to one capable of highly differentiated functions. The child's gross and fine motor development from birth through 18 years of age is outlined in Chapter 10.

Activity–Sleep

Activity, which includes both mobility and exercise, and sleep are essential for optimal development. The child's ability to be active depends upon intact neurological and musculoskeletal systems.

Activity/Mobility

The major parts of the musculoskeletal system arise from the embryonic mesoderm. Muscle development occurs concurrently with bone development, and new muscle fibers are formed until the fifth month of fetal life. Thereafter, muscle fibers increase in size but not in number.

The skeletal system undergoes two physiological processes during childhood growth: modeling and remodeling. During *modeling*, the bones lengthen and widen (bone growth). With the exception of long bones, modeling ends at puberty. *Remodeling* is the cyclical resorption of older bone and formation of new bone at the same surface (bone maturation). Skeletal maturation is complete when the epiphysis and diaphysis of the long bones fuse completely, generally between 18 and 21 years of age.

The child's skeletal system differs from the adult's in several important ways. The child's periosteum is thicker and the bones are more pliable, allowing for bending and buckling in response to stress. Thus, the young child's skeletal system is less susceptible to trauma because its flexibility absorbs and diffuses any forceful impact. The high level of osteogenic activity permits rapid healing of skeletal injuries.

Activity is essential for normal musculoskeletal and neurological development. A child's activity level (e.g., active, sedentary, hyperactive) and the types of activities in which the child engages vary with age, health, temperament, the child's interests, and childrearing practices. Thomas and Chess (1977) identify activity level as one component of the child's temperament, placing children on a continuum of high to low activity (see Chap. 12).

A child's activity level is most evident in play. Childhood play fosters sensorimotor and cognitive development and helps socialize children to the norms and roles of society. Play also allows the child an opportunity for creative expression and provides a socially acceptable way for children to release tension, anger, and anxiety. Trends in playing that should be evident at each developmental stage are highlighted in Table 22-10.

Unfortunately, many children today, especially those who watch television excessively, are physically inactive. Physical inactivity has been identified as a major factor contributing to childhood obesity (Becque, Rocchini, & Moorehead, 1988; Dennison, Straus, Mellits, & Charney, 1988). Establishing regular physical activity patterns in childhood may help foster a lifelong commitment to exercise and help reduce the risk of obesity and heart disease in adulthood (Becque et al., 1988).

The American Academy of Pediatrics (1987) recommends that children engage in nonstop activity or exercise at least three times weekly for a minimum of 20 minutes each.

Sleep

Sleep allows the child to maintain optimal physiological and cognitive functioning and a general sense of well-being. During periods of rapid growth, such as infancy and early childhood, sleep needs are greatest. Total daily sleep needs decrease throughout childhood (see Figure 22-3), although there is wide individual variation in amount and distribution of sleep time and sleep quality. Children spend most of their sleep time in stages III and IV, with progressive lengthening of the REM periods throughout the night. Night awakenings are infrequent.

Infants generally sleep 16 to 20 hours daily with no regard for day versus night. By 3 months of age, most infants have developed a nocturnal sleep pattern and stay awake for longer periods, with two or three naps, each day. Parents may express concern about their infant's sleep patterns. Generally, if the infant is active during wakeful periods and growing normally, sleep needs are being met sufficiently. Once a nocturnal sleeping pattern is established, night awakenings typically are related to separation from parents, unfamiliar sleep environment, or insufficient food intake to sustain the infant through the night.

Toddlers generally sleep 10 to 12 hours nightly, with one or two naps during the day. The most common sleep problem at this age is related to sep-

TABLE 22-10
Play Activity Characteristics Throughout Childhood

Age	Social Character of Play	Content of Play	Most Prevalent Type of Play	Characteristics of Spontaneous Activity	Purpose of Dramatic Play	Development of Ethical Sense
Infant	Solitary	Social–affective	Sensorimotor	Sense–pleasure	Self-identity	—
Toddler	Parallel	Imitative	Body movement	Intuitive judgment	Learning gender role	Beginning of moral values
Preschool	Associative	Imaginative	Fantasy Informal games	Concept formation Reasonably constant ideas	Imitating social life Learning social roles	Developing concern for playmates Learning to share and cooperate
School-age	Cooperative	Competitive games and contests Fantasy	Physical activity Gang activities Formal games Play acting	Testing concrete situations and problem solving Adding fresh information	Vicarious mastery	Peer loyalty Playing by the rules Hero worship

Note. From Wong, D.L., & Whaley, L.F. (1990). *Clinical manual of pediatric nursing* (3rd. ed.). St. Louis: Mosby, p. 202.

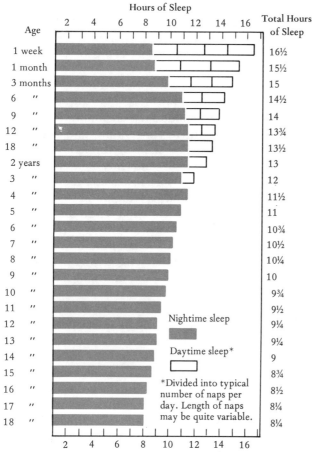

FIGURE 22-3. Sleep Patterns in Infancy and Childhood. (*Note.* From Ferber, R. [1985]. *Solve your child's sleep problems.* Copyright © 1985 by Richard Ferber, M.D. Reprinted by permission of Simon & Schuster, Inc.)

terrors upon awakening. In contrast, nightmares occur during REM sleep in the latter half of the sleep cycle. They are characterized by vivid visual images that fully arouse the child, who is frightened yet able to recall the images and events of the experience. Nightmares are most likely to occur when the child has had a particularly stressful or fatiguing day. Beltramini and Hertzig (1983) report that nearly two-thirds of preschoolers experience nightmares regularly during the preschool years.

After age 5, children require 9 to 11 hours of sleep daily and rarely nap. Somnambulism and soliloquy are seen most frequently in this age group. Boys experience these sleep disturbances, which are often associated with *enuresis* (bedwetting), more than girls. Like night terrors, they occur during the transition from stage IV to the first REM period. The child will sit up abruptly with eyes open but glassy and unseeing. If the child walks, the movements are clumsy and uncoordinated. Speech usually is mumbled, slurred, monosyllabic, and often incomprehensible. Nightmares may continue in this age group and usually are associated with fears or conflicts that have occurred during waking hours.

Illness and hospitalization disrupt a child's sleep pattern. Barndt-Maglio (1986) identifies intrinsic and extrinsic factors related to illness and hospitalization that interfere with normal sleep patterns. These factors include physiological alterations, anesthesia, medications, pain, psychological stress, unfamiliar environment, treatment protocols, routine care, lights, and noise, all of which desynchronize the child's body rhythms and established sleep patterns.

Oxygenation

Although structurally complete, the infant and young child's cardiorespiratory system is immature and differs physiologically in many respects from the adult's. The chest wall in infancy is thin and the rib cage is flexible. The chest is round, flattening gradually as the child grows older (see Figure 22-4). Diaphragmatic breathing is predominant in infancy and early childhood, owing to the horizontal position of the ribs in relation to the spine.

The nasal, tracheal, and bronchial pathways are narrow and there is less alveolar surface for gas exchange, thus increasing the infant's and young child's susceptibility to respiratory infection, obstruction, and atelectasis (collapse of lung). Young children also have far less oxygen reserve than adults. Their resting oxygen consumption is twice that of adults, which is reflected in their higher respiratory rate.

aration from parents at bedtime. The child is not able to differentiate between temporary and permanent separations and so may cling tightly to significant people or objects. Availability of a favorite object, such as a blanket or stuffed animal, and adhering to bedtime rituals become very important.

By age 5, children need 9 to 11 hours of sleep each night, with only one nap or rest period. During the preschool years, sleep disturbances, including *somnambulism* (sleepwalking), *somniloquy* (sleep talking), nightmares, and night terrors, are relatively common. These disturbances are thought to reflect the immaturity of the child's central nervous system and the fantasy thinking that characterizes this age.

Night terrors are most prevalent among 3- to 8-year-old children although they occur in fewer than 10% of all children (Beltramini & Hertzig, 1983). They tend to occur at the same point in the sleep cycle—at the transition from the first stage IV to the first REM period, about 90 to 100 minutes after going to sleep. Children typically do not recall night

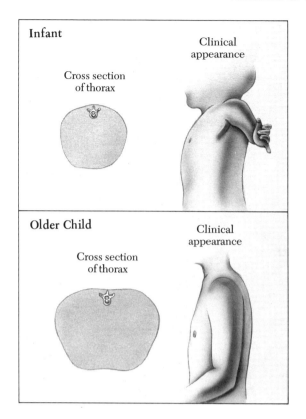

FIGURE 22-4. Chest Configuration in Infancy and Childhood.

The position of the cricoid cartilage moves from the level of the fourth cervical vertebra in infants to the fifth cervical vertebra in children. The number and size of the alveoli increase steadily until age 12, and collateral ventilatory structures develop. By late childhood, the respiratory system is functionally mature.

The infant's heart is large in proportion to total body size and lies at a transverse angle during infancy (see Figure 22-5). Sinus arrhythmia is common, with the heart rate increasing during inhalation and decreasing during exhalation. As the child grows and the lungs develop, the angle of the heart becomes oblique. The apical impulse, or point of maximal impulse (PMI), is usually visible in young infants and moves from the midclavicular line to the left by early school age. The size of the heart doubles in infancy and quadruples by 5 years of age. Because of the thin chest wall and changing relationships between the chest and internal organs as the child grows, heart murmurs are common in children, 50% of which are innocent and disappear as the child matures.

Physiological anemia is typical during the first months of life. A relatively high level of fetal hemoglobin is believed to depress the production of red blood cells for the first three months, until adult hemoglobin is produced. After 3 months of age, the red blood cell count gradually increases throughout childhood until adult levels are reached in adolescence (see Table 22-11). Blood gas values (PO_2, PCO_2, pH) in infancy and childhood are comparable to adult norms.

Nutrition and Dentition

Because of the tremendous changes in physical growth that occur throughout infancy and childhood, nutritional needs are great. Children must

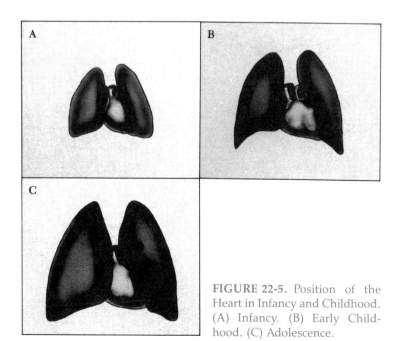

FIGURE 22-5. Position of the Heart in Infancy and Childhood. (A) Infancy. (B) Early Childhood. (C) Adolescence.

TABLE 22-11
Common Laboratory Values in Children

Test	Values
Cholesterol, serum	Infant 70–175 mg/dl
	Child 120–200 mg/dl
Glucose, serum	Infant 50–90 mg/dl
	Child 60–100 mg/dl
Hematocrit (Hct)	Infant 28–42%
	Child 35–45%
Hemoglobin (Hgb)	Infant 9.0–14.0 g/dl
	Child 10.5–15.5 g/dl
PCO$_2$ (arterial)	Infant 27–41 mm Hg
	Child 32–48 mm Hg
pH (arterial)	7.35–7.45
Platelet count	150,000–400,000/mm^3
PO$_2$ (arterial)	83–108 mm Hg
Potassium, serum	Infant 4.1–5.3 mmol/L
	Child 3.4–4.7 mmol/L
Red blood cell	1 month 3.0–5.4 million/mm^3
(RBC) count	6 months 3.1–4.5 million/mm^3
	1–2 years 3.7–5.3 million/mm^3
	4 years 3.9–5.3 million/mm^3
	6–12 years 4.0–5.2 million/mm^3
Sodium, serum	Infant 139–146 mmol/L
	Child 138–145 mmol/L
Urine specific gravity	1.002–1.025
White blood cell	Infant 5,000–19,500/mm^3
(WBC) count	1–3 years 6,000–17,500/mm^3
	4–7 years 5,500–15,500/mm^3
	8–12 years 4,500–13,500/mm^3

consume sufficient quantities of protein, carbohydrates, fats, vitamins, and minerals in order to grow and develop optimally. Protein, vitamins, and minerals are needed for tissue growth. Sufficient caloric intake is necessary to meet the child's needs for body functions, activity, and maturation of already developed tissue.

Good nutrition in childhood lays the foundation for a healthy adulthood. Overeating during childhood has been linked with such chronic diseases as hypertension, atherosclerosis, and diabetes in adulthood (American Academy of Pediatrics, 1987). Childhood obesity, especially beyond the age of 7 years, is likely to persist into adulthood, and may negatively influence the child's mental health and self-esteem as well as physical well-being (Alexander & Blank, 1988).

Nutritional requirements are influenced by the child's age and weight, gender, body type, metabolic rate, activity level, and general health. Illness places special demands on the child's metabolism, typically resulting in significant increases in nutritional requirements. Food intake is influenced by physiological requirements as well as complex psychosocial and cultural factors. Alexander and Blank (1988) note that a high proportion of Mexican-American preschool children are overweight, attributable to early feeding practices and cultural values about weight and weight control among Mexican-American mothers.

Because the rate of growth is most rapid in infancy, nutritional requirements per unit of body weight are greatest at this time. As children grow older, they require fewer calories per unit of body weight, although they require more total calories daily because of their increasing size (see Table 22-12). Energy requirements are thus greatest during infancy, declining gradually until adolescence (see chap. 23).

The Food and Nutrition Board of the National Research Council has established recommended daily allowances for children for protein, water- and fat-soluble vitamins, and for six minerals. These allowances are listed in Table 22-13.

TABLE 22-12
Recommended Energy Intakes for Children of Various Ages

Ranges	Age	Weight (kg)	Height (cm)	Average Energy Needs (kcal)
Infants	0.0–0.5	6	60	
	0.5–1.0	9	71	
Children	1–3	13	90	1300
	4–6	20	112	1800
	7–10	28	132	2000
Males	11–14	45	157	2500
	15–18	66	176	3000
Females	11–14	46	157	2200
	15–18	55	163	2200

Note. Reprinted with permission from *Recommended Dietary Allowances*, 10th edition, © 1989 by the National Academy of Sciences. Published by National Academy Press, Washington, DC.

Breast milk or commercial iron-fortified formula is sufficient for the infant's diet for the first six months. During the first year, 4 to 6 feedings daily are required. Breast-fed infants require fluoride supplementation, as do bottle-fed babies whose home water supply is not fluoridated.

Solid foods are not needed in the infant's diet until 6 months of age. Earlier introduction is not recommended because of the immaturity of the infant's digestive system. Developmental characteristics required for eating solid foods include the infant's ability to control head and neck muscles, tooth eruption, reaching and grasping, and beginning hand–eye coordination. Table 22-14 outlines the developmental milestones associated with infants' eating. Children with developmental disabilities may experience significant eating problems related to their inability to achieve the normal developmental milestones necessary for feeding themselves.

The first solid foods introduced to the infant are those that are least allergenic, such as cereals, fruits, and vegetables, progressing to more complex foods, such as meats, starches, and eggs. Infants begin to finger feed by 9 months of age and should be able to drink from a cup well by 12 months of age. By age 1, the child typically eats three meals and requires at least 32 oz of fluid daily.

During toddlerhood, fluid needs increase, although milk intake should be limited to less than a quart daily to assure sufficient intake of solids to meet dietary iron needs. Toddlers are able to feed themselves independently using their fingers and child-size utensils (Figure 22-6). They are often picky eaters, rejecting foods that don't smell or look appetizing. *Physiological anorexia* is a common problem during toddlerhood— the child's interest in eating declines and daily intake may seem insufficient. However, most toddlers consume sufficient calories and nutrients for growth as measured by standardized growth charts (see chap. 21).

Preschoolers often continue their picky eating habits, but may be more willing to try foods that are favored by the family or cultural group. They learn table manners, can assist with food preparation, are able to get snacks for themselves, and use eating utensils with ease.

School-age children eat increasing numbers of meals away from home, often at school or when visiting friends' homes, and assume greater responsibility for food purchase and preparation in today's busy families. Although school-age children generally understand the importance of nutrition to health, they tend to choose foods high in carbohydrates and fats (National Dairy Council,

1990). They are influenced by advertising gimmicks and succumb to eating junk foods such as candy, soda pop, and "munchies." Even when balanced meals are available at school, children often select or eat only those foods that appeal to them. Childhood obesity is a growing problem among American children, to whom "empty calorie" foods are available and who spend many sedentary hours watching television or playing video games. Breakfast is especially important to ensure the child begins each school day with sufficient energy to learn. Recommended daily servings for children from the four basic food groups are illustrated in the boxed insert that follows.

Tooth development begins in utero, although the teeth remain below the gum line until after birth. The deciduous (primary) teeth erupt during infancy and toddlerhood and are shed during the school years, when permanent teeth begin to replace them. The sequence of tooth eruption is similar for most children, although considerable variation occurs in the age of onset. Gradually, the lower central (medial) incisors erupt first, between 6 and 9 months of age, followed by the upper central incisors. There are 20 primary teeth. The shedding of the primary teeth and eruption of the permanent teeth follow a similar pattern. In addition, the permanent teeth include two sets of bicuspids (first and second premolars) and a third set of molars (wisdom teeth), for a total of 32 teeth. Figure 22-7 depicts the sequence and average ages of tooth eruption and shedding during childhood.

As the teeth erupt through the periodontal membrane, some inflammation occurs and the child may experience discomfort. Drooling, biting, and irritability often accompany teething. Rarely does the child experience fever or other symptoms of illness.

Fluid Requirements

As growth and maturation occur, the proportion of body fluid to body mass lessens gradually. During infancy, body water accounts for 70 to 75% of total body mass, decreasing to 65% in toddlerhood, and to 60% in childhood. A greater percentage of the infant and young child's fluid volume remains in the extracellular compartment—40% in the infant compared to 20% in the adult. Therefore, the infant must ingest and excrete proportionately more fluid than an adult in a 24-hour period. For example, a 1-month old infant requires 100 to 130 ml of water per kilogram of body weight in 24 hours, whereas an adult requires only 20 to 40 ml per kilogram of body weight. As the infant matures, daily fluid requirements decrease to 50 to 70 ml/Kg, depending

TABLE 22-13
Recommended Daily Dietary Allowances (RDAs) for Infants and Children (United States)

Age (Years)	Weight (kg)	Weight (lb)	Height (cm)	Height (in)	Protein (g)	Fat-Soluble Vitamins Vitamin A (μgRE)*	Vitamin D (μg)†	Vitamin E (mg α^{-TE})‡
Infants								
0.0–0.5	6	13	60	24	13	375	7.5	3
0.5–1.0	9	20	71	28	14	375	10	4
Children								
1–3	13	29	90	35	16	400	10	6
4–6	20	44	112	44	24	500	10	7
7–10	28	62	132	52	28	700	10	7

Note. The allowances are intended to provide for individual variations among most normal persons as they live in the United States under usual environmental stresses. Diets should be based on a variety of common foods in order to provide other nutrients for which human requirements have been less well defined.

*Retinol equivalents. 1 retinol equivalent = 1 μg of retinol or 6 μg of β-carotene.

†As cholecalciferol. 10 μg of cholecalciferol = 400 IU of vitamin D.

‡α-tocopherol equivalents. 1 mg of d-α-tocopherol = 1 α^{-TE}.

§1 NE (niacin equivalent) is equal to 1 mg of niacin or 60 mg of dietary tryptophan.

Note. Reprinted with permission from *Recommended Dietary Allowances*, 10th edition, © 1989 by the National Academy of Sciences. Published by National Academy Press, Washington, DC.

on age, weight, and body mass. Table 22-15 summarizes average daily water requirements by age and weight.

In addition, the infant's body surface area is greater in proportion to body weight, and the metabolic rate is higher than an adult's. The immature renal tubules cannot concentrate urine; thus, proportionately more water is required to excrete body wastes. Further, the infant's respiratory rate is higher, resulting in greater insensible fluid loss. All these factors increase the infant's susceptibility to fluid and electrolyte imbalances.

Elimination

During infancy, urinary and bowel elimination are involuntary and reflexive. As myelination of the spinal cord becomes complete, the child becomes physiologically able to voluntarily control the urinary and anal sphincters. Physiological readiness to achieve bowel and bladder control occurs between 15 and 24 months of age. Bowel control usually is accomplished before bladder control because bladder control requires the inhibition of a stronger neurological reflex. Most children accomplish bowel control before the third year. Daytime bladder control usually is achieved between 2½ and 3½ years of age, whereas complete nighttime control often is not accomplished until 4 to 5 years of age.

Physiological and psychosocial readiness to learn voluntary control of bowel and bladder elimination depends on several factors. Bowel movements must occur at regular times, and the child must show cognitive awareness that defecation or voiding is occurring. The child also must be able to follow directions, verbalize the need to defecate or void, and be capable of handling his or her clothing. The type and location of bathroom facilities also may influence the child's readiness. For some children, a child-size potty chair is helpful. Perhaps most important, however, is the interaction between the child and parent (or child and day care worker) as the child attempts to achieve independent control of elimination. Pressuring the child too early or when the child doesn't indicate interest can cause the child to resist toilet-training efforts.

The young child voids approximately 4 to 6 times daily. The 24-hour urine output increases steadily throughout childhood (see Table 22-16). The urine should be a clear, pale yellow. Urine pH ranges from 4.5 to 8.0, with an average of 6.0. Urine-specific gravity ranges from 1.002 to 1.025, depending on the child's age and fluid status.

The child's typical stool pattern (frequency, color, consistency) is established in early infancy and is influenced by diet and activity. In early infancy, the digestive system is immature. The gastrointestinal tract is permeable to large molecules, making it difficult for infants to digest complex foods and predisposing them to food allergy. High fiber foods, such as peas, corn, and carrots, are

Water-Soluble Vitamins							Minerals					
Vitamin C (mg)	Thiamin (mg)	Ribo-flavin (mg)	Niacin (mg NE)§	Vitamin B_6 (mg)	Folacin‖ (µg)	Vitamin B_{12} (µg)	Calcium (mg)	Phos-phorus (mg)	Mag-nesium (mg)	Iron (mg)	Zinc (mg)	Iodine (µg)
30	0.3	0.4	5	0.3	25	0.3¶	400	300	40	6	5	40
35	0.4	0.5	6	0.6	35	0.5	600	500	60	10	5	50
40	0.7	0.8	9	1.0	50	0.7	800	800	80	10	10	70
45	0.9	1.1	12	1.1	75	1.0	800	800	120	10	10	90
45	1.0	1.2	13	1.4	100	1.4	800	800	170	10	10	120

‖The folacin allowances refer to dietary sources as determined by *Lactobacillus casei* assay after treatment with enzymes (conjugases) to make polyglutamyl forms of the vitamin available to the test organism.

¶The recommended dietary allowance for vitamin B_{12} in infants is based on average concentration of the vitamin in human milk. The allowances after weaning are based on energy intake (as recommended by the American Academy of Pediatrics) and consideration of other factors, such as intestinal absorption.

Four Basic Food Groups—Daily Servings for Children

Food Group	Servings Per Day
Milk or equivalent ½ cup whole milk equals: ¾ ounce cheese ½ cup yogurt, milk pudding 1 cup cottage cheese ¾–1 cup ice cream	3 for child 4 for adolescent Usual serving: Toddler and preschooler—½ to ¾ cup School-age and older—1 cup
Meat, fish, poultry, or equivalent 1 ounce meat equals: 1 egg 1 ounce cheese 2 tablespoons peanut butter ¼ cup tuna fish ½ cup cooked legumes	2 for child and adolescent Usual serving: Toddler and preschooler— 1 egg, 1 to 2 ounces meat School-age and older—1 egg, 3 ounces meat
Vegetables and fruits Citrus equivalents: 1 orange or tomato ½ cup orange or grapefruit juice ¾ cup strawberries	4 for child and adolescent 1 citrus daily; 1 yellow or dark green vegetable 3 to 4 times weekly Usual serving: Toddler and preschooler—2 tablespoons to ¼ cup School-age and older—½ cup
Breads and cereals 1 slice enriched bread equals: ¾ cup dry cereal ½ cup cooked pasta, rice, or cereal ½ hamburger bun 1 small muffin or biscuit	4 for child and adolescent Usual serving: Toddler and preschooler—½ slice bread School-age and older—1 slice bread

Note. From Whaley, L.F., & Wong, D.L. (1991). *Nursing care of infants and children* (4th ed.). St. Louis: Mosby-Year Book, p. 143.

TABLE 22-14
Developmental Milestones Associated with Eating

Age (Months)	Development
Birth	Has sucking, rooting, and swallowing reflexes Feels hunger and indicates desire for food by crying; expresses satiety by falling asleep
1	Has strong extrusion reflex
3–4	Extrusion reflex is fading Begins to develop hand-eye coordination
4–5	Can approximate lips to the rim of a cup
5–6	Can use fingers to feed self a cracker
6–7	Chews and bites May hold own bottle, but may not drink from it (prefers for it to be held)
7–9	Refuses food by keeping lips closed; has taste preferences Holds a spoon and plays with it during feeding May drink from a straw Drinks from a cup with assistance
9–12	Picks up small morsels of food (finger foods) and feeds self Holds own bottle and drinks from it Drinks from a household cup without assistance but spills some Uses a spoon with much spilling
12–18	Drools less Drinks well from a household cup, but may drop it when finished Holds cup with both hands
24	Can use a straw Chews food with mouth closed and shifts food in mouth Distinguishes between finger and spoon foods Holds small glass in one hand; replaces glass without dropping
36	Spills small amount from spoon Begins to use fork; holds it in fist Uses adult pattern of chewing, which involves rotary action of jaw
48	Rarely spills when using spoon Serves self finger foods Eats with fork held with fingers
54	Uses fork in preference to spoon
72	Spreads with knife
84	Cuts tender food with knife

Note. From Wong, D.L., & Whaley, L.F. (1990). *Clinical manual of pediatric nursing* (3rd ed.). St. Louis: Mosby-Year Book, p. 168.

passed through the GI tract undigested. Peristalsis during infancy is relatively rapid, thus predisposing children to diarrhea. As a child grows, peristalsis slows and stomach capacity enlarges.

APPROACHES TO ASSESSING THE INFANT AND CHILD

Assessment of infants and young children typically requires that a parent or other familiar caregiver be present since children under the age of 7 usually are unable to provide accurate and reliable information about their health (Figure 22-8). Young children's cognitive immaturity and relative inexperience with the larger world influence their responses to a nurse or an unfamiliar health-care setting; their responses may range from overt fear and aggression to quiet retreat.

The child's age and developmental level influence responses to the assessment process. The nurse should be familiar with the developmental characteristics that affect the child's ability to participate in the interview and health examination. These characteristics are outlined in Table 22-17.

In order to conduct a comprehensive assessment of infants and young children, a nurse must be knowledgeable about their anatomical and physiological differences from adults (reviewed earlier in this chapter) and skilled in assessment techniques. Perhaps most important, a nurse must understand how to approach young children to gain their trust and cooperation. Generally, young

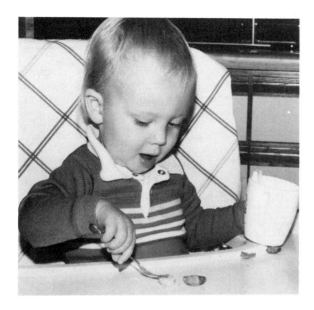

FIGURE 22-6. Assessing the toddler's self-feeding abilities is an important part of the nutritional assessment of children.

children are more sensitive to nonverbal messages, such as voice tone, movement, and eye contact, than verbal ones. Therefore, the nurse should speak to the child and parent in a soft, quiet, calm voice, and movements should be unhurried.

Honesty and predictability are critical to gaining, and keeping, a child's trust. If a procedure is going to hurt or be uncomfortable, the child should not be told otherwise. Nor should the nurse try to minimize the child's feelings or expressions of fear or pain. For example, if a child begins to cry loudly while being restrained for an examination of her ears, reassuring the child with, "You are trying so hard to help; I will be done soon" is better, and more realistic, than telling her to stop crying and hold still. Children should be praised for their cooperation, even when they aren't entirely successful.

The nurse should allow the young child to make the first overture rather than reaching out to the child with words, gestures, or even a smile. It is usually best to initiate contact with a young child's parent or caregiver in order to give the child an opportunity to "size up" the nurse. Most young children will initiate contact with a nurse by establishing eye contact, offering a toy for observation or comment, or with words ("I have a new dress"). If the child has a favorite stuffed animal or doll, the nurse can "talk" to it first or ask the child to share the doll or animal's name. A nurse should never try to separate a child from a parent by picking the child up or asking the parent to leave the room.

The environment in which the assessment is

conducted should be physically and psychologically comfortable for the child. Examination equipment should be kept out of sight until needed. Brightly colored walls or posters, soft music, and comfortable furniture create a conducive setting. Many children, especially infants and toddlers, are most comfortable on their parents' laps during the history and clinical appraisal (Figure 22-9).

During the examination, the nurse should proceed quickly yet calmly. Responding to a child's requests to "wait a minute" may actually increase the child's fear. It is usually best to continue the examination, even if restraining the child is necessary. However, if the child must be restrained, the nurse should explain by saying, "I'm (We are) going to help you hold still." Before proceeding with each step of the examination, the nurse should explain to the child in simple words what will be done— "I'm going to listen to your heart to see how strong it is." Lengthy, step-by-step explanations should be avoided.

If the child is unfamiliar with equipment to be used, such as a stethoscope, the child may be given an opportunity to play with it for a few seconds (Figure 22-10). Also, the child should be told what sensations are likely; use such words as "pushing," "cold," or "tight." The nurse should avoid using words that could be misinterpreted by the child, such as "take your temperature," because the child may think something will be taken away. Instead, the nurse can say, "Check your temperature."

When a nurse must enlist a child's involvement or cooperation, the request should be phrased as a statement rather than a question. For example, the nurse should say, "I need you to take off your shoes and socks so I can look at your feet," rather than "Can you take off your shoes and socks?" The child should not be offered choices when there are none.

Table 22-18 offers suggestions for facilitating the health examination of children at various developmental stages.

INFANT AND CHILD HEALTH HISTORY

Until early adolescence, a child's parent or reliable caregiver must provide most if not all of the historical information about the child's health. On occasion, the nurse also may need to interview other adults who know the child well, such as teachers, day care workers, or grandparents, in order to obtain a complete and accurate picture of a particular child or problem.

Once children reach early school-age, the

nurse should involve them as active participants in the nursing history interview. In fact, children who are older than 7 should have an opportunity to spend some time alone with the nurse to ask and answer health-related questions. Such an opportunity lays the foundation for children to become better informed about and take greater responsibility for their health.

Generally, the format of the nursing history is the same as that used with adults. Some additions are necessary, however, because of the importance of development to the child's health and well-being. Specifically, these additions include:

- Parental–neonatal history (children under age 3) [see chap. 10, Table 10-6]
- Developmental capabilities

TABLE 22-15
Daily Fluid Requirements by Age and Weight

Age	Daily Total	By Body Weight
1 year	1,150 to 1,300 ml	100 to 130 ml/Kg
2 years	1,350 to 1,500 ml	100 to 120 ml/Kg
4 years	1,600 to 1,800 ml	90 to 110 ml/Kg
10 years	2,000 to 2,500 ml	60 to 85 ml/Kg

TABLE 22-16
Average Daily Urine Output

Age	Amount
Infant	400 to 500 ml
1–3 years	500 to 600 ml
3–6 years	600 to 700 ml
6–9 years	700 to 1,000 ml
9–12 years	800 to 1,400 ml

- Child–parent relationship; child–sibling relationships
- Child–peer relationships
- School performance
- Play activities
- Immunization history
- Previous health-related experiences
- Daily patterns: eating, elimination, sleep

Also, the nurse should ascertain what recent events or changes have occurred that could contribute to childhood stress. Heisel and colleagues

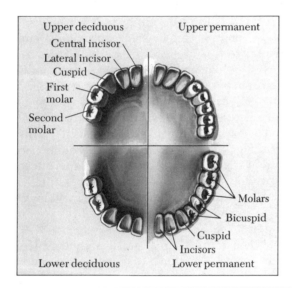

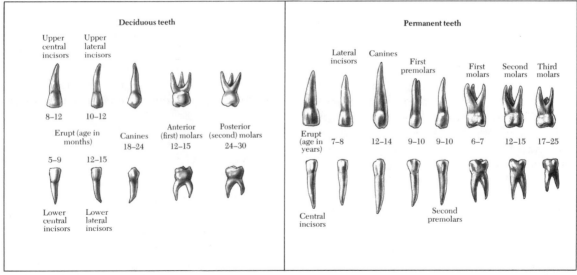

FIGURE 22-7. Position of Primary (Deciduous) and Permanent Teeth and Approximate Ages of Tooth Eruption.

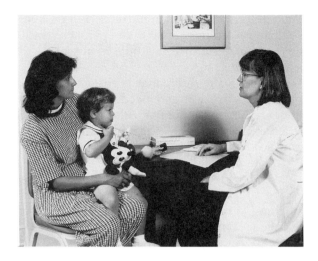

FIGURE 22-8. Young children cannot provide reliable information about their health. Therefore, the parent becomes the primary source of information for the health history.

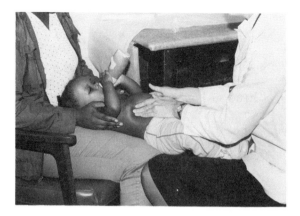

FIGURE 22-9. Allowing the infant to remain on the mother's lap during the clinical appraisal helps minimize fear and increase the infant's cooperation.

(1973) report on the significance of life events as factors contributing to illness in children. Different life events have varying impacts on children, depending on their developmental level. Table 22-19 depicts the Stress Scale for Children. This scale may be used to ask the child or parent about which life events the child has experienced within the previous year. The score should be totaled and compared with the mean score for healthy children (see Figure 22-11). Children who score more than one standard deviation above the mean are at

greater risk for illness than those who score less than one standard deviation above the mean.

When reviewing a child's physiological health, the nurse should pay special attention to sensory–neurological functioning, activity–mobility, oxygenation, and nutrition. Undetected problems in these areas can contribute to serious developmental consequences for the child.

Table 22-20 illustrates a child health history format.

CLINICAL APPRAISAL AND SCREENING

The usual head-to-toe approach is not always the best one to use with children, particularly infants

---

TABLE 22-17
Developmental Characteristics That Influence the Child's Responses to the Nursing Assessment

Children Under Age 7	Children Aged 7 to 12 Years
■ Egocentric—cannot see things from another's point of view; learns by first-hand experience only	■ Increased body awareness and knowledge of health and illness (see chap. 10)
■ Concept of time is poorly developed; may be able to differentiate past, present, and future, but is not able to understand specific differences (such as "yesterday" and "two months ago")	■ Able to participate in decision-making, such as choosing to receive immunization injection in arm or thigh
■ Cannot view things from another point in time, therefore is unable to provide accurate information concerning earlier or previous health-related experiences	■ Able to understand concrete explanations and learn correct medical terminology
■ Concept of causality is immature; events that occur in proximity are interpreted as related; as the child nears age 7, may comprehend *simple* cause and effect, such as "germs cause illness"	■ Increased ability to categorize and conceptualize (such as body systems)
■ Interpret words literally ("You're so sweet I could eat you up!" "You're going to cry your eyes out!")	■ Able to participate in portions of interview
	■ May be modest
	■ Better concept of time; more interested in own childhood health history

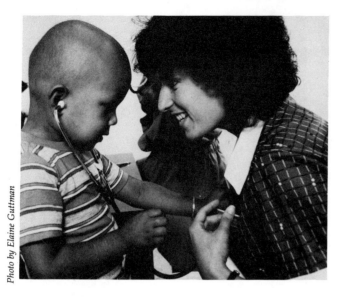

Photo by Elaine Guttman

FIGURE 22-10. Preschool children should be given an opportunity to play with unfamiliar equipment prior to the clinical appraisal to help decrease their fear and increase their cooperation. (*Note.* From Servonsky/Opas: *Nursing Management of Children,* © 1987. Boston: Jones and Bartlett Publishers, p. 363.)

and toddlers. Examining the ears and mouth is quite intrusive. If these areas are examined first, the child may resist, pull away, and fail to cooperate with other, less intrusive portions of the assessment.

When a child is anxious or fearful, many physiological responses occur, such as increased heart and respiratory rates, thus preventing the nurse from obtaining information about the child's typical patterns. Therefore, the nurse must use a flexible approach that will provide the most accurate and complete information about the child.

No single approach works best for all children. However, approaches based on the child's developmental level generally are most effective (see Table 22-18). Some portions of the clinical appraisal can be accomplished while gathering information during the nursing history. For example, the nurse can observe the child's general appearance, activity level, language, and fine and gross motor skills while collecting history. During the clinical appraisal, the nurse should be positioned as close to the child's eye level as possible (Figure 22-12). The nurse may have to sit or stoop to do so. Meeting the child at eye level helps foster trust and hold the child's attention.

When examining children, a nurse must take advantage of opportunities for assessment as they arise. When children remove their shoes and socks (which most will do readily), the opportunity to ex-

amine the child's feet should be used. If an infant is lying or sleeping quietly in the parent's arms or lap, the nurse can use this time to auscultate the heart and lungs.

Although the traditional head-to-toe order of the clinical appraisal may need to be altered, the sequence for examining particular areas should be systematic. For example, the nurse should use the same sequence consistently to auscultate the lungs or palpate the child's abdomen.

While the techniques used to examine children are the same as those used with adults, the nurse may have to modify them to assure the child's cooperation. Many children are ticklish and have difficulty cooperating when body parts, such as the abdomen or axillary lymph nodes, are palpated. By placing the child's hand under the nurse's, the child's ticklish response can be reduced. This approach also has the advantage of enlisting the child's active participation. When auscultating the heart, the nurse may find it helpful to place a hand on the child's back to keep the child from inadvertently leaning away from the pressure of the stethoscope.

The nurse should begin the clinical appraisal by examining the child's general appearance (see boxed insert). The child's physical condition (well or ill), general skin color and tone, alertness and activity level, speech or nature of the child's cry, the child's interaction with the parent or caregiver and response to the nurse, developmental level, general hygiene and dress, and neuromuscular functioning (posture, gait, coordination) all can be observed during the first few minutes of contact.

There are a number of aspects of the clinical appraisal that must be modified for assessing infants or children. Specifically, these include the measurement of physical growth and vital signs, vision and hearing screening, neurological and pain assessment, screening for impaired physical

---

Initial Appraisal of Infants and Children

Physical condition (well or ill)
Hygiene and dress
Skin color and tone
Alertness and activity level
Speech or nature of cry
Interaction with parent or caregiver
Response to environment and unfamiliar people
Developmental abilities
Neuromuscular functioning (posture, gait, coordination)

TABLE 22-18
Developmental Approaches to the Clinical Appraisal of Infants and Children

Infant	Toddler	Preschool Child	School-age Child
Perform most of exam while infant is held by parent.	Begin with nonthreatening interactions first, such as Denver II.	Begin with nonthreatening interactions, such as Denver II.	Show equipment and explain its use.
Avoid abrupt, sudden movements that may startle infant.	Examine while child is standing near parent or sitting on parent's lap.	Allow child opportunity to play with some equipment, such as stethoscope.	Allow child opportunity to ask questions and discuss feelings about examination.
Use toys, pacifier, or bottle to distract infant. Parent can assist with distraction.	Use toys or simple games to distract child. Parent can assist with distraction.	Allow child opportunity to ask questions and state feelings.	Give concrete answers to questions.
Perform intrusive tasks, such as taking rectal temperature or examining ears, after less intrusive ones, such as assessing heart and breath sounds.	Perform intrusive tasks, such as taking rectal temperature or examining ears, after less intrusive ones, such as assessing heart and breath sounds.	Give simple, honest answers to questions.	Determine if child will be more comfortable with parent present or absent during examination.
Examine skin color, respiration, and heart rate while infant is quiet or asleep.	Don't offer choices (negativism is characteristic of toddler).	Give choice of sitting/standing near parent or sitting on exam table.	Use head-to-toe approach.
Talk to infant in soft, soothing voice.	Provide an opportunity for child to play with or handle some equipment, such as stethoscope.	Indicate how and when child may help during examination, (e.g., undressing).	Indicate how and when child may help during examination.
Have parent assist with restraining infant to examine ears, mouth.	Remove one article of clothing at a time. Have parent assist child.	Use words that will decrease fantasies ("check blood pressure" instead of "take").	During examination, teach child how body functions.
	Give simple directions.	Give simple directions and feedback during examination.	Use correct medical and anatomical terminology.
	Restrain firmly and safely as needed. Praise child for cooperating.	Provide privacy while child undresses. Allow child to leave underwear on; pull underwear to side for genitalia exam.	Provide privacy while child undresses. Allow child to leave underwear on until it is necessary to examine abdomen and genitalia.
		Demonstrate techniques on a doll.	Examine genital area last.
		Praise child for cooperating.	Praise child for cooperating.

Note. Adapted from Servonsky/Opas: *Nursing Management of Children*, © 1987. Boston: Jones and Bartlett Publishers, p. 82.

mobility, and assessment of fluid–electrolyte balance. However, in order to ensure that no aspects are overlooked, Table 22-21 outlines a complete clinical appraisal of infants and children and indicates which parameters are covered in this chapter.

Measuring Physical Growth

Because of the rapid rate of growth throughout infancy and childhood, regular periodic screening of the child's physical growth provides important

TABLE 22-19
Children's Stress Scale (Life Event Changes)

Life Events	Pre-school	Ele-mentary	Junior High	Senior High
Beginning nursery school, first grade, seventh grade, or high school	42	46	45	42
Change to a different school	33	46	52	56
Birth or adoption of a brother or sister	50	50	50	50
Brother or sister leaving home	39	36	33	37
Hospitalization of brother or sister	37	41	44	41
Death of brother or sister	59	68	71	68
Change of father's occupation requiring increased absence from home	36	45	42	38
Loss of job by a parent	23	38	48	46
Marital separation of parents	74	78	77	69
Divorce of parents	78	84	84	77
Hospitalization of parent (serious illness)	51	55	54	55
Death of a parent	89	91	94	87
Death of a grandparent	30	38	35	36
Marriage of parent to stepparent	62	65	63	63
Jail sentence of parent for 30 days or less	34	44	50	53
Jail sentence of parent for 1 year or more	67	67	76	75
Addition of third adult to family (e.g., grandparent)	39	41	34	34
Change in parents' financial status	21	29	40	45
Mother beginning to work	47	44	36	26
Decrease in number of arguments between parents	21	25	29	27
Increase in number of arguments between parents	44	51	48	46
Decrease in number of arguments with parents	22	27	29	26
Increase in number of arguments with parents	39	47	46	47
Discovery of being an adopted child	33	52	70	64
Acquiring a visible deformity	52	69	83	81
Having a visible congenital deformity	39	60	70	62
Hospitalization of yourself (child)	59	62	59	58
Change in acceptance by peers	38	51	68	67
Outstanding personal achievement	23	39	45	46
Death of a close friend (child's friend)	38	53	65	63
Failure of a year in school		57	62	56
Suspension from school		46	54	50
Pregnancy in unwed teenager sister		36	60	64
Becoming involved with drugs or alcohol		61	70	76
Becoming a full-fledged member of a church/synagogue		25	28	31
Not making an extracurricular activity you wanted to be involved in (i.e., athletic team, band)			49	55
Breaking up with a boyfriend or girlfriend			47	53
Beginning to date			55	51
Fathering an unwed pregnancy			76	77
Unwed pregnancy			95	92
Being accepted to a college of your choice				43
Getting married				101

Note. From Heisel, J.S., Ream, S., Raitz, R., Rappaport, M., & Coddington, R.D. (1973). The significance of life events as contributing factors in the diseases of children. *Journal of Pediatrics, 83*(1), 120.

clues about the child's development and general well-being. Measurements of physical growth include height (length), weight, skinfold thickness, and head circumference (under age 3). Guidelines for measuring head circumference (Figure 22-13) may be found in Chapter 21. The technique for measuring skinfold thickness is the same as that used with adults (see chap. 18). Findings should be plotted on an anthropometric graph that indicates percentiles for triceps skinfold thickness in children at various ages (see Figure 22-14).

Height (Length)

Until age 3, recumbent (crown-to-heel) length of infants and toddlers is measured because 1) they cannot stand erect unassisted, and 2) the normal

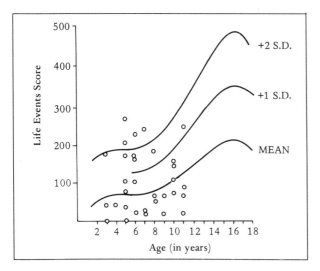

FIGURE 22-11. Healthy Children's Life Event Scores (Norms). (*Note.* From Heisel, J.S., et al. [1973]. The significance of life events as contributing factors in the diseases of children. *Journal of Pediatrics, 83,* 122.)

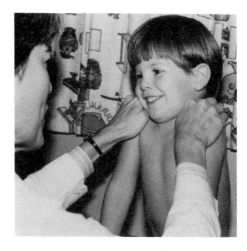

FIGURE 22-12. Approaching the child at eye level during the clinical appraisal helps foster trust and hold the child's attention.

flexion of the spine cannot be fully extended in a standing position. The infant or child should be placed in a supine position, with the head against a stationary board. The child's legs should be fully extended (with the examiner's hands placed over the child's knees to hold them straight) and the heel point marked. The child's heels should be pressed against the surface with the toes pointing toward the ceiling. The distance between crown and heel points then is measured and plotted on a standard growth chart appropriate to the child's gender (see Figures 21-18 and 21-19 in chap. 21).

Standing height is measured once the child reaches 3 years of age. The child is measured without shoes or socks and is directed to stand "as tall as possible" against a wall, pressing the shoulders, buttocks, and heels to the wall. Having the child stand against a wall instead of using a standard measuring scale is preferable because young children tend to stand more erect with wall support. The child may need assistance in holding the knees straight. A bar or ruler should be placed on the crown of the child's head perpendicular to the wall; the distance from crown to floor then is measured and plotted on a standard growth chart for the child's gender (see Figures 22-15 and 22-16). Also, the child's weight-for-stature is plotted to determine the relationship between the child's weight and height (see Figures 22-17 and 22-18).

Weight

Infants and young children should be weighed either sitting or lying on infant scales. Children older than 3 can be weighed on a standing platform scale. In each case, the scale should be balanced at zero before the child is weighed. Infants are weighed nude. Children should be weighed in their underwear (Figure 22-19). For consistency of measurement, it is important to use the same scale and measurement technique each time. An infant's weight should be recorded to the nearest 1/2 ounce (10 gm), while a child's weight should be recorded to the nearest 1/4 pound (100 gm). Findings are plotted on a standard growth chart (see Figures 22-15 and 22-16).

Interpretation of Growth Measurements

Certain principles should be kept in mind when interpreting growth measurements of children. In general, a child whose height (length) and weight fall between the 10th and 90th percentiles is likely to be growing normally. More important than any single measurement in evaluating a child's growth, however, is the overall *pattern* of growth. A series of measurements over time (longitudinal) are of greater value than a single (cross-sectional) measurement. Children should show a consistent progression in height and weight, often referred to as "following the growth curve." A child who "falls off the growth curve"—for example, one whose height (length) and weight have been at the 50th percentile and whose weight drops to the 25th percentile on a subsequent visit—should be evaluated more thoroughly to determine what may be contributing to the change. Also, children whose height (length) or weight falls below the 10th percentile or above the 90th percentile should be evaluated regularly.

The relationship between the child's weight and length (and head circumference in infants and

TABLE 22-20
Child Health History

Client Profile:
Child's name
Birthdate; current age
Gender
Race; ethnic/cultural group
Religious/spiritual affiliation
Grade/level in school; early childhood education experiences
Reason for health contact
Source(s) of information; reliability

Sociocultural History:
Family
Family members; birth order; significant others
Child's role(s) in family; interactions with parents and siblings
Child's responsibilities within family household
Child's participation in family decision-making
Family strengths; family coping
Family stressors/crises

Cultural
Health/illness beliefs
Value orientation (present/future)
Health-related customs: dietary practices/restrictions; treatment of illnesses (home, folk, traditional)
Religious affiliation, education, and practices
Child's understanding of family's cultural, spiritual, and religious beliefs and practices; family's responses to child's questioning of beliefs and practices

Environmental
Allergies—food, medication, other
Exposure to pollution hazards (air, water, noise)
Sensory stimulation in home, day care/school environments
Immunization history; childhood or recent illnesses/injuries; usual pattern of health care; use of medications (type, dose, frequency); experimentation with coffee, tea, alcohol, tobacco, drugs
Socioeconomic: family's employment and economic status; child—allowance, experiences with handling money; child–peer relationships; home environment—living space, study space, play space
Safety: actual or potential safety hazards in home, day care/school, neighborhood environments; child/parent knowledge of potential hazards and accident prevention; safety practices (e.g., use of auto restraints; others appropriate to child's age)

Developmental History:
Prenatal, perinatal, postnatal history (see chap. 10).
Achievement of developmental milestones (motor, language–cognition, personal–social)
Parents' perceptions of child's developmental progress; concerns

Psychosocial History:
Intrapersonal/Interpersonal
Body awareness; body image development and concerns; alterations in body image (recent, chronic)
Self-esteem (perception of self-worth)
Cognition: level of cognitive development, school achievement
Temperament: activity level, rhythmicity (regularity), adaptability, response to new situations (approach, withdrawal, variable), intensity of response (intense, mild, variable), level of sensory threshold (high, medium, low), mood (positive, negative), distractibility, persistence and attention span
Verbal and nonverbal communication; language development; speech articulation
Social interaction patterns; ability to get along with others
Stressors (life changes); responses to stress; coping strategies

Sexuality
Gender identity; onset of puberty
Sexual knowledge/education: sources of information, child's or parent's questions or concerns; parents' responses to child's sexual curiosity
Sexual activity: masturbation, exploration (occurrence, frequency, parents' responses); sexual abuse (occurrence, type, how managed)

TABLE 22-20 (Continued)

Physiological History:

Physical Integrity

Daily hygiene: bathing, hair and nail care, use of soaps, lotions; availability of bath facilities; child's self-care (bathing, grooming)

Growth patterns: recent weight loss or gain; increases in height; child or parent concerns

Skin: color changes, rashes or lesions; excessive dryness or oiliness; pruritus

Sensory–Neurological

Senses: problems with vision, hearing, taste/smell, touch; use of corrective aids

Neurological status: alertness, orientation (appropriate to age), coordination & balance, muscle tone; reflexes; any problems (seizures, weakness)

Pain—type, location, duration, intensity, associated factors; child's responses to pain, how managed

Activity–Sleep

Sleep patterns: number of hours, naps, bedtime rituals, use of attachment objects, sleep environment (where and with whom child sleeps; use of blankets, pillows), child's responses (avoidance behaviors, fears, nightmares, night terrors, somniloquy, somnambulism)—how managed; parent concerns about child's sleep

Play activities and interests; special abilities (creative, athletic)

Physical activity and fitness: muscle strength and endurance; problems with mobility (gait, posture, range of motion, movement); physical disability; use of assistive devices (crutches, braces, wheelchair, etc.)

Oxygenation

Exercise tolerance; ability to keep up with peers

Interferences with breathing, circulation; how managed

Nutrition

Dietary intake (24-hour recall or daily food record)—food types and amounts; use of vitamin and mineral supplements; food likes and dislikes; special dietary needs (special formula, food allergies, iron-rich foods, etc.)

Self-feeding practices: finger feeding, use of utensils, ability to drink from cup; food preparation activities

Teeth: number (primary, permanent), tooth eruption and shedding (sequence, age), teething discomfort; dental hygiene practices (including self-care abilities); visits to dentist; fluoridated water or use of fluoride supplements; orthodontic appliances

Fluid/Electrolytes and Elimination

Usual daily fluid intake and output; voiding and bowel patterns; constipation or diarrhea (frequency, how managed); regurgitation or vomiting (amount, color, consistency, frequency, associated factors); fluid or electrolyte imbalances (history of occurrence, how managed)

Diaper use: type, frequency, diaper rash—how managed

Toilet-training: parents' expectations; age initiated, method(s) used; ages at which bowel, daytime bladder, and nighttime bladder control achieved; enuresis or encopresis—frequency, how managed

---

young children) is significant. One study found that the weight and height of 72% of young Indochinese refugee children fell below the 10th percentile for their age on standardized American growth charts. Yet, when the children's weights-for-stature were compared, their growth was found to be within normal limits (Pickwell, 1982).

Growth measurements, therefore, must be considered in the context of all other available data, such as hereditary factors, the child's parents' growth patterns, the child's previous growth pattern, nutritional intake, and general health. Children who require specific attention to their physical growth include those:

1. Whose height (length) and weight percentiles show great disparity, such as a child whose weight is at the 5th percentile, but whose height is at the 50th percentile;

2. Who do not exhibit expected increases in height (length) and weight, especially during infancy and adolescence, when growth occurs rapidly;

3. Whose height (length) or weight suddenly increases (except during puberty) or decreases dramatically (Whaley & Wong, 1991).

Measuring Vital Signs

Generally, the same techniques used for adults are used for measuring vital signs in children. However, certain modifications may be necessary to ensure the child's cooperation and accuracy (Figure 22-20). Generally, it is best to obtain vital sign measurements in children in the following order:

1. Count respirations before disturbing the child.

TABLE 22-21
Clinical Appraisal Outline—Infants and Children

General Appearance

Physical Growth
  Height (length)*
  Weight*
  Head circumference (up to age 3) (see Chap. 21)
  Skinfold thickness (see Chap. 18)

Vital Signs
  Respiration*
  Pulse*
  Blood pressure*
  Temperature*

Skin Integrity (see Chap. 14)
  Color
  Turgor
  Texture, thickness, moisture
  Integrity
  Hair and nails
  Lymphatic system

Sensory–Perceptual Status
  Vision screening*
  Hearing screening*
  Speech/language screening*
  Smell/taste (see Chap. 15)
  Touch/proprioception (see Chap. 15)

Neurological Status
  Motor activities (see Chap. 10)
  Coordination/muscle tone (see Chap. 15)
  Level of consciousness*
  Increased intracranial pressure*
  Reflexes (see Chap. 15)

Pain Responses*

Activity
  Posture, gait (see Chap. 16)
  Musculoskeletal alignment*
  Range of motion (see Chap. 16)
  Physical fitness/endurance (see Chap. 16)

Oxygenation (see Chap. 17)
  Chest and lungs
  Heart
  Peripheral vascular system

Fluid Balance*

Elimination (see Chap. 19)
  Abdomen
  Urine, stool

Genitalia (see Chap. 13)

*Variations with infants and children reviewed in this chapter.

2. Obtain apical or radial pulse rate.
3. Measure blood pressure.
4. Measure temperature.

It is especially important to measure body temperature last if it must be taken rectally. If the child is active or crying during measurement of vital signs, it should be noted when the findings are recorded.

Measuring Respiration and Pulse

Respiration is assessed in the same way as for adults, although infants' respiration must be assessed by observing the rise and fall of the abdomen since infants are diaphragmatic breathers. Respirations should be counted for one full minute in infants and young children because of the irregularity of breathing at these ages. Findings should be compared with age norms (see Table 22-5).

An apical pulse should be measured in children younger than 3. As with respiration, the pulse should be counted for one full minute because sinus arrhythmia is common. A radial pulse may be obtained from children older than 3. Also, during early childhood, the child's radial and femoral pulses should be compared to rule out the possibility of coarctation of the aorta. The child's pulse rate

should be compared with norms (see Table 22-4), taking into account the child's behavior at the time the measurement is obtained.

Measuring Blood Pressure

Blood pressure should be measured routinely in children older than 3 and in younger children who have a family history of hypertension. Smith (1989) cautions that accurate and reliable measurement of blood pressure is one important index for determining cardiovascular risk in children. Accurate cuff size is essential. A cuff that is too small can give a falsely high reading. Cuff size should be approximately two-thirds the length of the upper arm or thigh to ensure an accurate reading, although in infants and young children the cuff may be slightly longer. The cuff bladder should completely encircle the extremity.

In older children, blood pressure can be measured with a mercury sphygmomanometer or aneroid manometer and auscultation (see chap. 14). The first Korotkoff sound is recorded as the systolic blood pressure, whereas the diastolic blood pressure in children is recorded as the fourth Korotkoff sound (muffling), believed to be a more reliable in-

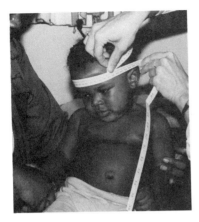

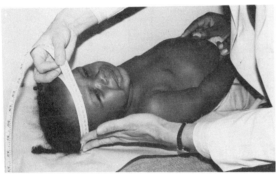

FIGURE 22-13. Measurement of head circumference is an important indicator of physical growth in children younger than 3. The frontal-occipital circumference should be measured with a paper tape and plotted on a standard growth chart.

dicator in children than the fifth sound (Smith, 1989).

In infants and very young children, it is sometimes not possible to obtain a blood pressure reading using auscultation. Instead, systolic blood pressure can be obtained by palpation. The cuff is inflated, and the brachial or radial arterial pulse is palpated. The pressure reading at which the pulse returns is recorded as the systolic blood pressure.

In early childhood, upper arm and thigh pressures should be measured and compared. Normally, a child's systolic blood pressure in the thigh is 10 mm Hg higher than in the upper arm. If the thigh pressure is lower, coarctation of the aorta should be suspected. Age norms (averages and ranges) for systolic and diastolic blood pressures may be found in Table 22-6.

Measuring Temperature

Generally, children cannot understand or fully cooperate with oral temperature measurements until the age of 5 or 6. However, certain electronic oral thermometers can be used with children because the child is not required to close the mouth completely and the plastic thermometer sheath is un-

breakable. These thermometers also can be used to measure axillary temperatures within seconds. Rectal temperatures should be taken only when oral and axillary methods cannot be used because of the intrusiveness of the procedure and the danger of perforating delicate rectal tissues. When a rectal temperature is indicated, the thermometer should be lubricated well and inserted to a maximum of 1 inch. Infants may be positioned on their backs with the legs flexed on the abdomen and the ankles held by the examiner. Children lie on their sides or in a prone position, with a hand placed on their waist or buttocks to remind them to be still.

Martyn, Urbano, Hayes, von Windeguth, and Sherrin (1988) compared rectal and axillary temperatures in preschool children with those obtained by a fever-detector strip (Clinitemp II), a heat sensitive method commonly referred to as a "forehead thermometer." The strip is designed to measure internal core temperature elevations. A reusable, inexpensive, plastic strip is pressed on the child's forehead and left in place for 1 to 2 minutes. Color changes are compared with a corresponding temperature guide. The investigators found that the fever-detector strip correlated positively with the rectal method and was more reliable than the axillary method.

The technique for measuring oral and axillary temperatures in children is the same as for adults, although children often need to be reminded to keep their mouths closed or assisted in holding their arms against their sides. Temperature findings should be recorded in the child's health record and interpreted according to age-appropriate norms (see Table 22-3).

Sensory Assessment

Periodic evaluation for sensory impairment is an important component of child health assessment. Techniques for assessing vision and hearing in the infant and child vary according to developmental level.

Reliability of screening findings depends largely on the degree to which the child is capable of understanding and cooperating with instructions. Generally, children have difficulty complying with vision and hearing screening procedures until the age of 4 or 5 (Sullivan, 1988). However, screening measures that do not require the child's cooperation can be employed with younger children or those who are mentally disabled.

Appraisal of Vision

Gortmaker and Sappenfield (1984) estimate that 20 to 35% of children experience some degree of vis-

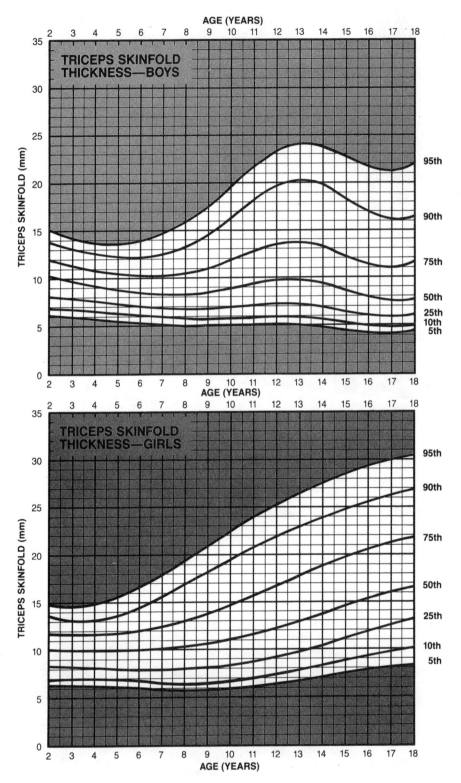

FIGURE 22-14. Triceps Skinfold Thickness in Childhood. (*Note.* Modified from Johnson, C.L. et al. [1981]. *Basic data on anthropometric measurements and angular measurements of the hip and knee joints for selected age groups, 1–74 years of age, United States, 1972–1975.* Vital and Health Statistics Series 11, No. 219. DHHS Publications No. [PHS] 81–1669. Provided as a service of Ross Laboratories, Copyright 1983, Columbus, Ohio 43216. May be copied for individual patient use.)

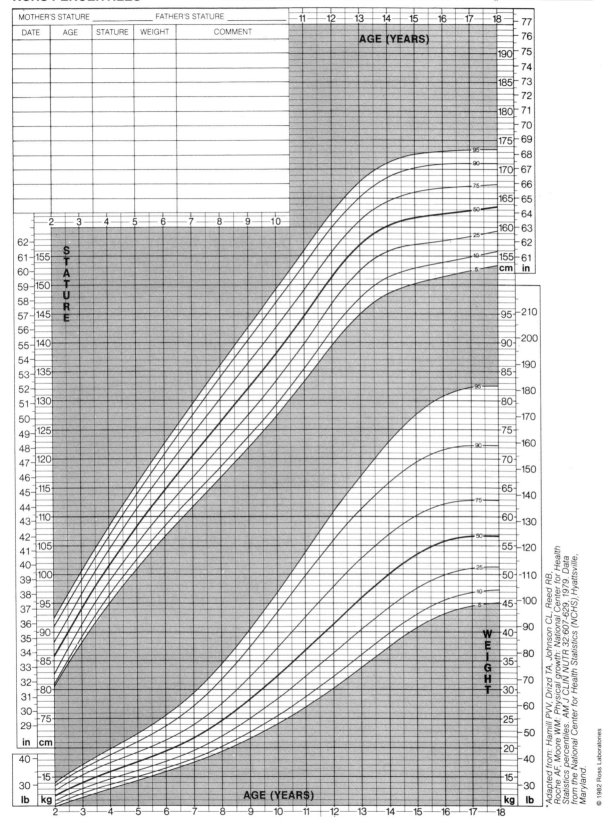

FIGURE 22-15. Girls: 2 to 18 years Physical Growth NCHS Percentiles. (*Note.* Adapted from Hamill, P.V.V., Drizd, T.A., Johnson, C.L., Reed, R.B., Roches, A.F., & Moore, W.M. Physical growth: National Center for Health Statistics percentiles. *American Journal of Clinical Nutrition* 32:607–629, 1979. Data from the National Center for Health Statistics [NCHS], Hyattsville, Maryland. © 1982 Ross Laboratories.)

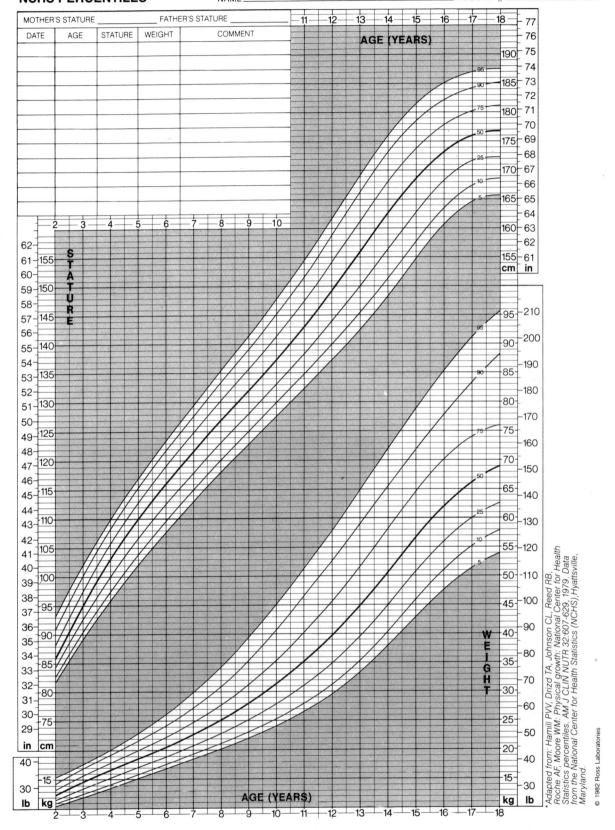

BOYS: 2 TO 18 YEARS
PHYSICAL GROWTH
NCHS PERCENTILES*

NAME _____ RECORD # _____

FIGURE 22-16. Boys: 2 to 18 Years Physical Growth NCHS Percentiles. (*Note.* Adapted from Hamill, P.V.V., Drizd, T.A., Johnson, C.L., Reed, R.B., Roches, A.F., & Moore, W.M. Physical growth: National Center for Health Statistics percentiles. *American Journal of Clinical Nutrition* 32:607–629, 1979. Data from the National Center for Health Statistics [NCHS], Hyattsville, Maryland. © 1982 Ross Laboratories.)

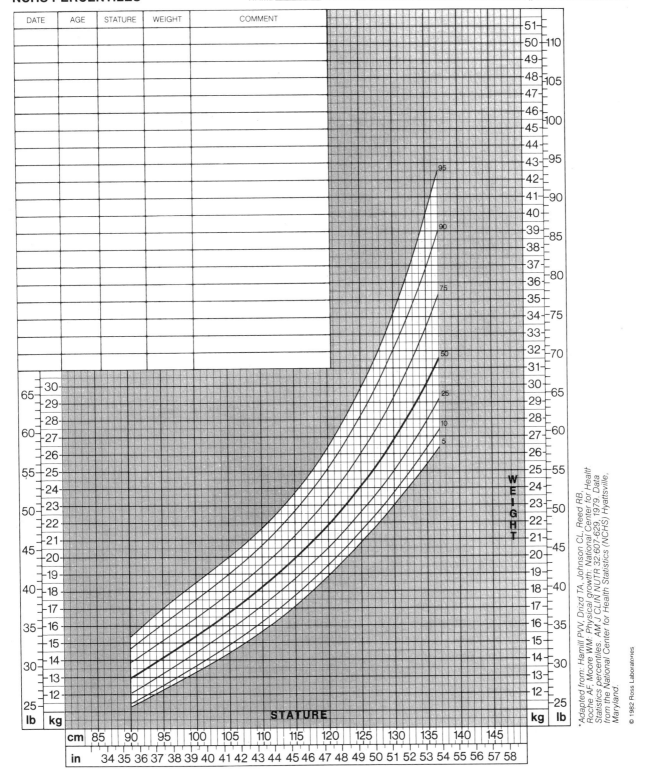

FIGURE 22-17. Girls: Prepubescent Physical Growth NCHS Percentiles. (*Note.* Adapted from Hamill, P.V.V., Drizd, T.A., Johnson, C.L., Reed, R.B., Roches, A.F., & Moore, W.M. Physical growth: National Center for Health Statistics percentiles. *American Journal of Clinical Nutrition* 32:607–629, 1979. Data from the National Center for Health Statistics [NCHS], Hyattsville, Maryland. © 1982 Ross Laboratories.)

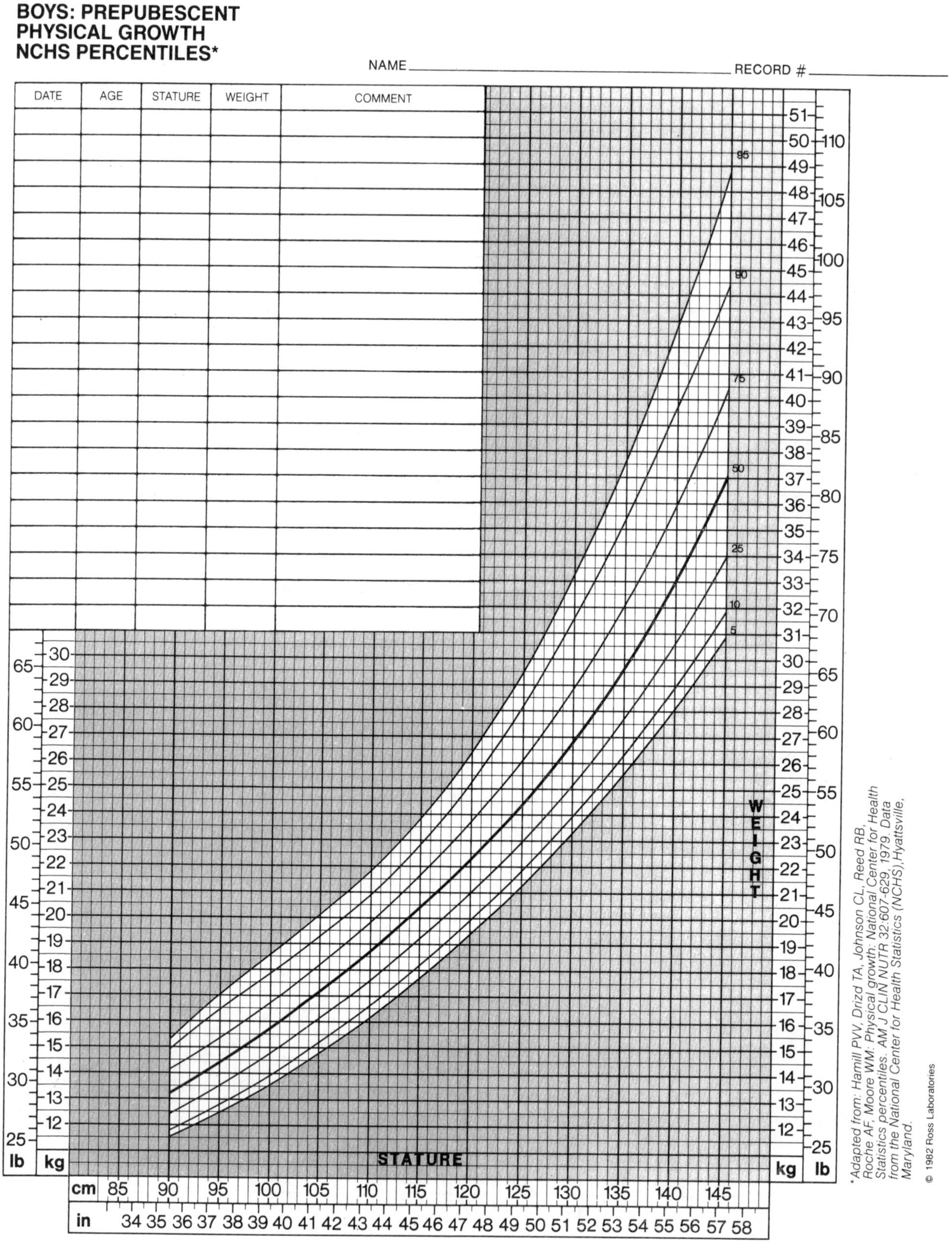

BOYS: PREPUBESCENT
PHYSICAL GROWTH
NCHS PERCENTILES*

FIGURE 22-18. Boys: Prepubescent Physical Growth NCHS Percentiles. (*Note.* Adapted from Hamill, P.V.V., Drizd, T.A., Johnson, C.L., Reed, R.B., Roches, A.F., & Moore, W.M. Physical growth: National Center for Health Statistics percentiles. *American Journal of Clinical Nutrition* 32:607–629, 1979. Data from the National Center for Health Statistics [NCHS], Hyattsville, Maryland. © 1982 Ross Laboratories.)

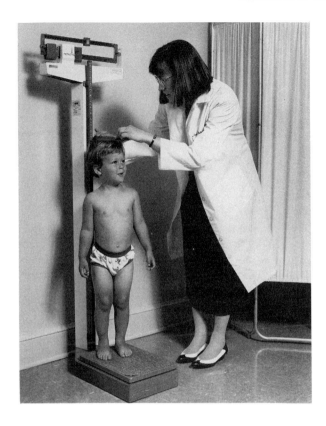

FIGURE 22-19. Young children can be weighed and measured in their underwear on a standing platform scale.

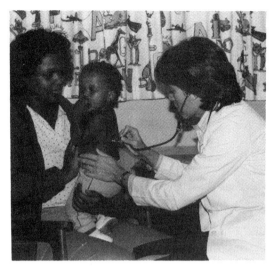

FIGURE 22-20. The infant's heart and lungs should be auscultated with the infant held quietly on the mother's lap.

ual impairment requiring corrective lenses. Early detection of visual impairment is essential for normal growth and development during childhood. Certain behaviors may indicate a problem with visual acuity or other vision problems, such as strabismus (abnormal alignment of the eyes) or congenital blindness. Visual acuity disturbances may be detected first by a child's parent or teacher when the child

- rubs the eyes excessively;
- sits close to a television or video game screen;
- holds books close to the eyes;
- holds the head close to paper when writing or coloring;
- bumps into objects;
- complains of inability to see objects clearly, or
- has difficulty with school work.

Squinting or tilting the head to one side may indicate strabismus or amblyopia (lazy eye). Children with visual impairment also may complain of headache, dizziness, or light sensitivity.

The techniques for screening vision in infants

and children vary according to the child's age. Table 22-22 summarizes techniques for evaluating visual ability (acuity, eye muscle balance, color vision) in children of different ages.

Clinical screening of vision in infants is difficult, although assessing the infant's pupil response to light, corneal light reflex, and ability to follow a light or brightly colored object provide a general measure of visual ability. The Denver Eye Screening Test (DEST) may be used with older infants and preschool children (see Figure 22-21). The DEST includes tests for visual acuity and strabismus. Infants as young as 6 months can be screened with the DEST. Parents are questioned about bilateral eye movement, although squinting is scored only if noted by the examiner. A cover–uncover test and pupillary light reflex test are performed as well (see chap. 15 for a description of these tests). Children aged 3 or older also are screened for visual acuity using the Snellen E chart (see Figure 22-22). Picture cards may be used for children $2^{1}/_{2}$ to $2^{11}/_{12}$ years or for those who cannot respond appropriately to the E.

When screening children for visual impairment, certain measures help ensure accuracy of test findings. Before beginning, the child should be observed for behavior that indicates the child might have difficulty cooperating. Patience, limiting the number of distractions, and incorporating techniques to hold the child's interest are necessary. Placing footprints on the floor for the child to stand on or a brightly marked line for the child to align the toes with can be useful. The child should be familiarized with what is to be done and what responses are expected. Symbols should be ex-

TABLE 22-22
Vision Screening Techniques for Infants and Children

Technique/Tool	Purpose	Age Group/Comments
Following an object	Visual acuity	Infants; refer if infant fails to follow object 180° 2 of 3 tries
STYCAR Chart (9 letters—H,C,O,L,U,T,X,V,A). Child has cards with same letters. Child instructed to point to letter on card that matches one on chart.	Visual acuity	Preschoolers
Allen Cards—series of cards with black and white pictures of familiar objects.	Visual acuity	Preschoolers. Refer if child has visual acuity difference between the right and left eye of 5 feet or more.
Snellen E chart*—Letter Es pointing in four directions; 8 lines of decreasing size	Visual acuity	Preschoolers; older children who are illiterate (see Table 22-23 for referral criteria)
Snellen alphabet chart*—various letters; 8 lines of decreasing size	Visual acuity	School-age children (see Table 22-23 for referral criteria)
Pupillary (corneal) light reflex test	To detect strabismus	Infants through school-age children; refer if results are abnormal
Cover–uncover test	To detect strabismus	Infants through school-age children; refer if results are abnormal
Ishihara plates	To detect color deficiency	School-age children; refer if results are abnormal

*May be tested with Titmus Vision Tester.

plained and the child given several trials to learn how to respond. The nurse should reassure the child that "all the answers are the right ones." During the test, the child should be observed for squinting, eye straining, or obvious distraction. Children who wear eyeglasses should be tested with and without them.

Several tips can help assure the child's cooperation with testing and thus increase reliability of the findings:

■ When screening groups of children, test each child individually, without other children present;

■ Have the child use a paper cup to occlude the eye that is not being tested (minimizes squinting of the test eye);

■ Begin the test with an easy-to-read line, so the child experiences some success, before moving on to more difficult lines.

Sometimes it is helpful to use two examiners—one to point to the letters or symbols while the other helps the child stand in place and cover one eye correctly.

Testing Distant Visual Acuity. The Snellen E (see Figure 22-22) chart can be used easily with children from preschool through age 6 or until the child is familiar with the alphabet. The nurse should de-

scribe the lines of the E as the legs of a table and ask the child to point in the same direction the table legs are pointing. Concrete terms such as "ceiling," "floor," "window," or "door" may be used to denote direction, instead of such abstract terms as "up," "down," "left," or "right." For some children, it is useful to provide a card with a large E. The child then can be asked to match directions of the legs of the E on the card with the E on the chart. Older children can be screened with the Snellen alphabet chart (see chap. 15).

At a distance of 20 feet, 3- and 4-year-old children should be exposed to individual letters, whereas 5- and 6-year-olds should be exposed to the entire line of letters and asked to respond. Each eye is tested separately and then both eyes are tested together.

Before the age of 6, visual acuity less than 20/20 is not considered abnormal. Children whose results are not within the expected range, however, should be rescreened within two weeks. If the results are still abnormal, the child should be referred for further evaluation. Referral guidelines are provided in Table 22-23.

The *Titmus vision tester* is a machine that projects letters of the alphabet or Es onto a screen. The child is asked to identify the symbols or letters. The advantages of this method include decreasing the likelihood of the child being distracted

Vision Tests	1ST SCREENING: Date Right Eye			Left Eye			RESCREENING: Date Right Eye			Left Eye			DENVER EYE SCREENING TEST
	Normal	Abnormal	Untestable	Normal	Abnormal	Untestable	Normal	Abnormal	Untestable	Normal	Abnormal	Untestable	
1. "E" (3 years and above - 3 to 5 trials).....	3P	3F	U	3P	3F	U	3P	3F	U	3P	3F	U	
2. Picture Card (2 1/2 - 2 11/12 years) (3 - 5 trials).......	3P	3F	U	3P	3F	U	3P	3F	U	3P	3F	U	
3. Fixation (6 mos.- 2 5/12 years).......	P	F	U	P	F	U	P	F	U	P	F	U	
4. Squinting		yes			yes			yes			yes		

Tests for Non-Straight Eyes	Normal	Abnormal	Untestable	Normal	Abnormal	Untestable	Name: Hospital No. Ward: Address:
1. Do your child's eyes turn in or out, or are they ever not straight?..............	No	Yes	U	No	Yes	U	
2. Cover Test	P	F	U	P	F	U	
3. Pupillary Light Reflex	P	F	U	P	F	U	

Total Test Rating (Both Eyes)		
Normal (passed vision test plus no squint, plus passed 2/3 tests for non-straight eyes)	Normal	Normal
Abnormal (abnormal on any vision test, squinting, or 2 of 3 procedures for non-straight eyes)	Abnormal	Abnormal
Untestable (untestable on any vision test or untestable on 2/3 tests for non-straight eyes)	Untestable	Untestable
Future Rescreening Appointment for Total Test Rating (Abnormal or Untestable)	Date:	Date:

FIGURE 22-21. Denver Eye Screening Test (DEST). (*Note.* From Frankenburg, W.K., University of Colorado Medical Center, Denver, CO. Reprinted with permission.)

and preventing the child from memorizing the chart in advance. This method also requires less space for conducting vision screening.

Picture cards, such as the *Allen cards*, sometimes are used with preschool children who are at least 2 years of age. The Allen cards are a series of familiar black and white pictures (birthday cake, car, horse and rider, house, teddy bear, telephone, and tree) that the child must identify. The examiner holds one card at a distance of 20 feet and walks slowly toward the child until the child identifies the picture. The distance at which the child correctly identifies a majority of the pictures is recorded as the numerator, with the denominator a constant 30. This method requires the child to be familiar with and able to remember and name each picture. Children who fail to identify a majority of pictures at a distance of 20 feet, or those who exhibit a difference between eyes of 5 feet or more, should be referred.

Another test of visual acuity that can be used easily with preschool children and mentally dis-

abled people is the STYCAR (Screening Test for Young Children and Retardates). The client is given cards with the letters H, C, O, L, U, T, X, V, and A, letters that they can recognize easily. The examiner points to one of the letters on a chart posted 20 feet away. The client must find the identical letter on one of the cards or name the letter.

Testing for Strabismus. Children with uncorrected strabismus may develop amblyopia and diminished visual acuity in the weaker eye. A two line or more difference between eyes on visual acuity testing is one means of screening for strabismus. The cover–uncover test is another method for detecting strabismus. The child is instructed to focus on a stationary object, and one eye is covered with a card. The uncovered eye should be observed for movement or inability to continue to focus. The card then is removed and the previously covered eye is observed for deviation from its focus on the object. The entire procedure is repeated for the other eye. No movement should be noted in either

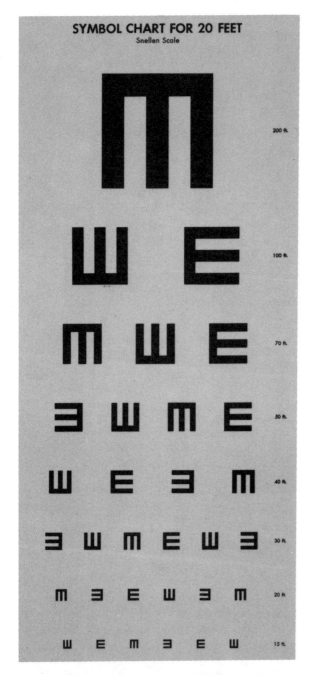

SYMBOL CHART FOR 20 FEET
Snellen Scale

FIGURE 22-22. Snellen E Chart. (*Note.* Provided courtesy of the National Society to Prevent Blindness, Inc., Schaumburg, IL.)

eye, covered or uncovered. Any deviation of the eye requires referral.

Testing for Color Vision. A test for color discrimination should be administered to all children at least once during the school-age years. The most accurate results seem to be obtained about sixth or seventh grade (National Society to Prevent Blindness, 1982). Color vision is a sex-linked recessive

TABLE 22-23
Visual Acuity Referral Criteria by Age

Age	Referral Criteria
3 years	20/50 or worse in one or both eyes
4–6 years	20/40 or worse in one or both eyes
Over 6 years	20/30 or worse in one or both eyes

Note. Any child with a difference of two lines or more between eyes should be referred: for example, a 5-year-old with 20/20 vision in the left eye and 20/40 vision in the right eye.

trait. Abnormalities of color vision occur in approximately 8% of males and 4% of females. Color deficiency is not correctable, but awareness is important because it influences driver and safety education and possibly career choice.

Ishihara plates, or similar pseudoisochromatic plates, can be used to screen color vision in children as young as 4. The plates consist of diagrams composed of colored dots superimposed over a field of dots of a confusion color. People with normal color vision can readily identify the diagrams.

Appraisal of Hearing, Speech, and Language

Significant hearing impairments occur in approximately 1% of all children and range from mild to extreme hearing loss. Behaviors that suggest the possibility of hearing impairment are outlined in Table 22-24. In addition, periodic screening of hearing should be conducted as part of routine child health checks.

Infants and toddlers can be screened for appropriate developmental responses to auditory stimuli. By 6 months of age, infants should be able to orient to and localize sound. Lack of a startle or blink in response to a loud sound, indifference to sound, or failure to respond to human voices may indicate hearing impairment. Language development is linked closely to hearing. Therefore, the infant who does not exhibit age-appropriate language development, such as imitating speech sounds by 6 to 8 months of age, or making talking sounds by 10 to 12 months of age, should be evaluated for hearing impairment.

The infant or toddler may be screened in a quiet room while sitting on the parent's lap. The examiner, out of the child's visual field, should produce sounds at various frequencies and observe the child's responses. A squeaky toy or a bell tests response to high frequency sounds; a rattle or crumpled tissue paper tests response to lower frequency sounds. The older toddler and preschooler should be capable of following directions, answering simple questions, and using purposeful sentences.

TABLE 22-24
Behaviors Suggesting Hearing Impairment

Responses to Auditory Stimuli
Failure to startle or blink in response to a loud sound
Generally inattentive to sound
Unable to localize sound by 6 months of age
Failure to respond to name or commands ("No!") by 9
    months of age
Failure to respond to verbal directions by 18 months of
    age

Vocalization
Few vocalizations during play ("talking," squealing) in
    infancy
Failure to imitate speech sounds by 7 months of age
Use of mostly vowel sounds after 12 months of age
Unintelligible speech after 24 months of age
Omission of initial consonants after age 3
Asks for statements to be repeated or responds incor-
    rectly
Use of gestures or yelling to express needs

Social Characteristics
Increased alertness to gestures and movement of others
Preference for solitary play
Overly reactive to tactile stimulation and physical affec-
    tion
Shy and timid in social situations

The Weber and Rinne tests provide gross measures of hearing ability. These tests can be administered to school-age and older preschool children who can understand the instructions (Figure 22-23). Directions for the Weber and Rinne tests are provided in Chapter 15.

Audiometric testing is a more refined method of testing for hearing loss and can be used with older preschool and school-age children. *Play audiometry* is useful with a child who is 3 or older and, because it is more enjoyable than conventional audiometry, the child is more likely to cooperate. The child is taught to perform a specified activity such as dropping a toy into a box in response to a verbal request or at a tone.

The *Denver Audiometric Screening Test* (DAST) is a 5- to 10-minute screening test with a pure tone audiometer designed for children 3 years of age or older. The test form (Figure 22-24) provides for screenings on three separate occasions.

Conventional, pure tone audiometry may be used with school-age children. With the child wearing earphones, each ear is tested separately at predetermined frequencies and decibels. The child is instructed to raise a hand upon hearing each sound. Pure tone audiometry permits a more precise measurement of the minimal level of hearing at varying frequencies. The *air conduction sweep check method* of audiometric screening is an economical and efficient way to screen for hearing loss in children (DiChiara, 1984). With this method, the child is tested only at 25 decibels (db), but at varying intensities of sound (250 Hz to 8000 Hz). If the child cannot hear two or more frequencies at 25 db in one or both ears, then a more complete *threshold acuity test* should be performed. This test evaluates the child's hearing at various decibels (5 db to 50 db) and frequencies (250 Hz to 8000 Hz). If the child is unable to hear the tone at 25 db or higher in the same ear at two consecutive frequencies, the child should be referred for a complete audiological evaluation.

Speech and language impairments may result from hearing loss, central nervous system dysfunction, emotional problems, or structural defects such as cleft palate. The sequence of normal language development is outlined in Chapter 10, Table 10-7.

Clinical appraisal of children for speech and language impairment focuses predominately on

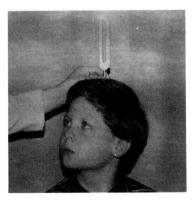 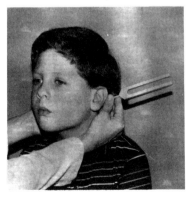 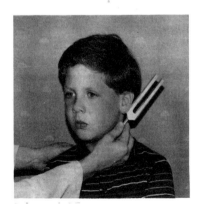

FIGURE 22-23. The Weber and Rinne tests for bone and air conduction can be administered to children who are old enough to understand and comply with instructions. (A) Weber test: Bone conduction. (B) Rinne test: Bone conduction. (C) Rinne test: Air conduction.

```
1ST SCREENING:  Date:                      RESULTS (Circle One):  P   F   U

Puretone Testing    Right Ear    Left Ear    Results
1000 Hz (25 dB)     P  F  U      P  F  U      Pass--Both ears, 3 correct responses, all frequencies.
2000 Hz (25 dB)     P  F  U      P  F  U      Fail--3 fails, any frequency.
4000 Hz (25 dB)     P  F  U      P  F  U      Uncertain--Test not completed or not sure of child's
                                                        responses
Comments:



2ND SCREENING:  Date:                      RESULTS (Circle One):  P   F   U

Puretone Testing    Right Ear    Left Ear    Results
1000 Hz (25 dB)     P  F  U      P  F  U      Pass--Both ears, 3 correct responses, all frequencies.
2000 Hz (25 dB)     P  F  U      P  F  U      Fail--3 fails, any frequency.
4000 Hz (25 dB)     P  F  U      P  F  U      Uncertain--Test not completed or not sure of child's
                                                        responses.
Comments:



3RD SCREENING:  Date:                      RESULTS (Circle One):  P   F   U

Puretone Testing    Right Ear    Left Ear    Results
1000 Hz (25 dB)     P  F  U      P  F  U      Pass--Both ears, 3 correct responses all frequencies.
2000 Hz (25 dB)     P  F  U      P  F  U      Fail--3 fails, any frequency.
4000 Hz (25 dB)     P  F  U      P  F  U      Uncertain--Test not completed or not sure of child's
                                                        responses.
Comments:
```

DENVER AUDIOMETRIC SCREENING TEST

Name:
Hospital No.:
Ward:
Address:

FIGURE 22-24. Denver Audiometric Screening Test (DAST). (*Note.* From Frankenburg, W.K., University of Colorado Medical Center, Denver, CO. Reprinted with permission.)

observations of behavior. Certain characteristics suggest specific types of disorders and may indicate the need to refer a child for a comprehensive speech and hearing evaluation. Language disorders include problems with assigning meaning to words (vocabulary), organizing words into sentences, or altering word forms. Speech disorders include stuttering (dysfluency), articulation deficiency (disarticulation), and voice disorders, such as hypernasality or deviations in pitch. Guidelines for referring children are delineated in Table 22-25.

The *Denver Articulation Screening Examination** (DASE) is a speech screening tool designed to discriminate reliably between significant delays and normal variations in the acquisition of speech sounds in children 2½ to 6 years of age. The DASE consists of 22 words containing 30 underlined consonants that the child is asked to repeat. Line-drawing picture cards that represent each word can be used for shy or hard-to-test children.

The child's raw score is the number of correctly

articulated sounds. The child's age is calculated to the *nearest previous half-year* and matched with the child's raw score to yield a percentile rank. The 15th percentile is the cut-off point for referral.

The child's intelligibility also is scored, using the chart on the back of the form (Figure 22-25). The test results are determined from the guidelines on the form. If the child scores "abnormal," the child should be rescreened in two weeks. If the results are again abnormal, the child should be referred for a comprehensive speech evaluation.

Neurological Assessment

The techniques for assessing a child's neurological functioning are the same as those used for adults and involve primarily observation and testing of pupil response, muscle tone, and reflexes. Observing an infant's or young child's motor activities is a useful way to assess neurological functioning (Figure 22-26). Age-appropriate items from the fine motor-adaptive and gross motor sections of the Denver II Screening Test (see chap. 10) can be administered to screen for potential problems. Other helpful techniques include offering the child a toy to determine the ability to reach and grasp, and in-

---

*Instruction manual, test forms, and picture cards are available from Denver Developmental Materials, Inc., P.O. Box 20037, Denver, CO 80220.

TABLE 22-25
Referral Guidelines for Speech/Language Disorders

Age	Assessment Findings
2 years	Failure to speak any meaningful words spontaneously
	Consistent use of gestures rather than vocalizations
	Difficulty in following verbal directions
	Failure to respond consistently to sound
3 years	Speech is largely unintelligible
	Failure to use sentences of three or more words
	Frequent omission of initial consonants
	Use of vowels rather than consonants
4 years	Frequent omission of final consonants
5 years	Stutters, stammers, or has any other type of dysfluency
	Sentence structure noticeably impaired
	Substitutes easily produced sounds for more difficult ones
	Omits word endings (plurals, tenses of verbs, and so on)
School age	Poor voice quality (monotonous, loud, or barely audible)
	Vocal pitch inappropriate for age
	Any distortions, omissions, or substitutions of sounds after age 7 years
	Connected speech characterized by use of unusual confusions or reversals
General	Any child with signs suggestive of a hearing impairment
	Any child who is embarrassed or disturbed by his speech
	Parents who are excessively concerned or who pressure the child to speak at a level above that appropriate for his age

Note. From Whaley, L.F., & Wong, D.L. (1991). *Nursing care of infants and children* (4th ed.). St. Louis: Mosby-Yearbook, p. 1118.

structing the child to squeeze the nurse's hand "as hard as you can" to determine bilateral muscle strength.

Infants may be evaluated for the presence of primitive reflexes such as Moro (startle), grasp, stepping, and Babinski. Reflexes that persist beyond the age they are expected to disappear (see Table 21-8) may indicate neurological dysfunction. Because the results of reflex tests are not reliable for young children, reflexes generally are not elicited routinely until the child reaches school age.

Assessing level of consciousness in infants and nonverbal children is difficult. Objective data related to an infant's responses to the environment must be relied upon. Changes in age-appropriate behaviors, such as recognizing the parent's face or familiar objects, or inappropriate behaviors such as lethargy, disinterest in eating, or difficulty awakening the infant or child are cause for concern.

For older children, level of consciousness can be evaluated by assessing the child's responses to questions about people, place, and time. Depending upon developmental level, the child may be able to give only a first name or nickname. Children younger than 7 or 8 may have difficulty stating the date, day of week, or month. A young child's response of "in my bed" is an acceptable answer for orientation to place.

A more objective method of assessing level of consciousness in infants and children is the *Pediatric Coma Scale* (Whaley & Wong, 1991). This scale is a modification of the commonly used Glasgow Coma Scale (GCS), developed to assess the degree of altered consciousness in adults. The Pediatric Coma Scale provides a guide for assessing a child's consciousness on three parameters: eyes opening, motor response, and verbal response. The child's parent should assist in eliciting the best responses since fear of an unfamiliar environment may inhibit the child. The child's scores on the three parameters are added. A child who receives a score of 7 or below is considered comatose, with the lowest score (3) indicating deep coma. The Pediatric Coma Scale is depicted in Table 22-26.

One of the most important aspects of assessing neurological functioning in infants and children is assessing for increased intracranial pressure. Common causes of increased intracranial pressure in infants and children include hydrocephalus, head trauma, intracranial tumors, or infections such as meningitis or encephalitis. Because the anterior fontanel does not close until 12 to 18 months of age, infants should be assessed for the following manifestations, any of which may indicate an increase in intracranial pressure:

- increased head circumference (see chap. 21)
- fullness and tension of the anterior fontanel
- irritability
- high-pitched cry
- eating difficulties

Once the cranial sutures have closed, children exhibit the same manifestations of increased intracranial pressure as adults (see chap. 15). Abnormal findings indicate the need for referral for a complete neurological evaluation.

Pain Assessment

Clinical assessment of pain in infants and children focuses predominantly on observation of their be-

DENVER ARTICULATION SCREENING EXAM
for children 2 1/2 to 6 years of age

Instructions: Have child repeat each word after
you. Circle the underlined sounds that he pro-
nounces correctly. Total correct sounds is the
Raw Score. Use charts on reverse side to score
results.

NAME

HOSP. NO.

ADDRESS

Date: _____ Child's Age: _____ Examiner: _____ Raw Score: _____
Percentile: _____ Intelligibility: _____ Result: _____

1. table   6. zipper   11. sock   16. wagon   21. leaf
2. shirt   7. grapes   12. vacuum   17. gum   22. carrot
3. door   8. flag   13. yarn   18. house
4. trunk   9. thumb   14. mother   19. pencil
5. jumping   10. toothbrush 15. twinkle   20. fish

Intelligibility: (circle one)   1. Easy to understand   3. Not understandable
                                 2. Understandable 1/2   4. Can't evaluate
                                    the time.

Comments:

Date: _____ Child's Age: _____ Examiner: _____ Raw Score _____
Percentile: _____ Intelligibility: _____ Result: _____

1. table   6. zipper   11. sock   16. wagon   21. leaf
2. shirt   7. grapes   12. vacuum   17. gum   22. carrot
3. door   8. flag   13. yarn   18. house
4. trunk   9. thumb   14. mother   19. pencil
5. jumping   10. toothbrush 15. twinkle   20. fish

Intelligibility: (circle one)   1. Easy to understand   3. Not understandable
                                 2. Understandable 1/2   4. Can't evaluate
                                    the time.

Comments:

Date: _____ Child's Age: _____ Examiner: _____ Raw Score _____
Percentile: _____ Intelligibility: _____ Result: _____

1. table   6. zipper   11. sock   16. wagon   21. leaf
2. shirt   7. grapes   12. vacuum   17. gum   22. carrot
3. door   8. flag   13. yarn   18. house
4. trunk   9. thumb   14. mother   19. pencil
5. jumping   10. toothbrush 15. twinkle   20. fish

Intelligibility: (circle one)   1. Easy to understand   3. Not understandable
                                 2. Understandable 1/2   4. Can't evaluate
                                    the time.

Comments:

FIGURE 22-25. Denver Articulation Screening Exam (DASE). (*Note.* Reprinted with permission, W.K. Frankenburg, University of Colorado Medical Center, Denver, 1971. Copyright 1971, Amelia F. Drumwright.)

To score DASE words: Note Raw Score for child's performance. Match raw score line (extreme left of chart) with column representing child's age (to the closest previous age group). Where raw score line and age column meet number in that square denotes percentile rank of child's performance when compared to other children that age. Percentiles above heavy line are ABNORMAL percentiles, below heavy line are NORMAL.

PERCENTILE RANK

Raw Score	2.5 yr.	3.0	3.5	4.0	4.5	5.0	5.5	6 years
2	1							
3	2							
4	5							
5	9							
6	16							
7	23							
8	31	2						
9	37	4	1					
10	42	6	2					
11	48	7	4					
12	54	9	6	1	1			
13	58	12	9	2	3	1	1	
14	62	17	11	5	4	2	2	
15	68	23	15	9	5	3	2	
16	75	31	19	12	5	4	3	
17	79	38	25	15	6	6	4	
18	83	46	31	19	8	7	4	
19	86	51	38	24	10	9	5	1
20	89	58	45	30	12	11	7	3
21	92	65	52	36	15	15	9	4
22	94	72	58	43	18	19	12	5
23	96	77	63	50	22	24	15	7
24	97	82	70	58	29	29	20	15
25	99	87	78	66	36	34	26	17
26	99	91	84	75	46	43	34	24
27		94	89	82	57	54	44	34
28		96	94	88	70	68	59	47
29		98	98	94	84	84	77	68
30		100	100	100	100	100	100	100

To Score intelligibility:

	NORMAL	ABNORMAL
2 1/2 years	Understandable 1/2 the time, or, "easy"	Not Understandable
3 years and older	Easy to understand	Understandable 1/2 time Not understandable

Test Result: 1. NORMAL on Dase and Intelligibility = NORMAL

2. ABNORMAL on Dase and/or Intelligibility = ABNORMAL

* If abnormal on initial screening rescreen within 2 weeks. If abnormal again child should be referred for complete speech evaluation.

FIGURE 22-25 Continued.

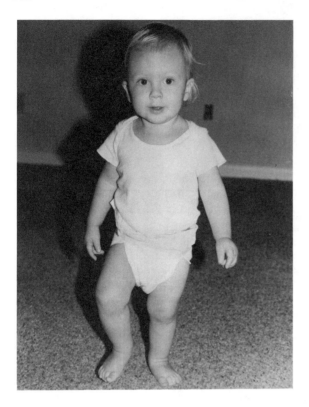

FIGURE 22-26. Observing a young child's posture, gait, coordination, and motor abilities is a useful way to assess neurological and musculoskeletal functioning.

havior (McGrath, 1989). Typical responses are outlined by age in Table 22-9. Knowledge of the child's usual responses to painful sensations provides a helpful basis for comparison. Hester and Barcus (1986) have developed a questionnaire for assessing children's pain experience (see Table 22-27). Children older than 3 or 4 usually can respond to the items.

Several pain rating scales have been developed for use with children (Ellis, 1988; Wong & Baker, 1988). These scales run from no pain to severe pain, using words, pictures, or other symbols a child can understand. Pain scales provide a simple way for children to describe their pain to others and for establishing the existence of a child's pain (Ellis, 1988). Commonly used pain scales include:

- A *simple descriptive scale* in which the child is asked to use adjectives to indicate the intensity of pain,

- A *numeric scale* in which the child is asked to rate the pain on a scale from 0 (no pain) to 10 (worst pain),

- A *faces scale*, which asks the child to choose one of six faces ranging from happy to crying to indicate the degree of pain,

- A *glasses scale*, depicting six glasses (empty =

TABLE 22-26
Pediatric Coma Scale*

	Score	Over 1 year	Less than 1 year	
Eyes opening	4	Spontaneously	Spontaneously	
	3	To verbal command	To shout	
	2	To pain	To pain	
	1	No response	No response	
		Over 1 year	**Less than 1 year**	
Best motor response	6	Obeys		
	5	Localizes pain	Localizes pain	
	4	Flexion withdrawal	Flexion withdrawal	
	3	Flexion—abnormal (decorticate rigidity)	Flexion—abnormal (decorticate rigidity)	
	2	Extension (decerebrate rigidity)	Extension (decerebrate rigidity)	
	1	No response	No response	
		Over 5 years	**2–5 years**	**0–23 months**
Best verbal	5	Oriented and converses	Appropriate words and phrases	Smiles, coos, cries appropriately
	4	Disoriented and converses	Inappropriate words	Cries
	3	Inappropriate words	Cries and/or screams	Inappropriate crying and/or screaming
	2	Incomprehensible sounds	Grunts	Grunts
	1	No response	No response	No response
Total		3–15		

*Modification of Glasgow Coma Scale.

Note. From Wong, D.L., & Whaley, L.F. (1990). *Clinical manual of pediatric nursing* (3rd ed.). St. Louis: Mosby, p. 393.

TABLE 22-27
Pain Experience Inventory

Questions for Parents

Describe any pain your child has had before.

How does your child usually react to pain?

Does your child tell you or others when he is hurting?

How do you know when your child is in pain?

What do you do to ease discomfort for your child when your child is hurting?

What does your child do to get relief when hurting?

Which of these actions work best to decrease or take away your child's pain?

Is there anything special that you would like me to know about your child and pain? (If yes, have parent[s] describe.)

Questions for Child

Tell me what pain is.

Tell me about the hurt you have had before.

What do you do when you hurt?

Do you tell others when you hurt?

What do you want others to do for you when you hurt?

What don't you want others to do for you when you hurt?

What helps the most to take away your hurt?

Is there anything special that you want me to know about you when you hurt? (If yes, have child describe.)

Note. From Hester, N., & Barcus, C. (1986). Assessment and management of pain in children. *Pediatrics: Nursing Update,* *1*(14), Princeton, NJ: Continuing Professional Education Center, Inc., p. 3.

no pain, full = worst pain) from which the child is asked to select the glass that best describes the pain,

■ A *chips scale* in which the child is asked to choose the number of chips equal to the pain (1 = a "little hurt," 5 = the "most hurt"), and

■ A *color scale*, which allows the child to rank six crayons of different colors (black, purple, blue, red, green, orange) and then to choose the color most like the pain the child is experiencing.

Wong and Baker (1988) investigated the validity, reliability, and children's preference for various pain rating scales with 3- to 18-year-old hospitalized children and adolescents. Their findings indicate that the chips scale is most valid for 3- to 12-year-olds, while the glasses scale has the most validity with adolescents. The chips scale was also the most reliable pain rating scale for all ages. Overall, however, children preferred the faces scale for rating their pain. The Faces Pain Scale is depicted in Figure 22-27.

Activity–Sleep Assessment

During early childhood, a child should be assessed periodically for abnormalities of the musculoskeletal system that can lead to impaired physical mobility and delays in motor development. Parents of toddlers may express concern about their children's "flat feet." The longitudinal arches of the feet do not develop until a child has been walking for one to two years. A fat pad under the medial arch gives the appearance of flat feet. Even if the child's longitudinal arches do not develop, however, treatment rarely is indicated unless the child experiences pain. To assess development of the foot arches, the nurse should observe the child's feet while the child is standing or examine an imprint of the child's feet.

Abnormalities in the positioning or shape of the feet and legs often become evident as the child begins to bear weight and walk. The child's lower extremities should be evaluated for alignment.

Instructions	Comments
Explain to child that each face is for a person who feels happy because there is no pain (hurt) or sad because there is some or a lot of pain. Face 0 is very happy because there is no hurt. Face 1 hurts just a little bit. Face 2 hurts a little more. Face 3 hurts even more. Face 4 hurts a whole lot, but Face 5 hurts as much as you can imagine, although you don't have to be crying to feel this bad. Ask child to choose face that best describes how the pain feels.	Can be used with children as young as 3 years.

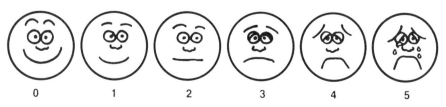

FIGURE 22-27. Faces Pain Rating Scale. (*Note.* From Whaley, L., & Wong, D.: *Nursing Care of Infants and Children,* ed. 4, 1991, p. 1148. Copyrighted by Mosby-Year Book, Inc. Reprinted by permission. The Wong-Baker Faces Pain Scale may be reproduced for clinical and research use, provided the copyright information is retained with the scale.)

When standing, the child's toes and feet should point directly forward. *Pes valgus* (toeing out) or *pes varus* (toeing in) may indicate an abnormality of the bones of the upper or lower leg (see Figure 22-28). Depending on the degree of misalignment and the parents' preferences, the child may need to be referred for a more complete evaluation.

Two other common problems of the legs are *genu varum* and *genu valgum*. *Genu varum* (bowlegs) is a condition in which the medial malleoli are touching and the knees are more than 1 inch apart. Also, the foot is medial to the midpatellar line. Genu varum is a normal finding until the child has been walking for about a year. In *genu valgum* (knock-knees), the foot is lateral to the midpatellar line and the medial malleoli are more than 1 inch apart when the knees are touching. This condition is considered normal in children 2 to 6 years of age. To assess for the presence of bowlegs or knock-knees, the nurse should observe the alignment of the leg between the pelvis and foot. An imaginary line should be drawn from the pelvis to the foot through the center of the patella, and the position of the foot in relation to the line observed to determine the presence of bowlegs or knock-knees (see Figure 22-29).

Toddlers also may exhibit an exaggerated lumbar curve and wide-based stance as they learn to walk and run. These characteristics are normal and may be evident until 30 months of age. Limping may indicate a congenital hip deformity that was missed during infancy (see chap. 21).

The activity–sleep patterns of infants and young children may be categorized according to state, or level of arousal. Two sleep states—quiet sleep and active sleep—and three awake states—quiet awake, active awake, and crying—have been identified (Keefe, Kotzer, Reuss, & Saunder, 1989). Each state is characterized by specific behavioral and physiological patterns. The infant and young child's sleep–wake cycle can be evaluated using certain behavioral criteria. Observation of the infant or young child's behavior while asleep and awake can be useful for validating parents' reports of concern about the child's sleep–activity patterns. Table 22-28 provides criteria that can be used to assess the sleep–wake patterns of infants and young children.

Assessing Fluid Balance

Objective assessment of fluid balance in infants and young children relies on observation of several factors, including body weight, skin color and turgor (Figure 22-30), urine output and specific gravity, and vital signs. The child's general appearance is of utmost importance. A healthy child is alert and active, with elastic skin tone and healthy color.

Infants are particularly susceptible to fluid loss, which can occur rapidly and without warning. If the child's previous weight is unknown, the nurse must rely on clinical signs that indicate loss of body fluid and resulting dehydration, which varies in degree depending on the amount of fluid

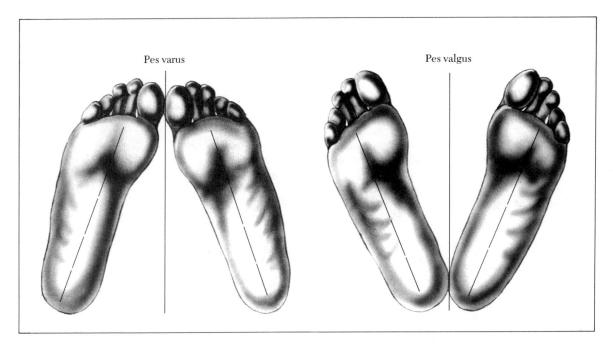

FIGURE 22-28. Pes Varus and Pes Valgus.

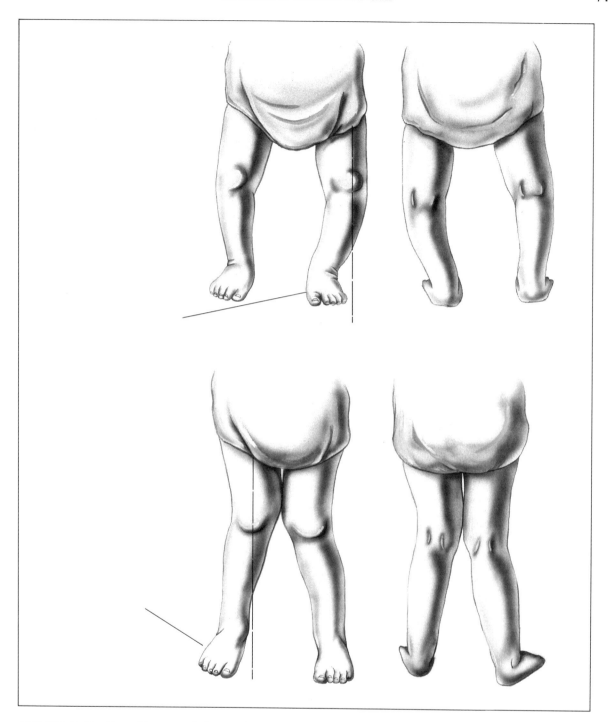

FIGURE 22-29. Genu Varum and Genu Valgum.

lost. Dehydration is most commonly *isotonic*, in which relatively equal proportions of water and sodium are lost. Isotonic dehydration is categorized according to the decrease in body weight: mild (5% weight loss), moderate (5–9% weight loss), and severe (10% or greater weight loss). Infants can progress rapidly from mild to severe dehydration in a matter of hours unless prompt measures are instituted to restore fluid balance.

Early manifestations of dehydration in infants and young children include:

- decreased urine output (dry diaper)
- increased urine specific gravity

TABLE 22-28
Behavioral State (Sleep–Wake) Criteria

State Categories	Behavioral Characteristics
Quiet or non-REM[a] sleep	Regular respiration; eyes closed; no facial movement; no vocalization; no motor activity except an occasional reflex movement (e.g., startle or sobbing inspiration)
Active or REM sleep	Irregular respiration; eyes closed with ocular motility; facial movement; vocalization can occur; peripheral movements
Awake	Irregular respiration; eyes open; facial movements and vocalization can occur; mild or gross motor activity
Transition	Within sleep from quiet to active sleep or vice versa; regular or irregular respirations; body movement; eyes closed; vocalization; no REM
Indeterminate	Infant behavior that does not fit in any of the above categories

[a]REM = rapid eye movement

Note. From Keefe, M.R., Kotzer, A.M., Reuss, J.L., & Sander, L.W. Development of a system for monitoring infant state behavior. Copyright 1989 American Journal of Nursing Company. Reprinted from *Nursing Research*, 1989, *38*, p. 345. Used with permission. All rights reserved.

- dry mucous membranes
- absence of tears
- irritability (indicates thirst)

If dehydration is not treated, additional clinical signs will appear, including:

- poor skin turgor (*tenting*)
- skin pallor progressing to mottling
- oliguria
- rapid, thready pulse
- sunken fontanel and eyeballs
- lethargy

Prompt assessment and early intervention are essential to prevent circulatory collapse and death.

NURSING DIAGNOSES RELATED TO THE INFANT AND CHILD

The findings of the nursing assessment will, in most instances, reveal that the infant or child is healthy and developing normally. In such instances, the findings can be used as a basis for anticipatory guidance and health teaching for parents and their children. Learning positive health habits in childhood contributes to the development of lifelong habits that enhance physical and mental well-

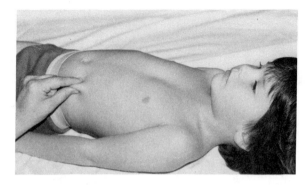

FIGURE 22-30. Elastic skin turgor indicates adequate hydration. The skin on the abdomen or thighs provides the most accurate site for skin turgor assessment.

being. Proper diet, physical activity, and safety practices in childhood provide an excellent foundation for a healthy adulthood. Healthy children are able to make the most of opportunities for enhancing their development as they grow from birth to adolescence.

Because of their unique characteristics and the dramatic changes that take place during infancy and childhood, certain nursing diagnoses occur with relative frequency among infants and children. Nursing diagnoses related to intrapersonal and interpersonal development, sexuality, and family, cultural, and environmental factors for infants and children are covered in earlier chapters. For example, "potential for injury or trauma" is commonly diagnosed in infants and children because of their developmental immaturity, which places them at risk for accidental injury. Children who are obese or who suffer physical disfigurement are at risk for "self-esteem disturbance" (see chap. 12). In this chapter, common nursing diagnoses that relate to physiological functioning in infants and children are considered (see Table 22-29).

Because of the dramatic physical changes of the developmental years, infants and children may be at risk of "altered physical growth and development" related to, for example, inadequate dietary intake, inadequate tissue perfusion (for example, children with congenital heart disease), or physical disability. Early detection of delays in physical growth and development is essential to prevent long-term consequences for the child's development and physical well-being. Children with short stature may have a previously undetected endocrine abnormality or, as is more often the case, a constitutional delay in achieving age-appropriate height. In the latter situation, the child's physical growth will catch up to age norms during puberty, but may adversely affect the child's self-esteem,

TABLE 22-29
Common Nursing Diagnoses Related to Infants and Children

Body temperature, altered, related to dehydration or infection

Communication, impaired verbal, related to hearing impairment, mental retardation, cleft palate, disarticulation, or stuttering

Diarrhea related to infection, overfeeding, food allergy, or excess dietary fiber

Fluid volume deficit related to vomiting, diarrhea, increased insensible water loss, or increased metabolic rate

Growth and development, altered physical, related to inadequate dietary intake, inadequate tissue perfusion, physical disability, or constitutional short stature

Mobility, impaired physical, related to physical injury, plaster cast or traction, or pain

Nutrition, altered (more or less than body requirements), related to excessive or inadequate dietary intake, physical inactivity, poverty, or decreased self-esteem

Pain related to health-related procedures (immunization injection, venipuncture, dressing change), surgical incision, trauma, or infection/inflammation

Self-care deficit: toileting, related to delayed opportunity or early parental pressure to learn bowel and bladder control, physiological factors (enuresis)

Sensory/perceptual alteration: visual or hearing, related to hereditary factors, trauma, or infection

Skin integrity, impaired, related to infection, inflammation, or trauma

Sleep pattern disturbance related to nightmares, night terrors, fear, unfamiliar environment, or overstimulation

sense of competence, and social interactions. Thus, early detection and referral are warranted.

Because of the susceptibility of a child's skin to bacterial invasion and inflammation, "impaired skin integrity" often is diagnosed in children suffering from a variety of skin disorders such as eczema, insect bites, or poison ivy, or from communicable diseases such as chicken pox or ringworm (*tinea capitas*). Impaired skin integrity also may result from trauma, including lacerations, puncture wounds, or burns.

Throughout childhood, children experience a variety of situations that may result in pain. These occurrences may be situational and acute, such as immunization injections or minor cuts and scrapes, or they involve pain of a longer duration, such as an earache caused by otitis media or postoperative pain from a surgical incision. Therefore, a nursing diagnosis of "pain" may be indicated.

Because of the high incidence of visual acuity disturbances (20 to 35% of children require corrective lenses) and other visual impairments, such as strabismus or color deficiency, children may be diagnosed with a "sensory–perceptual alteration: visual." Hearing impairments are much less common (1% of all children), although early diagnosis of "sensory–perceptual alteration: hearing" is critical for normal speech and language development. Children who do experience speech or language disorders resulting from hearing impairment or developmental delay, such as problems with sentence organization, fluency (stuttering), or articulation, may be diagnosed with "impaired verbal communication." Referral for comprehensive evaluation is essential for identifying intervention strategies to help the child develop optimally.

The high level of physical activity in which most children engage places them at risk for injury (Figure 22-31). Some of the most common injuries involve the musculoskeletal system and include muscle sprains, ligament tears, and fractures. School-age children who engage in sports and other activities, such as bicycle-riding, skateboarding, and climbing, are particularly at risk. Children who experience musculoskeletal injuries or altera-

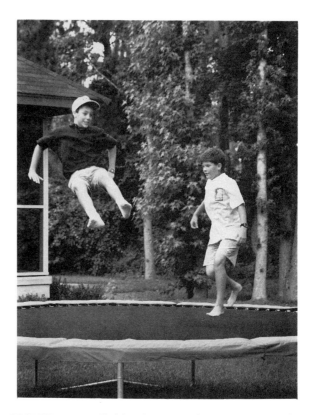

FIGURE 22-31. Children's sports place them at risk for injuries.

tions (e.g., Legg-Calvé-Perthes disease, congenital dislocated hip) often must be immobilized for a period of time, thus warranting a nursing diagnosis of "impaired physical mobility."

Because of the high incidence of sleep difficulties, especially during the preschool years, a nursing diagnosis of "sleep pattern disturbance" may be indicated. Hospitalized children also may be at risk for this diagnosis.

It has been estimated that 25% of U.S. children are obese (Rosenbaum & Leibel, 1988). Physical inactivity is one contributing factor but excess dietary intake, particularly of fats, is the major cause. A nursing diagnosis of "altered nutrition: more than body requirements" is indicated for children whose dietary history and physical growth measurements indicate overweight or obesity. Conversely, children whose dietary intake is insufficient for normal growth should be diagnosed as experiencing "altered nutrition: less than body requirements." Failure to thrive infants or children malnourished as a result of poverty are particularly at risk.

"Fluid volume deficit (active loss)" may result from vomiting or diarrhea, especially in infants. "Diarrhea" is a common alteration in bowel elimination, which may be caused by an infection, overeating, excess dietary fiber, food allergy, or a number of other factors.

A nursing diagnosis of "self-care deficit: delay in independent toileting" may be indicated for children who do not achieve voluntary control of bowel and bladder elimination by the expected ages or who experience bedwetting (enuresis) after bladder control has been achieved.

Adequate knowledge of the unique developmental and physiological characteristics of infants and children enables the nurse to conduct a comprehensive assessment. Findings from the nursing assessment should be analyzed to identify actual or potential responses to health problems or environmental factors that may require parental or nursing intervention. Early identification of nursing diagnoses and initiation of appropriate interventions are essential to enhance the infant or child's potential for optimal development and prevent serious delays or long-term consequences.

Chapter Highlights

■ Nursing assessment and diagnosis with children differ from their use with adults in two major ways: the knowledge needed to assess the child and the need for family involvement.

■ Infants and children have unique anatomical and physiological characteristics, developmental capabilities, and behavioral patterns that require modifications in the nursing assessment, particularly the approaches used and areas that are emphasized.

■ Until late childhood, the child's parent or reliable caregiver must provide most if not all the historical information about the child's health. However, once children reach school-age, the nurse should involve them as active participants in the nursing history interview.

■ Additions to the nursing history format for infants and children include parental–neonatal history, developmental milestones, child–parent and child–sibling relationships, child–peer relationships, school performance, play activities, and immunization history.

■ Children cooperate more readily when the sequence of the clinical appraisal proceeds from less intrusive (e.g., general appraisal, musculoskeletal assessment) to more intrusive procedures (e.g., temperature measurement, examination of the ears, nose, and mouth).

■ Aspects of the clinical appraisal that must be modified for infants and children include measuring physical growth and vital signs; vision, hearing, and speech/language screening; neurological assessment; pain assessment; evaluation of fluid balance; and assessment of mobility.

■ Common nursing diagnoses for infants and children include "potential for injury or trauma," "altered physical growth and development," "impaired skin integrity," "pain," "sensory–perceptual alteration (visual or auditory)," "impaired verbal communication," "impaired physical mobility," "sleep pattern disturbance," "altered nutrition," "fluid volume deficit (active loss)," "diarrhea," and "self-care deficit: delay in independent toileting."

Practice Activities

1. Observe children of various ages (infants, toddlers, preschoolers, school-age children) as they interact with others and with their environment. What age-typical characteristics (physical, intellectual, social) do they exhibit? What conclusions can you draw? What cultural and environmental fac-

tors are evident as forces influencing their development?

2. Obtain health histories (using the Child Health History format provided in this chapter) of an infant, a toddler or preschooler, and a school-age child (from different socioeconomic or cultural groups). Compare and contrast the differences in approaches you used to obtain the histories. Compare and contrast the findings, explaining the differences in terms of the children's physical, intellectual, and social development, and cultural background. What nursing diagnoses are suggested? How can you validate your judgments?

3. Measure the physical growth (height/length, weight, head circumference [if indicated], skinfold thickness) of at least one child in each of the following age groups: infancy, toddlerhood, preschool, school-age. What techniques did you use to ensure accuracy of the measurements? Plot your findings on the appropriate anthropometric charts, and interpret their meaning. What conclusions can you draw? What additional information is needed to validate your interpretations? What specific factors have contributed to each child's physical growth?

4. Measure vital signs (respiration, pulse, blood pressure, temperature) of at least one child in each of the different age groups. What factors influenced the measurement techniques you used? Compare findings with age norms. What conclusions can you draw?

5. Conduct vision (visual acuity, eye muscle balance, color vision [if indicated]) and hearing (audiometry, Weber and Rinne tests) screening of at least two preschool or school-age children. Interpret your findings. What conclusions can you draw?

6. Administer the Denver Articulation Screening Examination (DASE) to at least two children between the ages of 2½ and 6 years. Interpret the results. What conclusions can you draw?

7. Evaluate the neurological status of an infant, preschooler, and school-age child. What techniques/approaches did you use and why? Compare and contrast your findings. What conclusions can you draw? What additional information is needed to validate your conclusions?

8. Evaluate the behavioral responses of at least one preschool or school-age child who is experiencing pain. Use the Faces Pain Scale with the child. Describe your findings. What conclusions can you draw?

9. Perform a complete clinical appraisal of at least one infant, one toddler or preschooler, and one school-age child. Record and analyze your findings. What nursing diagnoses are suggested? What additional information is needed to validate your nursing diagnoses?

Recommended Readings

Carlson, K. (1989). Assessing a child's chest. *RN, 52*(11), 26–32.

DiChiara, E. (1984). A sound method for testing children's hearing. *American Journal of Nursing, 84,* 1104–1106.

Edgil, A.E., Wood, K.R., & Smith, D.P. (1985). Sleep problems of older infants and preschool children. *Pediatric Nursing, 11,* 87–89.

Ellis, J.A. (1988). Using pain scales to prevent undermedication. *MCN: The American Journal of Maternal–Child Nursing, 13,* 180–182.

Frappier, P.A., Marino, B.L., & Shishmanian, E. (1987). Nursing assessment of infant feeding problems. *Journal of Pediatric Nursing, 2,* 37–44.

Harris, J.A. (1986). Pediatric abdominal assessment. *Pediatric Nursing, 12*(5), 355–362.

Linley, J.F. (1987). Screening children for common orthopedic problems. *American Journal of Nursing, 87,* 1312–1316.

Martin, K.K., Urbano, M.T., Hayes, J.S., von Windeguth, B., & Sherrin, T. (1988). Comparison of axillary, rectal, and skin-based temperature assessment in preschoolers. *Nurse Practitioner, 13*(4), 31–36.

Moore, P.C. (1988). When you have to think small for a neurological exam. *RN, 51,* 38–43.

Rankin, W.W. (1988). Listening with the heart . . . to listen to a child. *Journal of Pediatric Nursing, 2,* 37–44.

Smith, B.A. (1989). Measurement of selected cardiovascular risk factors in children. *Applied Nursing Research, 2*(3), 143–146.

Wong, D.L., & Baker, C.M. (1988). Pain in children: Comparison of assessment scales. *Pediatric Nursing, 14*(1), 9–17.

References

Alexander, M.A., & Blank, J.J. (1988). Factors related to obesity in Mexican-American preschool children. *Image: Journal of Nursing Scholarship, 20,* 79–82.

American Academy of Pediatrics. (1987). *Fitness: The myths and facts.* Elk Grove Village, IL: Author.

American Academy of Pediatrics Committee on Nutrition. (1989). Indications for cholesterol testing in children. *Pediatrics, 83,* 141–142.

Barndt-Maglio, B. (1986). Sleep pattern disturbance. *Dimensions of Critical Care Nursing, 5*(6), 342–349.

Becque, M.D., Rocchini, A.P., & Moorehead, C. (1988). Coronary risk incidence of obese adolescents: Reduction by exercise plus diet intervention. *Pediatrics, 81,* 605–612.

Beltramini, A.U., & Hertzig, M.E. (1983). Sleep and bedtime behavior in preschool-aged children. *Pediatrics, 71,* 153–157.

Collins, J. (1985). *Persons injured and disability days due to injuries: United States, 1980–81,* Vital and Health Statistics (No. 149). Washington, DC: National Center for Health Statistics. (DHHS Pub. No. (PHS) 85–1577)

Dale, J.C. (1986). A multidimensional study of infants' responses to painful stimuli. *Pediatric Nursing, 12,* 27–31.

Dennison, B.A., Straus, J.H., Mellits, E.D., & Charney, E. (1988). Childhood physical fitness tests: Predictor of adult activity levels? *Pediatrics, 82,* 324–330.

DiChiara, E. (1984). A sound method for testing children's hearing. *American Journal of Nursing, 84,* 1104–1106.

Division of Injury Control, Centers for Disease Control (1990). Childhood injuries in the United States. *American Journal of Diseases of Children, 144(6),* 627–646.

Ellis, J.A. (1988). Using pain scales to prevent undermedication, *MCN: The American Journal of Maternal–Child Nursing, 13,* 180–182.

Eoff, M.J., & Joyce, B. (1981). Temperature measurements in children. *American Journal of Nursing, 81,* 1010–1011.

Eoff, M.J., Meier, R.S., & Miller, C. (1974). Temperature measurements in infants. *Nursing Research, 23,* 457–460.

Goldberg, I.R., Roghmann, K.J., McInerny, T.K., & Burke, J.D. (1984). Mental health problems among children seen in pediatric practice: Prevalence and management. *Pediatrics, 73,* 278–292.

Gortmaker, S.L., & Sappenfield, W. (1984). Chronic childhood disorders: Prevalence and impact. *Pediatric Clinics of North America, 31,* 3–18.

Guyer, B., & Gallagher, S.S. (1985). An approach to the epidemiology of childhood injuries. *Pediatric Clinics of North America, 32,* 163–174.

Heisel, J.S., Ream, S., Raitz, R., Rappaport, M., & Coddington, R.D. (1973). The significance of life events as contributing factors in the diseases of children. *Journal of Pediatrics, 83,* 119–123.

Hester, N., & Barcus, C. (1986). Assessment and management of pain in children. *Pediatrics: Nursing Update, 1(14),* 2–3.

Isaacs, P.C. (1989). Growth parameters and blood values in Arabic children. *Pediatric Nursing, 15,* 579–583.

Keefe, M.R., Kotzer, A.M., Reuss, J.L., & Sander, L.W. (1989). Development of a system for monitoring infant state behavior. *Nursing Research, 38,* 344–347.

Lewis, K.D., & Thompson, H.B. (1986). *Manual of school health.* Menlo Park, CA: Addison-Wesley.

Lieberman, E. (1978). Hypertension in childhood and adolescence. *CIBA Clinical Symposia, 30,* 1–30.

Martyn, K.K., Urbano, M.T., Hayes, J.S., von Windeguth, B., & Sherrin, T. (1988). Comparison of axillary, rectal and skin-based temperature assessment in preschoolers. *Nurse Practitioner, 13(4),* 31–36.

McGrath, P.A. (1989). Evaluating a child's pain. *Journal of Pain Symptom Management, 4,* 198–214.

Metcoff, J., Bentle, L., & Bodwell, C.E. (1981). Maternal nutrition and fetal outcome. *American Journal of Clinical Nutrition, 34,* 708–721.

Mills, N.M. (1989). Pain behaviors in infants and toddlers. *Journal of Pain Symptom Management, 4,* 184–190.

National Dairy Council. (1990). Children's health issues. *Dairy Council Digest, 61(6),* 31–36.

National Society to Prevent Blindness. (1982). *Children's eye health guide,* New York: Author.

Novello, A. (1989). Final report of the United States Department of Health and Human Services Secretary's workgroup on pediatric human immunodeficiency virus infection and disease: Content and implications. *Pediatrics, 84(3),* 547.

Peck, R.E., Marks, J.S., Dibley, M.J., Lee, S., & Trowbridge, F.L. (1987). Birth weight and subsequent growth among Navajo children. *Public Health Reports, 102,* 500–507.

Pickwell, S. (1982). Primary health care of Indochinese refugee children. *Pediatric Nursing, 8,* 104–106.

Rosenbaum, M., & Leibel, E.L., (1988). Pathophysiology of childhood obesity. *Advances in Pediatrics, 35,* 73–137.

Smith, B.A. (1989). Measurement of selected cardiovascular risk factors in children. *Applied Nursing Research, 2(3),* 143–146.

Sullivan, L. (1988). How effective is preschool vision, hearing, and developmental screening? *Pediatric Nursing, 14,* 181–183.

Thomas, A., & Chess, S. (1977). *Temperament and development.* New York: Brunner/Mazel.

Wegman, M. (1989). Annual summary of vital statistics—1988. *Pediatrics, 84(6),* 943–956.

Whaley, L.F., & Wong, D.L. (1991). *Nursing care of infants and children* (4th ed.). St. Louis: Mosby-Year Book.

Withrow, C., & Fleming, J.W. (1983). Pediatric social illness: A challenge to nurses. *Issues in Comprehensive Pediatric Nursing, 6,* 261–275.

Wong, D.L., & Baker, C.M. (1988). Pain in children: Comparison of assessment scales. *Pediatric Nursing, 14,* 9–17.

23

Assessment of the Adolescent

OBJECTIVES

Upon completion of this chapter, you should be
able to:

■ Delineate the biological, psychosocial, and
cultural characteristics of adolescence.

■ Compare and contrast the dimensions of
adolescent growth and development (physical
growth, cognition, identity, relationships with
others, sexuality, emotionality) according to early,
middle, and late phases of adolescence.

■ Trace the sequences of pubertal development
in males and females.

■ Describe the integumentary changes, activity–
sleep patterns, cardiorespiratory changes, nutritional requirements, and fluid–electrolyte needs
of adolescents.

■ Modify the approach to obtain the adolescent
health history and perform the clinical appraisal,
considering the unique characteristics of the adolescent client.

■ Evaluate the sexual maturity of the adolescent
client, interpreting and documenting findings
accurately.

■ Screen the adolescent client for scoliosis, using
correct techniques and documenting findings
accurately.

■ Perform a comprehensive assessment of
young, middle, and older adolescents, and analyze findings to formulate valid and appropriate
nursing diagnoses.

Adolescence is a biological, psychosocial, and cultural phenomenon characterized by dramatic changes in physical appearance, intellectual capacity, and personal and social behavior. At no other period in life, with the exception of infancy, do increases in physical growth occur so rapidly. Adolescence also is characterized by profound changes in psychosocial development.

Typically, the period of life known as adolescence begins with the physical transformation associated with the onset of puberty, or sexual maturation. The end of adolescence is less distinct and is characterized by the cessation of physical growth and a gradual assumption of adult roles and responsibilities.

Adolescence is largely a creation of post-industrial society (Coleman, 1974). Prior to the early 20th century, adolescence as a distinct period of development did not exist. Kett (1977) points out that the changes that occurred with industrialization of society prolonged the transition to adulthood, thus creating a rather lengthy period between the onset of sexual maturity (for centuries the "rite of passage" to adulthood) and full assumption of adult roles, privileges, and responsibilities. These social changes included the extension of legal protection to juveniles (child labor laws, juvenile justice system) and mandatory schooling, the dual purpose of which was to educate youth to participate in a democratic society and to keep them out of the labor market so they could not compete for scarce jobs. As a result, the adolescent period was significantly lengthened and became a distinct phase in human development.

Erikson (1980) characterizes contemporary adolescence as a period of "psychosocial moratorium," which has both advantages and disadvantages for today's youth (see Table 23-1). During adolescence, the individual generally enjoys freedom from the commitments associated with adulthood. Paradoxically, however, several experts (Elkind, 1981; Gilliam, 1983; Postman, 1982) note that while society grants youth certain freedoms from adult responsibilities, adolescents are being pushed more and more to look and behave like adults. Elkind (1981) refers to this phenomenon as the "hurried child syndrome." In today's society, with television and mass marketing, children are pressured to grow up sooner—to wear adult clothing, emulate adult behavior, and engage in adult activities. Thus, from a social and cultural perspective, the onset of adolescence occurs at an earlier age than it did a generation ago.

There are approximately 41 million adolescents in the United States (U.S. Bureau of the Census,

1987). Because of the aging of the general population, however, the proportion of the adolescent population is declining. In 1960, adolescents comprised slightly more than 15% of the population. As the baby boomers reached their teens in the 1960s, the adolescent population increased dramatically, to nearly 20% of the total population, which reflected a 48.5% increase in the number of people aged 14 to 24. In 1980, adolescents accounted for 20.4% of the population. By 1985, however, the number of adolescents began to decline and is projected to drop to 16.4% of the population in 1990.

Except for infancy, health risks are greatest during adolescence. Accidents are the leading cause of morbidity and mortality in the teen years, peaking between 15 and 24 years of age. Deaths from suicide and homicide also increase dramatically. Table 23-2 depicts causes of death and death rates for the 10 leading causes of death in young people.

There is little question that adolescence is a distinct developmental period that warrants special attention. When assessing adolescent clients, a nurse must be ever aware of their unique physical and behavioral characteristics. These characteristics necessitate modifications in how a nurse approaches, interacts with, and examines an adolescent client.

While many of the approaches and techniques the nurse uses to assess adults also can be employed successfully with adolescents, there are several areas of the nursing assessment that require special attention and would not necessarily be incorporated in a comprehensive assessment of an adult client.

This chapter focuses on those areas of the nursing assessment that should be modified or included when the client is an adolescent. When the approaches or techniques for assessing the adolescent are the same as those used with adult clients, they are not reviewed again in this chapter. However, an outline of a comprehensive clinical appraisal and screening of the adolescent client is provided (Table 23-10) to ensure that important areas of the assessment are not overlooked.

KNOWLEDGE NEEDED TO ASSESS THE ADOLESCENT

Nursing assessment of adolescent clients depends on a thorough understanding and appreciation of their unique and changing characteristics. Typically, adolescence is subdivided into three age groups: young, middle, and older adolescence. Adolescents in each of these subgroups share cer-

TABLE 23-1
Advantages and Disadvantages of Being an Adolescent

Advantages	Disadvantages
Freedom to explore new ideas, values, and roles	Isolation from the demands of real life
Longer period of schooling, which leads to better education, preparation for a career, and economic self-sufficiency	Enforced schooling for all youth, thus inhibiting early entry to the labor force for those who choose less skilled career paths
Development of a stronger independent identity	Prolonged dependence on adults (financial, emotional)
Acquisition of new privileges (driving, decision-making, holding a job, voting)	Creation of unrealistic expectations and a sense of entitlement ("getting" rather than "earning"), especially among affluent youth
	Value conflicts with family and community, creating problems between parents and adolescent
	Avoidance of commitment and assumption of adult responsibilities
	Pressure to experiment (sex, smoking, alcohol, drugs, fast driving)

tain physical, cognitive, and social qualities that distinguish them from each other.

Table 23-3 summarizes the various dimensions of adolescent development, by subgroup, that should be taken into account when assessing adolescent clients. The young adolescent, for example, differs dramatically from the middle or older adolescent in physical appearance, sexual maturity, cognitive ability, and social competence (Figure 23-1). Gender also plays a significant role in the maturation process, particularly with regard to physical growth, sexual maturity, and the development of

identity and a capacity for emotional intimacy. For instance, girls begin their physical growth spurt and achieve sexual maturity at an earlier age than boys. Psychosocially, the tasks of identity and intimacy are fused for females, while for males the development of a sense of identity necessarily precedes intimacy (Gilligan, 1982). Gilligan (1982) suggests that women come to know themselves through their relationships with others, whereas men must form separate, detached, autonomous selves before they become capable of forming intimate attachments with others.

TABLE 23-2
Deaths and Death Rates for the 10 Leading Causes of Death, Ages 15–24 Years: United States, 1988

Rank Order[1]	Cause of death (Ninth Revision International Classification of Diseases, 1975)	Number	Rate [Rates per 100,000 population in specified group]
———	All causes	38,167	102.1
1	Accidents and adverse effects	18,507	49.5
	Motor vehicle accidents	14,406	38.5
	All other accidents and adverse effects	4,101	11.0
2	Homicide and legal intervention	5,771	15.4
3	Suicide	4,929	13.2
4	Malignant neoplasms, including neoplasms of lymphatic and hemapoietic tissues	1,894	5.1
5	Diseases of heart	1,090	2.9
6	Human immunodeficiency virus infection	535	1.4
7	Congenital anomalies	474	1.3
8	Cerebrovascular diseases	266	0.7
8	Pneumonia and influenza	266	0.7
10	Chronic obstructive pulmonary diseases and allied conditions	178	0.5
———	All other causes	4,257	11.4

*Rank based on number of deaths.

TABLE 23-3
Developmental, Psychosocial, and Cultural Dimensions of Adolescence

Dimension	Early Adolescence 11–14 Years	Middle Adolescence 14–17 Years	Late Adolescence 17–20 Years
Growth	Rapidly accelerating growth Reaches peak velocity Secondary sex characteristics appear	Growth decelerating Stature reaches 95% of adult height Secondary sex characteristics well advanced	Physically mature Structure and reproductive growth almost complete
Cognition	Limited ability for abstract thinking Explores newfound ability for abstract thought Clumsy groping for new values and energies Comparison of "normality" with peers of same sex	Developing capacity for abstract thinking Enjoys intellectual powers, often in idealistic, altruistic terms Concern with philosophic, political, and social problems	Established abstract thought Can perceive and act on long-range options Able to view problems comprehensively Intellectual and functional identity established
Identity	Preoccupied with rapid body changes Trying out of various roles Measurement of attractiveness by acceptance or rejection of peers Conformity to group norms	Reestablishes body image as growth decelerates Very self-centered; increased narcissism Tendency toward inner experience and self-discovery Has a rich fantasy life Idealistic Able to perceive future implications of current behavior and decisions; variable application	Body image and gender role definition nearly secured Irreversible sexual identity Phase of consolidation of identity Stability of self-esteem Comfortable with physical growth Social roles defined and articulated
Relationships with parents	Defining independence-dependence boundaries Strong desire to remain dependent on parents while trying to detach No major conflicts over parental control	Major conflicts over independence and control Low point in parent-child relationship Greatest push for emancipation; disengagement Final and irreversible emotional detachment from parents; mourning	Emotional and physical separation from parents completed Independence from family and less conflict Emancipation nearly secured Extension of independence without conflict
Relationships with peers	Seeks peer affiliations to counter instability generated by rapid change Upsurge of close idealized friendships with members of the same sex Struggle for mastery takes place within peer group	Strong need for identity to affirm self-image Behavioral standards set by peer group Acceptance by peers extremely important—fear of rejection Exploration of ability to attract the opposite sex	Recedes in importance in favor of individual friendship Testing of male-female relationships against possibility of permanent alliance Relationships characterized by giving and sharing
Sexuality	Self-exploration and evaluation Limited dating Limited intimacy	Multiple plural relationships Decisive turn toward heterosexuality (if is homosexual, know by this time) Exploration of "sex appeal" Feeling of "being in love" Tentative establishment of relationships	Forms stable relationships and attachment to another Growing capacity for mutuality and reciprocity Preeminence of individual as dating partner Intimacy involves commitment rather than exploration and romanticism

TABLE 23-3 (Continued)

Dimension	Early Adolescence 11–14 Years	Middle Adolescence 14–17 Years	Late Adolescence 17–20 Years
Emotionality	Most ambivalence Wide mood swings Intense daydreaming Anger outwardly expressed with moodiness, temper outbursts, and verbal insults and name-calling	Tendency toward inner experiences; more introspective Tendency to withdraw when upset or feelings are hurt Vacillation of emotions in time and range Feelings of inadequacy common; difficulty in asking for help	More constancy of emotion Anger more apt to be concealed

Note. From Whaley, L.F., and Wong, D.L. (1991). *Nursing care of infants and children* (4th ed.). St. Louis: Mosby-Year Book, p. 891.

Physical Integrity

Today's youth, whether female or male, reach physical maturity earlier than children of previous generations. This worldwide trend has been attributed to improved nutrition and higher standards of living, as well as significant declines in infant mortality (Bullough, 1981; Tanner & Davies, 1985). North American males now reach their full stature at age 20 compared with age 25 in 1900. The average age of the first menstrual period in girls is 12.5 years compared with 13.5 years in 1950.

Puberty

The hallmark that heralds adolescence is the onset of *puberty*, a maturational and hormonal process by which the reproductive system begins to function.

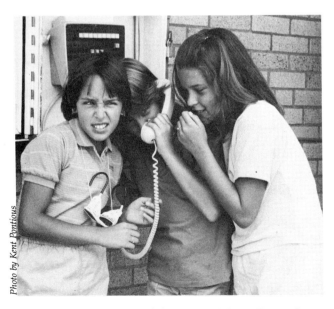

FIGURE 23-1. Early Adolescents. (*Note.* From Servonsky/Opas: *Nursing Management of Children*, © 1987. Boston: Jones and Bartlett Publishers, p. 255.)

The anterior pituitary gland secretes gonadotropins that stimulate the production of sperm in males and ovulation in females. Gonadotropins also stimulate the secretion of testosterone by the testes and estrogen and progesterone by the ovaries. These hormonal influences result in maturation of the reproductive system, the appearance of secondary sex characteristics, increases in height and weight, and integumentary changes.

Puberty sometimes is categorized in three phases: pubescence, puberty, and postpubescence. *Pubescence* begins approximately two years prior to puberty. This period is characterized by a growth spurt, most noticeable in the musculoskeletal system but involving other systems as well, such as endocrine, cardiorespiratory, and integumentary. Secondary sex characteristics also begin to appear, including the growth of pubic and axillary hair, breast development in girls, and enlargement of the external genitalia in boys. Pubescence culminates with puberty—marked by the first menstrual period in girls (*menarche*) and the production of spermatozoa in boys. The period of *postpubescence* lasts one to two years from the onset of menstruation or spermatogenesis and is characterized by a slowing of skeletal growth, the establishment of regular menstrual periods in girls, and achievement of full reproductive capability for both sexes.

There is wide individual variation in the onset of puberty (Figure 23-2). Differences are most pronounced between boys and girls. The onset of puberty occurs approximately two years earlier in girls than in boys. In girls, the first sign of puberty—beginning breast development—may appear between 9 and 11 years of age. The average age of menarche is 12.5 years among North American girls. Among boys, the first sign of puberty—enlargement of the penis and testes—begins at approximately 11.5 years of age, but may occur any time between 10 and 14 years of age. The average

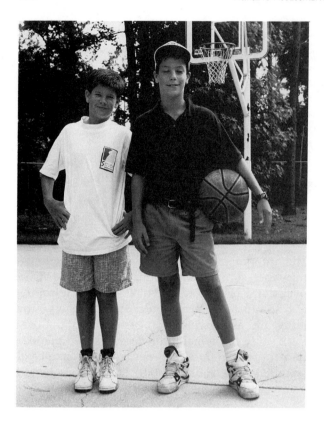

FIGURE 23-2. There is wide individual variation in the age at which the physical growth spurt occurs. Early- and late-maturing teens experience different types of problems, but often feel awkward with their peers.

age at which ejaculation occurs via masturbation or nocturnal emissions is 14.5 years, although it may occur somewhat earlier or several years later in some boys.

Table 23-4 outlines the specific sequence of pubertal development in males and females. While the sequence remains the same by gender for all, the rate is highly individual, governed predominantly by genetic factors, although environmental influences also play a role. For instance, improved nutrition and better disease control have allowed children to reach at an earlier age what some experts believe is the critical body weight needed to trigger the onset of puberty (Frisch, 1983). Climate also appears to play a role. Girls who live in extreme northern climates, such as Norway and Finland, begin their menstrual periods at older ages, on average, than girls who live in the United States and Great Britain (Tanner, 1973).

Physical Growth

The growth spurt associated with the onset of puberty is dramatic. During the school years, physical growth occurs at a relatively uniform and steady pace. During a two- to three-year period in early

adolescence, however, the final 25% of linear growth occurs. The increase in height is particularly rapid and extensive in boys. Boys may grow as much as 12 inches in height, whereas girls rarely gain more than 8 inches. Girls typically reach 95% of their adult height by age 16; boys continue to grow taller until 18 to 20 years of age. African-American adolescents attain a greater proportion of their adult height at an earlier age than white or Asian teens. Asian-American and Mexican-American adolescents tend to be smaller in stature than adolescents of other cultural groups. In all groups, linear growth precedes lateral growth: youth tend to grow taller before they fill out.

In addition to increases in height, other skeletal changes occur. The limbs lengthen and are longer in boys than in girls. Because the neck and limbs lengthen first, the early adolescent often has a gawky, long-legged, somewhat uncoordinated appearance. The shoulders and chest widen in boys whereas the pelvis and hips broaden in girls. The female pelvis assumes a *gynecoid* shape, becoming wider and shallower than the male's *android* pelvis, which is narrower and deeper.

The teenager's posture is affected by the rapid linear growth of the skeletal system and the lag in muscular growth, which leads to muscle weakness and, therefore, a slumped posture. This may be exacerbated in early-maturing teens, especially girls, who slump or hunch forward to avoid drawing attention to their height or breast development. Early-maturing adolescents tend to overcome poor posture as their peers catch up to them in growth and sexual development.

The head undergoes proportional changes during the adolescent growth spurt. The face and forehead lengthen and the forehead becomes wider. The jaw is the last structure of the head to achieve adult proportions. At the end of the pubertal growth period, the adolescent's head is approximately one-eighth of total body length (compared to one-fourth in infants).

The larynx and vocal cords hypertrophy during puberty, which causes the characteristic voice changes of adolescence. These changes are most noticeable among boys, whose voices may move from deep bass tones to squeaky high tones within a single phrase or sentence. Girls' voices become fuller and somewhat deeper, although the change tends to be more gradual.

Body composition also changes dramatically during early adolescence. Boys and girls both enter puberty with approximately the same proportion of body fat—15% in males, 19% in females. By the end of the growth spurt, body fat composition in girls is approximately 23%, whereas fat accounts

TABLE 23-4
Sequence of Pubertal Development

Female		
Average Age Onset	Physiologic Changes	Average Age Completion
9.0 to 11.0 years	*Breast development* Breast bud appears followed by general enlargement and raising of the breast and areola Areola and nipple are raised from breast Adult breast contour	14.0 to 17.0 years
About 1 year after breast buds appear	*Adrenarche* (growth of body hair) Pubic hair development	Late teens
About 1 year after onset of pubic hair growth	Axillary hair development	
10.5 years	*Growth spurt*—same sequence as male Height: increases 3–5 in/year at peak Weight: increases 15–50 pounds	16 years
12.5 years	*Menarche* (onset of menstruation) Initial cycles are usually anovulatory and irregular Ovulatory cycles usually occur within two years of menarche Dysmenorrhea more often associated with ovulatory cycles	

Male		
Average Age Onset	Physiologic Changes	Average Age Completion
11.5 years	*Genital development* Testicular volume increases Penile enlargement and lengthening	2–5 years after onset
12.5 years	*Adrenarche* (growth of body hair) Pubic hair development	Late teens
About 2 years after onset of pubic hair growth	Axillary and facial hair development	
13.5 years	*Growth spurt* Pattern: hands and feet, calves and forearms, hips, chest, shoulders, trunk Height: increases about 3–5 in/year at peak Weight: almost doubles between 12 and 16 years Larynx growth and voice deepening occur at end of penile growth	Late teens
About 3 years after onset of genital development	*Ejaculation* via masturbation or nocturnal emissions Mature sperm are produced between 14.5 and 17.5 years of age	14.5 to 17.5 years
	Breast development Areola darkens and enlarges Transient gynecomastia may occur between 10 and 16 years of age	

for about 12% of body composition in boys (Chumlea, 1981). Increases in body weight during the pubertal growth spurt range from 15 to 50 pounds in girls and typically occur in fat tissue, evident especially in the hips, thighs, buttocks, and breasts. Boys often double their weight between 12 and 16 years of age and may gain as much as 75 pounds,

most of which is muscle mass. The muscles of the thighs, buttocks, chest, and upper arms become particularly well developed in males.

Integumentary Changes

The hormones secreted during puberty produce significant changes in the integument. In girls, estrogen release causes the skin to soften and thicken while androgen release in boys thickens and darkens the skin. Sebaceous glands in both sexes become active, most noticeably on the face, shoulders, and upper trunk. Increased sebaceous activity may cause a flushed appearance over the face and upper torso and contributes to the occurrence of acne.

Acne vulgaris occurs predominantly during adolescence and is influenced by hormonal, immunological, genetic, and emotional factors. Nearly three-quarters of all adolescents experience some degree of acne, which can be mild to severe. Peak occurrence is among 16- to 18-year-olds. Acne is seen more commonly among boys than girls. Increased production of sebum, a secretion of the sebaceous glands, is responsible for the eruption of acne lesions. Factors that aggravate the condition include the use of oral contraceptives, oil-based cosmetics, and menstruation. Dietary factors, such as chocolate, iodine, or fatty foods, have not been substantiated.

The sweat glands of the body mature during puberty and may be stimulated by an increase in body or environmental temperature or by emotional responses. Boys tend to produce more sweat than girls. The *eccrine* sweat glands, functional throughout childhood, become fully mature and secrete sweat over the entire body surface, acting as a thermoregulator. *Apocrine* sweat glands first become functional during puberty and are located primarily in the axillae and genital areas. Apocrine glands produce thicker secretions than eccrine glands. The secretions interact with bacteria on the skin surface, causing an offensive odor. Apocrine glands respond to emotional stimulation as well as heat or exercise.

Changes in the distribution and texture of body hair also occur during puberty, owing primarily to the secretion of androgens. Body hair becomes thicker, darker, and coarser. Pubic and axillary hair appears and is typically thicker and more extensive in boys. Chest and facial hair appears in boys, although it may occur as well in some girls, depending on the level of androgen secretion, which is related primarily to genetic influences.

Sensory-Perceptual-Neurological Functioning

The adolescent's sensory–perceptual–neurological system is essentially fully mature. Visual refractive errors, however, are common at this age. Because of the demands that schoolwork places on the teenager's vision, visual problems first may be de-

tected during adolescence. Adolescents who must wear corrective lenses may have difficulty adapting to them because eyeglasses change their body image. Contact lenses are often a desirable alternative.

Adolescents who are exposed continuously to loud music are susceptible to sensorineural hearing loss (American Academy of Pediatrics, 1982). Because teenagers enjoy listening to rock and rap music (via radios, stereos, or rock concerts) at high decibel levels, they are at risk for hearing impairment. Use of earphones at loud volumes is particularly problematic. Adolescents, therefore, should be screened periodically for early detection of any hearing impairment (see chap. 22) and should be advised of the risk to hearing that loud noise levels create.

Activity-Sleep

As the adolescent's body systems mature, physical performance capabilities increase and often peak during the later adolescent years. Physiologically, the adolescent's body is able to adapt quickly to the demands of exercise or physical exertion. Muscle strength, coordination, and endurance improve. Most boys and an increasing number of girls enhance their athletic prowess through structured and informal activities such as team and individual sports (football, soccer, tennis, track), regular exercise (swimming, cycling, marching band, hiking), and physical conditioning (weight-lifting, aerobics). The drive to compete is strong among North American youth, instilled by society's preoccupation with physical fitness and competitive athletics (beginning with early school-age sports such as soccer and swimming, continuing with high school and college athletics, and culminating with professional sports).

Many of the activities that adolescents enjoy require high levels of energy. Although activity is beneficial for the adolescent because it provides for development of self-esteem and close relationships with peers, it is not without hazard. The musculoskeletal system grows rapidly in the postpubescent period, and muscles, ligaments, and tendon strength are not yet fully mature. These structures are susceptible to stressors and may be stretched, torn, or strained during vigorous activity (Figure 23-3) (Latinis, 1983).

Although adolescents often enjoy solitary time listening to music or watching television, they typically prefer to be involved in social activities. During early adolescence, boys are more interested in "hanging out with the guys," whereas girls prefer

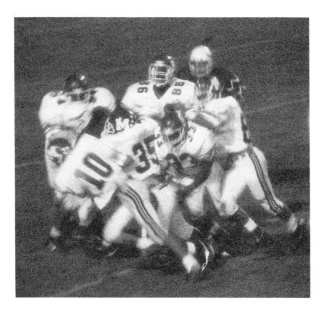

FIGURE 23-3. The adolescent's rapidly maturing musculoskeletal system is susceptible to trauma from too early or vigorous participation in sports.

social activities involving both boys and girls. As adolescents mature, going to the movies, shopping mall, dances, rock concerts, and parties occupy much of their social time.

Talking on the telephone is often a way for teenagers to connect with one another when they are unable to be together, and they may spend hours in lengthy conversation about their plans, dreams, and experiences or just gossiping. The telephone also provides a safe opportunity to begin or explore a romantic relationship.

Sleep needs and patterns vary considerably among adolescents. During the period of rapid physical growth in early adolescence, fatigue often occurs. The increased energy expenditure associated with sports, the lag in maturation of the cardiac and respiratory systems, and the tendency to stay up late also contribute to adolescent fatigue. Teenagers typically sleep late when they can. Napping during the early adolescent period of rapid physical growth is not uncommon.

Adolescents generally need 9 to 11 hours of sleep in a 24-hour period. The adolescent's sleep pattern is remarkably similar to that of adults with regard to the amount of sleep time spent in each stage of the sleep cycle (see chap. 16).

The cardiorespiratory system matures at a slower rate during puberty than the reproductive and musculoskeletal systems, contributing to fatigue during early adolescence before the cardiorespira-tory system catches up and assumes adult levels of capacity and functioning. During the period of rapid physical growth, the size and strength of the heart and lungs increase, especially in boys. The greater chest and shoulder size in boys contributes to a larger respiratory volume and vital capacity.

Blood volume and systolic blood pressure gradually increase to adult rates, while the pulse and respiratory rates decrease (see Table 23-5). Girls generally have slightly higher pulse and respiratory rates and lower systolic blood pressure than boys owing to their smaller stature and different body tissue composition.

The use of cigarettes among teenagers is on the rise and poses potentially serious threats to their respiratory and cardiovascular functioning (Figure 23-4). Smoking decreases breathing capacity and ventilatory muscle endurance, thus lowering exercise tolerance (Dessendorfer, Amsterdam, & Odland, 1983). Respiratory illnesses occur more frequently among teen smokers. The use of smokeless (chewing) tobacco contributes to serious dental disease and increases the risk of mouth cancer (Greer, 1983).

Contemporary teens begin smoking at earlier ages and more teens smoke now than in previous generations (U.S. Public Health Service, 1981). It has been established that 25% of today's teens are regular smokers. More than one-third of adolescent males also report using smokeless tobacco (Guggenheimer, Zullo, Kruper, & Verbin, 1986; Marty, McDermott, & Williams, 1986). Advertising by tobacco companies often targets young adolescents, associating smoking with maturity, sophistication, sexuality, and adventure (Staff Report on Cigarette Advertising Investigation, 1981). The U.S. Public Health Service (1981) points out that mortality is 50% higher among people who have been smoking since age 15 than among those who begin smoking in adulthood.

Nutrition and Dentition

The rapid growth spurt (height, weight, sexual maturity) of the early adolescent years is accompanied

TABLE 23-5
Pulse Rate, Respiratory Rate, and Blood Pressure
Norms in Adolescents

Age	Pulse Rate	Respiratory Rate	Blood Pressure
12–14 years	85/min	20/min	108/64
14–16 years	80/min	18/min	110/66
16–18 years	75/min	16/min	118/70

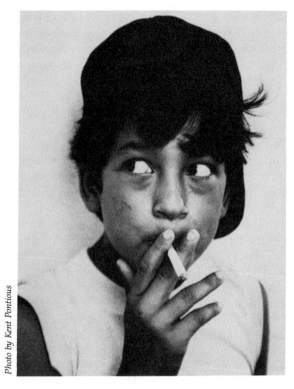

Photo by Kent Pontious

FIGURE 23-4. Smoking among teenagers is on the rise and poses serious threats to their respiratory and cardiovascular health. (*Note.* From Servonsky/Opas: *Nursing Management of Children,* © 1987. Boston: Jones and Bartlett Publishers, p. 446.)

by an increased need for calories, protein, and most vitamins and minerals. Nutritional requirements peak during the period of most rapid growth, typically between 10 and 12 years of age in girls and between 12 and 15 years of age in boys. Caloric and protein requirements during this period are proportionately greater than at nearly any other time in life. In fact, during the peak period of growth, nutritional requirements may be twice as great as they are at any other time during adolescence. There is also increased need for calcium for skeletal maturation, iron for muscle development and blood volume increase, and zinc for skeletal growth and sexual maturation (Marino & King, 1980).

Because boys experience proportionately greater growth in skeletal and muscle tissue, they have higher metabolic rates and basal energy expenditure than girls. Adolescent boys thus have greater needs than girls for calories, protein, and many minerals and vitamins. Needs for calcium, iron, zinc, and magnesium during the peak period of growth for both sexes are often twice as much as the usual requirement. For example, during peak growth girls need 240 mg of calcium compared to

110 mg during prepubescent and postpubescent periods. Girls nearly triple their need for iron intake during puberty (Forbes, 1981). However, at the end of the growth spurt, girls need proportionately fewer calories than boys to meet energy requirements (see Table 23-6). Protein, vitamin, and mineral requirements for adolescent males and females are shown in Table 23-7.

Iron deficiency anemia may occur in adolescents who do not increase their intake of iron during periods of greater need. Iron intake needs are influenced by the stage of sexual maturity (Table 23-12). Table 23-8 shows the hematocrit levels (by gender, race, and sexual maturity) below which anemia is considered to be present.

Nutritional requirements also are related to energy expenditure. Adolescents who engage in sports or strenuous exercise have greater caloric and vitamin needs. They may need as many as 5,000 calories per day and additional amounts of vitamins C and B complex during periods of peak physical activity (Lucas, Rees, & Mahan, 1985). Sedentary teens may be prone to obesity and thus require fewer calories.

Emotional factors also influence the adolescent's nutritional needs, but their role is not well defined. Eating disorders, such as anorexia and bulimia, are particularly likely to occur among teenage girls who are striving to achieve the slim figure that marks physical attractiveness in contemporary society. Excessive dieting can severely compromise the adolescent's health and development and, in extreme cases, may be life-threatening. Boys are less likely to undereat, but may lack certain essential nutrients in their diets.

Other common adolescent problems with nu-

TABLE 23-6
Recommended Energy (Caloric) Intake During Adolescence

	Daily Total (kcal)	
Age	Median*	Range*
Males		
11–14	2500	2000–3700
15–18	3000	2100–3900
Females		
11–14	2200	1500–3000
15–18	2200	1200–3000

*Median = median energy intake of children followed in longitudinal growth studies. Range = 10th and 90th percentiles, respectively, of the children's energy intake.

Note. Reprinted with permission from *Recommended Dietary Allowances*, 10th edition, © 1989 by the National Academy of Sciences. Published by National Academy Press, Washington, DC.

tritional implications are teenage pregnancy and use of oral contraceptives. For instance, a pregnant teenager not only has special nutritional needs related to the adolescent growth spurt but also the added demands of the developing fetus. Teenage girls who are taking oral contraceptives need additional vitamins B_6, B_{12}, and folic acid.

Because adolescents spend so much time away from home, much of their daily food intake is starchy cafeteria food, fast food, or easily accessible junk food. Therefore, their diets tend to be high in calories, carbohydrates, fat, and sodium, but low in fiber and essential minerals and vitamins, particularly vitamins A, B, and C. Further, many teenagers do not eat breakfast or, if they do, eat on-the-run breakfast foods, such as doughnuts, pastries, and sugar-coated cereals. Because adolescents' energy and growth requirements are so great, they should eat breakfast foods high in complex carbohydrates, protein, and calcium, and low in fat.

During adolescence, appetites become voracious, especially in boys. Food, particularly fast foods and snack foods, is an integral part of many adolescent social activities. Food habits are determined largely by family and cultural preferences, but are susceptible to influence by peers. Teens are often more willing than younger children to try new foods, especially if the food item is widely accepted among the peer group. Previous religious or cultural food taboos may be broken in order to gain social acceptance. For instance, a teenager raised in a Buddhist culture may accept a fast food hamburger, or an Orthodox Jewish adolescent may try a ham sandwich.

At the beginning of adolescence, most youngsters have 24 permanent teeth, including the first molars. By age 15 the second molars erupt. The third set of molars typically erupts between 17 and 25 years of age, resulting in a full set of 32 permanent teeth. Eruption of the second and third molars may be accompanied by some discomfort and mild gum inflammation. If the third molars fail to erupt or begin to displace the teeth in front of them, they may need to be extracted.

Dental caries are not as prevalent during adolescence as in earlier years, but good dental hygiene continues to be important. A hallmark of early adolescence, particularly among middle and upper middle class youth, is the wearing of corrective orthodontic braces. Although the adolescent may experience some initial embarrassment, the frequency with which braces are worn during the teenage years minimizes any serious threat to the youngster's self-concept. Careful and frequent toothbrushing and flossing are particularly important while orthodontic appliances are worn.

Fluid–Electrolytes and Elimination

The adolescent's fluid and electrolyte needs are essentially the same as the adult's (see chap. 19). Approximately 60% of body weight in the young adolescent is water. At the end of the growth spurt, girls' body weight is approximately 55% water, whereas in boys, water makes up 57% of body weight. Daily fluid requirements are 2,200 to 2,700 ml (30 to 50 ml/Kg of body weight).

Average daily urine output is 1,200 to 1,500 ml. Fluid also is excreted through sensible and insensible perspiration and through the lungs. Gastrointestinal function is fully mature, and elimination patterns depend on food and fluid intake, exercise patterns, physiological differences, and the availability of facilities.

APPROACHES TO ADOLESCENT ASSESSMENT

The adolescent's increased cognitive capacity and emotional maturity require a different approach to the health history and physical examination than is used with children. Each adolescent brings unique characteristics and capabilities to the health assessment situation. Depending on the phase of adolescence, individual growth patterns, cognitive development, and previous health-care experiences, the adolescent may respond more or less positively. Interactions with health-care providers are influenced heavily by cultural factors. Health beliefs and practices are fairly well established by adolescence and shaped by the attitudes, beliefs, and values of the adolescent's cultural group (see chap. 8). Therefore, the approach used must be adapted to each adolescent client and the particular context. As Bishop (1979) aptly notes, the "constant process of adjusting both tone [and content] of approach . . . to suit the adolescent *now* presents an enormous challenge for the health care professional" (p. xvi).

Depending on the reason for the adolescent's contact with the health-care provider, responses may range from genuine cooperativeness to bravado, hostility, or withdrawal. The nurse must be alert to the adolescent's moods and fears and adapt the approach to or sequence of the assessment in response. Generally speaking, most adolescents are cooperative, responsive, and keenly interested in their health and the findings of the assessment, although they may pretend they are not.

The adolescent client is usually willing to an-

TABLE 23-7
Recommended Daily Dietary Allowances for Adolescents[a]

	Age (yr)	Weight		Height		Pro-tein (gm)	Fat-Soluble Vitamins		
		(kg)	(lb)	(cm)	(in)		Vita-min A (μg RE)[b]	Vita-min D (μg)[c]	Vita-min E (mg α^{-TE})[d]
Females	11–14	46	101	157	62	46	800	10	8
	15–18	55	120	163	64	44	800	10	8
Males	11–14	45	99	157	62	45	1000	10	10
	15–18	66	145	176	69	59	1000	10	10

[a]The allowances are intended to provide for individual variations among most normal persons as they live in the United States under usual environmental stresses. Diets should be based on a variety of common foods in order to provide other nutrients for which human requirements have been less well defined.

[b]Retinol equivalents. 1 retinol equivalent equals 1 μg retinol or 6 μg β-carotene.

[c]As cholecalciferol. 10 μg cholecalciferol equal 400 IU of vitamin D.

Note. Reprinted with permission from *Recommended Dietary Allowances* 10th edition, © 1989 by the National Academy of Sciences. Published by National Academy Press, Washington, DC.

swer health-related questions, as long as they are asked in a nonjudgmental way and the nurse conveys interest in and acceptance of the responses. Adolescents want to feel respected, listened to, and accepted, even when their values conflict with those of the nurse. Creating a climate of acceptance fosters trust and encourages disclosure of information. Without such a climate, the adolescent is likely to withhold important information. When this occurs, the nurse gains an incomplete picture of the adolescent's health.

It is critical that the adolescent be viewed by the nurse as the *primary* source of information. Although adolescents often are accompanied by their parents for health visits, the nurse should provide time to interview the adolescent alone (Figure 23-5). The decision to initiate the interview alone with the adolescent, alone with the parent(s), or with the client and parent(s) together will depend upon the nature of the visit and the nurse's previous relationship (if any) with the client and fam-

TABLE 23-8
Hematocrit as Indicator of Anemia in Adolescents (at or below 15th percentile)

Sexual Maturity Stage	Black Males	White Males	Black Females	White Females
1	34.9	35.6	34.0	35.8
2	36.0	36.9	35.3	36.6
3	37.1	38.2	36.0	37.0
4	38.2	39.6	36.2	36.7
5	39.3	40.6	35.8	35.9

Note. Adapted with permission of Ross Laboratories, Columbus, OH 43216, from W.A. Daniel, *Dietetic Currents*, 3(4), 15, © 1976 Ross Laboratories.

ily. If possible, the nurse should try to incorporate time to meet separately with the adolescent and parent(s) and then with both together. Meeting with the teenager first can be especially helpful in establishing trust and conveying the message, "You are important and I value *your* thoughts and feelings about your health."

It is important to clarify with the adolescent and parent(s) that because the client is moving toward adulthood and has a clearer understanding of health and illness, interviewing the adolescent alone helps foster a sense of responsibility for his or her own health and the establishment of positive health habits for the future. This explanation helps prevent the parent(s) from misinterpreting the nurse's motives as "taking sides" with the adolescent. If the interview is conducted with the parent(s) present, the nurse should be careful to address questions directly to the adolescent, unless specific information is required from the parent's point of view.

The adolescent should be reassured that all information will be treated confidentially, within certain limits. The nurse should explain up front that information that indicates the client or others are at risk of harm, such as suicidal thoughts, threats against others, or criminal behavior, will be shared with appropriate people in the interest of the adolescent's welfare.

THE ADOLESCENT HEALTH HISTORY

The health history provides an opportunity to establish rapport with the teenage client. It also gives adolescents a chance to ask questions or express

Water-Soluble Vitamins							Minerals					
Vita-min C (mg)	Thia-min (mg)	Ribo-flavin (mg)	Niacin (mg NE)[e]	Vita-min B_6 (mg)	Fola-cin[f] (μg)	Vita-min B_{12} (μg)	Cal-cium (mg)	Phos-phorus (mg)	Mag-nesium (mg)	Iron (mg)	Zinc (mg)	Iodine (μg)
50	1.1	1.3	15	1.4	150	2.0	1200	1200	280	15	12	150
60	1.1	1.3	15	1.5	180	2.0	1200	1200	300	15	12	150
50	1.4	1.3	17	1.7	150	2.0	1200	1200	270	12	15	150
60	1.4	1.5	20	2.0	200	2.0	1200	1200	400	12	15	150

[d]α-Tocopherol equivalents. 1 mg d-α tocopherol equals 1 α-TE.

[e]1 NE (niacin equivalent) is equal to 1 mg of niacin or 60 mg of dietary tryptophan.

[f]The folacin allowances refer to dietary sources as determined by *Lactobacillus casei* assay after treatment with enzymes (conjugases) to make polyglutamyl forms of the vitamin available to the test organism.

concerns about their health in a relatively safe, un-threatening atmosphere. Because adolescents have developed the capacity for abstract thought, they are generally reliable sources of information. They usually are able to recall their own health history and have a fairly accurate perception of their current health. However, younger adolescents may need assistance from their parent(s) to provide specific details or validation of their recollections.

Adolescents have a fairly mature understanding of health and illness. Their increased knowledge results both from their intellectual capacity for abstract thought and from exposure to health information through school health programs and the media (e.g., television and movies). Most teen-agers also have had several personal experiences with minor illness and may know relatives or other close acquaintances who have serious acute or chronic illnesses. Some have dealt with the deaths of grandparents or others close to them.

Despite their greater knowledge of health and illness, adolescents may not relate their awareness to their own health. For instance, a teenager may have a grandparent who is dying from chronic lung disease due to smoking, yet chooses to smoke anyway. Such a response reflects the typical adolescent's sense of omnipotence and invulnerability, which leads to risk-taking behavior and the perception that "It won't happen to me."

The use of a health questionnaire, completed by the adolescent client prior to meeting with the nurse, is an excellent way to obtain information. Completion of a health questionnaire involves adolescents as active participants in their own health and increases their health awareness. A questionnaire also helps set the stage for the interview and may break the ice for potentially embarrassing topics, such as elimination and sexuality. Once the health questionnaire is completed, the nurse can matter-of-factly clarify, validate, or expand on the information provided.

When the health history is obtained by interview, the nurse should begin with factual, unembarrassing items. Careful listening for both feeling and content is essential. Prying should be avoided, and the nurse should be careful to respond in an accepting, supportive way. Initiating the interview by focusing on family, cultural, and environmental areas is generally unthreatening and encourages disclosure. The nurse then can move to asking

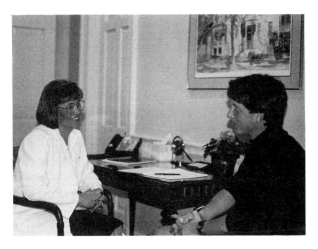

FIGURE 23-5. The nurse should create an opportunity to interview the adolescent alone during a health visit.

about the adolescent's childhood, school performance, relationships with friends and adults, current stressors, and coping patterns. Administration of the Stress Scale for Children (Heisel, Ream, Raitz, Rappaport, & Coddington, 1973) may be indicated and often serves as a helpful supplement to the nursing history (see Chap. 22, Table 22-19).

Questions about the client's physiological functioning, such as sensory status, activity–sleep patterns, and nutrition, should be introduced next. It is generally best to delay asking about sexuality until the end of the nursing history, following naturally from questions about elimination to questions related to puberty characteristics, knowledge of breast or testicular self-exam, sexual practices or activity, and concerns or questions about sex.

Focusing on the teenage client's health concerns is an excellent way to conclude the health history portion of the nursing assessment. Smith, Turner, and Jacobsen (1987) found that 12- to 15-year-old adolescents were most concerned about two health-related issues: personal concerns, such as worrying about the future, getting along with others, and emotions and feelings; and physical appearance, such as weight, skin problems, hair, and figure. Illness and social problems, such as drug abuse, sexually transmitted diseases, and pregnancy, were not reported to be of major concern.

The nurse can ascertain the client's particular health concerns by saying, "Many teenagers are concerned about [topics]—what concerns or questions do you have?" This gives the adolescent permission to introduce a particular topic that otherwise might seem too embarrassing to mention. Common health concerns of adolescents are outlined in Table 23-9.

The nurse should keep in mind that adolescents frequently use language or slang that may be unfamiliar to the nurse. Therefore, certain words and expressions may need to be clarified. The nurse simply should ask the client to explain what unfamiliar terms mean—"I haven't heard that one—what does it mean?"

A recommended format for the adolescent health history is presented in Table 23-10.

CLINICAL APPRAISAL AND SCREENING

Clinical examination of the adolescent should take into account the adolescent's emerging identity and independence. Therefore, examining the adolescent without the parent present usually is indicated. Some teenagers, however, may prefer to have their parent with them and should be given a choice. The need for a parent's presence may be

TABLE 23-9
Common Health Concerns of Adolescents

Body structure and function (scientific terminology, differences in male–female development, mental function)

Nutrition (requirements, muscle development, weight control)

Physical fitness; sports and injuries

Safety (driver education, first aid, CPR, common injuries)

Illness and disease (communicable diseases, AIDS, STDs, common ailments, cancer, heart disease)

Alcohol, drugs, tobacco (effects, hazards, alcoholism, addiction)

Sexuality (accurate and complete knowledge of human sexual function; decision-making—sexual relationships, contraception, "safe sex"; preparation for marriage and family life)

Self-awareness; values conflicts and clarification; handling life problems

Identity and independence; self-responsibility

Stress management

Mental illness

especially important when the adolescent is ill or has been injured.

Because of the teenager's self-consciousness and changing body image, modesty concerns are paramount. Assuring privacy while undressing and throughout the examination is essential to preserve the adolescent's dignity and trust in the nurse. Males should be instructed to keep their underwear on. Females may wear their bras and panties or patient gowns with Velcro front openings. Underclothing needs to be removed only for the examination of sexual maturity.

The clinical appraisal is an excellent time to teach adolescents about their body structure and function and answer health-related questions. Correct medical terminology should be used (for example, "abdomen" instead of "tummy," "urine" instead of "pee"), teaching the adolescent the proper terms for body parts and functions when they are unfamiliar.

Conversing in normal, relaxed tones throughout the examination helps put the client at ease. At each step of the appraisal, the nurse should explain what will be done and why, how the adolescent may help ("Breathe normally," "Raise your arms over your head") and the findings. Adolescents need assurance that they are developing and functioning normally.

The clinical examination of the adolescent client should follow the same sequence and guidelines as that used for adults (see Table 23-11). Three areas of the appraisal, however, deserve special

TABLE 23-10
Adolescent Health History

Client Profile:
Birthdate, current age
Grade in school/year in college; school performance; satisfaction with school
Employment (type, # hours/week); satisfaction with work

Sociocultural History:
Family
Family members; significant others (who does adolescent rely on for social support?)
Family interaction and communication patterns; conflicts—how handled.
Responsibilities within family (chores, caretaking for siblings or other family members)
Cultural
Value orientation (present/future)
Health/illness beliefs; importance of health to client
Health knowledge; health practices
Religious affiliation and practices
Environmental
Allergies (food, medication, other)
Exposure to pollutants (air, water, noise)
Use of tobacco (smoking, chewing), alcohol, marijuana, other substances; when initiated, frequency; knowledge of effects and long-term health hazards
Safety—driving (driver education, use of seatbelts, safe driving practices); safe use of firearms; swimming (ability, safe diving practices)
Home environment—own space for sleeping, studying/homework, leisure activities
Social network; participation in neighborhood and community life

Developmental History:
Family health history (risk factors)
Identity and intimacy concerns; satisfaction with own development (physical, cognitive, social)

Psychosocial History:
Intrapersonal/Interpersonal
Body image—satisfaction with; recent changes; concerns
Self-esteem—feelings about self; how negative feelings handled
Cognition—language, abstract reasoning ability, reading level, educational achievement
Affect/mood (general feeling; mood swings); feelings of anxiety, anger, depression; fears
Temperament—client's description of self
Spirituality—sources of hope
Relationships with peers, teachers/coaches, other adults; ability to get along with others; social support
Stressors; stressful life events; coping strategies (affective vs. cognitive)
Sexuality
Knowledge of puberty; awareness of own sexual devel-

opment; concerns about own sexual maturation (early, late)
Onset of menarche (females)—age, frequency/regularity, length of menstrual periods, use of sanitary pads or tampons; problems (e.g., menstrual cramps) or concerns
Nocturnal emissions (males)—age of onset, concerns
Knowledge and practice of breast self-exam (females) or testicular self-exam (males)
Sexual knowledge and education (sources of sexual information); questions or concerns about normality (sexual maturation; sexual impulses; masturbation)
Sexual activity; use of contraception; safe sex practices; problems or concerns

Physiological History:
Physical Integrity
Hygiene practices (bath/shower—frequency; use of deodorant; shaving—age begun, frequency; use of cosmetics—type, frequency; hair and nail care)
Growth patterns—onset of growth spurt; changes in height and weight; concerns
Skin—cleansing (agents used, frequency); acne—how managed
Sensory-Neurological
Vision or hearing problems; exposure to noise—decibel level, frequency
Neurological functioning—balance, coordination; problems
Pain—type, location, duration, intensity, precipitating and alleviating factors; how managed
Activity-Sleep
Daily sleep patterns (number of hours, naps); recent changes; fatigue (contributing factors)
Activity patterns—extracurricular activities, exercise (type, frequency), participation in sports (type, frequency); leisure activities; special abilities (artistic, athletic)
Muscle strength and endurance; problems with posture, range of motion, gait, mobility; physical fitness
Oxygenation
Interferences with breathing or circulation
Smoking, exposure to pollutants
Nutrition
Eating patterns—24-hour recall; food preferences; dietary restrictions for religious or health reasons
Eating problems—dieting, binging, purging, use of laxatives to control weight, overeating
Dentition—dental hygiene practices; eruption of molars; wearing of corrective orthodontic appliances; use of fluoride supplements
Fluid/Electrolytes and Elimination
Usual daily fluid intake (type, amounts)
Elimination patterns (urinary, bowel)—frequency; problems—how managed

Health Concerns: questions or concerns about own health

TABLE 23-11
Clinical Appraisal and Screening—The Adolescent

General Appearance

Physical Integrity
  Growth (height, weight)*
  Vital signs (temperature, pulse, respiration, blood
    pressure)
  Integument

Sensory–Neurological Status
  Vision screening
  Hearing screening
  Other senses
  Neurological functioning

Activity–Sleep Status
  Mobility
    Range of motion
    Scoliosis screening*
  Physical fitness

Oxygenation (chest and lungs, heart, peripheral vascular system)

Nutritional Status
  Clinical signs
  Anthropometric measurements

Elimination
  Urine and stool exam
  Anus and rectum

Sexual Maturity* (Tanner's stages)
*Reviewed in depth in this chapter.

mention: assessment of physical growth, appraisal of sexual maturity, and screening for scoliosis. The latter two are areas of the examination unique to the adolescent assessment.

Assessment of Physical Growth

Periodic evaluation of height and weight gains during adolescence provides important clues to physiological maturity and general well-being. During the pubertal growth spurt, the rate of growth accelerates dramatically during an 18- to 24-month period. Peak growth rate correlates positively with sexual maturity. Generally, girls achieve their peak growth rate during Tanner stage III, while boys do so during Tanner stage IV (Lee, 1980). (Tanner's criteria are used to stage sexual maturity, described in the next section.) Because there is wide variation in the ages at which adolescents mature sexually, there are also significant differences in physical growth among teens of the same chronological ages. Therefore, stage of sexual maturity is a more reliable correlate of physical growth than is chronological age (Lee, 1980).

The techniques for measuring height and weight in adolescents are the same as those used for adults. Measurements should be plotted on a standardized height and weight chart according to gender (see chap. 22). Interpretations of findings should take into account the teenager's previous growth pattern, family growth characteristics, ethnic/racial heritage (Asian adolescents are shorter and weigh less, on average, than white children, whereas African-American teenagers generally are taller and heavier), nutritional status, presence of any chronic health problems (e.g., insulin-dependent diabetes, asthma), and sexual maturity stage.

When findings reveal a concern about the adolescent's physical growth, referral for further evaluation is warranted. Late-maturing adolescents often express concern about their stature. Boys who have reached Tanner's sexual maturity stage 3 and girls who have reached stage 2 may be reassured that they can expect to achieve gains in height within the next 6 to 12 months. However, girls who have not begun their growth spurt by age 14 and boys who have not done so by age 15 should be referred for evaluation of delayed growth.

Appraisal of Sexual Maturity

Assessment of sexual maturity should be included in the examination of prepubescent, pubescent, and postpubescent clients. Because of the adolescent's extreme modesty and sensitivity, this portion of the clinical appraisal should be delayed until the end of the examination.

The nurse should explain to the adolescent the sequence of sexual changes that occurs during puberty and emphasize that the examination of sexual characteristics is performed to determine whether sexual maturation is progressing as expected. Because adolescents are concerned about their physical development and appearance, they usually are receptive to this portion of the examination, as long as it is conducted in a matter-of-fact, yet sensitive manner, and in a way that ensures their privacy.

The sexual maturity assessment primarily involves observation and inspection of visible secondary sex characteristics. The development of secondary sex characteristics proceeds through a series of clearly defined stages (Tanner, 1962), beginning two years earlier on the average in girls than in boys. Appraisal of sexual maturity using Tanner's stages as a guide enables the nurse to assess for normality or to screen for delayed onset of puberty, which requires further evaluation.

Tanner (1962) identifies four stages of pubic hair development in both males and females and five stages of female breast development and male genital development. The findings of the sexual maturity appraisal can be compared with Tanner's identified characteristics, which are illustrated in Figures 23-6 (female breast development), 23-7 (female pubic hair development), 23-8 (male genital development), and 23-9 (male pubic hair development). The stages are summarized in Table 23-12 as well.

Because there is a wide range of normal in the rate at which young adolescents mature sexually, adolescents often need reassurance that they are developing normally, even if they are maturing sexually at a faster or slower pace than their peers. Lee (1980) summarizes the mean ages of significant pubertal events in American adolescents (see Table 23-13), which are useful reference points. Findings that deviate from expected norms warrant referral for further evaluation and possibly intervention.

Findings of the sexual maturity appraisal should be recorded in the health record. Polaroid photographs of the breasts (girls), external genitalia (boys), and pubic hair development (both sexes) may be taken with the client's and parent's written permission, for inclusion in the health record and for future comparison on subsequent health visits. This practice is especially important when the adolescent is experiencing a delay in onset of secondary sex characteristics.

Appraisal of Females

When examining girls during this portion of the clinical appraisal, the nurse should begin with an appraisal of breast and axillary hair development. The client should be instructed to remove her clothing to the waist to enable adequate observation. With the client in a sitting or standing position, breast development should be staged using Tanner's criteria. For example, breasts with small raised breast buds should be classified as Tanner stage 2 (see Figure 23-6). The breasts should be examined with the same technique used for adult women (see chap. 13). This provides an excellent opportunity to teach the adolescent how to examine her own breasts, using the technique recommended by the American Cancer Society. Initiation of the practice of monthly breast self-examination during the teen years helps establish positive health habits early in life.

The presence, extent, and color of axillary hair also should be noted, although the nurse may have to base the assessment on the presence of hair stubble if the teenager has begun shaving under her arms. The practice of choosing to shave or not

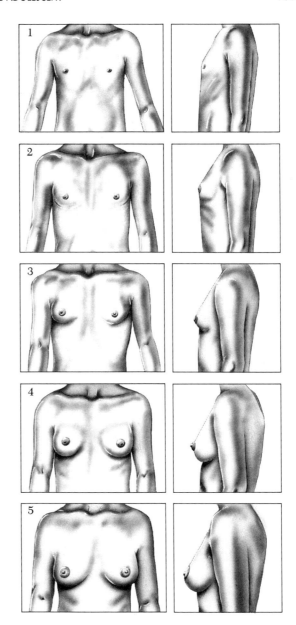

FIGURE 23-6. Stages of Breast Development in Adolescent Girls. (1) Prepubertal flat appearance like that of a child. (2) Small, raised breast bud. (3) General enlargement and raising of breast and areola. (4) Areola and papilla (nipple) form contour separate from that of breast. (5) Adult breast—areola is in same contour as breast. (*Note.* Adapted from Tanner, J.M. [1962]. *Growth in Adolescence* [2nd ed.]. Oxford: Blackwell. Used by permission of the author.)

shave axillary hair is determined culturally and often is influenced by religious beliefs.

Upon concluding the examination of the breasts and axillary region, the client should be instructed to dress from the waist up and undress from the waist down. With the teenager in a standing position, the nurse should observe the pres-

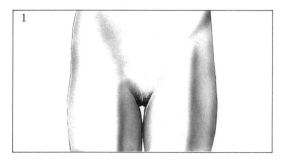

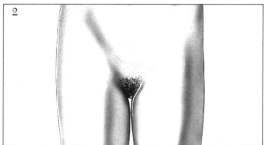

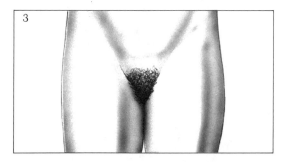

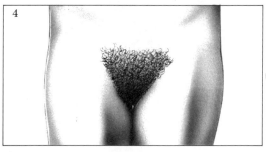

FIGURE 23-7. Stages of Pubic Hair Development in Adolescent Girls. (1) Sparse growth of downy hair mainly at sides of labia. (2) Pigmentation, coarsening, and curling, with an increase in the amount of hair. (3) Adult hair, but limited in area. (4) Adult hair with horizontal upper border. (*Note.* Adapted from Tanner, J.M. [1962]. *Growth in Adolescence* [2nd ed.]. Oxford: Blackwell. Used by permission of the author.)

ence, color, and distribution of pubic hair, noting the stage of pubic hair development according to Tanner's criteria. Sparse growth of downy hair on the labia, for example, indicates Tanner's stage 1 (see Figure 23-7). While the teenager is standing, the nurse also should look for broadening of the pelvis and fatty pad development, most noticeable in the hips, thighs, and buttocks.

Appraisal of Males

While obtaining the health history, voice pitch and fluctuations in voice tones can be assessed. The nurse should begin the clinical appraisal of sexual maturity in teenage boys by inspecting the distribution of hair on the face and chest and in the axillary region. Muscle development of the chest and upper arms should be noted as well.

The client should be asked to remove his underwear, and while he is in a standing position, the nurse should inspect the size of the penis (noting whether the client has been circumcised), the size and color of the scrotal sac, and the presence, color, and distribution of pubic hair. In uncircumcised clients, the foreskin of the penis should be retracted gently and the glans inspected. The scrotal sac should be palpated for texture, the presence and size of the testes, and any unusual findings such as fluid or a mass. Findings should be staged, using Tanner's criteria for genital and pubic hair development (see Figures 23-8 and 23-9). The nurse should use this opportunity to teach the adolescent how to perform testicular self-examination (see chap. 13).

Self-Assessment of Sexual Maturity

An alternative method of appraising sexual maturity is self-assessment of secondary sex characteristics. Self-assessment can be performed by showing the teenager body drawings of Tanner's stages (such as those depicted here) and asking the client to compare his or her own sexual maturation to the drawings. Duke, Litt, and Goss (1980) report a high correlation between adolescent self-assessments of sexual maturation and those performed by health-care providers.

Scoliosis Screening

Scoliosis, a lateral curvature of the spine, is a relatively common health problem in adolescence, particularly among girls. Approximately 25 adolescents per 1,000 require treatment for this disorder (Scoloveno, Yarcheski, & Mahon, 1990). Therefore, periodic assessment of the spine is a critical part of any adolescent health appraisal. Screening for scoliosis should be incorporated in the clinical appraisal of the adolescent's physical fitness and mobility.

Normally, the spine has an anteroposterior "S" curvature, with convex curves in the cervical and lumbar regions and concave curves in the thoracic and pelvic regions (see Figure 23-10). This curvature develops gradually from birth, at which time only the thoracic and pelvic curves are present.

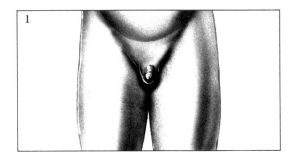
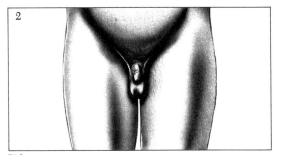
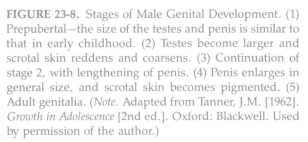
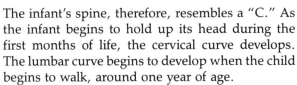
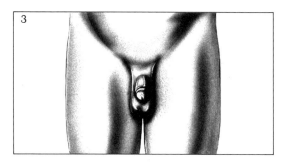

FIGURE 23-8. Stages of Male Genital Development. (1) Prepubertal—the size of the testes and penis is similar to that in early childhood. (2) Testes become larger and scrotal skin reddens and coarsens. (3) Continuation of stage 2, with lengthening of penis. (4) Penis enlarges in general size, and scrotal skin becomes pigmented. (5) Adult genitalia. (*Note.* Adapted from Tanner, J.M. [1962]. *Growth in Adolescence* [2nd ed.]. Oxford: Blackwell. Used by permission of the author.)

The infant's spine, therefore, resembles a "C." As the infant begins to hold up its head during the first months of life, the cervical curve develops. The lumbar curve begins to develop when the child begins to walk, around one year of age.

Idiopathic scoliosis is the most common type and a major health problem of adolescence. Routine annual screening for scoliosis should be conducted between the ages of 10 and 18, since early detection is essential for prevention of permanent deformity or disability. Mass screening can be performed effectively in the schools, thereby reducing cost and improving detection.

The procedure used to screen for scoliosis is a relatively simple one, relying on observation and inspection. Ideally, the adolescent should be undressed except for underwear, although when screening large school populations, the adolescent may undress only to the waist (girls may keep their bras on). With the adolescent in a standing position, the nurse should observe the posture while standing in front, to the side, and in back of the client. The shoulders and scapula should be observed for symmetry. The shoulder and scapula on the convex side of a scoliotic curve will be higher

than the opposite side. The rib cage also may be more prominent and the waist may appear fuller on the convex side of the curve. The iliac crest on the concave side may be elevated.

The client then should be instructed to bend forward halfway, with arms dangling in front, so the upper torso is perpendicular to the lower half of the body. When scoliosis is present, thoracic asymmetry often is more pronounced in this position, and a hump will be visible on the convex side of the curve owing to the elevation of the scapula and rib cage on that side. Alignment of the spine should be inspected for any deviation.

Figure 23-11 illustrates the screening procedure for detection of scoliosis. When performing mass screenings, efficiency can be increased with two examiners, one positioned in front of the client and the other behind the client.

NURSING DIAGNOSES RELATED TO THE ADOLESCENT

The findings of the nursing assessment may indicate that the adolescent is developing normally without notable health concerns or health prob-

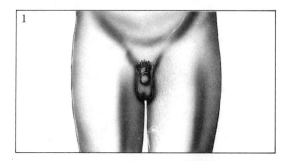
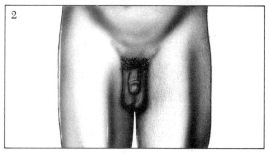
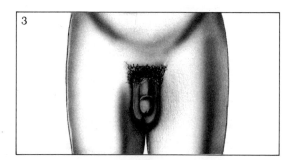
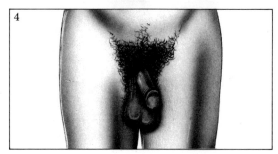

FIGURE 23-9. Stages of Pubic Hair Development in Adolescent Boys. (1) Sparse growth of downy hair mainly at base of penis. (2) Pigmentation, coarsening, and curling, with an increase in amount of hair. (3) Adult hair, but limited in area. (4) Adult hair with horizontal upper border and spread to thighs. (*Note.* Adapted from Tanner, J.M. [1962]. *Growth in Adolescence* [2nd ed.]. Oxford: Blackwell. Used by permission of the author.)

lems. In such instances, the assessment can be used as the basis for guidance and health teaching. Adoption or continuation of positive health practices during adolescence can contribute to the development of lifelong habits that maintain and improve the individual's health and well-being.

TABLE 23-12
Stages of Sexual Maturation

Stage	Pubic Hair	Genitalia/Breasts
Males		
Stage 1	Sparse growth of downy hair at base of penis	Prepubertal—size of penis and testes similar to early childhood
Stage 2	Darkens, coarsens, and curls	Testes enlarge (5 ml); scrotal skin reddens and thickens
Stage 3	Adult hair, but does not extend to thighs	Lengthening of penis and further enlargement of testes (10 ml)
Stage 4	Adult hair with horizontal upper border; spreads to thighs	Penis enlarges (width and length); testes 12 ml; scrotal skin darkens
Stage 5		Adult size; testes 15 ml
Females		
Stage 1	Sparse growth of downy hair at sides of labia	Prepubertal flat appearance
Stage 2	Darkens, coarsens, and curls	Small, raised breast bud
Stage 3	Adult hair, but limited in area	General enlargement and raising of breast and areola
Stage 4	Adult hair with horizontal upper border; spreads to thighs	Areola and nipple form contour separate from breast
Stage 5		Adult breasts; areola continues with breast contour

TABLE 23-13
Mean Ages of Significant Pubertal Events in American Adolescents

Pubertal Event*	Females	Males	Pubertal Event*	Females	Males
Br 2	11.2 ± 1.6		PH 3	12.7 ± 0.5	13.9 ± 0.9
G 2		11.9 ± 1.1	Voice change		14.1 ± 0.9
PH 2	11.9 ± 1.5	12.3 ± 0.8	Acne	13.2 ± 0.5	14.3 ± 1.3
G 3		13.2 ± 0.8	G 4		14.3 ± 0.8
Gynecomastia		13.2 ± 0.8	Regular menses	13.9 ± 1.0	
Voice break		13.5 ± 1.0	PH 4	13.4 ± 1.2	14.7 ± 0.9
Peak height velocity	12.5 ± 1.5	13.8 ± 1.1	Br 4	13.1 ± 0.7	
Peak weight gain	12.4 ± 1.4	13.9 ± 0.9	Facial hair		14.9 ± 1.1
Axillary hair	13.1 ± 0.8	14.0 ± 1.1	Br 5	14.5 ± 1.6	
Br 3	12.4 ± 1.2		G 5		15.1 ± 1.1
Menarche	13.3 ± 1.3		PH 5	14.6 ± 1.1	15.3 ± 0.8

*Br, breast; G, genital; PH, pubic hair; Br 2—breast development Tanner stage 2; G 4—genital development, Tanner stage 4

Reprinted by permission of Elsevier Science Publishing Co., Inc., from "Normal Ages of Pubertal Events Among American Males and Females," by P.A. Lee, *Journal of Adolescent Health Care*, 1(1), 28. Copyright 1980 by the Society for Adolescent Medicine.

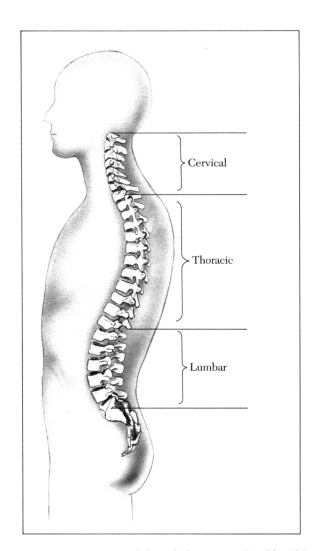

FIGURE 23-10. Normal Spinal Curvature (Double "S" Curve).

Proper diet, regular exercise, routine practice of breast or testicular self-examination, use of seatbelts, and avoidance of health hazards such as smoking, alcohol consumption, drug use, and sexually transmitted diseases, give the adolescent an excellent start on the path to adult health. Adolescents who are healthy and who establish positive health practices during their teenage years enjoy a sense of well-being, self-sufficiency, and personal competence that helps them cope with the new challenges and demands they face as they mature.

Because of their unique characteristics and the dramatic changes that take place during the teenage years, certain nursing diagnoses occur with relative frequency in adolescents. Adolescents who experience a delay in onset of puberty, for example, may be diagnosed with "altered growth and development." Those who encounter particular difficulty in coping with the demands placed on them as they grow older, and who resort to acting out behavior or use of drugs or alcohol, may be exhibiting "ineffective individual coping" related to, for example, value conflicts with parents or society, low self-esteem, or lack of social support.

Early or late-maturing teens may be at risk for "self-esteem disturbance." The psychosocial effects of early sexual maturation have been shown to be pronounced for some individuals, particularly late-maturing boys (Blyth, Bulcroft, & Simmons, 1981). Research has shown that late-maturing boys are at a disadvantage in sports competition and in relationships with girls, are less likely to assume leadership roles, and may feel inadequate in social situations (Livson & Peskin, 1980).

Because many adolescents develop acne, "im-

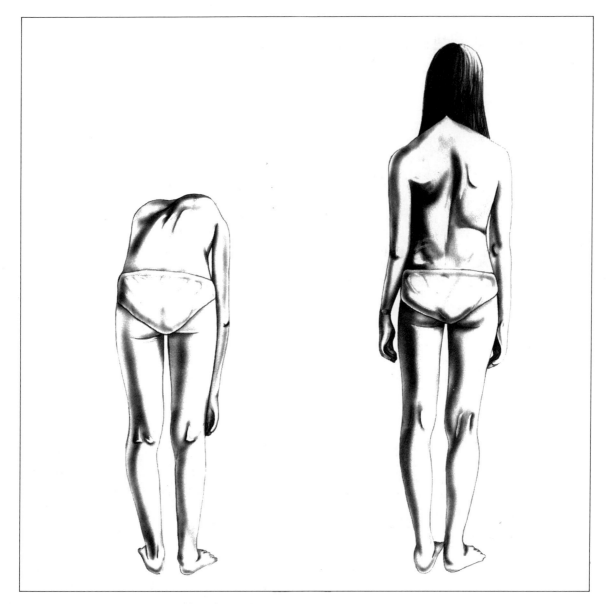

FIGURE 23-11. Screening Procedure for Scoliosis.

paired skin integrity" is a common nursing diagnosis. Impaired skin integrity may be related to excessive sebaceous gland secretions, use of oral contraceptives, or ineffective cleansing of the skin. Poor eating habits can lead to insufficient intake of minerals or vitamins or excessive intake of calories and fat. In such instances, a nursing diagnosis of "altered nutrition" should be formulated, specifying whether the problem is one of excessive (*more than body requirements*) or deficient (*less than body requirements*) intake. Eating behaviors, such as overeating, binge eating, purging, or excessive dieting, also can contribute to a diagnosis of "altered nutrition."

Detection of scoliosis during adolescence warrants a nursing diagnosis of "impaired physical mobility." Related factors may include bracing, surgery, or failure to adhere to the medical treatment plan. The presence of scoliosis or its various treatments also may affect the adolescent's self-concept, resulting in a diagnosis of "body image disturbance."

Adequate knowledge of adolescent characteristics and development, comprehensive assessment of the adolescent client, and careful analysis of all available information enable the nurse to identify actual or potential responses to adolescent health problems that require nursing intervention. Failure to address the unique and particular needs of the adolescent client for comprehensive, sensitive care

TABLE 23-14
Common Nursing Diagnoses Related to Adolescence

Altered nutrition (more or less than body requirements) related to excessive intake, binge eating, purging, or compulsive dieting

Impaired skin integrity (acne) related to ineffective cleansing of the skin, use of oral contraceptives, use of oil-based cosmetics, or excessive sebaceous secretions

Ineffective individual coping related to value conflicts with parents/society, low self-esteem, or lack of social support

Impaired physical mobility related to bracing or surgery for scoliosis, or failure to adhere to treatment plan for scoliosis

Altered growth and development related to delayed onset of puberty or physical disability

Self-esteem disturbance related to school failure, social inadequacy, or late maturation

can compromise the entire assessment, prevent accurate and timely identification of nursing diagnoses, and delay the initiation of appropriate interventions.

Chapter Highlights

■ Adolescence is a biological, psychosocial, and cultural phenomenon characterized by dramatic changes in physical appearance, intellectual capacity, and personal and social behavior.

■ Adolescents in each phase (young, middle, late) of this developmental period share certain physical, cognitive, and social characteristics that distinguish them from those in other phases.

■ The biological hallmark of adolescence is puberty, a maturational and hormonal process by which the reproductive system begins to function.

■ Puberty is distinguished by the appearance of secondary sex characteristics, dramatic increases in height and weight, integumentary changes, and increased nutritional requirements. Girls begin puberty and achieve sexual maturity approximately two years earlier on the average than boys.

■ The unique physical and behavioral characteristics of adolescents require modifications in how the nurse approaches, interacts with, and examines the adolescent client.

■ The adolescent should be the primary source for the nursing history, with parents or significant others providing supplemental information.

■ Because adolescents are concerned about their physical development and appearance, they usually are receptive to being examined, as long as the appraisal is performed in a matter-of-fact, yet sensitive manner and in a way that ensures their privacy.

■ Aspects of the clinical appraisal that should be part of the nursing assessment of every adolescent include examination for sexual maturity (Tanner's stages) and screening for scoliosis.

■ Common nursing diagnoses during adolescence include "impaired skin integrity" related to acne; "self-esteem disturbance" related to growth changes, delayed sexual development, or acne; "impaired physical mobility" related to bracing or spinal fusion surgery for scoliosis; and "altered nutrition" related to insufficient or excessive intake.

Practice Activities

1. Observe young (12–13 year olds), middle (14–16 year olds), and older (17–19 year olds) adolescents at a social event (dance, shopping mall, athletic event, movie theater, etc.). Compare and contrast their characteristics and behaviors: physical growth, appearance (skin, hair, clothing, grooming), interactions with others (peers of same and opposite sex, adults), and activities. What conclusions can you draw? What biological, psychosocial, and cultural forces play a role in shaping adolescent behavior at these different ages?

2. Obtain a health history (using the health history format provided in this chapter) from an early, middle, and older adolescent. Compare and contrast your findings. What conclusions can you draw? What nursing diagnoses are suggested? How can you validate your judgments?

3. Visit a high school classroom to ascertain:
   ■ health concerns ("What questions or concerns do you have about your health?")
   ■ health habits (nutrition, exercise, sleep, use of seatbelts, practice of BSE or TSE, dental hygiene, tobacco use)

What nursing diagnoses are suggested? Formulate a health teaching plan based on your findings. While at the high school, analyze the week's lunch menu for nutritional value. What are your findings? What are the implications for nursing care planning?

4. Perform scoliosis screening for at least 5 adolescents between 11 and 15 years of age. Interpret and record your findings. Report abnormal findings to parents or school personnel.

5. Perform a complete clinical appraisal of at least one male and one female adolescent between the ages of 12 and 17 years, including evaluation of sexual maturity (Tanner's stages). Record and analyze your findings. What nursing diagnoses are suggested?

Recommended Readings

Blum, R. (1987). Contemporary threats to adolescent health in the United States. *JAMA (Journal of the American Medical Association)*, 257, 3390–3395.

Elkind, D. (1984). Teenage thinking: Implications for health care. *Pediatric Nursing, 10*, 383–385.

Jack, M.S. (1989). Personal fable: A potential explanation for risk-taking behavior in adolescents. *Journal of Pediatric Nursing, 4*, 334–338.

Jordan, D., & Kelfer, L.S. (1983). Adolescent potential for participation in health care. *Issues in Comprehensive Pediatric Nursing, 6*, 147–156.

Kozinetz, C.A. (1986). Two noninvasive methods to measure female maturation. *Journal of School Health, 56*, 440–442.

Nelms, B.C. (1981). What is a normal adolescent? *MCN: The American Journal of Maternal-Child Nursing, 6*, 402–406.

Parker, F.C., Croft, J.B., Spuik, J.D., Webber, L.S., Hunter, S.M., & Berenson, G.S. (1986). Factors associated with adolescent participation in a cardiovascular risk factor assessment program. *Journal of School Health, 56*, 23–28.

Scoloveno, M.A., Yarcheski, A., & Mahon, N.E. (1990). Scoliosis treatment effects on selected variables among adolescents. *Western Journal of Nursing Research, 12*, 601–618.

Smith, K.L.D., Turner, J.G., & Jacobsen, R.B. (1987). Health concerns of adolescents. *Pediatric Nursing, 13*, 311–315.

Thomas, S.P., & Groer, M.W. (1986). Relationship of demographic, life-style, and stress variables to blood pressure in adolescents. *Nursing Research, 35*, 169–172.

Yoos, L. (1987). Adolescent cognitive and contraceptive behaviors. *Pediatric Nursing, 13*(4), 247–250.

References

American Academy of Pediatrics. (1982). Joint Committee on Infant Hearing: Position statement 1982. *Pediatrics, 70*, 496–497.

Bishop, B.E. (1979). Foreword. In R. T. Mercer (Ed.), *Perspectives on adolescent health care* (p. xvi). Philadelphia: Lippincott.

Blyth, D.A., Bulcroft, R., & Simmons, R.G. (1981, August). The impact of puberty on adolescents: A longitudinal study. Paper presented at the Annual Meeting of the American Psychological Association, Los Angeles, CA.

Bullough, V.L. (1981). Age at menarche: A misunderstanding. *Science, 213*, 365–366.

Chumlea, W.C. (1981). Size and number of adipocytes and measures of body fat in boys and girls 10 to 18 years of age. *American Journal of Clinical Nutrition, 34*, 1791.

Coleman, J.S. (Ed.). (1974). *Youth: Transition to adulthood.* Report of the Panel on Youth of the President's Science Advisory Committee. Chicago: University of Chicago Press.

Dessendorfer, E.A., Amsterdam, E.A., & Odland, T.M. (1983). Adolescent smoking and its effect on aerobic exercise tolerance. *Physical Sports Medicine, 11*, 109–119.

Duke, P.M., Litt, I.F., & Goss, R.T. (1980). Adolescents' self-assessment of sexual maturation. *Pediatrics, 66*, 918–920.

Elkind, D. (1981). *The hurried child.* Reading, MA: Addison-Wesley.

Erikson, E.H. (1980). *Identity and the life cycle.* New York: Norton.

Forbes, G.B. (1981). Nutritional requirements in adolescence. In R.M. Suskind (Ed.), *Textbook of pediatric nutrition.* New York: Raven.

Frisch, R.E. (1983). Fatness, puberty, and fertility. In J. Brooks-Gunn & A.C. Peterson (Eds.), *Girls at puberty: Biological, psychological, and social perspectives.* New York: Plenum.

Gilliam, D. (1983, September 27). Why do we insist on rushing kids into growing up? *The Philadelphia Inquirer.*

Gilligan, C. (1982). *In a different voice: Psychological theory and women's development.* Cambridge, MA: Harvard University Press.

Greer, R.O. (1983). Smokeless tobacco: An unheralded adolescent peril. *New York State Journal of Medicine, 83*, 1370–1371.

Guggenheimer, J., Zullo, T.G., Druper, D.C., & Verbin, R.S. (1986). Changing trends of tobacco use in a teenage population in Western Pennsylvania. *American Journal of Public Health, 76*, 196–197.

Heisel, J.S., Ream, S., Raitz, R., Rappaport, M., & Coddington, R.D. (1973). The significance of life events as contributing factors in the diseases of children. *Journal of Pediatrics, 83*, 119.

Kett, J.F. (1977). *Rites of passage: Adolescence in America 1790 to the present.* New York: Basic.

Latinis, B. (1983). Frequent sports injuries of children: Etiology, treatment, and prevention. *Issues in Comprehensive Pediatric Nursing, 6*, 167–178.

Lee, P.A. (1980). Normal ages of pubertal events among American males and females. *Journal of Adolescent Health Care, 1*, 28.

Livsin, N. & Peskin, H. (1980). Perspectives on adolescence from longitudinal research. In J. Adelson (Ed.), *Handbook of adolescent psychology*, New York: Wiley.

Lucas, B., Rees, J.M., & Mahan, L.K. (1985). Nutrition and the adolescent. In P.L. Pipes (Ed.), *Nutrition in infancy and childhood* (3rd ed.). St. Louis: Mosby.

Marino, D.D., & King, J.C. (1980). Nutritional concerns during adolescence. *Pediatric Clinics of North America, 27*, 125–140.

Marty, P.J., McDermott, R.J., & Williams, T. (1986). Patterns of smokeless tobacco use in a population of high school students. *American Journal of Public Health, 76*, 190–192.

Postman, N. (1982). *The disappearance of childhood.* New York: Delacorte.

Scoloveno, M.A., Yarcheski, A., & Mahon, N.E. (1990). Scoliosis treatment effects on selected variables among adolescents. *Western Journal of Nursing Research, 12*, 601–618.

Smith, K.L.D., Turner, J.G., & Jacobsen, R.B. (1987). Health concerns of adolescents. *Pediatric Nursing, 13*, 311–315.

Staff Report on Cigarette Advertising Investigation. (1981). Washington, DC: Federal Trade Commission.

Tanner, J.M. (1962). *Growth at adolescence* (2nd ed.). Oxford: Blackwell.

Tanner, J.M. (1973). Growing up. *Scientific American, 43*, 165–168.

Tanner, J.M., & Davies, P.S. (1985). Clinical longitudinal standards for height and height velocity of North American children. *Journal of Pediatrics, 107*, 317–329.

U.S. Bureau of the Census (1987). *Statistical abstract of the United States: 1987* (107th ed.). Washington, DC: U.S. Government Printing Office.

U.S. Public Health Service. (1981). *The health consequences of smoking: The changing cigarette: A report of the Surgeon General.* Washington, DC: U.S. Department of Health and Human Services.

Assessment of the Older Adult

OBJECTIVES

Upon completion of this chapter, you should be able to:

- Recognize the importance of using a multi-dimensional approach in the assessment of the older adult.
- Discuss the unique characteristics of the older adult.
- Describe the changes in body function and structure that commonly occur with aging.
- Describe the ways in which the nurse's approach to obtaining a nursing history should be modified for the older adult.
- Examine specific methods that are used to obtain a multidimensional nursing history of the older adult.
- Discuss modifications in the approach to the clinical appraisal of the older adult.
- Recognize the importance of screening as a component of the nursing assessment of the older adult.
- Delineate guidelines for health screening in the older adult.
- Conduct a comprehensive assessment of an older adult.
- Formulate appropriate nursing diagnoses for the older adult experiencing alterations in health.

The assessment of the older adult differs from that of the younger adult in many ways. Not only must one consider the changes that occur with aging and the interaction of these changes with acute and chronic illnesses, one must also be aware of the demands of the physical and social environment of the older person (Matteson & McConnell, 1988). Sickness, health, and normality all take on new dimensions when assessing the older adult. Assessment of the older individual is one of the most challenging tasks in clinical nursing because of the complex nature of the assessment process. It is clearly a multidimensional process involving mental health, physical health, functional health, and socioeconomic status.

Older adults are unique in that they may be harboring two or more chronic diseases, taking several medications, and still be functioning at a high level of health. The focus of the health assessment should be to identify those positive health practices that have enabled the older adult to maintain optimal health and functioning over the years and to determine the factors that influence or cause impairments or health problems. Approaching assessment in this manner enables the nurse to determine which practices could make a difference in the individual's health if they were modified or improved (Carotenuto & Bullock, 1980).

UNIQUE CHARACTERISTICS OF THE OLDER ADULT

People are living longer than ever before. The average life span has almost doubled since 1945. Those who are 85 and older are the fastest growing portion of the aging population. This group consists of frail elderly people who are often in need of health care and supportive living conditions. As this segment continues to grow and the baby boomers age, the nation will have a health-care problem greater than any problem previously faced. There will not only be an absence of dollars for health care, there will be an absence of people to care for the elderly people. The disproportionate growth in the older age group is shown in Figure 24-1.

Even more frightening are the statistics recently released by the Alzheimer's Disease Association (1990). The association states that 42% of those living past 85 have Alzheimer's disease. These Alzheimer patients have no private health insurance. Most private nursing home insurance policies exclude persons with Alzheimer's, leaving families with no recourse but to resort to Medicaid to care for their loved ones.

Heart disease and cancer are the leading causes of death for both men and women, followed by cerebrovascular diseases and pneumonia. All chronic diseases are more frequent in late life. Thus, as people grow older, they assess their health as poor. On the average, older people spend 32 days out of a year in restricted activity because of their health, leaving them 333 functional days for living out their lives (Beck, 1989). Most sick days are attributable to the 10 leading causes of death displayed in Table 24-1.

As Medicare costs rise, there is a tug of war for the health-care dollar between the young and the old. Callahan (1987) suggests that all medical treatments stop at the age of 85 as a way of controlling health-care costs. His statements have promoted great ethical discussions of health-care rationing. Horace Deets (1991), the director of American Association of Retired Persons (AARP), states that rationing health care defies American values.

On the bright side, many older people are leading healthier lives. They are exercising more, have more money for recreation, and enjoy their leisure time. The new Omnibus Budget Reconciliation Act (1987) provides the elderly with some additional protection. Those with higher incomes pay more for services. Those at the poverty level have greater benefits, such as having their Medicare B premiums paid. The bill also attends to women— all women over 65 receive regular mammograms.

To prepare for the future, nurses must focus on long-term care and nursing services provided in the home. Families may need to become more skilled in caregiving and assume much of the burden for care of their older relatives. They will, however, need continual teaching and counseling by nurses. Essentially, as the sick move out of the hospital into the home and extended care settings, nurses will be case managers more than care providers.

Older people's health will be judged by their ability to function rather than by the number of chronic illnesses housed in their bodies. The highest level of functioning possible will be the goal of care. Because chronic functional impairment increases with age, older people carry a disproportionate burden of disability. Disability and rehabilitation to increase functional ability will be the focus of federal funding. Nurses who promote independence and self-care will be the most effective caregivers for the elderly.

KNOWLEDGE NEEDED TO ASSESS THE OLDER ADULT

The process of aging begins the very day we are born. The rate at which one ages and the manifes-

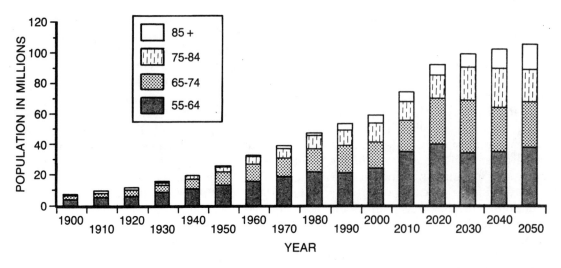

FIGURE 24-1. Population 55 Years and Over by Age: 1900–2050. (*Note.* From Taueber, C.M., U.S. Bureau of the Census. "America in Transition: An Aging Society." *Current Population Reports* Series P-23, No. 128 [September 1983] [for years 1900–1980]; and Spencer, G., U.S. Bureau of the Census. "Projections of the Population of the United States, by Age, Sex, and Race: 1983 to 2080." *Current Population Reports* Series P-25, No. 952 [May 1984] [for years 1990–2050]).

TABLE 24-1
Mortality, Ten Leading Causes of Death for Ages 75+ (1985)

Male	Female
All causes 421,525	All causes 566,374
Heart diseases 177,192	Heart diseases 258,426
Cancer 79,220	Cancer 78,921
Cerebrovascular diseases 34,934	Cerebrovascular diseases 68,278
Pneumonia, influenza 21,483	Pneumonia, influenza 27,518
Chronic obstructive lung diseases 21,366	Arteriosclerosis 13,265
Accidents 7,685	Chronic obstructive lung diseases 12,201
Arteriosclerosis 6,607	Diabetes 11,296
Diabetes 5,829	Accidents 8,703
Nephritis 5,808	Nephritis 6,874
Aortic aneurysm 4,424	Septicemia, pyemia 5,935

Note. From Vital Statistics of the United States, 1985.

tations of this process depend on genetic factors, environment, health, presence of illness, lifestyle, patterns of exercise and sleep, nutrition, stress, and a number of other factors (Eliopoulos, 1987).

As the nurse assesses the older adult, those 65 and older, some guidelines should be remembered. All functional changes are not necessarily related to disease. While many changes in biological function occur with aging (Table 24-2), other changes are associated with illness. Once diagnosed, these can be treated. Beginning students often have difficulty distinguishing normal age-related changes from pathological changes. In addition, because many variables influence the process of aging, assessment of older people is not only challenging but very complex (Rutledge, 1988). The ability to accurately and comprehensively assess the health needs of older individuals is "an art born of experience" (Ebersole & Hess, 1990).

With advancing age, the body has less reserve capacity and less resistance. Because compensatory mechanisms slow and sensory receptors decline, the body's response to injury or illness is not as vigorous. As a result, the body is less able to adapt and becomes more vulnerable to illness (Hudson, 1983). Because of these changes, it is often more difficult to diagnose disease in the older adult; the signs and symptoms may not be as obvious as they would be in a younger individual. In the older adult, both the quality and quantity of symptoms are modified (Burnside, 1988). Health

TABLE 24-2
Changes in Biological Function Between the Ages
of 30 and 70

Biological Function	Change
Work capacity (%)	Decreases 25–30
Cardiac output (%)	Decreases 30
Maximal heart rate (beats/min)	Decreases 24
Blood pressure (mm Hg)	
Systolic	Increases 10–40
Diastolic	Increases 5–10
Respiration (%)	
Vital capacity	Decreases 40–50
Residual volume	Increases 30–50
Basal metabolic rate (%)	Decreases 8–12
Musculature (%)	
Muscle mass	Decreases 25–30
Hand grip strength	Decreases 25–30
Nerve conduction velocity (%)	Decreases 10–15
Flexibility (%)	Decreases 20–30
Bone (%)	
Women	Decreases 25–30
Men	Decreases 15–20
Renal function (%)	Decreases 30–50

Note. From E.L. Smith and C. Gilligan, Physical activity prescription for the older adult. The *Physician and Sports Medicine,* 11(8): 91–101, copyright 1983. Reprinted by permission of McGraw-Hill, Inc.

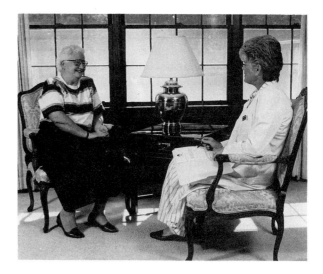

FIGURE 24-2. Older adults should be encouraged to discuss changes in their bodies to determine whether there is underlying disease or whether the changes are age-related.

problems in older individuals often come in clusters. While one problem may predominate, it can precipitate other problems (Hudson, 1983). Careful and thorough assessment is most important in order to determine whether specific signs and symptoms are related to a larger problem or indicate different health problems.

Older adults may hesitate to mention changes in their bodies because they perceive the changes to be a normal part of aging. Changes should be explored in order to determine whether there is an underlying illness or whether the changes are age-related (Burnside, 1988). An understanding of the structural and functional changes associated with aging will provide the nurse with the knowledge necessary for accurate and comprehensive assessment of the older adult.

Physical Integrity

Body temperature is maintained by the thermoregulatory center through the complex mechanisms of sweating, shivering, vasoconstriction and vasodilation, and chemical thermogenesis (Kane, Ouslander, & Abrass, 1989). Differences in body temperature regulation occur with aging. The el-

derly have a decreased ability to respond to changes in environmental temperature because sweat glands atrophy with age and the ability of the blood vessels to dilate or constrict declines. Shivering, the mechanism that produces heat in response to cold temperatures, is diminished. In addition, there is a general decrease in body temperature with age secondary to lowered metabolic rate and activity, decreased subcutaneous tissue, and poor circulation. Hypothermia and hyperthermia are of equal concern in the older adult. With age, the temperature regulator in the hypothalamus is not as effective. The loss of subcutaneous fat, with its insulating ability, further contributes to the older individual's decreased responsiveness to both hot and cold (see boxed insert).

The human body maintains normal temperature at approximately 98.6°F (plus or minus 1°F). Because older individuals have lower normal temperatures, accurate measurement of temperature is important. A study by Downton and colleagues (1987) examined the most accurate method for determining temperature in the older adult. The results indicated that the axillary and the oral methods of temperature measurement were not reliable indicators of core body temperature. Temperature measured with these methods was significantly lower than that obtained by the rectal method. This finding reflects the fact that differences between skin temperature and core temperature are greater in the older adult and more variable.

Because changes in temperature are less dramatic in the older adult, the nurse should be concerned about even a slight elevation in temperature. Infection in an older individual may not be accompanied by an elevated temperature and, therefore, a change in functioning may be a better indicator of illness than an elevated temperature (Miller, 1990). To accurately interpret temperature readings in the older adult, it is important to have some baseline measures. In addition, because normal temperature in the older adult tends to be below normal, it is important to use a thermometer that registers lower than 95°F.

The ability of the body to respond to antigens and protect against foreign cells and tumor formation is compromised due to structural and functional changes in the immune system of the older adult. As one ages, there is a decrease in natural antibodies and the body's response to antigenic stimuli. This occurs because the function of the thymus gland, which produces T lymphocytes (T cells) is greatly reduced. Only 5% to 10% of the gland functions at age 50. By age 60, thymic hormone production ceases. As a result of these changes, the older adult is less immunocompetent than younger individuals. Consequently, the older person is more vulnerable to illness.

A normal pulse usually ranges from 60 to 100 beats per minute. With aging, there is no change in the resting heart rate, but the heart takes longer to return to the resting state after activity. However, during strenuous activity the maximum heart rate achieved is decreased. Cardiac arrhythmias may occur with increasing frequency as one ages as a result of changes in the conduction mechanism of the heart. To determine an accurate reading, the pulse should be taken radially for one full minute. This then should be compared with the apical pulse to establish a baseline reading.

With aging, there is loss of arterial elasticity with a resulting increase in peripheral resistance. This causes a rise in systolic blood pressure with an accompanying slight rise in diastolic pressure. A systolic pressure of 160 over a diastolic pressure of 90 is considered within normal for the older adult. Research on the elderly has shown that systolic pressure increases more than diastolic pressure and that systolic pressure increases are greater in women than in men (Rowe & Lipsitz, 1988). A slight decrease in both systolic and diastolic pressure occurs in men and women after 75 years of age.

Structural and functional changes in the respiratory system occur gradually as one ages. This enables the older adult to maintain a relatively normal respiratory rate in the absence of any pathological process (Ebersole & Hess, 1990). However,

---

Physical Integrity

Temperature

- decreased ability to respond to changes in environmental temperature
- decrease in body temperature, subnormal not uncommon
- diminished sweating mechanism
- decreased febrile response to infection
- less dramatic changes in temperature

Pulse

- normal rate of 60–100 beats per minute in the resting state
- decrease in maximum heart rate during strenuous exercise
- increase in time required to return to resting state following exercise

Blood Pressure

- increase in systolic pressure
- slight increase in diastolic pressure

Respirations

- normal rate in the absence of any pathological process
- more abdominal movement than chest movement
- mouth breathing more common

Height

- loss of height anywhere from 2.5 cm to 10 cm, occurs gradually

Weight

- increases gradually until age 50 and then decreases
- accumulation of body fat particularly in the trunk

---

respiration may exhibit more abdominal movement than chest movement. This change is the result of a decrease in rib mobility, weakened intercostal muscles and diaphragm, increased calcification of the costal cartilages, and an increase in the anteroposterior diameter of the chest from degenerative changes in the thoracic spine (Yurick, Spier, Robb & Ebert, 1989). There is also a decrease in the number and size of alveoli (apical ventilation increases; basilar ventilation decreases). These factors, coupled with changes in ventilation, increase the occurrence of breathlessness with exercise commonly seen in older adults (Christ & Hohloch, 1988).

A loss of height is a normal age-related change. The spinal column shortens as a result of the thinning of the intervertebral discs. In addition, there is a reduction in the height of the individual vertebrae. Over time an adult may lose anywhere from 2.5 cm to 10 cm in total height.

During the adult years, weight increases gradually until one reaches the age of 50. After 50, weight begins to decrease due to the loss of body fluid and the replacement of the body's lean muscle mass by fat. "Thus, as the fluid parameters decrease relative to total weight, the percentage of fat increases," write Lamy and Vestal (1976, p. 113). The accumulation of body fat is accentuated in the trunk. By age 80, weight may decrease by as much as 30% (Christ & Hohloch, 1988).

As one ages, the overall appearance of the skin undergoes marked changes (see boxed insert). The rate at which the changes occur is influenced by health, diet, heredity, exposure, and drugs (Burnside, 1988). In the normal young adult, the epithelial skin layer is renewed every 20 days. The older individual requires 30 days or more to replace the epithelial layer due to decreased mitotic epidermal activity (Ebersole & Hess, 1990). This change in cellular activity results in delayed healing. The rate at which healing occurs in the older adult is considerably slower than the rate in a younger adult.

Exposure to environmental elements causes the skin to dry and the outer layer to become fragile. Sun-exposed skin looks weatherbeaten, exhibiting a thickened, yellowed, and deeply furrowed appearance. The skin thins with age due to the loss of elasticity and collagen. This becomes particularly noticeable on the backs of the hands, and forearms. In addition, the skin becomes paler and more opaque in white individuals as a result of the diminished vascularity of the dermis. The dermis is thinner in women than it is in men, which may explain why women appear to age more rapidly than men (Kligman, Grove, & Balin, 1985). As a result of these changes, the skin of the older adult becomes less elastic, more lax, lined, and wrinkled with age.

Pigmentation of the skin is altered with age because there are fewer melanocytes. However, in some areas of the skin melanin synthesis is increased, depositing more pigment. This results in the appearance of age spots, particularly on the backs of the hands and forearms. In addition to age spots (lentigines or "liver spots"), purpuric spots may appear on the skin. These result from the leakage of blood through weakened capillary structures within the dermis. The formation of purpuric spots, senile purpura, is more common in women than in men. There are a number of other commonly observed benign skin lesions in older cli-

---

Physical Integrity

Skin

- Delayed wound healing
- Increased dryness
- Exposed skin appears weather beaten, yellowed and deeply furrowed
- Loss of elasticity and collagen
- Diminished vascularity of the dermis (paler and more opaque)
- Increased wrinkling
- Appearance of age spots (lentigines) and purpuric spots (senile purpura)

---

ents, including skin (cutaneous) tags, sebaceous warts, cherry angiomas, and seborrheic keratosis. Seborrheic keratosis is a precancerous lesion and, therefore, should be evaluated.

The loss of pigment in the hair on the scalp causes graying as one grows older. Hair on the scalp also thins. This occurs more prominently in men than in women. In addition to the thinning of the hair on the scalp, overall body hair decreases as one ages, with the exception of the hair in the nose and ears, which thickens. Coarse facial hair may appear on the upper lip and chin of many women due to the decrease of estrogen and increase of androgen (see boxed insert).

The growth and strength of the nails decreases with age. The luster of the nails also diminishes. The nails thicken, develop longitudinal striations, and become more yellow, particularly on the toes.

Physical Integrity

Hair

- Loss of pigment; typical graying
- Thinning of scalp hair
- Decrease in overall body hair
- Appearance of coarse facial hair

Nails

- Decreased growth and strength
- Diminished luster
- Thickening and yellowing of nails, particularly on the toes

Glandular changes also occur with aging. The eccrine and apocrine glands, important in thermo-regulation and in the production of secretions creating body odor, diminish in number as well as functional ability with advancing age (Miller, 1990). While the sebaceous glands increase in size, the amount of sebum produced by the glands diminishes. As a result, there is less lubrication of the hair and skin and dryness results (Farrell, 1990).

Sensory-Perceptual-Neurological Status

Changes in sensory, perceptual and neurological status commonly occur with aging.

Sensory Functioning

"Each of the five senses becomes less efficient with advanced age, interfering in varying degrees with safety, normal activities of daily living and general well-being," writes Eliopoulis (1987, p. 62). The most significant changes probably occur in vision (see boxed insert). Visual acuity diminishes with age. There is a reduction in the size of the pupils (contraction of the iris muscle), opacification of the lens and vitreous, and a loss of photoreceptor cells in the retina (Miller, 1990). This makes it difficult for an older individual to distinguish the fine details of objects. Yurick and colleagues (1989) note that older individuals experiencing the normal age-related changes in visual acuity can be helped by providing more illumination in the environment.

Older individuals commonly develop *presbyopia* or farsightedness (loss of near vision) and require corrective lenses. This occurs because of a decrease in the ability of the lens to accommodate or focus quickly and clearly on objects in the visual field. In addition, the elasticity in the muscles of the eye diminishes. These combined changes have the overall effect of reducing the focusing power of the eye (Farrell, 1990). Senile macular degeneration (retinal disease) can occur with advancing age, causing blindness. Screening for macular degeneration is important because if discovered early enough, surgery can save the eyesight.

The ability to see peripherally also decreases due to rigidity of the iris and a narrowing of the visual field. The visual field is functionally important in performing tasks that require a broad perception of the environment (Miller, 1990). Shopping in department stores, walking in crowded places, and driving in high traffic areas are situations of daily living that rely on an individual's ability to perceive a broad visual field. Because of a narrowed visual field, older adults require more light and have difficulty seeing in dimly lit areas and at night. This is

Sensory-Perceptual Changes

Vision

- Diminished visual acuity
- Reduced pupillary size (constriction of the iris muscle)
- Decreased ability of the lens to accommodate
- Diminished elasticity of the eye muscles
- Decreased peripheral vision
- Atrophy of cones and rods
- Relaxation of the lower eye lid
- Decreased orbital fat
- Decreased tear production
- Thinning of the conjunctiva
- Yellowing of the sclera
- Development of arcus senilis (white ring around the sclera)
- Fading coloration of the iris
- Yellowing of the retina
- Narrowing of the retina arteries
- Altered depth perception

referred to as *dark and light adaptation*. The atrophy of light-sensitive cells (rods and cones) in the retina is primarily responsible for this change. As a result, older adults require more time to adapt visually when moving from different light levels, such as going from a darkened house to the bright outdoors. "This may be attributed to the decreased number of rods and cones, decreased accommodation, and decreased light filtering into the retina," according to Esberger and Hughes (1989, p. 67).

Sensitivity to glare and the time required to recover from glare are particularly problematic for the older adult (Yurick et al., 1989). In a study of visual changes in older adults, Kosnick and colleagues (1988) found that it took older adults longer to perform visual tasks. In addition, older adults had more difficulty with dim lighting and near visual tasks. Glare sensitivity results from changes in the opacity of the lens and turbidity of the vitreous. Older adults usually decrease their night driving because of the problem with glare.

Altered color perception or color discrimination is a normal age-related sensory change that results from decreased light filtering into the retina. Older individuals are less able to distinguish the cool color tones of the blues, greens, and violets. Reds and yellows, on the other hand, are readily distinguished. While color perception is not crucial in most activities of daily living, it becomes particularly important in distinguishing medications in the same color range or in detecting the color of spoiled food (Miller, 1990).

There are a number of additional normal changes in the eye that occur with aging. These include decreased tear production; decreased orbital fat, giving the eyes a hollowed appearance; thinned conjunctiva; decreased whiteness of the conjunctiva along with the development of *arcus senilis* (white ring around the cornea); yellowing of the sclera; and fading in the coloration of the iris. Relaxation of the lower eyelid can cause the conditions of *entropion* (lid falls away from conjunctiva) or *ectropion* (inversion of lower eyelid). The appearance of bags under the eyes is due to the herniation of fat under the lower eyelid (Burnside, 1988). Older individuals may also complain of "floaters" in their field of vision. These result from normal changes in the vitreous body of the eye. It is important, however, that an older individual be evaluated for this symptom in order to distinguish this benign condition from a retinal hemorrhage (Burnside, 1988).

Funduscopic changes also occur with aging. The fundus is more yellow in appearance and has less luster, while the retinal arteries are more opaque, narrower, and straighter.

A progressive loss of hearing, presbycusis, commonly occurs with aging. According to Farrell (1990) and Yurick and colleagues (1989), the functional abnormalities accompanying presbycusis include more loss of sensitivity to high frequency sounds than low frequency sounds; difficulty locating the direction of a sound; increased sensitivity to the intensity of sound (loudness); difficulty distinguishing sounds and the pitch of sound (tone perception); and reduced ability to process sound.

Changes in the structures of the inner ear, such as the loss of cells in the organ of Corti, diminished blood supply, and loss of neurons in the cochlea, are largely responsible for the gradual onset of presbycusis. The ability to transmit sound to the inner ear also is affected by changes in the structures of the middle ear. Thickening of the tympanic membrane, calcification of the ossicles, and accumulation of cerumen can result in a *conductive hearing loss,* which is a decrease in the transmission of sound waves to the inner ear. In a recent nursing study on the effect of cerumen removal on hearing ability of older clients, Lewis-Cullinan and Janken (1990) suggested that the health of older clients' ears can be promoted through assessment. Routine hearing and otoscopic evaluation in the acute care

---

Sensory-Perceptual Changes

Hearing

- Progressive loss of hearing
- Loss of sensitivity to high frequency sounds
- Difficulty locating direction of sound
- Increased sensitivity to the intensity of sound (loudness)
- Reduced ability to process and distinguish between sounds
- Thickening of tympanic membrane
- Calcification of ossicles
- Accumulation of cerumen

---

setting can identify the presence of cerumen, which can be removed with ear canal irrigations.

In contrast, changes in the inner ear, auditory nerve, or the brain can lead to *sensorineural hearing loss.* In this type of hearing loss, a person is able to hear but most of the words will be unintelligible (Yurick et al., 1989). When an older individual experiences a sensorineural hearing loss, the ability to perceive low frequency sounds is affected more than the ability to perceive high frequency sounds.

Further sensory changes also occur with aging (see boxed insert). The ability to distinguish taste diminishes as taste buds atrophy and decrease in number. The sense of smell also declines.

Vascular and tissue changes, along with the loss of neurons, result in a decrease in tactile sensation and the sense of touch. As a result, it is difficult for an older individual to discriminate temperatures,

---

Sensory-Perceptual Changes

Taste

- Taste buds atrophy and decrease in number
- Diminished ability to taste

Smell

- Decreased

Touch

- Decreased tactile sensation
- Difficulty discriminating temperatures (hot and cold) and sharp from dull

such as hot from warm. The ability to discriminate sharp from dull is also affected. Diminished tactile sensation also affects fine motor discrimination needed for hand-to-eye coordination (Esberger & Hughes, 1989). The older individual who has difficulty tying shoe laces, turning the pages of a newspaper, or opening a bottle cap exhibits a decrease in fine motor discrimination. A decrease in tactile sensitivity also affects the older individual's ability to sense pain, which raises many concerns for individual safety.

Perceptual Functioning

Perception is the awareness individuals have of their environment from the different senses visual, auditory, olfactory, kinesthetic, and gustatory. Individuals may experience distortions in one or several senses. The causes of these distortions may be *functional* (normal) or *organic* (pathological). The sensory changes associated with normal aging may alter the perception of one's surroundings.

For example, visual spatial ability is the ability to perceive the position of objects in visual space (Yurick et al., 1989). Environmental factors, such as the size of an object, its motion, and position, as well as its coloration and shading, cue the individual to an object's position spatially. Depth perception is the visual ability to estimate the relationship among objects in space, the depth of objects, and the dimensions of the objects. The ability to perceive depth involves both ocular and extraocular structures. "Eye changes or environmental conditions that reduce illumination of the retina thus decrease binocular depth perception in the elderly," note Yurick and colleagues (1989, p. 470).

An older individual may not be aware of the normal changes in sensory–perceptual ability that occur with aging. Consequently, the older person may not notice that the colors of the living room furniture do not match or that the colors of his or her clothing clash. Changes in visual field and depth perception may result in an older individual appearing suspicious of others, withdrawn, and antisocial. In actuality, the older individual is experiencing functional distortions in perceptual ability that affect the ways in which the individual behaves and responds.

Neurological Functioning

"Since the nervous system is affected by all other systems, it is difficult to identify specific changes due to aging," writes Farrell (1990, p. 83). However, there are a number of general structural and functional changes that occur (see boxed insert).

Neurological (General Changes)

- Decrease in brain size by approximately 7%
- Loss of neurons in the cortex
- Decreased cerebral blood flow and oxygen use
- Decrease in deep tendon reflexes
- Vascular and fibrotic changes in spinal cord and in peripheral nerves
- Decreased response to multiple stimuli
- Slowed reaction time
- Diminished functioning of the sympathetic and autonomic nervous systems

---

Due to atrophy, the size of the brain decreases by approximately 7%. A loss of neurons, particularly in the cerebral cortex, is apparent. Cerebral blood flow and oxygen use also are reduced (Christ & Hohloch, 1988). Vascular and fibrotic changes occur in the spinal cord and in the peripheral nerves. There is a general decrease in deep tendon reflexes and in peripheral nerve conduction. The ability to respond to multiple stimuli also is reduced and reaction time is slowed. Overall, sympathetic and autonomic nervous system function diminishes (Christ & Hohloch, 1988).

Changes in mental aging occur in both the cognitive and affective domains. In the cognitive domain, changes occur in intelligence, memory, and decision-making. A discussion of these changes is presented in the chapter on developmental assessment of the adult (see chap. 11).

Activity–Sleep Patterns

While the benefits of activity and exercise are numerous, Eliopoulos (1987) has noted that it is increasingly difficult not only for older adults but for adults in general to remain physically active. Technology has reduced the need for the performance of strenuous tasks and hard physical labor. Modern conveniences have reduced the amount of energy spent in household chores and the time and energy involved in commuting. Spectator sports and television further contribute to a growing sedentary lifestyle.

The physical changes associated with aging challenge the older individual's ability to remain active (Eliopoulos, 1987). Changes that occur in the musculoskeletal system (see boxed insert), as well as the changes that occur in many of the other body systems, affect the individual's ability to be mobile and active. While the older adult in good health has the stamina for the activities of daily living, there is a decline in overall stamina and endurance (Burnside, 1988).

With age, there is a loss of muscle mass due to muscle cell atrophy and the replacement of muscle tissue with fibrous tissue. The loss of muscle strength is more evident in the lower extremities than in the upper extremities. The arms and legs become noticeably thinner. In addition, the proportion of body fat to lean muscle mass increases (Christ & Hohloch, 1988). While marked wasting of the muscles of the hands can be observed, the older adult maintains a fairly firm grip. Farrell (1990) noted that the muscles of older individuals are not as effective in their use of oxygen. This fact, coupled with a loss of motor neurons, contributes to the diminished muscular functioning commonly seen with advanced age. It is also normal to observe slight tremors in an older adult due to the degenerative changes that occur in the nervous system.

"In contrast to the bones or muscles, which benefit from exercise, the joints show the effects of wear and tear, even in early adulthood," Miller writes (1990, p. 351). The synovial fluid thickens and the cartilage begins to erode. Joint capsules also may calcify. There is thinning of the intervertebral discs, and osteophytes can develop on the vertebrae, resulting in osteoarthritis.

Activity-Sleep Changes

Musculoskeletal System

- Loss of muscle mass and strength
- Atrophy of muscle cells
- Increased proportion of body fat to lean muscle mass
- Thickening of synovial fluid
- Eroding of cartilage
- Calcification of joint capsule
- Thinning of intervertebral discs
- Generalized posture of flexion
- Curvature of thoracic spine
- Decreased vibratory and position sense
- Altered proprioception
- Impaired righting reflex
- Increased body sway
- Decreased calcium absorption
- Accelerated bone loss

The posture of the aged individual is one of generalized flexion. Thoracic kyphosis, a curvature of the spine, occurs in varying degrees. With age, there is a widening of the pelvis, along with a slight flexion of the hips and knees. These changes, and the thinning of the intervertebral discs, contribute to the decrease in stature associated with aging. Changes in gait also occur. Women are particularly susceptible to falls and fractures because they develop a narrower stance, a narrower base of walking, and a waddling gait (Miller, 1990). Older individuals also can experience difficulty in maintaining balance due to decreased vibratory and position sense, altered proprioception, an impaired righting reflex, and increased body sway (Tideiksaar, 1989). These changes, coupled with a decrease in muscle control and strength, contribute to the risk of falls.

A variety of factors, including physical activity, hormonal changes, and diet, affect the rate of bone loss in the older adult (Christ & Hohloch, 1988). Bone is reabsorbed faster than it is formed and calcium absorption is decreased. The loss of trabecular bone (inner spongy matrix) is greater than the loss of cortical bone (outer hard surface). These age-related changes in bone that affect both men and women are classified as *type II osteoporosis* or *senile osteoporosis*. This type of osteoporosis occurs slowly and is age-dependent (Bellantoni & Blackman, 1988). *Type I osteoporosis*, or *menopausal osteoporosis* (Bellantoni & Blackman, 1988), occurs in women approximately 15 to 20 years after menopause. With this type of osteoporosis, bone loss is accelerated, the functioning of vitamin D is impaired, calcium absorption is diminished, and the secretion of parathyroid hormone is reduced (Miller, 1990). With normal aging, the parathyroid undergoes minimal atrophy or degeneration.

In addition to the changes that occur in the musculoskeletal system, Eliopoulos (1987) identified a variety of age-related factors that further affect the ability of the older adult to remain active. Intolerance for activity can result from a reduction in breathing capacity, cardiac output, or tissue perfusion. The individual may voluntarily limit mobility to the extent that the individual experiences social isolation or impaired social interaction. The presence of a short-term memory deficit also may affect social interaction and involvement in diversional activities. Financial constraints may limit available resources for leisure activities, transportation, and entertainment. This can further reduce the opportunities for social interaction.

Impaired mobility also is frequently an outcome of chronic and disabling diseases, the incidences of which are higher in the elderly population (Eliopoulos, 1987). The older individual, perhaps more than anyone in another age group, has to work hard at remaining active. Research has demonstrated the positive effects of movement and exercise in the elderly. In a nursing study on the use of a movement therapy group to enhance morale and self-esteem, Goldberg and Fitzpatrick (1980) found that the experimental group had improved morale and attitudes about their own aging. Similarly, exercise before bedtime was shown to reduce morning stiffness and improve joint function in clients with rheumatoid arthritis (Byers, 1985). Instructing older individuals on the benefits of activity and exercise and supporting them in their efforts to be active is essential in promoting the health of this population.

Activity and exercise also promote rest and sleep. This becomes particularly important to emphasize with older adults who experience a number of changes in sleep requirements and sleep patterns from earlier adult years (see boxed insert). The total sleep time of the older adult averages 6 to 7 hours. However, the hours of sleep do not always occur during the night. They also are distributed throughout the day. Unlike adults aged 20 to 50, who average approximately 6 to 9 hours of continuous sleep nightly, the total sleep time of the older adult is a combination of nighttime sleep and daytime naps.

In general, the quality of sleep of the older individual deteriorates with age. Older adults have more difficulty falling asleep and experience more frequent nightly awakenings (Matteson & McConnell, 1988). Older adults also spend less time in Stages III and IV (NREM) sleep. Consequently, the threshold for sleep is lower, and they are more easily aroused (Dement, Richardson, Prinz & Carskadon, 1985). While the length of time required for sleep is approximately the same as in earlier adult years, older adults require more rest.

Eliopoulos (1987) notes that a number of additional age-related changes interfere with the older individual's ability to achieve rest. For example, the older adult experiences an altered perception of night due to the changes in vision and hearing that occur with age. These sensory–perceptual alterations can lead to anxiety and fear, which can delay the onset of sleep. There is also an increased incidence of nocturia with aging. Thus, the older individual experiences more frequent nightly awakenings and a disturbance in sleep pattern. Older people may experience *restless leg syndrome*, a chronic disorder that is more common and more severe in the aged population (Esberger & Hughes,

---

Activity-Sleep Changes

Sleep and Rest

- Decrease in the quality of sleep
- Increased difficulty falling asleep
- Increased nightly awakenings
- Decrease in Stages III and IV (NREM) sleep
- Increased napping
- Altered perception of night environment
- Increased time in bed
- Increased need for rest

1989). With this disorder, the individual experiences a crawling or creeping sensation in the legs at the onset of sleep. These sensations are coupled with the urge to move. Massage and walking can bring temporary relief.

The use of sleep medications by this population should be avoided, according to Matteson and McConnell (1988), or used with extreme caution. Many medications used to promote sleep have longer half lives in older persons and therefore can accumulate over a number of days or weeks. Sleep problems should be thoroughly evaluated. Modifying the environment and encouraging activity and exercise are useful ways to promote sleep in the elderly.

Oxygenation Status

"The normal changes of aging produce a (respiratory) system still able to support the usual activities of an older person," Burnside says (1988, p. 165). The structural and functional changes (see boxed insert) that occur in this system are gradual and subtle. Usually, the older adult compensates well (Miller, 1990).

With age, the muscles of the pharynx and larynx atrophy. As a result, the voice softens and can be more difficult to understand (Burnside, 1988). Changes in the configuration of the chest also occur. The chest exhibits an increased anteroposterior diameter and an increased posterior thoracic curve, kyphosis. As a result, the chest may percuss more hyperresonantly than resonantly on examination. There may be less movement of the diaphragm with respiration. This should not be interpreted as pathological. Only after the history and clinical data indicate pulmonary changes consistent with disease would the client be referred for further evaluation.

Further age-related structural changes include increased rigidity of the rib cage and calcification of the costal cartilages. The skeletal muscles, connective tissue, and the smooth muscles also become more rigid. These changes reduce the efficiency of respiration and the force of inspiration and expiration (Miller, 1990). This results in a restriction of ventilation and a reduction in vital capacity. The lungs become smaller and less elastic with age. This further contributes to a decrease in vital capacity and an increase in residual volume (Burnside, 1988). There is also a decrease in the fluidity of the secretions of the respiratory tract. This can lead to obstruction and an increase in infection (Christ & Hohloch, 1988).

The age-related changes that occur in the lung parenchyma (terminal bronchioles, alveolar ducts, alveoli, and capillaries) have the most significant functional consequences for the older adult (Miller, 1990). The alveoli gradually enlarge, become thinner, and decrease in number, thus reducing the surface area of the lung. The vascular bed thickens, and there is a reduction in pulmonary capillary blood flow. There is also thickening of the mucosal bed where diffusion takes place, further reducing ventilatory capacity. With these changes, apical ventilation increases and basilar ventilation decreases resulting in poor ventilation of lung bases (Christ & Hohloch, 1988). Blood chemistries reveal that the pH, PaO_2, and $PaCO_2$ and bicarbonate levels remain the same, while the oxyhemoglobin saturation decreases approximately 5% (Christ & Hohloch, 1988).

Like the respiratory system, the cardiovascular system has a tremendous ability to adapt and to compensate for the changes associated with aging (see boxed insert). The most common changes occur in the myocardium and include hypertrophy, decreased elasticity, increased rigidity, and thickening of the left ventricle. The heart valves also become thicker and stiffen as a result of the degeneration of collagen and the accumulation of fat (Farrell, 1990). There is thickening of the endocardium from sclerosis and fibrosis. Connective tissue decreases and fat infiltrates (Christ & Hohloch, 1988). The heart becomes brown in color as the aging pigment, lipofuscin, is deposited in cardiac cells as a by-product of metabolism.

The ability of the heart to respond to stress decreases with age. After activity, it takes longer for the heart to return to the resting state. With age, the pulse rate slows, while the resting heart rate remains the same (Christ & Hohloch, 1988). It is not uncommon for pulse irregularities to occur in the older adult. This is due to the fact that the pacemaker cells in the right atrium decrease in number. Age-related changes also are observed on electrocardiogram (EKG). Recordings demonstrate that there is an increase in the PR, QRS, and QT intervals, with a decrease in the QRS complex (Christ &

Oxygenation

Respiratory

- Atrophy of muscles of the larynx and pharynx
- Softening of voice
- Increased anteroposterior diameter
- Increased posterior thoracic curvature
- More hyperresonance on percussion
- Decreased movement of diaphragm
- Increased rigidity of rib cage
- Calcification of costal cartilages
- Decrease in size and elasticity of lungs
- Decrease in vital capacity
- Increase in residual volume
- Decrease in fluidity of secretions
- Thinning and enlargement of alveoli
- Increased apical rather than basilar ventilation

Oxygenation

Cardiovascular

- Hypertrophy, decreased elasticity, and thickening of left ventricle
- Thickening and stiffening of heart valves
- Decreased connective tissue
- Increased fat infiltrates
- Decreased ability to respond to stress
- Decreased heart rate
- Increased pulse irregularities
- Decrease in stroke volume and cardiac output
- Decreased elasticity of arterial vessels
- Increased peripheral resistance
- Narrowing of blood vessels due to accumulation of calcium, cholesterol, and other lipids
- Increased prominence, tortuousness, and rupturing of veins
- Decreased hematocrit, hemoglobin, erythrocytes, and lymphocytes

Hohloch, 1988). Stroke volume and cardiac output decrease with age, as do coronary artery blood flow and blood flow to all organs.

Peripherally, the elasticity of arterial vessels decreases. This results in an increase in peripheral resistance. Blood vessels accumulate calcium, cholesterol, and other lipids, becoming narrower. Blood flow in the extremities meets increased resistance. With age, veins become tortuous and more prominent, particularly superficial veins. The valves in the veins are less efficient. Consequently, they can occlude and rupture more frequently (Eliopoulos, 1987). This reduces blood flow to the tissues dependent on those vessels.

Changes in lab values also occur with aging. There is a reduction in hematocrit, hemoglobin, erythrocytes, and lymphocytes. These changes explain the increased fatigue and reduced resistance to infection commonly observed in older adults (Matteson & McConnell, 1988).

Nutritional Requirements

"One of the most significant differences in nutrient requirements among people of different ages involves calorie intake," writes Eliopoulos (1987). In general, older adults require fewer calories. This is due to a number of factors. As one ages, the basal metabolic rate is reduced. This reduction, coupled with an overall decrease in physical activity, creates less energy demand as adults age (Williams & Worthington-Roberts, 1988). In addition, the older adult has more adipose tissue and less lean body mass. Metabolism is slower in adipose tissue. The Recommended Dietary Allowances (RDAs) specify calorie intake for men and women between the ages of 51 and 75 as well as those older than 76. While an overall decrease in caloric intake is noted with age, this can vary according to activity level, heredity, and environment.

A lower quantity and a higher quality of food should characterize the diet of an older adult (Eliopoulos, 1987). There is a need for fewer simple carbohydrates and fats. This is particularly important in light of the fact that older adults have difficulty maintaining regular blood glucose levels. A diet high in carbohydrates can cause an increased secretion of insulin and lead to hypoglycemia (Eliopoulos, 1987).

While differences exist among the nutritional requirements of the aging adult and those in other periods of the life cycle, recommendations cannot be made with certainty (Jenkins, 1988). If one examines the Recommended Dietary Allowances (RDA) for the older adult and compares them with

those for the younger adult, there are distinctions in only three areas. These are a decrease in caloric intake, decrease in B vitamin requirements, and a decrease in iron requirements for postmenopausal women (National Academy of Sciences/National Research Council, 1989). Miller (1990) notes that information on the nutritional needs of the older adult is limited by the lack of research.

According to the RDA, a 10% decrease in calories is recommended for people aged 51 to 75. An additional reduction of 10 to 15% is indicated after age 75 (National Academy of Sciences/National Research Council, 1989).

There is controversy about the amount of protein older individuals require (Jenkins, 1988). It has been suggested that older adults need more than the 0.8 grams per kilogram of body weight stipulated by the RDA. Others suggest that older adults need less. Until the controversy is resolved, older adults should take in at least the recommended daily amount. Older individuals may feel more comfortable taking in lower amounts of fat because digestion and absorption of fats may be delayed (Jenkins, 1988). An individual's daily intake of calories, however, should include no more than 25 to 30% from fats with equal amounts of saturated (animal fats and coconut oil), monounsaturated (peanut and olive oils) and polyunsaturated (most other vegetable oils) fats (Jenkins, 1988).

While the RDAs for vitamins and minerals are the same for all adults regardless of age, the minerals calcium and iron need to be emphasized. With age, calcium absorption decreases, the regulation of calcium balance is less efficient, and adaptation to lower calcium intake is altered (Miller, 1990). While the recommended standard is 800 mg per day, there is much support in the literature for 1,000 mg to 1,600 mg. Increasing daily levels of calcium above 1000 mg, however, can be problematic. Long-term use of calcium carbonate has been shown to increase one's risk of problems associated with hypercalcemia (Miller, 1990).

There is controversy about how widespread the problem of iron deficiency is in the older adult population. While a number of research studies on the intake of iron in this population have failed to demonstrate widespread deficiencies, certain high risk groups have been identified, such as those of low socioeconomic status (Miller, 1990). A deficiency of iron in the diet can lead to behavioral alterations and fatigue. Usually, a diet deficient in iron is also deficient in other minerals and vitamins, particularly vitamin C. Vitamin C is needed for iron absorption. Older individuals who rely on "tea and toast" diets may be at particular risk for iron deficiency. The tannins in the tea inhibit the absorption of whatever little iron there is in the toast or the bread (Jenkins, 1988).

There are a number of other gradual and subtle age-related changes that can interfere with the older adult's ability to maintain good nutrition. For example, the older adult has a considerable decrease in saliva, which can interfere with the chewing and mixing of food in the mouth. The loss of teeth or the poor condition of teeth can decrease chewing ability further. As one ages, the gag reflex becomes weaker. As a result, the potential for injury due to aspiration is increased. There is also a decrease in esophageal peristalsis, gastric motility, blood flow to the intestines, colonic peristalsis, and in the sensation that signals defecation. Many older individuals decrease their food (particularly bulk foods) and fluid intake. This, coupled with decreased bowel motility and a diminished signal for elimination, often leads to constipation. Laxative abuse is common among older adults (Eliopoulos, 1987).

In addition to these factors, financial constraints may limit the ability of the older adult to purchase foods high in quality. Functional limitations or the lack of transportation may prevent an individual from going to the grocery store. Living conditions may not be conducive to the storage and preparation of food. "Perhaps the lack of knowledge or experiences in cooking leads the person to depend on ready-to-eat foods of little nutritional value," Eliopoulos writes (1987, p. 89). The importance of a thorough nutritional history to evaluate all factors that influence nutrition cannot be emphasized enough.

Nutrition

- Decreased need for calories
- Decreased need for simple carbohydrates and fats
- Decreased calcium absorption
- Decreased saliva
- Loss of teeth
- Weakened gag reflex
- Decreased esophageal peristalsis
- Decreased gastric motility
- Decreased colonic peristalsis
- Decreased blood flow to intestines
- Decrease in sensation that signals defecation

Fluid/Electrolyte Requirements

The older adult usually is able to maintain fluid balance under normal conditions. However, when disease or environmental stress are introduced, the older adult does not respond as readily to changes in fluid balance, nor does the older individual have the fluid reserve. As a result, it may take longer for the older adult to adapt to fluid deficits and excesses (Metheny, 1987).

Multiple age-related changes affect fluid balance (see boxed insert). There is approximately an 8% decrease in body water by the age of 75. While the volume of extracellular water remains the same, there is a decrease in intracellular water. This is because there is less water in adipose tissue, which increases as one ages in comparison to lean muscle mass (Christ & Hohloch, 1988). As previously discussed, changes in body composition result in changes in weight for both men and women.

Not only is there a reduction in total body water and intracellular water, but the mechanisms that assist in maintaining fluid balance are less efficient. Because of changes in renal function, the body is less effective in concentrating urine and is slower to comply with conserving fluid in response to a restriction of fluid intake (Metheny, 1987). The older adult has a reduced ability to conserve sodium and potassium, as well as a diminished ability to adjust for acid-base imbalances. This is the result of age-related changes that affect the regulatory functions of the body. With age, Metheny notes, "skin is less effective in cooling body temperature" (1987, p. 347) due to the atrophy of the sweat glands and the loss of elasticity. The changes in the respiratory and cardiovascular systems result in the older individual's body being less able to respond quickly to blood loss, shock, acid-base imbalance, and fluid depletion (Metheny, 1987).

With aging, changes in body size and body composition have important implications for the distribution of drugs in the body. Because the elderly are usually smaller in size than younger adults (due to a decrease in height and loss of muscle mass), standard adult doses for a given medication may be excessive for the older client. If a dosage is excessive, the client may receive a higher concentration because the drug is distributed to a smaller amount of tissue (Simonson, 1984).

Similarly, older clients exhibit a higher percentage of body fat in comparison to body water. If a drug is distributed predominantly in water, the decreased percentage of body water will increase the concentration of the drug. In addition, Simonson notes, "medications that are fat soluble may actually be more widely distributed possibly resulting in a drug effect that is less intense owing to a lower blood concentration, but more prolonged as a result of the gradual release of the drug from the fatty tissue in which it is stored" (1984, p. 114).

Protein binding is also a factor in the distribution of drugs in the body. Most medications bind, to some extent, to protein. Older people have been shown to have a decrease in plasma protein (Simonson, 1984). This is believed to be due in part to a decrease in the production of albumin by the liver and a decrease in the dietary intake of protein by these clients. This results in a decrease in the percentage of protein-bound drug circulating in the body and an increase in the percentage of "free" drug that is not bound to protein. These changes can increase drug activity or toxicity. Additional age-related changes influence further the absorption, metabolism, and excretion of medications. These changes gradually occur over time and do not occur at the same time or at the same rate in all clients. It is, therefore, extremely important for the nurse to be knowledgeable of pharmacokinetics in this age group and to obtain detailed medication histories.

There is controversy over whether the thirst mechanism diminishes with age. While this is an issue, of equal and perhaps more concern is the fact that functional limitations or an alteration in mental status may prevent many older adults from taking in adequate fluids or recognizing thirst (Metheny, 1987). The daily intake of older adults should range from 2,500 to 3,000 ml. Therefore, it is important to evaluate the daily intake of older adults to determine if this fluid need is met. Eliopoulos (1987, p. 89) noted that older adults should be assessed for factors that may cause them to restrict their fluid intake, including:

Fluid–Electrolyte Balance

- Decreased ability to adapt to fluid deficits and excesses
- Decrease in body water, approximately 8% by age 75
- Decrease in intracellular water; extracellular remains the same
- Decreased ability to conserve sodium and potassium
- Decreased ability to adjust for acid-base imbalances

Lack of motivation

Desire to avoid nocturia or urinary frequency

Fear of incontinence

Inaccessibility of fluids

Inability to independently obtain or drink fluids

Altered mental status

Restricting fluids can cause serious fluid and electrolyte problems in the older adult. Dehydration and fluid overload threaten the lives of clients whose fluid regulating mechanisms are altered due to age.

Elimination Patterns

The excretory processes are natural and automatic and seldom are given any thought. As one ages, these processes become less efficient (see boxed insert). Conscious thought and assistance are required for these processes to occur satisfactorily in the later years (Eliopoulos, 1987).

There are a number of age-related changes that alter elimination. The structure and functions of the kidney and the bladder are altered. The size of the kidney decreases with age as a result of the reduction in renal tissue growth. Renal blood flow is decreased due to the decrease in cardiac output. The number of nephrons and glomeruli as well as the glomerular filtration rate decrease. These combined changes affect the excretion of drugs and the ability of the kidney to concentrate and dilute urine. The blood urea nitrogen level (BUN) normally increases with age up to 30 mg/dl. Also, the ability of the kidney to conserve sodium and potassium and adjust for acid-base imbalances is diminished (Christ & Hohloch, 1988). With age, there is a change in the renal threshold for substances such as glucose. It is not uncommon for an older adult with diabetes mellitus to have an elevated blood glucose and the absence of glycosuria, glucose in the urine.

The bladder also undergoes some age-related changes. The capacity of the bladder usually is reduced by approximately 50%. As a result, increased urinary frequency and nocturia occur in both men and women. With age, the shape of the bladder becomes more funnel-like, making bladder emptying more difficult. Consequently, large volumes of urine are retained (Christ & Hohloch, 1988). Multiple changes also occur in the gastrointestinal system, affecting bowel elimination, which was discussed in the section on nutrition.

Elimination

Urinary

- Decrease in size of the kidney
- Decreased renal blood flow
- Decrease in glomerular filtration rate
- Increase in blood urea nitrogen level
- Increased renal threshold for certain substances, such as glucose
- Reduced bladder capacity

Bowel

- Decreased blood flow to intestines
- Decreased gastric motility
- Decreased colonic peristalsis
- Decrease in sensation that signals defecation

The process of aging is complex. Most individuals adapt readily to the declines and losses associated with growing old (Eliopoulos, 1987). Understanding these changes and the challenges they present enables the nurse to creatively assist the older adult in maximizing the later years.

THE NURSING HISTORY

While preparing to take a history, the nurse should take full advantage of opportunities to observe as the client first walks into the room. Observe the client's affect, watch the client's gait, check the client's ease in getting on and off a bed or examining table. Excellent observation skills, coupled with precise history taking, provide a complete picture of the client before the clinical appraisal. Be sure not to interview the client while conducting the examination; do the interview separately. Talking and moving simultaneously often are difficult for older clients and cause them to tire more easily. A well-organized history will prevent fatigue of the client.

The nursing history includes an evaluation of physical and psychosocial parameters and uses all sources of information, including the client, the family, and old records. When taking the history, the nurse must listen to the client and take time. Thought and verbal processes are slower in the elderly and the history taker must be patient. Also, the history may be very lengthy because it covers many years. The evaluation should include key

TABLE 24-3
Key Aspects of the History in the Elderly

The nursing histories discussed in Chapters 14–19 will be helpful in obtaining a health history from the older client. Aspects of specific importance are listed below:

Parameters	Key Symptoms
Oxygenation	Increasing dyspnea
	Persistent cough
	Orthopnea
	Edema
	Angina
	Claudication
	Palpitations
	Dizziness
	Syncope
Nutrition	Difficulty chewing
	Dysphagia
	Abdominal pain
	Change in bowel habit
Fluid–Electrolyte Elimination	Altered mental status
	Thirst
	Frequency
	Urgency
	Nocturia
	Hesitancy, intermittent stream, straining to void
	Incontinence
	Hematuria
Activity–Sleep	Focal or diffuse pain or weakness
	Fatigue
	Difficulty sleeping
Neurological	Visual disturbances (transient or progressive)
	Progressive hearing loss
	Unsteadiness and/or falls
	Transient focal symptoms
Psychosocial	Depression
	Anxiety and/or agitation
	Paranoia
	Forgetfulness and/or confusion

symptoms. Table 24-3 lists key symptoms in older people.

Information on functional assessment is a vital component of the health picture of the older client and foundational for accurate assessment. Additional important aspects to assess include such areas as the skin, sensory impairment, mental status, nutritional intake, medications, and incontinence. The context of culture and environment also must be considered in any comprehensive assessment (see chaps. 8 and 9). Some tools that contribute to assessment follow.

Physical Integrity

The physical integrity history provides information on a number of important aspects that reflect the client's overall health. These include such aspects as skin integrity and vital signs.

While dry skin is a common finding in the older adult, disease and medication may exaggerate this tendency further. For example, hypothyroidism and anticholinergic drugs such as antidepressants increase the dryness of the skin (Gallo, Reichel, & Andersen, 1988). In obtaining a history, therefore, it would be important for the nurse to obtain baseline information about the client's skin and any changes in the skin, as well as the medications the client is taking.

Determining whether the client has a history of hypertension, an irregular heart rate, or chronic pulmonary problems is important. Difficulty with respirations may be readily apparent in the client who has to interrupt speaking to catch his or her breath during history taking (Gallo, Reichel, & Andersen, 1988). While temperature is often subnormal in the older adult, a variety of medications may interfere further with the body's thermoregulatory mechanism. For example, antidepressants, vasodilators, tranquilizers, and antihypertensives may increase the risk for hypothermia in the older adult with predisposing chronic health problems. Alcohol intake also can increase the risk for hypothermia (Reuler, 1978).

Sensory Functioning

A history of sensory functioning to detect possible impairment is also essential. It is particularly important to assess the impact of any impairment on the client's functioning. Function is the essential measure for older people because it is the link to independence. Older people often delete activities as they age without realizing they are doing so. For example, they tend to stop driving at night because of the changes they experience in visual accommodation. They may discontinue church meetings and other social activities because of difficulty hearing. In essence, the amount of impairment is not important, but the effect of the impairment on daily functioning is. An example of assessing sensory loss in terms of functional impairment is given in Table 24-4. This table displays a 9-item hearing handicap inventory that provides an in-depth assessment of a person's hearing loss and the effect of the loss. This inventory, combined with testing by a hand-held audiometer, is 74% accurate in predicting function (Gerety, 1988).

Mental Status

A history of mental status includes information about cognitive and affective functioning. Both need to be assessed to determine whether an impairment in intellectual ability or a depressive state exists (Kane et al., 1989). The recognition of mental impairment is essential to provide baseline data on clients as well as to predict incidents of confusion upon hospitalization. Often, clients are mistaken as confused and psychotic when they only may be responding to a new environment. Unfortunately, they may be labeled as confused and begin a downhill slide that might have been prevented with good baseline data. A complete mental status examination performed by a neurologist includes an assessment of such aspects as language, writing, and computation. Nurses can perform a less comprehensive exam, but one that includes most of the parts and still provides data on cognitive and affective functioning.

Cognitive Functioning

The cognitive assessment must be complete and in-depth. Cognitive function is complex and can be affected by age, stress, and disease. To help the client remain at the highest level of functioning, one must examine information processing, the ability to follow commands, the organization of thoughts, the use of abstract thinking, and judgment. These more in-depth assessments require more in-depth exams.

There are numerous tests of cognitive functioning. One of the most comprehensive is the Mini-Mental Status Exam (Andersen, 1988) and one of the quickest is the Mental Status Questionnaire (MSQ) (Kahn, Goldfarb, Pollack, & Peck, 1960). The MSQ consists of 10 questions and is particularly useful with dementia patients to classify their current stage of disease. Table 24-5 shows the MSQ and a legend for calculating the degree of deterioration that exists. The MSQ is limited, however, in that it only tests memory. Memory is only a small part of cognitive function.

The Folstein Mini-Mental Status Exam is more in-depth and tests the client in a number of areas (Folstein, Folstein, & McHugh, 1975). Two questions test orientation. The orientation questions are simple and not thought-provoking but are questions the client should be able to answer easily. In contrast, the MSQ questions (testing memory and orientation) are somewhat more difficult to answer. Not everyone keeps track of the former president of the United States.

TABLE 24-4
Hearing Inventory

A nine-item self-administered screening questionnaire, the Hearing Handicap Inventory for the Elderly—Screening Version detects functional impairment due to hearing loss.

A higher score indicates greater functional impairment.

No = 0   Sometimes = 2   Yes = 4

1. Does a hearing problem cause you to feel embarrassed when you meet new people?
   0 – No   2 – Sometimes   4 – Yes

2. Does a hearing problem cause you to feel frustrated when talking to members of your family?
   0 – No   2 – Sometimes   4 – Yes

3. Do you have difficulty hearing when someone speaks in a whisper?
   0 – No   2 – Sometimes   4 – Yes

4. Do you feel handicapped by a hearing problem?
   0 – No   2 – Sometimes   4 – Yes

5. Does a hearing problem cause you difficulty when visiting friends, relatives, or neighbors?
   0 – No   2 – Sometimes   4 – Yes

6. Does a hearing problem cause you to have arguments with family members?
   0 – No   2 – Sometimes   4 – Yes

7. Does a hearing problem cause you difficulty when listening to television or radio?
   0 – No   2 – Sometimes   4 – Yes

8. Do you feel that any difficulty with your hearing limits or hampers your personal or social life?
   0 – No   2 – Sometimes   4 – Yes

9. Does a hearing problem cause you difficulty when in a restaurant with relatives or friends?
   0 – No   2 – Sometimes   4 – Yes

   1–24 = 50% hearing loss
   26–40 = 84% hearing loss

Speech discrimination may be evaluated by speaking a series of words in a conversational tone three feet behind the patient. Have the patient repeat after you: Smart, Off, With, That, Within, That Chin, Will Cat, Room, All, Jaw, Does.

Note. Presented by Meghan Gerety, M.D. (1988, November). *Hearing Inventory—Screening Version.* Comprehensive Geriatric Assessment Seminar, San Francisco, CA.

Recalling three named objects tests registration. Registration is a part of memory and actually encompasses the act of paying attention. Many older people pay attention, but not with the intent to organize and retain the information. Consequently, they hear, but don't register; if the information is not registered, it will not be remembered.

Backward counting tests attention and calculation, a form of abstract thinking that is more difficult for older people. Older people have difficulty subtracting 7 from 100 in backward progression. It is easier to perform this test using a smaller number, such as 3. The individual's intellect and education affect this testing and the nurse should keep that in mind.

Language heads the next portion of the test. The language portion encompasses a three-stage command and the individual's ability to follow such a command. The command assesses information received, processed, and returned and therefore examines communication and its processes. The last three parts of the language portion are useful in testing visual/spatial ability and in examining losses encountered by victims of dementia. Victims of dementia have difficulty drawing the face of a clock and would find it even more difficult to copy a complex polygon.

The Folstein exam requires both oral and written responses. The maximum score for this test is 30. It is not timed and should be given in a non-threatening manner. Table 24-6 presents the Folstein exam.

In summary, each of these cognitive exams may be used for different reasons. Nurses should use

TABLE 24-5
Mental Status Questionnaire

1. What is this place?
2. Where is this place located?
3. What day in the month is it today?
4. What day of the week is it?
5. What year is it?
6. How old are you?
7. When is your birthday?
8. In what year were you born?
9. What is the name of the president?
10. Who was president before this one?

Score shows severity of brain syndrome

0–2 errors = none or minimal
3–8 errors = moderate
9–10 errors = severe

Note. Adapted from Kahn, R.L., Goldfarb, A.I., Pollack, M., & Peck, A. Brief objective measure for the determination of mental status in the aged. *American Journal of Psychiatry, 117,* 326, 1960. Copyright 1960, the American Psychiatric Association. Reprinted by permission.

them as screening tools for referral purposes and for establishing the best ways of working with clients. Other items falling under cognitive function that may need assessment are the client's psychomotor and perceptual abilities and problem-solving and learning abilities. In-depth assessment in these areas is best performed by a nurse practitioner working with a geriatrician, a physician specializing in the care of older adults.

Affect

Affect deals with feelings and perceptions of sadness and well-being. Though depression is a pervasive problem for the elderly, it often goes unrecognized. Older people view their own psychological problems as something they must conquer themselves and so don't always mention the problem during a history and clinical appraisal.

Depression is manifested in such a variety of ways in older people that identifying a depressive

TABLE 24-6
Folstein Mini–Mental Status Examination

Maximum score	
	Orientation
5	What is the (year) (season) (date) (day) (month)?
5	Where are we (state) (county) (town) (hospital) (floor)?
	Registration
3	Name three objects: *one second to say each*. Then ask the patient all three after you have said them. Give one point for each correct answer. Repeat them until he or she learns all three. Count trials and record number.
	Attention and Calculation
5	Begin with 100 and count backward by 7 (*stop after five answers*). Alternatively, spell "world" backward.
	Recall
3	Ask for the three objects repeated above.
	Language
2	Show a pencil and a watch and ask the patient to name them.
1	Repeat the following: "No ifs, ands, or buts."
3	A three-stage command: "Take a paper in your right hand, fold it in half, and put it on the floor."
1	Read and obey the following: (*show written item*) CLOSE YOUR EYES
1	Write a sentence.
1	Copy a design (*complex polygon*):
30	**Total score possible**

Note. Adapted by Gallo, J.J., Reichel, W., & Andersen, L. (1988). *Handbook of geriatric assessment.* Rockville, MD: Aspen, from Folstein, M.F., Folstein, S.E., & McHugh, P.R. (1975). Mini-mental state: a practical method for grading the cognitive state of patients for clinicians. *Journal of Psychiatric Research, 12,* 196–197.

condition, even a temporary one, is extremely important in helping the nurse understand the total patient. In an assessment, one screens for depression to detect illness, monitor treatment, evaluate the quality of care, and assess outcomes of chronic disease.

As one grows older, one incurs many losses: spouse, home, job, and social contacts. Any of these losses can set up a reactive depression in the older person. The reactive depression is transitory and can heal over time. However, often an older person is without resources or social contacts and so remains depressed. Depression causes forgetfulness and a lack of interest in life and must be identified before it clouds the mental health picture of the older client.

A paper and pencil test for a brief analysis of psychological well-being provides a glimpse of a client's feelings. The 10-question Affect Balance Scale (ABS) by Bradburn (1969) is one of the quickest and easiest measures and tests both positive and negative affect. The ABS tests current affect, how one feels today. The positive half of the test can be used separately to examine happiness and the negative half to examine sadness. An example of scoring follows: under positive feelings, three checks under "agree" are scored as +3 and two checks under "disagree" are scored as −2. Subtract −2 from +3 for +1. A zero signifies a steady state, a plus signifies a happy state and a minus a depressed state. The tool is fast and easy and

yields a concrete measure of well-being. This tool appears in Table 24-7.

Another scale designed to assess depression specifically in older adults is the Geriatric Depression Scale (GDS) presented in Table 24-8. The GDS is different from other depression scales in that it does not ask questions about somatic symptoms. A criticism of most geriatric scales is that the items representing depression also represent normal physical aging changes. For example, the Zung (1965) depression scale asks about early awakening (see chap. 12). Older peoples' sleep habits sometimes change and they awaken early. These changes can be misconstrued as signs of depression. The GDS has been tested and is valid and reliable with an older population (Norris, 1987).

Functional Assessment

The assessment of function in terms of performance is a vital component of the health picture of the aging client. One reason for this is that clients under-report symptoms of disease, but may acknowledge a limitation of function. Deterioration of functional independence in active, unimpaired older people may be the first sign of illness. When an older person begins to cut out previously enjoyed activities, the nurse should suspect an underlying cause. Function is a measurement of independence and health and is a better indicator

TABLE 24-7
Bradburn's Affect Balance Scale (ABS)

	Agree	Disagree
During the past few weeks, did you ever feel . . .		
Positive Feelings		
1. Pleased about having accomplished something?	[ ]	[ ]
2. That things were your way?	[ ]	[ ]
3. Proud because someone complimented you on something you had done?	[ ]	[ ]
4. Particularly excited or interested in something?	[ ]	[ ]
5. On top of the world?	[ ]	[ ]
Negative Feelings		
1. So restless that you couldn't sit long in a chair?	[ ]	[ ]
2. Bored?	[ ]	[ ]
3. Depressed or very unhappy?	[ ]	[ ]
4. Very lonely or remote from other people?	[ ]	[ ]
5. Upset because someone criticized you?	[ ]	[ ]

Note to Data Collector: WHEN YOU ASK THESE QUESTIONS, ROTATE BETWEEN POSITIVE AND NEGATIVE QUESTIONS.

Note. From Bradburn, N. (1969). *Structure of psychological well-being.* Chicago: Aldine.

TABLE 24-8
Geriatric Depression Scale

Choose the best answer for how you have felt over the past week:

1. Are you basically satisfied with your life? .... yes/no
2. Have you dropped many of your activities and interests? .... yes/no
3. Do you feel that your life is empty? .... yes/no
4. Do you often get bored? .... yes/no
5. Are you hopeful about the future? .... yes/no
6. Are you bothered by thoughts you can't get out of your head? .... yes/no
7. Are you in good spirits most of the time? .... yes/no
8. Are you afraid that something bad is going to happen to you? .... yes/no
9. Do you feel happy most of the time? .... yes/no
10. Do you often feel helpless? .... yes/no
11. Do you often get restless and fidgety? .... yes/no
12. Do you prefer to stay at home, rather than going out and doing new things? .... yes/no
13. Do you frequently worry about the future? .... yes/no
14. Do you feel you have more problems with memory than most? .... yes/no
15. Do you think it is wonderful to be alive now? .... yes/no
16. Do you often feel downhearted and blue? .... yes/no
17. Do you feel pretty worthless the way you are now? .... yes/no
18. Do you worry a lot about the past? .... yes/no
19. Do you find life very exciting? .... yes/no
20. Is it hard for you to get started on new projects? .... yes/no
21. Do you feel full of energy? .... yes/no
22. Do you feel that your situation is hopeless? .... yes/no
23. Do you think that most people are better off than you are? .... yes/no
24. Do you frequently get upset over little things? .... yes/no
25. Do you frequently feel like crying? .... yes/no
26. Do you have trouble concentrating? .... yes/no
27. Do you enjoy getting up in the morning? .... yes/no
28. Do you prefer to avoid social gatherings? .... yes/no
29. Is it easy for you to make decisions? .... yes/no
30. Is your mind as clear as it used to be? .... yes/no

Of the 30 questions selected for inclusion in the GDS, 20 indicated the presence of depression when answered positively while the others (Nos. 1, 5, 7, 9, 15, 27, 29, and 30) indicated depression when answered negatively. The questions were arranged in a 30-item, one-page format and ordered so as to maximize patient acceptance of the questionnaire.

Answer Key 0–10 = normal
              11–20 = mild depression
              21–30 = severe depression

Note. From Brink, T.L. (1983). Development and validation of a geriatric screening scale. *Journal of Psychiatric Research, 17*(1), 37–49.

of the older person's health than a report of the number of chronic illnesses.

What is functional assessment? Functional assessment is the systematic, multidimensional, detailed evaluation of an individual's abilities to perform various tasks associated with independent daily living (Beck, 1989). Function refers to physical, mental, socioeconomic, and activity factors. Functional assessment is time-consuming, but it is the best measure of the health of an older person. The purposes of functional assessment are to assess, screen, describe, monitor, and predict. Functional assessment, then, is a tool for disease prevention and health maintenance as well as for predicting clinical outcomes. No one functional test can serve the varied populations needing as-

sessment. As a result, the nurse must pick and choose those instruments that are most applicable to each client.

Activity

The client's ability to function independently depends on activity level. Functional activity is best understood if it is divided into three types: advanced, instrumental, and basic understanding. Table 24-9 shows the activity levels and types of activity at each level. These levels are important in making the assessment of function meaningful. For example, people who have full use of function can participate in sports, jog, and play tennis and have the greatest degree of choice. In assessing this person, the proper question to ask is: "Do you play as much tennis as you used to play? If not, why not?" If a question addresses basic levels of activity—"Do you bathe yourself?"—no additional information will be gleaned to help the nurse categorize the client's activity level.

It is also helpful to ask questions that incorporate "can" and "do." "Can you cook?" reveals nothing about activity level. "Do you cook?" is much more precise. Observation also contributes a great deal to an assessment of activity. If the client is arthritic and seems to have trouble opening her purse, then the client can't open medicine bottles or packages of food. A description of each activity level (advanced, instrumental, and basic) shown in Table 24-9 is important for accurate functional assessment.

Advanced Activity. People who are at the advanced level of activity are usually the young old. They may still be employed, participate actively in life, and enjoy a full recreational schedule. People at an advanced activity level are enjoying what has been called the golden years. Given the economic means, people at this activity level enjoy a time that is personally rewarding. Advanced activity is voluntary and may be characterized by participation in sports and other recreational activities. The nurse working in the community will see clients at this functional level. The client having problems at this functional level is still fully independent but anticipating a decline. The future decline and inability to function as freely as one did in the past

often requires an emotional adjustment. For some very active, athletic people this adjustment constitutes a difficult and trying time.

Instrumental Activity. Instrumental activity is the ability to care for oneself, do the shopping, handle finances, and so on. Instrumental activity often requires assessment when there is a life change, such as an illness or the death of a spouse. For example, a man who has had abdominal surgery may not be able to drive for some time afterward. If the man has no support systems, he may be unable to get food and medicine and take care of himself. Hence, he becomes more functionally dependent and requires more services than the client with built-in support systems.

The death of a spouse also can create functional changes. Usually, one partner handles the finances and the survivor must learn to do so. A functional assessment during a crisis will uncover hidden areas of need. Some people at the instrumental level may find it's too much work to live independently. They may prefer to relocate to a senior living complex where they can manage quite well with assistance. It is essential for the nurse to identify the assistance necessary for the most independent functioning and to inform clients of their choices.

Basic Activity. The third level of activity is basic: bathing, dressing, and using the toilet. At this level, the older person may need help with personal care. The person with these needs is usually

TABLE 24-9
Reuben's Model of Activity

Type	Activity	Need	Effect
AADL	Job Sports Recreation	Voluntary	1. Decreased self-esteem. 2. Worrying of future decline.
IADL	Shop Phone Cook Keep house Take medicine Handle finances	Semi-elective	1. Needs assistance. 2. Relocates.
BADL	Bathe Dress Toilet Transfer Feed	Mandatory	1. Needs help with personal care.

Key: AADL—Advanced activities of daily living
IADL—Instrumental activities of daily living
BADL—Basic activities of daily living

Note. Presented by David Reuben, M.D. (1988, November). *Functional Assessment.* Comprehensive Geriatric Assessment Seminar, San Francisco, CA.

found in a hospital or in a nursing home. Even in these settings, people who can function more independently are healthier and have higher self-esteem. The more personal care they manage, the longer they retain independence. Table 24-10 contains selected functional categories for assessing basic and instrumental activities of daily living. Additional tools can be added to answer the basic questions of what a client does and what the client is capable of doing. Conversation concerning the client's interests can be used to assess the more advanced activities of daily living.

Other very comprehensive functional assessment tools, such as Older American Resources and Services (OARS) and Patient Appraisal and Care Evaluation (PACE), can be found in their entirety in a series by Mangen and Peterson (1982). These tools (OARS & PACE) are lengthy and time-consuming; caregivers have been striving to develop shorter and simpler tools. Table 24-11 presents a shorter method of assessing instrumental activities of daily living.

Nutritional Intake

A nutritional history is important and should be more than a three-day diet recall. Many older people have excellent knowledge of nutrition, particularly if they are women who have cooked for families over the years. Often, the difficulty in eating well is economic, social, or functional rather than a lack of knowledge. Older people may no longer have the funds for food or the capabilities to fix the food. The nurse needs to consider all areas when interviewing the older client. Table 24-12 highlights areas to be covered in a nutritional history.

The history also should include a complete report of the client's medications. During this evaluation the nurse should assess the client's knowledge of the medication, ability to open the bottle, and method of remembering to take the medication. Noncompliance is one of the greatest sources of medication error in older people, but often noncompliance comes from misunderstanding directions or from functional or economic disability. Older clients are very creative in stretching their medications. For example, clients short on cash at the end of the month may compensate by taking medications every other day, instead of as prescribed. Table 24-13 provides a guideline for evaluating an older client's medication regimen. The regimen becomes more complicated as the number of medications increases. There is also a direct increase in the number of drug reactions in proportion to the number of medications taken.

Incontinence

Difficulty with incontinence is an area requiring specific evaluation. The prevalence of urinary incontinence is particularly high in the older, more

TABLE 24-10
Basic and Instrumental Activities of Daily Living

	Fully Independent*	Needs Some Human Assistance (including supervision)	Totally Dependent
Bathing	[ ]	[ ]	[ ]
Ambulation	[ ]	[ ]	[ ]
Transfer	[ ]	[ ]	[ ]
Dressing	[ ]	[ ]	[ ]
Personal grooming	[ ]	[ ]	[ ]
Toileting	[ ]	[ ]	[ ]
Eating	[ ]	[ ]	[ ]
Preparing meals	[ ]	[ ]	[ ]
Managing money	[ ]	[ ]	[ ]
Managing medications	[ ]	[ ]	[ ]
Using telephone	[ ]	[ ]	[ ]

Is the patient incontinent?
Bladder   [ ] Yes   [ ] No   Bowel   [ ] Yes   [ ] No

*Indicate whether mechanical aid used and what type(s).

Note. From Kane, R.L., Ouslander, J.G., & Abrass, I.B. (1989). *Essentials of clinical geriatrics* (2nd ed.). New York: McGraw-Hill, p. 478. Reprinted with permission of McGraw-Hill, Inc.

TABLE 24-11
Instrumental Activities of Daily Living (IADL) Scale

1. Can you use the telephone:
   3. without help
   2. with some help, or
   1. are you completely unable to use the telephone?

2. Can you get to places out of walking distance:
   3. without help,
   2. with some help, or
   1. are you completely unable to travel unless special arrangements are made?

3. Can you go shopping for groceries:
   3. without help
   2. with some help, or
   1. are you completely unable to do any shopping?

4. Can you prepare your own meals:
   3. without help,
   2. with some help, or
   1. are you completely unable to prepare any meals?

5. Can you do your own housework:
   3. without help,
   2. with some help, or
   1. are you completely unable to do any housework?

6. Can you do your own handyman work:
   3. without help,
   2. with some help, or
   1. are you completely unable to do any handyman work?

7. Can you do your own laundry:
   3. without help,
   2. with some help, or
   1. are you completely unable to do any laundry at all?

8a. Do you take medicines or use any medications?
   1. (If yes, answer Question 8b)   [ ] Yes
   2. (If no, answer Question 8c)   [ ] No

8b. Do you take your own medicine:
   3. without help (in the right doses at the right time),
   2. with some help (take medicine if someone prepares it for you or reminds you to take it) or
   1. (are you/would you be) completely unable to take your own medicine?

8c. If you had to take medicine, can you do it:
   3. without help (in the right doses at the right time),
   2. with some help (take medicine if someone prepares it for you or reminds you to take it), or
   1. (are you/would you be) completely unable to take your own medicine?

9. Can you manage your own money:
   3. without help,
   2. with some help, or
   1. are you completely unable to handle money?

Note. From Lawton, M.P., Moss, M., Fulcomer, M., et al. A research and service-oriented Multilevel Assessment Instrument. *Journal of Gerontology*, 1982, 37, 91–99. Copyright © The Gerontological Society of America. Reprinted with permission.

frail elderly. Elderly people may fail to report incontinence because of shame and the lack of knowledge that incontinence is a common problem. Incontinence needs to be evaluated specifically for its impact on the client. Does the incontinence cause social isolation and dependence that could lead to institutionalization? One should assess the frequency, amount, urge, stress, and stream strength. Table 24-14 provides additional questions that may be useful in gaining a history of incontinence. Incontinence is a treatable condition, and identifying the type of incontinence aids in choosing a treatment plan.

Because of the large amount of information needed for a complete assessment, the older patient may tire before it is completed. Choose those forms that are pertinent to the client you are interviewing. When the patient tires, end the interview and begin again upon completion of the clinical appraisal.

CLINICAL APPRAISAL AND SCREENING

Clinical appraisal of the older adult varies more in approach and focus than in technique. A number of factors, such as time, environment, and communication, warrant special consideration initially. These factors are also important throughout the

TABLE 24-12
Highlights of Nutritional History of the Elderly

Appetite
Access to food
Economic resources
Dietary knowledge
Dentition
Food preparation
Weight change
Intake change
Gastrointestinal symptoms

TABLE 24-13
Evaluating the Older Client's Medication Regimen

Number
  Prescription
  Over the counter
  "Natural preparations"

Source
  Single or multiple providers
    Physicians/pharmacies
  Sharing with family/friends

Drug Reactions
  Allergies
  Adverse drug reactions
  Prior drug treatment

Compliance
  Packaging
  Label reading (literacy/size of print)
  Timing
  Complexity of regimen
  Understanding of indications (control)
  Supervision/assistance needed
  Compliance aids

clinical appraisal and are useful in obtaining the nursing history as well.

As with the nursing history, the length of time to complete the clinical appraisal of older adults must be considered. The nurse first should determine the purpose of the assessment and then focus on those parameters that contribute to the total picture. The purpose of an assessment may be for a simple screening or for a complete evaluation of health. In the case of the latter, it is unrealistic to expect to cover all aspects of an assessment in one encounter. The reason for limiting the time of the assessment is to avoid fatigue. This is particularly a problem with the frail elderly. Plan for several sessions. The nurse should coordinate the assessment process by planning what is to be covered in one session or over several sessions (Rutledge, 1988). This gives the nurse adequate time for assessment. At the same time, it considers the special needs of the older individual.

Before beginning the examination, the nurse must make sure the environment is conducive to assessment. Rutledge (1988) suggests that the

TABLE 24-14
Urinary Incontinence Questionnaire

1. Have you ever experienced any involuntary leakage of urine?
2. Does the loss of urine ever keep you from leaving your home or participating in social events?
3. Do you ever have to schedule trips, social events, or errands around your toileting schedule?
4. Has the loss of urine caused you to change your intake of fluids?
5. Do you find that you must use special pads or other devices to protect yourself in case you do leak urine?
6. Do you experience burning or pain when you pass your urine?
7. How often do you urinate during the daytime hours?
   [ ] More than once an hour   [ ] Every couple of hours
   [ ] Three to four times a day   [ ] Once or twice a day
8. How many times do you get up to urinate (or experience loss of urine) at night?
   [ ] None   [ ] 1–2   [ ] 3–5   [ ] more than 5
9. Have you ever noticed blood in your urine or staining in the toilet water when you urinate?
10. When you try to urinate, does it take you a long time to get started?
11. Is your urinary stream as strong as it ever was?
12. Check the answer that best describes how often you experience this leakage of urine?
   [ ] Less than once a month   [ ] More than once a day
   [ ] Once or twice a month   [ ] Dribbling after each urination
   [ ] Once or twice a week   [ ] Dribbling all day long
   [ ] Daily   [ ] Can't really describe
13. Check the answer which best describes the amount of urine you lose each time that you lose urine.
   [ ] Amount which requires you to change your clothes, and more than could be contained by a sanitary napkin
   [ ] Amount which requires you to change your clothes but which could be contained by a sanitary napkin.
   [ ] Amount which wets your underwear but is not enough to make you immediately change your outer-wear.
   [ ] Can't really describe
14. At the time when you leak urine, are you aware of an urge to go to the bathroom?
15. Do you ever leak urine upon coughing, sneezing, laughing, or when you stand up?
16. Are you able to voluntarily stop urinating in mid-stream?

Presented by Meghan Gerety, M.D. (1988, November). *Incontinence.* Comprehensive Geriatric Assessment Seminar, San Francisco, CA.

nurse manipulate or modify the environment to correspond to the needs of the older client. A comfortable environment should be the initial concern. Adjust the temperature of the room: A room temperature of 75°F is generally comfortable for older persons and prevents chilling (Eliopoulos, 1987). Never expose the older client: Provide a modest gown for the examination. The furniture should be comfortable. Chairs with straight backs, short seats, and arms are preferable to low, soft chairs. Older individuals use their arms as leverage to raise themselves from chairs and the proper chair contributes to ease. The client should be allowed to sit comfortably in a chair for as much time as possible.

The light in the examination room should be indirect. Glare should be reduced. Older people have difficulty seeing in some types of overhead lighting and glare diminishes even more their abilities to see. If the nurse is sitting in front of a window facing the individual, the older person will not be able to see the nurse clearly due to the glare from the window. The nurse should do everything possible to facilitate the vision and hearing of the older person with diminished sensory function.

If possible, the environment should be quiet or the noise level of the surrounding environment reduced as much as possible. Noise generated by the telephone, activity in the halls, television, public address systems, intercoms, and loud conversation are distracting and make it much more difficult for an older person to discern the interviewer's questions. If the older adult uses a hearing aid or glasses, be sure they are in working order and the individual has them on during the assessment (Rutledge, 1988).

Positioning oneself in front of the older person and at the same level may reinforce hearing through lip reading. Lip reading is often an automatic response in older people when hearing begins to diminish. To facilitate lip reading, a female nurse can wear a brighter colored lipstick when interviewing older people so the lips are more visible. A male nurse who has a mustache should trim the mustache so the upper lip is easily visible (Burnside, 1988). If the older adult hears better in one ear than the other, the nurse should sit on that side of the person. When an older adult is very hard of hearing, a hand-held voice amplifier can be very helpful. If one is not available, the nurse can use a stethoscope by speaking into the bell and putting the ear pieces in the ears of the older person.

Communication is an essential aspect of the nurse–client interaction. For the older adult, both the ability to communicate and the opportunity for communication may be altered. This can occur as a result of the physiological changes associated with aging as well as the fact that age differences between people can be a natural barrier to communication. As a result, the nurse must bear in mind that communication with an older person may require some special considerations and modifications in approach.

When one is younger, one is more easily able to remember dates or a series of events and the details surrounding those events. When one is older, it is more difficult to pinpoint dates and events. Years and events have a tendency to run together because the perception of time is affected by age (Farrell, 1990). Recognizing this difference can decrease the nurse's frustration and prevent labeling the older adult as confused or a poor historian. To increase the accuracy of the data, the nurse should validate (Rutledge, 1988) the information obtained from the older individual with appropriate people and the client's medical record.

Changes in vision and hearing normally occur with aging. Older individuals have more difficulty understanding speech than younger individuals. The older person is able to hear, but often the words are not heard correctly. Presbycusis causes the older person to hear vowels more distinctly than consonants and consequently, words are garbled. Because of this difficulty a great deal of concentration is focused on listening to what is said. This can be tiring. Consequently, older people may resort to selective listening and hear what they want to hear.

Because of these normal changes, the nurse should not hesitate to ask an older client at the outset of the assessment about the quality of the client's hearing. Asking a client if you are speaking too loud or too fast or if the room is quiet enough is most appropriate and demonstrates attentiveness, respect, and concern for the individual.

The use of body language, gestures, and facial expressions may further help the older client to understand what is being communicated. Findings from a study on communicating with the elderly (Hollinger, 1986) indicates that nurses' use of touch increased the duration of verbal response in a sample of hospitalized elderly. Thus, nurses should use various forms of both nonverbal and verbal communication. Hollinger (1986) emphasizes that the need to communicate is even more paramount with clients experiencing impairments of more than one sense.

"When aging is not understood or is unacceptable, there is a tendency to talk at older persons or around them, rather than to them. If we think older persons cannot hear us or understand what we are saying, we talk as if they were not even present," Farrell notes (1990, p. 92). Mutual respect, caring, sincerity, and an awareness of the aging person as an individual become the basis for a trusting relationship and effective communication.

Burnside (1988) offers some additional helpful guidelines for assessing the very old. Because the effect of a day's events can be fatiguing, it is better to interview and examine the client in the morning. Also, the very old may give too much information in an attempt to be complete. In this instance, the nurse should set limits and gently guide the interaction to obtain the appropriate amount of detail. Also, the nurse should use terms that are familiar to the older person.

Approaches to Clinical Appraisal

While the head-to-toe approach is suggested for systemic clinical appraisal, it may have to be modified for the older adult to keep position changes and fatigue to a minimum. Above all, it is important for the nurse to be flexible and use the approach that will provide the most accurate and complete data without exhausting the client.

The nurse begins the clinical appraisal by observing the general appearance of the older adult. The client's physical condition (healthy or ill), general skin color and tone, alertness, body characteristics (size, shape, and movement), speech, general hygiene, and dress and the client's gait, coordination, and posture are observed. For each of these aspects, the nurse should be knowledgeable about the physical changes that occur with aging and compare what is observed and heard with what is normal for this age client. For example, posture and gait change as one ages. The general posture is one of flexion. The stance widens with toes pointed outward and the gait may evidence increased body sway. However, difficulty maintaining balance is not normal and may indicate a neurological problem.

Physical Integrity Assessment

Assessment of physical integrity covers a number of aspects, including temperature, pulse, blood pressure, respiration, height, weight, skin, hair, and nails. The approach to the assessment of these parameters is the same as that for a younger adult.

However, as the nurse performs the initial assessment of the client, the skin should be carefully evaluated. Turgor is best assessed by pinching the skin on the sternum or forehead, rather than on the arm. It is important to check under the breasts and in the perineal area for white patches (monilia), which may be the first indication of diabetes in the older adult. Because the elderly may develop a variety of skin lesions, it is important that any lesions be carefully evaluated and documented. Nurses should not overlook signs of abuse in the elderly. Bruises, lacerations, and swelling should alert the nurse to the possibility of abuse and therefore need to be thoroughly assessed.

Sensory–Perceptual–Neurological Functioning

Changes in sensory status, particularly vision and hearing, are among the most significant. While the assessment techniques are the same, there are a number of aspects that warrant careful evaluation. It is important for the nurse to assess the near vision by having the client read a newspaper, other printed material, or a standardized, hand-held chart. Older individuals are likely to develop presbyopia, farsightedness. In addition, they will report difficulty seeing objects at the peripheries of their visual fields. Careful evaluation will help the nurse determine the extent and degree of the deficit. Factors such as glaucoma also may cause visual field deficits, so evaluation is necessary. It is not uncommon to have to use prolonged stimulation to elicit the corneal light reflex. When the client does respond, the response is brisk. Evaluation of color discrimination and depth perception should be included as these become less acute with age.

The presence of cataracts to some degree is expected in this population. Therefore, the nurse should look carefully for this at the beginning of the ophthalmoscopic examination. Important to observe on fundoscopic examination is any evidence of macular degeneration.

Because loss of hearing is a normal age-related change, audiometric evaluation should be a routine aspect of the clinical appraisal of all older adults who report hearing difficulties. Similarly, a decrease in the sense of smell is common. Therefore, testing of the first cranial nerve should be done.

From a neurological perspective, the nurse would observe a decrease in deep tendon reflexes, diminished temperature and pain sensation, and a general slowing of reaction time in response to multiple stimuli. Because changes in mental aging occur in both the cognitive and affective areas, a careful examination of mental status should be performed. Due to the extensive nature of the neurological examination, it may be more difficult for the older individual to cooperate with all the aspects being tested. Scheduling a separate time for this exam may be necessary to avoid fatigue and enhance accuracy. The ways in which these are assessed, however, are the same as those for the younger adult.

Activity–Sleep Patterns

Changes in physical activity often result from changes in the musculoskeletal system. These changes are among the most noticeable and are assessed with the same techniques used for the younger adult. Particularly dramatic is the progressive loss of height that an individual may evidence, anywhere from 2.5 cm to 10 cm. It is important, therefore, to monitor height over time. Usually, there is a symmetrical decrease in muscle bulk, which should correlate with the amount of strength the client exhibits. Gait should be evaluated to distinguish normal, age-related changes from neurological problems. The older adult is particularly at risk for falls due to a variety of factors, so evaluation of the skeletal structure and joint range of motion, in addition to muscle strength, is important. As a result of a decrease in activity, sleep patterns change as discussed earlier in this chapter.

Oxygenation

As the nurse performs the respiratory and cardiac examinations of the older client, a number of differences may be noted in the findings. For example, the tonal quality of percussion changes due to the increased anteroposterior diameter of the chest. The percussion tone is more hyperresonant. As a result, auscultation of the lungs may reveal distant breath sounds. The same is true for the cardiac exam. Heart sounds may be difficult to hear and the increased incidence of arrhythmias in the elderly may make auscultating heart sounds that much more difficult.

Nutrition

A nutritional assessment of the older adult should use the ABCDEF approach outlined in Chapter 18. Careful dietary assessment will assist in identifying nutritional deficiencies, and laboratory data, and certain body measurements will complete the nutritional profile of the client. Particularly important is a careful examination of the mouth. The examination should be done without dentures in place and then with dentures in place (Figure 24-3). Weight loss and changes in facial muscles and

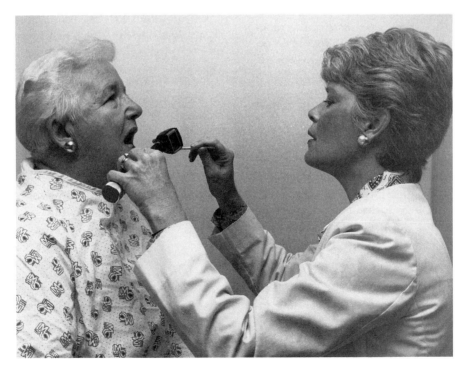

FIGURE 24-3. A careful examination of the mouth (with dentures in place and then without dentures in place) is an important aspect of nutritional assesssment. (*Note.* From Lee/Estes: *The Nation's Health,* Third Edition, © 1990. Boston: Jones and Bartlett Publishers, p. 68.)

structures can contribute to ill-fitting dentures, making it difficult for a person to chew food. Loss of teeth is problematic for the same reason. Any lesions or inflammation of the denture-bearing area should be noted.

Fluid–Electrolyte Balance

Laboratory values should be routinely obtained in the older client and compared with age-adjusted standard values. Changes in body size, body composition, and decreased plasma protein influence the distribution of medications in the body. The nurse should be particularly alert for signs and symptoms of drug side effects influenced by these age-related changes.

Elimination Patterns

The techniques used in an abdominal examination are the same for the older adult. However, the tonal quality of percussion may change, with the abdomen percussing less tympanic due to changes in muscle mass and connective tissue. Palpation should be performed more deeply in order to assess pain. This is due to the dulling of deep visceral pain as well as tactile sensation (Kelechi, 1989). Visible pulsations may be observed with the client in the supine position. Also, it is not uncommon for a client to complain of pain in the epigastrium when lying in the supine position.

Throughout the clinical appraisal of the older adult, the nurse should continually compare objective findings with those changes known to be associated with normal aging. Assessment of the older client is a multidimensional process, and the clinical appraisal is one aspect of that process.

Screening

Screening is an important component of the total nursing assessment of any client. The process of screening involves the identification of potential or probable health problems to promote early detection and intervention. The screening process must be used selectively and must be based on educated nursing judgment (see chap. 3).

A variety of screening approaches can be used with the older client population. Table 24-15 lists several techniques that are useful in obtaining information about a number of systems and integrated functions (Matteson & McConnell, 1988). While these techniques are very different from those used to screen for medical problems, they can be implemented quickly and can alert the nurse to problems requiring more thorough evaluation.

TABLE 24-15
Screening Techniques Useful in Various Settings

Technique	Purpose
"Take off your shoes"	Mobility, agility, vision, fine motor coordination, support network, complex task
"Show me your medicines"	Vision, over-the-counter med, prescription med, memory, literacy, compliance
Remember three objects	Cognition, alternate thought process
Genogram	Describe support network, altered family process
Orthostatic BPs	Potential for injury, fall
"What do you do for enjoyment?"	Anhedonia, depression
"Describe a typical day"	Diversional activities deficit, self-care deficit

Note. Adapted from Matteson, M.A., & McConnell, E. (1988). *Gerontological nursing practice.* Philadelphia: Saunders, p. 74.

Screening of older adults also may include screening for symptoms such as hearing difficulty, visual impairment, falls, pain, or forgetfulness. Using a symptom list, the nurse queries the client about whether the client has experienced any of the symptoms. In this manner, individual symptoms can be explored and subsequently managed.

Screening clients for medical problems is an important approach in health promotion and maintenance (Albert, 1987; Matteson & McConnell, 1988). Table 24-16 lists a number of screening activities that are recommended for the older adult. A combination of screening procedures is perhaps the most beneficial and helpful for this client population.

NURSING DIAGNOSES RELATED TO THE OLDER ADULT

A variety of nursing diagnoses that address problems in older people are presented in Table 24-17. These diagnoses from the *North American Nursing Diagnosis Association Taxonomy I— Revised* (NANDA, 1990) provide guidance in planning care. A common diagnosis for older people is "sensory–perceptual alteration" related to decreased visual acuity or diminished hearing.

Sensory–perceptual alteration is defined as a state in which the individual experiences, or is at

TABLE 24-16
Screening in the Elderly

History and Physical Exam
Cancer-related check-up: yearly after age 40, includes physical exam for cancer of the thyroid, breasts, testicles, prostate, lymph nodes, skin, and oral cavity; digital rectal exam; pelvic exam of all women; and health counseling
Assessment of physical, social, and psychological function; every two years until age 75, then annually

Tests and Procedures
Mammography: yearly at least through age 75
Pap smears: regularly until age 65, then every three to five years
Stools for occult blood; yearly; flexible sigmoidoscopy every three to five years for average risk individuals, barium enema every three to five years for those at high risk
Blood pressure: at every visit to provider, at least yearly
Vision exam and tonometry for glaucoma: every two years
Hearing exam: at every visit to provider
Thyroid assay: every two years
Measurement of height, weight: every visit to provider, at least yearly

Discretionary Studies
Blood hemoglobin
Serum protein and albumin
Tuberculin test
Urine cytology
Audiometry
Dental exam

Note. From Matteson, M.A. & McConnell, E. (1988). *Gerontological nursing practice*. Philadelphia: Saunders, p. 76. Adapted from Eddy D.M. (1986). Screening the "well elderly" (letter) *CA, 36,* 318–339; Sloane, P.D. (1984). How to maintain the health of the independent elderly. *Journal of American Geriatric Society, 39,* 93–104.

TABLE 24-17
Nursing Diagnoses for the Older Adult

Mobility, impaired physical, related to limited muscle strength and control or impaired coordination

Nutrition, altered, less than body requirements related to impaired swallowing

Role performance, altered, related to a disturbance in self-concept or change in physical capacity to resume role

Self-care deficit related to inability to put on or take off clothing or inability to bring food to mouth

Self-esteem, low situational, related to difficulty making decisions or evaluating self as unable to handle situations

Sensory–perceptual alteration related to decreased visual acuity or diminished hearing

Skin integrity, impaired, related to dehydration or use of restraints

Skin integrity, impaired potential related to immobility

Sleep pattern disturbance related to environmental changes or lack of exercise

Thought processes, altered, related to isolation or actual loss of significant others

Trauma, potential for, related to impaired sensory function or faulty judgment or dehydration

Urinary elimination, altered, related to functional incontinence associated with decreased attention to bladder cues or environmental barriers to the bathroom

risk of experiencing, a change in the amount, pattern, or interpretation of incoming stimuli. Sensory–perceptual alteration affects cognition but is the result of physiological, sensory, motor, and environmental disruptions rather than alterations in personality.

Sensory–perceptual alteration falls under the diagnostic category of perceiving. Assessment of sensory–perceptual alterations should include all five senses: visual, auditory, kinesthetic, gustatory, tactile, and olfactory. Normal aging causes changes in the senses and it can be generally stated that all senses are diminished. Pathophysiological causes of change include fluid and electrolyte imbalance, alterations in the organs themselves, malfunction of a prosthesis (hearing aid), or neurological and metabolic alterations, such as a CVA or diabetic acidosis.

In addition to maturational and pathophysiological causes, there are situational causes of sensory–perceptual alterations. These situational causes can be isolation, immobility, surgery, stress, noise pollution, pain, darkness, and even a different language or culture. Each of these contributing factors provides clues when looking for the cause of a sensory–perceptual alteration.

Characteristics that define a sensory–perceptual alteration are numerous. The individual can appear disoriented to time and place as well as people. There may be an altered ability to solve problems. People with sensory–perceptual alteration often change behavior and communication patterns. They may be restless and have sleep pattern disturbances. Reports of auditory and visual hallucinations are common, and older people may experience paranoid feelings and think people are talking about them. Along with these hallucinations, older people experience fear and anxiety and because of the difficulty they have communicating, they may withdraw and become apathetic.

When an older client exhibits such behaviors

as minimizing strengths, engaging in self-criticism or defeatist thinking, consistently underachieving, avoiding involvement, or exhibiting feelings of inferiority or loss of control of life, a nursing diagnosis of "situational low self-esteem" related to difficulty making decisions or handling situations may be made. The older client who is anticipating retirement or experiencing the normal physical changes associated with aging may feel out of control and unable to handle situations as in the past. Consequently, unrealistic goals may be established, further contributing to feelings of dissatisfaction with self.

A diagnosis of "sleep pattern disturbance" is categorized under the pattern of moving and implies the state in which disruption of sleep interferes with life style and causes discomfort. Defining characteristics may include verbal complaints of not feeling well rested or difficulty falling asleep. Daytime sleepiness, fatigue, and changes in behavior or performance also may be evident. The older client who continually naps during the day may find it difficult to fall asleep at night. This is due to the fact that late afternoon naps begin to approximate the normal nightly sleep pattern. Therefore, when it is time for sleep, the client is not sleepy. This is a common problem for older clients who are less active.

Another diagnosis categorized under the pattern of moving is "impaired physical mobility." This diagnosis describes the situation in which an individual experiences a limitation of ability to move independently. Changes in musculoskeletal, respiratory or psychosocial functioning may limit an individual's ability to be mobile. Decreased muscle strength, impaired coordination, hesitancy, or reluctance to attempt mobility may be among the defining characteristics. Thorough assessment of the client who exhibits impaired physical mobility enables the nurse to identify specific contributing factors, which can then be addressed in a plan of care.

Chapter Highlights

■ The health of older individuals is judged more by the individuals' abilities to function than by the number of their chronic illnesses.

■ With age, the body has less reserve capacity, less resistance, less ability to adapt to illness, and thus becomes more vulnerable to illness.

■ While all body systems are affected by age, the changes in sensory–perceptual and neurological function are among the most significant.

■ The physical changes associated with aging have important implications for the absorption, distribution, metabolism, and excretion of medications in the older adult.

■ Functional assessment is the systematic, multidimensional, detailed evaluation of an individual's abilities to perform various tasks associated with independent daily living.

■ The purposes of functional assessment are to assess, screen, describe, monitor, and predict.

■ Clinical appraisal of the older adult varies more in approach and focus than in technique.

■ Time, environment, and communication are important factors that should be considered throughout the clinical appraisal of the older adult.

■ A combination of screening procedures is the most beneficial and helpful for use with this client population.

Practice Activities

1. Role-play obtaining a functional assessment from the following clients:
   a. 65-year-old newly retired man.
   b. 75-year-old woman who has come for an annual physical examination.
   c. 85-year-old man living in a retirement home.
   d. 68-year-old man with a history of a stroke and resulting left-sided paresis.
What conclusions can you draw?

2. Review the medical record of an older hospitalized client and list all information that relates to sensory–perceptual–neurological status. What nursing diagnoses are indicated?

3. Perform a complete clinical appraisal of two older clients of differing ages, socioeconomic backgrounds, and diagnoses. Record your findings. What similarities and differences did you observe? What are the implications for nursing care of these individuals?

4. Identify appropriate screening procedures that would be incorporated in the assessments of the following clients:
   a. 75-year-old man with chronic obstructive pulmonary disease.

b. healthy 80-year-old woman.

c. 71-year-old woman with rheumatoid arthritis.

d. 60-year-old woman with a family history of breast cancer and colon cancer.

Recommended Readings

Applegate, W.B. (1987). Use of assessment instruments in clinical settings. *Journal of the American Geriatric Society, 35*(1), 45–50.

Becker, P.M., & Cohen, H.J. (1984). The functional approach to the care of the elderly: A conceptual framework. *Journal of the American Geriatric Society, 32*(12), 923–929.

Brown, M.D. (1988). Functional assessment of the elderly. *Journal of Gerontological Nursing, 14*(5), 13–17.

Burggraf, V., & Donlon, B. (1985). Assessing the elderly, Part I: System by system. *American Journal of Nursing, 85*(9), 974–984.

Carpenito, L.J. (1985). Altered thoughts or altered perceptions? *American Journal of Nursing, 85*(11), 1283.

Gomez, G., Otto, D., & Blattstein, E. (1985). Beginning nursing students can change attitudes about the aged. *Journal of Gerontological Nursing, 11*(1), 6–11.

Hallal, J. (1985). Nursing diagnosis: An essential step to quality care. *Journal of Gerontological Nursing, 11*(9), 35–38.

Henderson, M. (1985). Assessing the elderly, Part II: Altered presentation. *American Journal of Nursing, 85*(10), 1103–1111.

Lenihan, A.A. (1988). Identification of self-care behaviors in the elderly: A nursing assessment. *Journal of Professional Nursing, 4*(4), 285–288.

Molde, S. (1986). Understanding patients' agendas. *Image, 18*(4), 145–147.

Pace, W. (1989). Geriatric assessment in the office setting. *Geriatrics, 44*(6), 29–35.

Robbins, L. (1989). Evaluation of weight loss in the elderly. *Geriatrics, 44*(4), 31–37.

Walker, S.N. (1988). Health-promoting life styles of older adults: Comparisons with young and middle-aged adults, correlates and patterns. *Advances in Nursing Science, 11*(1), 76–90.

References

Advisory Panel on Alzheimer's Disease. (1989). *Report of the Advisory Panel on Alzheimer's Disease.* (DHHS Publication No. ADM 89–1644). Washington, DC: U.S. Government Printing Office.

Albert, M. (1987). Health screening to promote health for the elderly. *Nurse Practitioner, 12*(5), 42–56.

Andersen, L. (1988). *Handbook of geriatric assessment.* Rockville, MD: Aspen.

Beck, J.C. (1989). *Geriatrics review syllabus: A core curriculum in geriatric medicine.* New York: American Geriatrics Society.

Bellantoni, M.F., & Blackman, M.R. (1988). Osteoporosis: Diagnostic screening and its place in current care. *Geriatrics, 43*(2), 63–70.

Bradburn, N. (1969). *Structure of psychological well-being.* Chicago, IL: Aldine.

Brink, T.L. (1983). Development and validation of a geriatric screening scale. *Journal of Psychiatric Research, 17*(1), 37–49.

Burnside, I. (1988). *Nursing and the aged.* (3rd ed.). New York: McGraw-Hill.

Byers, P. (1985). Effect of exercise on morning stiffness and mobility in patients with rheumatoid arthritis. *Research in Nursing and Health, 8*(3), 275–281.

Callahan, D. (1987). *Setting limits: Medical goals in an aging society.* New York: Simon & Schuster.

Carotenuto, R., & Bullock, J. (1980). *Physical assessment of the gerontologic client.* Philadelphia: Davis.

Christ, M.A., & Hohloch, F. (1988). *Gerontologic nursing.* Springhouse, PA: Springhouse.

Deets, H. (1991). Rationing health care defies American values. *AARP Bulletin, 31*(11), 3.

Dement, W., Richardson, G., Prinz, P., & Carskadon, M.A. (1985). Changes of sleep and wakefulness with age. In C.E. Finch & E.L. Schneider (Eds.), *Handbook of the biology of aging* (2nd ed.). New York: Van Nostrand Reinhold.

Downton, J.H., Andrews, K., & Puxty, J.A.H. (1987). "Silent" pyrexia in the elderly. *Age and Aging, 16*, 41–44.

Ebersole, P., & Hess, P. (1990). *Toward healthy aging.* St. Louis: Mosby.

Eliopoulos, C. (1987). *Gerontological nursing.* Philadelphia: Lippincott.

Esberger, K., & Hughes, S. (1989). *Nursing care of the aged.* Norwalk, CT: Appleton & Lange.

Farrell, J. (1990). *Nursing care of older persons.* Philadelphia: Lippincott.

Folstein, M.F., Folstein, S., & McHugh, P.R. (1975). Minimental state: A practical method for grading the cognitive state of patients for the clinician. *Journal of Psychiatric Research, 12*, 189–198.

Gallo, J.J., Reichel, W., & Andersen, L. (1988). *Handbook of geriatric assessment.* Rockville, MD: Aspen.

Gerety, M. (1988, November). *Incontinence.* Geriatric Assessment Symposium, San Francisco, CA.

Goldberg, W., & Fitzpatrick, J. (1980). Movement therapy with the aged. *Nursing Research, 29*(6), 339–346.

Hollinger, L.M. (1986). Communicating with the elderly

. . . Nurses' touch and the verbal responses of the hospitalized elderly. *Journal of Gerontological Nursing, 12*(3), 8–13.

Hudson, M.F. (1983). Safeguard your elderly patient's health through accurate physical assessment. *Nursing, 13*(11), 58–64.

Jenkins, C.H. (1988). *Nutrition and the older adult: Nursing update.* Princeton, NJ: Continuing Professional Education Center.

Kahn, R.L., Goldfarb, A.I., Pollack, M., & Peck, A. (1960). Brief objective measure for the determination of mental status in the aged. *American Journal of Psychiatry, 117,* 326.

Kane, R.L., Ouslander, J.G., & Abrass, I.B. (1989). *Essentials of clinical geriatrics* (2nd ed.). New York: McGraw-Hill.

Kligman, A.M., Grove, G.L., & Balin, A.U. (1985). Aging of human skin. In C.E. Finch & E.L. Schneider (Eds.), *Handbook of the biology of aging.* New York: Van Nostrand Reinhold.

Kosnik, W., Winslow, L., Kline, D., Rabinski, K., & Sekuler, R. (1988). Visual changes in daily life throughout adulthood. *Journal of Gerontology, 43*(3), 63–70.

Lamy, P., & Vestal, R. (1976). Drug prescribing for the elderly. *Hospital Practice, 11*(1), 111–118.

Lewis-Cullinan, C., & Janken, J. (1990). Effect of cerumen removal on the hearing ability of geriatric patients. *Journal of Advanced Nursing, 15,* 594–600.

Mangen, D.J., & Peterson, W.A. (1982abc). *Research instruments in social gerontology: Clinical and social psychology* (Vols. 1–3). Minneapolis: University of Minnesota Press.

Matteson, M.A., & McConnell, E.S. (1988). *Gerontological nursing: Concepts & practice.* Philadelphia: Saunders.

Metheny, N. (1987). *Fluid and electrolyte balance.* Philadelphia: Lippincott.

Miller, C. (1990). *Nursing care of older adults: Theory and practice.* Glenview, IL: Scott, Foresman/Little, Brown.

National Academy of Sciences/National Research Council (1989). *Diet and health.* Washington, DC: National Academy Press.

Norris, J.T., Gallagher, D., Wilson, A., & Winograd, C.H. (1987). Assessment of depression in geriatric medical outpatients: The validity of two screening measures. *Journal of the American Geriatric Society, 35*(11), 989–995.

Reichel, W. (1989). *Clinical aspects of aging.* Baltimore: Williams & Wilkins.

Rowe, J.W., & Lipsitz, L.A. (1988). Altered blood pressure. In J.W. Rowe & R.W. Besdine (Eds.), *Geriatric medicine.* Boston: Little, Brown.

Rueben, D. (1988, November). *Functional Assessment.* Geriatric Assessment Symposium, San Francisco, CA.

Rueler, J.B. (1978). Hypothermia: Pathophysiology, clinical settings, and management. *Annals of Internal Medicine, 89,* 519–527.

Rutledge, D. (1988). Functional assessments. In M.A. Matteson & E.S. McConnell, (Eds.), *Gerontological nursing: Concepts & practice.* Philadelphia: Saunders.

Simonson, W. (1984). *Medications and the elderly: A guide for promoting proper use.* Rockville, MD: Aspen.

Tideiksaar, R. (1989). *Falling in old age: Its prevention and treatment.* New York: Springer.

Williams, S., & Worthington-Roberts, S. (1988). *Nutrition throughout the life cycle.* St. Louis: Times Mirror/Mosby College.

Yurick, A., Spier, B., Robb, S., & Ebert, N. (1989). *The aged person and the nursing process.* Norwalk, CT: Appleton & Lange.

Zung, W.W.K. (1965). A self-rating depression scale. *Archives of General Psychiatry, 12.* 63–70.

Integrating the Nursing Assessment

OBJECTIVES

Upon completion of this chapter, you should be able to:

■ Integrate the various dimensions of a comprehensive, multidimensional nursing assessment.

■ Select key aspects of a client's health that warrant special attention during the nursing assessment.

■ Perform a comprehensive, multidimensional nursing assessment of selected clients of varying ages, ethnic/cultural groups, and states of health.

■ Analyze and synthesize nursing assessment data to formulate valid and appropriate nursing diagnoses.

Health is multidimensional. Family, cultural, environmental, developmental, psychosocial, and physiological factors all must be considered when assessing a client's health. A comprehensive nursing assessment incorporates each dimension in order to gain a complete and accurate understanding of a given client's health. Such understanding enables the nurse to formulate appropriate and valid nursing diagnoses as a basis for planning nursing care.

In order to acquire the knowledge and skills needed to conduct a comprehensive nursing assessment, the nurse should study and practice each component in depth. Chapters 7 through 19 focused on assessing the various dimensions of health and formulating nursing diagnoses specific to those dimensions. Assessment of special clients was considered in chapters 20 through 24. Special clients include the pregnant woman, the neonate, the infant and child, the adolescent, and the older adult. This final chapter illustrates how the many dimensions of health are integrated in a comprehensive nursing assessment of an adult client. Interpretation of assessment data and formulation of nursing diagnoses also are illustrated.

The nurse's responsibility for a client's care does not end with the formulation of nursing diagnoses, however. Instead, nursing diagnoses give direction and focus for planning nursing care. For each nursing diagnosis, goals or objectives should be developed, accompanied by delineation of nursing interventions to accomplish each goal or objective. Projected outcomes allow the nurse to evaluate achievement of each nursing goal or objective. Ongoing evaluation also allows for revision to reflect the client's changing responses to actual or potential health alterations. Ultimately, of course, the nurse is concerned with ensuring that the client achieves, maintains, or is restored to an optimal level of health or assisted to die peacefully and with dignity.

Today's busy practice settings require that nursing care, including assessment and diagnosis, be efficient, cost-effective, and outcome-oriented. Therefore, assessment cannot be performed to the full depth and extent suggested in chapters 7 through 19 for each and every client the nurse cares for. Instead, the nurse must determine which aspects of a particular client's health merit special attention. For example, general information that should be obtained about all clients includes age, gender, ethnic/cultural/religious affiliation, family structure, educational level, employment, and reason for health contact. Also, *some* data should be collected in all areas—developmental, psychosocial, family–cultural, environmental, and physio-

logical—of a client's health. The depth of the nursing assessment and the emphasis given to each, however, will vary according to the nature of the client's contact with the nurse, the duration of contact, and the particular health-care setting. The assessment also is influenced by the client's developmental level, ethnic/cultural identity, and health. For example, the very young and the very old require more frequent assessment, the former because of their rapid rate of development, the latter because of aging and the prevalence of chronic health problems.

Within the context of each nurse–client encounter, the nurse decides which information to collect. The ability to determine which aspects of the assessment require special focus depends on the nurse's knowledge and expertise in making clinical judgments (see chap. 5). For example, knowledge of the special needs of a pregnant client mandates that sufficient information be collected about nutritional status, health risks, and family needs. Other examples of special emphasis include developmental assessment for children, pain assessment for postoperative clients, and activity and self-esteem assessment for clients with physical disabilities.

The following example illustrates how the nurse integrates the various dimensions of a client's health in order to perform a comprehensive nursing assessment and identify valid nursing diagnoses. Practice activities are incorporated throughout the chapter to encourage active involvement in the diagnostic reasoning process as it relates to this client's situation:

> Kay R. is a 42-year-old black female who is seeking health care at Women's Care Clinic for severe headaches.

CUE IDENTIFICATION

A nurse begins to attend to relevant cues even before meeting with the client on the basis of certain pre-encounter data. For example, before seeing the client the nurse knows from the appointment book that she is a 42-year-old black woman named Kay whose major health complaint is severe headaches. The nurse reviews Kay's health record and determines that she has not been to the clinic for 2 years, when she sought care for a flu-like illness. A review of Kay's health record also reveals the following:

> Kay is divorced, with 3 children (ages 19, 17, 14 years—the 2 youngest live at home. Kay is of African-American ancestry and is a southern Baptist. She holds a B.S. degree in math education and is

employed full-time (academic year) as a 6th & 7th grade math and algebra teacher at a local middle school.

■ *Identify the variables that may influence the nurse's collection of information (include diagnostician and environmental variables), and explain how they may apply to this particular client and health-care context.*[1]

At the time of initial contact with Kay, the nurse observes the following:

Black adult female wearing a tailored dress sitting in chair next to desk in examination room; purse on lap, legs crossed; brows drawn together and shoulders slumped; hair and nails well groomed; taller than average, medium body frame; slightly overweight; establishes immediate eye contact with nurse, attempts to smile, and says, "Hi."

■ *Which of the information above is a cue and which is an inference? Which cues and inferences are likely to be valid? Reliable? Relevant? What additional cues should the nurse note in the initial general appraisal of this client?*

Following an introduction, the nurse asks Kay what brought her to the clinic.

Kay states that she has been having severe headaches "off and on" for the past several months. Her headaches are unrelieved by over-the-counter remedies. She also has experienced occasional episodes of dizziness and complains of feeling exhausted much of the time. She has missed several days of work and is worried she has "high blood pressure like my mother."

The nurse proceeds to obtain a complete nursing history.

■ *As the nursing history is revealed, pay attention to how you cluster or "chunk" the information. What patterns begin to emerge? What tentative inferences or diagnostic hypotheses are suggested?*

NURSING HISTORY[2]

SOCIOCULTURAL HISTORY

Family

Family health hx reveals:
Mother—61 yrs, hx of hypertension "since I can remember"; obese

Father—died 54 yrs from complications of diabetes
Sibs—brother, 43 yrs, diabetes controlled c̄ oral meds.
  brother, 39 yrs, A&W
  sister, 36 yrs, A&W, overweight
  sister, 34 yrs, A&W
Grandparents
  maternal grandmother—died 72 yrs, cervical cancer, hypertension
  maternal grandfather—died 66 yrs, stroke
  paternal grandmother—died 78 yrs, "natural causes"
  paternal grandfather—died 52 yrs, diabetes

Denies family history of coronary artery disease, anemia, sickle cell disease, TB, kidney disease, thyroid disease, mental illness.

Lives c̄ 17 y.o. daughter and 14 y.o. son; 19 y.o. daughter attends college 200 miles from home, home for holidays and summers; ex-husband lives in town and sees children regularly; states they are "good friends" and he is a "good provider" for the children. Gets along well c̄ her children although says son is "strong-willed" and often defies family rules. She responds by "yelling and screaming," and sometimes feels unable to control him—"his father handles him better than I do." Shares household maintenance responsibilities with children; involves them in family decisions when possible. Has been unable to "keep up" with home responsibilities lately because of headaches. Describes relationships with siblings (all live in town) as positive—"we help each other out."

Cultural

Considers self "African-American"; attends church services Wednesday evenings and Sundays; gets much support from God, church, and her minister; reads the Bible daily "for strength." Prays that God will help her get well; is fearful of having a stroke "like my grandfather." Rarely seeks health care "unless I can't take care of it myself."

Environmental

No known allergies, except hay fever during summer months; takes OTC remedies for relief. Usual childhood illnesses and full series of immunizations; tetanus booster 3 yrs ago; PPD 6 months ago—negative. Hospitalizations—age 3, T&A; ages 23, 25, & 28 for childbirth—no complications. Bilateral tubal ligation following last child's birth. No history of accidents/injuries.

Seeks health care at Women's Care Clinic when necessary; last health check 2 yrs ago for severe flu-like illness; last dental visit 18 mos ago. Drinks coffee (2 cups at breakfast; 1 cup mid-morning, 1 cup after lunch). Does not smoke or drink alcohol. Wears auto seat belt "most of the time." Insists that her children wear them.

---

[1]See Chapter 5 for a discussion of the variables that may influence the collection and interpretation of clinical information.

[2]The nursing history appears here as it should be recorded in the client's health record. Abbreviations used in the history may be found in Table 4-3.

Extra-strength acetaminophen (2 tabs) and ibuprofen (2 tabs) alternated every 4 hours for headache, c̄ minimal or no relief. Gets information about health from reading magazines and from school nurse, who "pushed me to come here." Considers self in good health except for headaches.

Enjoys job as schoolteacher; tutors "for extra money" during school year, summers. Family income approximately $41,000 (includes salary, child support, tutoring income). 17 y.o. daughter works 10 hrs./wk. at fast food restaurant to earn spending money. Able to meet living expenses, but feels she "has to watch it pretty close." Health insurance through employer; $200 deductible per family member. Denies safety hazards in home or work environment. Buying older 1-story, 3-bedroom home in suburban neighborhood; modern conveniences; new gas heating system recently installed; "adequate" yard, quiet road; satisfied c̄ living environment.

DEVELOPMENTAL HISTORY

Satisfied c̄ life achievements and lifestyle; job is challenging and rewarding; stays busy c̄ church activities, work responsibilities, and children's activities (marching band, debate team, athletics). Teaches Sunday school class. No problems c̄ physical, psychological, or intellectual development as a child or adult.

PSYCHOSOCIAL HISTORY

Intrapersonal/Interpersonal

Describes self as "usually happy, outgoing, easy to get along with"; occasionally has "the blues" about her weight and when she feels overworked; generally feels "positive" about herself. Wants to begin taking courses toward her master's degree but says she is already trying to cope c̄ "too much." Prefers to be c̄ others most of the time; also needs some time to herself each day or she gets "bitchy." Favorite activities are church choir, reading, listening to music (gospel, jazz). Has two very close female friends who are also divorced single mothers—"we help each other a lot." Has been dating one man "off and on" for the last two years—states "neither one of us wants to get married again."

No problems c̄ oral or written communication. Describes self as "open, willing to tell others how I feel and what I'm thinking"; says others sometimes perceive her as "aggressive, opinionated." Sources of stress are classroom discipline problems, uninterested parents of her students, her teenage son, and occasional financial strain. Younger sister was recently divorced; client has spent much time helping her sister "get through it." Usual ways of coping are "talking it over c̄ my friends or just being by myself until I feel better."

Sexuality

Gr$_3$ P$_3$ Ab$_0$; menses at age 12; LMP 1/18/92; menstrual periods regular every 26–28 days, 1 day heavy flow, 3 days moderate to light flow; severe menstrual cramps 1st or 2nd day, relieved by heating pad and ibuprofen, 2 tabs. Last Pap smear 2 1/2 yrs ago. No history of STDs or vaginal infections. Sexually active; has intercourse "several times a month"; same partner last 2 years; uses latex condoms. Minimal interest in sex for the past "several months." Performs breast self-exam sporadically; not sure she "does it the right way; most of the time I forget"; wants to learn correct technique.

PHYSIOLOGICAL HISTORY

Physical Integrity

Height 5'7"; weighs "about 160 lbs." Has gradually gained weight over the past 10 yrs. Occasional high blood pressure; most recently 160/110 (by school nurse). Showers daily in the morning c̄ deodorant soap; shampoos hair 3 X/wk. Does not shave legs or axillae; uses roll-on antiperspirant (c̄ aluminum hydroxide) daily but has been experiencing a mild axillary rash and itching for the past month. Uses makeup sparingly; manicures nails weekly. Brushes teeth 2 X/day; flosses 2 X/wk. Gums bleed c̄ flossing. Third molars extracted in 1975. Numerous cavities as a child, but none in past 10 years.

Sensory-Perceptual-Neurological

Senses—recent difficulty c̄ reading and other close work; last eye exam "years ago." Denies hearing impairment; no problems c̄ taste/smell; c/o seasonal sinus congestion and hay fever—watery eyes, nasal congestion, sneezing; takes OTC antihistamines for relief.

Neurological status—Denies problems c̄ coordination, balance, reflexes, muscle weakness. Recent difficulties c̄ concentration when preparing class lessons or grading papers.

Pain—Severe headaches 3–4 times/wk for past several months; worsen c̄ activity and premenstrually. OTC meds offer little or no relief. Lying down c̄ cold cloth on forehead in completely quiet room provides moderate relief. Monthly menstrual cramps. Denies other pain.

Activity-Sleep

Able to carry out ADLs s̄ difficulty except c̄ headaches. Does not exercise "at all"; daily activity is work-related and "carrying the kids everywhere." Sleeps alone in own room; needs 7 hours of sleep/night to feel rested. Retires at 11:00 p.m. although in past month has "fallen into bed exhausted" at 9:00–

9:30 p.m. on work nights; arises at 6:00 a.m. Sleeps later on weekends. Occasionally wakens during night, but usually able to get back to sleep s̄ difficulty. Does not nap—"no time." Lately has been so tired she's been unable to "keep up c̄ the housework." Has overslept twice in past month and been late to work.

Oxygenation

Denies any problems c̄ circulation or respiration, except "high blood pressure" in family. Occasional palpitations, especially on exertion or p̄ meals.

Nutrition

Typical daily diet:

Breakfast

> 2 oz dry cereal c̄ 1 tsp sugar
> 6 oz 2% milk
> 1 slice whole wheat toast c̄ 1 tsp margarine
> coffee (2 cups) c̄ cream

Lunch (at school cafeteria)

> Pizza, hamburger, spaghetti, tacos, or grilled cheese sandwich
> French fries, corn, or green vegetable
> Dessert (ice cream, brownie, cake, cookies)
> 8 oz whole milk

Dinner

> 6–8 oz meat (beef, ham, pork) roasted or pan fried, or chicken (fried, roasted)
> 1 medium potato (baked, mashed, homefries) c̄ margarine
> 1 c. green vegetable c̄ margarine
> 8–12 oz cola

Uses vegetable oil margarine. 1 cup coffee c̄ cream mid-morning and p̄ lunch. Late evening snack while grading papers—microwave popcorn, 6–8 pretzels, 1–2 oz peanuts (salted), or 2 scoops ice cream. Uses salt in cooking and at table. Says she knows she should "cut down" on salt and sugar. No supplemental vitamins or minerals. No cultural or religious food restrictions. Able to meet family food expenses. Prepares most meals at home herself, although children help some. Eats lunch or dinner at fast food restaurants 2–3 times/wk.

Fluid/Electrolytes and Elimination

Fluid intake 8–10 full glasses/day. Voids approx. 4–6 X/day; no difficulties c̄ urination. Bowel habits—daily or qod usually in a.m.; soft, formed, brown. Occasional (2–3 X/month) problem c̄ constipation (no BM for 3–4 days) accompanied by flatulence, rectal pressure, straining on defecation, hard stools;

relieved c̄ 1–2 tbsp Milk of Magnesia. Prefers to have BM in privacy of own bathroom; sometimes ignores urge to defecate when at work or away from home.

■ *Which data from the above nursing history do you consider to be valid? Invalid? Reliable? Unreliable? Relevant? Irrelevant? Current? Historical? Diagnostic? Supporting? What inferences have you formulated? What preliminary nursing diagnoses are suggested by the information available to this point?*

While obtaining the history, the nurse formulates the following general impression:

> Alert, responsive, cooperative. Answers questions readily and volunteers information without hesitation. Maintains eye contact. Advanced vocabulary; intelligible speech. Conveys thoughts clearly. Manner is assertive, yet calm.

■ *Differentiate cues from inferences in this impression.*

Upon completion of the nursing history, the nurse explains to Kay that additional information will be obtained by physical examination and some laboratory tests. Kay is given a gown and provided with privacy for undressing. The nurse returns to conduct the clinical appraisal. The findings are recorded as follows:

CLINICAL APPRAISAL

Physical Integrity

> Well-developed, well-nourished BF. Well dressed and well groomed; drawn facial expression. Wt 162 lbs. Ht 5'6 1/2" (s̄ shoes).
>
> 37.4° C. (oral); P—84, regular, bounding; R—26, regular, slightly shallow; BP 169/108 left arm.

Full set of permanent teeth minus third molars. Teeth straight; some plaque visible on molar surfaces. Multiple silver fillings in molars. Gums and mucous membranes pink and moist. Skin dry, warm, firm, reddish brown. Skin clear except for papular rash in axillary region (8–10 reddened, raised lesions, 3–4 mm diameter, on each axilla at base of hair follicles). Axillae unshaved. No palpable lymph nodes. Small varicose vessels over posterior thighs and popliteal areas.

Sensory-Neurological

PERRLA; visual acuity 20/20 O.U. (Snellen). Unable to read book passage at 12–14 inches. Corneal, blink, and red reflexes present. Responsive to normal voice tones. Weber & Rinne WNL. Peripheral vision: temporal 90°, nasal 60°, upward 50°, downward 70°. Able to discriminate smells and tastes. Alert, oriented X 3 (time, person, place).

Hand grip strong & equal bilaterally. Able to discriminate touch & temperature. Biceps, triceps, patellar, Achilles, plantar reflexes 2+ bilaterally. Babinski ↓. Cranial nerves I–XII intact. Follows commands readily. Unsteady while standing c̄ eyes closed. Winces and holds hand to forehead when moving.

Activity

Full, active, symmetrical ROM. Muscle mass, tone, and strength equal bilaterally and age-appropriate.

Oxygenation

Chest symmetrical; excursion even. Breath sounds clear bilaterally. PMI 5th ICS; apical pulse 84, regular. Carotid, temporal, and brachial pulses regular and bounding.

Elimination

Straie visible over lower abdomen and upper thighs. Abdomen slightly protruberant. Bowel sounds diminished; present all 4 quadrants. No masses palpated. Rectum patent; formed stool present.

Sexuality

Breasts symmetrical; striae present; no visible abnormalities; no masses palpated. Mature female pubic hair texture and distribution.

Routine laboratory tests, including hematocrit, hemoglobin, serum cholesterol, urinalysis, and stool hemoccult are performed, revealing the following findings:

LABORATORY DATA

> Hematocrit—38%
> Hemoglobin—14.2 g/dl
> Serum cholesterol—220 mg/dl
> Urine pale yellow, clear, sp. gr. 1.016; negative for protein, S&A
> Stool hemoccult—negative

CUE CLUSTERING

As clinical information is obtained, the nurse begins to sort myriad cues into categories or clusters of related information. For instance, the following data all relate to health maintenance and thus form a cue cluster:

> Family history of hypertension, stroke, cervical cancer, obesity, diabetes

Last health visit 2 years ago for illness
Last dental visit 18 months ago
Flosses 2X weekly
Gums bleed when flossed
Plaque visible on molar surfaces
Last Pap smear 2½ years ago
Performs breast self-exam "sporadically"
Fear of having a stroke like her grandfather
Drinks 4 cups of coffee daily
Weight 162 lbs; height 5'7"
Blood pressure 168/108
Last eye exam "years ago," recent difficulty with reading
Does not exercise
Dietary intake (see client's 24-hour recall)
Knows she should "cut down" on salt and sugar intake

- *Which of the above cues are subjective? Objective?*

The cue cluster relates to Kay's general health and suggests certain health risks. The various cues also concern her failure to seek preventive health care or engage in a healthy lifestyle (see Figure 25-1).

Another cue cluster is somewhat easier to identify because it is more circumscribed. Consider the following data:

> Showers daily, using deodorant soap
> Uses daily roll-on antiperspirant containing aluminum hydroxide
> Complaint of mild axillary rash and itching for past month
> Papular rash in axillae (8–10 reddened, raised lesions, 3–4 mm diameter, on each axilla at base of hair follicles)

None of the other data from the history or clinical appraisal fit this particular cue cluster.

- *What other cue clusters can you identify from the available data?*

As cue clusters form, they suggest patterns. Recognition of cue patterns allows the nurse to begin formulating *inferences* (diagnostic hypotheses).

INFERENCING AND HYPOTHESIS ACTIVATION

As clustering occurs, the nurse narrows the realm of nursing diagnoses that are possible. Aware that many are possible, the nurse begins to rule in some diagnoses and rule out others. For instance, when gathering information about Kay's elimination pat-

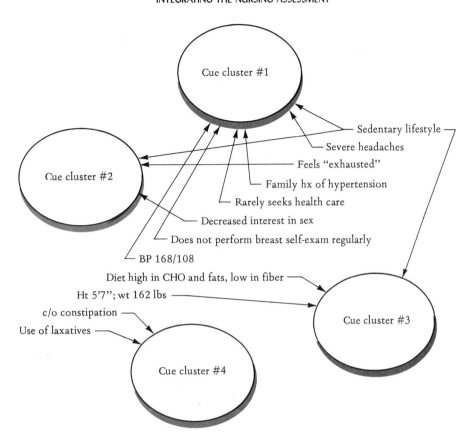

FIGURE 25-1. Cue Clustering. As cues emerge from the nursing history and clinical appraisal, the nurse begins to mentally form cue clusters.

terns, the information seems to suggest a diagnosis of *constipation*. The cue cluster that supports this diagnosis includes Kay's report of constipation one to two times each month, accompanied by flatulence, rectal pressure, straining on defecation, and hard stools. Additional cues include ignoring the urge to defecate when away from home, and reliance on a laxative for relief. The diagnosis is substantiated further by the clinical findings of diminished bowel sounds on auscultation (see defining characteristics for this diagnosis in chap. 6). The data also allow a diagnosis of *diarrhea* to be ruled out because there is no information, such as increased frequency of stool, hyperactive bowel sounds, or intestinal cramping, to suggest it.

Figure 25-2 illustrates a cue cluster and hypotheses related to another possible nursing diagnosis.

In some instances, information may fit more than one cue cluster and thus may indicate more than one diagnostic possibility. For example, Kay's complaint of exhaustion may suggest a diagnosis of *fatigue* (when combined with such cues as lack of interest in sex and difficulty concentrating) or may be a manifestation (defining characteristic) of another diagnosis such as *sleep pattern disturbance* or

anxiety. Her loss of interest in sexual intimacy may lend further weight to a diagnosis of fatigue or it may indicate an *altered sexuality pattern.* Until the data and the nurse's inferences are validated, the possibilities must remain open. Premature acceptance of one diagnosis over another can lead to diagnostic errors and, ultimately, an inappropriate or even harmful plan of care.

- *What additional inferences or diagnostic hypotheses are suggested by the available information?*

HYPOTHESIS VALIDATION

As various diagnostic hypotheses are developed, the nurse must try to confirm (validate) or rule out each one. This process involves systematic, focused collection of additional information that supports or disconfirms the hypothesis. For instance, one diagnostic hypothesis is that Kay's dietary intake exceeds that required for her age, gender, and activity level (see Figure 25-3). In order to validate this hypothesis, the nurse can analyze and compare Kay's dietary intake with dietary recommendations for her age, gender, and activity level to

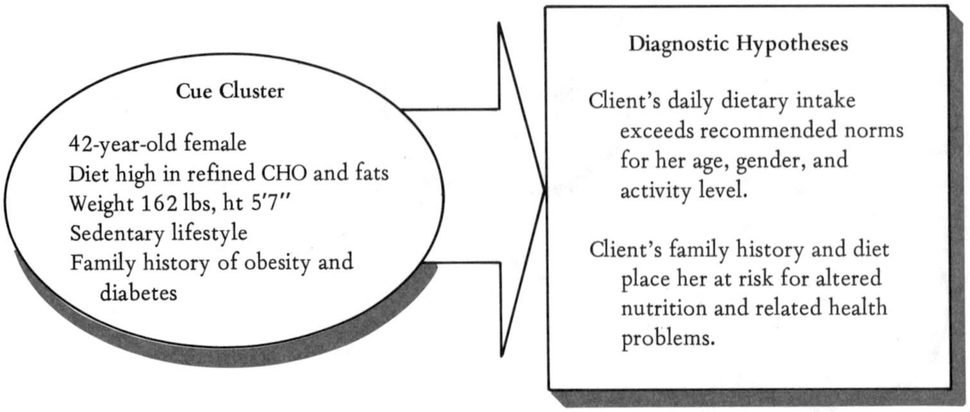

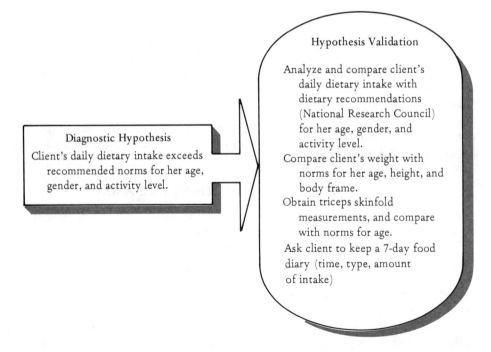

FIGURE 25-2. Hypothesis Activation. As cues are clustered, the nurse begins to form diagnostic hypotheses.

confirm or disconfirm that her intake is excessive. The nurse also can validate this diagnostic hypothesis by comparing Kay's weight with recommended norms for her age, height, and body frame. Additional data that could help further confirm the diagnosis include obtaining triceps skinfold measurements and attempting to determine Kay's responses to internal and external cues that affect her food intake. For example, Kay could be asked to keep a 7-day food diary to provide more detailed information.

Another means of validating diagnostic hypotheses involves referring to the defining charac-

teristics for the diagnosis approved by the North American Nursing Diagnosis Association that most closely approximates the diagnostic hypothesis. A review of the NANDA-approved diagnoses indicates a nursing diagnosis of *altered nutrition: more than body requirements.* Defining characteristics for this diagnosis include:

- Weight 10–20% over ideal for height and frame
- Triceps skinfold greater than 25 mm in women

FIGURE 25-3. Hypothesis Validation. For each diagnostic hypothesis, the nurse attempts to collect additional data to support or disconfirm the hypothesis.

■ Measured food consumption exceeds ADA recommendations for activity level, age, sex

■ Reported or observed dysfunctional eating patterns:

Pairing food with other activities

Concentrating food intake at end of day

Eating in response to external cues such as time of day

Eating in response to internal cues other than hunger, e.g., anxiety

Sedentary activity level

■ *Which of these defining characteristics are reflected in the data for Kay's situation? For the other inferences/hypotheses you identified earlier, what additional data are needed for validation? Do the NANDA defining characteristics support or disconfirm your inferences/hypotheses?*

The nurse's inferences also should be validated with the client when possible. For example, the nurse might say to Kay, "From the information you've given me and the findings of the physical examination, it appears that your dietary intake is excessive for your age, body frame, and activity level, and that you are overweight as a result. Is this how you see the problem?"

■ *Suggest ways you would validate your other inferences/hypotheses with Kay. What would you say to her?*

FORMULATING NURSING DIAGNOSES

Once tentative diagnostic hypotheses have been validated, the nurse draws on previous knowledge and experience to formulate the best possible or *most probable* nursing diagnoses for a particular client, taking into account all that is known.

■ *Given all possible diagnostic hypotheses for Kay, which nursing diagnoses are most probable (validated by the data and confirmed with all else that is known about the situation)?*

The following nursing diagnoses are formulated for Kay:

1. Constipation

2. Fatigue

3. Altered health maintenance

4. Altered nutrition: more than body requirements

5. Pain

6. Potential sensory–perceptual alteration: vision

7. Impaired skin integrity

Other diagnoses that were considered but ruled out because (1) there was insufficient information or (2) the data did not match the defining characteristics include *activity intolerance, anxiety, parental role conflict, ineffective individual coping, fear, hopelessness, altered sexuality patterns,* and *sleep pattern disturbance.*

IDENTIFYING RELATED FACTORS

After formulating the most probable nursing diagnoses, the nurse also must specify the factors that have contributed to each diagnosis. Related factors may be environmental, cultural, psychosocial, developmental, or physiological. The NANDA list of approved nursing diagnoses also includes "related factors" for each diagnosis (see chap. 6). The nurse should refer to them when formulating each diagnostic statement. Based on the data provided, the nurse specifies the related factors for Kay's nursing diagnoses. These are illustrated in Figure 25-4.

■ *Identify defining characteristics and supportive data for each of Kay's nursing diagnoses. Do the data suggest additional (or different) nursing diagnoses? List Kay's nursing diagnoses in order of priority and provide rationale for doing so.*

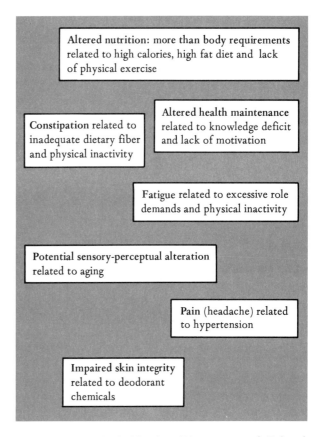

Altered nutrition: more than body requirements related to high calories, high fat diet and lack of physical exercise

Constipation related to inadequate dietary fiber and physical inactivity

Altered health maintenance related to knowledge deficit and lack of motivation

Fatigue related to excessive role demands and physical inactivity

Potential sensory-perceptual alteration related to aging

Pain (headache) related to hypertension

Impaired skin integrity related to deodorant chemicals

FIGURE 25-4. Kay's Nursing Diagnoses and Related Factors.

TABLE 25-1
Sample Nursing Care Plan for Kay's Nursing Diagnosis: Constipation

Nursing Diagnosis: Constipation related to inadequate dietary fiber and physical inactivity

Supporting Data:

Subjective: Does not exercise "at all"
24-hour recall dietary history
Usually has BM qd or qod, soft, formed, brown
Occasional problem (1–2 X/month) c̄ constipation (no BM for 3–4 days) accompanied by flatulence, rectal pressure, straining on defecation, hard stools
Prefers privacy of own bathroom; sometimes ignores urge to defecate when at work or away from home
Relieved c̄ 1–2 tbsp Milk of Magnesia

Objective: Abdomen slightly protruberant
Diminished bowel sounds
Formed stool in rectum

Interpretation/Validation of Data:

Analysis of dietary intake reveals diet high in refined carbohydrates and fat, low in dietary fiber (see chap. 18). Lack of physical activity contributes to decreased peristalsis (see chaps. 16 and 19). Ignoring urge to defecate contributes to decreased anal sphincter tone (see chaps. 16 and 19). Dependence on laxatives may contribute to recurrence of constipation (see chap. 19). Diminished bowel sounds confirm decreased peristalsis (see chap. 19).

NANDA defines *constipation* as "the state in which the individual experiences decreased number of bowel movements in relation to normal elimination pattern." Decreased frequency of bowel movements, hard stools, straining at stool, decreased bowel sounds, flatulence, and rectal pressure are listed as defining characteristics for the NANDA-approved diagnosis of constipation (see chap. 6). Related factors for this diagnosis include less than adequate dietary bulk, less than adequate physical activity, chronic use of laxatives, and ignoring the urge to defecate (see chap. 6).

Goal: Kay's daily or qod bowel elimination pattern will be maintained.

Nursing Interventions:

- Teach Kay about the relationship between dietary fiber and maintenance of normal bowel elimination.
- Plan with Kay ways she can increase her daily intake of dietary fiber and decrease refined CHO and fats in her diet.
- Teach Kay about the relationship between chronic use of laxatives and recurrence of constipation. Emphasize the importance of adequate intake of dietary fiber and sufficient daily physical activity as ways to avoid her perceived need to use Milk of Magnesia to relieve constipation.
- Involve Kay in identifying acceptable ways to increase her daily physical activity. Help her identify and choose motivational strategies to ensure adequate daily physical activity.
- Emphasize the importance of responding to the urge to defecate. Work with Kay to show her how she might overcome her reluctance to respond to the urge to defecate when she is away from home.

Evaluation (client outcomes):

Kay has a soft formed bowel movement daily or qod.

ESTABLISHING DIAGNOSTIC PRIORITIES

Once the nurse has formulated Kay's nursing diagnoses, a judgment must be made concerning their relative importance to Kay's health and well-being. By establishing diagnostic priorities, the nurse is able to determine the most responsive, feasible, efficient, and cost-effective plan of care.

As discussed in Chapter 1, several factors should be considered when establishing diagnostic priorities. These include (1) the hierarchy of human needs (see chap. 12), (2) the urgency of the diagnosis, (3) the client's perceptions and values, (4) the human and material resources needed to re-

solve the diagnosis, and (5) the nature of the nurse–client relationship.

When each of these variables is considered as an *independent* guide for ranking the priority of Kay's diagnoses, a different picture emerges than when her nursing diagnoses are considered within the context of these variables operating *interdependently*. For example, if Kay's diagnoses are ranked only in light of the hierarchy of human needs, "impaired skin integrity" would probably be given the highest priority because the skin is the body's first line of defense against infection. This diagnosis also requires a minimal investment of human and material resources to resolve it. If urgency is considered as the sole variable, "pain" would be given the highest priority. "Impaired skin integrity" is less urgent because it does not interfere with Kay's daily functioning to the extent that her painful headaches do.

■ *Rank Kay's nursing diagnoses in order of priority. Explain your reasons for doing so. Compare your listing with that of a colleague or classmate. Working with your colleague or classmate, try to achieve a consensus on the final ranking for Kay's nursing diagnoses. Provide rationale for your decisions.*

Determining the priority of Kay's nursing diagnoses enables the nurse to decide which ones require immediate attention and which can be put on hold temporarily. Once diagnostic priorities have been established, the nurse proceeds to develop a plan of nursing care to address each of Kay's diagnoses.

NURSING CARE PLANNING

Nursing care planning involves developing goals, identifying nursing interventions to achieve the client's goals, and specifying desired outcomes. A sample nursing care plan for Kay's nursing diagnosis of "constipation" related to inadequate dietary fiber and physical inactivity is outlined in Table 25-1.

■ *Develop goals, identify possible nursing interventions, and specify outcomes for at least two of Kay's remaining nursing diagnoses. What human and material resources are needed to accomplish the goals and achieve the specified outcomes? What factors might facilitate or inhibit achievement of the desired outcomes? How will you evaluate Kay's nursing care? Discuss the immediate and long-term consequences for Kay's health should her nursing diagnoses not be resolved.*

SUMMARY

The importance of considering all dimensions of human functioning that affect health and well-being when performing a nursing assessment cannot be overstated. If the nurse's attention is focused too narrowly, the risk of overlooking key variables that contribute to or interfere with a client's health is great. Too often, attention is paid to the obvious physiological manifestations of health or illness while the more subtle dimensions, such as culture, environment, interpersonal functioning, and development are minimized or, worse, neglected entirely.

A person's responses to actual or potential health alterations cannot be categorized neatly. Rather, human responses to health and illness must be considered from a multidimensional perspective that takes into account family, cultural, environmental, developmental, psychosocial, and physiological forces that together shape the individual. Just as a single musical instrument cannot provide full knowledge of and appreciation for an entire symphony orchestra, neither can one dimension of human health acquaint the nurse with a client as a multidimensional, holistic being. In order to understand and fully appreciate the complexity of any client's health and functioning, the nurse must collect sufficient information about the many dimensions of health in order to form a valid and reliable picture of each client as a unique biopsychosocial being within an equally unique family–cultural–environmental context.

Chapter Highlights

■   Human responses to health and illness must be considered from a multidimensional perspective that takes into account the family, cultural, environmental, developmental, psychosocial, and physiological forces that shape the individual.

■   The emphasis given to each factor of a client's health varies according to the client's developmental level, ethnic/cultural identity, and health, as well as the nature of the client's contact with the nurse, the duration of contact, and the particular health-care setting.

■   Within the context of each nurse–client encounter, the nurse decides which data to collect. The ability to determine which aspects of the assessment require special focus depends on the nurse's knowledge and expertise in making clinical judgments.

■   If the nursing assessment is focused too narrowly, the risk of overlooking key variables that contribute to or interfere with the client's health is great.

■   Nursing assessment and diagnosis provide the basis for nursing care planning, which involves developing goals, identifying possible nursing interventions, and specifying desired outcomes.

■   Evaluation of the plan of care provides an ongoing means for revising the plan of care to reflect the client's changing responses to actual or potential health alterations.

■   Ultimately, the nurse is concerned with ensuring that the client achieves, maintains, or is restored to an optimal level of health or helped to die peacefully and with dignity.

Practice Activities

1. Develop goals, identify possible nursing interventions, and specify outcomes for at least two of Kay's remaining nursing diagnoses.

2. Conduct a comprehensive, multidimensional assessment of at least two clients. Select clients who are of different ethnic/cultural backgrounds and in different types of health-care settings (e.g., hospital, clinic, home), such as:

    a. a newborn infant
    b. an infant or preschool child
    c. a school-age child or adolescent
    d. a pregnant woman
    e. a young adult
    f. a middle-aged adult
    g. an older adult

Formulate valid and appropriate nursing diagnoses, and develop a plan of care for at least one nursing diagnosis for each client.

Index

Index of Official Nursing Diagnoses
Taxonomy I Revised—1990
North American Nursing Diagnosis Association (NANDA)

*These terms are duo-referenced for ease and speed in locating the correct diagnosis.